2005 Publications

Critical coding and reim information you need on the same page as the code you want!

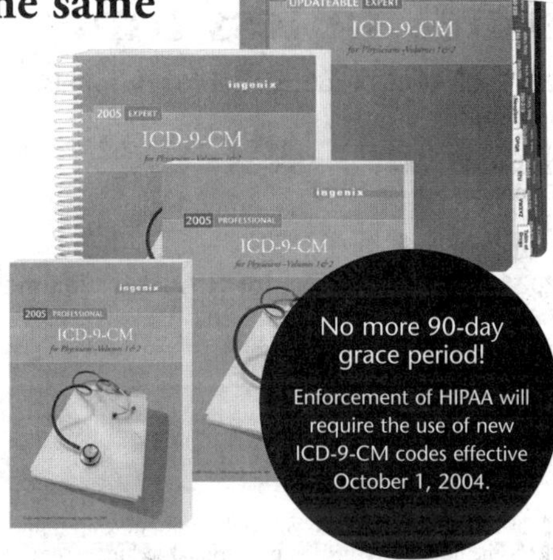

2005 ICD-9-CM Professional for Physicians, Volumes 1 & 2

Softbound
Item No.: 6361 — Available: September 2004
ISBN: 1-56337-582-6 — **$74.95**

Compact
Item No.: 6362 — Available: September 2004
ISBN: 1-56337-583-4 — **$69.95**

2005 ICD-9-CM Expert for Physicians, Volumes 1 & 2

Spiral
Item No.: 6363 — Available: September 2004
ISBN: 1-56337-584-2 — **$84.95**

Updateable
Item No.: 3534 — Available: Now
ISBN: 1-56329-594-X — **$149.95**

Save time and help reduce errors with the 2005 *ICD-9-CM Expert* or *Professional* code books. Inside each edition, essential coding references, edit details, and guidelines are all provided on the same pages as the codes themselves for greater ease and efficiency.

- **Completely HIPAA compliant.** Review the official coding guidelines, current code set, and AHA's *Coding Clinic for ICD-9-CM* references—all in one book!
- **EXCLUSIVE! Assign V codes with confidence.** V code symbols identify when V codes can be used only as a primary or only as a secondary diagnosis.
- **EXCLUSIVE! Symbols located in the tabular section and in the index remind you when a code requires a 4th or 5th digit.**
- **Confirm coding selection with clinically-oriented illustrations and definitions.** In-depth visual references and descriptions are included.
- **Be aware of the etiology/manifestation code convention.** Codes representing manifestations of underlying disease that should not be assigned a principal diagnosis are identified.
- **Prevent denials due to restrictions based on age or sex.** Edit symbols distinguish codes that detect inconsistencies between age or sex and diagnosis.

100% Money Back Guarantee:
If our merchandise* ever fails to meet your expectations, please contact our Customer Service Department toll-free at 1.800.INGENIX (464.3649), option 1, for an immediate response.
**Software: Credit will be granted for unopened packages only.*

Exclusive to the Expert Editions:

- **EXCLUSIVE! Easily verify the validity of a three-digit code.** The three-digit code list identifies whether or not a code is valid for submitting a claim.
- **EXCLUSIVE! Simplify complex coding issues with intuitive tables.** Complex coding issues are presented in an understandable table format.
- **EXCLUSIVE! Keep current with special reports.** Alerts sent via e-mail inform you of important developments posted on our web site.

The *Updatedable Expert* Edition offers even more!:

- **EXCLUSIVE! Updated three times a year.** In September, in February and in July.
- **EXCLUSIVE! Browse AHA's *Coding Clinic* topics quickly.** A summary of the official coding advice is part of your subscription.

CMS proposes semi-annual ICD-9-CM changes effective April 1 and October 1. As always, Ingenix strives to keep you up-to-date on possible new changes that could affect your bottom line. If an April 2005 update does occur, we are willing to provide you with the update information at no additional charge. Just visit www.ingenixonline.com and look for the ICD-9-CM update icon to review the latest available update.

SAVE 5% when you order at www.ingenixonline.com (reference source code FOBW5)

or call toll-free 1.800.INGENIX (464.3649), option 1.

Also available from your medical bookstore or distributor.

FOBA5

2005 Publications

ingenix

Code it right the first time...in less time!

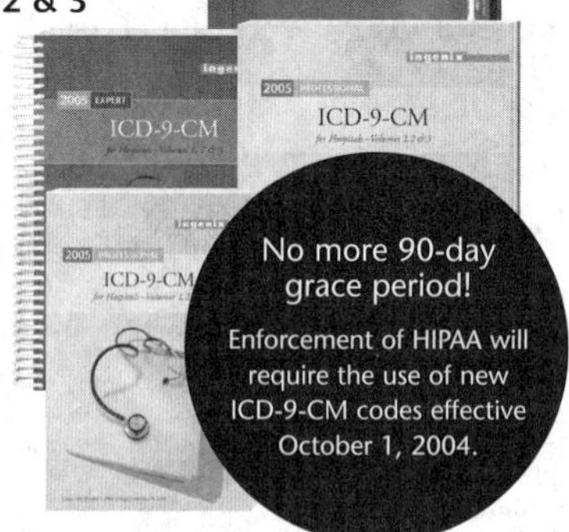

2005 ICD-9-CM Professional for Hospitals, Volumes 1, 2 & 3

Softbound

Item No.: 6365 — Available: September 2004
ISBN: 1-56337-586-9 — **$84.95**

Compact

Item No.: 6366 — Available: September 2004
ISBN: 1-56337-587-7 — **$79.95**

2005 ICD-9-CM Expert for Hospitals, Volumes 1, 2 & 3

Spiral

Item No.: 6367 — Available: September 2004
ISBN: 1-56337-588-5 — **$94.95**

Updateable

Item No.: 3539 — Available: Now
ISBN: 1-56329-595-8 — **$159.95**

Be HIPAA compliant with code books developed for the health information professional seeking a comprehensive coding and reimbursement solution. Do it right...in less time!

- **Comply with HIPAA regulations.** The official coding guidelines, current code set, and AHA's *Coding Clinic for ICD-9-CM* references—all in one book!
- **Affirm coding selection with clinically-oriented illustrations and definitions.** Visual references and descriptions are included.
- **Avoid claim inaccuracies with Medicare Code Edit Alerts.** Color-coding and symbols identify Nonspecific Dx, Unacceptable PDx, Complex and Major Cardiovascular Dx, age, sex, HIV-related Dx, CC, Questionable Admission PDx, etiology/manifestation convention and all major Medicare procedure code edits.
- **Easily recognize complication or comorbidity diagnoses along with the excluded principal diagnoses.** A CC exclusion list with each CC diagnosis shows those principal diagnoses for which the CC code does not affect DRG assignment.
- **Symbols in tabular sections and indexes remind you when a code requires a 4th or 5th digit.**
- **Be alert to the etiology/manifestation code convention.** Color-coding identifies mandatory dual coding situations (two codes required for reporting).
- **Know when a PDx requires specific documentation to support a DRG assignment.** Icons identify codes that group to targeted DRGs.

Exclusive to the *Expert* Editions:

- **Verify the validity of a three-digit code with ease.** The three-digit code list indicates if a code is valid for submitting a claim.
- **Reduce the risk of lost revenue.** The list of Complications and Comorbidities and the Pharmacological Listing help identify conditions that may affect DRG assignment.
- **Quick DRG Verification.** The PDx/MDC/DRG list confirms that the PDx matches the Major Diagnostic Category and DRG assigned.
- **Stay up-to-date with late-breaking news.** Alerts are e-mailed regarding important news on our web site.

The *Updatedable Expert* Edition offers even more!:

- **Review AHA *Coding Clinic* topics quickly.** A summary of the official coding advice on topics is provided.
- **Updated three times a year.** In September, in February and in July.

CMS proposes semi-annual ICD-9-CM changes effective April 1 and October 1. As always, Ingenix strives to keep you up-to-date on possible new changes that could affect your bottom line. If an April 2005 update does occur, we are willing to provide you with the update information at no additional charge. Just visit www.ingenixonline.com and look for the ICD-9-CM update icon to review the latest available update.

100% Money Back Guarantee:
If our merchandise* ever fails to meet your expectations, please contact our Customer Service Department toll-free at 1.800.INGENIX (464.3649), option 1, for an immediate response.
**Software: Credit will be granted for unopened packages only.*

SAVE 5% when you order at www.ingenixonline.com (reference source code FOBW5)

or call toll-free 1.800.INGENIX (464.3649), option 1.

Also available from your medical bookstore or distributor.

FOBA5

2005 Publications

ingenix®

The official source for procedural codes and guidelines—the 2005 AMA CPT® books

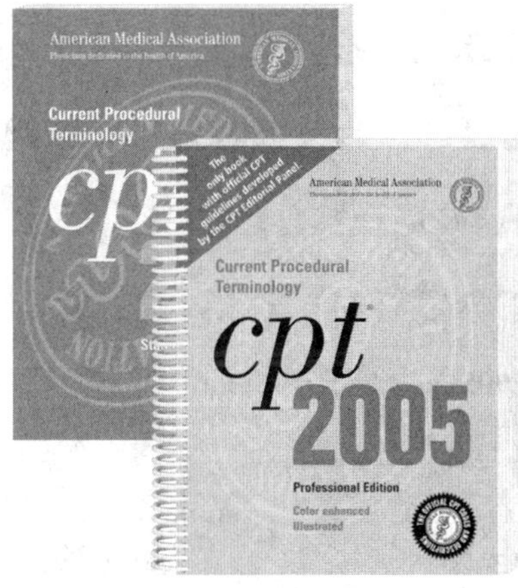

2005 CPT® Standard (Perfect Bound)

Item No.: 4474 **$62.95**

Available: October 2004 ISBN: 1-57947-578-7

2005 CPT® Professional (Spiral)

Item No.: 4457 **$86.95**

Available: October 2004 ISBN: 1-57947-579-5

The American Medical Association (AMA) makes hundreds of CPT® code changes each year. Coders need the official, comprehensive resource to help them avoid using the wrong codes and prevent potential delays in reimbursement.

The *CPT® Standard* and the *CPT® Professional*, published by the AMA, are the official sources of this information. Easy-to-use and easy-to-understand, each reference provides over 7,000 official CPT® codes and the rules you need to know to use them efficiently for optimal reimbursement.

- **EXCLUSIVE to the 2005 CPT® Professional book! Access the latest official codes.** Use of the official codes is required by CMS to be in compliance with HIPAA regulations.
- **EXCLUSIVE to the 2005 CPT® Professional book! Improve efficiency when searching for specific CPT® codes.** Each page includes color-coding, icons, and bars—all designed to help you code with increased speed and proficiency.
- **EXCLUSIVE to the 2005 CPT® Professional book! Locate descriptions, tips, and rulings regarding specific CPT® codes with ease.** *CPT® Assistant* references are included to help provide guidance and practical advice.
- **Stay up-to-date on hundreds of code changes.** All of the CPT® codes, their descriptions, and the official rules and guidelines are included.
- **Quickly find the CPT® code you need.** A comprehensive index—by procedure, service, organ, condition, eponym, synonym, and abbreviation—makes searching fast.
- **Better understand rules and procedures.** Refer to the visual references for help with coding selection.

100% Money Back Guarantee:
If our merchandise* ever fails to meet your expectations, please contact our Customer Service Department toll-free at 1.800.INGENIX (464.3649), option 1, for an immediate response.
*Software: Credit will be granted for unopened packages only.

CPT is a registered trademark of the American Medical Association.

SAVE 5% when you order at www.ingenixonline.com (reference source code FOBW5)

or call toll-free 1.800.INGENIX (464.3649), option 1.

Also available from your medical bookstore or distributor.

FOBA5

2005 Publications

ingenix

Expedite claim submission with an enhanced CPT® coding resource

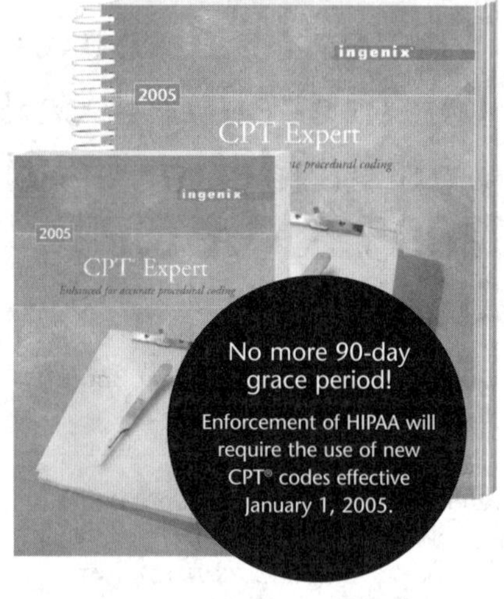

2005 CPT® Expert (Spiral)

Item No.: 4566 **$94.95**
Available: December 2004 ISBN: 1-56337-562-1

2005 CPT® Expert (Compact)

Item No.: 4565 **$79.95**
Available: December 2004 ISBN: 1-56337-563-X

Interpret annual CPT® code changes, understand their implications, and apply them appropriately to expedite claim submission with the *CPT® Expert.* A one-of-a-kind resource, the *CPT® Expert* provides not only 2005 CPT® codes, but guidance on how to improve your coding precision and increase coding efficiency. Stop searching through more complicated code books and software for answers to easily solvable coding questions—reach for the *CPT® Expert.*

- **NEW! Find out how to best apply a CPT® code.** *CPT® Assistant* references are included to help provide guidance and practical advice.
- **EXCLUSIVE! Improve the precision of CPT® coding selection.** Information from the AMA, CMS, the *Medicare Coverage Manual,* the *Coverage Issues Manual* and Ingenix experts helps you better understand the rules, regulations, and guidelines that affect your CPT® code selection.
- **Access a complete, comprehensive listing of CPT® codes.** All 2005 CPT® codes are included, along with their official, full descriptions.
- **Determine which codes are payable under OPPS and how.** APC status indicators are included.
- **Know which codes can be billed using ASC groupings.** ASC designation symbols are provided.
- **Complete unfinished claims requiring deleted 2004 CPT® codes.** Deleted codes from 2004 and their complete descriptions are included, but denoted with strike-outs.
- **Easily identify commonly miscoded codes, unlisted codes, and codes not covered by Medicare.** Color keys mark the CPT® codes that can affect your Medicare reimbursement.
- **Know how to best report particular codes.** Icons identify the codes that are affected by Medicare rules.
- **Increase claim submission speed.** Short, simple introductions to each chapter provide tips and instruction.
- **Save time locating the information you need.** An extensive index helps you code with increased speed and proficiency.
- **Keep current with corrections to CPT® codes and other late-breaking news.** Alerts are sent via e-mail to provide valuable code change information.

100% Money Back Guarantee:
If our merchandise* ever fails to meet your expectations, please contact our Customer Service Department toll-free at 1.800.INGENIX (464.3649), option 1, for an immediate response.
*Software: Credit will be granted for unopened packages only.

The *CPT® Expert* is not a replacement for the American Medical Association's *CPT® Standard* and *Professional* code books. CPT is a registered trademark of the American Medical Association.

SAVE 5% when you order at www.ingenixonline.com (reference source code FOBW5)

or call toll-free 1.800.INGENIX (464.3649), option 1.

Also available from your medical bookstore or distributor.

FOBA5

2005 Publications

ingenix

Answers to the toughest coding questions

2005 Coders' Desk References

Coders' Desk Reference for Procedures
Item No.: 5764 — Available: December 2004
ISBN: 1-56337-598-2 — **$119.95**

Coders' Desk Reference for Diagnoses
Item No.: 5766 — Available: September 2004
ISBN: 1-56337-599-0 — **$119.95**

Coders' Desk Reference for HCPCS Level II
Item No.: 4975 — Available: December 2004
ISBN: 1-56337-600-8 — **$119.95**

With the nationwide shortage of coders continuing, new coders are expected to be proficient right away...while experienced coders are under pressure to be more productive than ever before. That's why Ingenix has created a comprehensive *Coders' Desk Reference* suite for all three code sets, creating an essential power suite for every health care professional.

- **Decrease coding time with comprehensive lay descriptions.** Clinical explanations clarify procedures in *Coders' Desk Reference for Procedures,* indicate the disease processes and causes of conditions in *Coders' Desk Reference for Diagnoses* and simplify HCPCS Level II codes by describing supplies and services in *Coders' Desk Reference for HCPCS.*
- **Reduce costly claim delays and denials by always using the latest code sets.** All *Coders' Desk References* conform to standard code book organization and use updated codes for 2005.
- **New coders: Master the intricacies of coding, documentation, and billing. Veteran health care professionals: Code faster and more efficiently.** The suite offers advice to avoid common coding errors and includes anatomical charts, eponyms, acronyms and medical abbreviations.

100% Money Back Guarantee:
If our merchandise* ever fails to meet your expectations, please contact our Customer Service Department toll-free at 1.800.INGENIX (464.3649), option 1, for an immediate response.
*Software: Credit will be granted for unopened packages only.

CPT is a registered trademark of the American Medical Association.

SAVE 5% when you order at www.ingenixonline.com (reference source code FOBW5)

or call toll-free 1.800.INGENIX (464.3649), option 1.

Also available from your medical bookstore or distributor.

FOBA5

2005 Publications

ingenix

Essential Coding and Payment Resources for Your Specialty

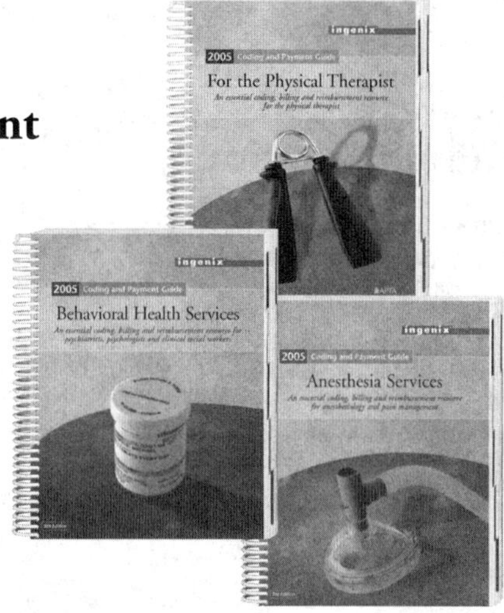

2005 Coding and Payment Guides

Coding and Payment Guide for the Physical Therapist
Item No.: 1543 Available: December 2004
ISBN: 1-56337-616-4 **$179.95**

Coding and Payment Guide for Behavioral Health Services
Item No.: 1545 Available: December 2004
ISBN: 1-56337-618-0 **$179.95**

Coding and Payment Guide for Anesthesia Services
Item No.: 1544 Available: December 2004
ISBN: 1-56337-617-2 **$179.95**

Stop searching through separate references to code claims for your specialty! With the 2005 *Coding and Payment Guides*, ICD-9-CM, CPT® and HCPCS Level II codes relevant to your specialty are compiled into one easy-to-use resource. Indexed, fully referenced and complete with up-to-date information for 2005, these comprehensive guides will help you reduce errors and code with assurance.

- **Reinforce coding selection with simple descriptions.** Easy-to-understand descriptions of the procedures represented by each CPT® code are included, as well as clinical definitions and ICD-9-CM code explanations, specific to your specialty.
- **Stay up-to-date with Medicare Correct Coding Initiative (CCI) edits with updates delivered via e-mail.** Identify which coding combinations cannot be billed together to reduce the risk of audit.
- **Prevent claim delays or denials by using only current code sets.** Find the updated 2005 specialty codes you need all in this one, comprehensive resource.
- **Improve the precision of ICD-9-CM code selection.** ICD-9-CM codes with icons allow users to identify the most accurate application of ICD-9-CM codes.
- **Improve efficiency with a readable format.** An innovative, two-column layout makes it easy to find the information needed when coding for your specialty.
- **Continuing Education Units (CEUs).** Earn 5-6 CEUs from AAPC.

100% Money Back Guarantee:
If our merchandise* ever fails to meet your expectations, please contact our Customer Service Department toll-free at 1.800.INGENIX (464.3649), option 1, for an immediate response.
*Software: Credit will be granted for unopened packages only.

CPT is a registered trademark of the American Medical Association.

SAVE 5% when you order at www.ingenixonline.com (reference source code FOBW5)

or call toll-free 1.800.INGENIX (464.3649), option 1.

Also available from your medical bookstore or distributor.

FOBA5

2005 Publications

ingenix

Specialty-Specific Comprehensive Illustrated Guides to Coding and Reimbursement

2005 Coding Companions

$189.95 each

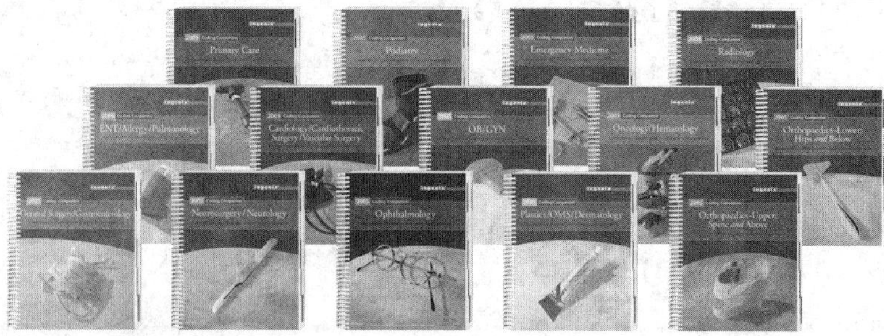

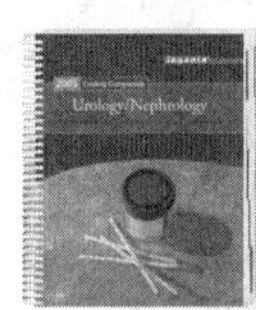

ISBN No.	Item Description	Item No.	Available
1-56337-601-6	Coding Companion for Cardiology/Cardiothoracic Surgery/Vascular Surgery	1528	December 2004
1-56337-602-4	Coding Companion for ENT/Allergy/Pulmonology **Special discount for AAO-HNS members**	1529	December 2004
1-56337-603-2	Coding Companion for General Surgery/ Gastroenterology	1530	December 2004
1-56337-604-0	Coding Companion for Neurosurgery/Neurology	1531	December 2004
1-56337-605-9	Coding Companion for OB/GYN	1532	December 2004
1-56337-606-7	Coding Companion for Ophthalmology **Special discount for ASOA members**	1533	December 2004
1-56337-607-5	Coding Companion for Orthopaedics—Lower: Hips & Below	1534	December 2004
1-56337-608-3	Coding Companion for Orthopaedics—Upper: Spine & Above	1535	December 2004
1-56337-609-1	Coding Companion for Plastics/OMS/Dermatology	1536	December 2004
1-56337-610-5	Coding Companion for Urology/Nephrology	1537	December 2004
1-56337-611-3	Coding Companion for Oncology/Hematology	1538	January 2005
1-56337-612-1	Coding Companion for Primary Care **NEW!**	1539	January 2005
1-56337-615-6	Coding Companion for Podiatry **NEW! Special discount for APMA members**	1542	December 2004
1-56337-613-X	Coding Companion for Emergency Medicine **NEW!**	1540	January 2005
1-56337-614-8	Coding Companion for Radiology **NEW!**	1541	December 2004

Coding Companions provide the comprehensive information a coder/biller needs—CPT codes with ICD-9-CM, HCPCS Level II, and anesthesia crosswalks—along with procedural definitions, coding and reimbursement tips, clinical and procedural information, CCI edits, Pubs 100 issues and illustrations—all in a one-page format for surgical codes, along with most medicine codes, related to each specific specialty.

- **New!—Pubs 100 references (formerly known as MCM/CIM references).** Keep current with Medicare coverage issues with Pubs 100 information specific to your specialty.
- **Submit claims with current, comprehensive code sets.** Updated 2005 surgery, medicine, E/M, radiology and lab/path CPT® codes are included.
- **Facilitate your coding with helpful illustrations.** Medical illustrations help link operative report language to code definitions.
- **Prevent unbundling mistakes by staying current with CCI edits.** Updates sent quarterly via e-mail help identify which code combinations cannot be billed together. A set of CCI edits is published in the guide, followed by three FREE quarterly e-mail updates.

100% Money Back Guarantee:
If our merchandise* ever fails to meet your expectations, please contact our Customer Service Department toll-free at 1.800.INGENIX (464.3649), option 1, for an immediate response.
*Software: Credit will be granted for unopened packages only.

CPT is a registered trademark of the American Medical Association.

SAVE 5% when you order at www.ingenixonline.com (reference source code FOBW5)

or call toll-free 1.800.INGENIX (464.3649), option 1.

Also available from your medical bookstore or distributor.

FOBA5

2005 Publications

ingenix

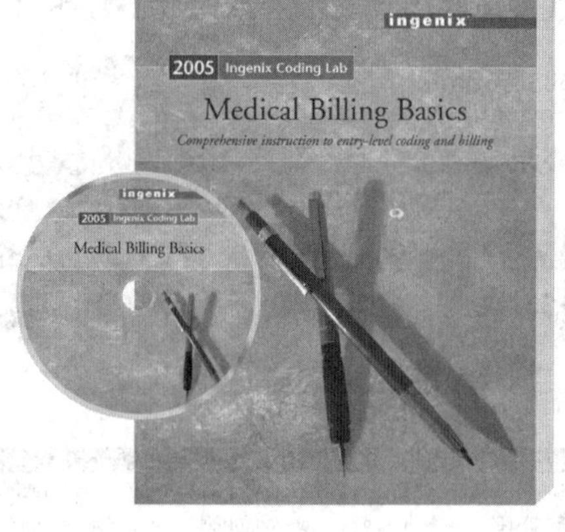

Master the Skills Needed to Be an Effective Coder!

2005 Ingenix Coding Lab: Medical Billing Basics

Item No.: 5788 **$74.95**

Available: December 2004 ISBN: 1-56337-633-4

This comprehensive entry-level education module helps beginning and aspiring coders in the office or the classroom. Designed to allow the user to understand and master the basic skills needed to be an effective coder, this module includes a CD containing a student workbook and a teacher's guide.

- **New!—Understand the intricacies behind billing.** Learn how to read an EOB/EOMB, how to conduct write-offs, how to track payments, and how to process overpayments. ABN issues with a new and improved billing chapter included.
- **New!—Conduct self audits effectively and efficiently to ensure compliance.** New chapter on Post Payment Reviews and Audits included.
- **Understand key terms and the human anatomy through detailed illustrations.** Anatomy and Terminology chapter included.
- **Learn the foundation of coding and billing.** Broad overview of coding, payers, and the reimbursement process for the entry-level coder or billing professional.
- **Test your coding knowledge.** Chapter quizzes available on the Student Guide CD.
- **Allows an instructor to better tutor and challenge students.** Teacher's Guide on CD available.
- **Make the complex world of medical reimbursement real and easier to understand.** Review simple coding scenarios and real-life case studies.
- **Learn the words that only the reimbursement process uses.** Review a full glossary of coding and reimbursement terms.
- **Three-Month *EncoderPRO* demo included on Student CD.** *EncoderPRO* look-up includes the latest CPT®, HCPCS, and ICD-9-CM codes.
- **Earn CEUs from AAPC.** Earn up to 5 CEUs awarded by AAPC.

100% Money Back Guarantee:
If our merchandise* ever fails to meet your expectations, please contact our Customer Service Department toll-free at 1.800.INGENIX (464.3649), option 1, for an immediate response.
*Software: Credit will be granted for unopened packages only.

CPT is a registered trademark of the American Medical Association.

SAVE 5% when you order at www.ingenixonline.com (reference source code FOBW5)

or call toll-free 1.800.INGENIX (464.3649), option 1.

Also available from your medical bookstore or distributor.

FOBA5

2005 Software Products

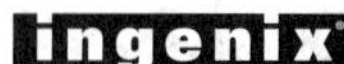

Make the Right Coding Decisions the First Time!

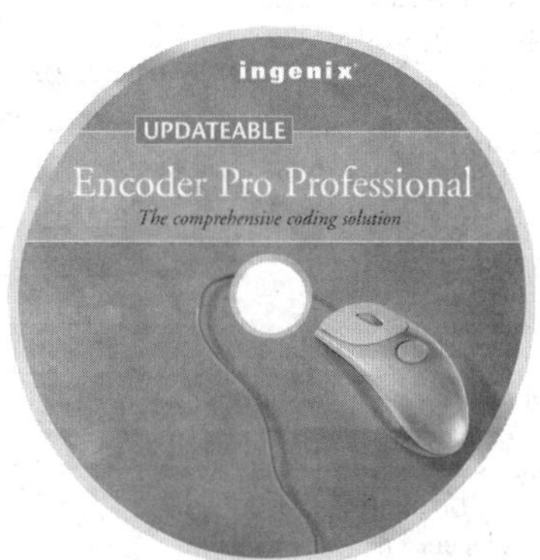

Encoder Pro Professional

Item No.: 2717 **$499.95***

Available: Now *Call for multi-user pricing.

Improve your reimbursement and your staff's productivity by increasing coding efficiency and accuracy. Powered by the CodeLogic™ Search Engine, you and your coders get lightning fast search results that return relevant code edit content; allowing your staff to make speedy and accurate code selection.

- **Exclusive—Easily search all three code sets simultaneously.** Powerful Code Lookup across CPT®, HCPCS, and ICD-9-CM code sets with Ingenix Code Logic™ Search Engine. Search using multiple lay terms, acronyms, abbreviations, and even misspelled words.
- **Exclusive—Enhance your understanding of procedures with easy-to-understand Ingenix lay descriptions.**
- **Stay in compliance with quarterly releases of Medicare's national and local coverage determinations.** Receive quarterly updates to Medicare coverage guidelines.
- **Reference coding rules and billing combinations for procedures and services and their commercially acceptable modifiers.**
- **Quickly check your selected code for proper reporting.** Access Ingenix references and Medicare color code edits for instant validation on gender, age, unbundles, and more.
- **Customize your coding experience.** Use sticky notes and bookmarks to help you set reminders and establish relationships among codes.

100% Money Back Guarantee:
If our merchandise* ever fails to meet your expectations, please contact our Customer Service Department toll-free at 1.800.INGENIX (464.3649), option 1, for an immediate response.
*Software: Credit will be granted for unopened packages only.

CPT is a registered trademark of the American Medical Association.

SAVE 5% when you order at www.ingenixonline.com (reference source code FOBW5)

or call toll-free 1.800.INGENIX (464.3649), option 1.

Also available from your medical bookstore or distributor.

FOBA5

Four simple ways to place an order.

Call

1.800.ingenix (464.3649), option 1. Mention source code FOBA5 when ordering.

Mail

PO Box 27116
Salt Lake City, UT 84127-0116
With payment and/or purchase order.

Fax

801.982.4033
With credit card information and/or purchase order.

Click

www.ingenixonline.com
Save 5% when you order online today—use source code FOBW5.

ingenix esmart
ingenix online frequent buyer program

GET REWARDS FOR SHOPPING ONLINE!
To find out more, visit IngenixOnline.com

E-Smart program available only to Ingenix customers who are not part of Medallion, Gold Medallion or Partner Accounts programs. You must be registered at Ingenix Online to have your online purchases tracked for rewards purposes. Shipping charges and taxes still apply and cannot be used for rewards. Offer valid online only.

100% Money Back Guarantee

If our merchandise* ever fails to meet your expectations, please contact our Customer Service Department toll-free at 1.800.ingenix (464.3649), option 1 for an immediate response.

*Software: Credit will be granted for unopened packages only.

Customer Service Hours

7:00 am - 5:00 pm Mountain Time
9:00 am - 7:00 pm Eastern Time

Shipping and Handling

no. of items	fee
1	$10.95
2-4	$12.95
5-7	$14.95
8-10	$19.95
11+	Call

ingenix

Order Form

Information

Customer No. ________________ Contact No. ________________

Source Code ________________

Contact Name ________________

Title ________________ Specialty ________________

Company ________________

Street Address ________________
NO PO BOXES, PLEASE

City ________________ State ________ Zip ________

Telephone (   ) ________________ Fax (   ) ________________
IN CASE WE HAVE QUESTIONS ABOUT YOUR ORDER

E-mail ________________ @ ________________
REQUIRED FOR ORDER CONFIRMATION AND SELECT PRODUCT DELIVERY.

Ingenix respects your right to privacy. We will not sell or rent your e-mail address or fax number to anyone outside Ingenix and its business partners. If you would like to remove your name from Ingenix promotion, please call 1.800.ingenix (464.3649), option 1.

Product

Item No.	Qty	Description	Price	Total

Subtotal ________

UT, OH, & VA residents, please add applicable Sales tax ________

(See chart on the left). Shipping & handling charges ________
All foreign orders, please call for shipping costs

Total ________

Payment

○Please bill my credit card ○MasterCard ○VISA ○Amex ○Discover

Card No. ________________ Expires ____ | ____
MONTH YEAR

Signature ________________

○Check enclosed, made payable to: Ingenix, Inc. ○Please bill my office

Purchase Order No. ________________
ATTACH COPY OF PURCHASE ORDER

©2004 Ingenix, Inc. All prices subject to change without notice.

FOBA5

ingenix™

Coders' Desk Reference *for* Diagnoses

Property of Lahey Clinic
Coding Department

2005

2nd Edition

Notice

Coders' Desk Reference for Diagnoses was conceived to be an accurate and authoritative source of information about coding and reimbursement issues. Every effort has been made to verify accuracy and information is believed reliable at the time of publication. Absolute accuracy cannot be guaranteed, however. This publication is made available with the understanding that the publisher is not engaged in rendering legal or other services requiring a professional license. Please address questions regarding this product to the Ingenix customer service department at:

1-800-INGENIX (464-3649) option 1
or e-mail us at
customerservice@ingenix.com

Acknowledgments

The following staff contributed to the development and/or production of this book:

Bonnie G. Schreck, CCS, CPC, CPC-H, CCS-P, *Product Manager*
Sheri Poe Bernard, CPC, *Product Director*
Karen Schmidt, BSN, *Clinical/Technical Director*
Lynn Speirs, *Senior Director, Publishing Services Group*
Wendy McConkie, CPC, CPC-H, *Clinical/Technical Editor*
Kate Holden, *Project Editor*
Kerrie Hornsby, *Desktop Publishing Manager*
Gregory A. Kemp, *Desktop Publishing Specialist*

Copyright

Copyright ©2004 Ingenix, Inc.

All rights reserved. No part of this publication may be reproduced or transmitted in any form or by any means, electronic or mechanical, including photocopy, recording, or storage in a database or retrieval system, without the prior written permission of the publisher. Printed in the United States of America.

Made in the USA

First printing – August 2004

ISBN 1-56337-599-0

About the Technical Editors

Wendy McConkie, CPC, CPC-H

Ms. McConkie has more than 20 years of experience in the health care field. She has extensive background in CPT/HCPCS and ICD-9-CM coding. She served several years as a coding consultant. Her areas of expertise include physician and hospital CPT coding assessments, chargemaster reviews, and the Outpatient Prospective Payment System (OPPS). She is a member of the American Academy of Professional Coders (AAPC).

Bonnie G. Schreck, CCS, CCS-P, CPC, CPC-H

With over 15 years' experience in the health care industry, Ms. Schreck is an expert in Medicare reimbursement and regulations, CPT-4 and ICD-9-CM coding, compliance, and medical insurance billing procedures. She is currently Product Manager of essential regulatory specialty products for Ingenix, where she manages a line of books for medical specialties.

Contents

© 2004 Ingenix, Inc.

 © 2004 Ingenix, Inc.

 © 2003 Ingenix, Inc.

Introduction

Coders' Desk Reference for Diagnoses is a comprehensive ICD-9-CM coding reference designed for medical offices, hospitals, health insurance companies, educators, and students who seek to expand their understanding of diagnostic coding. Its goal is to enrich the user's clinical understanding of ICD-9-CM, so code selection becomes more accurate.

Unlike other ICD-9-CM references, *Coders' Desk Reference for Diagnoses* includes numeric codes in ICD-9-CM, from 001 to 999. In some cases, its narrative discusses clinical issues affecting code selection for comprehensive categories (diabetes, fractures) and in other cases provides code-specific information (sudden infant death syndrome, hydatidiform mole). Because the book does not include the comprehensive index found in the official ICD-9-CM, it does not replace use of an official code book. However, used in conjunction with a code book, *Coders' Desk Reference for Diagnoses* will provide an unparalleled clinical roadmap to code selection.

Format

Coders' Desk Reference for Diagnoses begins with sections on the history of diagnostic coding; ICD-9-CM conventions, ICD-9-CM coding guidelines; ICD-10-CM conventions; syndromes; common prefixes and suffixes; common abbreviations, acronyms, and symbols; reimbursement terms; and anatomy charts. It then follows the organization of ICD-9-CM, looking at diseases and their codes beginning with Infectious and Parasitic Diseases (Chapter 1) through Injury and Poisoning (Chapter 17), in numeric order. The basic format of the book is to provide clinical coding support, with illustrations, narrative, definitions, and other resources that will help the user working from the medical record.

ICD-9-CM Codes and Descriptions

The codes in *Coders' Desk Reference for Diagnoses* are organized in hierarchical context, appearing within an appropriate three-digit rubric. All three-digit rubrics appear in a capitalized format. If the three-digit code is valid, an icon (OK) appears next to the code to indicate it is a valid code for use on a claim form. For example:

129 Intestinal parasitism, unspecified OK

Note that (OK) next to the description with 129 indicates that code 129 represents a valid ICD-9-CM code. There are fewer than 100 valid three-digit codes in ICD-9-CM.

Though all three-digit categories appear in *Coders' Desk Reference for Diagnoses*, invalid four-digit categories have been eliminated to reduce confusion regarding code choices. With the exception of valid three-digit codes, which are displayed above, all other valid codes in *Coders' Desk Reference for Diagnoses* appear at the same indent, unlike the presentation in ICD-9-CM itself. For example, all valid codes that occur in rubric 088 *Other Arthropod-borne diseases*, appear as follows:

088.0 Bartonellosis — Bartonella bacilliformis; sandflies; Andes

088.81 Lyme disease — *Borrelia burgdorferi*; ticks, United States

AHA: 4Q, '91, 15; 3Q, '90, 14; 2Q, '89, 10

088.82 Babesiosis — *Babesia*; ticks

AHA: 4Q, '93, 23

088.89 Other specified arthropod-borne diseases — not elsewhere classified

088.9 Arthropod-borne disease, unspecified — unknown

Note that some valid codes in rubric 088 are four-digit codes and some valid codes in this rubric are five-digit codes. Only valid codes are included.

Should there be information within a four-digit subclassification that applies to all five-digit codes within that subclassification, the invalid four-digit code will appear with a 5th icon, to differentiate it from the valid five-digit codes that follow. For example:

722.8 5th Postlaminectomy syndrome

Postlaminectomy syndrome is a complex of symptoms following laminectomy surgery. It includes conditions and syndromes described as postfusion, postmicrosurgery, and postchemonucleolysis.

722.80 Postlaminectomy syndrome, unspecified region — unknown site on spine

722.81 Postlaminectomy syndrome, cervical region — neck, C1-C7

722.82 Postlaminectomy syndrome, thoracic region — upper back, T1-T12

722.83 Postlaminectomy syndrome, lumbar region — lower back, L1-L5

Because the elimination of invalid four-digit codes could compromise the completeness of the code descriptions as they appear in ICD-9-CM, complete descriptions are used with each code in *Coders' Desk Reference for Diagnoses*. Therefore, while a code would read in an ICD-9-CM book like this:

239 Neoplasms of unspecified nature

239.0 Digestive system

In *Coders' Desk Reference for Diagnoses*, the codes would read like this:

239 Neoplasms of unspecified nature

239.0 Neoplasms of unspecified nature of digestive system

Note that the information from ICD-9-CM's description for 239 has been combined with the information from ICD-9-CM's description for 239.0 to create the description for *Coders' Desk Reference for Diagnoses* 239.0.

Additional Descriptors

Following most codes in *Coders' Desk Reference for Diagnoses* are brief descriptors that help differentiate the codes and determine which code is best suited for each clinical situation. For example:

701.9 Unspecified hypertrophic and atrophic condition of skin — skin tag, atrophoderma, pendulous abdomen, redundant skin, or unknown

In this example, the term "atrophoderma" appears as a descriptive term under 701.9 in ICD-9-CM; and the other terms are indexed to 701.9 in the official ICD-9-CM alphabetic index. In other cases, clinical research has provided the synonyms or support information that appears following the dash after a code, as in the case of:

001.0 Cholera due to Vibrio cholerae — Inaba, Ogawa, Hikojima serotypes; classical

001.1 Cholera due to Vibrio cholerae el tor — commonly less severe or asymptomatic

001.9 Cholera, unspecified — unknown whether *V. cholerae* or *V. cholerae el tor*

None of the supporting information appears in the official ICD-9-CM code text.

Narrative

Coders' Desk Reference for Diagnoses provides valuable background information on thousands of medical conditions. Information that appears directly after a three-digit category applies to all codes within that rubric. Information that appears following a four-digit subclassification applies to all codes in that subclassification, and information following a five-digit code applies only to that code.

Coding Clinic References

Listed with the ICD-9-CM codes are the AHA (American Hospital Association) *Coding Clinic* references. These identify diagnostic coding issues and answers on how to code for them properly, based on a patient situation (e.g., inpatient, outpatient). For example:

345 Epilepsy

AHA: 1Q, '93, 24; 2Q, '92, 8; 4Q, '92, 23

1Q indicates 1st Quarter, '93 is the year, and 24 is the page number in *Coding Clinic*.

Documentation Issues

This section indicates specific documentation issues that may arise while coding. For example:

> The terms grand mal and tonic-clonic seizures in the documentation do not establish the diagnosis of epilepsy.

Coding Clarification

These assist the user in clarifying coding problems and issues that may come up. For example:

> Recurrent Seizures: Recurrent seizures are not epilepsy, although all seizures in an epileptic patient are recurrent.

Coding Scenarios

The coding scenarios will assist the user in understanding how to code in particular situations. For example:

> A patient with known epilepsy is admitted after having experienced a grand mal seizure.
>
> Code assignment: 345.10, Epilepsy, grand mal status, without mention of intractable epilepsy

Illustrations

Illustrations provide users a better understanding of the anatomical nuances associated with specific codes. The illustrations usually include a labeled anatomical view, and may include narrative that discusses specific conditions or anatomic sites. The illustrations are almost always simplified schematic representations. In many instances, some detail is eliminated in order to make a clear point about the anatomic site that is the focus of the depiction.

© 2004 Ingenix, Inc.

ICD-9-CM Conventions

ICD-9-CM Conventions

The following section summarizes the coding conventions found in ICD-9-CM and the coding conventions that will be found in ICD-10-CM. In ICD-9-CM, the overview compares the following features:

1. Format
2. Typeface
3. Punctuation
4. Notes
5. Instructional notes
6. Modifiers
7. Abbreviations
8. Cross-references

Three Volume Set

1. Volume 1 of ICD-9-CM is a tabular listing of disease and injury divided into 17 sections, generally along anatomic sites. Two supplementary classifications contain alphanumeric codes to report factors influencing health status and other contact with health services (V codes) and causes of injury and poisoning (E codes). Appendixes to Volume 1 provide additional information and references.
2. Volume 2 is an alphabetic index of codes contained in Volume 1 and is important in locating proper diagnoses. An index to external causes of injury (E codes) is included. Three tables are included to assist in the selection of proper codes for hypertension, neoplasms, and drugs and chemicals.
3. A third volume of ICD-9-CM contains codes developed for coding inpatient facility procedures and is not ordinarily consulted for physician or outpatient services. Volume 3 contains both a tabular listing, arranged along anatomic lines, and an alphabetic index. Volume 3 coding issues are outside the framework of this reference manual.

Supplemental Classifications

Volume 1 contains two supplemental code classifications: V codes and E codes. V codes can be used as primary diagnoses when reporting services not related to current medical problems or conditions such as periodic or routine medical exams. E codes are never used as primary diagnoses, providing supplemental information only on the causes of injury and poisoning. See the individual listings for more information.

V codes (V01-V83), describe circumstances that influence a patient's health status and identify reasons for medical encounters resulting from circumstances other than a disease or injury classified in the main part of ICD-9-CM.

V codes are generally used in three instances:

- When a physician identifies a circumstance or problem in a person who is not currently sick but has nonetheless come in contact with health services (to act as an organ donor or to receive a prophylactic vaccination, for example)
- When an ill or injured patient requires specific treatment (such as chemotherapy for malignancy or removal of pins or rods in postoperative orthopedic care)
- When a problem or circumstance that influences the patient's health is not itself a current illness but may affect future medical treatment

The second set of supplemental codes in Volume 1 is the *Supplementary Classification of External Causes of Injury and Poisoning* (E800-E999), also known as E codes. The E codes are never listed as the primary diagnosis; they are adjunctive. More than one E code may be needed to describe fully the circumstances of an accident. Use them to establish medical necessity to indicate a secondary payer responsible for payment of the service, identify causes of injury and poisoning, and to identify drugs. The index for the E codes is found in Volume 2, following the Table of Drugs and Chemicals.

Approaches to ICD-9-CM Coding

Determining a diagnostic code begins with analysis of the encounter form, operative report, or diagnostic statement for those words or main terms that best identify the patient's current condition or symptoms. Once the current condition or symptom is identified, consult Volume 2, the alphabetic index, to identify the main term associated with the condition or symptom. Next, identify any modifying terms listed below the main term to more specifically describe the condition or symptom. After the most specific main term and modifiers have been identified, look up the corresponding code in Volume 1, the tabular list. Follow any instructions or notes in both the alphabetic index and the tabular list.

Rules of ICD-9-CM Reference

An ironclad rule in diagnostic coding is to never derive a code by consulting only the Volume 2 alphabetic index. It is a reference index to the full tabular listing of Volume 1, which often yields a different code, additional codes, or a more specific code.

The six-step process for assigning diagnostic codes can be summarized as follows:

1. Determine the main terms that describe the patient's condition or symptoms.
2. Look up the main term in Volume 2 where the condition is alphabetized as a noun or adjective.
3. If indicated, follow cross-references such as *see*, *see also*, and see category to find the correct code.
4. Review subterms and modifying words. Refer to any indented terms under the main term to further clarify the code selection.
5. Verify the code as listed in Volume 2, the alphabetic index, by checking it against Volume 1, the tabular listing.
6. Review all instructions and notes in Volume 1 such as *includes*, *excludes*, *code first underlying disease*, or *use additional code* to assure that the correct code has been selected.

In outpatient coding, do not attempt to code "rule out," "probable," "suspect," or "questionable" descriptions in the documentation. While acceptable in a patient's medical record and for inpatient coding, coding rules do not allow their use in outpatient coding. Rather, code the condition, symptoms, signs, test results, or other reasons that can be documented for the medical encounter. (See "Official ICD-9-CM Coding Guidelines" chapter for specifics on inpatient hospital coding.)

Format

ICD-9-CM has an indented format. Subterms are indented two spaces to the right of the term to which they are linked. Continuations of lines too long for columns are indented four spaces.

251.2 Hypoglycemia, unspecified

Hypoglycemia:	Hypoglycemia:
NOS	spontaneous
reactive	

Typeface

Bold type identifies all codes and main terms in the Tabular List (Volume 1), separating them from subordinate information or notes.

Italicized type identifies those categories that cannot be reported as a primary diagnosis and also for all exclusion notes.

Punctuation

- Braces (}) enclose a series of terms modified by the statement or terms appearing to the right of the brace.
- Brackets ([ ]) enclose synonyms, alternative wordings, or explanatory phrases. The brackets may be square [ ] or italicized *[ ]*.
- Colon (:) is used in Volume 1 of ICD-9-CM to identify a term that is incomplete without one or more of the descriptors following it. Do not assign the code unless one or more of the descriptors is present in the physician's diagnostic statement.
- Parentheses ( ) enclose supplementary (nonessential) modifiers and do not generally affect code assignment. However, they do serve to confirm for the user that the correct code was selected when the nonessential modifier is present in both ICD-9-CM and the physician's documented diagnosis. Parentheses also enclose many *see also* references.

Notes

Notes are found in Volumes 1 and 2 and have no fixed length. They give general coding instructions. Notes in Volume 1 are indented and printed in plain type, while those in Volume 2 are boxed and italicized. The placement of these notes is as important as their content. Notes at the beginning of a section apply to all categories within the section. Those at the beginning of a subsection apply to all categories within the subsection. Likewise, notes preceding three-digit categories apply to all fourth-digit and fifth-digit codes within that category.

- *Code Also* dictates the use of two diagnostic codes. List the etiology (cause) first, followed by the manifestation. The two codes combined represent the primary diagnosis.
- *Code First Underlying Disease* identifies diagnoses that are not primary and are incomplete when used alone. In such cases the code, its title, and instructions are italicized. This type of instructional note appears only in Volume 1. A code with this instructional note should be recorded second, with the underlying cause recorded first. Italicized brackets identify this situation in Volume 2.

Instructional Notes

To assign diagnostic codes at the highest level of specificity, there are additional notes to follow.

- Excludes indicates terms that are not ordinarily coded under the referenced term. The word "Excludes" is surrounded by a box for easy identification and the corresponding note is italicized. This note does not prevent you from using the excluded code in addition to the code

 © 2004 Ingenix, Inc.

from which it was excluded when both conditions are present.

- Includes appear immediately under a three-digit code title to provide further definition or to give an example of the category contents.
- Use Additional Code in Volume 1 indicates those categories where an additional code is available to provide further information and to give a more complete picture of the diagnosis. The additional code should identify other aspects of the disease, including manifestation, cause, associated condition, and nature of the condition itself.

Modifiers

Essential modifiers are indented two spaces just below the main terms. They are generally presented in alphabetical order, with the exceptions of with and without, which appear before the alphabetized modifiers. Each additional essential modifier clarifies the previous one and is indented two additional spaces to the right. These descriptive terms affect code selection since they describe essential differences in site, etiology, and symptoms. When a main term in the tabular Volume 1 has only one essential modifier, it appears on the same line as the main term, separated by a comma.

Nonessential modifiers are listed immediately to the right of the main term and are enclosed in parentheses. They serve as examples to help translate written terminology into numeric codes and may be present or absent in the diagnostic without affecting code assignment.

Abbreviations

NEC (not elsewhere classifiable) indicates the main term is broad or not well defined or simply that even though the condition is identified, there is no other specific code provided for it. Use an NEC code only when more information is unavailable or a more specific code is not available. This term is used only in Volume 2.

NOS (not otherwise specified) is the equivalent of "unspecified" and is used only in Volume 1. NOS means there is a lack of information and documentation to support a specific code selection.

Cross-references

In Volume 2, several types of cross-references are encountered:

- *See* indicates that you should see the condition listed instead of the term you've found in order to assign the correct diagnostic code.
- *See also* indicates that additional information is available. This cross-reference may provide a more specific code or an additional code.
- *See category* directs the user to an additional three-digit category, not just a single code. Again, an appropriate code cannot be assigned unless you follow this instruction.

© 2004 Ingenix, Inc.

Official ICD-9-CM Coding Guidelines

ICD-9-CM Official Guidelines For Coding and Reporting

Effective Oct. 1, 2002

The Centers for Medicare and Medicaid Services (CMS) and the National Center for Health Statistics (NCHS), two departments within the Department of Health and Human Services (DHHS) present the following guidelines for coding and reporting using the *International Classification of Diseases, 9th Revision, Clinical Modification* (ICD-9-CM). These guidelines should be used as a companion document to the official version of the ICD-9-CM as published on CD-ROM.

These guidelines for coding and reporting have been developed and approved by the Cooperating Parties for ICD-9-CM: the American Hospital Association, the American Health Information Management Association, CMS, and the NCHS. These guidelines, published by the Department of Health and Human Services have also appeared in the Coding Clinic for ICD-9-CM, published by the American Hospital Association.

These guidelines have been developed to assist the user in coding and reporting in situations where the ICD-9-CM does not provide direction. Coding and sequencing instructions in Volumes I, II, and III of ICD-9-CM take precedence over any guidelines. The conventions, general guidelines, and chapter-specific guidelines apply to the proper use of ICD-9-CM, regardless of the health care setting. A joint effort between the attending physician and coder is essential to achieve complete and accurate documentation, code assignment, and reporting of diagnoses and procedures. These guidelines have been developed and approved by the Cooperating Parties to assist both the physician and the coder in identifying those diagnoses that are to be reported. The importance of consistent, complete documentation in the medical record cannot be overemphasized. Without such documentation the application of all coding guidelines is a difficult, if not impossible, task.

These guidelines are not exhaustive. The cooperating parties are continuing to conduct reviews of these guidelines and develop new guidelines as needed. Users of the ICD-9-CM should be aware that only guidelines approved by the cooperating parties are official. Revision of these guidelines and new guidelines will be published by the U.S. Department of Health and Human Services when they are approved by the cooperating parties. The term "admitted" is used generally to mean a health care encounter in any setting.

The guidelines have been reorganized into several new sections including an enhanced introduction that provides more detail about the structure and conventions of the classification usually found in the classification itself. The other new section, General Guidelines, brings together overarching guidelines that were previously found throughout the various sections of the guidelines. The new format of the guidelines also includes a resequencing of the disease-specific guidelines. They are sequenced in the same order as they appear in the tabular list chapters (Infectious and Parasitic diseases, Neoplasms, etc.).

These changes will make it easier for coders, experienced and beginners, to more easily find the specific portion of the coding guideline information they seek.

Table of Contents

ICD-9-CM Coding Guidelines

© 2004 Ingenix, Inc.

Section I Conventions, General Coding Guidelines and Chapter-Specific Guidelines

The conventions, general guidelines and chapter-specific guidelines are applicable to all health care settings unless otherwise indicated.

A. Conventions for the ICD-9-CM

The conventions for the ICD-9-CM are the general rules for use of the classification independent of the guidelines. These conventions are incorporated within the index and tabular of the ICD-9-CM as instructional notes. The conventions are as follows:

1. Format: The ICD-9-CM uses an indented format for ease in reference
2. Abbreviations
   a. Index Abbreviations

      NEC "Not elsewhere classifiable" This abbreviation in the index represents "other specified" When a specific code is not available for a condition the index directs the coder to the "other specified" code in the tabular.

   b. Tabular Abbreviations

      NEC "Not elsewhere classifiable" This abbreviation in the tabular represents "other specified" When a specific code is not available for a condition the tabular includes an NEC entry under a code to identify the code as the "other specified" code. (see "Other" codes)

      NOS "Not otherwise specified" This abbreviation is the equivalent of unspecified. (see "Unspecified" codes)
3. Punctuation

   [ ] Brackets are used in the tabular list to enclose synonyms, alternative wording or explanatory phrases. Brackets are used in the index to identify manifestation codes. (see etiology/manifestations).

   ( ) Parentheses are used in both the index and tabular to enclose supplementary words which may be present or absent in the statement of a disease or procedure without affecting the code number to which it is assigned. The terms within the parentheses are referred to as nonessential modifiers.

   : Colons are used in the Tabular list after an incomplete term which needs one or more of the modifiers following the colon to make it assignable to a given category.
4. Includes and Excludes Notes and Inclusion terms

   Includes:

   This note appears immediately under a three-digit code title to further define, or give examples of, the content of the category.

   Excludes:

   An excludes note under a code indicate that the terms excluded from the code are to be coded elsewhere. In some cases the codes for the excluded terms should not be used in conjunction with the code from which it is excluded. An example of this is a congenital condition excluded from an acquired form of the same condition. The congenital and acquired codes should not be used together.

© 2004 Ingenix, Inc.

ICD-9-CM Coding Guidelines

In other cases, the excluded terms may be used together with an excluded code. An example of this is when fractures of different bones are coded to different codes. Both codes may be used together if both types of fractures are present.

Inclusion terms:

List of terms are included under certain four and five digit codes. These terms are the conditions for which that code number is to be used. The terms may be synonyms of the code title, or, in the case of "other specified" codes, the terms are a list of the various conditions assigned to that code. The inclusion terms are not necessarily exhaustive. Additional terms found only in the index may also be assigned to a code.

5. Other and Unspecified codes

   a. "Other" codes
   Codes titled "other" or "other specified" (usually a code with a 4th digit 8 or fifth-digit 9 for diagnosis codes) are for use when the information in the medical record provides detail for which a specific code does not exist. Index entries with NEC in the line designate "other" codes in the tabular. These index entries represent specific disease entities for which no specific code exists so the term is included within an "other" code.

   b. "Unspecified" codes
   Codes (usually a code with a 4th digit 9 or 5th digit 0 for diagnosis codes) titled "unspecified" are for use when the information in the medical record is insufficient to assign a more specific code.

6. Etiology/manifestation convention ("code first", "use additional code" and "in diseases classified elsewhere" notes)

   Certain conditions have both an underlying etiology and multiple body system manifestations due to the underlying etiology. For such conditions the ICD-9-CM has a coding convention that requires the underlying condition be sequenced first followed by the manifestation. Wherever such a combination exists there is a "use additional code" note at the etiology code, and a "code first" note at the manifestation code. These instructional notes indicate the proper sequencing order of the codes, etiology followed by manifestation.

   In most cases the manifestation codes will have in the code title, "in diseases classified elsewhere." Codes with this title are a component of the etiology/ manifestation convention. The code title indicates that it is a manifestation code. "In diseases classified elsewhere" codes are never permitted to be used as first listed or principal diagnosis codes. They must be used in conjunction with an underlying condition code and they must be listed following the underlying condition.

   There are manifestation codes that do not have "in diseases classified elsewhere" in the title. For such codes a "use additional code" note will still be present and the rules for sequencing apply.

   In addition to the notes in the tabular, these conditions also have a specific index entry structure. In the index both conditions are listed together with the etiology code first followed by the manifestation codes in brackets. The code in brackets is always to be sequenced second.

   The most commonly used etiology/ manifestation combinations are the codes for Diabetes mellitus, category 250. For each code under category 250 there is a use additional code note for the manifestation that is specific for that particular diabetic manifestation. Should a patient have more than one manifestation of diabetes more than one code from category 250 may be used with as many manifestation codes as are needed to fully describe the patient's complete diabetic condition. The 250 diabetes codes should be sequenced first, followed by the manifestation codes.

   "Code first" and "Use additional code" notes are also used as sequencing rules in the classification for certain codes that are not part of an etiology/ manifestation combination. See - Other multiple coding for a single condition in the General Guidelines section.

B. General Coding Guidelines

1. Use of Both Alphabetic Index and Tabular List
   Use both the Alphabetic Index and the Tabular List when locating and assigning a code. Reliance on only the Alphabetic Index or the Tabular List leads to errors in code assignments and less specificity in code selection.

2. Locate each term in the Alphabetic Index and verify the code selected in the Tabular List. Read and be guided by instructional notations that appear in both the Alphabetic Index and the Tabular List.

3. Level of Detail in Coding
   Diagnosis and procedure codes are to be used at their highest number of digits available.

   ICD-9-CM diagnosis codes are composed of codes with either 3, 4, or 5 digits. Codes with three digits are included in ICD-9-CM as the heading of a category of codes that may be further subdivided by the use of fourth and/or fifth digits, which provide greater detail.

   A three-digit code is to be used only if it is not further subdivided. Where fourth-digit subcategories and/or fifth-digit subclassifications are provided, they must be assigned. A code is invalid if it has not been coded to the full number of digits required for that code. For example, Acute myocardial infarction, code 410, has fourth digits that describe the location of the

© 2004 Ingenix, Inc.

infarction (e.g., 410.2, Of inferolateral wall), and fifth digits that identify the episode of care. It would be incorrect to report a code in category 410 without a fourth and fifth digit.

ICD-9-CM Volume 3 procedure codes are composed of codes with either 3 or 4 digits. Codes with two digits are included in ICD-9-CM as the heading of a category of codes that may be further subdivided by the use of third and/or fourth digits, which provide greater detail.

4. The appropriate code or codes from 001.0 through V83.89 must be used to identify diagnoses, symptoms, conditions, problems, complaints or other reason(s) for the encounter/visit.
5. The selection of codes 001.0 through 999.9 will frequently be used to describe the reason for the admission/encounter. These codes are from the section of ICD-9-CM for the classification of diseases and injuries (e.g., infectious and parasitic diseases; neoplasms; symptoms, signs, and ill-defined conditions, etc.).
6. Codes that describe symptoms and signs, as opposed to diagnoses, are acceptable for reporting purposes when a related definitive diagnosis has not been established (confirmed) by the physician. Chapter 16 of ICD-9-CM, Symptoms, Signs, and Ill-defined conditions (codes 780.0 -799.9) contain many, but not all codes for symptoms.
7. Conditions that are an integral part of a disease process

   Signs and symptoms that are integral to the disease process should not be assigned as additional codes.
8. Conditions that are not an integral part of a disease process

   Additional signs and symptoms that may not be associated routinely with a disease process should be coded when present.
9. Multiple coding for a single condition

   In addition to the etiology/manifestation convention that requires two codes to fully describe a single condition that affects multiple body systems, there are other single conditions that also require more than one code. "Use additional code" notes are found in the tabular at codes that are not part of an etiology/ manifestation pair where a secondary code is useful to fully describe a condition. The sequencing rule is the same, "use additional code" indicates that a secondary code should be added.

   For example, for infections that are not included in chapter 1, a secondary code from category 041, Bacterial infection in conditions classified elsewhere and of unspecified site, may be required to identify the bacterial organism causing the infection. A "use additional code" note will normally be found at the infection code indicates a need for the organism code to be added as a secondary code.

   "Code first" notes are also under certain codes that are not specifically manifestation codes but may be due to an underlying cause. When a "code first" note is present and an underlying condition is present the underlying condition should be sequenced first.

   "Code, if applicable, any causal condition first", notes indicate that this code may be assigned as a principal diagnosis when the causal condition is unknown or not applicable. If a causal condition is known, then the code for that condition should be sequenced as the principal or first-listed diagnosis.

   Multiple codes may be needed for late effects, complication codes and obstetric codes to more fully describe a condition. See the specific guidelines for these conditions for further instruction.
10. Acute and Chronic Conditions

    If the same condition is described as both acute (subacute) and chronic, and separate subentries exist in the Alphabetic Index at the same indentation level, code both and sequence the acute (subacute) code first.
11. Combination Code

    A combination code is a single code used to classify: two diagnoses, or

    A diagnosis with an associated secondary process (manifestation)

    A diagnosis with an associated complication

    Combination codes are identified by referring to subterm entries in the Alphabetic Index and by reading the inclusion and exclusion notes in the Tabular List.

    Assign only the combination code when that code fully identifies the diagnostic conditions involved or when the Alphabetic Index so directs. Multiple coding should not be used when the classification provides a combination code that clearly identifies all of the elements documented in the diagnosis. When the combination code lacks necessary specificity in describing the manifestation or complication, an additional code may be used as a secondary code.
12. Late Effects

    A late effect is the residual effect (condition produced) after the acute phase of an illness or injury has terminated. There is no time limit on when a late effect code can be used. The residual may be apparent early, such as in cerebrovascular accident cases, or it may occur months or years later, such as that due to a previous injury. Coding of late effects generally requires two codes sequenced in the following order: The

© 2004 Ingenix, Inc.

condition or nature of the late effect is sequenced first. The late effect code is sequenced second.

An exception to the above guidelines are those instances where the code for late effect is followed by a manifestation code identified in the Tabular List and title, or the late effect code has been expanded (at the fourth and fifth-digit levels) to include the manifestation(s). The code for the acute phase of an illness or injury that led to the late effect is never used with a code for the late effect.

13. Impending or Threatened Condition

Code any condition described at the time of discharge as "impending" or "threatened" as follows: If it did occur, code as confirmed diagnosis. If it did not occur, reference the Alphabetic Index to determine if the condition has a subentry term for "impending" or "threatened" and also reference main term entries for "Impending" and for "Threatened." If the subterms are listed, assign the given code. If the subterms are not listed, code the existing underlying condition(s) and not the condition described as impending or threatened.

C. Chapter-Specific Coding Guidelines

In addition to general coding guidelines, there are guidelines for specific diagnoses and/or conditions in the classification. Unless otherwise indicated, these guidelines apply to all health care settings.

C1. Infectious and Parasitic Diseases

A. Human Immunodeficiency Virus (HIV) Infections

1. Code only confirmed cases of HIV infection/illness. This is an exception to the hospital inpatient guideline Section II, H.

   In this context, "confirmation" does not require documentation of positive serology or culture for HIV; the physician's diagnostic statement that the patient is HIV positive, or has an HIV-related illness is sufficient.

2. Selection and sequencing

   a. If a patient is admitted for an HIV-related condition, the principal diagnosis should be 042, followed by additional diagnosis codes for all reported HIV-related conditions.

   b. If a patient with HIV disease is admitted for an unrelated condition (such as a traumatic injury), the code for the unrelated condition (e.g., the nature of injury code) should be the principal diagnosis. Other diagnoses would be 042 followed by additional diagnosis codes for all reported HIV-related conditions.

   c. Whether the patient is newly diagnosed or has had previous admissions/encounters for HIV conditions is irrelevant to the sequencing decision.

   d. V08 Asymptomatic human immunodeficiency virus [HIV] infection, is to be applied when the patient without any documentation of symptoms is listed as being "HIV positive," "known HIV," "HIV test positive," or similar terminology. Do not use this code if the term "AIDS" is used or if the patient is treated for any HIV-related illness or is described as having any condition(s) resulting from his/her HIV positive status; use 042 in these cases.

   e. Patients with inconclusive HIV serology, but no definitive diagnosis or manifestations of the illness, may be assigned code 795.71, Inconclusive serologic test for Human Immunodeficiency Virus [HIV]

   f. Previously diagnosed HIV-related illness

      Patients with any known prior diagnosis of an HIV-related illness should be coded to 042. Once a patient had developed an HIV-related illness, the patient should always be assigned code 042 on every subsequent admission/encounter. Patients previously diagnosed with any HIV illness (042) should never be assigned to 795.71 or V08.

   g. HIV Infection in Pregnancy, Childbirth and the Puerperium

      During pregnancy, childbirth or the puerperium, a patient admitted (or presenting for a health care encounter) because of an HIV-related illness should receive a principal diagnosis of 647.6X, Other specified infectious and parasitic diseases in the mother classifiable elsewhere, but complicating the pregnancy, childbirth or the puerperium, followed by 042 and the code(s) for the HIV-related illness(es). Codes from Chapter 15 always take sequencing priority.

      Patients with asymptomatic HIV infection status admitted (or presenting for a health care encounter) during pregnancy, childbirth, or the puerperium should receive codes of 647.6X and V08.

   h. Encounters for Testing for HIV

      If a patient is being seen to determine his/her HIV status, use code V73.89, Screening for other specified viral disease. Use code V69.8, Other problems related to lifestyle, as a secondary code if an asymptomatic

ICD-9-CM Coding Guidelines

© 2004 Ingenix, Inc.

patient is in a known high risk group for HIV. Should a patient with signs or symptoms or illness, or a confirmed HIV related diagnosis be tested for HIV, code the signs and symptoms or the diagnosis. An additional counseling code V65.44 may be used if counseling is provided during the encounter for the test.

When a patient returns to be informed of his/her HIV test results use code V65.44, HIV counseling, if the results of the test are negative.

If the results are positive but the patient is asymptomatic use code V08, Asymptomatic HIV infection. If the results are positive and the patient is symptomatic use code 042, HIV infection, with codes for the HIV related symptoms or diagnosis. The HIV counseling code may also be used if counseling is provided for patients with positive test results.

B. Septicemia and Septic Shock

1. When the diagnosis of septicemia with shock or the diagnosis of general sepsis with septic shock is documented, code and list the septicemia first and report the septic shock code as a secondary condition. The septicemia code assignment should identify the type of bacteria if it is known.
2. Sepsis and septic shock associated with abortion, ectopic pregnancy, and molar pregnancy are classified to category codes in Chapter 11 (630-639).
3. Negative or inconclusive blood cultures do not preclude a diagnosis of septicemia in patients with clinical evidence of the condition.

C2. Neoplasms

Chapter 2 of the ICD-9-CM contains the code for most benign and all malignant neoplasms. Certain benign neoplasms, such as prostatic adenomas, may be found in the specific body system chapters. To properly code a neoplasm it is necessary to determine from the record if the neoplasm is benign, in-situ, malignant, or of uncertain histologic behavior. If malignant, any secondary (metastatic) sites should also be determined.

The neoplasm table in the Alphabetic Index should be referenced first. If the histological term is documented, that term should be referenced first, rather than going immediately to the Neoplasm Table, in order to determine which column in the Neoplasm Table is appropriate. For example, if the documentation indicates "adenoma," refer to the term in the Alphabetic Index to review the entries under this term and the instructional note to "see also neoplasm, by site, benign." The table provides the proper code based on the type of neoplasm and the site. It is important to select the proper column in the table that corresponds to the type of neoplasm. The tabular should then be referenced to verify that the correct code has been selected from the table and that a more specific site code does not exist.

A. If the treatment is directed at the malignancy, designate the malignancy as the principal diagnosis.

B. When a patient is admitted because of a primary neoplasm with metastasis and treatment is directed toward the secondary site only, the secondary neoplasm is designated as the principal diagnosis even though the primary malignancy is still present.

C. Coding and sequencing of complications associated with the malignant neoplasm or with the therapy thereof are subject to the following guidelines:

1. When admission/encounter is for management of an anemia associated with the malignancy, and the treatment is only for anemia, the anemia is designated at the principal diagnosis and is followed by the appropriate code(s) for the malignancy.
2. When the admission/encounter is for management of an anemia associated with chemotherapy or radiotherapy and the only treatment is for the anemia, the anemia is sequenced first followed by the appropriate code(s) for the malignancy.
3. When the admission/encounter is for management of dehydration due to the malignancy or the therapy, or a combination of both, and only the dehydration is being treated (intravenous rehydration), the dehydration is sequenced first, followed by the code(s) for the malignancy.
4. When the admission/encounter is for treatment of a complication resulting from a surgical procedure performed for the treatment of an intestinal malignancy, designate the complication as the principal or first-listed diagnosis if treatment is directed at resolving the complication.

D. When a primary malignancy has been previously excised or eradicated from its site and there is no further treatment directed to that site and there is no evidence of any existing primary malignancy, a code from category V10, Personal history of malignant neoplasm, should be used to indicate the former site of the malignancy. Any mention of extension, invasion, or metastasis to another site is coded as a secondary malignant neoplasm to that site. The secondary site may be the principal or first-listed with the V10 code used as a secondary code.

E. Admissions/Encounters involving chemotherapy and radiation therapy

1. When an episode of care involves the surgical removal of a neoplasm, primary or secondary site, followed by chemotherapy or radiation treatment, the neoplasm code should be assigned as principal or first-listed diagnosis. When an episode of inpatient care involves surgical removal of a primary site or secondary site malignancy followed by adjunct chemotherapy or radiotherapy, code the malignancy as the principal or first-listed diagnosis, using codes in the 140-198 series or where appropriate in the 200-203 series.

2. If a patient admission/encounter is solely for the administration of chemotherapy or radiation therapy code V58.0, Encounter for radiation therapy, or V58.1, Encounter for chemotherapy, should be the first-listed or principal diagnosis. If a patient receives both chemotherapy and radiation therapy both codes should be listed, in either order of sequence.

3. When a patient is admitted for the purpose of radiotherapy or chemotherapy and develops complications such as uncontrolled nausea and vomiting or dehydration, the principal or first-listed diagnosis is V58.0, Encounter for radiotherapy, or V58.1, Encounter for chemotherapy.

F. When the reason for admission/encounter is to determine the extent of the malignancy, or for a procedure such as paracentesis or thoracentesis, the primary malignancy or appropriate metastatic site is designated as the principal or first-listed diagnosis, even though chemotherapy or radiotherapy is administered.

G. Symptoms, signs, and ill-defined conditions listed in Chapter 16 characteristic of, or associated with, an existing primary or secondary site malignancy cannot be used to replace the malignancy as principal or first-listed diagnosis, regardless of the number of admissions or encounters for treatment and care of the neoplasm.

C3. Endocrine, Nutritional, and Metabolic Diseases and Immunity Disorders

Reserved for future guideline expansion

C4. Diseases of Blood and Blood Forming Organs

Reserved for future guideline expansion

C5. Mental Disorders

Reserved for future guideline expansion

C6. Diseases of Nervous System and Sense Organs

Reserved for future guideline expansion

C7. Diseases of Circulatory System

A. Hypertension

The Hypertension Table, found under the main term, "Hypertension", in the Alphabetic Index, contains a complete listing of all conditions due to or associated with hypertension and classifies them according to malignant, benign, and unspecified.

1. Hypertension, Essential, or NOS Assign hypertension (arterial) (essential) (primary) (systemic) (NOS) to category code 401 with the appropriate fourth digit to indicate malignant (.0), benign (.1), or unspecified (.9). Do not use either .0 malignant or .1 benign unless medical record documentation supports such a designation.

2. Hypertension with Heart Disease

Heart conditions (425.8, 429.0-429.3, 429.8, 429.9) are assigned to a code from category 402 when a causal relationship is stated (due to hypertension) or implied (hypertensive). Use an additional code from category 428 to identify the type of heart failure in those patients with heart failure. More than one code from category 428 may be assigned if the patient has systolic or diastolic failure and congestive heart failure.

The same heart conditions (425.8, 428, 429.0-429.3, 429.8, 429.9) with hypertension, but without a stated casual relationship, are coded separately. Sequence according to the circumstances of the admission/encounter.

3. Hypertensive Renal Disease with Chronic Renal Failure

Assign codes from category 403, Hypertensive renal disease, when conditions classified to categories 585-587 are present. Unlike hypertension with heart disease, ICD-9-CM presumes a cause-and-effect relationship and classifies renal failure with hypertension as hypertensive renal disease.

4. Hypertensive Heart and Renal Disease

Assign codes from combination category 404, Hypertensive heart and renal disease, when both hypertensive renal disease and hypertensive heart disease are stated in the diagnosis. Assume a relationship between the hypertension and the renal disease, whether or not the condition is so designated. Assign an additional code from category 428, to identify the type of heart failure. More than one code from category 428 may be assigned if the patient has systolic or diastolic failure and congestive heart failure.

5. Hypertensive Cerebrovascular Disease

© 2004 Ingenix, Inc.

First assign codes from 430-438, Cerebrovascular disease, then the appropriate hypertension code from categories 401-405.

6. Hypertensive Retinopathy

   Two codes are necessary to identify the condition. First assign the code from subcategory 362.11, Hypertensive retinopathy, then the appropriate code from categories 401-405 to indicate the type of hypertension.

7. Hypertension, Secondary

   Two codes are required: one to identify the underlying etiology and one from category 405 to identify the hypertension. Sequencing of codes is determined by the reason for admission/encounter.

8. Hypertension, Transient

   Assign code 796.2, Elevated blood pressure reading without diagnosis of hypertension, unless patient has an established diagnosis of hypertension. Assign code 642.3x for transient hypertension of pregnancy.

9. Hypertension, Controlled

   Assign appropriate code from categories 401-405. This diagnostic statement usually refers to an existing state of hypertension under control by therapy.

10. Hypertension, Uncontrolled

    Uncontrolled hypertension may refer to untreated hypertension or hypertension not responding to current therapeutic regimen. In either case, assign the appropriate code from categories 401-405 to designate the stage and type of hypertension. Code to the type of hypertension.

11. Elevated Blood Pressure

    For a statement of elevated blood pressure without further specificity, assign code 796.2, Elevated blood pressure reading without diagnosis of hypertension, rather than a code from category 401.

B. Late Effects of Cerebrovascular Disease

Category 438 is used to indicate conditions classifiable to categories 430-437 as the causes of late effects (neurologic deficits), themselves classified elsewhere. These "late effects" include neurologic deficits that persist after initial onset of conditions classifiable to 430-437. The neurologic deficits caused by cerebrovascular disease may be present from the onset or may arise at any time after the onset of the condition classifiable to 430-437.

Codes from category 438 may be assigned on a health care record with codes from 430-437, if the patient has a current cerebrovascular accident (CVA) and deficits from an old CVA. Assign code V12.59 (and not a code from category 438) as an additional code for history of cerebrovascular disease when no neurologic deficits are present.

C8. Diseases of Respiratory System

Reserved for future guideline expansion

C9. Diseases of Digestive System

Reserved for future guideline expansion

C10. Diseases of Genitourinary System

Reserved for future guideline expansion

C11. Complications of Pregnancy, Childbirth, and the Puerperium

A. General Rules for Obstetric Cases

1. Obstetric cases require codes from chapter 11, codes in the range 630-677, Complications of Pregnancy, Childbirth, and the Puerperium. Should the physician document that the pregnancy is incidental to the encounter, then code V22.2 should be used in place of any chapter 11 codes. It is the physician's responsibility to state that the condition being treated is not affecting the pregnancy.
2. Chapter 11 codes have sequencing priority over codes from other chapters. Additional codes from other chapters may be used in conjunction with chapter 11 codes to further specify conditions. For example, sepsis and septic shock associated with abortion, ectopic pregnancy, and molar pregnancy are classified to category codes in Chapter 11 (630-639).
3. Chapter 11 codes are to be used only on the maternal record, never on the record of the newborn.
4. Categories 640-648, 651-676 have required fifth-digits, which indicate whether the encounter is antepartum, postpartum and whether a delivery has also occurred.
5. The fifth-digits, which are appropriate for each code number, are listed in brackets under each code. The fifth-digits on each code should all be consistent with each other. That is, should a delivery occur all of the fifth-digits should indicate the delivery.
6. For prenatal outpatient visits for patients with high-risk pregnancies, a code from category V23, Supervision of high-risk pregnancy, should be used as the principal or first-listed diagnosis. Secondary chapter 11 codes may be used in conjunction with these codes if appropriate. A thorough review of any pertinent excludes note is necessary to be certain that these V codes are being used properly.
7. An outcome of delivery code, V27.0-V27.9, should be included on every maternal record

when a delivery has occurred. These codes are not to be used on subsequent records or on the newborn record.

8. For routine outpatient prenatal visits when no complications are present codes V22.0, Supervision of normal first pregnancy, and V22.1, Supervision of other normal pregnancy, should be used as the first-listed diagnoses. These codes should not be used in conjunction with chapter 11 codes.

B. Selection of OB Principal or First-listed Diagnosis

1. In episodes when no delivery occurs, the principal diagnosis should correspond to the principal complication of the pregnancy, which necessitated the encounter. Should more than one complication exist, all of which are treated or monitored, any of the complications codes may be sequenced first.

2. When a delivery occurs, the principal diagnosis should correspond to the main circumstances or complication of the delivery.

   In cases of cesarean delivery, the selection of the principal diagnosis should correspond to the reason the cesarean delivery was performed unless the reason for admission/encounter was unrelated to the condition resulting in the cesarean delivery.

C. Fetal Conditions Affecting the Management of the Mother

Codes from category 655, Known or suspected fetal abnormality affecting management of the mother, and category 656, Other fetal and placental problems affecting the management of the mother, are assigned only when the fetal condition is actually responsible for modifying the management of the mother, i.e., by requiring diagnostic studies, additional observation, special care, or termination of pregnancy. The fact that the fetal condition exists does not justify assigning a code from this series to the mother's record.

D. HIV Infection in Pregnancy, Childbirth and the Puerperium

During pregnancy, childbirth or the puerperium, a patient admitted because of an HIV-related illness should receive a principal diagnosis of 647.6X, Other specified infectious and parasitic diseases in the mother classifiable elsewhere, but complicating the pregnancy, childbirth or the puerperium, followed by 042 and the code(s) for the HIV-related illness(es). This is an exception to the sequencing rule found in above.

Patients with asymptomatic HIV infection status admitted during pregnancy, childbirth, or the puerperium should receive codes of 647.6x and V08.

E. Normal Delivery, 650

1. Code 650 is for use in cases when a woman is admitted for a full-term normal delivery and delivers a single, healthy infant without any complications antepartum, during the delivery, or postpartum during the delivery episode.

2. Code 650 may be used if the patient had a complication at some point during her pregnancy but the complication is not present at the time of the admission for delivery.

3. Code 650 is always a principal diagnosis. It is not to be used if any other code from chapter 11 is needed to describe a current complication of the antenatal, delivery, or perinatal period. Additional codes from other chapters may be used with code 650 if they are not related to or are in any way complicating the pregnancy.

4. V27.0, Single liveborn, is the only outcome of delivery code appropriate for use with 650.

F. The Postpartum Period

1. The postpartum period begins immediately after delivery and continues for six weeks following delivery.

2. A postpartum complication is any complication occurring within the six-week period.

3. Chapter 11 codes may also be used to describe pregnancy-related complications after the six-week period should the physician document that a condition is pregnancy related.

4. Postpartum complications that occur during the same admission as the delivery are identified with a fifth digit of "2." Subsequent admissions/encounters for postpartum complications should identified with a fifth digit of "4."

5. When the mother delivers outside the hospital prior to admission and is admitted for routine postpartum care and no complications are noted, code V24.0, Postpartum care and examination immediately after delivery, should be assigned as the principal diagnosis.

6. A delivery diagnosis code should not be used for a woman who has delivered prior to admission to the hospital. Any postpartum procedures should be coded.

G. Code 677, Late effect of complication of pregnancy, childbirth, and the puerperium

1. Code 677, Late effect of complication of pregnancy, childbirth, and the puerperium is for use in those cases when an initial complication of a pregnancy develops a

 © 2004 Ingenix, Inc.

sequelae requiring care or treatment at a future date.

2. This code may be used at any time after the initial postpartum period.
3. This code, like all late effect codes, is to be sequenced following the code describing the sequelae of the complication.

H. Abortions

1. Fifth-digits are required for abortion categories 634-637. Fifth-digit 1, incomplete, indicates that all of the products of conception have not been expelled from the uterus. Fifth-digit 2, complete, indicates that all products of conception have been expelled from the uterus prior to the episode of care.
2. A code from categories 640-648 and 651-657 may be used as additional codes with an abortion code to indicate the complication leading to the abortion.

   Fifth digit 3 is assigned with codes from these categories when used with an abortion code because the other fifth digits will not apply. Codes from the 660-669 series are not to be used for complications of abortion.
3. Code 639 is to be used for all complications following abortion. Code 639 cannot be assigned with codes from categories 634-638.
4. Abortion with Liveborn Fetus.

   When an attempted termination of pregnancy results in a liveborn fetus assign code 644.21, Early onset of delivery, with an appropriate code from category V27, Outcome of Delivery. The procedure code for the attempted termination of pregnancy should also be assigned.
5. Retained Products of Conception following an abortion.

   Subsequent admissions for retained products of conception following a spontaneous or legally induced abortion are assigned the appropriate code from category 634, Spontaneous abortion, or legally induced abortion, with a fifth digit of "1" (incomplete). This advice is appropriate even when the patient was discharged previously with a discharge diagnosis of complete abortion.

C12. Diseases Skin and Subcutaneous Tissue

Reserved for future guideline expansion

C13. Diseases of Musculoskeletal and Connective Tissue

Reserved for future guideline expansion

C14. Congenital Anomalies

Reserved for future guideline expansion

C15. Newborn (Perinatal) Guidelines

For coding and reporting purposes the perinatal period is defined as birth through the 28th day following birth. The following guidelines are provided for reporting purposes. Hospitals may record other diagnoses as needed for internal data use.

A. General Perinatal Rule

All clinically significant conditions noted on routine newborn examination should be coded. A condition is clinically significant if it requires: clinical evaluation; or therapeutic treatment; or diagnostic procedures; or extended length of hospital stay; or increased nursing care and/or monitoring; or has implications for future health care needs.

Note: The perinatal guidelines listed above are the same as the general coding guidelines for "additional diagnoses," except for the final point regarding implications for future health care needs. Whether or not a condition is clinically significant can only be determined by the physician.

B. Use of Codes V30-V39

When coding the birth of an infant, assign a code from categories V30-V39, according to the type of birth. A code from this series is assigned as a principal diagnosis, and assigned only once to a newborn at the time of birth.

C. Newborn Transfers

If the newborn is transferred to another institution, the V30 series is not used at the receiving hospital.

D. Use of Category V29

1. Assign a code from category V29, Observation and evaluation of newborns and infants for suspected conditions not found, to identify those instances when a healthy newborn is evaluated for a suspected condition that is determined after study not to be present. Do not use a code from category V29 when the patient has identified signs or symptoms of a suspected problem; in such cases, code the sign or symptom.
2. A V29 code is to be used as a secondary code after the V30, Outcome of delivery, code. It may also be assigned as a principal code for readmissions or encounters when the V30 code no longer applies. It is for use only for healthy newborns and infants for which no condition after study is found to be present.

E. Maternal Causes of Perinatal Morbidity

Codes from categories 760-763, Maternal causes of perinatal morbidity and mortality, are assigned only when the maternal condition has actually affected the fetus or newborn. The fact that the mother has an associated medical condition or experiences some complication of pregnancy, labor or delivery does not justify the routine assignment of codes from these categories to the newborn record.

F. Congenital Anomalies

Assign an appropriate code from categories 740-759, Congenital Anomalies, as an additional diagnosis when a specific abnormality is diagnosed for an infant. Congenital anomalies may also be the principal or first listed diagnosis for admissions/encounters subsequent to the newborn admission. Such abnormalities may occur as a set of symptoms or multiple malformations. A code should be assigned for each presenting manifestation of the syndrome if the syndrome is not specifically indexed in ICD-9-CM.

G. Coding of Additional Perinatal Diagnoses

1. Assign codes for conditions that require treatment or further investigation, prolong the length of stay, or require resource utilization.
2. Assign codes for conditions that have been specified by the physician as having implications for future health care needs.

   Note: This guideline should not be used for adult patients.
3. Assign a code for Newborn conditions originating in the perinatal period (categories 760-779), as well as complications arising during the current episode of care classified in other chapters, only if the diagnoses have been documented by the responsible physician at the time of transfer or discharge as having affected the fetus or newborn.

H. Prematurity and Fetal Growth Retardation

Codes from category 764 and subcategories 765.0 and 765.1 should not be assigned based solely on recorded birthweight or estimated gestational age, but on the attending physician's clinical assessment of maturity of the infant. NOTE: Since physicians may utilize different criteria in determining prematurity, do not code the diagnosis of prematurity unless the physician documents this condition.

A code from subcategory 765.2, Weeks of gestation, should be assigned as an additional code with category 764 and codes from 765.0 and 765.1 to specify weeks of gestation as documented by the physician.

C16. Signs, Symptoms and Ill-Defined Conditions

Reserved for future guideline expansion

C17. Injury and Poisoning

A. Coding of Injuries

When coding injuries, assign separate codes for each injury unless a combination code is provided, in which case the combination code is assigned. Multiple injury codes are provided in ICD-9-CM, but should not be assigned unless information for a more specific code is not available. These codes are not to be used for normal, healing surgical wounds or to identify complications of surgical wounds.

The code for the most serious injury, as determined by the physician, is sequenced first.

1. Superficial injuries such as abrasions or contusions are not coded when associated with more severe injuries of the same site.
2. When a primary injury results in minor damage to peripheral nerves or blood vessels, the primary injury is sequenced first with additional code(s) from categories 950-957, Injury to nerves and spinal cord, and/or 900-904, Injury to blood vessels. When the primary injury is to the blood vessels or nerves, that injury should be sequenced first.

B. Coding of Fractures

The principles of multiple coding of injuries should be followed in coding fractures. Fractures of specified sites are coded individually by site in accordance with both the provisions within categories 800-829 and the level of detail furnished by medical record content. Combination categories for multiple fractures are provided for use when there is insufficient detail in the medical record (such as trauma cases transferred to another hospital), when the reporting form limits the number of codes that can be used in reporting pertinent clinical data, or when there is insufficient specificity at the fourth-digit or fifth-digit level. More specific guidelines are as follows:

1. Multiple fractures of same limb classifiable to the same three-digit or four-digit category are coded to that category.
2. Multiple unilateral or bilateral fractures of same bone(s) but classified to different fourth-digit subdivisions (bone part) within the same three-digit category are coded individually by site.
3. Multiple fracture categories 819 and 828 classify bilateral fractures of both upper limbs (819) and both lower limbs (828), but without any detail at the fourth-digit level other than open and closed type of fractures.
4. Multiple fractures are sequenced in accordance with the severity of the fracture and the physician should be asked to list the fracture diagnoses in the order of severity.

C. Coding of Burns

Current burns (940-948) are classified by depth, extent and by agent (E code). Burns are classified by depth as first degree (erythema), second degree (blistering), and third degree (full-thickness involvement).

 © 2004 Ingenix, Inc.

1. Sequence first the code that reflects the highest degree of burn when more than one burn is present.
2. Classify burns of the same local site (three-digit category level, (940-947) but of different degrees to the subcategory identifying the highest degree recorded in the diagnosis.
3. Non-healing burns are coded as acute burns.

   Necrosis of burned skin should be coded as a non-healed burn.
4. Assign code 958.3, Posttraumatic wound infection, not elsewhere classified, as an additional code for any documented infected burn site.
5. When coding burns, assign separate codes for each burn site. Category 946 Burns of Multiple specified sites, should only be used if the location of the burns are not documented.

   Category 949, Burn, unspecified, is extremely vague and should rarely be used.
6. Assign codes from category 948, Burns classified according to extent of body surface involved, when the site of the burn is not specified or when there is a need for additional data. It is advisable to use category 948 as additional coding when needed to provide data for evaluating burn mortality, such as that needed by burn units. It is also advisable to use category 948 as an additional code for reporting purposes when there is mention of a third-degree burn involving 20 percent or more of the body surface.

   In assigning a code from category 948: Fourth-digit codes are used to identify the percentage of total body surface involved in a burn (all degree).

   Fifth-digits are assigned to identify the percentage of body surface involved in third-degree burn.

   Fifth-digit zero (0) is assigned when less than 10 percent or when no body surface is involved in a third-degree burn.

   Category 948 is based on the classic "rule of nines" in estimating body surface involved: head and neck are assigned nine percent, each arm nine percent, each leg 18 percent, the anterior trunk 18 percent, posterior trunk 18 percent, and genitalia one percent. Physicians may change these percentage assignments where necessary to accommodate infants and children who have proportionately larger heads than adults and patients who have large buttocks, thighs, or abdomen that involve burns.
7. Encounters for the treatment of the late effects of burns (i.e., scars or joint contractures) should be coded to the residual condition (sequelae) followed by the appropriate late effect code (906.5-906.9). A late effect E code may also be used, if desired.
8. When appropriate, both a sequelae with a late effect code, and a current burn code may be assigned on the same record.

D. Coding of Debridement of Wound, Infection, or Burn

Excisional debridement may be performed by a physician and/or other health care provider and involves an excisional, as opposed to a mechanical (brushing, scrubbing, washing) debridement.

For coding purposes, excisional debridement, 86.22.

Nonexcisional debridement is assigned to 86.28.

Modified based on Coding Clinic, 2nd Quarter 2000, p. 9.

E. Adverse Effects, Poisoning and Toxic Effects

The properties of certain drugs, medicinal and biological substances or combinations of such substances, may cause toxic reactions. The occurrence of drug toxicity is classified in ICD-9-CM as follows:

1. Adverse Effect

   When the drug was correctly prescribed and properly administered, code the reaction plus the appropriate code from the E930-E949 series. Codes from the E930-E949 series must be used to identify the causative substance for an adverse effect of drug, medicinal and biological substances, correctly prescribed and properly administered. The effect, such as tachycardia, delirium, gastrointestinal hemorrhaging, vomiting, hypokalemia, hepatitis, renal failure, or respiratory failure, is coded and followed by the appropriate code from the E930-E949 series.

   Adverse effects of therapeutic substances correctly prescribed and properly administered (toxicity, synergistic reaction, side effect, and idiosyncratic reaction) may be due to (1) differences among patients, such as age, sex, disease, and genetic factors, and (2) drug-related factors, such as type of drug, route of administration, duration of therapy, dosage, and bioavailability.
2. Poisoning
   a. When an error was made in drug prescription or in the administration of the drug by physician, nurse, patient, or other person, use the appropriate

poisoning code from the 960-979 series.

b. If an overdose of a drug was intentionally taken or administered and resulted in drug toxicity, it would be coded as a poisoning (960-979 series).

c. If a nonprescribed drug or medicinal agent was taken in combination with a correctly prescribed and properly administered drug, any drug toxicity or other reaction resulting from the interaction of the two drugs would be classified as a poisoning.

d. When coding a poisoning or reaction to the improper use of a medication (e.g., wrong dose, wrong substance, wrong route of administration) the poisoning code is sequenced first, followed by a code for the manifestation. If there is also a diagnosis of drug abuse or dependence to the substance, the abuse or dependence is coded as an additional code.

C18. Classification of Factors Influencing Health Status and Contact with Health Service

A. ICD-9-CM provides codes to deal with encounters for circumstances other than a disease or injury. The Supplementary Classification of Factors Influencing Health Status and Contact with Health Services (V01.0 - V83.89) is provided to deal with occasions when circumstances other than a disease or injury (codes 001-999) are recorded as a diagnosis or problem.

There are four primary circumstances for the use of V codes:

1. When a person who is not currently sick encounters the health services for some specific reason, such as to act as an organ donor, to receive prophylactic care, such as inoculations or health screenings, or to receive counseling on health related issue.

2. When a person with a resolving disease or injury, or a chronic, long-term condition requiring continuous care, encounters the health care system for specific aftercare of that disease or injury (e.g.,dialysis for renal disease; chemotherapy for malignancy; cast change). A diagnosis/symptom code should be used whenever a current, acute, diagnosis is being treated or a sign or symptom is being studied.

3. When circumstances or problems influence a person's health status but are not in themselves a current illness or injury.

4. For newborns, to indicate birth status.

B. V codes are for use in both the inpatient and outpatient setting but are generally more applicable to the outpatient setting. V codes may be used as either a first listed (principal diagnosis code in the inpatient setting) or secondary code depending on the circumstances of the encounter. Certain V codes may only be used as first listed, others only as secondary codes.

C. V Codes indicate a reason for an encounter. They are not procedure codes. A corresponding procedure code must accompany a V code to describe the procedure performed.

D. Categories of V Codes

1. Contact/Exposure

Category V01 indicates contact with or exposure to communicable diseases. These codes are for patients who do not show any sign or symptom of a disease but have been exposed to it by close personal contact with an infected individual or are in an area where a disease is epidemic. These codes may be used as a first listed code to explain an encounter for testing, or, more commonly, as a secondary code to identify a potential risk.

2. Inoculations and vaccinations

Categories V03-V06 are for encounters for inoculations and vaccinations. They indicate that a patient is being seen to receive a prophylactic inoculation against a disease. The injection itself must be represented by the appropriate procedure code. A code from V03-V06 may be used as a secondary code if the inoculation is given as a routine part of preventive health care, such as a well-baby visit.

3. Status

Status codes indicate that a patient is either a carrier of a disease or has the sequelae or residual of a past disease or condition. This includes such things as the presence of prosthetic or mechanical devices resulting from past treatment. A status code is informative because the status may affect the course of treatment and its outcome. A status code is distinct from a history code. The history code indicates that the patient no longer has the condition.

The status V codes/categories are:

V02 Carrier or suspected carrier of infectious diseases
Carrier status, indicates that a person harbors the specific organisms of a disease without manifest symptoms and is capable of transmitting the infection.

V08 Asymptomatic HIV infection status
This code indicates that a patient has tested positive for HIV but has manifested no signs or symptoms of the disease.

V09 Infection with drug-resistant microorganisms

ICD-9-CM Coding Guidelines

© 2004 Ingenix, Inc.

This category indicates that a patient has an infection which is resistant to drug treatment. Sequence the infection code first.

V21 Constitutional states in development

V22.2 Pregnant state, incidental
This code is a secondary code only for use when the pregnancy is in no way complicating the reason for visit. Otherwise, a code from the obstetric chapter is required.

V26.5x Sterilization status

V42 Organ or tissue replaced by transplant

V43 Organ or tissue replaced by other means

V44 Artificial opening status

V45 Other postsurgical states

V46 Other dependence on machines

V49.6 Upper limb amputation status

V49.7 Lower limb amputation status

V48.81 Postmenopausal status

V49.82 Dental sealant status

V58.6 Long-term (current) drug use
This subcategory indicates a patient's continuous use of a prescribed drug (including such things as aspirin therapy) for the long-term treatment of a condition or for prophylactic use. It is not for use for patients who have addictions to drugs.

V83 Genetic carrier status Categories V42-V46, and subcategories V49.6, V49.7 are for use only if there are no complications or malfunctions of the organ or tissue replaced, the amputation site or the equipment on which the patient is dependent. These are always secondary codes.

4. History (of)

There are two types of history V codes, personal and family. Personal history codes explain a patient's past medical condition that no longer exists and is not receiving any treatment but that has the potential for recurrence, and, therefore, may require continued monitoring. The exceptions to this general rule are category V14, Personal history of allergy to medicinal agents and subcategory V15.0, Allergy, other than to medicinal agents. A person who has had an allergic episode to a substance or food in the past should always be considered allergic to the substance.

Family history codes are for use when a patient has a family member(s) who has had a particular disease that causes the patient to be at higher risk of also contracting the disease.

Personal history codes may be used in conjunction with follow-up codes and family history codes may be use in conjunction with screening codes to explain the need for a test or procedure. History codes are also acceptable on any medical record regardless of the reason for visit. A history of an illness, even if no longer present, is important information that may alter the type of treatment ordered.

The history V code categories are:

V10 Personal history of malignant neoplasm

V12 Personal history of certain other diseases

V13 Personal history of other diseases
Except: V13.4, Personal history of arthritis, and V13.6, Personal history of congenital malformations. These conditions are life-long so are not true history codes.

V14 Personal history of allergy to medicinal agents

V15 Other personal history presenting hazards to health
Except: V15.7, Personal history of contraception.

V16 Family history of malignant neoplasm

V17 Family history of certain chronic disabling diseases

V18 Family history of certain other specific diseases

V19 Family history of other conditions

5. Screening

Screening is the testing for disease or disease precursors in seemingly well individuals so that early detection and treatment can be provided for those who test positive for the disease. Screenings that are recommended for many subgroups in a population include: routine mammograms for women over 40, a fecal occult blood test for everyone over 50, an amniocentesis to rule out a fetal anomaly for pregnant women over 35, because the incidence of breast cancer and colon cancer in these subgroups is higher than in the general population, as is the incidence of Down's syndrome in older mothers.

The testing of a person to rule out or confirm a suspected diagnosis because the patient has some sign or symptom is a diagnostic examination, not a screening. In these cases, the sign or symptom is used to explain the reason for the test.

A screening code may be a first listed code if the reason for the visit is specifically the screening exam. It may also be used as an additional code if the screening is done during an office visit for other health problems. A screening code is not necessary if the screening is inherent to a routine examination, such as a pap smear done during a routine pelvic examination.

Should a condition be discovered during the screening then the code for the condition may be assigned as an additional diagnosis.

The V code indicates that a screening exam is planned. A procedure code is required to confirm that the screening was performed.

The screening V code categories:

V28 Antenatal screening

V73-V82 Special screening examinations

6. Observation

There are two observation V code categories. They are for use in very limited circumstances when a person is being observed for a suspected condition that is ruled out. The observation codes are not for use if an injury or illness or any signs or symptoms related to the suspected condition are present. In such cases the diagnosis/symptom code is used with the corresponding E code to identify any external cause.

The observation codes are to be used as principal diagnosis only. The only exception to this is when the principal diagnosis is required to be a code from the V30, Live born infant, category. Then the V29 observation code is sequenced after the V30 code. Additional codes may be used in addition to the observation code but only if they are unrelated to the suspected condition being observed.

The observation V code categories:

V29 Observation and evaluation of newborns for suspected condition not found
A code from category V30 should be sequenced before the V29 code.

V71 Observation and evaluation for suspected condition not found

7. Aftercare

Aftercare visit codes cover situations when the initial treatment of a disease or injury has been performed and the patient requires continued care during the healing or recovery phase, or for the long-term consequences of the disease. The aftercare V code should not be used if treatment is directed at a current, acute disease or injury, the diagnosis code is to be used in these cases. Exceptions to this rule are codes V58.0, Radiotherapy, and V58.1, Chemotherapy. These codes are to be first listed, followed by the diagnosis code when a patient's encounter is solely to receive radiation therapy or chemotherapy for the treatment of a neoplasm. Should a patient receive both chemotherapy and radiation therapy during the same encounter code V58.0 and V58.1 may be used together on a record with either one being sequenced first.

The aftercare codes are generally first listed to explain the specific reason for the encounter. An aftercare code may be used as an additional code when some type of aftercare is provided in addition to the reason for admission and no diagnosis code is applicable. An example of this would be the closure of a colostomy during an encounter for treatment of another condition.

Certain aftercare V code categories need a secondary diagnosis code to describe the resolving condition or sequelae, for others, the condition is inherent in the code title.

Additional V code aftercare category terms include, fitting and adjustment, and attention to artificial openings.

The aftercare V category/codes:

V52 Fitting and adjustment of prosthetic device and implant

V53 Fitting and adjustment of other device

V54 Other orthopedic aftercare

V55 Attention to artificial openings

V56 Encounter for dialysis and dialysis catheter care

V57 Care involving the use of rehabilitation procedures

V58.0 Radiotherapy

V58.1 Chemotherapy

V58.3 Attention to surgical dressings and sutures

V58.41 Encounter for planned post-operative wound closure

V53.42 Aftercare, surgery, neoplasm

V53.43 Aftercare, surgery, trauma

V58.49 Other specified aftercare following surgery

V53.71-V53.78 Aftercare following surgery

V58.81 Fitting and adjustment of vascular catheter

V58.82 Fitting and adjustment of non-vascular catheter

V53.83 Monitoring therapeutic drug

V58.89 Other specified aftercare

© 2004 Ingenix, Inc.

8. Follow-up

The follow-up codes are for use to explain continuing surveillance following completed treatment of a disease, condition, or injury. They infer that the condition has been fully treated and no longer exists. They should not be confused with aftercare codes which explain current treatment for a healing condition or its sequelae. Follow-up codes may be used in conjunction with history codes to provide the full picture of the healed condition and its treatment. The follow-up code is sequenced first, followed by the history code.

A follow-up code may be used to explain repeated visits. Should a condition be found to have recurred on the follow-up visit, then the diagnosis code should be used in place of the follow-up code.

The follow-up V code categories: V24 Postpartum care and evaluation V67 Follow-up examination

9. Donor

Category V59 is the donor codes. They are for use for living individuals who are donating blood or other body tissue. These codes are only for individuals donating for others, not for self donations. They are not for use to identify cadaveric donations.

10. Counseling

Counseling V codes are for use for when a patient or family member receives assistance in the aftermath of an illness or injury, or when support is required in coping with family or social problems. They are not necessary for use in conjunction with a diagnosis code when the counseling component of care is considered integral to standard treatment.

The counseling V categories/codes:

- V25.0 General counseling and advice for contraceptive management
- V26.3 Genetic counseling
- V26.4 General counseling and advice for procreative management

V61 Other family circumstances

- V65.1 Person consulted on behalf of another person
- V65.3 Dietary surveillance and counseling
- V65.4 Other counseling, not elsewhere classified

11. Obstetrics and related conditions

See the Obstetrics guidelines for further instruction on the use of these codes.

V codes for pregnancy are for use in those circumstances when none of the problems or complications included in the codes from the Obstetrics chapter exist (a routine prenatal visit or postpartum care) V22.0, Supervision of normal first pregnancy, and V22.1, Supervision of other normal pregnancy, are always first listed and are not to be used with any other code from the OB chapter.

The outcome of delivery, category V27, should be included on all maternal delivery records. It is always a secondary code.

V codes for family planning (contraceptive) or procreative management and counseling should be included on an obstetric record either during the pregnancy or the postpartum stage, if applicable.

Obstetrics and related conditions V code categories:

V22 Normal pregnancy

V23 Supervision of high-risk pregnancy
Except: V23.2, Pregnancy with history of abortion. Code 646.3, Habitual aborter, from the OB chapter is required to indicate a history of abortion during a pregnancy.

V24 Postpartum care and evaluation

V25 Encounter for contraceptive management
Except V25.0x (See counseling above)

V26 Procreative management
Except V26.5x, Sterilization status, V26.3 and V26.4 (Counseling)

V27 Outcome of delivery

V28 Antenatal screening
See Screening - see section 5 of this article

12. Newborn, infant and child

See the newborn guidelines for further instruction on the use of these codes.

Newborn V code categories:

V20 Health supervision of infant or child

V29 Observation and evaluation of newborns for suspected condition not found-see Observation, section 6 of this article.

V30-V39 Liveborn infant according to type of birth

13. Routine and administrative examinations

The V codes allow for the description of encounters for routine examinations, such as, a general check-up, or, examinations for administrative purposes, such as, a pre-employment physical. The codes are for use as first listed codes only and are not to be used if the examination is for diagnosis of a suspected condition or for treatment

ICD-9-CM Coding Guidelines

purposes. In such cases the diagnosis code is used. During a routine exam, should a diagnosis or condition be discovered, it should be coded as an additional code. Pre-existing and chronic conditions, and history codes may also be included as additional codes as long as the examination is for administrative purposes and not focused on any particular condition.

Pre-operative examination V codes are for use only in those situations when a patient is being cleared for surgery and no treatment is given.

The V codes categories/code for routine and administrative examinations:

- V20.2 Routine infant or child health check
  Any injections given should have a corresponding procedure code.
- V70 General medical examination
- V72 Special investigations and examinations
  Except V72.5 and V72.6

14. Miscellaneous V codes

The miscellaneous V codes capture a number of other health care encounters that do not fall into one of the other categories. Certain of these codes identify the reason for the encounter, others are for use as additional codes which provide useful information on circumstances which may affect a patient's care and treatment.

Miscellaneous V code categories/codes:

- V07 Need for isolation and other prophylactic measures
- V50 Elective surgery for purposes other than remedying health states
  - V58.5 Orthodontics
- V60 Housing, household, and economic circumstances
- V62 Other psychosocial circumstances
- V63 Unavailability of other medical facilities for care
- V64 Persons encountering health services for specific procedures, not carried out
- V66 Convalescence and Palliative Care
- V68 Encounters for administrative purposes
- V69 Problems related to lifestyle

15. Nonspecific V codes

Certain V codes are so non-specific, or potentially redundant with other codes in the classification that there can be little justification for their use in the inpatient setting. Their use in the outpatient setting should be limited to those instances when there is no further documentation to permit more precise coding. Otherwise, any sign or symptom or any other reason for visit which is captured in another code should be used.

Nonspecific V code categories/codes:

- V11 Personal history of mental disorder
  A code from the mental disorders chapter, with an in remission fifth-digit, should be used.
  - V13.4 Personal history of arthritis
  - V13.6 Personal history of congenital malformations
  - V15.7 Personal history of contraception
  - V23.2 Pregnancy with history of abortion
- V40 Mental and behavioral problems
- V41 Problems with special senses and other special functions
- V47 Other problems with internal organs
- V48 Problems with head, neck, and trunk
- V49 Problems with limbs and other problems
  Exceptions: V49.6 Upper limb amputation status V49.7 Lower limb amputation status V49.81 Postmenopausal status V49.82 Dental sealant status
- V51 Aftercare involving the use of plastic surgery
  - V58.2 Blood transfusion, without reported diagnosis
  - V58.9 Unspecified aftercare
  - V72.5 Radiological examination, NEC
  - V72.6 Laboratory examination
    Codes V72.5 and V72.6 are not to be used if any sign or symptoms, or reason for a test is documented. See section K and L of the outpatient guidelines.

C19. Supplemental Classification of External Causes of Injury and Poisoning (E-codes)

Introduction: These guidelines are provided for those who are currently collecting E codes in order that there will be standardization in the process. If your institution plans to begin collecting E codes, these guidelines are to be applied. The use of E codes is supplemental to the application of ICD-9-CM diagnosis codes. E codes are never to be recorded as principal diagnosis (first-listed in noninpatient setting) and are not required for reporting to CMS.

External causes of injury and poisoning codes (E codes) are intended to provide data for injury research and evaluation of injury prevention strategies. E codes capture how the injury or poisoning happened (cause), the intent

 © 2004 Ingenix, Inc.

(unintentional or accidental; or intentional, such as suicide or assault), and the place where the event occurred. Some major categories of E codes include:

- transport accidents
- poisoning and adverse effects of drugs, medicinal substances and biologicals
- accidental falls
- accidents caused by fire and flames
- accidents due to natural and environmental factors
- late effects of accidents, assaults or self injury
- assaults or purposely inflicted injury
- suicide or self inflicted injury

These guidelines apply for the coding and collection of E codes from records in hospitals, outpatient clinics, emergency departments, other ambulatory care settings and physician offices, and nonacute care settings, except when other specific guidelines apply. (See Section III, Reporting Diagnostic Guidelines for Hospital-based Outpatient Services/Reporting Requirements for Physician Billing.)

A. General E Code Coding Guidelines

1. An E code may be used with any code in the range of 001-V83.89, which indicates an injury, poisoning, or adverse effect due to an external cause.
2. Assign the appropriate E code for all initial treatments of an injury, poisoning, or adverse effect of drugs.
3. Use a late effect E code for subsequent visits when a late effect of the initial injury or poisoning is being treated. There is no late effect E code for adverse effects of drugs.
4. Use the full range of E codes to completely describe the cause, the intent and the place of occurrence, if applicable, for all injuries, poisonings, and adverse effects of drugs.
5. Assign as many E codes as necessary to fully explain each cause. If only one E code can be recorded, assign the E code most related to the principal diagnosis.
6. The selection of the appropriate E code is guided by the Index to External Causes, which is located after the alphabetical index to diseases and by Inclusion and Exclusion notes in the Tabular List.
7. An E code can never be a principal (first listed) diagnosis.

B. Place of Occurrence Guideline

Use an additional code from category E849 to indicate the Place of Occurrence for injuries and poisonings. The Place of Occurrence describes the place where the event occurred and not the patient's activity at the time of the event.

Do not use E849.9 if the place of occurrence is not stated.

C. Adverse Effects of Drugs, Medicinal and Biological Substances Guidelines

1. Do not code directly from the Table of Drugs and Chemicals. Always refer back to the Tabular List.
2. Use as many codes as necessary to describe completely all drugs, medicinal or biological substances.
3. If the same E code would describe the causative agent for more than one adverse reaction, assign the code only once.
4. If two or more drugs, medicinal or biological substances are reported, code each individually unless the combination code is listed in the Table of Drugs and Chemicals. In that case, assign the E code for the combination.
5. When a reaction results from the interaction of a drug(s) and alcohol, use poisoning codes and E codes for both.
6. If the reporting format limits the number of E codes that can be used in reporting clinical data, code the one most related to the principal diagnosis. Include at least one from each category (cause, intent, place) if possible.

   If there are different fourth digit codes in the same three digit category, use the code for "Other specified" of that category. If there is no "Other specified" code in that category, use the appropriate "Unspecified" code in that category.

   If the codes are in different three digit categories, assign the appropriate E code for other multiple drugs and medicinal substances.
7. Codes from the E930-E949 series must be used to identify the causative substance for an adverse effect of drug, medicinal and biological substances, correctly prescribed and properly administered. The effect, such as tachycardia, delirium, gastrointestinal hemorrhaging, vomiting, hypokalemia, hepatitis, renal failure, or respiratory failure, is coded and followed by the appropriate code from the E930-E949 series.

D. Multiple Cause E Code Coding Guidelines

If two or more events cause separate injuries, an E code should be assigned for each cause. The first listed E code will be selected in the following order:

E codes for child and adult abuse take priority over all other E codes - see Child and Adult abuse guidelines.

E codes for terrorism events take priority over all other E codes except child and adult abuse.

E codes for cataclysmic events take priority over all other E codes except child and adult abuse and terrorism.

E codes for transport accidents take priority over all other E codes except cataclysmic events and child and adult abuse and terrorism.

The first-listed E code should correspond to the cause of the most serious diagnosis due to an assault, accident, or self-harm, following the order of hierarchy listed above.

E. Child and Adult Abuse Guideline

1. When the cause of an injury or neglect is intentional child or adult abuse, the first listed E code should be assigned from categories E960-E968, Homicide and injury purposely inflicted by other persons, (except category E967). An E code from category E967, Child and adult battering and other maltreatment, should be added as an additional code to identify the perpetrator, if known.
2. In cases of neglect when the intent is determined to be accidental E code E904.0, Abandonment or neglect of infant and helpless person, should be the first listed E code.

F. Unknown or Suspected Intent Guideline

1. If the intent (accident, self-harm, assault) of the cause of an injury or poisoning is unknown or unspecified, code the intent as undetermined E980-E989.
2. If the intent (accident, self-harm, assault) of the cause of an injury or poisoning is questionable, probable or suspected, code the intent as undetermined E980-E989.

G. Undetermined Cause

When the intent of an injury or poisoning is known, but the cause is unknown, use codes: E928.9, Unspecified accident, E958.9, Suicide and self-inflicted injury by unspecified means, and E968.9, Assault by unspecified means.

These E codes should rarely be used, as the documentation in the medical record, in both the inpatient outpatient and other settings, should normally provide sufficient detail to determine the cause of the injury.

H. Late Effects of External Cause Guidelines

1. Late effect E codes exist for injuries and poisonings but not for adverse effects of drugs, misadventures and surgical complications.
2. A late effect E code (E929, E959, E969, E977, E989, or E999.1) should be used with any report of a late effect or sequela resulting from a previous injury or poisoning (905-909).
3. A late effect E code should never be used with a related current nature of injury code.

I. Misadventures and Complications of Care Guidelines

1. Assign a code in the range of E870-E876 if misadventures are stated by the physician.
2. Assign a code in the range of E878-E879 if the physician attributes an abnormal reaction or later complication to a surgical or medical procedure, but does not mention misadventure at the time of the procedure as the cause of the reaction.

J. Terrorism Guidelines

1. When the cause of an injury is identified by the Federal Government (FBI) as terrorism, the first-listed E-code should be a code from category E979, Terrorism. The definition of terrorism employed by the FBI is found at the inclusion note at E979. The terrorism E-code is the only E-code that should be assigned. Additional E codes from the assault categories should not be assigned.
2. When the cause of an injury is suspected to be the result of terrorism a code from category E979 should not be assigned. Assign a code in the range of E codes based circumstances on the documentation of intent and mechanism.
3. Assign code E979.9, Terrorism, secondary effects, for conditions occurring subsequent to the terrorist event. This code should not be assigned for conditions that are due to the initial terrorist act.
4. For statistical purposes these codes will be tabulated within the category for assault, expanding the current category from E960-E969 to include E979 and E999.1.

Section II Selection of Principal Diagnosis(es) for Inpatient, Short-term, Acute Care Hospital Records

The circumstances of inpatient admission always govern the selection of principal diagnosis. The principal diagnosis is defined in the Uniform Hospital Discharge Data Set (UHDDS) as "that condition established after study to be chiefly responsible for occasioning the admission of the patient to the hospital for care."

The UHDDS definitions are used by acute care short-term hospitals to report inpatient data elements in a standardized manner. These data elements and their definitions can be found in the July 31, 1985, Federal Register (Vol. 50, No, 147), pp. 31038-40.

© 2004 Ingenix, Inc.

In determining principal diagnosis the coding conventions in the ICD-9-CM, Volumes I and II take precedence over these official coding guidelines. (See Section IA).

The importance of consistent, complete documentation in the medical record cannot be overemphasized. Without such documentation the application of all coding guidelines is a difficult, if not impossible, task.

A. Codes for symptoms, signs, and ill-defined conditions

Codes for symptoms, signs, and ill-defined conditions from Chapter 16 are not to be used as principal diagnosis when a related definitive diagnosis has been established.

B. Two or more interrelated conditions, each potentially meeting the definition for principal diagnosis

When there are two or more interrelated conditions (such as diseases in the same ICD-9-CM chapter or manifestations characteristically associated with a certain disease) potentially meeting the definition of principal diagnosis, either condition may be sequenced first, unless the circumstances of the admission, the therapy provided, the Tabular List, or the Alphabetic Index indicate otherwise.

C. Two or more diagnoses that equally meet the definition for principal diagnosis

In the unusual instance when two or more diagnoses equally meet the criteria for principal diagnosis as determined by the circumstances of admission, diagnostic workup and/or therapy provided, and the Alphabetic Index, Tabular List, or another coding guidelines does not provide sequencing direction, any one of the diagnoses may be sequenced first.

D. Two or more comparative or contrasting conditions

In those rare instances when two or more contrasting or comparative diagnoses are documented as "either/or" (or similar terminology), they are coded as if the diagnoses were confirmed and the diagnoses are sequenced according to the circumstances of the admission. If no further determination can be made as to which diagnosis should be principal, either diagnosis may be sequenced first.

E. A symptom(s) followed by contrasting/comparative diagnoses

When a symptom(s) is followed by contrasting/comparative diagnoses, the symptom code is sequenced first. All the contrasting/comparative diagnoses should be coded as additional diagnoses.

F. Original treatment plan not carried out

Sequence as the principal diagnosis the condition, which after study occasioned the admission to the hospital, even though treatment may not have been carried out due to unforeseen circumstances.

G. Complications of surgery and other medical care

When the admission is for treatment of a complication resulting from surgery or other medical care, the complication code is sequenced as the principal diagnosis. If the complication is classified to the 996-999 series, an additional code for the specific complication may be assigned.

H. Uncertain Diagnosis

If the diagnosis documented at the time of discharge is qualified as "probable", "suspected", "likely", "questionable", "possible", or "still to be ruled out", code the condition as if it existed or was established. The bases for these guidelines are the diagnostic workup, arrangements for further workup or observation, and initial therapeutic approach that correspond most closely with the established diagnosis.

Section III Reporting Additional Diagnoses for Inpatient, Short-term, Acute Care Hospital Records

GENERAL RULES FOR OTHER (ADDITIONAL) DIAGNOSES

For reporting purposes the definition for "other diagnoses" is interpreted as additional conditions that affect patient care in terms of requiring: clinical evaluation; or therapeutic treatment; or diagnostic procedures; or extended length of hospital stay; or increased nursing care and/or monitoring.

The UHDDS item #11-b defines Other Diagnoses as "all conditions that coexist at the time of admission, that develop subsequently, or that affect the treatment received and/or the length of stay. Diagnoses that relate to an earlier episode which have no bearing on the current hospital stay are to be excluded." UHDDS definitions apply to inpatients in acute care, short-term, hospital setting The UHDDS definitions are used by acute care short-term hospitals to report inpatient data elements in a standardized manner. These data elements and their definitions can be found in the July 31, 1985, Federal Register (Vol. 50, No, 147), pp. 31038-40.

The following guidelines are to be applied in designating "other diagnoses" when neither the Alphabetic Index nor the Tabular List in ICD-9-CM provide direction. The listing of the diagnoses in the patient record is the responsibility of the attending physician.

A. Previous conditions

If the physician has included a diagnosis in the final diagnostic statement, such as the discharge summary or the face sheet, it should ordinarily be coded. Some physicians include in the diagnostic statement resolved conditions or diagnoses and status-post procedures from previous admission that have no bearing on the current stay. Such conditions are not to be reported and are coded only if required by hospital policy.

However, history codes (V10-V19) may be used as secondary codes if the historical condition or family history has an impact on current care or influences treatment.

B. Abnormal findings

Abnormal findings (laboratory, x-ray, pathologic, and other diagnostic results) are not coded and reported unless the physician indicates their clinical significance. If the findings are outside the normal range and the attending physician has ordered other tests to evaluate the condition or prescribed treatment, it is appropriate to ask the physician whether the abnormal finding should be added.

Please note: This differs from the coding practices in the outpatient setting for coding encounters for diagnostic tests that have been interpreted by a physician.

C. Uncertain Diagnosis

If the diagnosis documented at the time of discharge is qualified as "probable", "suspected", "likely", "questionable", "possible", or "still to be ruled out", code the condition as if it existed or was established. The bases for these guidelines are the diagnostic workup, arrangements for further workup or observation, and initial therapeutic approach that correspond most closely with the established diagnosis.

Section IV Diagnostic Coding and Reporting Guidelines for Outpatient Services

These coding guidelines for outpatient diagnoses have been approved for use by hospitals/physicians in coding and reporting hospital-based outpatient services and physician office visits.

Information about the use of certain abbreviations, punctuation, symbols, and other conventions used in the ICD-9-CM Tabular List (code numbers and titles), can be found in Section IA of these guidelines, under "Conventions Used in the Tabular List." Information about the correct sequence to use in finding a code is also described in Section I.

The terms encounter and visit are often used interchangeably in describing outpatient service contacts and, therefore, appear together in these guidelines without distinguishing one from the other.

Though the conventions and general guidelines apply to all settings, coding guidelines for outpatient and physician reporting of diagnoses will vary in a number of instances from those for inpatient diagnoses, recognizing that:

The Uniform Hospital Discharge Data Set (UHDDS) definition of principal diagnosis applies only to inpatients in acute, short-term, general hospitals.

Coding guidelines for inconclusive diagnoses (probable, suspected, rule out, etc.) were developed for inpatient reporting and do not apply to outpatients.

A. Selection of first-listed condition

In the outpatient setting, the term first-listed diagnosis is used in lieu of principal diagnosis.

In determining the first-listed diagnosis the coding conventions of ICD-9-CM, as well as the general and disease specific guidelines take precedence over the outpatient guidelines.

Diagnoses often are not established at the time of the initial encounter/visit. It may take two or more visits before the diagnosis is confirmed.

The most critical rule involves beginning the search for the correct code assignment through the Alphabetic Index. Never begin searching initially in the Tabular List as this will lead to coding errors.

B. The appropriate code or codes from 001.0 through V83.89 must be used to identify diagnoses, symptoms, conditions, problems, complaints, or other reason(s) for the encounter/visit.

C. For accurate reporting of ICD-9-CM diagnosis codes, the documentation should describe the patient's condition, using terminology which includes specific diagnoses as well as symptoms, problems, or reasons for the encounter. There are ICD-9-CM codes to describe all of these.

D. The selection of codes 001.0 through 999.9 will frequently be used to describe the reason for the encounter. These codes are from the section of ICD-9-CM for the classification of diseases and injuries (e.g. infectious and parasitic diseases; neoplasms; symptoms, signs, and ill-defined conditions, etc.).

E. Codes that describe symptoms and signs, as opposed to diagnoses, are acceptable for reporting purposes when a diagnosis has not been established (confirmed) by the physician. Chapter 16 of ICD-9-CM, Symptoms, Signs, and Ill-defined conditions (codes 780.0 - 799.9) contain many, but not all codes for symptoms.

F. ICD-9-CM provides codes to deal with encounters for circumstances other than a disease or injury. The Supplementary Classification of factors Influencing Health Status and Contact with Health Services (V01.0- V83.89) is provided to deal with occasions when circumstances other than a disease or injury are recorded as diagnosis or problems.

 © 2004 Ingenix, Inc.

G. Level of Detail in Coding

1. ICD-9-CM is composed of codes with either 3, 4, or 5 digits. Codes with three digits are included in ICD-9-CM as the heading of a category of codes that may be further subdivided by the use of fourth and/or fifth digits, which provide greater specificity.
2. A three-digit code is to be used only if it is not further subdivided. Where fourth-digit subcategories and/or fifth-digit subclassifications are provided, they must be assigned. A code is invalid if it has not been coded to the full number of digits required for that code. See also discussion under Section I, General Coding Guidelines, Level of Detail.

H. List first the ICD-9-CM code for the diagnosis, condition, problem, or other reason for encounter/visit shown in the medical record to be chiefly responsible for the services provided. List additional codes that describe any coexisting conditions.

I. Do not code diagnoses documented as "probable", "suspected," "questionable," "rule out," or "working diagnosis". Rather, code the condition(s) to the highest degree of certainty for that encounter/visit, such as symptoms, signs, abnormal test results, or other reason for the visit.

Please note: This differs from the coding practices used by hospital medical record departments for coding the diagnosis of acute care, short-term hospital inpatients.

J. Chronic diseases treated on an ongoing basis may be coded and reported as many times as the patient receives treatment and care for the condition(s).

K. Code all documented conditions that coexist at the time of the encounter/visit, and require or affect patient care treatment or management. Do not code conditions that were previously treated and no longer exist. However, history codes (V10-V19) may be used as secondary codes if the historical condition or family history has an impact on current care or influences treatment.

L. For patients receiving diagnostic services only during an encounter/visit, sequence first the diagnosis, condition, problem, or other reason for encounter/visit shown in the medical record to be chiefly responsible for the outpatient services provided during the encounter/visit. Codes for other diagnoses (e.g., chronic conditions) may be sequenced as additional diagnoses.

For outpatient encounters for diagnostic tests that have been interpreted by a physician, and the final report is available at the time of coding, code any confirmed or definitive diagnosis(es) documented in the interpretation. Do not code related signs and symptoms as additional diagnoses.

Please note: This differs from the coding practice in the hospital inpatient setting regarding abnormal findings on test results.

M. For patients receiving therapeutic services only during an encounter/visit, sequence first the diagnosis, condition, problem, or other reason for encounter/visit shown in the medical record to be chiefly responsible for the outpatient services provided during the encounter/visit. Codes for other diagnoses (e.g., chronic conditions) may be sequenced as additional diagnoses.

The only exception to this rule is that when the primary reason for the admission/encounter is chemotherapy, radiation therapy, or rehabilitation, the appropriate V code for the service is listed first, and the diagnosis or problem for which the service is being performed listed second.

N. For patient's receiving preoperative evaluations only, sequence a code from category V72.8, Other specified examinations, to describe the pre-op consultations. Assign a code for the condition to describe the reason for the surgery as an additional diagnosis. Code also any findings related to the pre-op evaluation.

O. For ambulatory surgery, code the diagnosis for which the surgery was performed. If the postoperative diagnosis is known to be different from the preoperative diagnosis at the time the diagnosis is confirmed, select the postoperative diagnosis for coding, since it is the most definitive.

P. For routine outpatient prenatal visits when no complications are present codes V22.0, Supervision of normal first pregnancy, and V22.1, Supervision of other normal pregnancy, should be used as principal diagnoses. These codes should not be used in conjunction with chapter 11 codes.

Diagnosis Related Groups

Diagnosis Related Groups

Diagnosis related groups (DRGs) are a prospective payment system (PPS) in which patient categories are defined by diagnoses and/or procedures, and modified by age, complications, co-existing conditions, or discharge status. Each DRG groups similar patients with similar ailments, and anticipates the level of care required during hospitalization. Under the DRG prospective payment system, the facility is paid what the hospitalization was expected to cost, instead of its actual cost. The hospital may keep any excess payments, but also risks underpayment. DRGs are assigned to report inpatient services to Medicare, Medicaid, and some private payers. Case mix is the distribution of a hospital's inpatients across various diagnoses that create different DRGs. Case mix is a major factor in the rate-setting process for hospitals.

Annual Changes to DRGs

The government revises the Medicare hospital inpatient prospective payment system every year in reaction to its continuing experience with the system. Proposed changes are published in the *Federal Register* and the public is invited to comment on the rules before they are adopted. Usually, the final rules are published in August for the following year. They are effective Oct. 1 of every year.

The Importance of DRGs

DRGs provide the basis for payment to hospitals for care of Medicare, Medicaid, and an increasing number of commercially insured patients. The federal government adopted DRGs more than a decade ago to curb rising hospital costs associated with reasonable cost and line-item reimbursement methods. Through the DRG-based Prospective Payment System (PPS), hospitals are reimbursed a flat-rate based on a patient's diagnosis and treatment. On the assumption that patients with similar illnesses undergoing similar procedures will require similar care, each category of illness/treatment is assigned a DRG that is the main factor in determining reimbursement.

Before DRGs, hospitals itemized services following treatment and release. The payer and provider tallied the costs in retrospect — after the care was provided. Because DRG payments are standardized by illness and treatment, DRGs allow payers and providers to predict reimbursement prospectively — before the care is provided.

The scope of DRGs has expanded far beyond Medicare and private payer costs and claims. Personnel in health information management departments now influence the financial health of hospitals, as DRGs are based on patient records that list principal and secondary diagnoses, age, complications, discharge status, and comorbidities. Documentation is crucial. Hospital personnel closely evaluate case mix — the patients the hospital serves — since the nature and severity of overall patient illnesses play heavily in budget projections. DRGs affect literally everyone within a hospital — from nurses to department heads, social workers to utilization review coordinators, physicians to patients — because some standardization of treatments is necessary to keep costs in line with flat-rate reimbursements.

DRG Histories and Hierarchies

The Medicare program began in 1965 to pay a portion of the cost of health care for its beneficiaries. Until 1982, the method of payment for eligible Medicare beneficiaries was based on costs reported by the hospitals to the government. In 1982, a section of the Tax Equity and Fiscal Responsibility Act (TEFRA) mandated limits on Medicare payments to hospitals. Medicare began using PPS in late 1983.

CMS, the agency responsible for the administration of Medicare, funded studies seeking ways to decrease the cost of health care. One of the studies was based on DRGs, originally developed by Yale University researchers for utilization review purposes in the late 1960s. It was this revised study of DRGs, updated and changed to an ICD–9-CM version by Yale, that became the Medicare PPS. Today, correct assignment of DRGs is still dependent on ICD-9-CM diagnosis and procedure codes. CMS remains the lead agency for the maintenance and modification of DRGs; revisions have been contracted to 3M Health Information Systems (HIS).

Researchers at Yale University developed the early application of the ICD-9-CM version of DRGs based on the concept of patient case mix complexity. The researchers identified patient attributes that contributed most to resource demands. Key among them were the following:

- Severity of illness
- Prognosis
- Treatment difficulty
- Need for intervention

- Resource intensity

Researchers next sought to classify patients based on information routinely collected in hospital medical records. The goal was to identify a manageable number of patient groups that shared demographic, diagnostic, and therapeutic attributes. The classifications that resulted were of clinically comparable patients that consume hospital resources in a comparable fashion.

The revised DRGs developed at Yale divided all possible principal diagnoses into 25 mutually exclusive categories, referred to as major diagnostic categories (MDCs). The MDCs were further subdivided into DRGs:

- First — Principal diagnosis linked to anatomical system (MDC)
- Second — Patient's surgical status
  - principal diagnosis (nonsurgical DRG)
  - extent of surgical procedure (surgical DRG)
- Third — Comorbidities, complications, age, discharge status

Diagnosis Linked To Anatomical System

The MDC classification of diagnoses typically grouped by anatomic system is the basis for the DRG prospective payment system; each DRG falls into an MDC category.

The diagnoses and procedures in each MDC fall under the umbrella of a single organ system or etiology and are usually grouped by medical specialty, as in MDC 19 Mental Diseases and Disorders or MDC 14 Pregnancy, Childbirth and the Puerperium. In recent years, two new MDCs have been added to the original list to cover multiple trauma and HIV infections.

MDC Categories

MDC 1 Diseases and Disorders of the Nervous System (DRGs 1–35, 524, 528-534)

MDC 2 Diseases and Disorders of the Eye (DRGs 36–48)

MDC 3 Diseases and Disorders of the Ear, Nose, Mouth and Throat (DRGs 49–74, 168–169, 185–187)

MDC 4 Diseases and Disorders of the Respiratory System (DRGs 75–102, 475)

MDC 5 Diseases and Disorders of the Circulatory System (DRGs 104–145, 478–479, 514–518, 525-527, 535-536)

MDC 6 Diseases and Disorders of the Digestive System (DRGs 146–167, 170–184, 188–190)

MDC 7 Diseases and Disorders of the Hepatobiliary System and Pancreas (DRGs 191–208, 493–494)

MDC 8 Diseases and Disorders of the Musculoskeletal System and Connective Tissue (DRGs 209–213, 216–220, 223–256, 471, 491, 496–503, 519–520, 537-538)

MDC 9 Diseases and Disorders of the Skin, Subcutaneous Tissue and Breast (DRGs 257–284)

MDC 10 Endocrine, Nutritional and Metabolic Diseases and Disorders (DRGs 285–301)

MDC 11 Diseases and Disorders of the Kidney and Urinary Tract (DRGs 302–333)

MDC 12 Diseases and Disorders of the Male Reproductive System (DRGs 334–352)

MDC 13 Diseases and Disorders of the Female Reproductive System (DRGs 353–369)

MDC 14 Pregnancy, Childbirth and the Puerperium (DRGs 370–384)

MDC 15 Newborns and Other Neonates with Conditions Originating in the Perinatal Period (DRGs 385–391, 469–470)

MDC 16 Diseases and Disorders of the Blood and Blood Forming Organs and Immunological Disorders (DRGs 392–399)

MDC 17 Myeloproliferative Diseases and Disorders, and Poorly Differentiated Neoplasms (DRGs 400–414, 473, 492, 539-540)

MDC 18 Infectious and Parasitic Diseases (Systemic or Unspecified Sites) (DRGs 415–423)

MDC 19 Mental Diseases and Disorders (DRGs 424–432)

MDC 20 Alcohol/Drug Use and Alcohol/Drug Induced Organic Mental Disorders (DRG 433, 521–523)

MDC 21 Injury, Poisoning and Toxic Effects of Drugs (DRGs 439–455)

MDC 22 Burns (DRGs 504–511)

MDC 23 Factors Influencing Health Status and Other Contacts with Health Services (DRGs 461–467)

MDC 24 Multiple Significant Trauma (DRGs 484–487)

MDC 25 Human Immunodeficiency Virus Infections (DRGs 488–490)

© 2004 Ingenix, Inc.

Pre-MDC

Pre-MDCs originated in the eighth edition of DRGs. They are a departure from the traditional way DRGs had been determined (by principal diagnosis). In Pre-MDCs, the initial assignment of the DRG is based on a procedure. The Pre-MDCs are:

Heart Transplant or Implant of Heart Assist System (DRG 103)

Liver Transplant (DRG 480)

Bone Marrow Transplant (DRG 481)

Tracheostomy (DRGs 482, 541-542)

Lung Transplant (DRG 495)

Simultaneous Pancreas/Kidney Transplant (DRG 512)

Pancreas Transplant (DRG 513)

They allow patient assignment to these DRGs independent of the MDC of the principal diagnosis, and take into consideration the resource intensity of these procedures.

Patient's Surgical Status:

Surgery performed in an operating room (OR) is the principal deciding factor in consumption of hospital resources. The performance of OR procedures brings into play a host of inpatient resources, including anesthesia, nursing care, recovery room, and the operating suite. As a result, DRGs are separated into categories of surgical or medical (nonsurgical) cases.

Surgical Patients

Surgical DRGs are chosen based on the ICD-9-CM Volume 3 procedural code assigned. For example, DRG 191 includes 50. 0 *Hepatotomy* and 52.6 *Total pancreatectomy*. Both fall under MDC 7 Diseases and Disorders of the Hepatobiliary System and Pancreas. For patients undergoing multiple procedures, the most complex, applicable DRG in the hierarchy of major surgery, minor surgery, other surgery, and surgery unrelated to principal diagnosis that applies is chosen.

Medical Patients

Medical diagnoses are divided into categories in the medical DRGs. These categories include neoplasms and symptoms and conditions related to a single anatomical system. The level of service required for medical DRGs is generally less resource-intense than that for patients who undergo surgery.

Other Factors

A patient's age can occasionally be a defining factor in DRG assignment. Patients younger than 17 or older than 70 years of age are often assigned age-sensitive DRGs. For instance, DRG 342 is assigned to a patient older than 17 undergoing a circumcision. A male age 17 or younger would be assigned DRG 343 instead.

The patient's status upon discharge from the hospital is also considered a variable in the definition of a DRG. Burn patients transferred to another facility, for example, are designated a unique DRG. Separate DRGs were designed for patients who leave the hospital against medical advice (AMA).

Complications and Comorbidities (CCs)

A comorbidity, by DRG definition, is a condition existing prior to hospitalization, such as diabetes mellitus in a cancer patient. A complication, by DRG definition, is a new illness occurring during the hospitalization, as in postoperative pneumonia. A CC results in at least one extra day of hospitalization 75 percent of the time, and may be factored into the DRG to reflect a need for a higher level of care. CCs generally adjust reimbursement upward.

Both medical and surgical classes are sometimes further subdivided if complications or comorbidities (CCs) could affect the consumption of hospital resources. For example, patients admitted for congestive heart failure may exhibit numerous CCs, such as kidney failure or urinary retention, and their length of stay in the hospital and use of other services could be higher than other patients with congestive heart failure but functioning kidneys.

However, the validity of CCs is dependent on the principal diagnosis or procedure. The government has developed a list of CC exclusions for inappropriate associations with the principal diagnoses.

Assigning DRGs

There are 25 major diagnostic categories (MDCs) that are mutually exclusive groups based upon principal diagnosis. MDCs are subdivided primarily into medical and surgical DRGs. There are, however, two groups of DRGs that are not assigned to an MDC. The first are those DRGs that may be associated with all MDCs and reflect admission with an invalid principal diagnosis into a facility, have operating room procedures unrelated to the principal diagnosis, or are otherwise ungroupable. The other DRGs not assigned to an MDC are called pre-MDC DRGs and are grouped by surgical procedure rather than principal diagnosis.

Exempt Providers

There are some hospitals and hospital units that are exempt from the inpatient prospective payment system (IPPS), including rehabilitation, psychiatric, pediatric, and other units or facilities that deliver long-term care. Teaching facilities receive a larger payment than non-teaching facilities.

Patients are defined according to principal diagnosis or principal procedure after study. Once a surgical category is established for a patient, further definition is based on the type of procedure performed — the surgical/medical hierarchies. Special circumstances, such as age and complications, play a role in DRG assignment.

ICD-9-CM Coding Accuracy

Correct ICD-9-CM coding is essential for correct DRG assignment. Coding references, whether hard copy or electronic, will probably feature some level of support material to steer the individual coding toward the most specific code selection. The Ingenix hospital edition of Volume 1 ICD-9-CM features indicators for codes that affect DRG assignments, including unacceptable principal diagnoses, complications and comorbidities (CC), questionable admissions, and nonspecific diagnoses. Volume 3 tabular references also usually feature an indicator for codes that affect DRG assignments, including operating room (OR) or non-OR procedures, noncovered procedures, or nonspecific OR procedures.

Principal diagnosis

The principal diagnosis is the condition established after study to be chiefly responsible for occasioning the admission of the patient to the hospital.

To assign a DRG, first determine and code the principal diagnosis, then all secondary diagnoses, complications, and comorbidities. With the principal and secondary diagnoses in mind, consult Volume 3 to assign any procedure code that might apply to the patient's case.

Principal procedure

The principal procedure is the procedure that was performed for definitive treatment, rather than for diagnostic or exploratory purposes, or necessary to address a complication. It is the procedure most closely related to the principal diagnosis. If two procedures seem to meet the principal procedure definition, the one most closely related to the principal diagnosis should be designated as the principal procedure.

GMLOS

GMLOS (geometric mean length of stay) is a statistical tool used to compute reimbursement for a given DRG. An adjusted value of all cases, making allowances for outliers, transfer cases, and negative outlier cases that normally skew data. The GMLOS is calculated by CMS and announced yearly in the *Federal Register*.

AMLOS

AMLOS (arithmetic mean length of stay) is the average number of days a patient is expected to be hospitalized under a given DRG. Payment may be adjusted if hospitalization varies significantly from the AMLOS. AMLOS is calculated by CMS and announced yearly in the *Federal Register*.

RW

RW (relative weight) is an assigned weight that reflects the relative resource consumption associated with each DRG. The higher the relative weight, the greater the payment.

Outliers

Outliers are patients who fall outside the norm for a DRG, because they have an atypical length of stay (too short or too long), they die during their stay, or they leave against medical advice.

Medical partition

If no procedures were performed, a medical DRG is assigned. Secondary diagnosis codes, such as comorbidities and complications and discharge status, must be taken into consideration.

The Future

Refinements that would further divide DRGs by degrees of severity are being considered by CMS. While plans are made to launch a new system of expanded DRGs, other changes in current coding systems could require a complete overhaul of the DRG system within a few years. CMS intends to implement ICD-10-CM, a new alphanumeric coding system for diseases and procedures, by mid decade.

Since DRGs are all based on ICD-9-CM codes, the change to ICD-10-CM and ICD-10-PCS would greatly affect DRG decision trees and assignments. The same issues of mapping will be at work when ICD-10-CM and PCS are adopted. Once CMS formally presents the proposed DRG and ICD-10-CM and PCS changes, the hospital industry can begin to analyze the effects these changes will have upon their businesses.

Under Medicare PPS, any revision of the DRG system must redistribute reimbursement among hospitals according to the case mix, but may not increase or decrease aggregate Medicare payments to hospitals. Individual hospitals, however, could see significant changes in reimbursement under the new DRGs depending on their case mix as generated by the new DRGs.

Private payers may lag Medicare in the adoption of the new DRG system. If hospitals use both old and new systems concomitantly, their information systems will be challenged to differentiate between the old and new. This difficulty is inherent in assimilating the mammoth code changes involved in ICD-10-CM into a new set of DRG algorithms, whose DRG numbers may overlap wth old DRG numbers with the same or different meaning. The alphanumeric nature of ICD-10-CM is a challenge in itself for hospital information systems, since most are designed to accept either an alpha or numeric entry per field, but not a combination of the two. The ability to map from the old system to the new one would also be critical for utilization, finance, quality assurance, and case-mix analysis.

 © 2004 Ingenix, Inc.

ICD-10-CM Conventions

ICD-10-CM Conventions

Three Volume Set

Similar to ICD-9-CM, the tenth revision is divided into three volumes:

1. Volume 1 (Tabular List) is comprised of 21 chapters that contain the listing of alphanumeric codes. The same hierarchical organization of ICD-9-CM applies to ICD-10-CM: All codes with the same first three characters have common traits. Each character beyond three adds more specificity. In ICD-10-CM, valid codes may contain a seventh character.
2. If Volume 2 remains the title of the instructional manual after clinical modification in the United States, coders will need to remember that Volume 2 in ICD-10-CM refers to instructions, and not the index, as ICD-9-CM.
3. Volume 3 provides the index to the codes in the Tabular List. As in the ICD-9-CM index, terms in the ICD-10-CM index are found alphabetically, by diagnosis.

All codes in ICD-10-CM are alphanumeric (i.e., one letter followed by two numbers at the three-character level) as opposed to three numeric characters in the main classification of ICD-9-CM. Of the 26 available letters, all but the letter U is used. Some three-character categories have been left vacant for future expansion and revision.

Axis of Classification

ICD-10-CM is an arrangement of similar entities, diseases, and other conventions on the basis of specific criteria. Diseases can be arranged in a variety of ways, according to etiology, anatomy, or severity. The particular criteria chosen is called the axis of classification. Anatomy is the primary axis of classification of ICD-10-CM.

Different axes, such as etiology, site, type, or morphology, are used in classifying different diseases within the same chapters. The choice is based upon the most important aspects of the disease from both a statistical and clinical point of view. For example:

- Pneumonia: etiology of the pneumonia
- Malignant neoplasm: site
- Cardiac arrhythmia: type
- Leukemia: morphology

Supplemental Classifications

Many of the chapters in ICD-10-CM classify diseases of an organ system. Others are devoted to specific types of conditions grouped according to etiology or nature, e.g., neoplasms, referred to in ICD-10 as "special group" chapters. Three chapters do not fall into either of these categories: Symptoms, Signs and Abnormal Clinical and Laboratory Findings, Not Elsewhere Classified; External Causes of Morbidity and Mortality; and Factors Influencing Health Status and Contact with Health Services.

A residual category is a place for classifying a specified form of a condition that does not have its own specific subdivision.

Format

Similar to ICD-9-CM, the format in ICD-10-CM depends on indentation. For example, individual five-character subdivisions of four-character subcategories represent the etiology of the disease and, as such, appear like the following:

A02.2 Localized salmonella infections
  A02.20 Localized salmonella infection, unspecified
  A02.21 Salmonella meningitis
  A02.22 Salmonella pneumonia
  A02.23 Salmonella arthritis
  A02.24 Salmonella osteomyelitis
  A02.25 Salmonella pyelonephritis

ICD-10-CM also includes a sixth character for classification for the most precise subdivision, which appears like the following:

S61.4 Open wound of hand
  S61.40 Unspecifed open wound of hand
    S61.401 Unspecified open wound, right hand
    S61.402 Unspecified open wound, left hand
    S61.403 Unspecified open wound, unspecified hand

Typeface

Codes and titles in the Tabular List and main terms in the Alphabetic Index are in bold typeface. Exclusion notes and rubrics not used for primary tabulations of disease are in an italicized typeface.

Punctuation

The ICD-10-CM Tabular List uses certain punctuation. These include:

- Brace (}) enclose a series of terms, each of which is modified by the words following the brace.
- Brackets ([ ]) enclose synonyms, alternative wordings, or explanatory phrases.
- Colon (:) is applied rather than a comma for a term that has more than one essential modifier.
- Comma (,) distinguishes modifiers. Words following a comma are essential modifiers.
- Parentheses ( ) enclose supplementary words that are present or absent in the statement of a disease or procedure, but do not affect the code.
- Point Dash (.-) instructs you to turn to the category or subcategory referenced to review the subdivisions available for coding.

Notes

The tenth revision contains notes that describe the general content of the succeeding categories and provide instructions for using the codes. These include:

- A *code first* note tells you that two codes are necessary to describe the condition. *Code first* notes may identify the added code — or examples of the added code — required, a range of codes, or instructions to code the underlying disease.
- A *use* note gives specific instructions for using an additional code to completely describe a condition. Depending on the additional information to be encoded, a *use* note may apply to a specific code or range of codes. No codes may be specified though the notes describe the information to be encoded.

Instructional Notes

Throughout the Tabular List in ICD-9-CM, notes describe the general content of the succeeding categories and provide instructions for using codes. The same holds true for ICD-10-CM.

- Inclusion terms carry the same meaning in ICD-10-CM as they do in ICD-9-CM. The Tabular List contains inclusion notes to clarify the content of the chapter, subchapter, three-character, four-character, or five-character category to which the note applies. The inclusion terms describe other conditions classified to that code, such as synonyms of the condition listed in the code title or for an entirely different condition.
- Exclusion notes always appear with the word "excludes" and, similar to ICD-9-CM, the instructional exclusion note prevents a code from being applied incorrectly. ICD-10-CM expands the usage of exclusion notes, which are found at the beginning of a chapter, block, or category title. For example, exclusion notes are found in certain categories that represent diseases in combination and instruct the user not to use the code if the condition mentioned in the exclusion note is also present.

After the appropriate instructional notes, each chapter in ICD-10-CM begins with a list of subchapters or "blocks" of three-character categories. These blocks provide an overview of the structure of the chapter.

Modifiers

Two types of descriptors, called modifiers, are found in the Alphabetic Index:

- Essential modifiers affect code selection for a given diagnosis, due to the axis of classification.
- Non-essential modifiers may be present or absent for the diagnosis to be coded. Either way, the code stays the same.

Abbreviations

Two abbreviations are found in the tabular list:

NEC means "not elsewhere classified" and tells the coder when certain specified forms are classified elsewhere.

NOS means "not otherwise specified" and applies to residual categories that do not appear in sequence with (i.e., immediately following) the pertinent specific categories. These residual categories are entitled "Other specified." The abbreviation is equivalent to "unspecified." The term is assigned when documentation does not provide the detail for a specific code.

Cross-references

In the Alphabetic Index, cross-references point to all the possible information for a term or its synonyms.

 © 2004 Ingenix, Inc.

Syndromes

The term syndrome is commonly misused by the lay public to embrace a very broad spectrum of diseases and illnesses, many of which are not accepted by the traditional western medical fraternity. A syndrome is the composite of signs and symptoms that give a picture of the disease process. In genetics, a syndrome constitutes a pattern of related abnormalities that may be genetically related.

Syndromes may be eponymic — named for an individual, or several individuals (e.g., Tourette's, Ostrum-Furst). Others may be simply descriptive (e.g., cat-cry, acquired immune deficiency); some names are associated with several unrelated syndromes (see Weber). Other syndromes may be referenced by either description or eponym (e.g., bruising syndrome, or Diamond-Gardner syndrome).

The symptoms that comprise a syndrome may be singular or plural, specific, or broadly outlined. Syndromes may be physical or behavioral, congenital, or found later in life; and while syndromes are not diseases, they are used to describe diseases seen daily by health care givers. Commonly known diseases may be known by their accompanying syndromes, which complicates proper coding of ICD-9-CM codes.

ICD-9-CM contains a list of nearly 1,500 syndromes cross-referenced under its numeric system. The following list contains most of those syndromes, explained and cross-referenced by number and name. Many syndromes carry a number of names, which are noted within parenthesis in each entry. Similar syndromes with negligible differences are also grouped together to ease use.

13

758.1 (Patau's, trisomy D, D1) Variable symptoms of newborns with an extra chromosome in group D. Condition is usually fatal within two years and includes mental retardation and malformed ears, cardiac defects, convulsions, and others.

16-18 or E

758.2 (Edward's, trisomy E, E3) Congenital malformations in which extra chromosome is group E. Includes mental retardation, abnormal skull shape, malformed ears, small mandible, cardiac defects, short sternum, and other symptoms.

21 or 22

758.0 (Down, G, mongolism) Retardation with numerous markers varying from one person to another. Symptoms include retarded growth, flat face with short nose, epicanthic skin folds, protruding lower lip, rounded ears, thickened tongue, pelvic dysplasia, broad hands and feet, stubby fingers, and absence of Moro reflex.

Abercrombie's

277.3 One of a group of syndromes characterized by accumulation of insoluble fibrillar proteins in various organs and tissues of the body.

Achard-Thiers

255.2 Aranodactyly with small, receding mandible, broad skull, and laxity of joints in hands and feet.

Acid pulmonary aspiration

997.3 (Mendelson's) Pulmonary disorder resulting from aspirating the contents of stomach following vomiting or regurgitation.

Acquired immune deficiency

042 (AIDS) A contagious retroviral disease resulting from infection with human immunodeficiency virus (HIV) that can, in severe cases, suppress vital immunity. Several opportunistic infections, such as Kaposi's sarcoma and pneumocystitis pneumonia, are associated with this syndrome.

Acrocephalosyndactylism

755.55 (Aperts) A chromosomal condition with webbing of digits and a pointed head and variety of defects. Often associated with other chromosomal abnormalities.

Acute psycho-organic

293.0 Describes a mental health patient who chooses not to participate in day-to-day activities or therapy as a a result of emotional, organic, or chemical causes.

Adair-Dighton

756.51 (van der Hoeve's) Hereditary condition with symptoms including blue sclera, little growth, brittle bones, and deafness.

© 2004 Ingenix, Inc.

Adams-Stokes (-Morgagni)

426.9 (Stokes-Adams, Morgagni's disease, and Spens) Heart block often causing slow or absent pulse, vertigo, syncope, convulsions, and sometimes Cheyne-Stokes respiration.

Addisonian

255.4 (Bernard-Sergent) Acute adrenal insufficiency caused by illness, trauma, or large amounts of hormones used as therapy. Symptoms include hypotension, hyperthermia, hyponatremia, hyperkalemia, hypoglycemia, nausea, and vomiting.

Adie (-Holmes)

379.46 Paralysis of conjugate movement of eyes without paralysis of convergence. Caused by lesions of midbrain.

Adiposogenital

253.8 (Babinski-Frohlich, Frohlich) Obesity and hypogonadism in adolescent boys. Rare accompanying dwarfism is thought to indicate hypothyroidism.

Adrenogenital

255.2 (Achard-Thiers) Aranodactyly with small, receding mandible, broad skull, and joint laxity in hands and feet.

Adult maltreatment

995.8x Maltreatment (abuse) of an adult with emotional or physical violence. Most often committed against spouses and elders.

Adult respiratory distress

518.5 Respiratory distress following surgery, shock, or trauma; similar to, but not caused by, adult respiratory distress system.

Affective NEC

293.83 (affective organic NEC) Organic disorder in which the patient exhibits a number of changes in personality such as amotivation, depression, outbursts, and poor social judgment.

Afferent loop NEC

537.89 (Gastrojejunal loop obstruction) Distended afferent loop with illness and pain caused by acute or chronic obstruction of the duodenum and jejunum proximal to a gastrojejunostomy.

African macroglobulinemia

273.3 (Waldenström's) Earmarked by an increase in macroglobulins in the blood with symptoms of hyperviscosity such as weakness, fatigue, bleeding disorders, and visual disturbances.

Ahumada-Del Castillo

253.1 (Argonz-Del Castillo) Lactation and amenorrhea not following pregnancy characterized by hyperprolactinemia and pituitary adenoma.

Albright (-Martin)

275.49 (Martin-Albright, Seabright-Bantam) Similar to hypoparathyroidism and caused by a failure to respond to parathyroid hormone. Short stature, obesity, short metacarpals, and ectopic calcification.

Albright-McCune-Sternberg

756.59 (McCune-Albright, Albright's hereditary osteodystrophy) Patchy skin pigmentation, endocrine dysfunctions, and polyostotic fibrous dysplasia.

Alcohol withdrawal

291.81 (alcohol) Absence of alcohol in an alcohol-dependent individual with physiological and psychological symptoms. Severity may result in death.

Alcoholic amnestic

291.1 Physical and emotional symptoms resulting from profound ingestion of alcohol.

Alder's

288.2 Polymorphonuclear leukocytes, or white blood cells.

Aldrich (-Wiskott)

279.12 (Wiskott-Aldrich) Inherited immunodeficiency with eczema, thrombocyopenia, recurrent pyogenic infection, and increased susceptibility to infection with encapsulated bacteria.

Alibert-Bazin

202.1x Malignant neoplasm resembling a fungus and growing outside of the body.

Alice in Wonderland

293.89 Organic disorder with patient presenting an illusion of dreams, feelings of levitation, and alteration of passage of time. Associated with epilepsy, migraines, and other problems of the parietal part of brain.

Allen-Masters

620.6 Pelvic pain resulting from old laceration of broad ligament received during delivery.

Alport's

759.89 Progressive sensorineural hearing loss, ocular defects, and glomerulonephritis, or pyelonephritis. Cause is inherited.

Alveolar capillary block

516.3 (Hamman-Rich) Chronic inflammation and progressive fibrosis of pulmonary alveolar

© 2004 Ingenix, Inc.

walls, with progressive dyspnea leading to death by oxygen deprivation or right heart failure.

Amnestic

294.0 Amnestic dementia in which the patient has no short-term or long-term memories but is not delirious.

Amotivational

292.89 Patient who chooses not to participate in day-to-day activities or therapy as a a result of emotional, organic, or chemical causes.

Amyostatic

275.1 Accumulation of copper in the brain, cornea, kidney, liver, and other tissues causing cirrhosis of the liver and deterioration in the basal ganglia of the brain.

Angelman

759.89 Emergence in early childhood of a pattern of interrupted development, stiff, jerky gait, absence or impairment of speech, excessive laughter, and seizures.

Angina

413.9 Acute, choking pain most notable in the pectoral region of the chest and implying the onset of a heart attack.

Angina cruris

443.9 (Charcot's) Number of symptoms in a moving limb including pain, tension, and weakness but absent at rest. Caused by occlusive arterial diseases of the limbs.

Antimongolism

758.3 Mental and growth retardation, hypertonia, high-arched palate, micrognathia, microcephaly and an anti-mongoloid obliquity of the palpebral fissures.

Anton (-Babinski)

307.9 A form of cortical blindness caused by damage to the occipital lobe and where the patient denies the visual impairment.

Apert's

755.55 Chromosomal condition with webbing of digits, a pointed head, and varieties of defects. Often associated with other chromosomal abnormalities.

Apert-Gallais

255.2 Type I acrocephalosyndactyly with a peaked head, fusion of digits (specifically the second through fifth digits), and severe acne vulgaris of forearms.

Aphasia-apraxia-alexia

784.69 (Bianchi's) Sensory aphasic condition with alexia and apraxia associated with lesions in the left parietal lobe.

Arc-welders'

370.24 Temporary or permanent spot blindness resulting from observing bright light unprotected.

Arch

446.7 (Marorell-Fabre, Raed-Harbitz, Takayasu-Onishi) Progressive obliteration of brachiocephalic trunk and left subclavian and left common carotid arteries above their source in the aortic arch. Symptoms include ischemia, transient blindness, facial atrophy, and many others.

Arcuate ligament

447.4 Compression of the celiac artery by the median arcuate ligament in the diaphragm.

Argentaffin, argintaffinoma

259.2 (Bjorck-Thorson, Cassidy-Scholte, Hedinger's) Carcinoid tumors causing severe attacks of cyanotic flushing of the skin, diarrhea watery stools, bronchoconstrictive attacks, hypotension, edema, and ascites.

Argonz-Del Castillo

253.1 (Ahumada-Del Castillo) Lactation and amenorrhea not following pregnancy and characterized by hyperprolactinemia and pituitary adenoma.

Argyll Robertson

094.89 (syphilitic), 379.49 (nonsyphilitic) A condition where the pupil of the eye is small and unresponsive to changes in light intensity.

Arm-shoulder

337.9 (Claude Bernard-Horner, Reilly's, Steinbrocker's) Disorder following a heart attack with pain and stiffness in the shoulder and swelling and pain in the hand.

Arnold-Chiari

741.0 Cerebellomedullary malformation syndrome. Displacement of the caudal spinal cord due to tethering with or without spina bifida and other problems such as meningomyelocele.

Arrillaga-Ayerza

416.0 (arteriosclerosis) Cyanosis and hypertension resulting from sclerosis of the pulmonary arteries.

Arteriomesenteric duodenum occlusion

537.89 (Gastrojejunal loop obstruction) Distended afferent loop with illness and pain caused by acute or chronic obstruction of the

© 2004 Ingenix, Inc.

duodenum and jejunum proximal to a gastrojejunostomy.

Arteriosclerosis depressive
293.83 Organic disorder in which the patient exhibits changes in personality such as amotivation, depression, outbursts, poor social judgment, etc. Caused by constriction of the arteries to the brain.

Artery compression
447.4 Compression of the celiac artery by the median arcuate ligament in the diaphragm.

Artery entrapment
447.8 Malignant atrophic papulosis.

Artery, superior
557.1 (Wilkie's) Complete or partial block of the superior mesenteric artery with vomiting, pain, blood in the stool, distended abdomen, and resulting in bowel infarction.

Asherman's
621.5 Adhesions in the endometrial cavity causing amenorrhea and infertility.

Aspiration
770.1 Intrauterine fetal aspiration of amniotic fluid contaminated by meconium.

Ataxia-telangiectasia
334.8 (Boder-Sedgwick, Louis-Bar) Gonadal hypoplasia, insulin resistance and hyperglycemia, liver function problems, increased sensitivity to ionizing radiation, ataxia, and nystagmus.

Audry's
757.39 Increased thickening of the skin on extremities and face with clubbing of fingers and deformities in bone of the limb.

Auriculotemporal
350.8 (Frey's) Localized sweating and flushing of the cheek and ear in response to chewing.

Automatism
348.8 Infarction of the postero-inferior thalamus causing transient hemiparesis, severe loss of sensation with crude pain in the limbs, or vasomotor or trophic disturbances.

Avellis'
344.89 (Babinski-Nageotte, Benedikt's, Brown-Sequard, Cestan's, Cestan-Chenais, Foville's, Gubler-Millard, Jackson's, Weber-Leyden) Paraplegia and anesthesia over part of the body caused by lesions in the brain or spinal cord.

Axenfeld's
743.44 A dysgenesis of the eye marked through widened trabecular meshwork, large iridial bands, and glaucoma.

Ayerza (-Arrillaga)
416.0 Cyanosis and hypertension, resulting from sclerosis of the pulmonary arteries.

Baader's
695.1 Necrolysis of the skin caused by toxins.

Baastrup's
721.5 Kissing spine. Malformation of the spine in which kyphosis becomes so great nonadjacent vertebrae touch.

Babinski-Fröhlich
253.8 (Frölich) Obesity and hypogonadism in adolescent boys with rare accompanying dwarfism, thought to indicate hypothyroidism.

Babinski-Nageotte
344.89 (Avellis, Benedikt's, Brown-Sequard, Cestan's, Cestan-Chenais, Foville's, Gubler-Millard, Jackson's, Weber-Leyden) Paraplegia and anesthesia over part of the body caused by lesions in the brain or spinal cord.

Baby or child maltreatment
995.5 Maltreatment of a child (child abuse) through physical violence, emotional violence, or starvation.

Bagratuni's
446.5 (Horton's, giant cell arteritis) Temoral arteritis.

Balint's
368.16 (Balint's, Holmes', Riddoch's) Cortical paralysis of visual fixation, optic ataxia, and disturbance of visual attention with normal eye movements.

Ballantyne (-Runge)
766.2 Placental dysfunction occurring in postmature fetuses.

Ballooning posterior leaflet
424.0 (Barlow's) "Mid-late" systolic click of the heart due to massive protrusion of the mitral valvular leaflet in the left atrial cavity.

Barlow's
424.0 "Mid-late" systolic click of the heart due to massive protrusion of the mitral valvular leaflet in the left atrial cavity.

Baron Munchausen's
301.51 (see Munchausen's)

 © 2004 Ingenix, Inc.

Barraquer (-Simon)

272.6 Progressive lipodystrophy, a progressive atrophy of the subcutaneous fat of the face.

Barré-Guillain

357.0 (Guillain-Barre, Landry, Fisher's, Strohl, Miller) Disorder of the immune system with paraplegia of limbs, flaccid paralysis, ophthalmoplegia, ataxia, and areflexia.

Barré-Liéou

723.2 Irritation of the nerve roots emanating from the posterior cervical spinal cord.

Barrett's

530.2 Gastrointestinal reflux in the esophagus associated heartburn and regurgitation caused by stricture constructed of epithelium.

Bársony-Polgár

530.5 (Barsony-Teschendorf) Strong, uncoordinated contraction of the esophagus evoked by deglutition in the elderly. Appears as a series of concentric narrows or as spiral on an x-ray.

Bartter's

255.1 Found in children with hypokalemic alkalosis, elevated renin or angiotensin levels, low or normal blood pressure, no edema, and retarded growth.

Basedow's

242.0x (Basedow, Parry's, Grave's disease) Fatigue, nervousness, emotional lability and irritability, heat intolerance and increased sweating, weight loss, palpitation, and tremor of hands and tongue. May be autoimmune in etiology.

Basilar artery

435.0 (Raymond-Cestan) Quadriplegia, anesthesia, and nystagmus. Due to obstruction of twigs of the basilar artery, causing lesions in the pontine region.

Basofrontal

377.04 (Foster-Kennedy, Gowers-Paton-Kennedy) Meningioma of the optic nerve, marked by central scotoma and contralateral choked disk.

Bassen-Kornzweig

272.5 Retinal pigmentary degeneration, malabsorption, engorgement of upper intestinal cells with triglycerides, neuromuscular abnormalities, and an absence from plasma of low density lipoproteins.

Batten-Steinert

359.2 Condition in which the peritoneal cover of the liver converts to a white mass resembling cake icing.

Battered child (baby)

995.54 Injuries sustained by a baby or child from physical abuse, usually inflicted by a caregiver; also known as shaken baby syndrome.

Baumgarten-Cruveilhier

571.5 Cirrhosis of the liver with patent paraumbilical, varicose periumbilical, or umbilical veins.

Bearn-Kunkel (-Slater)

571.49 Chronic hepatitis with autoimmune manifestations.

Beau's

429.1 Cardiac arrest.

Bechterew-Strümpell-Marie

720.0 Rheumatoid inflammation of the vertebrae.

Beck's

433.8x Occlusion of the spinal artery as result of injury, disk damage, or cardiovascular disease.

Beckwith (-Wiedemann)

759.89 Congenital disorder with macroglossia, gigantism, dysplasia of the renal medulla, visceromegaly, adrenocortical cytomegaly, and exomphalos.

Bekhterev-Strümpell-Marie

720.0 Rheumatoid inflammation of the vertebrae.

Behcet's

136.1 A chronic condition linked to disturbances in the immune system where small blood vessels become locally Inflammed, causing ulcerations of the oral and pharyngeal mucous membranes, skin lesions, and Inflammation of joints.

Benedikt's

344.89 (Avellis, Babinski-Nageotte, Benedikt's, Brown-Sequard, Cestan's, Cestan-Chenais, Foville's, Gubler-Millard, Jackson's, Weber-Leyden) Paraplegia and anesthesia over part of the body caused by lesions in the brain or spinal cord.

Bernard-Horner

337.9 Claude Bernard-Homer, Reilly's, Steinbrocker's) Disorder following a heart attack with pain and stiffness in the shoulder, and swelling and pain in the hand.

Bernard-Sergent

255.4 Acute adrenal insufficiency caused by illness or trauma or by large amounts of hormones used as therapy. Symptoms include hypotension, hyperthermia, hyponatremia, hyperkalemia, hypoglycemia, nausea, and vomiting.

Bernhardt-Roth

355.1 Tingling, formication, itching, and other symptoms on the outer side of the lower part of the thigh. Caused by lateral femoral cutaneous nerve.

Bernheim's

428.0 Right heart failure accompanied by enlarged liver, distended neck veins, and edema without pulmonary congestion, caused by hypertrophied septum.

Bertolotti's

756.15 Fusion of the bottom lumbar vertebra to the top sacral vertebra, making a sixth sacral vertebra accompanied by sciatica and scoliosis.

Bianchi's

784.69 Sensory aphasic condition with alexia and apraxia and lesions in the left parietal lobe.

Biedl-Bardet

759.89 (Biemond's) Mental retardation, pigmentary retinopathy, obesity, polydactyly, and hypogonadism.

Biemond's

759.89 Mental retardation, pigmentary retinopathy, obesity, polydactyly, and hypogonadism.

Bifurcation

444.0 (Leriche's) Obstruction of the terminal aorta causing fatigue in the hips, thighs, or calves and pallor of lower extremities and impotence in exercising males.

Big Spleen

289.4 (hypersplenism) Enlarged spleen caused by cirrohsis of liver or portal or splenic vein thrombosis causing anemia, hyperplasia of marrow precursers of deficient cell type.

Bilateral polycystic ovarian

256.4 Acute adrenal insufficiency caused by illness, trauma, or by large amounts of hormones used as therapy with hypotension, hyperthermia, hyponatremia, hyperkalemia, hypoglycemia, nausea, and vomiting.

Bing-Horton's (cluster headache)

346.2 Idiopathic unilateral headaches that reoccur in brief, sudden attacks that may disappear entirely over time.

Biörck (-Thorson)

259.2 (Cassidy-Scholte, Hedinger's) Carcinoid tumors that cause cyanotic flushing of the skin, diarrhea watery stools, bronchoconstrictive attacks, hypotension, edema, and ascites.

Blackfan-Diamond

284.0 (Diamond-Blackfan, Fanconi, Kaznelson's) Congenital anemia that manifests during infancy and requires a number of blood transfusions to maintain life.

Black lung

500 (coal miner's pneumoconiosis, anthracosis) Blockage of bronchioles by "coal machules" brought about by aspiration of coal dust.

Blind loop

579.2 Loop of small intestine detached surgically or detaching itself and, in the former case, becomes bacterial, and, in the latter case, accepts feces but cannot discharge it, becoming infected.

Bloch-Siemens

757.33 (Block-Sulzberger) Pigmented lesions appear in linear, zebra stripe, and other configurations and preceded by vesicles and bullae and followed by verrucal lesions.

Bloch-Sulzberger

757.33 (Block-Siemens) Pigmented lesions appear in linear, zebra stripe, and other configurations and preceded by vesicles and bullae and followed by verrucal lesions.

Bloom (-Machacek) (-Torre)

757.39 Butterfly-shaped lesions on the face and hands, dolichocephalic skull and narrow face, and dwarfism with normal body proportions.

Blount-Barber

732.4 Bow-legs in children.

Blue toe

445.02 A complication of pancreatitis characterized by tissue ischemia secondary to cholesterol crystal or atherothrombotic embolization, which leads to occlusion of small vessels that may present as cyanosis of digits, such as the toes.

Boder-Sedgwick

334.8 (Boder-Sedgwick, Louis-Bar) Gonadal hypoplasia, insulin resistance and hyperglycemia, liver function problems, increased sensitivity to ionizing radiation, ataxia, and nystagmus.

 © 2004 Ingenix, Inc.

Body or sinus, carotid
337.0 (Charcot-Weiss-Baker, Sluder's) Stimulation of an overactive carotid sinus, causing a marked drop in blood pressure, which, in turn, may stop the heart.

Bonnevie-Ullrich
758.6 Short stature, webbed neck, congenital heart disease, and mental retardation.

Bonnier's
386.19 Ocular disturbances, deafness, nausea, thirst, anorexia, and symptoms resulting from a lesion of Deiters' nucleus and its connections.

Bouveret (-Hoffmann)
427.2 Rapid action of the heart with sudden onset and cessation.

Bowel
579.3 Hypoglycemia and malabsorption following surgery.

Bowel distress
564.1 Abdominal pain, watery stools, and gas.

Brachial plexus
353.0 (Naffziger's) Anesthesis and vascular contraction in extremities caused by pressure of brachial plexus and subclavian artery against first thoracic rib.

Bradycardia-tachycardia
427.81 Rapid action of the heart followed by protracted or transient stopping of the heart.

Brailsford-Morquio
277.5 Accumulation of mucopolyscharide sulfates affecting the eye, ear, skin, teeth, skeleton, joints, liver, spleen, cardiovascular system, respiratory system, and central nervous system.

Brandt's
686.8 (Danbolt) Zinc metabolism defect in young children with blisters, crusting, oozing eruptions, loss of hair, and diarrhea.

Brennemann's
289.2 Lymphadenitis in the mesentery and retroperitoneal area as a sequel of throat infection.

Briquet's (Brissaud-Marie)
300.81 Personality disorder more prevalent among women involving concurrent alcoholism and somatisation whereby the patient reports physical complaints absent of medical indication.

Brissaud-Meige
244.9 Hypothyroidism resulting from acquired injury of thyroid gland or presence of cretinism.

Brock's
518.0 Incomplete expansion of the right middle lobe of a lung with chronic pneumonitis.

Brown spot
756.59 (McCune-Albright, Albright's hereditary osteodystrophy) Patchy skin pigmentation, endocrine dysfunctions, and polyostotic fibrous dysplasia.

Brown's tendon sheath
378.61 Limited elevation of eye, marked by paresis of inferior oblique muscle.

Brown-Séquard
344.89 (Avellis, Babinski-Nageotte, Benedikt's, Cestan's, Cestan-Chenais, Foville's, Gubler-Millard, Jackson's, Weber-Leyden) Paraplegia and anesthesia over part of the body caused by lesions in the brain or spinal cord.

Bruck-de Lange
759.89 Congenital cerebral condition involving dwarfism, mental deficiency, and brachycephaly.

Brugsch's
757.39 Increased thickening of the skin on extremities and face with clubbing of fingers and deformities in bone of the limb.

Brugada
746.89 A congenital heart anamoly in which the hypertrophy (enlargement) is localized to the left ventricle.

Bruising
287.2 (Diamond-Gardner, Gardner-Diamond) Bruising occurring easily and large in women, involving surrounding tissues, resulting in pain, and spawning others.

Bubbly lung
770.7 Intrauterine fetal aspiration of amniotic fluid contaminated by meconium.

Buchem's
733.3 Multiple fractures and bowing of all extremities, thickening of skull bones, and osteoporosis beginning in childhood.

Budd-Chiari
453.0 Thrombosis of the hepatic vein with enlargement of the liver and severe hypertension.

Büdinger-Ludloff-Läwen
717.89 An old disruption of ligaments in the knee.

© 2004 Ingenix, Inc.

Bulbar
335.22 (Duchenne's) Paralysis-based symptoms from defects in the medulla oblongata.

Bundle of Kent
426.7 Muscular bundle forming a direct connection between the ventricle and atrial walls.

Bürger-Grütz
272.3 Abdominal pain, hepatosplenomegaly, pancreatitis, and eruptive zanthomas in a genetic condition.

Burke's
577.8 (Burke's, Clarke-Hadfield, Cystic Fibrosis) Obstruction of mucosal passageways, poor growth, chronic bronchitis, recurrent pneumonia, emphysema, clubbing of fingers, and salt depletion with abnormal secretions in exocrine glands.

Burnett's
999.9 Disorder of the kidneys induced by ingestion of large amounts of alkali and calcium in the therapy of a peptic ulcer. Reversible in the early stages, but can lead to renal failure.

Burnier's
253.3 (Levi, Lorain-Levi) Dwarfism resulting from malfunction of the pituitary gland.

Burning feet
266.2 (Gopalan's) Severe discomfort of the feet and other extremities with excessive sweating and elevated skin temperature, and believed to be caused by a riboflavin deficiency.

Bywaters'
958.5 Traumatic anuria following crushing, especially of kidneys.

Caffey's
756.59 Soft tissue swelling over the affected bones, irritability, and fever, and running periods of exacerbation and remission.

Calvé-Legg-Perthes
732.1 Disease of the growth centers, especially the top of the femur, in which the epiphyses is replaced by new calcification.

Carcinogenic thrombophlebitis
453.1 Spontaneous development of thromboses in the upper and lower limbs because of visceral neoplasm.

Carcinoid
259.2 (Bjorck-Thorson, Cassidy-Scholte, Hedinger's) Carcinoid tumors causing cyanotic flushing of the skin, diarrhea watery stools, bronchoconstrictive attacks, hypotension, edema, and ascites.

Cardiacos negros
416.0 (Arrilaga-Ayerza) Cyanosis and hypertension resulting from sclerosis of the pulmonary arteries.

Cardiopulmonary obesity
278.8 (Pickwick) Obesity, hypoventilation, somnolence, and erythrocytosis.

Cardiorespiratory distress (idiopathic), newborn
769 (Hyaline membrane) Respiratory distress resulting from reduced amounts of lung surfactant in premature infants. Frequently fatal.

Cardiovasorenal
272.7 Abnormal accumulations of neutral glycolipids in histiocytes in blood vessel walls, cornea verticillata, parasthesia in extremities, cataracts, and angioperatomas on the thighs, buttocks, and genitalia.

Carini's
757.1 Scaling of skin accompanying other congenital syndromes.

Carpal tunnel
354.0 Pain and tingling, numbness, or burning in the hand resulting from compression of the median nerve by tendons. Often called a repetitive motion injury.

Carpenter's
759.89 Small head with mental retardation as result of genetic disorder.

Cassidy (-Scholte)
259.2 (Bjorck-Thorson, Hedinger's) Carcinoid tumors that cause cyanotic flushing of the skin, diarrheal watery stools, bronchoconstrictive attacks, hypotension, edema, and ascites.

Cat-cry
758.3x (Cri-du-chat) Microcephaly, antimongoloid palpebral fissures, epicanthal folds, micrognathia, strabismus, mental and physical retardation, and a cat-like whine.

Cauda equina
344.60 Aching pain of the perineum, bladder, and sacrum, radiating in a sciatic fashion, due to compression of spinal nerve roots.

Cerebellomedullary malformation
741.0x (Arnold-Chiari) Displacement of the caudal spinal cord due to tethering with or without spina bifida and meningomyelocele.

 © 2004 Ingenix, Inc.

Cerebrohepatorenal
759.89 Craniofacial abnormalities, hypotonia, hepatomegaly, polycystic kidneys, jaundice, and death in infancy.

Cervical paralysis
337.0 (Charcot-Weiss-Baker, Sluder's) Overactive carotid sinus, causing a marked drop in blood pressure stopping or blocking the heart.

Cervical (root) (spine) NEC
723.8 Symptoms originating form the cervical spine.

Cervical sympathetic
723.2 (cervicocranial) Irritation of nerve roots emanating from posterior cervical spinal cord.

Cervicodorsal outlet
353.2 Pain or anesthesis affecting the neck and the upper back.

Céstan (-Raymond)
433.8x Quadriplegia, anesthesia, and nystagmus caused by obstruction of twigs of the basilar artery and lesions in the pontine region.

Céstan's
344.89 (Avellis, Babinski-Nageotte, Benedikt's, Brown-Sequard, Cestan-Chenais, Foville's, Gubler-Millard, Jackson's, Weber-Leyden) Paraplegia and anesthesia over part of the body caused by lesions in the brain or spinal cord.

Céstan-Chenais
344.89 (Avellis, Babinski-Nageotte, Benedikt's, Brown-Sequard, Cestan's, Foville's, Gubler-Millard, Jackson's, Weber-Leyden) Paraplegia and anesthesia over part of the body caused by lesions in the brain or spinal cord.

Chancriform
114.1 Symptoms resembling a chancre.

Charcot's
443.9 Pain, tension, and weakness in a moving limb but absent at rest and caused by occlusive arterial diseases of the limbs.

Charcot-Marie-Tooth
356.1 Pain across the shoulder and upper arm.

Charcot-Weiss-Baker
337.0 (Sluder's) Overactive carotid sinus, causing a marked drop in blood pressure stopping or blocking the heart.

Cheadle (-Möller) (-Barlow)
267 Anemia, spongy gums, weakness, induration of leg muscles, and mucocutaneous hemorrhages.

Chédiak-Higashi (-Steinbrinck)
288.2 (Chediak-Higashi, Dohle body, Hegglin, Jordan's, May) Hepatosplenomegaly, lymphadenopathy, anemia, thrombocytopenia and changes in the bones, cardiopulmonary system, skin, psychomotor skills, abnormalities of granulation, and nuclear structure of white cells open the patient to infection.

Chiari's
453.0 Thrombosis of the hepatic vein with enlargement of the liver and severe hypertension.

Chiari-Frommel
676.6x Unphysiological lactation and amenorrhea following pregnancy caused by hyperprolactinemia and a pituitary adenoma.

Chiasmatic
368.41 Impairment of vision, limitations of the field of vision, scotoma, headache, syncope, and vertigo.

Chilaiditi's
751.4 Interposition of the colon between the liver and diaphragm.

Child maltreatment
995.5 (child abuse) Maltreatment of a child through physical violence, emotional violence, or starvation.

Chondroectodermal dysplasia
756.55 (Ellis-van Creveld) Congenital dwarfism with defective development of the cardiac septum, skin, hair, and teeth.

Chorea-athetosis-agitans
275.1 Accumulation of copper in the brain, cornea, kidney, liver, and other tissues causing cirrhosis of the liver and deterioration in the basal ganglia of the brain.

Christian's
277.8 (Hand-Schüller-Christian) Multiple-system defects of the membranous bones, exophthalmos, diabetes insipidus, soft tissues, and bone involvement.

Chromosome 4 short arm deletion
758.3 (Cri-du-chat) Microcephaly, antimongoloid palpebral fissures, epicanthal folds, micrgnathia, strabismus, mental and physical retardation, and a cat-like whine.

© 2004 Ingenix, Inc.

Chronic alcoholic
291.2 Numerous symptoms caused by constant, long-time ingestion of alcohol affecting the nervous and gastrointestinal systems.

Chronic fatigue
780.71 Persistent fatigue that significantly reduces daily activity with chronic sore throat, mild fever, muscle weakness, myalgia, headaches, and neurological problems.

Chronic mesenteric
557.1 (Wilkie's) Complete or partial block of the superior mesenteric artery with symptoms of vomiting, pain, blood in the stool, and distended abdomen resulting in bowel infarction.

Churg-Strauss
446.4 Form of systemic inflammation and cell death of vessels with prominent lung involvement, manifested by severe asthma, among other respiratory disorders.

Clarke-Hadfield
577.8 (Burke's, Cystic Fibrosis) Obstructions of mucosal passageways, poor growth, chronic bronchitis, recurrent pneumonia, emphysema, clubbing of fingers, salt depletion, and abnormal secretions of exocrine glands.

Claude Bernard-Horner
337.9 (Reilly's, Steinbrocker's) Disorder following a heart attack with pain and stiffness in the shoulder, and swelling and pain in the hand.

Clerambault's
297.8 The delusional belief that someone, often a person of high social status, is in love with the patient.

Clifford's
766.2 Placental dysfunction occurring in postmature fetuses.

Climacteric
627.2 Chills, depression, hot flashes, headache, and irritability in menopausal women.

Clouston's
757.31 Congenital thickened nails and sparse or absent scalp hair, often accompanied by keratoderma of the palms and soles.

Coagulation-fibrinolysis (ICF)
286.6 (coagulopathy) Decrease of elements needed for coagulation of blood causing profuse bleeding.

Cockayne's
759.89 Dwarfism with deafness, retinal atrophy, mental retardation, and photo sensitivity.

Cockayne-Weber
757.39 Dwarfism with a precociously senile appearance, pigmentary degeneration of the retina, optic atrophy, deafness, sensitivity to sunlight, and mental retardation.

Coffin-Lowry
759.89 A genetic disorder characterized by craniofacial and skeletal abnormalities, mental retardation, short stature, and hypotonia (skeletal muscle weakness).

Cogan's
370.52 Abrupt onset of interstitial keratitis, tinnitus, and vertigo followed by deafness.

Cold injury (newborn)
778.2 Birth injury resulting from hypothermia.

Collet (-Sicard)
352.6 Unilateral lesions of the ninth, tenth, eleventh, and twelfth cranial nerves producing paralysis of the vagal, glossal, and other nerves and the tongue on the same side.

Compartment(al) (anterior) (deep) (posterior) (tibial)
958.8 Early complication of trauma.

Compression, cervical
721.1 Cervical spondylosis.

Compression, crushing
958.5 Traumatic anuria following crushing.

Concussion
310.2 Persistent personality disturbance following a blow to the head featuring affective instability, bursts of aggression, apathy and indifference, impaired social judgment, and suspiciousness or paranoid ideation.

Congenital muscle hypoplasia
756.89 Dysplasia of the fingernails and toenails, hypoplasia of the patella, iliac horns, thickening of the glomerular lamina densa, and a flask-shaped femur.

Congenital oculofacial paralysis
352.6 (Collet-Sicard) Unilateral lesions of the ninth, tenth, eleventh, and twelfth cranial nerves producing paralysis of the vagal, glossal, and other nerves and the tongue on the same side.

Conjunctivourethrosynovial
099.3 A symptom of Reiter's disease.

Conn (-Louis)
255.1 Headaches, nocturia, plyuria, fatigue, hypertension, hypokalemic alkalosis, potassium depletion, hyperfolemia, and

 © 2004 Ingenix, Inc.

decreased renin activity, caused by a benign pituitary tumor.

Conradi (-Hünermann)

756.59 Asymmetric shortening of the limbs and scoliosis. Caused by both genetic and maternal medication sources.

Conus medullaris

336.8 (Froin's) Cerebral spinal fluid of a yellowish hue signaling neoplastic or inflammatory obstruction.

Cooke-Apert-Gallais

255.2 Type I acrocephalosyndactyly with peak head and fusion of digits (specifically the second through fifth digits) and severe acne vulgaris of forearms.

Cornelia de Lange's

759.8x Mental retardation, eyebrows across bridge of nose, hairline well down on forehead, uptilted tip of nose with depressed bridge of nose, and small head with low-set ears.

Corticosexual

255.2 (Apert-Gallais, Cooke) Type I acrocephalosyndactyly with peak head and fusion of digits, specifically the second through fifth digits fused and severe acne vulgaris of forearms.

Costochondral junction

733.6 (Tietze's) Painful swelling of costal cartilages, especially of the second rib and interpreted as coronary artery disease.

Costovertebral

253.0 Arthritis of spine accompanying acromegaly, resembling rheumatoid arthritis and progressing to bony ankylosis with lipping of vertebral margins.

Cotard's

297.1 Paranoia marked by sensory disturbances, delusions of negation, and suicidal ideations.

Cowden

759.6 (multiple hamartoma) inherited disorder characterized by hamartomas of stomach and gastrointestinal tract, breast, thyroid carcinoma, and brain. An increased incidence of malignant tumors of the breast, endometrial tissues, and thyroid gland is also described.

Craniovertebral

723.2 Nerve root irritation emanating from posterior cervical spinal cord.

Creutzfeldt-Jakob

046.1 Progressive destruction of the pyramidal and extrapyramidal systems with progressive dementia, wasting of muscles, tremor, and other symptoms leading to death.

Cri-du-chat

758.3 (Cat-cry) Microcephaly, antimongoloid palpebral fissures, epicanthal folds, micrgnathia, strabismus, mental and physical retardation, and a cat-like whine.

Crib death

798.0 (Sudden infant death) Unexpected death of healthy infant under 12 months old.

Crocodile tears

351.8 (Melkersson-Rosenthal) Facial paralysis with dramatic lacrimation during eating prompted by lesion on the seventh cranial nerve, causing impulses to be misdirected from salivary glands to lacrimal glands.

Croup

464.4 Obstruction of the larynx caused by allergy, foreign body, infection, or new growth in infants and children.

CRST

710.1 Induration and thickening of the skin with circulatory and organ changes in the face and hands. The name is an acronym for calcinosis, usually of the fingers, Raynaud's, sclerodactyly (hardened skin and bone deformity of the fingers), and telangiectasia (microvascular red spotting of the skin). Esophageal involvement is termed CREST syndrome.

Cruveilhier-Baumgarten

571.5 Cirrhosis of the liver with patent paraumbilical, varicose periumbilical, or umbilical veins.

Cubital tunnel

354.2 Lesion of the ulnar nerve, affecting movement and feeling of hand.

Cuiffini-Pancoast

162.3 (Hare's) Neoplasm of upper lobe of lung.

Curschmann (-Batten) (-Steinert)

359.2 Condition in which the peritoneal cover of the liver converts into a white mass resembling cake icing.

Cushing's

255.0 Abdominal striae, acne, hypertension decreased carbohydrate tolerance, moon face, obesity, protein catabolism, and psychiatric disturbances resulting from increased adrenocortical secretion of cartisol caused by ACTH-dependent adrenocortical hyperplasia or tumor, or by effects of steriods.

© 2004 Ingenix, Inc.

Cutaneocerebral angioma
759.6 (Kalischer's) Formation of multiple angiomas in skin of head and scalp.

Cutaneous nerve of thigh
355.1 Tingling, formication, itching, and other symptoms on lower part of the thigh. Caused by lateral femoral cutaneous nerve.

Cystic duct stump
576.0 Recurrence of gall bladder pain following removal of the organ.

D_1
758.1 (Patau's, trisomy D) Extra chromosome in group D. Condition is usually fatal within two years and includes mental retardation, malformed ears, cardiac defects, convulsions, and other symptoms.

Dameshek's
282.4 One of hemolytic anemias that share a common decreased rate of synthesis of hemoglobin polypeptide chains and classified according to chain involved.

Dana-Putnam
281.0 [336.2] Numbness, tingling, weakness, a sore tongue, dyspnea, faintness, pallor of the skin and mucous membranes, anorexia, diarrhea, loss of weight, and fever. Strikes in the fifth decade.

Danbolt (-Closs)
686.8 (Brandt's) Zinc metabolism defect in young children with blisters, crusting, oozing eruptions, loss of hair, and diarrhea.

Dandy-Walker
742.3 Hydrocephalus with atresia of the foramina of Luschka and Magendie.

Danlos'
756.83 (Meekeren, Ehlers) Group of congenital connective tissue diseases with overly elastic skin, hyperextensive joints, and fragility of blood vessels and arteries.

Davies-Colley
733.99 (Cyriax's) Arthritis with degeneration of cartilage leading to collapse of the ears, nose, and tracheobronchial tree. Death may occur as the respiratory system is affected.

De Lange's
759.89 Inherited deformity with impaired development, mental retardation, eyebrows growing across bridge of nose, hairline well down on forehead, uptilted tip of nose with depressed bridge of nose, and small head with low-set ears.

De Toni-Fanconi (-Debré)
270.0 (Harts) Renal tubular malfunction, including cytinosis and osteomalacia and caused by inherited disorders or resulting from multiple myeloma or proximal epithelial growth.

Dead fetus
641.3x Loss of non-clotting blood and lengthy retention of dead fetus following tachycardia and related symptoms.

Death, sudden (SIDS)
798.0 Unexpected death of healthy infant typically under 12 months old.

Debré
270.0 (Harts) Renal tubular malfunction, including cytinosis and osteomalacia and caused by inherited disorders or resulting from multiple myeloma or proximal epithelial growth.

Defeminization
255.2 Mature masculine somatic characteristics by prepubescent male, girl, or woman showing at birth or developing later as result of adrenocortical dysfunction.

Defibrination
286.6 Dilution of fibrin by enzyme action.

Deficiency
260 Any syndrome resulting from deficiencies in proteins, hormones, carolies, trace minerals, vitamins, and other chemicals necessary for function or growth.

Degos'
447.8 Malignant atrophic papulosis.

Deiters' nucleus
386.19 (Bonnier) Ocular disturbances, deafness, nausea, thirst, anorexia, and symptoms traced to vagus centers resulting from lesion of Deiters' nucleus and its connections.

Déjérine-Roussy
348.8x Infarction of the postero-inferior thalamus causing transient hemiparesis, severe loss of superficial and deep sensation with crude pain in the limbs, and vasomotor or trophic disturbances.

Déjérine-Thomas
333.0 (Hallervorden-Spatz) Nerves between the striatum and pallidum are completely demyelinated.

Del Castillo's
606.0 Cessation of menses not associated with pregnancy.

 © 2004 Ingenix, Inc.

Deletion chromosomes
758.3 General description of syndromes such as antimongolism and cat-cry in which chromosomes are missing rather than duplicated.

Delusional
293.81 Organic disorder including hallucinations, beliefs about being followed, being poisoned, etc., and not meeting criteria for schizophrenia.

Dementia-aphonia, of childhood
299.1x Dementia in which child becomes mute.

Depersonalization
300.6 Patient feels detached from his or her body and experiences the feeling of being an automaton or in a dream-like state. Depersonalization must be a primary symptom and not part of schizophrenia or another disorder.

Dercum's
272.8 (Ander's) Deposits of painful symmetrical nodular or pendulous masses of fat in various body regions.

Diabetes-dwarfism-obesity
258.1 Endocrine dysfunction causing diabetes and affecting growth and weight.

Diabetes mellitus-hypertension-nephrosis
250.4x [581.81] High blood pressure and kidney failure resulting from diabetes in which carbohydrate utilization is reduced and lipid and protein use is enhanced.

Diabetes mellitus in newborn infant
775.1 Diabetes mellitus

Diabetes-nephrosis
250.4x [581.81] High blood pressure and kidney failure resulting from diabetes in which carbohydrate utilization is reduced and lipid and protein use is enhanced.

Diabetic amyotrophy
250.6x [358.1] Muscular atrophy resulting from diabetes

Diamond-Blackfan
284.0 (Blackfan-Diamond, Fanconi, Kaznelson's) Congenital anemia of infancy requiring a number of blood transfusions to maintain life.

Diamond-Gardener
287.2 Bruising occuring easily and large, involving surrounding tissues, resulting in pain, and spawning others. Assumed to be a form of autoimmune problem.

Diaper
270.0 Infantile form of Fanconi's syndrome with cytinosis.

DIC
286.6 Decrease of elements needed for coagulation of blood causing profuse bleeding.

Diencephalohypophyseal
253.8 Problem with the thalamus or pituitary gland not otherwise specified.

DiGeorge's
279.11 Hypoplasia or aphasia of the thymus and parathyroid gland with congenital heart defects, anomalies of the great vessels, esophageal atresia, seizures, and facial deformities.

Dighton's
756.51 (van der Hoeve's) Blue sclera, little growth, brittle bones, and deafness.

Di Guglielmo's
207.0 Condition characterized by large numbers of nucleated red cells appearing in the bone marrow and blood.

Disseminated platelet thrombosis
446.6 Fatal disease with central nervous system involvement due to formation of fibrin or platelet thrombi in arterioles and capillaries in many organs.

Doan-Wiseman
288.0 (Kostmann's, Schultz, Shwachman) Inherited bronchiectasis and pancreatic insufficiency resulting in malnutrition, sinusitis, short stature, and bone abnormalities.

Döhle body
288.2 (Chediak-Higashi, Hegglin, Jordan's, May) Hepatosplenomegaly, lymphadenopathy, anemia, thrombocytopenia, changes in the bones, cardiopulmonary system, skin, and psychomotor skills. Granulation and nuclear structure of white cells opens patient to infection and results in death.

Donohue's
259.8 Slow physical and mental development, elfin facial features such as wide-set eyes and low-set ears, and severe endocrine disorders indicated by enlarged sexual organs. Rare and fatal.

Double whammy
360.81 Dislocation of eye ball.

Down's
758.0 (Trisomy 21) Retardation with numerous markers varying from one person to another.

© 2004 Ingenix, Inc.

Symptoms include retarded growth, flat face with short nose, epicanthic skin folds, protruding lower lip, rounded ears, thickened tongue, pelvic dysplasia, broad hands and feet, stubby fingers, and absence of Moro reflex.

Dressler's
411.0 Fever, leukocytosis, chest pain, evidence of pericarditis, pleurisy, and pneumonia occurring days or weeks after a myocardial infarction.

Drug
292.0 A number of physical symptoms resulting from long-time ingestion of, and dependence on, therapeutic and illicit drugs.

Drug withdrawal, infant, of dependent mother
779.5 A number of physical symptoms suffered by newborns whose drug-dependent mothers allowed drugs to cross the placenta.

Drug-induced
292.84 Description of symptoms, physiological and psychological, produced by drug abuse or dependence.

Drum
381.02 Symptom of a number of syndromes affecting the ear.

Dry skin
701.1 Keratosis producing lesions appearing as dry skin.

DSAP
692.75 (Disseminated Superficial Actinic Porokeratosis) Skin disorder occurring on sun-exposed skin and characterized by numerous superficial, keratotic, brownish-red macules.

Duane's
378.71 (Still-Turk-Duane, Duane-Stilling-Turk) Simultaneous retraction of eye muscles causing an inability to abduct the affected eye with retraction of the globe.

Dubin-Johnson
277.4 (Dubin-Sprinz) Nonhemilitic jaundice thought as a defect in concentrated bilirubin and other organs causing a brown granular pigment in the hepatic duct.

Duchenne's
335.22 Paralysis symptoms caused by medulla oblongata.

Due to mesenteric artery insufficiency
557.1 (Wilkie's) Blocked superior mesenteric artery with vomiting, pain, blood in the stool, distended abdomen, and bowel infarction.

Dumping
564.2 Emptying of contents of jejunum with nausea, sweating, weakness, palpitation, syncope, warmth, and diarrhea. Occurs after eating in patients who have had partial gastrectomy and gastrojejunostomy.

Duplay's
726.2 Inflammation of subacromial or subdeltoid bursa.

Dupré's
781.6 Irritation of spinal cord and brain mimicking meningitis, but in which there is no swelling of membranes.

During labor
668.0x (Mendelson's) Disorders of lung following vomiting and regurgitation by obstetric patients.

Dyke-Young
283.9 (Hayem-Widal) Anemia caused by exposure to trauma, poisons,and other causes.

Dyspraxia
315.4 Organic disorder affecting patient's ability to perform coordinated acts and not due to psychotic diagnosis.

Dyssynergia cerebellaris myoclonica
334.2 (Hunt's) Disorder marked by myoclonus epilepsy and muscular tremors associated with disturbance of muscle tone and coordination.

E_3
758.2 (Edward's, trisomy E) Congenital malformations in which extra chromosome is group E. Includes mental retardation, abnormal skull shape, malformed ears, small mandible, cardiac defects, short sternum, and other symptoms.

Eagle-Barrett
756.71 (Prune belly) Congenital absence of muscles of abdomen and genitourinary anamolies.

Eale's
362.18 Retinal vasculitis marked by phlebitis, arteritis, and endarteritis.

Eaton-Lambert
199.1 [358.1] (Lambert-Eaton) Progressive proximal muscle weakness resulting from antibodies directed against motor-nerve axon terminals.

Ebstein's
746.7 (Hypoplastic left heart) Hypoplasia or atresia of the left ventricle and aorta or mitral valve

© 2004 Ingenix, Inc.

with respiratory distress and extreme cyanosis. Cardiac failure and death often result in early infancy.

Ectopic ACTH secretion
255.0 (Cushing) Abdominal striae, acne, hypertension decreased carbohydrate tolerance, moon face, obesity, protein catabolism, and psychiatric disturbances resulting from increased adrenocortical secretion of cortisol caused by ACTH-dependent adreocortical hyperplasia or tumor, or administration of steriods.

Eczema-thrombocytopenia
279.12 (Aldrich, Wiskott-Aldrich) Immunodeficiency shown by eczema, thrombocyopenia, and recurrent pyogenic infection with increased susceptibility to infection from encapsulated bacteria.

Eddowes'
756.51 (Ekman's, Spurway's) Blue sclera, little growth, brittle and malformed bones, and malformed teeth.

Edwards'
758.2 (E, trisomy E) Congenital malformations in which extra chromosome is group E. Includes mental retardation, abnormal skull shape, malformed ears, small mandible, cardiac defects, short sternum, and other symptoms.

Efferent loop
537.89 (Gastrojejunal loop obstruction) Distended efferent loop with illness and pain caused by acute or chronic obstruction of the duodenum and jejunum proximal to a gastrojejunostomy.

Ehlers-Danlos
756.83 (Meekeren, Ehlers, Danlos) Congenital connective tissue diseases with overly elastic skin, hyperextensive joints, and fragility of blood vessels and arteries.

Eisenmenger's
745.4 Pulmonary hypertension with congenital communication between two circulations so that a right to left shunt results.

Ekman's
756.51 (Eddowes', Spurway's) Blue sclera, little growth, brittle and malformed bones, and malformed teeth.

Electric feet
266.2 (Gopalan's) Discomfort of feet and other extremities, excessive sweating, elevated skin temperature, and riboflavin deficiency.

Ellis-van Creveld
756.55 Dwarfism with defective development of cardiac septum, skin, hair, and teeth.

Ellison-Zollinger
251.5 (Zollinger-Ellison) Peptic ulceration with gastric hypersecretion, tumor of the pancreatic islets, and hypoglycemia.

Embryonic fixation
270.2 (Mendes, van der Hoeve-Halbertsma-Waardenburg, Waardenburg-Klein) Eyebrow or upper or lower eyelid sags.

Empty sella
253.8 Sella turcica containing no pituitary gland caused by herniating arachnoid, radiotherapy, or surgery.

Endocrine-hypertensive
255.3 (Schroeder's, Slocumb's) Disorder of adrenal medullary tissue with hypertension, attacks of palpitation, headache, nausea, dyspnea, anxiety, pallor, and profuse sweating.

Engel-von Recklinghausen
252.0 (Jaffe-Lichtenstein-Uehlinger) Osteitis with fibrous degeneration and formation of cysts with fibrous nodules on affected bones.

Enteroarticular
099.3 (Fiessinger-Leroy-Reiter) Association of arthritis, iredocyclitis, urethritis, and diarrhea.

Eosinophilia myalgia
710.5 Painful muscles resulting from accumulation of a large number of granular leukocytes.

Epidemic vomiting
078.82 (Winter's disease) Nausea and vomiting attacking a group of people suddenly without prior illness or malaise. Headache, vomiting, abdominal pain, and giddiness end quickly.

Erb (-Oppenheim) - Goldflam
358.0 (Goldflam, Erb, Hoppe) Myoneural conduction-caused progressive muscular weakness beginning in face and throat.

Erdheim's
253.0 Arthritis of spine accompanying acromegaly, resembling rheumatoid arthritis and progressing to bony ankylosis with lipping of vertebral margins.

Erlacher-Blount
732.4 Disease causing bow-legs in children.

Erythrocyte fragmentation
283.19 (Lederer-Brill) Fragmentation of red blood cells.

© 2004 Ingenix, Inc.

Evans'
287.3 Condition where number of platelets in circulating blood increases, causing bruising.

Exhaustion
300.5 Hypersomatic disorder.

Eye, dry
375.15 Lacrimal glands are unable to provide enough moisture to cover the eye.

Eye retraction
378.71 (Duane, Still-Turk-Duane) Retraction of eye muscles with inability to abduct the affected eye with retraction of the globe.

Eyelid-malar-mandible
756.0 (Franceschetti's) Malformations of derivatives of the first branchial arch, with pallpebral fissures sloping outward and downward with notches in the outer third of the lower lids, defects of malar bones and zygome, hypoplasia of the jawbone, high or cleft palate, low-set ears, unusual hair growth, and pits between mouth and ear.

Faber's
280.9 (Hayem-Faber) Central pallor in the red blood cells caused by lack of red cell hemoglobin in blood.

Fabry (-Anderson)
272.7 Neutral glycolipids in histiocytes in blood vessel walls, cornea verticillata, parasthesia in extremities, cataracts and angioperatomas on the thighs, buttocks, and genitalia. Death comes from cardiac, cerebrovascular, and renal complications.

Facial diplegia
352.6 (Collet-Sicard) Unilateral lesions of the ninth, tenth, eleventh, and twelfth cranial nerves producing paralysis of the vagal, glossal, other nerves, and the tongue on the same side. Most usually result of injury.

Fallot's
745.2 Also called tetralogy of Fallot. Congenital cardiac defects with pulmonary stenosis, intervetricular septal defect, dextroposeptum and venous as well as arterial blood, and right ventricular hypertrophy.

Familial acanthosis nigricans
701.2 Velvety acanthosis with gray, black, or brown pigmentation on axillae and other body folds. In adults, it results from internal carcinoma. In children, it results from obesity-producing endocrine disturbance.

Familial eczema-thrombocytopenia
279.12 (Aldrich, Wiskott-Aldrich) Eczema, thrombocyopenia, and recurrent pyogenic infection with increased susceptibility to infection from encapsulated bacteria.

Fanconi
759.81 Rounded face, almond-shaped eyes, strabismus, low forehead, hypogonadism, hypotomia, mental retardation, and an insatiable appetite.

Fanconi (-de Toni) (-Debré)
270.0 (Harts) Renal tubular malfunction, including cytinosis and osteomalacia caused by inherited disorders, the result of multiple myeloma, or proximal epithelial growth.

Fanconi's
284.0 (Blackfan-Diamond, Kaznelson's) Anemia of infancy requiring a number of blood transfusions to maintain life.

Farber (-Uzman)
272.8 Swollen joints, lymphadenopathy, subcutaneous nodules, and accumulation in lyosomes of affected cells of PAS-positive lipid consisting of ceramide. Begins soon after birth and caused by deficiency of ceramidase.

Fatigue NEC
300.5 Hypersomatic disorder with no identifiable pathology.

FDH
757.39 Linear areas of dermal hyperplasia with soft yellow nodules of fat. Areas are widely distributed and resemble striae distensae.

Feet, burning
266.2 (Gopalan's) Severe discomfort of feet and other extremities associated with excessive sweating and elevated skin temperature; believed to be caused by a riboflavin deficiency.

Feil-Klippel
756.16 Shorter than average neck and a low hairline. Caused by fewer than average cervical vertebrae or fusion of hemivertebrae into one bony mass.

Felty's
714.1 Splenomegaly, leukopenia, arthritis, hypersplenism, anemia and other symptoms.

Feminizing
255.2 (Achard-Thiers) Aranodactyly with small, receding mandible, broad skull, and joint laxity in hands and feet.

Fertile eunuch
257.2 Hypogonadism with gynecomastia, hypospadias, and pospubertal testicular atrophy. Caused by an inherited defect of

© 2004 Ingenix, Inc.

androgen receptors and insensitivity to testosterone.

Fetal alcohol

760.71 Growth deficiency, craniofacial anomalies, and limb defects among offspring of mothers who are chronic alcoholics.

Fiedler's

422.91 Isolated infection of heart muscle.

Fiessinger-Leroy (-Reiter)

099.3 (Fiessinger-Leroy-Reiter) An association of arthritis, iredocyclitis, and urethritis, sometimes with diarrhea. While symptoms may recur, the arthritis is constant.

Fiessinger-Rendu

695.1 Necrolysis of the skin caused by toxins.

First arch

756.0 (Franceschetti's) Malformations of the first branchial arch with pallpebral fissures sloping outward and downward with notches in the outer third of the lower lids, defects of malar bones and zygoma, hypoplasia of the jawbone, high or cleft palate, low-set ears, unusual hair growth, and pits between mouth and ear.

Fisher's

357.0 (Guillain-Barre, Landry, Strohl, Miller) Paraplegia of limbs, flaccid paralysis, ophthalmoplegia, ataxia, and areflexia caused by disorder of immune system.

Fitz-Hugh and Curtis

098.86 Peritonitis of the upper abdominal region in persons with a history of gonorrheal or other infections.

Fitz's

577.0 Acute infection of the pancreas with the formation of necrotic areas, bleeding in the gland, fever, leukocytosis, nausea, and pain.

Flajani (-Basedow)

242.0x (Basedow, Parry's, Grave's disease) Fatigue, nervousness, emotional lability and irritability, heat intolerance and increased sweating, weight loss, palpitation, and tremor of hands and tongue caused by excess thyroidal hormones.

Flush

259.2 (Bjorck-Thorson, Cassidy-Scholte, Hedinger's) Carcinoid tumors causing severe attacks of cyanotic flushing of the skin, diarrheal watery stools, bronchoconstrictive attacks, hypotension, edema, and ascites.

Foix-Alajouanine

336.1 Ophthalmoplegia, paresis of the sympathetic nerves, and neuroparalytic keratitis from compression of lateral wall of the cavernous sinus.

Following crush injury

958.5 Traumatic anuria following crushing by a heavy object.

Following delivery

674.8x Hepatorenal syndrome, cardiomyopathy, uterine hypertrophy, and other symptoms following childbirth.

Fong's

756.89 Dysplasia of the fingernails and toenails, hypoplasia of patella, iliac horns, thickening of the glomerular lamina densa, and a flask-shaped femur.

Foramen magnum

348.4 Compression of brain from the space above.

Forbes-Albright

253.1 Persistent lactation and amenorrhea caused by pituitary tumor, marked by secretion of excessive amounts of prolactin.

Fossa compression

348.4 Compression of brain from the fossa underneath.

Foster-Kennedy

377.04 (Gowers-Paton-Kennedy) Meningioma of optic nerve with central scotoma and contralateral choked disk.

Foville's

344.89 (Avellis, Babinski-Nageotte, Benedikt's, Brown-Sequard, Cestan's, Cestan-Chenais, Gubler-Millard, Jackson's, Weber-Leyden) Paraplegia and anesthesia over part of the body caused by lesions in the brain or spinal cord.

Fragile X

759.83 Mental retardation, enlarged testes, big jaw, high forehead, and long ears in males. In females, fragile X presents mild retardation and heterozygous sexual structures. In some families, males have shown no symptoms but carry the gene.

Franceschetti's

756.0 Malformations of derivatives of the first branchial arch, marked by pallpebral fissures sloping outward and downward with notches in the outer third of the lower lids, defects of malar bones and zygome, hypoplasia of the jawbone, high or cleft palate, low-set ears, unusual hair growth, and pits between mouth and ear.

Fraser's
759.89 Cyptophthalmus with ear malformations, cleft palate, laryngeal deformity, displacement of umbilicus and nipples, digital malformation, separation of symphysis pubis, maldeveloped kidneys, and masculine female genitals.

Freeman-Sheldon
759.89 (Whistling face syndrome) Deviation of hands and face with protrusion of lips as in whistling, sunken eyes, and small nose.

Frey's
350.8 Localized sweating and flushing of cheek and ear in response to chewing.

Friderichsen-Waterhouse
036.3 Fulminating meningococcal septicemia in children below 10 years of age with vomiting, cyanosis, diarrhea, purpura, convulsions, circulatory collapse, meningitis, and hemorrhaging into the adrenal glands.

Friedrich-Erb-Arnold
757.39 Thickening of skin on extremities and face with clubbing of fingers and deformities in bone of the limb.

Fröhlich's
253.8 (Babinski-Frohlich, Launois-Cleret, Renon-Delille) Obesity and hypogonadism in adolescent boys. Dwarfism indicates hypothyroidism.

Froin's
336.8 (Froin's) Alteration in the cerebral spinal fluid resulting in a yellowish hue and indictive of neoplastic or inflammatory obstruction.

Frommel-Chiari
676.6x Hyperprolactinemia and a pituitary adenoma causing unphysiological lactation and amenorrhea following pregnancy.

Frontal Lobe Syndrome
310.0 Changes in behavior following damage to the frontal areas of the brain including reduction in self-control, foresight, creativity, spontaneity, emotional vivaciousness, and empathy.

Fuller Albright's
756.59 (McCune-Albright; Albright's hereditary osteodystrophy) Patchy skin pigmentation, endocrine dysfunctions, and polyostotic fibrous dysplasia.

Functional, hyperinsulinism
251.1 (Harris', organic hyperinsulinism) Hyperinsulinism due to organic endogenous factors with hypoglycemia, weakness, perspiration, jitteriness, tachycardia, mental confusion, and vision disturbances.

Gaisböck's
289.0 Associated with hypertension, but without hyposplenomegaly.

Ganser's, hysterical
300.16 Psychotic-like condition (but without symptoms and signs of a traditional psychosis) occurring in prisoners who feign insanity or who suffer head injury.

Gardner-Diamond
287.2 Bruising occurring easily and large, involving surrounding tissues, resulting in pain, and spawning others. Assumed to be a form of autoimmune deficiency.

Gastrojejunal loop obstruction
537.89 (Gastrojejunal loop obstruction) A distended afferent loop marked by illness and pain. Caused by acute or chronic obstruction of the duodenum and jejunum proximal to a gastrojejunostomy.

Gayet-Wernicke's
265.1 Thiamine deficiency, disturbances in ocular motility, pulpillary alterations, nystagmus, ataxia with tremors, and co-existing organic toxic psychosis. Most often due to alcoholism.

Gee-Herter-Heubner
579.0 Catarrhal dysentery. Malabsortion syndrome of all ages precipitated by gluten-containing foods. Wasting and fatigue in both adults and children. Children suffer growth retardation and irritability. Adults suffer difficulty in breathing and clubbing of fingers.

Gélineau's
347 Narcolepsy, a form of epilepsy where the patient abruptly falls asleep rather than suffering grand or petite mals.

Geniculate ganglion
053.11 (Hunt's) Facial paralysis, otalgia, and herpes zoster caused by viral infection in seventh cranial nerve and genticulate ganglion.

Gerhardt's
478.30 Paralysis of vocal cords causing inspiratory dyspnea.

Gerstmann's
784.69 Right-left disorientation, finger agnosia, agraphia, and constructional apraxia, due to lesion in the angular gyrus of the dominant hemisphere of the brain.

© 2004 Ingenix, Inc.

Gilbert's
277.4 Benign elevation of unconjugated bilirubin with no liver damage or other deformities.

Gilford (-Hutchinson)
259.8 (Hutchinson-Gilford) Precocious senility with death from coronary artery disease occurring before 10 years of age.

Gilles de la Tourette's
307.23 Motor and vocal tics occurring many times a day beginning before age 21 and in which the type of tic changes over time.

Gillespie's
759.89 Congenital dysplasia of the eyes, teeth, and extremities.

Glénard's
569.89 Bloating, gas, pain, and fullness experienced in left upper abdominal quadrant with pain sometimes radiating up into left chest. Downward displacement of viscera may cause bulging of abdomen and other symptoms.

Glinski-Simmonds
253.2 Wasting of pituitary gland as result of some other condition or affliction.

Glucuronyl transferase
277.4 Benign elevation of unconjugated bilirubin with no liver damage or other deformities.

Glue ear
381.20 Painless secretion of mucoid fluid in the middle ear, stopping up the eustachian tube and causing hearing loss.

Goldberg (-Maxwell) (-Morris)
257.8 (Morris, hairless women, Goldberg-Maxwell) Male pseudohermaphroditism with incompletely developed vagina with rudimentary uterus and fallopian tubes, scanty or absent axillary/public hair, and amenorrhea.

Goldenhar's
756.0 Epibulbar dermoid cysts, preauricular appendages, micrognathia, and vertebral anomalies.

Goldflam-Erb
358.0 (Goldflam, Erb, Hoppe) Progressive muscular weakness beginning in face and throat caused by a defect in myoneural conduction.

Goltz-Gorlin
757.39 Irregular linear streaks of skin atrophy, skeletal malformations, papillomas of the lips and labia, and occassional alopecia.

Goodpasture's
446.21 Renal condition where nephritis progresses rapidly to death, leaving lungs showing extensive hemosiderosis or bleeding.

Gopalan's
266.2 Severe discomfort of the feet and other extremities associated with excessive sweating and elevated skin temperature; believed to be caused by a riboflavin deficiency.

Gorlin-Chaudhry-Moss
759.89 Congenital lesion of the basal cells.

Gougerot (-Houwer) - Sjögren
710.2 (Sicca) Complex of symptoms of unknown source in middle aged women in which following triad exists: keratoconjunctivitis sicca, zerostomia, and connective tissue disease (usually rheumatoid arthritis but sometimes systemic lupus erythematosus). Cause may be abnormal immune response.

Gougerot-Blum
709.1 Purpuric skin eruption seen on the legs, thighs, and lower trunk of men 40 to 60 years of age and characterized by minute rust-colored papules that fuse into plaques.

Gougerot-Carteaud
701.8 Benign neoplasm producing fingerlike projections from epithelial surface in girls nearing puberty. Papillas begin on back and between breasts, eventually spreading over the torso and throughout the body.

Gouley's
423.2 Restrictive pericarditis.

Gowers'
780.2 Fall in blood pressure, slow pulse, and convulsions. Believed to be sudden stimulation of vagal nerve by receptors in heart, carotid sinus, or aortic arch.

Gowers-Paton-Kennedy
377.04 (Foster-Kennedy, Gowers-Paton-Kennedy) Meningioma of optic nerve with central scotoma and contralateral choked disk.

Gradenigo's
383.02 Localized meningitis in fifth and sixth cranial nerves, causing paralysis and pain in the temporal region.

Gray or grey
779.4 Effects of chloramphenicol taken by mother during gestation on the newborn.

Greig's
756.0 Abnormal increase in the interorbital distance with cleidcranial or craniofacial

© 2004 Ingenix, Inc.

malformations, along with occasional mental deficiencies.

Gubler-Millard

344.89 (Avellis, Babinski-Nageotte, Benedikt's, Brown-Sequard, Cestan's, Cestan-Chenais, Foville's, Jackson's, Weber-Leyden) Paraplegia and anesthesia over half or part of the body caused by lesions in the brain or spinal cord.

Guérin-Stern

754.89 Congenital immobility of most joints, fixed in various postures, with little muscle development and growth.

Guillain-Barré (-Strohl)

357.0 (Landry, Fisher's, Strohl, Miller) Often follows viral infections and may be a disorder of immune system with paraplegia of limbs, flaccid paralysis, ophthalmoplegia, ataxia, and areflexia.

Gunn's

742.8 (jaw-winking) Eyelids widen during chewing, sometimes with an elevation of the upper lid when the mouth is open and closing of the lid when the mouth is closed.

Günther's

277.1 Cutaneous photosensitivity leading to mutilating skin lesions, homlytic anemia and splenomegaly, and greatly increased urinary excretion of uroporphyrin.

Gustatory sweating

350.8 (Frey's) Localized sweating and flushing of cheek and ear in response to chewing.

H3O

759.81 Rounded face, almond-shaped eyes, strabismus, low forehead, hypogonadism, hypotomia, mental retardation, and an insatiable appetite.

Hadfield-Clarke

577.8 (Burke's, Clarke-Hadfield, Cystic Fibrosis) Abnormal secretions of exocrine glands, obstructions of mucosal passageways, poor growth, chronic bronchitis, recurrent pneumonia, emphysema, clubbing of fingers, and salt depletion.

Haglund-Läwen-Fründ

717.89 Traumatic separation of the cartilage of the patella with fissures.

Hairless women

257.8 (Morris, Goldberg, Goldberg-Maxwell) Male pseudohermaphroditism with incompletely developed vagina, rudimentary uterus and fallopian tubes, scanty or absent axillary/public hair, and amenorrhea.

Hallervorden-Spatz

333.0 (Dejerine-Thomas) Nerves between the striatum and pallidum are completely demyelated.

Hallucinatory type

293.82 (hallucinosis) Organic disorder in which the patient exhibits chronic hallucinations not occuring during the course of delirium.

Hamman's

518.1 Pneumothorax or pneumopericardium resulting from presence of air or gas in the mediastinum beginning spontaneously or from trauma or disease. Sometimes induced to aid in diagnosis.

Hamman-Rich

516.3 Chronic inflammation, progressive fibrosis of the pulmonary alveolar walls, and progressive dyspnea leading to death by oxygen deprivation or right heart failure.

Hand-foot

282.61 (Herrick's) Sickle cell anemia.

Hand-Schüller-Christian

277.8 (Christian) Histiocytosis with an occasional accumulation of cholesterol, defects of the membranous bones, exophthalmos, diabetes insipidus, and multiple-system, soft tissue, and bone involvement.

Hanot-Chauffard (-Troisier)

275.0 Hypertrophic cirrhosis with pigmentation and diabetes mellitus.

Hare's

162.3 (Cuiffini-Pancoast) Neoplasm of upper lobe of lung.

Harkavy's

446.0 (MCLS) Fever, conjunctival injection reddening of the oral cavity, ulcerative gingivitis, cervical lymph nodes, and skin eruptions that cover the hands and feet. Skin becomes puffy and sloughs off.

Harris'

251.1 Hyperinsulinism due to organic endogenous factors, hypoglycemia, weakness, perspiration, jitteriness, tachycardia, mental confusion, and vision disturbances.

Hart's

270.0 Renal tubular malfunction, cytinosis, and osteomalacia caused by inherited disorders or the result of multiple myeloma or proximal epithelial growth.

 © 2004 Ingenix, Inc.

Hayem-Faber
280.9 (Faber) Central pallor in red blood cells caused by lack of red cell hemoglobin in blood.

Hayem-Widal
283.9 (Dyke-Young, Widal) One of a group of anemic syndromes caused by exposures to trauma, poisons, and other causes that decreases the number of red blood cells.

Heat exhaustion or prostration
992.4 Salt depletion following exposure to sunlight and heat, causing heat exhaustion.

Heberden's
413.9 (angina pectoris) Severe pain in the chest caused by ischemia of the heart prompted by coronary artery disease.

Hedinger's
259.2 (Bjorck-Thorson, Cassidy-Scholte) Carcinoid tumors causing severe attacks of cyanotic flushing of skin, diarrheal watery stools, bronchoconstrictive attacks, hypotension, edema, and ascites.

Hegglin's
288.2 (Chediak-Higashi, Dohle body, Jordan's, May) Hepatosplenomegaly, lymphadenopathy, anemia, thrombocytopenia, and changes in the bones, cardopulmonary system, skin, and psychomotor skills. Abnormalities of granulation and nuclear structure of white cells open patients to infection and result in death.

Heller's
299.1x Dementia in which a child becomes mute with irritability, tantrums, and other behavioral disorders.

Hemoglobinuria
283.2 (Marchiafava-Micheli) Acquired blood cell dysplasis in which there are many clones of stem cells producing red blood cells, platelets, and granulocytes.

Hemolytic-uremic
283.11 Enlargement of liver and spleen and many erythroblasts in circulation.

Hemorrhage
036.3 (Friderichsen-Waterhouse, Waterhouse, 036.3) Fulminating meningococcal septicemia occurring in children below 10 years of age with vomiting, cyanosis, diarrhea, purpura, convulsions, circulatory collapse, meningitis, and hemorrhaging into adrenal glands.

Hench-Rosenberg
719.3x Repeated episodes of arthritis and periarthritis without fever or changes in joints.

Henoch-Schönlein
287.0 Eruption of purpuric lesions with joint pain and swelling, colic, passage of bloody stools, and glomerulonephritis in young children.

Hepatorenal
572.4 (Heyd's, hepatourologic) Acute renal failure in patients with disease of the biliary or liver tract. Caused by decreased renal blood flow, damaging both organs.

Hercules
255.2 (Apert-Gallais, Cooke) Type I acrocephalosyndactyly with peaked head, fusion of digits (specifically the second through fifth digits), and severe acne vulgaris of forearms.

Herpetic geniculate ganglionitis
053.11 (Hunt's) Facial paralysis, otalgia, and herpes zoster caused by viral infection in seventh cranial nerve and genticulate ganglion.

Herrick's
282.61 Sickle cell anemia.

Herter (-Gee)
579.0 (Heubner-Herter) Catarrhal dysentery. Inherited malabsortion syndrome of all ages precipitated by gluten-containing foods with wasting and fatigue. Children suffer growth retardation and irritability. Adults suffer difficulty in breathing and clubbing of fingers.

Heyd's
572.4 Acute renal failure with disease of the biliary or liver tract. Cause is decreased renal blood flow, damaging both organs.

HHHO
759.81 (H3O) Rounded face, almond-shaped eyes, strabismus, low forehead, hypogonadism, hypotomia, mental retardation, and an insatiable appetite.

Hoffa (-Kastert)
272.8 Traumatic proliferation of fatty tissue on knee joint.

Hoffmann's
244.9 [359.5] Hypothyroidism beginning during infancy as result of acquired injury of thyroid gland or presence of cretinism.

Hoffmann-Bouveret
427.2 Rapid action of the heart having sudden onset and cessation.

© 2004 Ingenix, Inc.

Holländer-Simons
272.6 Loss of subcutanious fat of the upper torso, the arms, the neck, and face but with an increase in fat on and below the pelvis.

Holmes'
368.16 (Balint's, Riddoch's) Corical paralysis of visual fixation, optic ataxia, and disturbance of visual attention. Eye movements are normal.

Holmes-Adie
379.46 (Adie, Holmes, Markus, Saenger's) Pathological reaction in which the pupil does not react to changes in light and changes if focus is changed. Cause is certain tendon deficiency.

Hoppe-Goldflam
358.0 (Goldflam, Erb, Hoppe) Progressive muscular weakness beginning in face and throat caused by a defect in myoneural conduction.

Horner's
337.9 (Claude Bernard-Homer, Reilly's, Steinbrocker's) Pain and stiffness in the shoulder, with puffy swelling and pain in the hand following a heart attack.

Hospital addiction
301.51 (Multiple operations, Munchhausen) Description of psychoxomatic behavior with physical symptoms exhibited by some patients with histrionic personality disorder.

Hunt's
053.11 (Ramsey-Hunt) Facial paralysis, otalgia, and herpes zoster caused by viral infection in seventh cranial nerve and genticulate ganglion.

Hunter (-Hurler)
277.5 Mucopolysccharide sulfates affecting the eye, ear, skin, teeth, skeleton, joints, liver, spleen, cardiovascular system, respiratory system, and central nervous system.

Hutchinson-Boeck
135 (Lofgren's, Schaumann's, Besnier-Boeck-Schaumann) Disorder with fibrosis, lymph nodes, skin, enlarged liver, eyes, enlarged spleen, phalangeal bones, parotid glands, and systemic granulomas composed of epithelioid and multinucleated giant cells.

Hutchinson-Gilford
259.8 (Gilford) Precocious senility with death from coronary artery disease occurring before 16 years of age.

Hyperabduction
447.8 Malignant atrophic papulosis.

Hyperactive bowel
564.1 Abdominal pain, watery stools, and gas.

Hyperaldosteronism with hypokalemic alkalosis
255.1 (Bartter's) Low or normal blood pressure, no edema, retarded growth, hypokalemic alkalosis, and elevated renin or angiotensin levels.

Hypercalcemic
275.42 (Albright-Martin, Seabright-Bantam) Similar to hypoparthyroidism, Failure to repond to parathyroid hormone causing short stature, obesity, short metacarpals, and ectopic calcification.

Hypersomnia-bulimia
349.89 (Kleine-Levin, Parry-Romberg) Hypersomnia associated with bulimia and occurring in males between 10 to 25 years of age. Ravenous appetite is followed by prolonged sleep, along with behavioral disturbances, impaired thought processes, and hallucinations.

Hypersympathetic
337.9 (Claude Bernard-Homer, Reilly's, Steinbrocker's) Pain and stiffness in the shoulder and swelling and pain in the hand following heart attack.

Hypertransfusion, newborn
776.4 Polycythemia of newborn resulting from blood flow from mother.

Hyperviscosity
273.3 Increase in macroglobulins in the blood, hyperviscosity, weakness, fatigue, bleeding disorders, and visual disturbances.

Hypoglycemic
251.2 (idiopathic familial hypoglycemia) Hypoglycemia described as unspecified

Hypoperfusion
769 (Hyaline membrane) Respiratory distress in premature neonates associated with reduced amounts of lung surfactant. Frequently fatal.

Hypophyseal
253.8 Relating to hyphysis.

Hypophyseothalamic
253.8 Relating to thalamus.

Hypopituitarism
253.2 Decreasing production of pituitary hormones caused by lessening activity of of the anterior lobe of the hypophysis.

© 2004 Ingenix, Inc.

Hypoplastic left heart
746.7 Hypoplasia or atresia of the left ventricle and aorta or mitral valve with respiratory distress and extreme cyanosis. Cardiac failure and death often result in early infancy.

Hypotension, maternal
669.2x Significantly reduced blood pressure during pregnancy.

Hypotonia-hypomentia-hypogonadism-obesity
759.81 (Prader-Willi) Rounded face, almond-shaped eyes, strabismus, low forehead, hypogonadism, hypotomia, mental retardation, and an insatiable appetite.

ICF
286.6 Decrease of elements needed for coagulation of blood and profuse bleeding.

Idiopathic cardiorespiratory distress, newborn
769 (Hyaline membrane, respiratory distress) Respiratory distress in premature neonates associated with reduced amounts of lung surfactant. Frequently fatal.

Idiopathic nephrotic
581.9 Affects the kidneys of a child with unknown cause.

Immobility
728.3 Paralysis of legs and lower part of body.

Immunologic deficiency
279.00 (Antibody deficiency) Inherited immune deficiencies characterized by insufficient antibodies.

Inappropriate secretion of antidiuretic hormone
253.6 (Schwartz-Bartter) Low or normal blood pressure, no edema, and retarded growth found in children with hypokalemic alkalosis and elevated renin or angiotensin levels.

Induced by drug
292.11 Description of symptoms, physiological and psychological, produced by drug abuse or dependence.

Infantilism
253.3 Profound retardation of mental and physical development

Inferior vena cava
459.2 Obstruction of the vena cava.

Inspissated bile, newborn
774.4 Biliary obstruction in newborn resulting from plugging of outflow tract.

IRDS (infant reflex distress)
769 (Hyaline membrane) Respiratory distress in premature neonates associated with reduced amounts of lung surfactant. Frequently fatal.

Itsenko-Cushing
255.0 (Cushing) Increased adrenocortical secretion of cortisol caused by ACTH-dependent adrenocortical hyperplasia or tumor with abdominal striae, acne, hypertension decreased carbohydrate tolerance, moon face, obesity, protein catabolism, and psychiatric disturbances.

IVC (intravascular coagulopathy)
286.6 Decrease of elements needed for coagulation of blood. Later stages are marked by profuse bleeding.

Ivemark's
759.0 Organs of left side of the body are a mirror image of organs on right side. Splenic agenisis and cardiac malformation are associated.

Jaccoud's
714.4 Post rheumatic fever arthritis with fibrous changes in the joint capsules and tendons. Malformation of the joints resembles rheumatoid arthritis.

Jackson's
344.89 (Avellis, Babinski-Nageotte, Benedikt's, Brown-Sequard, Cestan's, Cestan-Chenais, Foville's, Gubler-Millard, Weber-Leyden) Paraplegia and anesthesia over part of the body. Caused by lesions in the brain or spinal cord.

Jadassohn-Lewandowski
757.5 Abnormal thickness and elevation of nail plates with palmar and plantar hyperkeratosis. The tongue is whitish.

Jaffe-Lichtenstein (-Uehlinger)
252.0 (Engel-von Recklinghausen) Osteitis with fibrous degeneration and formation of cysts, along with fibrous nodules on affected bones due to misfunctioning parathyroid gland.

Jahnke's
759.6 Angioma in trigeminal nerve, homolateral meningeal angioma with intracranial calcification, and/or angioma of choroid.

Jakob-Creutzfeldt
046.1 Progressive dementia, wasting of muscles, tremor, and other symptoms. Communicable, rare spongiform encephalopathy occurring in middle life with progressive destruction of the pyramidal and extrapyramidal systems to death.

© 2004 Ingenix, Inc.

Jaksch (-Hayem-Luzet)

285.8 An anemic disorder among children under age three characterized by acute hemolytic anemia, infections, and gastrointestinal disorders.

Jaw-winking

742.8 Eyelids widen during chewing, sometimes with an elevation of upper lid when mouth is open and closing of the lid when mouth is closed.

Jejunal

564.2 (dumping) Emptying of contents of jejunum with nausea, sweating, weakness, palpitation, syncope, warmth, and diarrhea occurring after eating in patients who have had partial gastrectomy and gastrojejunostomy.

Jet lag

307.45 Imbalance of the normal circadian rhythm resulting from airplane travel through a number of time zones. Leads to fatigue, irritability, and other consitutional disturbances.

Jeune's

756.4 (ATD) Pelvis and phalanges are malformed, and cartilage of rib cage is unable to support breath action, leading to asphyxia.

Job's

288.1 Autosomal disorder of neutrophils with abnormal or absent chemotactic responses, eczema, and staphylococcal abcesses on the skin. Patients tend to be females with fair skin and red hair.

Jordan's

288.2 (Chediak-Higashi, Dohle body, Hegglin, May) Hepatosplenomegaly, lymphadenopathy, anemia, and thrombocytopenia with changes in the bones, cardiopulmonary system, skin, and psychomotor skills. Abnormalities of granulation and nuclear structure of white cells opens patient to infection and results in death.

Joseph-Diamond-Blackfan

284.0 (Fanconi's, Blackfan-Diamond, Kaznelson's) Congenital anemia of infancy requiring a number of blood transfusions to maintain life.

Jugular foramen

352.6 (Collet-Sicard) Unilateral lesions of the ninth, tenth, eleventh, and twelfth cranial nerves producing paralysis of the vagal, glossal, and other nerves and the tongue on the same side resulting from injury.

Kahler's

203.0x Malignant neoplasm associated with anemia, hemorrhages, recurrent infections, and weakness that originates in bone marrow.

Kalischer's

759.6 Multiple angiomas in skin of head and scalp.

Kallmann's

253.4 Failure of sexual development resulting from inadequate secretion of pituitary gonadotropines. Associated with anosmia due to agenisis of the olfactory lobes in the brain, a product of X-linked inheritance.

Kartagener's

759.3 Reversal of the position or location of organs or viscera.

Kasabach-Merritt

287.3 Small number of platelets in circulating blood, causing bruising.

Kast's

756.4 (Maffucci's) Benign cartilaginous growths in bones with bleeding in viscera and skin.

Kaznelson's

284.0 (Diamond-Blackfan, Fanconi's, Joseph) Congenital anemia of infancy and requiring a number of blood transfusions to maintain life.

Kelly's

280.8 (Paterson-Brown-Kelly, Plummer-Vinson) Condition in middle-aged women with hypochronic anemia, cracks or fissures at the corners of the mouth, painful tongue, and dysphagia due to esophageal stenosis or webs.

Kimmelstiel-Wilson

250.4x [581.81] High blood pressure and kidney failure resulting from a form of diabetes in which carbohydrate utilization is reduced and lipid and protein enhanced.

Klauder's

695.1 Necrolysis of skin caused by toxins.

Klein-Waardenburg

270.2 (Mendes, van der Hoeve-Halbertsma-Waardenburg, Waardenburg-Klein) Eyebrow or upper or lower eyelid sags.

Kleine-Levin

349.89 (Parry-Romberg) Hypersomnia with bulimia occurring in males between 10 to 25 years of age. Ravenous appetite is followed by prolonged sleep, along with behavioral disturbances, impaired thought processes, and hallucinations.

 © 2004 Ingenix, Inc.

Klinefelter's
758.7 (XXY) Male in development, but with seminal tube dysgenisis, gynecomastia, and urinary gonadotropins.

Klippel-Feil
756.16 Shorter than average neck and a low hairline caused by fewer than average cervical vertebrae or fusion of hemivertebrae into one bony mass.

Klippel-Trenaunay
759.89 One extremity with hypertrophy of bone and soft tissues, hemangiomas on the skin, and port-wine stain over the bone.

Klumpke (-Déjérine)
767.6 Atrophic paralysis of forearm and hand as result of birth trauma to brachial plexus.

Klüver-Bucy (-Terzian)
310.0 Bilateral temporal lobe ablation with psychic hyperreactivity to visual stimuli or blindness, increased oral and sexual activity, and depressed drive and emotional reactions.

Köhler-Pellegrini-Stieda
726.62 Calcification of medial collateral ligament of the knee.

König's
564.89 Alternating constipation and diarrhea with pain meteorism and gurgling sounds in the right illiac fossa.

Korsakoff (-Wernicke)
294.0 Amnestic dementia in which the patient cannot remember short-term or long-term memories but is not delirious.

Kostmann's
288.0 (Doan-Wiseman, Schultz, Schwachman) Bronchiectasis and pancreatic insufficiency, resulting in malnutrition, sinusitis, short stature, and bone abnormalities.

Kunkel
571.49 (lupid hepatitis) Chronic hepatitis with autoimmune manifestations.

Langdon Down
758.0 (mongolism) Congenital retardation with retarded growth, flat face with short nose, epicanthic skin folds, protruding lower lip, rounded ears, thickened tongue, pelvic dysplasia, broad hands and feet, stubby fingers, and absence of Moro reflex.

Larsen's
755.8 Numerous congenital dislocations with anomalies of the bones and flattened facial features.

Late effect
760.71 Late effects of fetal malformation resulting among offspring of mothers who are chronic alcoholics. Symptoms include growth deficiency, craniofacial anomalies, and limb defects.

Launois'
253.0 Pituitary secretions causing gigantism beginning before puberty with eosinophilic cell hyperplasia, eosinophilic adenoma, or chromophobe adenoma.

Launois-Cléret
253.8 (Babinski-Frolich, Renon-Delille) Marked by obesity and hypogonadism in adolescent boys with dwarfism indicating hypothyroidism.

Laurence-Moon (-Bardet) - Biedl
759.89 Retardation, pigmentary retinopathy, obesity, polydactyly, and hypogonadism.

Lawford's
759.6 (Kalischer's) Formation of multiple angiomas in skin of head and scalp.

Lederer-Brill
283.19 Anemic syndrome noted for fragmentation of red blood cells.

Legg-Calvé-Perthes
732.1 Disease of children in growth centers, especially at top of femur, in which the epiphyses is replaced by new calcification.

Lennox's
345.0x Childhood epilepsy with slow brain waves.

Lenticular
275.1 Accumulation of copper in the brain, cornea, kidney, liver, and other tissues causing cirrhosis of the liver and deterioration in the basal ganglia of the brain.

Lepore hemoglobin
282.4 Cardiac defects, coarse facial features, multiple lentigines, pulmonary stenosis, abnormalities of the genitalia, sensorineural deafness, and skeletal changes.

Léri-Weill
756.59 Dorsal dislocation of the distal ulna and carpal bones, bowing of the radius, and mesomelic dwarfism.

Leriche's
444.0 Obstruction of the terminal aorta causing fatigue in the hips, thighs, and calves; pallor of lower extremities; and impotence of exercising males.

Lermoyez's
386.00 Vertigo, nausea, vomiting, tinnitus, and progressive deafness caused by endolymphatic hydrops.

Lesch-Nyhan
277.2 Physical and mental retardation, compulsive self-mutilation of the lips and fingers through biting, impaired renal function, choreoathetosis, spastic cerebral palsy, and purine synthesis and consequent hyperuricemia and uricaciduria.

Leukocyte
288.0 (Doan-Wiseman, Schultz, Schachman) Bronchiectasis and pancreatic insufficiency, resulting in malnutrition, sinusitis, short stature, and bone abnormalities.

Lev's
426.0 (Rytand-Lipstitch) Bundle branch block in patient with normal coronary arteries and myocardium resulting from calcification of the conducting system.

Levi's
253.3 (Burnier, Lorain-Levi) (pituitary dwarfism) Dwarfism resulting from the absence of functional anterior pituitary gland.

Lichtheim's
281.0 [336.2] Numbness and tingling, weakness, a sore tongue, dyspnea, faintness, pallor of the skin and mucous membranes, anorexia, diarrhea, loss of weight, and fever. Most often strikes in the fifth decade.

Lightwood's
588.8 Variety of syndromes resulting from metabolic acidosis springing from renal misfunction.

Lignac (-Fanconi)
270.0 Metabolic disorder of kidney, involving failure to reabsorb water, minerals, and other substances as well as failure to transport.

Likoff's
413.9 Severe pain in the chest caused by ischemia of heart prompted by coronary artery disease.

Liver-kidney
572.4 (Heyd's) Acute renal failure in patients with disease of biliary or liver tract. Cause seems to be decreased renal blood flow, damaging both organs.

Lloyd's
258.1 Endocrine dysfunction causing diabetes and affecting growth and weight.

Lobe (lung) (right)
518.0 (Brock) Incomplete expansion of right middle lobe of lung with chronic pneumonitis.

Lobectomy behavior
310.0 Symptomatic description of Kluver-Bucy syndrome.

Löffler's
518.3 Transient infiltrations of lungs by eosinophilia resulting in coughing, fever, and dyspnea.

Löfgren's
135 (Hutchinson-Boeck, Schaumann's, Besnier-Boeck-Schaumann) Involves fibrosis in lungs, lymph nodes, skin, liver, eyes, spleen, phalangeal bones, and parotid glands. Identified by systemic granulomas composed of epithelioid and multinucleated giant cells.

Long arm 18 or 21 deletion
758.3 Autosomal deletion causing a variety of symptoms.

Looser (-Debray) - Milkman
268.2 (Milkman) Osteoporosis with frequent fractures striking middle-aged women.

Lorain-Levi
253.3 (Burnier, Levi) Dwarfism resulting from absence of functional anterior pituitary gland.

Louis-Bar
334.8 (Boder-Sedgwick) Gonadal hypoplasia, insulin resistance and hyperglycemia, liver function problems, ataxia, nystagmus, and increased sensitivity to ionizing radiation.

Lowe's
270.8 (Lowe-Terrey-MacLachlan) Aminoaciduria, cataracts, mental retardation, hydrophthalmia, rickets, and reduced ammonia production by the kidney.

Lower radicular, newborn
767.4 Damage of nerve root during birth.

Lown (-Ganong)-Levine
426.81 Electrocardiographic disorder indicated by a short P-R interval with normal duration of the QRS complex.

Lucey-Driscoll
774.30 Retention jaundice in newborn infants resulting from defective bilirubin conjugation, a product of a steroid in mother's blood being transferred to the infant.

© 2004 Ingenix, Inc.

Lung
518.5 Respiratory distress following surgery, shock or trauma, similar to but not caused by, adult respiratory distress system.

Lutembacher's
745.5 Atrial septal defect associated with mitral stenosis.

Lyell's
695.1 Necrolysis of skin caused by toxins.

MacLeod's
492.8 (Swyer-James) Acquired unilateral hyperlucent lung with severe airway obstruction during expiration.

Macrogenitosomia praecox
259.8 1) Excessive bodily development with unusual growth of sexual organs; 2) a description of symptoms indicating Donohue's and other syndromes.

Macroglobulinemia
273.3 (Waldenström's) Earmarked by increase in macroglobulins in the blood. Has symptoms of hyperviscosity such as weakness, fatigue, bleeding disorders, and visual disturbances.

Maffucci's
756.4 (Maffucci's) Benign cartilaginous growths in bones with bleeding in viscera and skin.

Magnesium-deficiency
781.7 Tetany. Any number of syndromes affecting newborns and others. Hyperexcitability of nerve and muscles due to decrease in concentration of extracellular ionized calcium, resulting in calcium and magnesium deficiency.

Malabsorption
579.9 A number of syndromes in which the body does not adequately absorb dietary constituents and loses nonabsorbed substances in the stool. Due to muscle, digestive, or lymphactic defect.

Malignant carcinoid
259.2 (Bjorck-Thorson, Cassidy-Scholte, Hedinger's) Carcinoid tumors causing cyanotic flushing of skin, diarrheal watery stools, bronchoconstrictive attacks, hypotension, edema, and ascites.

Mallory-Weiss
530.7 A tear in esophagus following several hours or days of vomiting, marked by vomiting of blood.

Mandibulofacial
756.0 (Franceschetti's, mandibulofacial dysostosis) Malformations of derivatives of the first branchial arch, marked by pallpebral fissures sloping outward and downward with notches in the outer third of the lower lids, defects of malar bones and zygome, hypoplasia of the jawbone, high or cleft palate, low-set ears, unusual hair growth, and pits between mouth and ear.

Manic depression
296.80 (bipolar) Alternating major depressive and manic periods.

Mankowsky's
731.2 (Pierre Marie-Bamberger) Symmetrical osteitis of limbs localized to phalanges and terminal epiphyses of the long bones of forearm and leg. Symptoms include kyphosis of spine and affection of joints.

Maple syrup
270.3 Anomaly in amino acid metabolism marked by urine and perspiration odor, hypertonicity, convulsions, coma, and death.

Marable's
447.4 Compression of celiac artery by median arcuate ligament in diaphragm.

Marchesani (-Weill)
759.89 Short stature, heavy musculature, reduced joint mobility, myopic, glaucoma, and many other symptoms.

Marcus Gunn's
742.8 (jaw-winking) Eyelids widen during chewing, sometimes with elevation of upper lid when the mouth is open and closing of lid when mouth is closed.

Marfan's
759.82 Unusually long extremities, subluxation of the lens, dilation of the aorta, and other symptoms.

Marie-Bamberger
731.2 (Hagner's) A condition characterized by clubbed fingers and toes, vasomotor disturbances of the hands and feet; it occurs in association with pulmonary diseases. Also known as hypertrophic pulmonary osteoarthropathy.

Marie's
253.0 Secondary to chronic conditions in lung and heart, localized to phalanges and terminal epiphyses of long bones of arm and leg, and accompanied by kyphosis. Caused by pituitary disorder.

Markus-Adie
379.46 Paralysis of conjugate movement of eyes without paralysis of convergence. Caused by lesions of midbrain.

© 2004 Ingenix, Inc.

Maroteaux-Lamy
277.5 Accumulation of mucopolysaccharide sulfates affecting eye, ear, skin, teeth, skeleton, joints, liver, spleen, cardiovascular system, respiratory system, and central nervous system.

Martin-Albright
275.49 (Albright-Martin, Seabright-Bantam) Short stature, obesity, short metacarpals, and ectopic calcification. Similar to hypoparathyroidism and caused by failure to repond to parathyroid hormone.

Martorell-Fabré
446.7 (Marorell-Fabre, Raed-Harbitz, Takayasu-Onishi) Ischemia, transient blindness, facial atrophy, and many others. Progressive obliteration of the brachiocephalic trunk and the left subclavian and common carotid arteries above their source in the aortic arch.

Massive aspiration of newborn
770.1 Intrauterine aspiration of amniotic fluid contaminated by meconium.

Masters-Allen
620.6 Pelvic pain resulting from old laceration of broad ligament received during delivery.

Mastocytosis
757.33 Inherited disorder of skin (and sometimes other structures) in which pigmented lesions appear in linear, zebra stripe, and other configurations and are preceded by vesicles and bullae and followed by verrucal lesions.

Maternal hypotension
669.2x Significantly reduced blood pressure during pregnancy.

Maternal obesity
646.1x Edema or excessive weight gain in pregnancy with no hypertension.

May (-Hegglin)
288.2 (Chediak-Higashi, Dohle body, Hegglin, Jordan's, May) Hepatosplenomegaly, lymphadenopathy, anemia, thrombocytopenia, along with changes in the bones, cardiopulmonary system, skin, and psychomotor skills. Abnormalities of granulation and nuclear structure of white cells open child to infection and result in death.

McArdle (-Schmid) (-Pearson)
271.0 Glucose-6-phosphatase deficiency due to inherited defects of glycogen metabolism resulting in excess accumulation of glycogen in muscle, characterized by myopathies and hepatorenal effects.

McCune-Albright
756.59 (Albright's hereditary osteodystrophy) Patchy skin pigmentation, endocrine dysfunctions, and polyostotic fibrous dysplasia.

McQuarrie's
251.2 Hypoglycemia described as primary and unspecified, reactive, or spontaneous.

Median arcuate ligament
447.4 Compression of celiac artery by median arcuate ligament in diaphragm.

Meekeren-Ehlers-Danlos
756.83 (Meekeren, Ehlers, Danlos) Group of congenital connective tissue diseases with overly elastic skin, hyperextensive joints, and fragility of blood vessels and arteries.

Meige
757.0 (Nonne-Milroy-Meige) Lymphatic edema of the legs (and face and arms in severe cases) caused by obstruction of lymphatic ducts.

Melkersson (-Rosenthal)
351.8 (crocodile tears) Facial paralysis with dramatic lacrimation during eating. Caused by lesion on seventh cranial nerve, prompting impulses to be misdirected from salivary glands to lacrimal glands.

Mende's (ptosis-epicanthus)
270.2 (Mendes, van der Hoeve-Halbertsma-Waardenburg, Waardenburg-Klein) Eyebrow or upper or lower eyelid sags.

Mendelson's
997.3 Pulmonary disorders caused by aspirating of lung following vomiting or regurgitation during medical procedure.

Ménétrier's
535.2x Giant hypertrophy of gastric mucosa.

Ménière's
386.00 Vertigo, nausea, vomiting, tinnitus, and progressive deafness caused by endolymphatic hydrops.

Meningo-eruptive
047.1 Enteric cytopathogenic human orphan (ECHO) virus. Common form of virus (which has many variations) is meningo-eruptive, with fever and aseptic meningitis.

Meningococcic
036.3 (Friderichsen-Waterhouse, Waterhouse,) Acute fulminating meningococcal septicemia occurring in children below 10 years of age with vomiting, cyanosis, diarrhea, purpura, convulsions, circulatory collapse, meningitis, and hemorrhaging into adrenal glands.

 © 2004 Ingenix, Inc.

Menkes'
759.89 Congenital abnormality in copper absorption characterized by severe cerebral degeneration and arterial changes resulting in death in infancy.

Menopause
627.2 Chills, depression, hot flashes, headache, and irritability.

Menstruation
625.4 (Premenstrual, PMS) Monthly physiological and emotional distress during the several days preceding menses with symptoms of nervousness, fluid retention, weight gain, and depression.

Mesenteric artery
557.1 (Wilkie's) Complete or partial block of the superior mesenteric artery with symptoms of vomiting, pain, blood in the stool, and distended abdomen. Results in bowel infarction.

Metastatic carcinoid
259.2 (Bjorck-Thorson, Cassidy-Scholte, Hedinger's) Carcinoid tumors that causes cyanotic flushing of skin, diarrheal watery stools, bronchoconstrictive attacks, hypotension, edema, and ascites.

Meyenburg-Altherr-Uehlinger
733.99 Arthritis with degeneration of cartilage leading to collapse of ears, nose, and tracheobronchial tree. Death may occur as respiratory system is affected.

Meyer-Schwickerath and Weyers
759.89 Abnormally small nose with anteverted nostrils, dental anomalies, and missing phalanges of toes.

Micheli-Rietti
282.4 Hemolytic anemias that share a common decreased rate of synthesis of one or more hemoglobin polypeptide chains and are classified according to the chain involved.

Michotte's
721.5 Kissing spine. Malformation of spine in which kyphosis becomes so great nonadjacent vertebrae touch.

Micrognathia-glossoptosis
756.0 Description of anomalies of face and skull.

Microphthalmos
759.89 Reduction in the size of the eye, opacities of the cornea and lens, and scarring of the retina.

Midbrain
348.8 Infarction of postero-inferior thalamus causing transient hemiparesis, severe loss of superficial and deep sensation with crude pain in the hypalgic limbs, vasomotor, or trophic disturbances.

Mieten's
759.89 Affects multiple systems.

Mikity-Wilson
770.7 Symptoms include hypercapnia and cyanosis of rapid onset during first month of life and frequently result in death. Rare pulmonary insufficiency in newborn babies, especially those with low birth weight.

Mikulicz's
527.1 Complex of lacrimal and salivary gland swelling, which may include enlargement associated with other syndromes, such as Sjogren's.

Milk alkali
999.9 (Burnett's) (milk drinkers) Disorder of kidneys induced by ingestion of large amounts of alkali and calcium in therapy of a peptic ulcer. While reversable in the early stages, it can lead to renal failure.

Milkman (-Looser-Debray)
268.2 Osteoporosis striking middle-aged women with frequent fractures.

Millard-Gubler
344.89 (Avellis, Babinski-Nageotte, Benedikt's, Brown-Sequard, Cestan's, Cestan-Chenais, Foville's, Gubler-Millard, Jackson's, Weber-Leyden) Paraplegia and anesthesia over half or part of the body. Caused by lesions in brain or spinal cord.

Miller Fisher's
357.0 (Guillain-Barre, Landry, Fisher's, Strohl, Miller) Often follows viral infections and may be a disorder of the immune system with symptoms of paraplegia of limbs, flaccid paralysis, ophalmoplegia, ataxia, and areflexia.

Milles'
759.6 (Kalischer's) Formation of multiple angiomas in skin of head and scalp.

Milroy
757.0 (Nonne-Milroy-Meige) Lymphatic edema of the legs (and face and arms in severe cases) caused by obstruction of lymphatic ducts.

Minkowski-Chauffard
282.0 Hemolytic anemia with spherocytosis, fragility of erthrocytes, splenomegaly, and jaundice.

© 2004 Ingenix, Inc.

Mirizzi's

576.2 Stone in cystic duct and chronic cystitis leading to spasms and scarring of connective tissue and obstruction of hepatic ducts.

Mohr's

759.89 (Oral-Fascial-Digital) Cranial, facial, lingual, mandibular, digital, and palatal abnormalities.

Monofixation

378.34 Strabismus of slight degree.

Moore's

345.5x Epilepsy with unilateral clonic movements starting in one group of muscles and spreading to adjacent groups, following the movement of the epilepsy through the contralateral motor cortex.

Morel-Moore

733.3 (Morel-Morgagni, -Stewart-Morel) Thickening of the inner table of the frontal bone related to obesity in women nearing menopause.

Morgagni-Adams-Stokes

426.9 (Stokes-Adams; Morgagni's disease; and Spens) Heart block causing slow or absent pulse, vertigo, syncope, convulsions, and Cheyne-Stokes respiration.

Morquio (-Brailsford) (-Ullrich)

277.5 Accumulation of mucopolysccharide sulfates affecting the eye, ear, skin, teeth, skeleton, joints, liver, spleen, cardiovascular system, respiratory system, and central nervous system.

Morris

257.8 (Morris, hairless women, Goldberg, Goldberg-Maxwell) Male pseudohermaphroditism with incompletely developed vagina, rudimentary uterus, fallopian tubes, scanty or absent axillary/public hair, and amenorrhea.

Morton's

355.6 Pain in the forefoot caused by a lesion of the plantar nerve.

Moschcowitz (-Singer-Symmers)

446.6 Central nervous system involvement due to formation of fibrin or platelet thrombi in arterioles and capillaries in many organs.

Mounier-Kuhn

494 Tracheobronchomegaly.

Mucha-Haberman

696.2 Chronic dermatosis of unknown origin with scaling lesions that produce small pox-like scars. Recurrence of attacks are common, but disease is self-limiting.

Mucocutaneous lymph node

446.1 (Harkavy) Fever, conjunctival injection reddening of the oral cavity, ulcerative gingivitis, cervical lymph nodes, skin eruptions that cover the hands and feet, and skin becoming puffy and sloughs off.

Munchhausen's

301.51 (Hospital addiction, Multiple operations) Emotional condition in which patient exhibits physical, but psychosomatic, symptoms.

Münchmeyer's

728.11 Diffuse progressive ossifying polymyositis.

Muscle deficiency

756.71 (Prune Belly, Eagle-Barrett) Absence of muscles of abdomen and genitourinary anomalies. Intestinal outlines are visible on patient's skin.

Myelodysplastic

238.7 Neoplasm of lymphatic and hematopoietic tissues, affecting the spinal cord.

Myeloproliferative

238.7 Unusual proliferation of myelopoietic tissue.

Naffziger's

353.0 Raynaud-like symptoms of vascular contractions caused by pressure of brachial plexus and subclavian artery against first thoracic rib.

Nager-de Reynier

756.0 Franceschetti's syndrome with limb deformities consisting of absence of the radius, radioulnar synostosis, and hypoplasia or absence of thumbs.

Nail-patella

756.89 Dysplasia of the fingernails and toenails, hypoplasia of the patella, iliac horns, thickening of the glomerular lamina densa, and a flask-shaped femur.

Nebécourt's

253.3 (Burnier, Lorain-Levi) Dwarfism resulting from absence of functional anterior pituitary gland.

Neill-Dingwall

759.89 Small head and dwarfism. One of many syndromes affecting several body systems, but not elsewhere specified.

Nerve compression

354.8 Pain in upper and posterior part of the shoulder radiating into neck and occiput, down the arm, and around the chest. Caused

 © 2004 Ingenix, Inc.

by abnormal positioning between the scapula and thorax, pain includes tingling in the fingers.

Netherton's
757.1 Scaling of skin showing a peripheral double margin in and around the vagina.

Neurocutaneous
759.6 Occurance of nevi and skeletal deformities as result of gliosis and abiotrophy of central nervous system.

Neuroleptic malignant
333.92 Description of the effects of antipsychotic drugs on behavior and cognition.

Newborn distress
770.6 Intrauterine fetal aspiration of amniotic fluid contaminated by meconium.

Niemann-Pick
272.7 Accumulation of phospholipid in histiocytes in the bone marrow, liver, lymph nodes, and spleen, cerebral involvement, and red macular spots similar to Tay-Sachs disease. Most commonly found in Jewish infants.

Nonne-Milroy-Meige
757.0 (Milroy) Lymphatic edema of the legs (and face and arms in severe cases) caused by obstruction of lymphatic ducts.

Nonpsychotic
310.2 Persistent personality disturbance of nonpsychotic origin following blow to the head with affective instability, bursts of aggression, apathy and indifference, impaired social judgment, and suspiciousness or paranoid ideation.

Noonan's
759.89 (Ulrich-Turner) Ptosis, hypogonadism webbed, neck, congenital heart disease, short stature; once diagnosed as Turner's syndrome until this female component was identified.

Nucleus ambiguous-hypoglossal
352.6 (Collet-Sicard) Unilateral lesions of the ninth, tenth, eleventh, and twelfth cranial nerves producing paralysis of vagal, glossal, other nerves, and tongue on the same side. Most usually result of injury.

OAV (oculoauriulovertebral dysplasia)
756.0 (Goldenhar's) Number of anomalies, including epibulbar dermoids, preauricular appendages, micrognathia, and vertebral.

Oculocutaneous
364.24 (Vogt-Koyanagi) Uveomeningitis with patchy depigmentation of hair, eyebrows, and lashes; retinal detatchment, deafness, and tinnitus may also result.

Oculoglandular
372.02 Syndrome of the eyes and glands.

Oculomotor
378.81 (Parinaud's) Paralysis of conjugate movement of the eyes without paralysis of convergence. Caused by lesions of the midbrain.

Of diabetic mother
775.0 Maternal diabetes mellitus affecting fetus or newborn with hypoglycemia.

Ogilvie's
560.89 Colonic obstruction with symptoms of persistent contraction of intestinal musculature. Caused by defect in sympathetic nerve supply.

Ophthalmica
053.19 Any symptoms of herpes arising in eye.

Ophthalmoplegia-cerebellar ataxia
378.52 Paralysis of one or more optic muscles or failure to control muscles.

Ophthalmoplegic migraine
346.8x Migraine headache accompanied by amblyopia and other visual disturbances.

Oppenheim-Urbach
250.8x [709.3] Diabetes with skin disorder.

Oral-facial-digital
759.89 (Papillon-Leage and Psaume) Defects of the oral cavity, face, and hands including bifid tongue, cleft palate, missing teeth, pug-nose, depressed nasal bridge, mental retardation, and others. Syndrome is lethal in males.

Organic affective
293.83 Patient may exhibit a number of changes in personality such as amotivation, depression, outbursts, poor social judgment, and others.

Organic personality
310.1 Persistent personality disturbance of nonpsychotic origin featuring affective instability, bursts of aggression, apathy and indifference, impaired social judgment, and suspiciousness or paranoid ideation.

Ormond's
593.4 (Ormond's) Retroperitoneal structures involving and often obstructing ureters sometimes following certain types of chemical treatment; there is no identified cause.

© 2004 Ingenix, Inc.

Orthostatic hypotensive-dysautonomic dyskinetic
333.0 (Hallervorden-Spatz, Dejerine-Thomas) Nerves between the striatum and pallidum are completely demyelated.

Osler-Weber-Rendu
448.0 A post-pubescent disorder with small telangiectasia and dilated venules developing slowly on the skin and mucus membranes of the lips, nasopharynx, and tongue.

Osteodermopathic hyperostosis
757.39 Irregular linear streaks of skin atrophy, skeletal malformations, and papillomas of lips.

Osteoporosis-osteomalacia
268.2 (Milkman, Looser, Debray) Osteoporosis striking middle-aged women with frequently-suffered fractures.

Österreicher-Turner
756.89 Dysplasia of the fingernails and toenails, hypoplasia of the patella, iliac horns, thickening of the glomerular lamina densa, and a flask-shaped femur.

Ostrum-Furst
756.59 Deformities of neck, platybasia, and Sprengel's neck.

Otolith
386.19 (Bonnier) Ocular disturbances, deafness, nausea, thirst, anorexia, and symptoms traced to vagus centers as result of a lesion of Deiters nucleus and its connections.

Otopalatodigital
759.89 Defects of ear, oral cavity, face, and hands.

Outlet
353.0 (Naffziger's) Vascular contractions of the digits similar to Raynaud's, caused by pressure of brachial plexus and subclavian artery against first thoracic rib.

Ovarian remnant
620.8 Pelvic pain typically occurring several weeks or several months following surgical removal of the ovaries, often due to the survival of an ovarian fragment after the operation.

Ovarian vein
593.4 (Ormond's) Retroperitoneal structures involving and often obstructing the ureters following certain types of chemical treatment; there is no identified cause.

Owren's
286.3 (Stewart-Prower) Deficiencies of clotting factors noticable from birth.

P-R interval
426.81 (Lown-Ganong) Electrocardiographic disorder indicated by a short P-R interval with normal duration of the QRS complex.

Pacemaker
429.4 Functional deficiency following heart surgery in which the triggering mechanism of the heart may be irregular.

Paget-Schroetter
453.8 Stress thrombosis of subclavian or axillary vein.

Pancoast's
162.3 (Hare's, Cuiffini) Neoplasm of upper lobe of the lung.

Panhypopituitary
253.2 Secretion of all anterior pituitary hormones is inadequate or absent after childbirth.

Parabiotic (transfusion) donor (twin)
772.0 Transfusion of blood from one fetus to another.

Parabiotic (transfusion) recipient (twin)
776.4 Polycythemia of newborn as result of blood flow from mother.

Paranoid type
293.81 Organic disorder with hallucinations, beliefs about being followed, being poisoned, etc.; and not meeting criteria for schizophrenia.

Parinaud's
378.81 Paralysis of conjugate movement of eyes without paralysis of convergence caused by lesions of the midbrain.

Parkes Weber and Dimitri
759.6 (Kalischer's) Formation of multiple angiomas in skin of head and scalp.

Parry's
242.0x (Basedow, Grave's disease) Fatigue, nervousness, emotional lability and irritability, heat intolerance and increased sweating, weight loss, palpitation, and tremor of hands and tongue. Autoimmune in etiology and caused by excess thyroidal hormones.

Parry-Romberg
349.89 (Kleine-Levin) Hypersomnia associated with bulimia and occurring in males between 10 to 25 years of age with ravenous appetite followed by prolonged sleep, along with behavioral disturbances, impaired thought processes, and hallucinations.

© 2004 Ingenix, Inc.

Parsonage-Aldren-Turner
353.5 Paroxysmal pain extending length of one of many nerves.

Patau's
758.1 (Patau's, trisomy D) Variety of symptoms in newborns with extra chromosome in group D and number of symptoms, including mental retardation and malformed ears, cardiac defects, convulsions, and others.

Paterson (-Brown) (-Kelly)
280.8 (Kelly, Plummer-Vinson) Condition in middle-aged women with hypochronic anemia of cracks or fissures at the corners of the mouth, painful tongue, and dysphagia due to esophageal stenosis or webs.

Payr's
569.89 Bloating, gas, pain, and fullness experienced left upper abdominal quadrant with pain sometimes radiating up into left chest.

Pectoral girdle
447.8 Malignant atrophic papulosis.

Pelger-Huët
288.2 (Chediak-Higashi, Dohle body, Hegglin, Jordan's, May) Patients present hepatosplenomegaly, lymphadenopathy, anemia, thrombocytopenia, along with changes in bones, cardopulmonary system, skin, and psychomotor skills. Abnormalities of granulation and nuclear structure of white cells open child to infection and result in death.

Pellagra-cerebellar ataxia-renal aminoaciduria
270.0 (Harts, Toni, Fanconi, Debre) Renal tubular malfunction, including cytinosis and osteomalacia, caused by inherited disorders or the result of multiple myeloma or proximal epithelial growth.

Pellagroid
265.2 Resembling pellagra or a description of pellagra.

Pellegrini-Stieda
726.62 (Kohler-Pellegrini-Stieda) Calcification of medial collateral ligament of knee.

Pellizzi's
259.8 Precocious development of external sexual organs, precocious development of long bones, and hydrocephalus indicating lesion of pineal body.

Pendred's
243 Familial goiter paired with congenital nerve deafness due to defective organic binding of iodine in the thyroid.

Penfield's
345.5x Epilepsy with unilateral clonic movements starting in one group of muscles and spreading to adjacent groups, following the movement of the epilepsy through the contralateral motor cortex.

Penta X
758.81 Pentasomy. Presence of three additional chromosomes of one type.

Perabduction
447.8 Malignant atrophic papulosis.

Periurethral fibrosis
593.4 (Ormond's) Retroperitoneal structures involving and often obstructing the ureters.

Petges-Cléjat
710.3 (Unverricht-Wagner) Polymyositis occurring with characteristic skin changes including rash on upper eyelids with edema, a rash on the forehead, neck, shoulders, trunk, and arms, and papules on knuckles.

Peutz-Jeghers
759.6 Formation of multiple hematomas.

Phantom limb
353.6 Itching, dull ache, or sharp, shooting pains mimicking the nerves of amputated limb.

Pharyngeal pouch
279.11 (DiGeorge's) Hypoplasia or aphasia of the thymus and prathyroid gland with congenital heart defects, anomalies of the great vessels, esophageal atresia, and facial deformities result from aphasia or hypoplasia of thymus and parathyroid glands. Seizures may accompany most severe cases.

Pick-Herxheimer
701.8 Atrophy of skin throughout body and of unknown cause.

Pickwickian
278.8 Obesity, hypoventilation, somnolence, and erythrocytosis. After Pickwick, Dicken's character.

PIE
518.3 (Loffler's) Transient infiltrations of lungs by eosinophilia, resulting in coughing, fever, and dyspnea.

Pierre Marie-Bamberger
731.2 (Mankowsky's) Symmetrical osteitis of limbs localized to phalanges, terminal epiphyses of long bones of forearm and leg, kyphosis of the spine, and affection of the joints.

Pierre Mauriac's
258.1 Endocrine dysfunction causing diabetes and affecting growth and weight.

Pigment dispersion, iris
364.53 Lack of pigment in iris.

Pineal
259.8 (Pellizi's) Precocious development of external sexual organs, precocious development of long bones, and hydrocephalus indicating lesion of pineal body.

Pink puffer
492.8 (Swyer-James) Acquired unilateral hyperlucent lung with severe airway obstruction during expiration, oligemia, and a small hilum.

Pituitary
253.0 Excessive pituitary secretions causing gigantism and beginning before puberty.

Placental dysfunction
762.2 (placental insufficiency) Fetal hypoxia and malnutrition resulting from lack of nutrition and oxygen transferred from mother. Due to degeneration of placenta and identified by yellow vernix.

Placental transfusion
762.3 Birth of one anemic twin and one plethoric twin due to forcing of blood of one twin into other.

Plantar fascia
728.71 Disorder of the fascia at the bottom of the foot.

Plug (newborn) NEC
777.1 Meconium obstruction of newborn's intestines, resulting from unusually thick or hard meconium.

Plummer-Vinson
280.8 (Kelly, Paterson-Brown-Vinson) Condition in middle-aged women with hypochronic anemia, marked by cracks or fissures at the corners of mouth, painful tongue, and dysphagia due to esophageal stenosis or webs.

Polycythemic
289.0 Gaisbock's syndrome.

Polysplenia
759.0 Organs of left side of body are mirror image of organs on right side. Splenic agenisis and cardiac malformation are associated.

Pontine
433.8x Quadriplegia, anesthesia, and nystagmus due to the obstruction of twigs of the basilar artery, causing lesions in pontine region.

Post-gastric surgery
564.2 (Dumping) Emptying of contents of jejunum with nausea, sweating, weakness, palpitation, syncope, warmth, and diarrhea. Occurs after eating in patients who have had partial gastrectomy and gastrojejunostomy.

Postartificial
627.4 Menopausal symptoms suffered by some women following destruction of their ovaries, including chills, depression, hot flashes, headache, and irritability.

Postcholecystectomy
576.0 Recurrence of gall bladder pain following removal of organ.

Postconcussional
310.2 (postcontusional, postencephalitic) Persistent personality disturbance of nonpsychotic origin following blow to head and featuring affective instability, bursts of aggression, apathy and indifference, impaired social judgment, and suspiciousness or paranoid ideation.

Posthepatitis
780.7x Chronic Fatigue Syndrome. Marked by persistent or relapsing fatigue not resolved by bed rest that significantly reduces daily activity. Other symptoms include chronic sore throat, mild fever, muscle weakness, myalgia, headaches, and neurological problems. Patients are primarily women. The syndrome arises sporadically with no confirmed etiology but is known to occur in clusters.

Postherpetic
053.19 Description of any symptoms of herpes arising in parts of body.

Postinfarction
411.0 (Dressler) Fever, leukocytosis, chest pain, evidence of pericarditis, pleurisy and pneumonia occurring days or weeks after a myocardial infarction.

Postleukotomy
310.0 Kluver-Bucy or postlobotomy syndrome.

Postmastectomy lymphedema
457.0 Edema of arms and hands following a mastectomy requiring removal of adjacent lymph nodes.

 © 2004 Ingenix, Inc.

Postmature
766.2 Placental dysfunction occurring in postmature fetuses.

Postmyocardial infarction
411.0 (Dressler) Fever, leukocytosis, chest pain, evidence of pericarditis, pleurisy, and pneumonia occurring days or weeks after myocardial infarction.

Postpartum panhypopituitary
253.2 Secretion of all anterior pituitary hormones is inadequate or absent after childbirth.

Postphlebitic
459.1x Deep vein thrombosis with edema, pain, purpua, and increased cutaneous pigmentation, eczema dermatitis, pruritus, ulceration, and cellulitis.

Postpolio
138 Inflammation of spinal cord following polio. Symptoms vary.

Postsurgical
579.3 Hypoglycemia and malabsorption following surgery.

Posttraumatic
294.0 Amnestic dementia in which patient cannot remember short-term or long-term memories but is not delirious.

Postvagotomy
564.2 (dumping) Emptying of contents of jejunum with nausea, sweating, weakness, palpitation, syncope, warmth, and diarrhea. Occurs after eating in patients who have had partial gastrectomy and vagotomy.

Potain's
536.1 Dilation of stomach with indigestion.

Potassium intoxication
276.7 (potassium overload) Excessive potassium, causing a number of symptoms.

Potter's
753.0 Renal agenesis with hypoplastic lungs and associated neonatal respiratory distress, hemodynamic instability, acidosis, cyanosis, edema, and characteristic facial features. Death usually occurs from lack of oxygen.

Premenstrual tension
625.4 (Premenstrual, PMS) Monthly physiological and emotional distress during the days preceding menses with symptoms of nervousness, fluid retention, weight gain, and depression.

Pre-ulcer
536.8 (Reichmann's) Excessive secretion of gastric juice either constantly or during digestion only.

Primary or idiopathic
757.39 Increased thickening of skin on extremities and face with clubbing of fingers and deformities in bone of limb.

Prinzmetal
786.52 Chest pain secondary to large vessel spasm that may interfere with breathing.

Profichet's
729.9 Calcareous nodules in the subcutaneous tissues primarily around larger joints. The nodules ulcerate and exhibit nervous symptoms.

Progeria
259.8 (Hutchinson-Gilford) Precocious senility with death from coronary artery disease occurring before 10 years of age.

Progressive pallidal degeneration
333.0 (Hallervorden-Spatz, Dejerine-Thomas) Condition in which the nerves between the striatum and pallidum are completely demyelated.

Prolonged gestation
766.2 Gestation beyond 42 completed weeks.

Prune belly
756.71 (Eagle-Barrett) Congenital absence of muscles of abdomen and genitourinary anomalies. Intestinal outlines are visible on skin.

Prurigo-asthma
691.8 Several itchy skin eruptions of unknown cause accompanying asthma.

Pseudocarpal tunnel
354.0 Pain and tingling, numbness, or burning in the hand as result of compression of median nerve by tendons.

Pseudohermaphroditism-virilism-hirsutism
255.2 Possession of mature masculine somatic characteristics by a prepubescent male, girl, or woman. This syndrome may show at birth or develop later as result of adrenocortical dysfunction.

Pseudoparalytica
358.0 (Goldflam, Erb, Hoppe) Progressive muscular weakness beginning in face and throat and caused by a defect in myoneural conduction.

Pseudo-Turner's
759.89 (Bonnevie-Ullrich) Congenital disorder with short stature, mental retardation, and a webbed neck but, unlike Turner's, patients can be of either sex and have normal chromosomes and no renal abnormalities.

Pterygolymphangiectasia
758.6 (XO) Congenital disorder characterized by short stature and webbed neck. Patients of either sex suffer congenital heart disease, mental retardation, and other symptoms.

Ptosis-epicanthus
270.2 (Mendes, van der Hoeve-Halbertsma-Waardenburg, Waardenburg-Klein) Eyebrow or upper or lower eyelid sags.

Pulmonary sulcus
162.3 (Cuiffini-Pancoast, Hare's) Neoplasm of upper lobe of lung.

Putnam-Dana
281.0 [336.2] Numbness and tingling, weakness, a sore tongue, dyspnea, faintness, pallor of the skin and mucous membranes, anorexia, diarrhea, loss of weight, and fever. Strikes in fifth decade.

Pyloroduodenal
537.89 (Gastrojejunal loop obstruction) Distended efferent loop causing illness and pain with acute or chronic obstruction of the duodenum and jejunum proximal to a gastrojejunostomy.

Pyriformis
355.0 Lesion on the sciatica nerve causing a pear shaped area of pain and parasthesia.

Q-T interval prolongation
794.31 (Romano-Ward) Prolonged Q-T interval and syncope, sometimes leading to ventricular fibrillation and sudden death.

Radicular
353.0 (Naffziger's) A disorder presenting symptoms similar to Raynaud's, caused by pressure of brachial plexus and subclavian artery against first thoracic rib.

Raeder-Harbitz
446.7 (Marorell-Fabre, Takayasu-Onishi) Progressive obliteration of brachiocephalic trunk and left subclavian and left common carotid arteries above their source in the aortic arch. Symptoms include ischemia, transient blindness, facial atrophy, and many others.

Rapid time-zone change
307.45 (jet lag) Imbalance of normal circadian rhythm resulting from airplane travel through a number of time zones. Leads to fatigue, irritability, and other consitutional disturbances.

Raymond (-Céstan)
433.8x Identified through symptoms of quadriplegia, anesthesia, and nystagmus due to the obstruction of twigs of the basilar artery, causing lesions in the pontine region.

Raynaud's
443.0 (Patriots disease) Constriction of the arteries of the digits caused by cold or emotion. Temperature drops in extremities as much as 30 degrees Farenheit, and skin turns white with red and blue mottling. Caused by nerve or arterial damage and can be prompted by stress.

RDS
769 (Hyaline membrane) Reduced amounts of lung surfactant in premature neonates with respiratory distress. Frequently fatal.

Recipient twin
776.4 Polycythemia of newborn as result of blood flow from mother.

Refsum's
356.3 Deafness, retinitis pigmentosa, polyneuritis, nystagmus, and cerebellar signs.

Reichmann's
536.8 Excessive secretion of gastric juice either constantly or during digestion only.

Reifenstein's
257.2 Hypogonadism with gynecomastia, hypospadias, and pospubertal testicular atrophy. Caused by inherited defect of androgen receptors and insensitivity to testosterone.

Reilly's
337.9 (Claude Bernard-Homer, Steinbrocker's) Pain and stiffness in the shoulder, with puffy swelling and pain in the hand following a heart attack.

Reiter's
099.3 (Fiessinger-Leroy-Reiter) Arthritis, iredocyclitis, and urethritis, sometimes with diarrhea. While symptoms may recur, arthritis is constant.

Renal
446.21 (Goodpasture's) Renal condition in which nephritis progresses rapidly to death, with lungs showing extensive hemosiderosis or bleeding.

© 2004 Ingenix, Inc.

Renal glomerulohyalinosis-diabetic
250.4x [581.81] High blood pressure and kidney failure resulting from a form of diabetes in which carbohydrate utilization is reduced and that of lipid and protein enhanced.

Rendu-Osler-Weber
448.0 Post-pubescent disorder with small telagiectases and dilated venules developing slowly on skin and mucus membranes of lips, tongue, nasopharynx, tongue, and face.

Renofacial
753.0 Renal agenesis with hypoplastic lungs and associated neonatal respiratory distress, hemodynamic instability, acidosis, cyanosis, edema, and characteristic facial features. Death usually occurs from lack of oxygen.

Rénon-Delille
253.8 (Babinski-Frolich, Launois-Cleret) Obesity and hypogonadism in adolescent boys. Rare accompanying dwarfism is thought to indicate hypothyroidism.

Respiratory distress
769 (Hyaline membrane) Premature neonates with respiratory distress and associated with reduced amounts of lung surfactant. Frequently fatal.

Restless leg
333.99 (Ekborn's) Indescribable uneasiness, restlessness, or twitching in the legs after going to bed. Often caused by poor circulation or antipsychotic medications, it can lead to insomnia.

Retraction
378.71 (Still-Turk-Duane) Simultaneous retraction of eye muscles causing an inability to abduct the affected eye with retraction of the globe.

Retroperitoneal fibrosis
593.4 (Ormond's) Retroperitoneal structures obstructing ureters following certain types of chemical treatment; there is no identified cause.

Rett's
330.8 Progressive disease affecting grey matter of the brain, where infant females present ataxia, autism, dementia, seizures, loss of purposeful use of the hands, and cerebral atrophy.

Reye's
331.81 Condition of childhood spawned by a spirochetic or viral disease of the upper respiratory system. Symptoms include recurrent vomiting, brain swelling, disturbances of consciousness, and seizures. Often fatal. Can be prompted by use of aspirin.

Reye-Sheehan's
253.2 (Sheehan's) Secretion of all anterior pituitary hormones is inadequate or absent presenting after childbirth.

Riddoch's
368.16 (Balint's, Holmes', Riddoch's) Corical paralysis of visual fixation, optic ataxia, and disturbance of visual attention. Eye movements are normal.

Ridley's
428.1 Left heart failure marked by acute edema of lung.

Rieger's
743.44 Dysgenesis of eye marked through widened trabecular meshwork, large iridial bands, and glaucoma.

Rietti-Greppi-Micheli
282.4 One of a group of hemolytic anemias sharing a common decreased rate of synthesis of one or more hemoglobin polypeptide chains and are classified according to chain involved.

Riley-Day
742.8 Eyelids widen during chewing, sometimes with an elevation of the upper lid when mouth is open and closing of lid when mouth is closed.

Robin's
756.0 (Pierre Robin's) Brachygnathia and cleft palate, upward displacement of the larynx, and angulation of the manubrium sterni. May be paired with others or the sole hyperplasia.

Rokitansky-Kuster-Hauser
752.49 Absence of vagina and uterus with normal karyotype and ovaries. Amenorrhea.

Romano-Ward
794.31 Prolonged Q-T interval and syncope, sometimes leading to ventricular fibrillation and sudden death.

Romberg's
349.89 (Kleine-Levin, Parry-Romberg) Hypersomnia associated with bulimia and occurring in males between 10 to 25 years of age. Ravenous appetite following prolonged sleep, along with behavioral disturbances, impaired thought processes, and hallucinations.

Rosen-Castleman-Liebow
516.0 Chronic disease of lungs marked by chest pain, weakness, hemoptysis, dyspnea, and

productive cough. Ventilation of affected areas is prevented by a proteinaceous material.

Roth's

355.1 Feeling of tingling, formication, itching, and other symptoms on the outer side of the lower part of the thigh caused by lateral femoral cutaneous nerve.

Rothmund's

757.33 Pigmentation and atrophy of the skin, along with cataracts, saddle nose, bone defects, disturbance of hair growth, and hypogonadism.

Rotor's

277.4 Nonhemolytic jaundice differing from Dubin-Johnson syndrome in that it does not produce liver pigmentation.

Rubella

771.0 Developmental abnormalities of newborn baby as resulting from transplacental transference of rubella during the first trimester of pregnancy. Symptoms include ocular and cardiac lesions, deafness, microcephaly, mental retardation, hepatitis, encephalitis, and others.

Rubinstein-Taybi's

759.89 Congenital defects including broad thumb and great toe, antimongloid slant to the eyes, beaked nose, prominent forehead, low set ears, high arched palate, mental retardation, and cardiac defects.

Rud's

759.89 Dwarfism, hypogonadism, and epilepsy with scaly skin as result of inherited disorder.

Ruiter-Pompen (-Wyers)

272.7 (Fabry's) Corneal opacities; burning pain in palms, soles, and abdomen; chronic paresthesia on hands and feet; cardiopulmonary involvement; edema of the legs; osteoporosis; retarded growth; and delayed puberty. Patients die of renal, cardiac, or cerebrovascular failure.

Runge's

766.22 (Ballantyne) Placental dysfunction occurring in postmature fetuses.

Russell (-Silver)

759.89 Suprasellar lesions in anterior third ventricle, hampering a child's ability to thrive. Despite elevated growth hormones, child is emaciated and looses body fat.

Rytand-Lipsitch

426.0 (Lev's) Bundle branch block in a patient with normal coronary arteries and myocardium resulting from calcification of conducting system.

Sacralization-scoliosis-sciatica

756.15 (Bertolotti's) Fusion of bottom lumbar vertebra to top sacral vertebra, making a sixth sacral vertebra. Other symptoms include sciatica and scoliosis.

Saenger's

379.46 Paralysis of conjugate movement of eyes without paralysis of convergence. Caused by lesions of midbrain.

Sanfilippo's

277.5 Results from accumulation of mucopolysaccharide sulfates affecting the eye, ear, skin, teeth, skeleton, joints, liver, spleen, cardiovascular system, respiratory system, and central nervous system.

Scaglietti-Dagnini

253.0 Arthritis of spine accompanying acromegaly, resembling rheumatoid arthritis, and progressing to bony ankylosis with lipping of vertebral margins.

Scalded skin

695.1 Necrolysis of skin caused by toxins.

Scalenus anticus

353.0 (Naffziger's) A disorder presenting symptoms similar to Raynaud's, caused by pressure of brachial plexus and subclavian artery against first thoracic rib.

Scapulocostal

354.8 Pain in upper and posterior part of the shoulder radiating into neck and occiput, down the arm, and around the chest. Caused by abnormal positioning between scapula and thorax, pain can include tingling in the fingers.

Scapuloperoneal

359.1 A position of fetus in which the scapula rests closest to the perineal area.

Schaumann's

135 (Hutchinson-Boeck, Lofgren's, Besnier-Boeck-Schaumann) Involves the lungs with resulting fibrosis, lymph nodes, skin, liver, eyes, spleen, phalangeal bones, and parotid glands. Identified by systemic granulomas composed of epithelioid and multinucleated giant cells.

Scheie's

277.5 Accumulation of mucopolysaccharide sulfates affecting the eye, ear, skin, teeth, skeleton, joints, liver, spleen, cardiovascular system, respiratory system, and central nervous system.

© 2004 Ingenix, Inc.

Scheuthauer-Marie-Sainton

755.59 Defective bone formation in skull, often associated with other symptoms.

Schirmer's

759.6 (Kalischer's) Formation of multiple angiomas in skin of the head and scalp.

Schizophrenic, of childhood

299.9x Description of schizophrenia occurring in childhood.

Schmidt's

258.1 Hypofunction of endocrine glands involving Hashimoto's thyroiditis, hypoparathyroidism, adrenal insufficiency, and underfunctioning gonads.

Schneider's

047.9 Viral meningitis that is unspecified.

Scholte's

259.2 (Bjorck-Thorson, Cassidy-Scholte, Hedinger's) Carcinoid tumors causing cyanotic flushing of skin, diarrheal watery stools, bronchoconstrictive attacks, hypotension, edema, and ascites.

Scholz (-Bielschowsky-Henneberg)

330.0 Metachromatic leukodystrophy, a disturbance of white substance of brain.

Schroeder's

255.3 (Slocumb's) Disorder of adrenal medullary tissue resulting in hypertension accompanied with attacks of palpitation, headache, nausea, dyspnea, anxiety, pallor, and profuse sweating.

Schüller-Christian

277.8 (Hand-Schuller-Christian) Histiocytosis with occasional accumulation of cholesterol. Symptoms include defects of the membranous bones, exophthalmos and diabetes insipidus. There is often also a multiple-system, soft tissue, and skeletal involvement.

Schultz's

288.0 (Doan-Wiseman, Kostmann, Schwachman) Bronchiectasis and pancreatic insufficiency, resulting in malnutrition, sinusitis, short stature, and bone abnormalities.

Schwartz (-Jampel)

756.89 Dysplasia of fingernails and toenails, hypoplasia of patella, iliac horns, thickening of glomerular lamina densa, and flask-shaped femur.

Schwartz-Bartter

253.6 Found in children with hypokalemic alkalosis and elevated renin or angiotensin levels with low or normal blood pressure, no edema, and retarded growth.

Scimitar

747.49 Venous drainage of right lung into the inferior vena cava with hypoplasia of the right lung. Name comes from the convex shadow of the anomalous vein to the right of the lower border of the heart in an x-ray.

Sclera

756.51 (van der Hoeve's) Blue sclera, little growth, brittle bones, and deafness.

Sclerocystic ovary

256.4 (Stein, Stein-Leventhal) Oligomenorrhea or amenorrhea, anovulation and infertility, and hirsutism. Most often caused by bilateral polycystic ovaries.

Sea-blue histiocyte

272.7 (Ruiter-Pompen-Wyers, Fabry's) Corneal opacities; burning pain in palms, soles, and abdomen; chronic paresthesia of hands and feet; cardiopulmonary involvement; edema of the legs; osteoporosis; retarded growth; and delayed puberty. Patients die of renal, cardiac, or cerebrovascular failure.

Seabright-Bantam

275.49 (Albright-Martin, Martin-Albright) Similar to hypoparathyroidism, caused by failure to repond to parathyroid hormone with short stature, obesity, short metacarpals, and ectopic calcification.

Seckel's

759.89 Dwarfism with low birth weight, microcephaly, large eyes, beaked nose, receding mandible, and moderate mental retardation.

Secondary

731.2 Symmetrical osteitis of limbs localized to phalanges and terminal epiphyses of long bones of forearm and leg. Symptoms include kyphosis of the spine and affection of joints.

Secretan's

782.3 Traumatic, recurrent edema or hemorrhage of the back of the hand.

Secretoinhibitor

710.2 (Gougerot-Houwer, Sjogren) Complex of symptoms of unknown source in middle aged women in which the following triad exists: keratoconjunctivitis sicca, zerostomia, and connective tissue disease (usually rheumatoid arthritis but sometimes systemic lupus erythematosus. Cause may be an abnormal immune response.

© 2004 Ingenix, Inc.

Senear-Usher

694.4 Eruption of the skin on the face, scalp, and trunk with lesions scaling erthymatosus.

Senilism

259.8 Progeria syndrome which includes marked senility by 10 years of age.

Serous meningitis

348.2 Meningitis with serious inflammation in subarachnoid and ventricle spaces and little change in cerebrospinal fluid.

Sertoli cell

606.0 Congenital germinal epithelium absence of the testes.

Shaver's

503 Condition resulting from the ingestion of bauxite fumes and fine particles of alumina and silica in the aluminum mining and manufacturing process. Symptoms include pulmonary emphysema and pneumothorax.

Sheehan's

253.2 (Reye-Sheehan) Secretion of all anterior pituitary hormones is inadequate or absent; presenting after childbirth.

Shoulder-arm

337.9 (Claude Bernard-Homer, Reilly's, Steinbrocker's, shoulder-hand) Clinical disorder following a heart attack, marked by pain and stiffness in the shoulder, with puffy swelling and pain in the hand.

Shwachman's

288.0 (Doan-Wiseman, Kostmann, Schultz) Bronchiectasis and pancreatic insufficiency, resulting in malnutrition and sinusitis. Other symptoms include short stature and bone abnormalities.

Shy-Drager

333.0 (Hallervorden-Spatz, Dejerine-Thomas) Condition in which the nerves between the striatum and pallidum are completely demyelated.

Sicard's

352.6 (Collet-Sicard) Unilateral lesions of ninth, tenth, eleventh, and twelfth cranial nerves producing paralysis of the vagal, glossal, and other nerves and tongue on same side. Usually result of injury.

Sicca

710.2 (Gougerot-Houwer, Sjogren) Complex of symptoms of unknown source in middle-aged women in which the following triad exists: keratoconjunctivitis sicca, zerostomia, and connective tissue disease (usually rheumatoid arthritis but sometimes systemic lupus erythematosus). Cause may be an abnormal immune response.

Sideropenic

280.8 Eczema, thrombocyopenia, and recurrent pyogenic infection. Patients suffer an increased susceptibility to infection with encapsulated bacteria.

Siemens' ectodermal dysplasia

757.31 Congenitally absent sweat glands, smooth finely wrinkled skin, sunken nose, malformed teeth, sparse hair, and deformed nails. Sometimes absent breast tissue, mental retardation, or syndactyly.

Siemens' keratosis follicularis spinulosa

757.39 Inherited condition in which the hair follicles are replaced by keratosis.

Silfverskiöld's

756.50 A dominant inherited disease with skeletal changes in extremities.

Silver's

759.89 Dwarfism marked by late closure of anterior fontanel, bilateral body asymmetry, low birth weight, clinodactyly of the fifth fingers, triangular facial shape, and carp mouth.

Silvestroni-Bianco

282.4 One of a group of hemolytic anemias that shares common decreased rate of synthesis of one or more hemoglobin polypeptide chains and are classified according to chain involved.

Simons'

272.6 (Hollander-Simons) Characterized by loss of subcutaneous fat of upper torso, the arms, the neck, and the face but with an increase in fat on and below the pelvis.

Sinus tarsi

726.79 Caused by posterior tibial nerve at ankle, syndrome can produce significant neuropathy.

Sinusitis-bronchiectasis-situs inversus

759.3 (Kartagener's) Transposition or misplacement of organs or viscera.

Sipple's

193 Familial endocrine adenomatosis

Sjögren (-Gougerot)

710.2 (Gougerot-Houwer) Complex of symptoms of unknown source in middle aged women in which the following triad exists: keratoconjunctivitis sicca, zerostomia, and connective tissue disease (usually rheumatoid arthritis but sometimes systemic

© 2004 Ingenix, Inc.

lupus erythematosus). Cause may be an abnormal immune response.

Sjögren-Larsson
757.1 Congenital malformation of the skin with scaling and spastic paraplegia.

Slocumb's
255.3 (Schroeder's) Disorder of adrenal medullary tissue resulting in hypertension accompanied with attacks of palpitation, headache, nausea, dyspnea, anxiety, pallor, and profuse sweating.

Sluder's
337.0 (Charcot-Weiss-Baker) Stimulation of an overactive carotid sinus, causing a marked drop in blood pressure, which, in turn, may stop or block the heart.

Smith-Lemli-Opitz
759.89 Mental retardation, small stature, ptosis, male genital anomalies, anteverted nostrils, and syndactyly of the second and third toes.

Sneddon-Wilkinson
694.1 Non-inflammatory intimal hyperplasia of medium-sized vessels.

Sotos'
253.0 Increased birth weight and length, accelerated growth rate for the first four or five years with no elevation of serum growth hormone levels, followed by revision to normal growth rate, antimongoloid slant, prognathism, hypertelorism, dolichocephalic skull, impaired coordination, and moderate mental retardation may be present.

Specified focal (partial)
310.8 Persistent personality disturbance of nonpsychotic origin with one of the following symptoms: affective instability, bursts of aggression, apathy and indifference, impaired social judgment, and suspiciousness or paranoid ideation.

Spens'
426.9 (Stokes-Adams; Morgagni's disease) Heart block often causing slow or absent pulse, vertigo, syncope, convulsions, and Cheyne-Stokes respiration.

Sphallo-pharyngo-laryngeal hemiplegia
352.6 (Collet-Sicard) Unilateral lesions of the ninth, tenth, eleventh, and twelfth cranial nerves producing paralysis of the vagal, glossal, and other nerves and the tongue on the same side. Most usually result of injury.

Spherophakia-brachymorphia
759.89 (Weill-Marchesani) Abnormally round and small lens of the eyes, short stature, and brachydactyly.

Spinal artery
433.8x (Beck's) Occlusion of spinal artery as result of injury, disk damage, or cardiovascular disease.

Splenic agenesis
759.0 Congenital disorder in which organs of left side of body are a mirror image of the organs on the right side. Splenic agenesis and cardiac malformation are associated.

Splenic flexure
569.89 Bloating, gas, pain, and fullness experienced in left upper abdominal quadrant with pain sometimes radiating up into left chest.

Splenic neutropenia
288.0 Inherited disorder with bronchiectasis and pancreatic insufficiency, resulting in malnutrition, sinusitis, short stature, and bone abnormalities.

Spousal abuse
995.8x Maltreatment (abuse) of spouses and elders with emotional or physical violence.

Spurway's
756.51 (Ekman's, Eddowes') Blue sclera, little growth, brittle and malformed bones, and malformed teeth.

Staphylococcal scalded skin
695.1 Necrolysis of skin caused by toxins.

Steal
435.1 A number of symptoms in a moving limb including pain, tension, and weakness but absent at rest. Caused by occlusive arterial diseases of limbs.

Stein's
256.4 (Stein-Leventhal) Oligomenorrhea or amenorrhea, anovulation and infertility, and hirsutism. Most often caused by bilateral polycystic ovaries.

Steinbrocker's
337.9 (Claude-Bernard-Homer, Reilly's) Pain and stiffness in the shoulder with puffy swelling and pain in the hand following a heart attack.

Stevens-Johnson
695.1 Necrolysis of skin caused by toxins.

© 2004 Ingenix, Inc.

Stewart-Morel
733.3 Thickening of inner table of the frontal bone associated with obesity in women nearing menopause.

Stiff-man
333.91 Increasing but fluctuating rigidity of upper limb and axial muscles and increasing cerebral and spinal disease but with increased electrical activity.

Still-Felty
714.1 Splenomegaly, leukopenia, arthritis, hypersplenism, anemia and other symptoms.

Stilling-Türk-Duane
378.71 (Duane) Simultaneous retraction of eye muscles causing an inability to abduct affected eye with retraction of globe.

Stokes (-Adams)
426.9 (Morgagni's disease, and Spens) Heart block often causing slow or absent pulse, vertigo, syncope, convulsions, and Cheyne-Stokes respiration.

Straight-back
756.19 Loss of the anterior concavity in the upper thoracic vertebrae causing spine to move forward and compress the heart between sternum and vertebral body.

Sturge-Kalischer-Weber
759.6 Subclavian steal

Subclavian-carotid obstruction
446.7 (Marorell-Fabre, Raed-Harbitz, Takayasu-Onishi) Occurs in the brachiocephalic trunk and the left subclavian and left common carotid arteries above their source in the aortic arch. Symptoms include ischemia, transient blindness, facial atrophy, and many others.

Subcoracoid-pectoralis minor
447.8 Malignant atrophic papulosis.

Subperiosteal hematoma
267 (Barlow, Moller, Cheadle) Anemia, spongy gums, weakness, induration of leg muscles, and mucocutaneous hemorrhages.

Subphrenic interposition
751.4 Interposition of colon between liver and diaphragm.

Sudden infant death
798.0 (crib death) Unexpected death of healthy infant typically under 12 months old.

Sudeck's
733.7 (Sudeck-Leriche) Post-traumatic osteoporosis associated with vasospasm.

Suprarenal cortical
255.3 (Schroeder's, Slocumb's) Disorder of adrenal medullary tissue resulting in hypertension with attacks of palpitation, headache, nausea, dyspnea, anxiety, pallor, and profuse sweating.

Supraspinatus
726.10 Pain on abduction of shoulder and tenderness upon deep pressure of supraspinatus tendon.

Swallowed blood
777.3 Swallowed blood syndrome in the newborn, causing hematemesis and melena.

Sweet
695.89 Disease of women marked by plaque-like lesions on face, neck, and upper extremities and conjunctivitis, mucosal lesion, malaise, fever, and arthralgia.

Swyer-James
492.8 (MacLeod's) Acquired unilateral hyperlucent lung with severe airway obstruction during expiration, oligemia, and a small hilum.

Symonds'
348.2 (Symonds') Meningitis with serious inflammation in subarachnoid and ventricle spaces and little change in the cerebrospinal fluid.

Sympathetic paralysis
337.0 (Charcot-Weiss-Baker, Sluder's) Stimulation of overactive carotid sinus, causing a marked drop in blood pressure, which, in turn, may stop or block the heart.

Syndactylic oxycephaly
755.55 (Aperts) Chromosomal condition with primary symptoms including webbing of digits and a pointed head with variations of defects. Often associated with other chromosomal abnormalities.

Systemic fibrosclerosing
710.8 Widespread formation of fibrous tissue.

Tachycardia-bradycardia
427.81 Rapid action of heart followed by protracted or transient stopping of heart.

Takayasu (-Onishi)
446.7 (Marorell-Fabre, Raed-Harbitz) Brachiocephalic trunk and the left subclavian and left common carotid arteries above their source in the aortic arch. Symptoms include ischemia, transient blindness, facial atrophy, and many others.

© 2004 Ingenix, Inc.

Tapia's
352.6 (Collet-Sicard) Unilateral lesions of ninth, tenth, eleventh, and twelfth cranial nerves producing paralysis of vagal, glossal, and other nerves and tongue on the same side. Usually a result of injury.

Tarsal tunnel
355.5 Caused by posterior tibial nerve at the ankle, syndrome can produce significant neuropathy.

Taussig-Bing
745.11 Complete transposition of aorta, with major vessels transposed, high septral ventricular defect, and other symptoms.

Taybi's
759.89 Condition affecting ears, palate, mouth, and fingers.

Teething
520.7 Eruption of teeth in small child.

Tegmental
344.89 (Avellis, Babinski-Nageotte, Benedikt's, Brown-Sequard, Cestan's, Cestan-Chenais, Foville's, Gubler-Millard, Jackson's, Weber-Leyden) Paraplegia and anesthesia over part of the body. Caused by lesions in the brain or spinal cord.

Telangiectasis-pigmentation-cataract
757.33 (Rothmund's) An inherited disorder marked by pigmentation and atrophy of skin, along with cataracts, saddle nose, bone defects, disturbance of hair growth, and hypogonadism.

Temporal
383.02 (Gradenigo's) Localized meningitis in fifth and sixth cranial nerves, causing paralysis and pain in temporal region.

Temporomandibular joint-pain-dysfunction [TMJ]
524.60 Headache, dizziness, tinnitis, and other symptoms resulting from dysfunction of the mandibular joint.

Terry's
362.21 Retinopathy occurring in premature infants treated with high amounts of oxygen. Retina converts into a fibrous mass stunting growth of eye, resulting in blindness.

Testicular feminization
257.8 (Morris, hairless women, Goldberg, Goldberg-Maxwell, testis, nonvirilizing) Male pseudohermaphroditism marked by female external genitalia. This includes incompletely developed vagina with rudimentary uterus and fallopian tubes, scanty or absent axillary/public hair, and amenorrhea.

Tethered (spinal) cord
742.59 Adhesions distorting spinal cord in the caudal area and associated with Arnold-Chiari syndrome and spina bifida.

Thalamic
348.8 Infarction of postero-inferior thalamus causing transient hemiparesis and severe loss of superficial and deep sensation with crude pain in the limbs. Limbs frequently have vasomotor or trophic disturbances.

Thibierge-Weissenbach
710.1 Systemic disorder of connective tissue marked by induration and thickening of the skin, with circulatory and organ changes. May reside in the face and hands for some time. Also includes Raynaud's phenomenon and, in some cases, esophageal problems.

Thoracic outlet
353.0 (Naffziger's) Disorder presenting symptoms similar to Raynaud's, caused by pressure of brachial plexus and subclavian artery against first thoracic rib.

Thoracogenous rheumatic
731.2 (Mankowsky's, Pierre Marie-Bamberger) Symmetrical osteitis of the limbs localized to the phalanges and terminal epiphyses of the long bones of the forearm and leg. Symptoms include kyphosis of the spine and affection of the joints.

Thorson-Biörck
259.2 (Cassidy-Scholte, Hedinger's) Carcinoid tumors causing cyanotic flushing of skin, diarrheal watery stools, bronchoconstrictive attacks, hypotension, edema, and ascites.

Thrombopenia-hemangioma
287.3 Small number of platelets in circulating blood, causing bruising.

Thyroid-adrenocortical insufficiency
258.1 Insufficient production of hormones by the pituitary and thyroid glands.

Tibial
958.8 Early complication of trauma.

Tietze's
733.6 Painful swelling of unknown origin of one or more costal cartilages, especially of second rib. Patients may interpret chest pain as coronary artery disease.

Time-zone
307.45 (jet lag) Imbalance of the normal circadian rhythm resulting from airplane travel

© 2004 Ingenix, Inc.

through a number of time zones. Leads to fatigue, irritability, and other consitutional disturbances.

Tobias'
162.3 (Cuiffini-Pancoast, Hare's) Neoplasm of the upper lobe of the lung.

Tolosa-Hunt
378.55 Cavernous sinus syndrome produced by idiopathic granuloma.

Toni-Fanconi
270.0 (Harts) Renal tubular malfunction, including cytinosis and osteomalacia that may be caused by inherited disorders or may be the result of multiple myeloma or proximal epithelial growth.

Touraine's
756.89 Dysplasia of the fingernails and toenails, hypoplasia of the patella, iliac horns, thickening of the glomerular lamina densa, and a flask-shaped femur.

Touraine-Solente-Golé
757.39 Thickening of the skin on extremities and face with clubbing of fingers and deformities in bone of limb.

Toxic oil
710.5 Pain in muscles as a result of accumulation of a large number of granular leukocytes.

Toxic shock
040.2 Staphylococci producing an endotoxin, presenting a high fever, vomiting and diarrhea, decreasing blood pressure, a skin rash, and shock. Hyperemia of several mucous membranes also occurs.

Transfusion donor
772.0 Transfusion of fetus's blood across the placenta to mother's blood supply.

Transfusion recipient
776.4 Polycythemia of newborn as result of blood flow from mother.

Traumatic (acute)
847.0 Acute cervical sprain caused by hyperextension of the neck (C4-C5) during an accident, usually in an automobile.

Traumatic shock
958.4 Particularly dangerous state of shock following a traumatic injury.

Treacher Collins'
756.0 (Franceschetti's) Malformations of derivatives of the first branchial arch, marked by palpebral fissures sloping outward and downward with notches in the outer third of the lower lids, defects of malar bones and zygome, hypoplasia of the jawbone, high or cleft palate, low-set ears, unusual hair growth, and pits between mouth and ear.

Trigeminal plate
259.8 Progeria, which includes marked senility by 10 years of age.

Triplex X female
758.81 Three X chromosomes where the only confirmed symptom is the occurrence of twin Barr bodies in a typical cell.

Troisier-Hanot-Chauffard
275.0 Hypertrophic cirrhosis with pigmentation and diabetes mellitus.

Trousseau's
453.1 Spontaneous development of thromboses in upper and lower limbs as a result of visceral neoplasm.

Türk's
378.71 (Duane, Still-Turk-Duane) Simultaneous retraction of eye muscles causing an inability to abduct affected eye with retraction of the globe.

Turner's
758.6 (XO, Turner-Varny) Congenital disorder characterized by short stature, webbed neck, congenital heart disease, mental retardation, and other symptoms.

Twin-to-twin transfusion
762.3 The birth of one anemic twin and one plethoric twin due to the forcing of blood of one twin into the other.

Type I
348.4 Brain damage as result of compression.

Uehlinger's
757.39 Thickening of skin on extremities and face with clubbing of fingers and deformities in bone of limb.

Ullrich (-Bonnevie) (-Turner)
758.6 (XO, Turner-Varny) Congenital disorder characterized by short stature, webbed neck, congenital heart disease, mental retardation, and other symptoms.

Ullrich-Feichtiger
759.89 Congenital abnormalities, depressed nose, small eyes, hypertelorism, and protuberant ears.

Universal joint, cervix
620.6 (Allen-Masters, Masters-Allen) Pelvic pain resulting from old laceration of broad ligament received during delivery.

 © 2004 Ingenix, Inc.

Unverricht-Wagner

710.3 (Petges-Clejat) Polymyositis occurring with characteristic skin changes that include a rash on upper eyelids with edema, a rash on the forehead, neck, shoulders, trunk, and arms, and papules on the knuckles.

Upward gaze

378.81 (Parinaud's) Paralysis of conjugate movement of eyes without paralysis of convergence. Caused by lesions of the midbrain.

Urbach-Oppenheim

250.8x [709.3] Diabetes with skin disorder.

Urbach-Wiethe

272.8 Deposition of hyaline material in the skin and mucosa of mouth, pharynx, hypopharynx, and larynx. Skin lesions as pustules on faces and exposed surfaces of arms and legs, which heal and form scars.

Urethro-oculoarticular

099.3 (Fiessinger-Leroy-Reiter, urethro-oculosynovial) Association of arthritis, iridocyclitis, and urethritis, sometimes with diarrhea. While symptoms may recur, the arthritis is constant.

Urohepatic

572.4 (Heyd's) Acute renal failure in patients with disease of biliary or liver tract. Cause seems to be decreased renal blood flow, damaging both organs.

Uveocutaneous

364.24 (Vogt-Koyanagi) Uveomeningitis marked by patchy depigmentation of hair, eyebrows, and lashes. Retinal detatchment, deafness, and tinnitus may also result.

Vagoaccessory

352.6 (Collet-Sicard, vagohypoglossal) Unilateral lesions of the ninth, tenth, eleventh, and twelfth cranial nerves producing paralysis of the vagal, glossal, and other nerves and the tongue on the same side. Most usually result of injury.

Valve prolapse

424.0 (Barlow's) "Mid-late" systolic click due to massive protrusion of mitral valvular leaflet in left atrial cavity.

Van Buchem's

733.3 Multiple fractures and bowing of all extremities, thickening of skull bones, and osteoporosis.

Van der Hoeve's

756.51 Blue sclera, little growth, brittle bones, and deafness.

Van der Hoeve-Halbertsma-Waardenburg

270.2 (Mendes, Waardenburg-Kleinvan, der Hoeve-Waardenburg-Gualdi, ptosis-epicanthus) Eyebrow or upper or lower eyelid sags.

Van Neck-Odelberg

732.1 Disease of growth centers, especially at the top of the femur [illegible]ich the epiphyses is replaced by new [illegible]cation.

Vascular insufficiency

557.1 (Wilkie's) Complete or partial block of the superior mesenteric artery with symptoms of vomiting, pain, blood in the stool, and distended abdomen. Results in bowel infarction.

Vascular splanchnic

557.0 Visceral circulation syndrome.

Vasomotor

443.9 (Charcot's) Symptoms in a moving limb including pain tension, and weakness but absent at rest. Caused by occlusive arterial diseases of the limbs.

Vasomotor acroparesthesia

443.89 (Nothnagels Type) Parasthesia of the tips of the extremities or attacks of tingling resulting from nerve compression at several levels, and cyanosis. May result in gangrene of the affected areas.

Vasovagal

780.2 (Gower's) Fall in blood pressure, slow pulse, and convulsions. Believed to be sudden stimulation of the vagal nerve by receptors in the heart, carotid sinus, or aortic arch.

VATER

759.89 Vertebral defects, anal atresia, tracheoesophageal fistula with esophageal atresia, and radial and renal anomalies.

Vena cava

459.2 Obstruction of the vena cava.

Verbiest's

435.1 (Charcot's) Symptoms in a moving limb including pain, tension, and weakness but absent at rest. Caused by occlusive arterial diseases of the limbs.

Vernet's

352.6 (Collet-Sicard) Unilateral lesions of the ninth, tenth, eleventh, and twelfth cranial nerves producing paralysis of the vagal, glossal, and other nerves and the tongue on the same side. Most usually result of injury.

© 2004 Ingenix, Inc.

Video display tube
723.8 (VDT) Chronic neck and back pain developing from sitting at a computer.

Villaret's
352.6 (Collet-Sicard) Unilateral lesions of the ninth, tenth, eleventh, and twelfth cranial nerves producing paralysis of the vagal, glossal, and other nerves and the tongue on the same side. Most usually result of injury.

Vinson-Plummer
280.8 (Kelly, Plummer-Vinson, Paterson-Brown-Vinson) Condition in middle-aged women with hypochromic anemia, marked by cracks or fissures at the corners of the mouth, painful tongue, and dysphagia due to esophageal stenosis or webs.

Virilism
255.2 (virilizing adrenocortical hyperplasia, congenital) Mature masculine somatic characteristics by a prepubescent male, girl, or woman. This syndrome may show at birth or develop later as result of adrenocortical dysfunction.

Visceral larval migrans
128.0 Prolonged migration of nematode larvae in the viscera, which can cause hyperosinophilia, hepatomegaly, and pneumonitis.

Visual disorientation
368.16 (Balint's, Holmes', Riddoch's) ACorical paralysis of visual fixation, optic ataxia, and disturbance of visual attention. Eye movements are normal.

Vitamin B6 deficiency
266.1 Pellagra, a deficiency-caused syndrome exhibiting gastrointestinal disturbance, erythema, nervous disorders, and mental disturbances.

Vogt's
333.7 Spastic diplegia with athetosis and pseudobulbar paralysis found with a lesion of the caudate nucleus and putamen.

Vogt-Koyanagi (-Harada)
364.24 Uveomeningitis marked by patchy depigmentation of hair, eyebrows, and lashes. Retinal detatchment, deafness, and tinnitus may also result.

Von Bechterew-Strümpell
720.0 Rheumatoid infllammation of vertebrae.

Von Graefe's
378.72 Progressive external ophthalmoplegia, a slowly progressive bilateral myopathy only affecting the muscles around the eye, including lids. Paralysis of the muscles around the eye results.

Von Hippel-Lindau
759.6 Formation of multiple angiomas on the retina.

Von Schroetter's
453.8 Stress thrombosis of the subclavian or axillary vein.

Waardenburg-Klein
270.2 (Mendes, van der Hoeve-Halbertsma-Waardenburg) Eyebrow or upper or lower eyelid sags.

Wagner (-Unverricht)
710.3 (Petges-Clegat, Unverricht-Wagner) Polymyositis occurring with characteristic skin changes that include a rash on the upper eyelids with edema, a rash on the forehead, neck, shoulders, trunk, and arms, and papules on the knuckles.

Waldenström's
273.3 Increase in macroglobulins in the blood. Has symptoms of hyperviscosity such as weakness, fatigue, bleeding disorders, and visual disturbances.

Waldenström-Kjellberg
280.8 (Kelly, Plummer-Vinson, Paterson-Brown-Vinson) Condition in middle-aged women with hypochronic anemia, marked by cracks or fissures at the corners of the mouth, painful tongue, and dysphagia due to esophageal stenosis or webs.

Water retention
276.6 Fluid overload caused by electrolyte and acid-base imbalance.

Waterhouse (-Friderichsen)
036.3 Acute fulminating meningococcal septicemia occurring in children below 10 years of age. Symptoms include vomiting, cyanosis, diarrhea, purpura, convulsions, and circulatory collapse. The patient will often display meningitis and hemorrhaging into the adrenal glands.

Weakness
300.5 Hypersomatic disorder with no idenfiable pathology.

Web
756.89 Dysplasia of the fingernails and toenails, hypoplasia of the patella, iliac horns, thickening of the glomerular lamina densa, and a flask-shaped femur.

 © 2004 Ingenix, Inc.

Weber's
344.89 (Avellis, Babinski-Nageotte, Benedikt's, Brown-Sequard, Cestan's, Cestan-Chenais, Foville's, Gubler-Millard, Jackson's, Weber-Leyden) Paraplegia and anesthesia over half or part of the body. Caused by lesions in the brain or spinal cord.

Weber-Christian
729.30 Relapsing febrile nodular nonsuppurative panniculitis with development of nodules that spread centrifugally with erythematous borders and clearing centrally to form pigmented plaques.

Weber-Cockayne
757.39 Dwarfism with a precociously senile appearance, pigmentary degeneration of the retina, optic atrophy, deafness, sensitivity to sunlight, and mental retardation.

Weber-Dimitri
759.6 (Kalischer's) Formation of multiple angiomas in the skin of the head and scalp.

Weber-Gubler
344.89 (Avellis, Babinski-Nageotte, Benedikt's, Brown-Sequard, Cestan's, Cestan-Chenais, Foville's, Gubler-Millard, Jackson's, Weber-Leyden) Paraplegia over half or part of the body. Caused by lesions in the brain or spinal cord.

Weber-Osler (-Rendu)
448.0 Small telangiectasias and dilated venules that develop slowly on the skin and mucus membranes of the lips, tongue, nasopharynx, tongue, and the face.

Wegener's
446.4 Necrotizing granulomatous vasculitis involving the upper and lower respiratory tracts, which is thought to be a hypersensitivity to unknown antigens.

Weill-Marchesani
759.89 Abnormally round and small lens, short stature, and brachydactyly.

Weingarten's
518.3 Transient infiltrations of lungs by eosinophilia, resulting in night coughing, fever, and dyspnea.

Weiss-Baker
337.0 (Charcot-Weiss-Baker, Sluder's) Stimulation of an overactive carotid sinus, causing a marked drop in blood pressure, which, in turn, may stop or block the heart.

Weissenbach-Thibierge
710.1 Systemic disorder of the connective tissue marked by induration and thickening of the skin, with circulatory and organ changes. May reside in the face and hands for some time. Also includes Raynaud's phenomenon and, in some cases, esophageal problems.

Werlhof-Wichmann
287.3 Small number of platelets in circulating blood, causing bruising.

Wermer's
258.0 Tumors in more than one endocrine gland, including the pancreatic islets and parathyroid glands. Syndrome is inherited.

Werner's
259.8 Premature aging in the adult as result of genetic trait and characterized by sclerodermal skin changes, cataracts, muscular atrophy, diabetes mellitus, baldness, and high incidence of neoplasm.

Wernicke's
265.1 (Gayet-Wernicke) Thiamine deficiency, disturbances in ocular motility, pupillary alterations, nystagmus, and ataxia with tremors. Organic toxic psychosis often co-exists. Most often due to alcoholism.

Wernicke-Korsakoff
294.0 Amnestic dementia where the patient cannot remember short-term or long-term memories but is not delirious.

Westphal-Strümpell
275.1 (Wilson) Defect in the metabolism of copper. Marked by accumulation of copper in the brain, cornea, kidney, liver, and other tissues causing cirrhosis of the liver and deterioration in the basal ganglia of the brain.

Wet brain
303.9x Description of chronic alcoholism.

Wet feet
991.4 (immersion foot, trench foot) Blotchy cyanosis, increased sweating, parasthesia, and edema. Caused by hypothermia.

Whiplash
847.0 Acute cervical sprain caused by hyperextension of the neck (C4-C5) during an accident, usually in an automobile.

Whipple's
040.2 Radical removal of the head of the pancreas, duodenum, and distal third of the stomach. Jejunum is connected to the stomach, pancreas, and bile duct.

"Whistling face"
759.89 (Freeman-Sheldon) Deviation of hands and face, with protrusion of lips as in whistling, sunken eyes, and small nose.

Widal (-Abrami)
283.9 (Dyke-Young, Hayem-Widal) One of anemic syndromes caused by exposures to trauma, poisons, and other causes that decreases the number of red blood cells.

Wilkie's
557.1 Complete or partial block of the superior mesenteric artery with symptoms of vomiting, pain, blood in the stool, and distended abdomen. Results in bowel infarction.

Wilkinson-Sneddon
694.1 Non-inflammatory intimal hyperplasia of medium sized vessels.

Willan-Plumbe
696.1 Eruption of circumscribed, discrete, reddish, silvery-scaled maculopapules on the knees, elbows, scalp, and trunk.

Willi-Prader
759.81 Rounded face, almond-shaped eyes, strabismus, low forehead, hypogonadism, hypotomia, mental retardation, and an insatiable appetite.

Wilson's
275.1 (Westphal-Strumpell) Defect in the metabolism of copper with accumulation of copper in the brain, cornea, kidney, liver, and other tissues causing cirrhosis of the liver and deterioration in the basal ganglia of the brain.

Wilson-Mikity
770.7 Pulmonary insufficiency in newborn babies, especially those with low birth weight with hypercapnia and cyanosis of rapid onset during the first month of life and resulting frequently in death.

Winking
307.20 Tic motor disorder not otherwise specified.

Wiskott-Aldrich
279.12 Immunodeficiency shown by eczema, thrombocytopenia, and recurrent pyogenic infection. Patients suffer an increased susceptibility to infection with encapsulated bacteria.

With neurogenic bladder
344.61 Aching pain of the perineum, bladder, and sacrum, radiating in a sciatic fashion, due to compression of spinal nerve roots. Symptoms include paralysis of organs and limbs served by those roots, including the bladder.

With spina bifida
741.0x (Arnold-Chiari) Displacement of the caudal spinal cord due to tethering with or without spina bifida and other problems such as meningomyelocele.

Woake's
471.1 (polypoid sinus degeneration) Polyp-like growths that hamper sinus function.

XO
758.6 (Turner's) Short stature, webbed neck, congenital heart disease, mental retardation, and other symptoms.

Yellow vernix
656.7 (placental dysfunction) Marked by placental dysfunction, infarction, and insufficiency.

Zahorsky's
074.0 (herpangina) Vesicular pharyngitis caused by Coxsackie virus.

Ziere's
571.1 Acute hepatitis or cirrhosis of the liver associated with alcoholism.

Zollinger-Ellison
251.5 (Ellison-Zollinger) Peptic ulceration with gastric hypersecretion, tumor of the pancreatic islets, and hypoglycemia.

Zuelzer-Ogden
281.2 Folate-deficiency anemia caused by a drug, congenital, dietary, or other reason.

© 2004 Ingenix, Inc.

Prefixes and Suffixes

The uniquely efficient language of medicine is possible thanks to the prefixes and suffixes attached to roots. Changing prefixes and suffixes allows subtle and overt changes in meaning of the terms. The following prefixes and suffixes are paired with their meanings.

Prefixes

Prefixes are one half of the medical language equation and are attached to the beginning of words. For example, the prefix "eu-," meaning good or well, combined with the Greek word for death, "thanatos," produces euthanasia — a good death.

a-, an-	without, away from, not
ab-	from, away from, absent
acro-	extremity, top, highest point
ad-	indicates toward, adherence to, or increase
adeno-	relating to a gland
adip-	relating to fat (*also* adipo-)
aero-	relating to gas or air
all-	meaning another, other, or different
allo-	indicates difference or divergence from the norm
ambi-	both sides; about or around (*also* amphi-)
an-	without
angi-	relating to a vessel
aniso-	dissimilar, unequal, or asymmetrical
ankylo-	bent, crooked, or two parts growing together
ante-	in front of, before
antero-	before, front, anterior
anti-	in opposition to, against
antro-	relating to a chamber or cavity
arch-	beginning, first, principal (*also* arche-, archi-)
archo-	relating to the rectum or anus
arterio-	relating to an artery
arthro-	relating to a joint
astro-	star-like or shaped
atelo-	incomplete or imperfect
auto-	relating to the self
axio-	relating to an axis (*also* axo-)
balano-	relating to the glans penis or glans clitoridis
baro-	relating to weight or heaviness
basi-	relating to the base or foundation (*also* basio-)
bi-	double, twice, two
blasto-	relating to germs
blenn-	relating to mucus (*also* blenno-)
blepharo-	relating to the eyelid
brachi-	relating to the arm (*also* brachio-)
brachy-	short
brady-	meaning slow or prolonged
broncho-	relating to the trachea
cac-	meaning diseased or bad (*also* caci-, caco-)
cardio-	relating to the heart
carpo-	relating to the wrist
cata-	down from, down, according to
celo-	indicating a tumor or hernia; cavity
cervico-	relating to the neck or neck of an organ
chilo-	relating to the lip (*also* cheilo-)
chole-	relating to the gallbladder
cleido-	relating to the clavicle
cyst-	relating to the urinary bladder or a cyst (*also* cysto-)
cyto-	in relation to cell
dacry-	pertaining to the lacrimal glands
dactyl-	relating to the fingers or toes
demi-	half the amount
desmo-	relating to ligaments

© 2004 Ingenix, Inc.

deuter-	secondary or second
dextro-	meaning on or to the right
dorsi-	relating to the back (*also* dorso-)
dys-	painful, bad, disordered, difficult
echo-	reverberating sound
ecto-	external, outside
ectro-	congenital absence of something
endo-	within, internal
entero-	relating to the intestines
epi-	on, upon, in addition to
eu-	well, healthy, good, normal
exo-	outside of, without
fibro-	relating to fibers or fibrous tissue
galacto-	relating to milk
gastro-	relating to the stomach and abdominal region
genito-	relating to reproduction
gono-	relating to the genitals, offspring, origination
gyn-	relating to the female gender
hema-	relating to blood (*also* hemato-)
hemi-	half
hepato-	relating to the liver
histo-	relating to tissue
homeo-	indicates resemblance or likeness (*also* homo-)
hydro-	relating to fluid, water, or hydrogen
hyper-	excessive, above, exaggerated
hypo-	below, less than, under
hyster-	relating to either the womb or hysteria (*also* hystero-)
idio-	distinct or individual characteristics
ileo-	relating to the ileum (part of the small intestine)
ilio-	relating to the pelvis
infra-	meaning inferior to, beneath, under
irid-	relating to the iris
ischio-	relating to the hip
iso-	equal
jejuno-	relating to the jejunum (part of the small intestine)
juxta-	next to, near
karyo-	relating to the nucleus of a cell
kerato-	relating to the cornea or horny tissue
laparo-	flank, loins; operations through the abdominal wall
laryngo-	relating to the larynx
lien-	relating to the spleen
lip-	relating to fat (*also* lipo-)
lith-	relating to a hard or calcified substance (*also* litho-)
lumbo-	relating to the loin region
macro-	meaning oversized, large
mal-	bad, poor, ill
melano-	dark or black in color
meningo-	relating to membranes covering the brain and spine
mesio-	toward the middle; secondary (*also* meso-)
meta-	indicates a change
mis-	bad, improper
my-	relating to muscle (*also* myo-)
myc-	relating to fungus (*also* myco-)
myelo-	relating to bone marrow or the spinal cord
narco-	indicates insensate condition or numbness
necro-	indicates death or dead tissue
nephr-	relating to the kidney
noci-	relating to injury or pain
nycto-	relating to darkness or night
odont-	relating to the teeth
oligo-	indicates few or small
omo-	relating to the shoulder
omphalo-	relating to the navel
onco-	relating to a mass, tumor, or swelling
onycho-	relating to the finger- or toenails
oophor-	relating to the ovaries
opistho-	indicates behind or backwards
orchi-	relating to the testicles (*also* orchido-)
oscheo-	relating to the scrotum

 © 2004 Ingenix, Inc.

osteo-	having to do with bone
oto-	relating to the ear
pachy-	indicates heavy, large, or thick
pali-	repetition, back again, recurring (*also* palin-)
panto-	indicates the whole or all
para-	indicates near, similar, beside, or past
patho-	indicates sensitivity, feeling, or suffering
ped-	relating to the foot (*also* pedi-)
peri-	about, around, or in the vicinity
pero-	indicates being maimed or deformed
phaco-	relating to the lens of the eye
phago-	relating to eating and ingestion
pharyngo-	relating to the pharynx
phlebo-	relating to the vein
phreno-	relating to the diaphragm; head or mind
pimel-	relating to fat
platy-	indicates wide or broad
pleio-	more, additional
pleur-	relating to the side or ribs
pneum-	relating to respiration, air, the lungs
pod-	relating to the feet (*also* podo-)
poly-	indicates much or many
procto-	relating to the rectum and/or anus
proso-	indicates toward the front, anterior, forward
pseudo-	indicates false or imagined
pulmo-	relating to the lungs and respiration
pyelo-	relating to the pelvis
pygo-	relating to the buttocks or rump
pyle-	relating to an opening/orifice of the portal vein
pyloro-	relating to the pylorus, the stomach opening into the duodenum
pyo-	relating to pus
pyreto-	indicates a fever, heat
rachi-	relating to the spine (*also* rachio-)
recto-	meaning straight or relating to the rectum
retro-	indicates behind, backward, in a reverse direction
rheo-	indicates a flow or stream of fluid
rhino-	relating to the nose
sacro-	relating to the sacrum, the base of the vertebral column
salpingo-	relating to the fallopian or eustachian tubes
sarco-	relating to flesh
scapho-	indicates deformed condition, shaped like a boat
scapulo-	relating to the shoulder
schisto-	indicates cleft or split; a fissure
scoto-	relating to darkness; visual field gap
sial-	relating to saliva
sinistro-	meaning on or to the left
somato-	relating to the body
spheno-	relating to the sphenoid bone at the base of the skull
sphygmo-	relating to the pulse
splanch-	relating to the intestines; viscera
steato-	relating to fat
stetho-	relating to the chest
stomato-	relating to the mouth
sym-	indicates together with, along with, beside
syn-	indicates being joined together
tachy-	indicates swift or fast
tarso-	relating to the foot; margin of the eyelid
teleo-	indicates complete or perfectly formed
teno-	relating to tendons
terato-	indicates being seriously deformed, esp. a fetus
thalamo-	relating to the thalamus, origin of nerves in the brain
thanato-	relating to death
thoraco-	relating to the chest
thrombo-	relating to blood clots
thymo-	relating to the thymus
toco-	relating to birth
trachelo-	relating to the neck

Prefixes and Suffixes

trichi-	relating to hair; hair-like shape (*also* tricho-)
tympano-	relating to the eardrum
typhlo-	relating to the cecum; relating to blindness
vaso-	relating to blood vessels
ventro-	relating to the abdomen; anterior surface of the body
vesico-	relating to the bladder
viscero-	relating to the abdominal organs
xeno-	relating to a foreign substance
xero-	indicates a dry condition

Suffixes

Suffixes are the other half of the equation. These are attached to the ends of words.

-agra	indicating severe pain
-algia	pain
-ase	denoting an enzyme
-blast	incomplete cellular development
-centesis	puncture
-cephal	having to do with the head
-cle	meaning small or little (*also* -cule)
-cyte	having to do with cells
-dactyl	having to do with fingers
-desis	binding or fusion
-ectomy	excision, removal
-ferous	produces, causes, or brings about
-fuge	drive out or expel
-genic	indicates production, causation, generation
-gram	drawn, written, and recorded
-graphic	written or drawn
-ia	state of being, condition (abnormal)
-iasis	condition
-itis	inflammation
-lysis	release, free, reduction of
-metry	scientific measurement
-odynia	indicates pain or discomfort
-oid	indicates likeness or resemblance
-ology	study of
-oma	tumor
-orraphy	suturing
-oscopy	to examine
-osis	condition, process
-ostomy	indicates a surgically created artificial opening
-otomy	indicates a cutting
-pagus	indicates fixed or joined together
-pathic	indicates a feeling, diseased condition, or therapy
-penia	indicates a deficiency; less than normal
-pexy	fixation
-philia	inordinate love of or craving for something
-phobia	abnormal fear of or aversion to something
-plasty	indicates surgically formed or molded
-plegia	indicates a stroke or paralysis
-poietic	indicates producing or making
-praxis	indicates activity, action, condition, or use
-rhage	indicates bleeding or other fluid discharge (*also* -rhagia)
-rhaphy	indicates a suture or seam joining two structures
-rrhagia	indicates an abnormal or excessive fluid discharge
-rrhexis	splitting or breaking
-spasm	contraction
-taxy	arrangement, grouping (*also* -taxis)
-tomy	indicates a cutting
-trophy	relating to food or nutrition
-tropic	indicates an affinity for or turning toward
-tropism	responding to an external stimulus

© 2004 Ingenix, Inc.

Abbreviations, Acronyms, and Symbols

The acronyms, abbreviations, and symbols used by health care providers speed communications. The following list includes the most often seen acronyms, abbreviations, and symbols. In some cases, abbreviations have more than one meaning. Multiple interpretations are separated by a slash (/). Abbreviations of Latin phrases are punctuated.

<	less than
>	greater than
@	at
A	assessment/blood type
a (ante)	before
a fib	atrial fibrillation
a flutter	atrial flutter
A2	aortic second sound
a.a.	of each
AA	Alcoholics Anonymous
AAHP	American Association of Health Plans
AAL	anterior axillary line
AAMT	American Association for Medical Transcription
AAPCC	adjusted average per capita cost
AAPPO	American Association of Preferred Provider Organizations
AAROM	active assistive range of motion
ab	abortion
AB	blood type
abd	abdomen
ABE	acute bacterial endocarditis
ABG	arterial blood gas
abn.	abnormal
ABO	referring to ABO incompatibility
abs. fev.	without fever
a.c.	before eating
ACD	absolute cardiac dullness
ACE	angiotensin converting enzyme/adrenal cortical extract
ACL	anterior cruciate ligament
ACLS	advanced cardiac life support
ACP	acid phosphatase
acq.	acquired
ACTH	adrenocorticotropic hormone
ACVD	acute cardiovascular disease
ad lib	as desired, at pleasure
ad part. dolent.	to the aching parts
a.d.	right ear/to, up to
ad. us. ext.	for external use
ADA	American Dental Association, or Americans with Disabilities Act
ADH	antidiuretic hormone
ad. hib.	to be administered
ADL	activities of daily living
ad. lib.	as desired
adm	admission, admit
ADM	alcohol, drug or mental disorder
ADP	adenosine diphosphate
ADS	alternative delivery system
adst. feb.	when fever is present
AE	above the elbow
AF	atrial fibrillation
AFB	acid fast bacilli
A/G	albumin-globulin ratio
AGA	appropriate (average) for gestational age
AgNO3	silver nitrate
AHA	American Hospital Association
AHC	alternative health care
AHIMA	American Health Information Management Association
AI	aortic insufficiency
AICD	automatic implant cardioverter defibrilator
AID	artificial insemination donor/acute infectious disease

AIDS	acquired immunodeficiency syndrome
AIH	artificial insemination by husband
AK	above the knee
AKA	above knee amputation
ALA	aminolevulinic acid
alb. (albus)	white
alk. phos.	alkaline phosphatase
ALL	acute lymphocytic leukemia
ALP	alkaline phosphatase
ALS	advanced life support
ALT	alanine aminotransferase
alt. dieb.	every other day
alt. hor.	every other hour
alt. noc.	every other night
a.m.	morning
ama	against medical advice
AMA	American Medical Association
amb	ambulate
AMGA	American Medical Group Association
AMI	acute myocardial infarction
AML	acute myelogenous leukemia
AMML	acute myelomonocytic leukemia
AMP	adenosine monophosphate/ampule
ANA	American Nursing Association, or antinuclear antibodies
ANS	autonomic nervous system
ANSI	American National Standards Institute
ANSI/HISB	ANSI Health Information Standards Board
ant	anterior
AOD	arterial occlusive disease
AODM	adult onset diabetes mellitus
A&P	auscultation and percussion
A-P	anterior posterior
Ap	apical
AP	antepartum/anterior-posterior
APC	Ambulatory Payment Classification
APM	arterial pressure monitoring
approx	approximately
appy.	appendectomy
aq.	water (aqua)
ARC	AIDS-related complex
ARD	Acute respiratory disease
ARDS	adult respiratory distress syndrome
ARF	acute respiratory/renal failure
AROM	active range of motion/artificial rupture of membranes
art.	artery, arterial
AS	aortic stenosis/ arteriosclerosis
a.s.	left ear
ASAP	as soon as possible
ASC	ambulatory surgery center
ASCVD	arteriosclerotic cardiovascular disease
ASCX12N	American Standard Committee standard for claims and reimbursement
ASD	atrial septal defect
ASHD	arteriosclerotic heart disease
ASO	administrative services only
ASR	age/sex rate
Asst	assistance (min= minimal; mod= moderate)
AST	aspartate aminotransferase
ATP	adenosine triphosphate
a.u.	each ear, both ears
AUR	ambulatory utilization review
A-V	arterioveneous
AV	atrioventricular
AVF	arteriovenous fistula
ax	auxiliary
AZT	azidothymidine
Ba	barium
bal.	bath
B&B	bowel and bladder
BB	blow bottles
BBA	Balanced Budget Act of 1997
BBB	bundle branch block
BCC	basal cell carcinoma
BCP	birth control pill
BE	barium enema/below the elbow
BI	biopsy
bib.	drink
b.i.d.	two times a day
b.i.n.	twice a night
b.i.s.	twice
BK	below the knee
BKA	below knee amputation
BLS	basic life support
BM	bowel movement

Abbreviations

© 2004 Ingenix, Inc.

BMR	basal metabolic rate
BMT	bone marrow transplant
BO	body order
BOW	bag of water
BP	blood pressure
BPD	bronchopulmonary displasia
BPH	benign prostatic hypertrophy
Br	breastfeeding
BrC	breast care
BS	bachelor of surgery/breath sounds/bowel sounds
BSA	body surface area
BSC	bedside commode
BSD	bedside drainage
BUN	blood urea nitrogen
BUR	back-up rate (ventilator)
BUS	Bartholin urethra skenes
bx	biopsy
C&S	culture and sensitivity
C	centigrade/complements/cervical vertebrae
c	with
C-collar	cervical collar
CA	cancer
Ca	calcium/cancer
CABG	coronary artery bypass graft
CAD	coronary artery disease
CAPD	continuous ambulatory peritoneal dialysis
caps.(capsula)	capsule
CAT	computerized axial tomography
cath	catheterize
CBC	complete blood count
CBR	complete bed rest
cc	chief complaint
CCPD	continuous cycling peritoneal dialysis
CCU	coronary care unit
CDC	Centers for Disease Control
CDH	congenital dislocation of hip
CE	cardiac enlargement
CEA	carcinoembryonic antigen
CF	cystic fibrosis
CH,Chol	cholesterol
CHD	congenital heart disease/congestive heart disease
CHF	congestive heart failure
CI	confidence interval/chloride
CIS	carcinoma in situ
cl liqs	clear liquids
CLD	chronic lung disease/chronic liver disease
CLL	chronic lymphatic leukemia
c.m.	tomorrow morning
cm	centimeter
cm2	square centimeters
CMC	carpometacarpal
CMG	cystometrogram
CMHC	community mental health center
CML	chronic myelogenous leukemia
CMP	competitive medical plan
CMRI	cardiac magnetic resonance imaging
CMS	circulation motion sensation
CMS	Centers for Medicare and Medicaid Services
CMS-1500	a universal billing form developed by CMS
CMV	cytomegalovirus
cn	cranial nerves
c.n.	tomorrow night
CNM	certified nurse midwife
CNP	continuous negative airway pressure
CNS	central nervous system
co	cardiac output
c/o	complaints of
CO2	carbon dioxide
COB	coordination of benefits
COBRA	Consolidated Omnibus Budget Reconciliation Act
COC	certificate of coverage
COLD	chronic obstructive lung disease
CON	certificate of need
conc.	concentration
cont.	continue
COPD	chronic obstructive pulmonary disease
CP	cerebral palsy
CPAP	continuous positive airway pressure
CPB	cardiopulmonary bypass
CPD	cephalopelvic disproportion
CPK	creatine phosphokinase
CPM	continuous passive motion

Abbreviations

CPR	cardiopulmonary resuscitation, or computer-based patient record
CPT	chest physical therapy
CPT	Physicians' Current Procedural Terminology
CQI	Continuous Quality Improvement
CR	creatine
CRC	community rating by class
CRF	chronic renal failure
CRH	corticotropic releasing hormone
crit.	hematocrit
CROS	contralateral routing of signals
CRP	C-reactive protein
C/S	cesarean section
CS	central service
CSF	cerebrospinal fluid
CT	computerized tomography/corneal thickness/ carpal tunnel syndrome
CTLSO	cervical-thoracic-lumbar-sacral-orthosis
CTZ	chemoreceptor trigger zone
cu	cubic
CV	cardiovascular
CVA	cerebral vascular accident/cerebrovascular accident/costovertebral angle
CVD	cardiovascular disease, cerebrovascular disease
CVI	chronic venous insufficiency
CVL	central venous line
CVMS	clean voided midstream urine
CVP	central venous pressure
CVU	cerebrovascular unit
CW	closed ward
CXR	chest x-ray
cysto	cystoscopy
D	day/diopter
DAW	dispense as written
D&C	dilation and curettage
D/C	discharge/discontinue
dc	discontinue
DC	dual choice
DCíd	discharged/discontinued
DCA	deferred compensation administrator
DCI	duplicate coverage inquiry
DCR	dacrocytstorhinostomy
DDST	Denver Developmental Screening Test
DE	dose equivalent
decem	ten
decub.	decubitus ulcer/lying down
def.	deficient, deficiency
del	delivery
dep.	dependent
det.	let it be given
DEXA	dual energy x-ray absorptiometry
dexter, dextra	the right
DHEA	dehydroepiandrosterone
DHHS	Department of Health and Human Services
DHT	dihydrotestosterone
DIC	disseminated intravascular coagulopathy
DIF	direct immunofluorescence
disp	disposition
DJD	degenerative joint disease
DKA	diabetic ketoacidosis
DM	diabetes mellitus
DMD	Duchenne muscular dystrophy
DME	durable medical equipment
DNA	deoxyribonucleic acid
DNP	do not publish
DNR	do not resuscitate
DO	Doctor of Osteopathy
DOA	dead on arrival
DOB	date of birth
DOE	dyspnea on exertion
DOH	Department of Health
DOS	date of service
DPR	drug price review
DPT	days per thousand
DPT	diphtheria - pertussis - tetanus
D/R	dayroom
DR	delivery room
Dr	doctor
DRG	diagnosis related group
Dsg	dressing
DSM-IV	Diagnostic and Statistical Manual of the American Psychiatric Association's Task Force on Terminology, Fourth Edition
DSS	dioctyl sulfosoccinate

Abbreviations

© 2004 Ingenix, Inc.

DTs	delirium tremens
DTRs	deep tendon reflexes
DUE	drug use evaluation
duo	two
DVT	deep vein thrombosis
D/W	dextrose in water
dx	diagnosis
DX	diagnosis code
dz	disease
ead.	the same
EBL	estimated blood loss
EBV	Epstein-Barr virus
ECCE	extracapsular cataract extraction
ECF	extended care facility, extracellular fluid
ECG	electrocardiogram
ECHO	enterocytopathogenic human orphan virus/echocardiogram
ECMO	extracorporeal membrane oxygenation
ECT	electro-convulsive therapy/emission computerized tomography
ectopic	ectopic pregnancy (OB)
ED	emergency department/effective dose
EDC	estimated date of confinement/ expected date of confinement
EDI	electronic data interchange
EEG	electroencephalogram
EENT	eye, ear, nose, and throat
EGA	estimated gestational age
EGD	esophagus, stomach and duodenum
EKG	electrocardiogram
E/M	evaluation and management
EMG	electromyograme.m.p. as directed
en	an enema, a clyster
en bloc	in total
eng.	engorged
ENG	electronystagmogram
ENT	ear, nose, and throat
EO	elbow orthosis
EOB	explanation of benefits
EOG	electrooculography
EOM	end of month
EOM	extraocular motion
EOMB	explanation of Medicare benefits
EOMI	extraocular motion intact
EOP	external occipital protuberance
Epis.	episiotomy
EPO	epoetin alfa
EPS	electrophysiologic stimulation
EPSDT	early periodic screening, diagnosis and treatment
ER	emergency room
ERC	endoscopic retrograde cholangiography
ERCP	endoscopic retrograde cholangiopancreatography
ERG	electroretinogram
ERISA	Employee Retirement Income Security Act of 1974
ESR	erythrocyte sedimentation rate
ESRD	end stage renal disease
EST	electroshock therapy
ESWL	extracorporeal shockwave lithotripsy
et	and
ET	endotracheal
ETOH	alcohol
Ex	examination
ext.	extremity
F (on OB)	firm
F	Fahrenheit/female
FAS	fetal alcohol syndrome
FB (fb)	fingerbreadth
FB	foreign body
FBR	foreign body removal
FBS	fasting blood sugar
FDP	fibrin degradation products
Fe	female/iron
FEV	forced expiratory volume
FFP	fresh frozen plasma
FFS	fee for service equivalency
FFS	fee for service reimbursement
FH	family history
FHR	fetal heart rate
FHT	fetal heart tone
FI	firm one finger down from umbilicus
fl	fluid
fluro	fluoroscopy
FM	face mask
FNP	family nurse practitioner

Abbreviations

FP	family planning/family practitioner
FR	family relationship
FSA	flexible spending account
FSE	fetal scalp electrode
FSH	follicle stimulating hormone
FTND	full term normal delivery
FTSG	full thickness skin graft
FTT	failure to thrive
F/U	follow-up
FUO	fever of unknown origin
fx	fracture
G	gram
GA	gastric analysis
gav.	gavage
GB	gallbladder
GDM	gestational diabetes mellitus
GFR	glomerular filtration rate
GH	growth hormone
GI	gastrointestinal
GIFT	gamete intrafallopian transfer
GLC	gas liquid chromatography
GMP	guanosine monophosphate
GnRH	gonadotropin-releasing hormone
GP	general practitioner
gr.	grain
grav	number of pregnancies
GS	general surgeon
gsw	gunshot wound
gt./gtt.	drop/drops
GU	genitourinary
Gu	guiac
GxT	graded exercise test
gyn	gynecology
h (hora)	hour
H2O	water
H2O2	hydrogen peroxide
HA	headache/hearing aide
HAA	hepatitis antigen B
HAAb	hepatitis antibody A
HaAg	hepatitis antigen A
HAI	hemaglutination test
HAV	hepatitis A virus
HB	headbox/hepatitis B
HBsAb	hepatitis surface antibody B
HBcAg	hepatitis antigen B
HBD	hydroxybutyril dehydrogenase
Hbg	hemoglobin
HBO	hyperbaric oxygen
HbO2	oxyhemoglobin
HBP	high blood pressure
HBsAg	hepatitis antigen B
HBV	hepatitis B vaccine
HCFA	Health Care Financing Administration. See CMS
HCFA-1500	see CMS-1500
HCG	human chorionic gonadotropin
HCl	hydrochloric acid
HCPCS	Healthcare Common Procedural Coding System
Hct	hematocrit
Hctz	hydrochlorothiazide
HCVD	hypertensive cardiovascular disease
HD	hip disarticulation
h.d.	at bedtime
HDL	high-density lipoproteins
HEDIS	Health Plan Employer Data and Information Set
HEENT	head, eyes, ears, nose, and throat
HGH	human growth hormone
Hg/Hgb	hemoglobin
HH	hard of hearing
HHA	home health agency
HHS	Department of Health and Human Services
HIAA	hydroxyindolacetic acid
Hib	Hemophilus influenzae vaccine
HIPAA	Health Insurance Portability and Accountability Act of 1996
HIV	human immunodeficiency virus
HLV	herpes-like virus
HMD	hyaline membrane disease
HMO	health maintenance organization
HMS	hepatosplenomegaly
H.O.	house officer
HORF	high output renal failure
H&P	history and physical
HPs	hot packs
HPF	high power field
HPG	human pituitary gonadotropin
HPI	history of present illness

© 2004 Ingenix, Inc.

HPV	human papilloma virus
HR	Harrington rod/heart rate/hour
HRT	hormone replacement therapy
HS	heelstick/hour of sleep
HSBG	heelstick blood gas
HSG	hysterosalpingogram
HSP	health service plan
HSV	herpes simplex virus
ht.	height
HTLV/III	human T-cell lymphotropic virus /three
HTN	hypertension
HVA	homovanillic acid
Hx	history
hypo	hypodermic injection
IA	intra-arterial
IAB	intra-aortic balloon
IABC	intra-aortic balloon counterpulsation
IABP	intra-aortic balloon pump
IBS	irritable bowel syndrome
IBW	ideal body weight
ICCE	intracapsular cataract extraction
ICD-9-CM	International Classification of Diseases, Ninth Revision, Clinical Modification
ICD-10	International Classification of Diseases, Tenth Revision
ICD-10-PCS	International Classification of Diseases, Tenth Revision, Procedural Coding System
ICF	intermediate care facility
ICH	intracranial/cerebral hemorrhage
ICP	intracranial pressure
ICS	intercostal space
ICSH	interstitial cell stimulating hormone
ICU	intensive care unit
ID	infective dose
I& D	incision and drainage
Id31	radioactive iodine
IDDM	insulin dependent diabetis mellitis
IDH	isocitric dehydrogenase
IDM	infant of diabetic mother
Ig	immunoglobulin, gamma
IH	infectious hepatitis
IM	internal medicine/intramuscular/infectious mononucleosis
IMC	intermediate care
IME	independent medical evaluation
IMO	integrated multiple option
IMV	intermittent mandatory ventilation
inc.	incision
indep	independent
INF	inferior, infusion
INH	inhalation solution
INJ	injection
instill	instillation
I& O	intake and output
IOL	intraocular lens
IOP	intraocular pressure
IP	intraperitoneal/interphalangeal
IPA	individual practice association
IPD	intermittent peritoneal dialysis
IPPB	intermittent positive pressure breathing
IQ	intelligence quotient
ISC	infant servo-control
ISG	immune serum globulin
ISN	integrated service network
IT	intrathecal administration
ITP	idiopathic thrombocytopenia purpura
IU	international units
IUD	intrauterine device
IV	intravenous
IVC	inferior vena cava, intravenous cholangiogram
IVF	in vitro fertilization
IVH	intraventricular hemorrhage
IVP	intravenous pyelogram
JCAHO	Joint Commission on Accreditation of Healthcare Organizations
JODM	juvenile onset diabetes mellitus
JVP	jugular venous pressure
K	potassium
Kcal	kilocalorie
KCL	potassium chloride
kg	kilogram
KO	keep open/knee orthosis
KUB	kidneys, ureters, bladder
KVO	keep vein open
L	left/lumbar vertebrae

L&A	light and accommodation
LA	left atrium
LAD	left anterior descending
LAP	leucine aminopeptidase
LAT	lateral
LAV	lymphadenopathy associated virus
LAVH	laparascopic assisted vaginal hysterectomy
LB	legbag
LBB	left bundle branch
LBBB	left bundle branch block
LBP	lower back pain
LCP	licensed clinical psychologist
LCSW	licensed clinical social worker
LD	lethal dose
LDH	lactate dehydrogenase
LDL	low-density lipoproteins
LE	lower extremity/lupus erythematosis
LEEP	loop electrocautery excision procedure
LGA	large for gestational age
LH	luteinizing hormone
LHF	left heart failure
LHR	leukocyte histamine release
Li	lithium
lido	lidocaine
liq.	solution (liquor)
LKS	liver, kidneys, spleen
LLL	left lower lobe
LLQ	left lower quadrant
LMD	local medical doctor
LML	left medio lateral position
LMP	last menstrual period
LMS	left mentum anterior position (chin)
LMT	left mentum transverse position
LOA	leave of absence
LOC	level of consciousness/loss of consciousness
LOM	limitation of motion
LOP	left occiput posterior position
LOT	left occiput transverse position
LP	lumbar puncture
LPM	liters per minute
LR	lactated Ringer's/log roll
LS fusion	lumbar sacral fusion
LSA	left sacrum anterior position
LSB	left sternal border
LSO	lumbar sacral orthosis
LT	left
LTC	long term care
lul	left upper lobe
luq	left upper quadrant
LV	left ventricle
lymphs	lymphocytes
lytes	electrolytes
M	manifest refraction/male
M1	mitral first sound
M2	mitral second sound
MA1	volume respirator
MAC	maximum allowable cost
MAD	monoamine oxidase (inhibitor)
MAP	mean arterial pressure
MASER	microwave amplification by stimulated emission of radiation
MBC	minimum bactericidal concentration/maximum breathing capacity
MBD	minimal brain dysfunction
mcg	microgram
MCH	mean corpuscular hemoglobin
MCL	midclavicular line
MCP	metacarpophalangeal
MCR	modified community rating
MCT	mediastinal chest tube
MCV	mean corpuscular volume
MD	medical doctor
MD	muscular dystrophy/myocardial disease/manic depression
MDC	major diagnostic category
MDD	manic-depressive disorder
Mec	meconium
MED	minimal effective dose
med/surg	Medical, surgical
Medigap	Medicare supplemental insurance
meds	medications
Medsupp	Medicare supplemental insurance
mEq	milliequivalent
mEq/l	milliequivalent per liter
MFD	minimum fatal dose
MFT	muscle function test
mg	milligram

Abbreviations

© 2004 Ingenix, Inc.

Mg	magnesium
MHC	mental health clinic
MH/CD	mental health/chemical dependency
MH/SA	mental health/substance abuse
MI	myocardial infarction
min	minimum/minimal/minute
misce.	miscellaneous
ML	midline
ml	milliliter
MLC	midline catheter
mm	millimeter
mmHg	millimeters of mercury
MMPI	Minnesota Multiphasic Personality Inventory
MMRV	measles, mumps, rubella vaccine
MOM	milk of magnesia
mono	monocyte/mononucleosis
MPD	maximum permissible dose
MR	mitral regurgitation
MRA	magnetic resonance angiography
MRI	magnetic resonance imaging
MS	morphine sulfate/multiple sclerosis
MSLT	multiple sleep latency testing
MSO	management service organization
MSS	medical social services
MSW	masterís in social work
MTD	right eardrum
MTM	metamucil
MTP	metatarsophalangeal
MTS	left eardrum
multip.	multipara - pregnant woman who has more than one child
MVP	mitral valve prolapse
MWS	Mickety-Wilson syndrome
N	nitrogen
N2O	nitrous oxide
Na	sodium
NaCl	sodium chloride (salt)
NAD	no appreciable disease
NAT	nonaccidental trauma
NB	newborn
NBICU	newborn intensive care unit
NBT	nitroblue tetrazolium
NCA	neurocirculatory asthenia
NCHS	National Center for Health Statistics
NCPR	no cardiopulmonary resuscitation
NCQA	National Committee on Quality Assurance
NCR	no cardiac resuscitation
NCV	nerve conduction velocity
NCVHS	National Committee on Vital Health Statistics
NDC	national drug code
NEC	necrotizing enterocolitis/not elsewhere classified
neg.	negative
NF	National Formulary
NG	nasogastric
NGU	nongonococcal urethritis
NIDDM	non-insulin dependent diabetes mellitus
NJ	nasojejunal
NKA	no known allergies
NKMA	no known medical allergies
NNR	new and nonofficial remedies
NOS	not otherwise specified
novem.	nine
NP	neuropsychiatry/nurse practitioner
NP-CPAP	nasopharyngeal continuous positive airway pressure
NPN	Non-par Not Approved/nonprotein nitrogen
n.p.o.	nothing by mouth
npt	normal pressure and temperature
NS	normal saline/not significant
NSAID	nonsteroidal anti-inflammatory drug
NSD	nominal standard dose
NSR	normal sinus rhythm
NST	nonstress test
NSVB	normal spontaneous vaginal bleeding
NSVD	normal spontaneous vaginal delivery
NT	nasotracheal/nontender
NTE	neutral thermal environment
NTP	normal temperature and pressure
N&V	nausea and vomiting
o	no information
O	blood type/oxygen
O2	oxygen
OA	open access
OA	osteoarthritis
OAG	open angle glaucoma

OB	obstetrics
OB-GYN	obstetrics and gynecology
OC	open crib/oral contraceptive/ office call
OCT	ornithine carbamyl transterase/oxytocin challenge test
octo.	eight
o.d.	right eye
OFC	occipitofrontal circumference
oint	ointment
OJ	orange juice
o.m.	every morning/otitis media
OMS	oralmaxillary surgery
OMT	osteopathic manipulation therapy
o.n.	every night
ONH	optic nerve head
O&P	ova and parasites
OPD	outpatient department
OPG	oculoplethysmography
ophth	ophthalmology
OPV	oral polio vaccine
OR	operating room
ORIF	open reduction internal fixation
ortho.	orthopedics
o.s.	left eye
os, oris	mouth
OSA	obstructive sleep apnea
OST	oxytocin stress test
OT	occupational therapy
OTC	over-the-counter
OTD	organ tolerance dose
OTH	other routes of administration
o.u.	each eye, both eyes
ov.	ovum/office visit
OW	open ward
oz.	ounce
P	plan/after/pulse, phosphorus
P2	pulmonic 2nd sound
PA	physician assistant/posteroanterior/pulmonary artery
PAB	premature atrial beats
PAC	pre-admission certification
PAC	premature atrial contraction
PACU	post anesthesia care unit
PAD	pulmonary artery diastolic
PAP	Papanicolaou test or smear/pulmonary artery pressure
Par	participating provider
PAR	post anesthesia recovery/parenteral
para	along side of/number of pregnancies, as para 1, 2, 3, etc
PARR	post anesthesia recovery room
part. vic.	in divided doses
PAT	paroxysmal atrial tachycardia
path	pathology
PBI	protein-bound iodine
PC	packed cells
p.c.	after eating
PCA	patient controlled analgesia
PCD	polycystic disease
PCG	phonocardiogram
PCN	penicillin
PCN	primary care network
PCP	primary care physician
PCPM	per contract per month
PCTA	percutaneous transluminal angioplasty
PCV	packed cell volume
PCW	pulmonary capillary wedge
PD	postural drainage/Parkinsonís disease
PDA	patent ductus arteriosus
PE	physical examination/pulmonary embolism/pulmonary edema
PEC	pre-existing condition
Peds	pediatrics
PEG	pneumoencephalogram
PEN	parenteral and enteral nutrition
PENS	percutaneous electrical nerve stimulation
PERRLA	pupils equal, regular, reactive to light and accommodation
PET	positron emission tomography
PFC	persistent fetal circulation
PFT	pulmonary function test
PG	prostaglandin
PH	past history
PharmD	Doctor of Pharmacy
pH	potential of hydrogen
PI	present illness
PICC	peripherally inserted central catheter
PID	pelvic inflammatory disease

© 2004 Ingenix, Inc.

PKU	phenylketonuria
PMG	primary medical group
PMHx	past medical history
PMI	point of maximum intensity
PMPM	per member per month
PMPY	per member per year
PMN	polvmorphonuclear neutrophil leukocytes
PMS	premenstrual syndrome
PNC	premature nodal contraction
PND	paroxysmal nocturnal dyspnea/ post nasal drip
PNS	peripheral nervous system
p/o	by mouth
PO	(per os) by mouth/post operative
POD	post operative day
polys	polymorphonuclear neutrophil leukocytes
POR	problem oriented record
POS	place of service/point of service/point of sale
pos.	positive
post or PM	postmortem exam or autopsy
PP	postprandial
p.p.	near point of visual accommodation
PPD	percussion and postural drainage
PPH	post partum hemorrhage
PPO	preferred provider organization
PPP	protamine paracoagulation
p.r.	far point of visual accommodation/through the rectum
pr	per return
PRBC	packed red blood cells
PREs	progressive resistive exercises
preg	pregnant
previa	placenta previa
primip	primipara - a woman having her first child
p.r.n.	as needed for
PRO	professional (or peer) review organization
PROM	premature rupture of membranes
PSA	prostate specific antigen
PSP	phenolsulfonphthalein
PsyD	Doctor of Psychology
PT	physical therapy/prothrombin time

Pt	patient/prothrombin time
PTA	prior to admission/percutaneous transluminal angioplasty
PTB	patellar tendon bearing (cast)
PTCA	percutaneous transluminal coronary angioplasty
PTH	parathyroid hormone
PTT	partial thromboplastin time
PUD	peptic ulcer disease
pulv.	powder
PVC	premature ventricular contraction
PVD	premature ventricular depolarization
PVL	paraventricular leukomalasia
Px	prognosis
Q.	every
q.2h	every two hours
QA	quality assurance
q.a.m.	every morning
q.d.	every day
q.h.	every hour
q.h.s.	every night
q.i.d.	four times daily
QM	quality management
q.n.	every night
qns	quantity not sufficient
q.o.d.	every other day
q.q.h.	every four hours
qs	quantity sufficient
quotid	daily
R	respiration/right atrium
r	roentgen units (x-rays)
R&C	reasonable and customary
RA	rheumatoid arthritis
RBB	right bundle branch
RBBB	right bundle branch block
RBC	red blood cell
RBOW	ruptured bag of water
RBRVS	resource based relative value scale
RCD	relative cardiac dullness
RDS	respiratory distress syndrome
REM	rapid eye movement
RESA	radial cryosurgical ablation
resp	respiration, respiratory
Retro	retrospective rate derivation
rev.	revise, revision

Rh	Rhesus
Rh neg	Rhesus factor negative
RHD	rheumatic heart disease
RHF	right heart failure
RIA	radioimmunoassay
RL	Ringer's lactate
RLE	right lower extremity
RLF	rentrolental fibroplasia
RLL	right lower lobe
rlq	right lower quadrant
RML	right middle lobe
RN	registered nurse
RNA	ribonucleic acid
R/O	rule out
ROA	right occiput anterior position
ROM	range of motion
ROP	right occiput posterior position
ROS	review of systems
RPG	retrograde pyelogram
RR	recovery room
RRA	registered record administrator
R,R,& E	round, regular, and equal
RRR	regular rate and rhythm
RS	reducing substances
RSV	respiratory syncytial virus
RT	recreational therapist/respiratory therapist/resting tracing/right
RUL	right upper lobe
ruq	right upper quadrant
RV	right ventricle
Rx	take (prescription; treatment)
RxN	reaction
s	without
SAH	subarachnoid hemorrhage
SALT	serum alanine aminotransferase
SAST	serum aspartate aminotransferase
SB	sinus bradycardia
SBFT	small bowel follow through
s.c.	subcutaneous
S-C disease	sickle cell hemoglobin-c disease
SCI	spinal cord injury
SCR	standard class rate
sed rate	sedimentation rate of erythrocytes
SEM	systolic ejection murmur
sex	six
SG	Swan-Ganz
SGA	small for gestational age
SGOT	serum glutamic oxaloacetic acid
SH	social history
SHBG	sex hormone binding globulin
SIADH	syndrome of inappropriate antidiuretic hormone
SIDS	sudden infant death syndrome
sine	without
SISI	short increment sensitivity index
s.l.	under the tongue, sublingual
SLE	systemic lupus erythematosus
SMI	supplementary medical insurance program
SNF	skilled nursing facility
SNS	sympathetic nervous system
SOAP	subjective objective assessment plan
SOB	shortness of breath
sol.	solution
SOP	standard operation procedure
S.O.S.	if necessary (si opus sit)
S/P	status post
SPD	summary plan description
SQ	status quo/subcutaneous
SROM	spontaneous rupture of membranes
ss	half
ST	sinus tachycardia
staph	staphylococcus
stat	immediately
STD	sexually transmitted disease
STH	somatotrophic hormone
strep	streptococcus
STS	serology test for syphilis
STSG	split thickness skin graft
STU	skin test unit
subcu	subcutaneous
supp	suppository
Sv	scalp vein
SVC	service
SVCS	superior vena cava syndrome
Sx	sign/symptom
T	temperature/tender/thoracic vertebrae
T3	triiodothyronine
T4	thyroxine

Abbreviations

© 2004 Ingenix, Inc.

T&A	tonsils and adenoids
TAH	total abdominal hysterectomy
TAT	tetanus antitoxin/turnaround time
Tb	tubercule bacillus
TB	tuberculosis
TBA	to be arranged
TBG	thyroxine/thyroid binding globulin
TBI	total body irradiation
TBSA	total body surface area
TC&DB	turn, cough, and deep breathe
Td	tetanus
TEFRA	Tax Equity and Fiscal Responsibility Act
temp	temperature
TENS	transcutaneous electrical nerve stimulation
TFT	transfer factor test
THA	total hip arthroplasty
Thal	Thalassemia
THC	tetrahydrocannabinol
TI	tricuspid insufficiency
TIA	transient ischemic attack
t.i.d.	three times daily
TKA	total knee arthroplasty
TM	tympanic membrane
TMJ	temporomandibular joint
TNS	transcutaneous nerve stimulator/stimulation
TO	telephone order
TOA	tubo-ovarian abscess
TORCH	Toxoplasmosis, Other (includes syphilis), Rubella, Cytomegalo virus, and Herpes virus
TP	total protein
TPN	total parenteral nutrition
TPR	temperature, pulse, respiration
Tr	tinctura, tincture/trace
TRAM	transverse rectus abdominos musculocutaneous
trans	transverse
TRF	thyrotropin releasing factor
TRH	thyrotropin releasing hormone
Ts	tension by Schiotz
TSA	tumor specific antigen
TSD	Tay-Sachs disease
TSE	testicular self-exam
TSH	thyroid stimulating hormone
TSS	toxic shock syndrome
TTN	transient tachypnea of newborn
TULIP	transurethral ultrasound guided laser induced prostate
TUR	transurethral resection
TURP	transurethral resection of prostate
Tx	treatment
U	unit
U/A	urinalysis
UAC	umbilical artery catheter/catheterization
UB-92	Uniform Billing Code of 1992
U&C	usual and customary
UC	unit clerk
UCHD	usual childhood diseases
UCR	usual, customary and reasonable
UE	upper extremity
UFR	uroflowmetry
UGI	upper gastrointestinal
UMN	upper motor neuron
UPIN	universal physician identification number
UPP	urethra pressure profile
ur.	Urine
UR	utilization review
URI	upper respiratory infection
URN	utilization review nurse
UR/QA	utilization review/quality assurance
US	unstable spine/ultrasound
UTI	urinary tract infection
UV	ultraviolet light
UVC	umbilical vein catheter
V Fib	ventricular fibrillation
V tach	ventricular tachycardia
Va	visual acuity
VA	Veterans Administration
VBAC	vaginal birth after cesarean
VC	vena cava
VCG	vectorcardiogram
VD	venereal disease
VDH	valvular disease of the heart
VDRL	venereal disease report
VEP	visual evoked potential

Abbreviations

VF	visual field/ventricular fibrillation
VIP	vasoactive intestinal peptide
Vit	vitamin (followed by specific letter)
VO	verbal order
VO2	maximum oxygen consumption
VP	vasopressin/voiding pressure
VPC	ventricular premature contraction
VPRC	volume of packed red cells
VS	vital signs/vesicular sound
VSD	ventricular septal defect
vv	veins
WB	whole blood
WBC	white blood count
WC	wheelchair
WCC	well child care
WD	well developed
W-D	wet to dry (dressings)
WHO	World Health Organization
w/HSBH	warmed heelstick blood gas
WLS	wet lung syndrome
WN	well nourished
WNL	within normal limits
Wt	weight
x	except
YTD	year-to-date
ZIFT	zygote intrafallopian transfer

© 2004 Ingenix, Inc.

Reimbursement Terms

An increasingly complex reimbursement climate means new terminology develops every year. The following glossary includes terms not only used when coding, it includes terms used by major insurers and the federal government.

AAPA — American Academy of Physician Assistants.

AAPC — American Academy of Professional Coders.

AAPCC — Adjusted average per capita cost. The best estimate of the amount of money it costs to care for Medicare recipients in a given area.

AAPPO — American Association of Preferred Provider Organizations.

Abstractor — Selects and extracts data from the medical record entered into computer files. The data and coded diagnoses track morbidity and mortality, infectious disease, and index disease. Information may be gathered to track data for departments such as quality assurance and utilization review within the facility.

Accrual — The amount of money set aside to cover the benefit plan's expenses. It is estimated using a combination of data including the claims system and plan's prior history.

ACLS — Advanced Cardiac Life Support. A certification often required of professionals who serve seriously injured or ill patients.

ACR — Adjusted community rate. A calculation of what premium the plan charges to provide Medicare-covered benefits for greater frequency of use by participants.

ACS contract — *See* ASO

Activities of daily living — Activities often used to determine eligibility for long-term care. They include bathing, dressing, using a toilet, transferring in and out of bed or chair, continence, eating, and walking.

Actuarial assumptions — Characteristics used in calculating the risks and costs of a plan. Assumptions include age, sex, and occupation of enrollees; location; utilization rates; and service costs.

Adjudication — The judging of a claim.

Admission — Registration of a patient for services in a health care facility.

ADS — Alternative delivery system. Any method of providing health care benefits that differs from traditional indemnity methods.

Adverse selection — The risk of enrolling members who are sicker than assumed and who will utilize more expensive services more frequently.

Age restriction — Limitation of benefits when a patient reaches a certain age.

Age/sex rating — Structuring capitation payments based on members' ages and genders.

Aggregate amount — The maximum for which a member is insured for any single event.

AHA — American Hospital Association.

AHIMA — American Health Information Management Association.

Al-Anon, Alateen — Alcoholic support groups.

ALOS — Average length of stay. A benchmark average used for analysis of utilization.

AMA — American Medical Association.

Ambulatory surgery — Surgical procedure in which the patient is admitted, treated, and released on the same day.

AMCRA — American Managed Care Review Association.

AMLOS — Arithmetic mean length of stay — Average numbers of days within a given DRG stay in the hospital.

ANA — American Nursing Association.

AOA — American Osteopathic Association.

APA — American Psychiatric Association.

AP-DRG — All Patient Diagnostic Related Group. 3M HIS made revisions and adjustments to the DRG system, now referred to as the All Patient DRGs (AP-DRGs). Early features of AP-DRGs included MDC 24, specifically devoted to the human immunodeficiency virus (HIV), and restructuring of the MDC governing newborns.

APG — Ambulatory patient group. A reimbursement methodology developed for the Centers for Medicare and Medicaid Services.

Appeal — A request for reconsideration of a negative claim decision.

Appropriateness of care — Term often used to denote proper setting of medical care that best meets the patient's diagnosis.

APR — Average payment rate. The amount of money the Centers for Medicare and Medicaid Services could pay a Health Maintenance Organization for service to Medicare recipients under a risk contract.

ART — Accredited Record Technician. *See* RHIT.

AS — Associate of Science.

ASN — Associate of Science, Nursing.

ASO — Administrative service only. A contract stipulation between a self-funded plan and an insurance company in which the insurance company assumes no risk and provides administrative services only.

Assignment — An arrangement in which the provider submits the claim on behalf of the patient and is reimbursed directly by the patient's plan. By doing so, the provider agrees to accept what the plan pays.

Assignment of benefits — Payment of benefits directly to the provider of the services rather than to the member who received the benefits.

At risk — A contract between Medicare and a payer or a payer and a provider in which the payer (in the case of Medicare) and the provider (in the case of the payer contracts) gets paid a set amount for care of a patient base. If costs exceed the amount the payer or provider were paid, the patients still receive care during the term of the contract.

Attained age — The age of the member as of the last birthday.

Auditor — A professional who evaluates a provider's utilization, quality of care, or level of reimbursement.

AWP — 1) Average wholesale price. A pharmaceutical price based on common data that is included in a pharmacy provider contract. 2) Any willing provider. Statutes requiring a provider network to accept any provider who meets the network's usual selection criteria.

Backlog — The queue of claims that have not been adjudicated.

Balance billing — When providers charge the patient the amount not paid by the insurance carrier above the agreed deductible.

Basic coverage — Insurance providing coverage for hospital care.

Basic health services — Benefits all federally qualified HMOs must offer.

Board certification — A certification in a particular specialty based on the physician's expertise and experience.

Boarder — An individual who receives lodging — a parent, caregiver, or other family member — who is not a patient but may wish or need to be near the patient.

Boarder baby — 1) A newborn who remains in the nursery following discharge because the mother is still hospitalized; 2) A premature infant who no longer needs intensive care but who remains for observation.

Book of business — A payer's list of clients and contracts.

BSN — Bachelor of Science, Nursing

Bundled — 1) The gathering of several types of health insurance policies under a single payer; 2) The inclusive grouping of codes related to a procedure when submitting a claim.

Business coalition — Employers who form a cooperative to purchase health care less expensively.

Cafeteria plan — A benefit by an employer where various services of many payers are offered to members as separate elements in the health care plan.

Cap — Contract maximum.

Capitation — A system in which a set amount of money is received or paid out based on membership rather than on a number of services rendered.

Care unit — A specific department or facility within a hospital or long-term care facility designed and staffed for the treatment of a particular type of patient.

Carrier — Insurance company responsible for processing claims.

Carve-out — 1) Term often used when referring to the integrated plan method of providing coverage to Medicare-eligible employees; 2) Medical benefits for a specific type of care that are not provided by the carrier of the members' insurance (e.g., Mental/Nervous provided by company A while company B carries the medical plan).

Case management — The ongoing review of cases by professionals to assure the most appropriate utilization of services.

Case manager — A medical professional (usually a nurse or social worker) who reviews cases every few days to determine necessity of care and to advise provider on payer's utilization restrictions. Certifies ongoing care.

Case-mix index — Sum of all DRG relative weights, divided by number of Medicare cases.

Catastrophic case management — Also called large case management. A method of review of ongoing cases in which the patient sustains catastrophic or extremely costly medical problems.

Catchment area — The geographical area from which a health care organization draws its members.

CC — Complication or comorbidity affecting payment.

CCU — Coronary Care Unit. A facility dedicated to patients suffering from heart attack, stroke, or other serious cardiopulmonary problems.

CDC — Center for Disease Control.

Census — The number and demographics of patients or members.

Certification — Approval by a payer's case manager to continue care for a given number of days or visits.

Cherry picking — Practice of enrolling only healthy individuals and excluding those with existing problems.

 © 2004 Ingenix, Inc.

Chief complaint — The presenting problem.

Churning — 1) A performance-based reimbursement system emphasizing provider productivity; 2) When a provider sees a patient more than medically necessary with the intent of generating more revenue.

CLA — Certified Laboratory Assistant.

Claim — Statement of medical services rendered requesting payment from an insurance company or a government entity.

Claim lag — 1) The time between the incurred date of the claim and its submission; 2) The time between the incurred date of the claim and its payment.

Claim manual — The administrative guidelines used by claims processors to adjudicate claims according to company policy and procedure.

Claims manager — Payer's manager who oversees the employee who processes routine claims.

Claims reviewer —Payer employee who reviews claims like an auditor, looking at coding, prior authority, contract violations, etc.

CLIA — Clinical Laboratory Improvement Amendments. Requirements set in 1988, CLIA imposes varying levels of federal regulations on clinical procedures. Few laboratories, including those in physician offices, are exempt. Adopted by Medicare and Medicaid, CLIA regulations redefine laboratory testing in regard to laboratory certification and accreditation, proficiency testing, quality assurance, personnel standards, and program administration.

Closed claim — A claim for which all apparent benefits have been paid.

Closed panel — An arrangement in which a managed care organization contracts providers on an exclusive basis, restricting the providers from seeing patients enrolled in other payers' plans.

Closed treatment — A fracture site that is not surgically opened. There are three methods of closed treatment of fractures: without manipulation, with manipulation, and with or without traction.

CMA — Certified Medical Assistant.

CMI — Case mix index. Sum of all DRG relative weights, divided by the number of Medicare cases.

CMP — Competitive medical plan. A federal designation allowing plans to obtain eligibility to receive a Medicare risk contract without having to qualify as an HMO.

CMS — Centers for Medicare and Medicaid Services. The federal agency that administers the public health programs.

CMS-1500 — A standard claim form.

CMT — Certified Medical Transcriptionist.

COA — Certificate of authority. A state license to operate as an HMO.

COB — Coordination of benefits. An agreement that prevents double payment for services when the member is covered by two or more sources. The agreement dictates which organization is primarily and secondarily responsible for payment.

COBRA — Consolidated Omnibus Reconciliation Act. Legislation that in part requires employers to offer terminated employees the opportunity to continue buying coverage as part of the employer's group.

Coder — Professional who translates documented, written diagnoses and procedures into numeric and alphanumeric codes.

Coding conventions — Each space, type face, indentation, and punctuation mark determining how ICD-9-CM codes are interpreted. These "conventions" were developed to help match correct codes to the diagnoses that are encountered.

Coinsurance — A limitation of the amount payable by the payer to the provider or member for care in traditional plans or in parts of managed care plans. For example, most traditional plans only pay 80 percent of care costs.

Commercial carriers — For-profit insurance companies issuing health coverage.

Common working file — All beneficiary entitlement information (Part A, Part B, Medicare Secondary Payer, and Health Maintenance Organization), deductible status, and all Part A and Part B claims history are maintained in CWF.

Community rating — Methodology of state and federal governments that requires qualified HMOs to request the same amount of money for each member in a plan.

Comorbidity — Preexisting condition that causes an increase in length of stay by at least one day in around 75 percent of cases. Used in DRG reimbursement.

Comparative performance reports — CPRs. CPRs annually compare a physician's services and procedures to those of physicians in the same specialty and geographic area.

Complex repair — The repair of wounds requiring reconstructive surgery, complicated wound closure, debridement, skin grafting, or intricate, unusual, and time-consuming techniques to obtain the maximum functional and cosmetic result. Complex repairs include the creation of a defect (e.g., extending excisions), necessary preparations for repairs, and moderate debridement of complicated lacerations, avulsions, and other wounds.

Complication — From an insurer's point of view, this is a condition that arises during a hospital stay prolonging patients' stays by at least one day in 75 percent of the cases.

Component code — In CCI, the code following the comprehensive code that cannot be charged to Medicare when the comprehensive code is charged.

Component coding — Standardizes the reporting of interventional radiological services. Component coding allows a physician, regardless of specialty, to specifically identify and report those aspects of the service he or she provided, whether the procedural component, the radiological component, or both.

Comprehensive codes — The code behind which component codes fall. *See also* CCI.

Consultation — Advice or an opinion rendered by a medical professional at the request of the primary care provider.

Continuity of coverage — Transfer of benefits from one plan to another without a lapse of coverage.

Conversion — Shifting of a member under a group contract to an individual contract.

Conversion factors — National multipliers that convert the geographically adjusted relative value units into Medicare Fee Schedule dollar amounts and applies to all services paid under the MFS.

Coordinated care — *See* managed care.

Copayment — A portion of the medical expense the member must pay out of pocket. In managed care plans, the member pays the copayment while checking in for his or her appointment.

Correct Coding Initiative — CCI. Provides edits that determine the appropriateness of CPT code combinations in Medicare billing. Updated quarterly.

Corridor deductible — A fixed out-of-pocket amount that the member must pay before benefits are available. Also called simply "deductible."

COT — Certified Ophthalmic Technician.

COTA — Certified Occupational Therapy Assistant.

Counseling — A discussion with a patient and/or family concerning one or more of the following areas: diagnostic results, impressions, and/or recommended diagnostic studies; prognosis; risks and benefits of management (treatment) options; instructions for management (treatment) and/or follow-up; importance of compliance with chosen management (treatment) options; risk factor reduction; patient and family education.

Coverage issues manual — CIM. The CIM is a CMS publication containing national coverage decisions and presenting specific medical items, services, treatment procedures, or technologies paid for under the Medicare program. The CIM is used by Part A Intermediaries, Part B Carriers, and Peer Review Organizations (PROs).

Covered charges — Charges for medical care and supplies that the insurance plan will pay.

Covered person — Any person entitled to benefits under the policy, whether a member or dependent.

CPR — Computerized patient record — A computer application that allows all or most elements of a patient's medical record to be stored in a computerized database.

CPT — *Physicians' Current Procedural Terminology, Fourth Edition*. The American Medical Association's list of five-digit codes used to report medical services. A standard reference for billing.

CPT code — A descriptor of a procedure with a five-digit identifying code number. CPT codes are developed, maintained, and copyrighted by the American Medical Association.

CPT modifiers — Additional codes to indicate that a service was altered in some way from the stated CPT code description without actually changing the basic definition of the service. Modifiers can indicate a service or procedure has both a professional and a technical component, a service or procedure was performed by more than one physician, only part of a service was performed, an adjunctive service was performed, a bilateral procedure was performed, a service or procedure was provided more than once, unusual events occurred, or a procedure or service was altered in some way. A complete listing of modifiers is located in an appendix of the CPT book.

Credentialing — Reviewing the medical degrees, licensure, malpractice, and any disciplinary record of medical providers for panel and quality assurance purposes.

Critical care — The care of critically ill patients in a variety of medical emergencies that requires the constant attendance of the physician (e.g., cardiac arrest, shock, bleeding, respiratory failure, postoperative complications, critically ill neonate).

CRNA — Certified Registered Nurse Anesthetist.

Crosswalk — The cross-referencing of CPT codes with ICD-9-CM, anesthesia, dental, or HCPCS codes.

CRT — 1) Cathode ray tube. An old term for the computer used by coders. Refers specifically to the monitor; 2) Certified Respiratory Therapist.

CSO — Clinical service organization — Health care organization developed by academic medical centers to integrate medical school, faculty practice plan, and hospital.

CST — Certified Surgical Technologist.

Cutback — Reduction of the amount or type of insurance for a member who attains a specified age or condition (e.g., age 65, retirement).

Daily benefit — A specified maximum benefit payable for room and board charges at a hospital.

Database — The electronic store of utilization information used by payers to pay claims, negotiate contracts, and track utilization and cost of services.

Date of Service — *See* Service date

DAW — Dispense as written. The notation from a physician to a pharmacist requesting that the brand-name medication be given in lieu of a generic medication.

Days per thousand — A standard unit of measurement of utilization determined by calculating

 © 2004 Ingenix, Inc.

the number of hospital days used in a year for each thousand covered lives.

DC — Doctor of Chiropractic medicine.

Decapitation — Inadequate capitation.

Deductible — Member's medical services that must be paid out of pocket before the payer begins to pay.

Diagnosis — Determination of condition, disease, or syndrome and its implications.

Diagnostic — Services provided to determine the nature of the member's complaints.

Direct claim payment — A method where members deal directly with the payer rather than submitting claims through the employer.

Direct contract model — A plan that contracts directly with individual private practice physicians rather than through an intermediary.

Discharge plan — A plan submitted by a provider to the case manager as part of the treatment plan that details follow-up care after discharge.

Discharge status — Circumstance of patient at discharge. Examples include "expired," "transferred to another facility," "left against medical advice."

Discharge transfer — Discharge of a patient from one facility to another.

Disposition of patient — A term used for data and quality assurance purposes that is accompanied by a description of the patient's status and destination at discharge (for example, "discharged to home").

DME — Durable medical equipment. Permanent equipment meant for medical treatment.

DO — Doctor of Osteopathy.

DOS — Date of service. The date on which care was provided.

DPM — Doctor of Podiatric Medicine.

DRG — Diagnosis Related Groups. The method CMS uses to pay hospitals for Medicare recipients based on a statistical system of classifying any inpatient stay into one of 25 groups. It is a classification scheme whose patient types are defined by patients' diagnoses or procedures and in some cases, by the patient's age or discharge status. Each DRG is intended to be medically meaningful and would ordinarily require an approximately equal resource consumption as measured by length of stay and cost.

Drug formulary — *See* Formulary.

DSM-IV-TR — *Diagnostic and Statistical Manual of Mental Disorders, Fourth Edition, Text Revision*. The manual used by mental health workers as the diagnostic coding system for substance abuse and mental health patients.

Dual option — The offering of an HMO and traditional plan by one carrier.

DUR — Drug utilization review. A review to assure prescribed medications are medically necessary and appropriate.

DVM — Doctor of Veterinary Medicine.

E codes — ICD-9-CM codes describing circumstances of an injury or illness. Their use establish medical necessity, identify causes of injury and poisoning, and identify medications. Their use can also be pivotal in reimbursements from payers such as medical insurance plans, car insurers, home insurers, or workers' compensation programs. Also known as the Supplementary Classification of External Causes of Injury and Poisoning (E800—E999) The index for the E codes is found in Volume 2, following the Table of Drugs and Chemicals.

EAP — Employee assistance program. Short-term counseling offered to members to quickly resolve transient emotional problems and to identify on-going mental or substance abuse problems for subsequent referral. Often limited to a handful of visits.

EdD — Doctor of Education.

EDI — Electronic data interchange. The transference of claims, certifications, quality assurance reviews, and utilization data via computer.

EHO — Emerging healthcare organizations — Hospitals and other providers that are emerging or affiliating.

Elective admission — An admission made at the discretion of the patient and facility based on available resources.

ELOS — Estimated length of stay. The average number of days of hospitalization required for a given illness or procedure. Base on prior histories of patients who have been hospitalized for the same illness or procedure.

E/M — Evaluation and management services. Contacts with the patient for assessment, counseling, and other services provided to a patient and reported through CPT-4 codes.

E/M service components — The key components in determining the correct level of E/M codes are history, examination, and medical decision making.

Emergency admission — An admission in which the patient requires immediate medical or psychiatric attention because of life-threatening, severe, and potentially disabling conditions.

Emergency department — An organized hospital-based facility for the provision of unscheduled episodic services to patients who present for immediate medical attention. The facility must be available 24 hours a day.

Emergency outpatient — A patient admitted for diagnosis and treatment of a condition requiring immediate attention but who will not stay at that facility or be transferred to another.

EMT — Emergency medical technician.

EMT-P — Paramedic.

Encoder — A computer application that helps assign a DRG.

Encounter — Contact with a patient.

Enrollee — A person who subscribes to a specific health plan.

Enrollment — The number of lives covered by the plan.

EOB — Explanation of benefits. A statement mailed to member (and sometimes provider) explaining claim adjudication and payment.

Episode of care — One or more health care services received during a period of relatively continuous care by a hospital or health care provider.

EPO — Exclusive provider organization. Similar to an HMO but the member must remain within the provider network to receive benefits. EPOs are regulated under insurance statutes rather than HMO legislation.

ERISA — Employee Retirement Income Security Act. An act with several provisions protecting both payer and member, including requiring that payers send the member an EOB when a claim is denied.

Established patient — An individual who has received professional services from the physician, or another physician of the same specialty who belongs to the same group practice, within the past three years.

Exclusions — Also called exceptions, services excluded from a plan's coverage by the employer or payer because of risk or cost.

Experience rating — The designation of a group's previous claims history to help determine premium rates.

Extramural birth — An infant born outside of a sterile environment.

Facility — A place of patient care, including inpatient and outpatient, acute or long term.

Facility of payment — A contractual relationship that permits the payer to pay someone other than the member or provider.

Fact-oriented V codes — Do not describe a problem or a service; they simply state a fact. These generally do not serve as an outpatient primary or inpatient principal diagnosis.

FAR — Federal Acquisition Regulations. Regulations of the federal government's acquisition of services.

FDA — Food and Drug Administration.

Federal Register — A government publication listing all changes in regulations and federally-mandated standards, including HCPCS and ICD-9-CM.

Federally qualified HMO — An HMO that meets CMS guidelines for Medicare reimbursement.

Fee schedule — The maximum fees a plan will pay for services, primarily listed by CPT codes.

FEHBARS —Federal Employee Health Benefits Acquisition Regulations. Federal regulations for acquisition of health services used by government agencies and subcontractors.

FEHBP — Federal Employee Health Benefits Program. Provides health plans to federal workers.

FFS — Fee for service. Situation in which payer pays full charges for medical services.

Formulary — A listing of drugs providers may prescribe as dictated by the plan or Medicare. Prescription of a medication not included in the formulary usually is not reimbursed.

FPP — Faculty practice plan. A form of group practice developed around a teaching program or medical school.

Fragmentation — *See* unbundling.

Fraternal insurance — A cooperative plan provided to members of an association or fraternal group.

FTE — Full time employee. The accounting equivalent of one full time employee that includes wages, benefits, and other costs.

Gatekeeper — A practice in which a member's care must be provided by a primary care physician, unless the physician refers the member to a specialist or approves the care provided by a specialist.

GHAA — Group Health Association of America — An HMO trade organization.

Global surgery package — A code denoting a normal surgical procedure with no complications that includes all of the elements needed to perform the procedure.

GMLOS — Geometric mean length of stay. A component that figures in the reimbursement calculation for a DRG.

Government mandates — Services mandated by state or federal law. In government claims, the correct use of ICD-9-CM codes is required by law. In 1988, Congress passed the Medicare Catastrophic Coverage Act. Although the act itself was later repealed, the mandate requiring ICD-9-CM codes on all physician-submitted Part B claims was upheld. Medicare's rules changed again in 1996, when it began to reject any claim that did not assign the most specific ICD-9-CM code available.

Grace period — The period after a member has terminated employment for which he or she is still covered.

Group model — An HMO that contracts with a group of providers.

Group practice — A group of providers that shares facilities, resources, and staff, and who may represent a single unit in a managed care network.

Grouper — Computer application that assigns DRGs.

 © 2004 Ingenix, Inc.

Guidelines — Information appearing at the beginning of each of the six major sections of the CPT book. They also may appear at the beginning of subsections and code ranges. The information contained in the guidelines provides definitions, explanations of terms, and factors relevant to the section.

HCPCS — Healthcare Common Procedural Coding System. Codes used by Medicare and other payers to describe procedures and supplies.

HCPCS modifiers — Modifiers should, or in some cases must, be used to identify circumstances that alter or enhance the description of a service or supply. Level II/HCPCS modifiers are two alphabetic digits (AA–ZZ). They are recognized by carriers nationally and are updated annually by CMS. Level III /Local modifiers are assigned by individual Medicare carriers and are distributed to physicians and suppliers through carrier newsletters. The carrier may change, add, or delete these local modifiers as needed.

HHS — Health and Human Services. The cabinet department that oversees CMS, Medicare, and other entities.

HIAA — Health Insurance Association of America. A trade organization for payers.

Hierarchy — The rank or order of codes. Numerical hierarchy plays a key role in ICD-9-CM coding because each digit beyond three adds more detail.

HMO — Health maintenance organization. A health plan that uses primary care physicians as gatekeepers. Emphasis is on preventive care.

Hold harmless — The contractual clause stating that if either party is held liable for malpractice, the other party is absolved.

Home health — Palliative and therapeutic care and assistance in the activities of daily life to home bound Medicare and private plan members.

Hospice — A service program, either inpatient or outpatient, that offers palliative support, counseling, and daily resources to the terminally ill and their family members.

Hospital admission plan — Used to facilitate admission to the hospital and to assure prompt payment to the hospital.

IBNR — Incurred but not reported. The amount of money the payer's plan accrues to forestall unknown medical expenses.

ICD-9-CM — *International Classification of Diseases, Ninth edition, Clinically Modified* for use in reimbursement and statistical reporting in the United States. Classification is primarily numeric.

ICD-10 — *International Classification of Diseases, Tenth Revision.* Classification of diseases by alphanumeric code, used by the World Health Organization but not yet adopted in the United States.

ICD-10-CM — Clinical modification of ICD-10 developed for use in the United States.

ICF — Intermediate care facility. A step-down facility for patients leaving the hospital but who cannot be discharged to home because of continuing medical needs.

ID card — The wallet card carried by the member providing name, member number, group number, effective dates, deductibles, and other information.

Immediate maternity — Coverage provided for pregnancies that began prior to the date the member became insured.

In plan — Services chosen from a network provider.

Incontestable clause — A provision in a policy that prohibits the plan from disputing coverage for certain conditions after a specified period of time.

Inpatient hospitalization — A period in which a patient is housed in a single hospital usually without interruption.

Inpatient reimbursement — The payment to hospital for the costs incurred to treat a patient.

Intermediate repair — Repair performed for wounds and lacerations where one or more of the deeper layers of subcutaneous tissue and non-muscle fascia are repaired in addition to the skin and subcutaneous tissue. Single-layer closure can also be coded as an intermediate repair if the wound is heavily contaminated and requires extensive cleaning or removal of particulate matter.

Internal skeletal fixation — Repair involves wires, pins, screws, and/or plates placed through or within the fractured area to stabilize and immobilize the injury.

IPA — Individual practice association. An organization made up of providers who along with the rest of a group contract with payers at a discounted fee-for-service or capitated rate.

IPO — Individual practice organization. *See* IPA.

IS — Information services. The administrators of the computer systems used by payers and providers.

JCAHO — Joint Commission for the Accreditation of Health Organizations. The primary accrediting body for hospitals, out-patient facilities, and other facilities. This non-profit organization audits these facilities and was previously known as the Joint Commission for the Accreditation of Hospitals.

JD — Doctor of Jurisprudence.

Key Components — The three components of history, examination, and medical decision making are considered the keys to selecting the correct level of E/M codes. In most cases, all three components must be addressed in the documentation. However, in established, subsequent, and follow-up categories, only two of the three must be met or exceeded for a given code.

Lag study — A report used by plan managers to determine how long claims are pending and how much is paid out each month.

Lapse — A terminated policy.

Late effect — A residual condition occurring after the acute phase of an illness or injury has terminated. The original illness or injury is healed, but a chronic or long-term condition remains.

LCSW — Licensed Clinical Social Worker.

Limiting charge — The maximum amount a nonparticipating physician can charge for services to a Medicare patient.

Limits — The ceiling for benefits payable under a plan.

Line of business — Different health plans offered by a larger insurer or insurance broker as a product line.

Lives — The unit of measurement used by plans to determine the number of people covered. Calculated by multiplying the number of members by 2.5.

Local medical review policy — A policy that is carrier specific and used in the absence of a national coverage policy and is used to make local Medicare medical coverage decisions when needed. Developing local Medicare policy includes creating a draft policy based on review of medical literature, understanding local practice, soliciting comments from the medical community and Carrier Advisory Committee, responding to and incorporating into final local policy comments received, and notifying providers of the policy effective date.

Long-term care facility — A nursing home or, more specifically, a facility offering extended, non-acute care to a resident patient whose illness does not require acute care.

Loss ratio — The ratio between the cost to deliver medical care and the amount of money taken in by the plan.

LPN — Licensed Practical Nurse.

LVN — Licensed Vocational Nurse/Licensed Visiting Nurse.

MA — Master of Arts degree/Medical Assistant.

MAC — Maximum allowable charge. The maximum a pharmacy vendor can charge for something.

Malingering — The feigning of illness, either as the result of intentional deceit or as the result of mental illness.

Managed health care — 1) The concept of managing cases while in progress to assure care is the most appropriate, efficient, and effective; 2) A system of health care meant to manage overall cost; 3) A method of health care where contracted physicians participate in the management of health care costs.

Mandated benefits — Services mandated by state or federal law such as in child abuse or rape, not necessarily covered by insurers.

Maximum allowable charge — Amount set by insurer as highest amount to be charged for a particular medical service.

MCE — Medical care evaluation. A part of the quality assurance program that reviews the process of medical care.

MCO — Managed care organization. A generic term for EPA, IPO, HMO, and others.

MD — Medical Doctor.

MDC — Major diagnostic category — Classification of diagnoses typically grouped by body system. Used in DRG reimbursement.

ME — Medical Examiner.

MEd — Master of Education.

Medicaid — Federal-state health insurance for qualified low-income people.

Medical consultation — Advice or an opinion rendered by a physician at the request of the primary care provider.

Medical loss ratio — *See* loss ratio.

Medical meaningfulness — Patients in the same DRG can be expected to evoke a set of clinical responses which result in a similar pattern of resource use.

Medicare — A national program that provides medical care to the elderly, people with disabilities, and those who have End Stage Renal Disease (ESRD).

Medicare Carriers Manual — MCM. The manual CMS provides to Medicare carriers. It contains instructions for processing and payment of Medicare claims, preparing reimbursement forms, billing procedures, and Medicare regulations. As processes and regulations change, CMS issues revisions to the manual.

Medicare Fee Schedule — MFS. A fee schedule designed to slow the rise in cost for services and standardizes payment to physicians regardless of specialty or location. Payments vary through geographic adjustments. Different payment for the same service performed by physicians of different specialties is eliminated. The MFS is based on the Resource Based Relative Value Scale (RBRVS). A national total relative value unit (RVU) is given for each procedure (HCPCS Level I [CPT], Level II codes) by a physician. Each total RVU has three components: physician work, practice expense, and malpractice insurance.

Medicare Part A — Coverage includes hospital, nursing home, hospice, home health, and other inpatient care. Claims are submitted to intermediaries for reimbursement. Ten regional offices provide the Centers for Medicare and Medicaid Services (CMS) with a decentralized administration and delivery of Medicare programs. Each regional office manages private insurance companies that contract with the government to process and make payment for Medicare services.

Medicare Part B — Coverage provides payment for physician and outpatient services. Physicians submit

 © 2004 Ingenix, Inc.

their claims to carriers for reimbursement. Regional offices provide the Centers for Medicare and Medicaid Services (CMS) with a decentralized administration and delivery of Medicare programs. Each regional office manages private insurance companies that contract with the government to process and make payment for Medicare services.

Medicare Secondary Payer — MSP. Medicare becomes secondary when patients are 65 or older and have group health benefits through their own employer or their spouse's. Also covered under the MSP program are patients of any age who have End-Stage Renal Disease (ESRD), are covered by an employer group plan, and are in the first 18 months of treatment. Variables apply to this program.

Medicare supplement — Private insurance coverage that pays costs of services not covered by Medicare.

Medigap policy — A health insurance or other health benefit plan offered by a private company to those entitled to Medicare benefits. The policy provides payment for Medicare charges not payable because of deductibles, coinsurance amounts, or other Medicare imposed limitations.

Member — A subscriber of a health plan.

Member months — Total of months each member was covered.

Member services — A payer department that works as a patient advocate to solve problems. The department also works with the patient to take claims appeals to a final committee after all other processes have been exhausted.

Mental health/Substance abuse — A payer term for services rendered to members for emotional problems or chemical dependency.

Mental/Nervous — *See* Mental health/Substance abuse.

MeSH — Medical Staff-Hospital Organization. Organization that bonds hospital and attending medical staff as a network.

MET — Multiple employer trust. A group of employers that joins together to purchase health insurance on a self-funded approach. This approach lowers cost by preventing an adverse selection by broadening the membership pool.

MEWA — Multiple Employer Welfare Association. *See* MET.

MHA — Master of Health Administration.

Minor procedures — Procedures considered by many payers to be part of the package for a primary surgical service.

MIS — Management information system. Hardware and software that facilitates claims management.

Mixed model — An HMO that includes both an open panel and closed panel option.

MLP — Midlevel practitioners. Professionals such as nurse practitioners, nurse midwives, physical therapists, physician assistants, and others who provide medical care but do so with physician input.

MLT — Medical Laboratory Technician.

Modality — 1) A form of imaging. These include x-ray, fluoroscopy, ultrasound, nuclear medicine, duplex Doppler, CT, and MRI; 2) Any physical agent applied to produce therapeutic changes to biologic tissue; includes but is not limited to thermal, acoustic, light, mechanical, or electric energy.

Modifier — A descriptive code attached to a CPT code as a suffix.

Morbidity rate — Actuarial term describing predicted medical expense rate.

MPH — Master of Public Health.

MSA — Medical savings account.

MSN — Master of Science in Nursing.

MSW — Master of Social Work.

MT — Medical Technologist.

Multiple birth — Two or more infants delivered with no complications.

Multiple employer group — A group of employers who contract together to subscribe to a plan, broadening the risk pool and saving money. Different from a multiple employer trust.

NA — Nurse Assistant.

NAHMOR — National Association of HMO Regulators.

NAIC — National Association of Insurance Commissioners. An organization of state insurance regulators.

National coverage policy — Policy outlining Medicare coverage decisions that apply to all states and regions. National coverage policy indicates whether and under what circumstances items/services are covered. These policies are published in CMS regulations in the *Federal Register*, contained in CMS rulings, or issued as program memorandums, manual issuances to Coverage Issues Manual, or the Medicare Carriers Manual.

NBICU — Newborn Intensive Care Unit. A special care unit for premature and seriously ill infants.

NCHS — National Center for Health Statistics.

NCQA — National Committee on Quality Assurance. The organization that accredits payers' quality assurance programs.

ND — Doctor of Naturopathy.

NEC — Not elsewhere classifiable. Indicates that the main term in ICD-9-CM is broad or ill-defined. Use an NEC code only when you lack the information necessary to code to a more specific category. This term is used only in Volume 2.

Neonatal period — The period of an infant's life from birth to the age of 27 days, 23 hours, and 59 minutes.

Network model — A plan that contracts with multiple groups of providers, or networks, to provide care.

New patient — Patient who is receiving care from the provider for the first time within three years.

Newborn admission — An infant born in the facility.

Normal delivery — A baby delivered without complication.

NOS — Not otherwise specified. The equivalent of NEC, indicating that the main term in ICD-9-CM is broad or ill-defined. Use an NOS code only when you lack the information necessary to code to a more specific category. NOS is used only in Volume 1.

NP — Nurse practitioner.

OB — Obstetrician.

Observation patient — A patient who needs to be monitored and assessed for inpatient admission or referral to another site for care.

Occupational therapy — Therapy meant to help a member who is recovering from a serious illness or injury retain activities of daily life.

OL — Outlier threshold. A component that figures in the reimbursement calculation for a DRG.

Open enrollment period — A period of usually one month annually during which members can revise their medical coverage.

Open panel — An arrangement in which a managed care organization that contracts providers on an exclusive basis is still seeking providers.

OPL — Other party liability. In COBs, the decision that the other plan is the primary plan.

Orthotics — Braces and other appliances worn to alleviate a medical condition.

OTR — Occupational Therapist Registered.

Out of plan— Choosing a provider who is not a member of the preferred provider network.

Out of service area — Medical care received out of the geographic area that may or may not be covered, depending on the plan.

Outliers — Medical cases that statistically fall outside of established parameters of length of stay or cost.

Outpatient — A patient who receives care without being admitted for inpatient or resident care.

Outpatient visit — A patient's visit to a recognized outpatient facility or service.

Overutilization — Services rendered by providers more frequently than desired by payers.

PA — 1) Physician's Assistant. 2) Physician Association.

Paneled — A provider contracted with an HMO.

Par provider — Shorthand for a provider who is participating in the plan.

Partial disability — Inability to perform part of one's job.

Partial hospitalization — A situation in which the patient only stays part of each day over a long period. Cardiac, rehabilitation, and chronic pain patients, for example, could use this service.

Partial payment — A payment to the provider or member in which it is expected that other payments will be made before the claim is closed.

PAS norms — Professional acuity study. Based on a professional activity study performed regularly by the Commission Professional and Hospital Activities and broken out by average length of stay (ALOS) by region.

PBM — Prescription benefit managers — HMO staff who monitor amount and use of drugs prescribed.

PCP — Primary care physician. The physician who makes initial diagnosis and referral and retains control over the patient and utilization of services both in and outside the plan.

Pediatric patient — A patient usually younger than 14 years of age.

Peer review — Evaluation of physician's performance by his or her peers.

PEPM — Per employee per month.

PEPP — Payment error prevention program. Program to help reduce Medicare PPS inpatient hospital payment errors.

Per diem reimbursement — Reimbursement to an institution based on a set rate per day rather than on a charge by charge basis.

Percutaneous skeletal fixation — Describes a fracture treatment that is neither open nor closed. Fixation, such as pins, is placed across the fracture site, usually under x-ray imaging.

Perinatal death — Refers to both stillborn births and neonatal deaths.

PharmD — Doctor of Pharmacy.

PhD — Doctor of Philosophy.

PHO — Physician-hospital organization. *See* MeSH.

Physician assistant — A medical professional who receives additional training and can assess, treat, and prescribe medications under a physician's review. *See also* PA.

PIN — Physician identification number.

Plan manager — Payer employee managing all of the contracts and contract negotiations for one or more specific plans.

PMPM — Per member per month.

PMPY — Per member per year.

Pooling — Health payers' practice of combining risk.

 © 2004 Ingenix, Inc.

POS — Point of service. A plan in which members do not have to choose services (HMO vs. traditional) until they need them. Benefits may differ by choice and members may be financially motivated to choose managed care plans.

Posting date —The date a charge is posted to a patient account by the provider. The posting date is frequently not the same as the actual date of service, but usually within five days of the actual date of service. Some providers list the posting date and the actual date of service for a charge.

PPA — Preferred provider arrangement. Similar to a PPO.

PPO — Preferred provider organization. A plan contracting with providers to provide services on a discounted basis. Members must stay within the plan or pay a greater copay.

PPS — Prospective payment system. A payment system, such as DRGs, that pays on historical data of case mix and regional differences.

Pre-existing condition — A condition that existed prior to the effective date of the plan. There is often a short-term or permanent limitation to reimbursement for care of this condition.

Precertification — Preadmission certification. The approval of a procedure or hospital stay before the act by a payer employee, who considers the diagnosis, the planned treatment, and expected length of stay.

Premature delivery — An infant delivered with weight and time of gestation qualifying it as premature.

Presenting problem — A disease, condition, illness, injury, symptom, sign, finding, complaint, or other reason for the patient encounter.

Primary care — First contact and continuing care, including diagnosis and treatment. *See* PCP.

Primary diagnosis — The code reflecting the current, most significant reason for the services or procedures provided. If the disease or condition has been successfully treated and no longer exists, it is not billable and should not be coded.

Principal diagnosis — The condition established after study to be chiefly responsible for occasioning the admission of the patient to the hospital of care.

Principal procedure — The procedure performed for definitive treatment rather than one performed for diagnostic or exploratory purposes, or was necessary to take care of a complication. If there appears to be two procedures that are principal, then the one most related to the principal diagnosis should be selected as the principal procedure.

PRO — Peer review organization. An organization that reviews costs charges in Medicare reimbursement.

Problem-oriented V codes — ICD-9-CM codes that identify circumstances that could affect the patient in the future but are neither a current illness or injury. Use these codes to describe an existing circumstance or problem that may influence future medical care.

Professional association plans — A plan provided by a professional association that affords self-employed professionals (e.g., physicians, CPAs, lawyers) less expensive coverage.

Provider — A business entity that furnishes health care to a consumer.

PT — Physical Therapy. Physical Therapist.

PTA — Physical Therapy Assistant.

PTMPY — Per thousand members per year.

QA — Quality assurance. Monitoring and maintenance of established standards of quality for patient care.

QM — Quality management. Monitoring and maintenance of established standards of quality using techniques proposed by Crosby, Demming, and Juran. *See* TQM.

RBRVS — Resource-based relative value study. A relative value scale originally developed by Harvard for use in Medicare. The scale assigns value to procedures based on the related resources rather than based on historical data.

Reasonable and customary — The prevailing fees for services in a given geographical area.

Referral — In managed care, the primary care physician's act of sending a member to a specialist within or outside the panel.

Regional Medical Center — A descriptive term for a hospital that provides comprehensive services to a large regional area but that may not be a tertiary care facility. Largely used in the west where facilities may serve hundreds of square miles.

Rehabilitation — Physical and mental restoration of disabled members.

Reimbursement — Payment of actual charges incurred as a result of accident or illness.

Reinsurance — Insurance purchased by a payer to protect itself from extremely high losses.

Relative weight — Assigned weight intended to reflect relative resource consumption associated with each DRG.

Review committee — A multidisciplinary committee that considers denied cases being appealed, catastrophic cases, or fee-for-service cases.

RHIA — Registered Health Information Administrator. Formerly known as RRA (Registered Record Administrator). An accreditation for health information administrators.

RHIT — Registered Health Information Technologist. Formerly known as ART (Accredited Records Technician). An accreditation for health information practitioners.

Risk contract — *See* At risk.

Risk factor reduction — The reduction of risk in the pool of members.

Risk manager — The person charged with keeping financial risk low, including malpractice cases.

Risk pool — The pool of people who will be in the insured group, their medical and mental histories, other factors such as age, and their predicted health.

RN — Register nurse.

RPh — Registered Pharmacist.

RPT — Registered Physical Therapist.

RRA — Registered Records Administrator. *See* RHIA.

RRT — Registered Respiratory Therapist.

Rush charge — A charge for expeditious test results.

RVS — Relative value study. A guide that shows the relationship between the time, resources, competency, experience, severity, and other factors necessary to perform procedures.

RVU — Relative value unit. A value assigned a procedure based on difficulty and time consumed used for computing relative value study.

Sanction — Imposition of penalties or exclusion of a provider for infractions such as using services inappropriately, using procedures that are harmful to the patient, and using a technique that is inferior in quality. Fraud will also earn a sanction for the provider.

Schedule — The listing of amounts payable for specific procedures.

Second opinion — Another professional's opinion to help determine the necessity of a medical procedure. This is often required by plans before a surgical procedure.

Secondary insurer — In a COB arrangement, the insurer that reimburses for benefits pending after payment by the primary insurer.

Self-insured or self-funded plan — A plan where the risk is assumed by the employer rather than an insurer.

Self-pay patients — Patients who pay for medical care out-of-pocket.

Separate procedures — Services that are commonly carried out as an integral part of a total service, and as such do not warrant a separate identification. These services are noted in the CPT book with the parenthetical phrase *(separate procedure)* at the end of the description. When this phrase appears before the semicolon, all indented descriptions that follow are covered by it.

Service date — The date a charge is incurred for a service.

Service-oriented V codes — ICD-9-CM codes that identify or define examinations, aftercare, ancillary services, or therapy. Use these V codes to describe the patient who is not currently ill but seeks medical services for some specific purpose such as follow-up visits. You can also use this type of V code as a primary diagnosis for outpatient services when the patient has no symptoms that can be coded and screening services are provided.

Service plan — 1) A plan that has contracts with providers but is not a managed care plan; 2) Another name for Blue Cross/Blue Shield plans.

Shadow pricing — Setting rates just below a competitor's rates. This procedure maximizes profits but raises medical costs.

Short stay patients — In-patients admitted for 48 hours or less, or outpatients who stay 24 hours or less.

Sick baby — An infant with medical complications not resulting from premature birth.

Simple repair — Performed when the wound is superficial, e.g., involving partial or full thickness damage to the skin and/or subcutaneous tissues. There is no significant involvement of deeper structures and only simple, primary suturing is required.

Skeletal traction — The application of a force to a limb segment through a wire, pin, screw, or clamp attached to bone.

Skin traction — The application of a force to a limb using felt or strapping applied directly to skin only.

Small subscriber group aggregate — An aggregate of professional associations, small business, or other entities formed to be considered a single, large subscriber group.

SNF — Skilled nursing facility. A facility that cares for long-term patients with acute medical needs.

Specimen — Tissue submitted for individual and separate attention, requiring individual examination and pathologic diagnosis.

SSN — Social security number.

Staff model — An HMO that employs its own providers.

Standard anesthesia formula — Reimbursement formula that consists of basic value (units) + time units + modifying units (e.g., physical status and qualifying circumstances) + other allowed unit/charges. An abbreviation is B + T + M (basic + time + modifying circumstances). The formula may also include O (other) for other allowed unit charges.

Starred procedure — Identified surgical procedures in the CPT book.

Stat charge — A charge for expeditious test results.

State insurance commission — The state group that approves insurance certificates for each state and regulate the industry based on statutes.

Steering — The act of providing financial incentives to members to use the managed care provider panel.

 © 2004 Ingenix, Inc.

Stop loss — A form of reinsurance that protects health insurance above a certain limit and minimizes risks for providers.

Subrogation — Recovery of monies or benefits from a third party who is liable for the payment.

Subsidiary "In Addition To" codes — Services not included as part of the primary procedure. Key phrases are used throughout the CPT book to indicate that a code is to be used "in addition" to the primary code. Phrases that help identify subsidiary codes include, but are not limited to: each additional, list in addition to, and done at time of other major procedure.

Substantial co-morbidity — A pre-existing condition that will, because of its presence with a specific principle diagnosis, cause an increase in the length of stay by at least one day in approximately 75 percent of the cases.

Substantial complication — A condition that arises during the hospital stay that prolongs the length of stay by at least one day in approximately 75 percent of the cases.

Subtraction — The removal of an overlying structure in order to better visualize the structure in question. This is done in a series by imposing one x-ray on top of another.

Supplemental health services — Benefits HMOs offer in addition to base services.

Surgical package — A normal, uncomplicated performance of specific surgical services, with the assumption that on average, all surgical procedures of a given type are similar with respect to skill-level, duration, and length of normal follow-up care.

Swing beds — Hospital beds designated to serve varying needs, depending on census. This is usually done to convert acute care beds to long-term care to meet a rural community's needs.

TCC — Transitional care center. Used in lieu of extended care facility or prior to discharge to an extended care facility.

Technical component — A part of a radiology service that includes the provision of the equipment, supplies, technical personnel, and costs attendant to the performance of the procedure other than the professional services.

TEFRA — Tax Equity and Fiscal Responsibility Act. An act that protects the rights of full-time employees to remain on the company's plan to age 69.

Tertiary care facility — A hospital providing specialty care to patients referred from other hospitals because of the severity of their injuries or illnesses.

Therapeutic — An act meant to alleviate a medical or mental condition.

Therapeutic procedures — A manner of effecting change through the application of clinical skills and/or services that attempt to improve function.

Therapeutic services — Services performed for treatment of a specific diagnosis. These services include performance of the procedure, various incidental elements, and normal, related follow-up care.

Third party payer — Payer responsible for claims paid by a health plan or member for claims incurred for which the health plan or member should not have primary liability.

Three-digit diagnostic codes — Codes used only when no fourth or fifth digit is available. There are only about 100 codes at the highest level of specificity in the three-digit form. Many payers, including Medicare, do not accept three-digit codes when higher levels of specificity exist.

Time limit — Set number of days in which a claim can be filed.

TPA — Third party administrator. A firm that performs administrative functions for a self-funded plan but assumes no risk.

TPL — The third party payer liable for the cost of an illness or injury, such as auto or homeowner insurer.

TQM — Total quality management. The concept that quality is an organic part of a plan's service and a provider's care and can be quantified and constantly improved.

Transfer — Movement of a patient from one treatment service or location to another.

Treatment plan — The plan of care submitted by the provider to the case manager when seeking certification for a member.

Triage — 1) Medical screening of patients to determine priority of treatment based on severity of illness or injury and resources at hand; 2) Charge levied by health care facilities for emergency and other patients.

Triple option — The offering of an HMO, indemnity plan, and PPO by one insurance firm.

UB-92 — The common claim form used by facilities to bill for services.

UCR — Usual, customary, and reasonable. The prevailing fees for services in a given geographical area.

Unbundling — Breaking a single service into its multiple components to increase total billing charges.

Underwriting — Evaluating and determining the financial risk a member or member group will have on an insurer.

Unlisted procedures — Procedural descriptions in each section of the CPT book used when the overall procedure and outcome of the surgery is not adequately described by an existing CPT code. Use unlisted procedures as a last resort in finding an appropriate CPT code.

Unspecified — A term in ICD-9-CM that indicates more information is necessary to code the term to further specificity. In these cases, the fourth digit of the code is always 9. Fourth digits 0 through 7 identify more specific information of the main term or condition. The fourth-digit number 8 is reserved for identifying other information.

Upcoding — Provider billing for a procedure that reimburses more than the procedure actually performed.

UPIN — Unique physician identification number.

URAC — Utilization Review Accreditation Commission. The accrediting body of case management.

Urgent admission — An admission in which the patient requires immediate attention for treatment of a physical or psychiatric problem.

USP — United States Pharmacopeia.

USPHS — United States Public Health Service.

Utilization review — Review of the utilization of medical services based on the diagnosis, site, ALOS, and other factors in each case.

Utilization review nurse — A nurse who evaluates cases for appropriateness of care and length of service and can plan discharge and services needed after discharge in home health appointments.

V codes — Also known as The Supplementary Classification of Factors Influencing Health Status and Contact with Health Services (V01—V82), V codes describe circumstances that influence a patient's health status and identify reasons for medical encounters resulting from circumstances other than a disease or injury already classified in the main part of ICD-9-CM.

Volume — 1) The number of services performed; 2) The number of patients; 3) The number of patients in a DRG during a specific time.

Weighting — The practice of assigning more worth to a fee based on the number of times it is charged, "weighting" the RBRVS fees for an area.

Well-baby care — Medical services, immunizations, and regular provider visits considered routine for an infant.

Withhold — Percentage of payment to providers held by HMO until cost of referral or services has been determined. If the provider goes over the amount determined appropriate, that amount is kept by the HMO.

Workers' Compensation — Laws requiring employers to furnish care to employees injured on the job.

Wraparound plan — Insurance or health plan coverage for copays and deductibles not covered under a member's base plan.

© 2004 Ingenix, Inc.

Anatomy Charts

Skeletal System

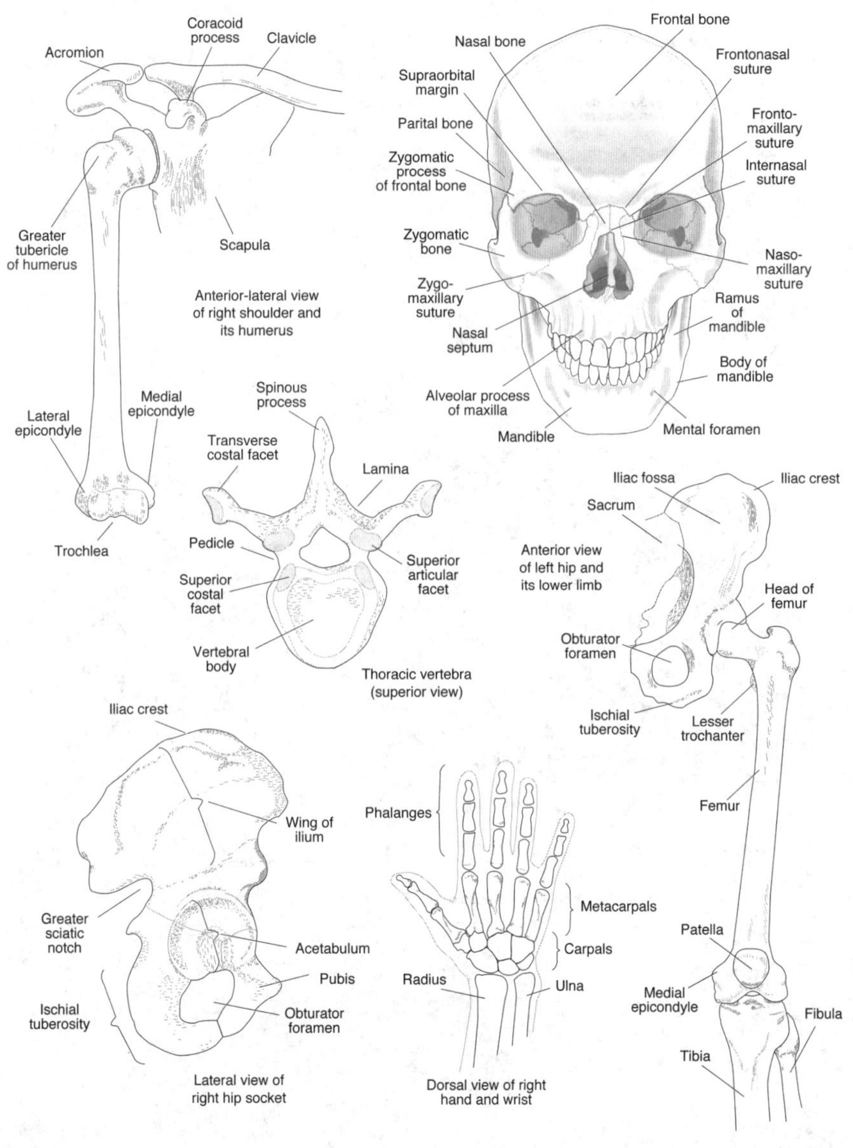

Lympahatic System

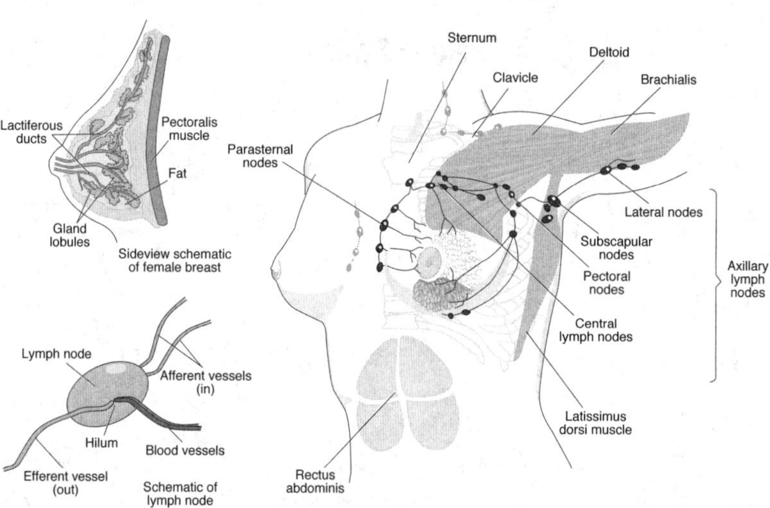

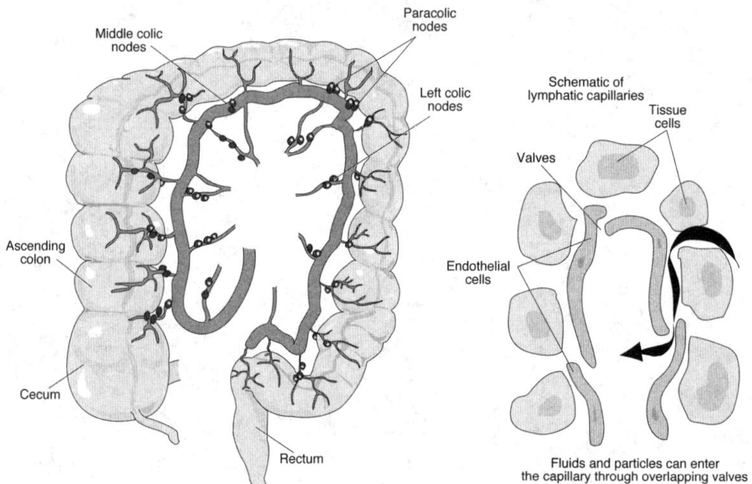

Lymphatic drainage of the colon follows blood supply

 © 2004 Ingenix, Inc.

Endocrine System

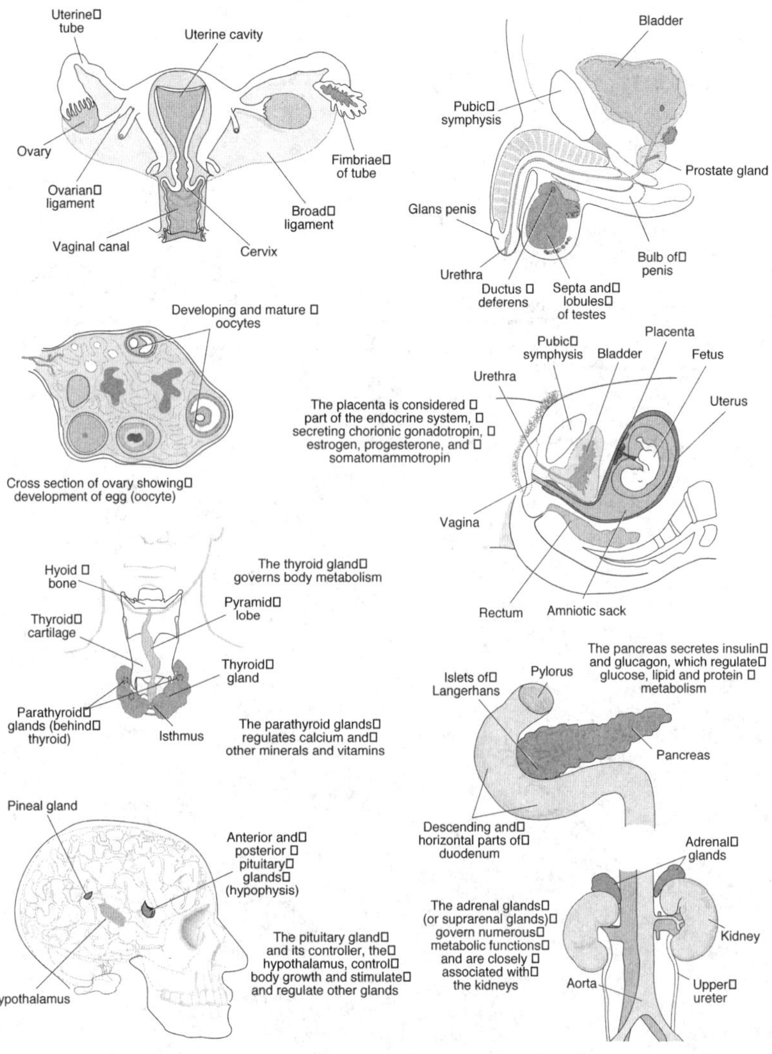

Digestive System

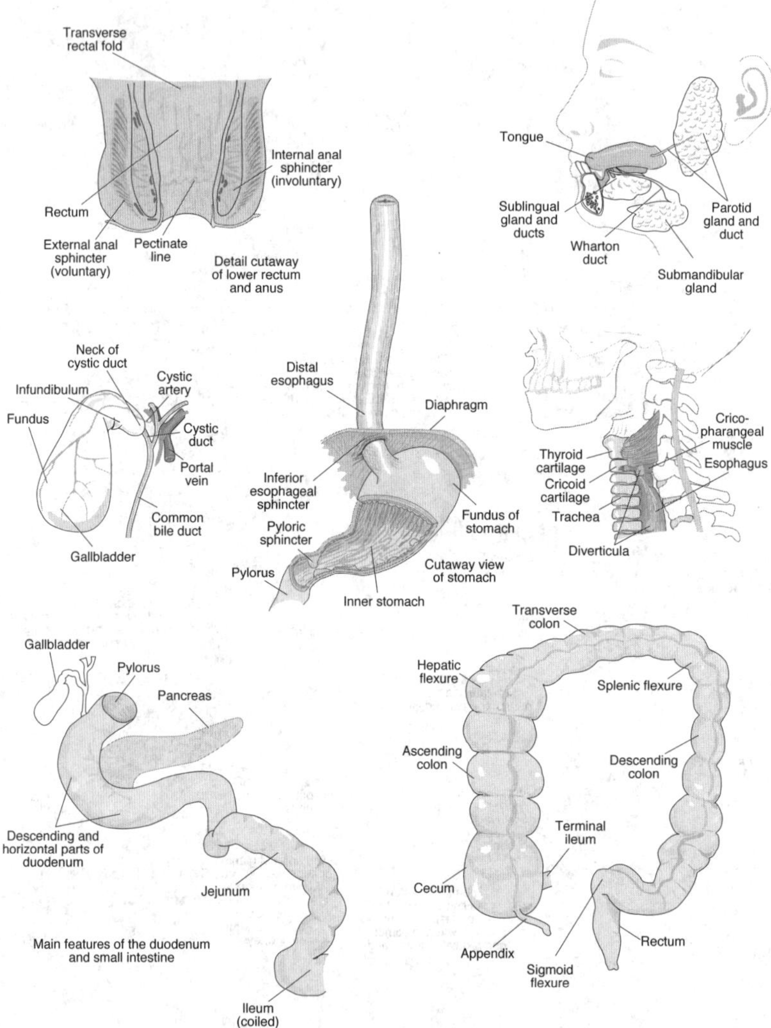

 © 2004 Ingenix, Inc.

Nervous System

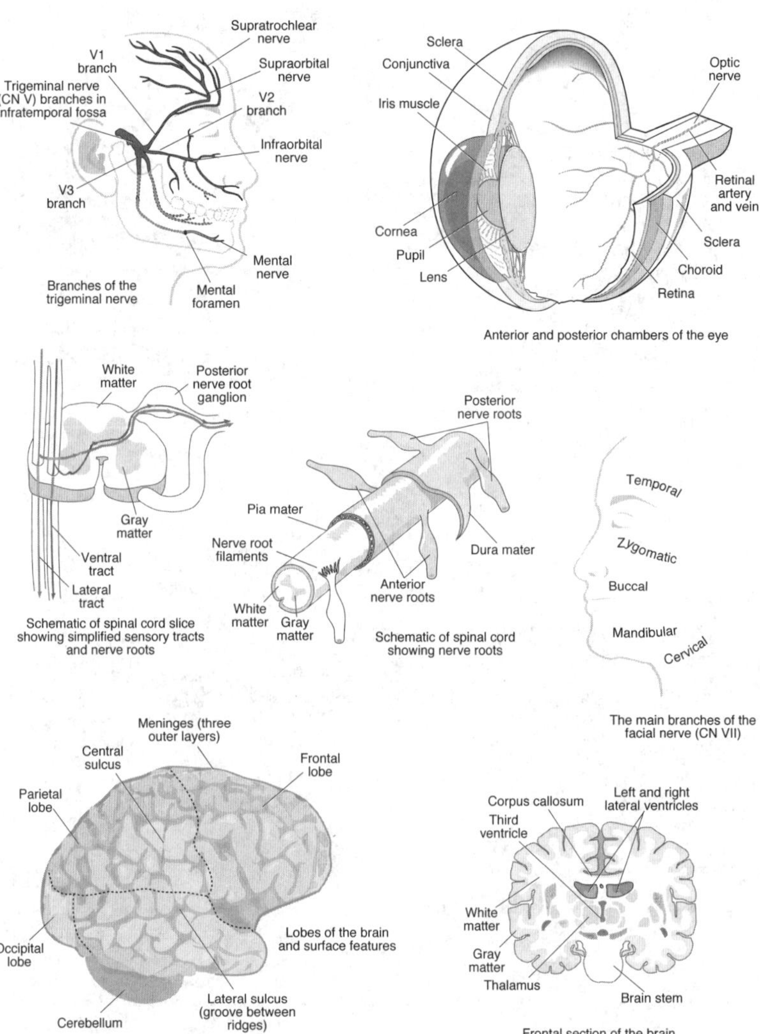

Branches of the trigeminal nerve

Anterior and posterior chambers of the eye

Schematic of spinal cord slice showing simplified sensory tracts and nerve roots

Schematic of spinal cord showing nerve roots

The main branches of the facial nerve (CN VII)

Lobes of the brain and surface features

Frontal section of the brain

© 2004 Ingenix, Inc.

Circulatory System: Arterial

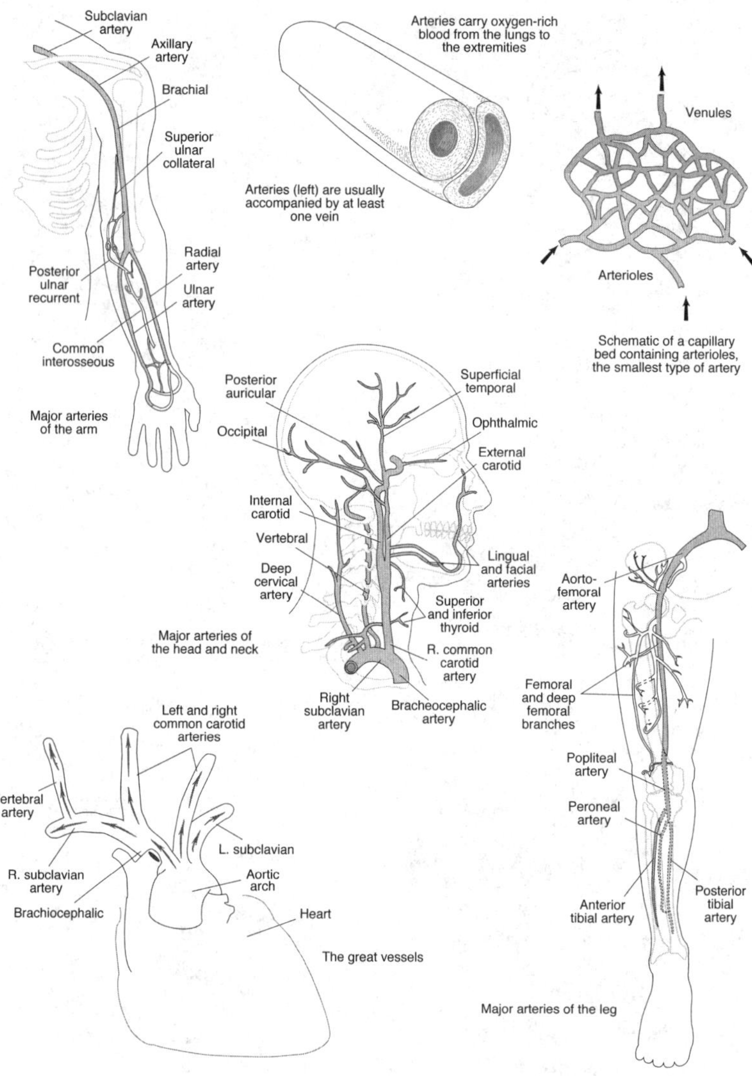

© 2004 Ingenix, Inc.

Circulatory System: Venous

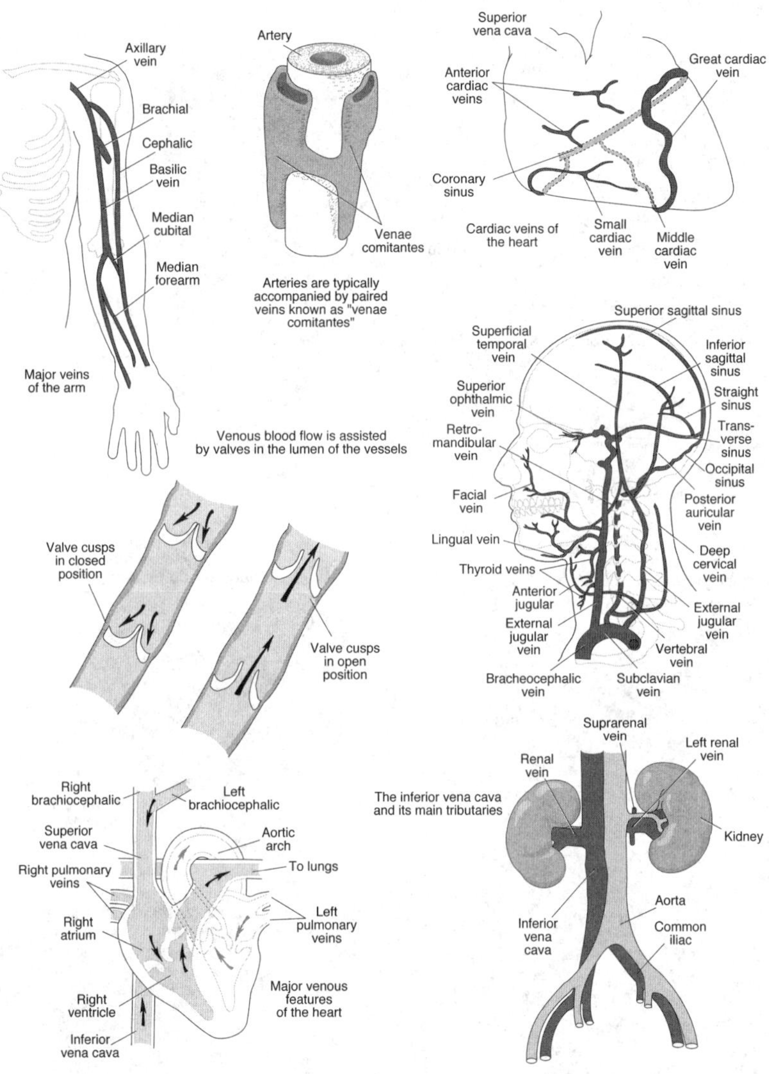

© 2004 Ingenix, Inc.

Urogenital Tracts

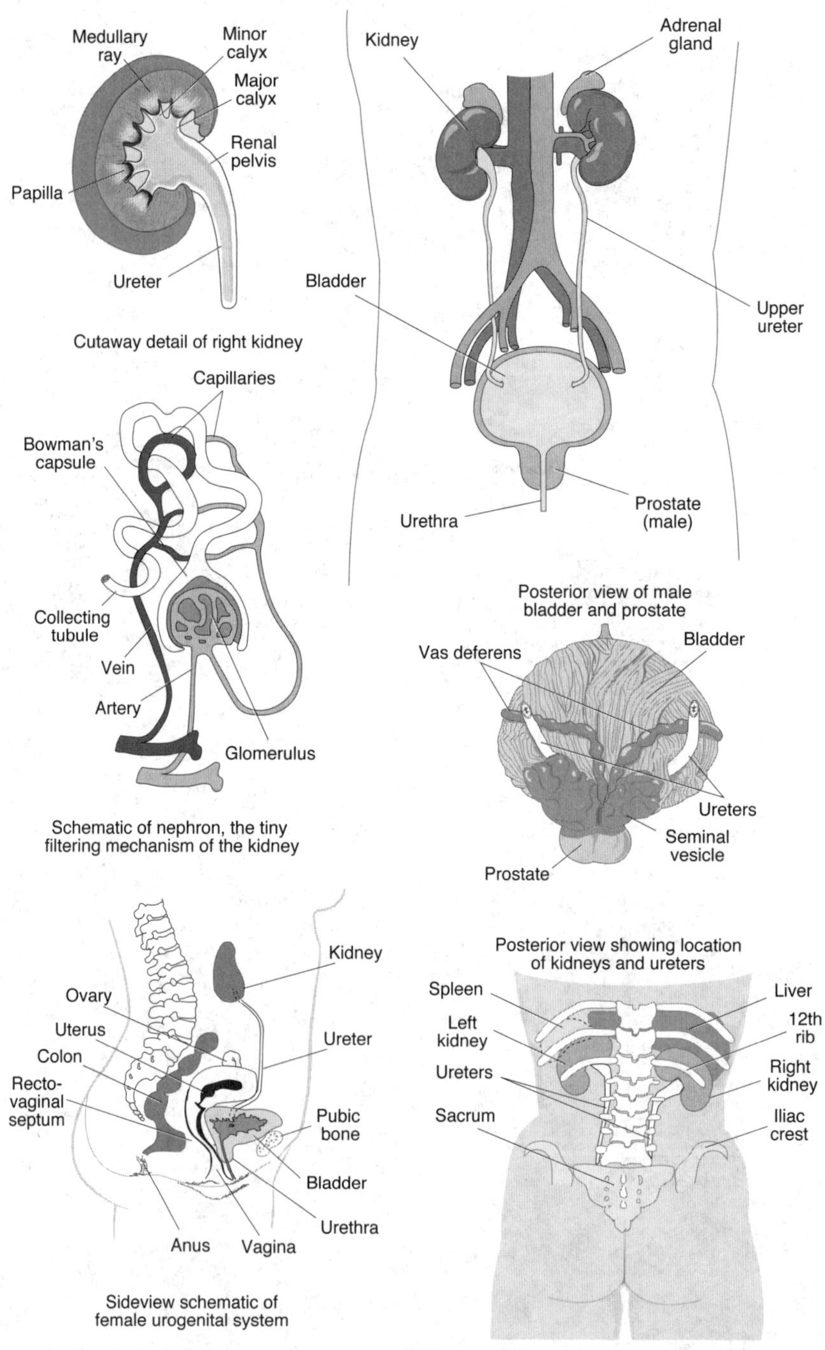

Anatomy Charts

© 2004 Ingenix, Inc.

Respiratory System

The bronchi (dark below) branch further into bronchioles and then into alveolar sacs where venous blood is aerated

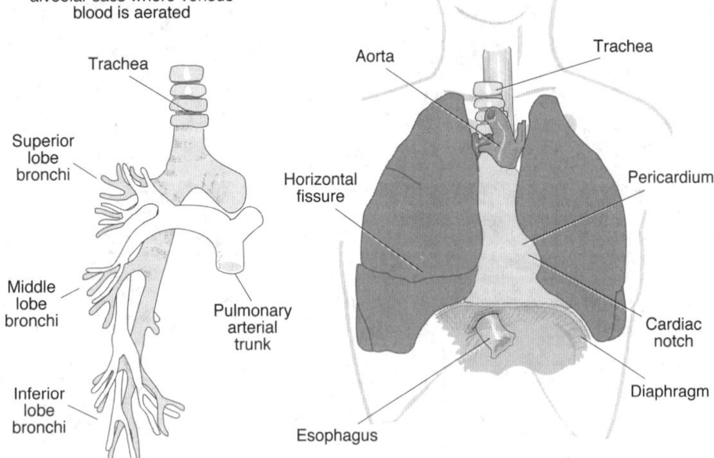

The pulmonary arteries (white above) deliver venous blood to the lungs where it is oxygenated and converted into arterial blood

The right lung is larger and heavier than its counterpart due to space lost to the bulge of the heart at the cardiac notch

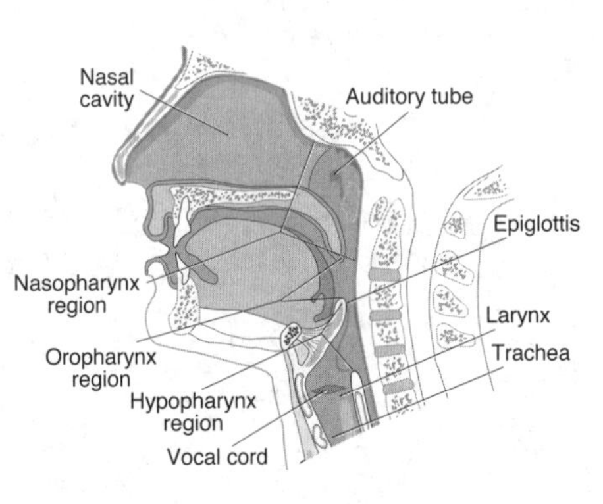

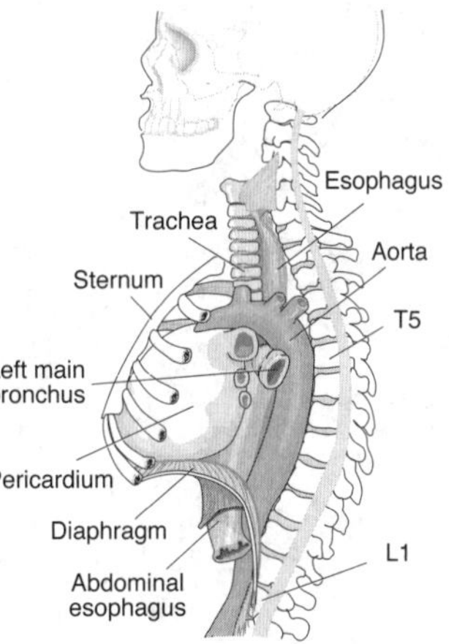

© 2004 Ingenix, Inc.

001–139
Infectious and Parasitic Diseases

This section of ICD-9-CM includes communicable diseases, as well as disease of unknown origin but possibly due to infectious organisms. Infective organisms classified to this chapter include bacteria, chlamydia, fungi, helminths, mycoplasmas, protozoans, rickettsias, and viruses. The diseases may be further divided in ICD-9-CM by anatomic site.

Infectious and parasitic agents live in soil, water, and in the air — virtually everywhere. When these agents infect a host, there are three possible outcomes. The host's immune system can successfully defeat the infective agent. In this outcome, the host may test positive for exposure to the infective agent, but show no symptoms of active disease. In the second outcome, the host can lose ground against the agent, and an equalized state in which the host cannot eradicate the low-grade infection stabilizes. This is generally considered a chronic condition. In its acute form of infection, the infective agent can prevail, causing a multiplication of organisms and an overwhelming infection in the patient. Care must be taken to determine the status of the host before assigning codes. A patient testing positive for tuberculosis, for instance, but exhibiting no symptoms of active disease, would be classified to 795.5 *Nonspecific reaction to tuberculin skin test without active tuberculosis,* rather than to an active TB infection in the 010-018 (active tuberculosis) codes.

In some cases, infectious and parasitic diseases are classified by anatomical site rather than source of infection and found in other chapters of ICD-9-CM. Examples of this include pneumonia and other respiratory infections (460-466), influenza (487), and certain other localized infections. Also, codes reporting contact with infectious diseases, suspected carriers of infectious diseases, and prophylactic vaccination against infectious disease can be found in the supplementary classification of factors influencing health status (V01-V06).

001–009 Intestinal Infectious Diseases

001 Cholera

Cholera is an infection of the entire bowel due to *Vibrio cholerae* and presents with profuse diarrhea, cramps, and vomiting. It is spread through the ingestion of food or water contaminated with feces of an infected person. Cholera is endemic to parts of Asia, Africa, the Middle East, and also portions of the Gulf Coast of the United States. In endemic areas, outbreaks are usually limited to warm seasons. If the infection is imported to other locales, an outbreak can occur in any season.

Symptoms of cholera can be mild or life threatening. Hypovolemia poses the greatest risk, as it can lead to severe metabolic acidosis and possibly renal tubular necrosis. Cholera responds to antibiotics, and with treatment, the mortality rate from cholera is less than one percent.

A toxic effect of antimony is called "antimonial cholera," but has no relation to a *V. cholerae* infection.

001.0 Cholera due to Vibrio cholerae — *Inaba, Ogawa, Hikojima serotypes; classical*

001.1 Cholera due to Vibrio cholerae el tor — *commonly less severe or asymptomatic*

001.9 Unspecified cholera — *unknown whether V. cholerae or V. cholerae el tor*

Coding Clarification

Antimonial cholera is reported with 985.4. Report suspected carrier of cholera with V02.0, and exposure to cholera with V01.0. Vaccination against cholera is reported with V03.0.

002 *Typhoid and paratyphoid fevers*

Typhoid fever is a systemic bacterial disease caused by the unique human strain of salmonella, *Salmonella typhi*. Outbreaks of typhoid are rare, because most of the cases are acquired during foreign travel to underdeveloped countries. Paratyphoid is similar in presentation to typhoid, though usually milder, caused by any of several organisms: *S. paratyphi* (paratyphoid A), *S. schottmulleri* (paratyphoid B), or *S. hirschfeldii* (paratyphoid C). The means of infection, clinical course, pathology, and treatment are similar to those for typhoid.

Typhoid and paratyphoid cause high fever, abdominal pain, and rash. Intestinal hemorrhage may occur in severe cases of typhoid. The bacilli are generally transmitted by the ingestion of food or water that is contaminated with feces from an infected person. While typhoid and paratyphoid A are strictly human diseases, paratyphoid B and C have been found in other animals and fowl. Contamination of food and water by infected animals or fowl can spread paratyphoid B and C. In either case, the organism moves through the gastrointestinal tract and enters the bloodstream through the lymphatic system.

002.0 Typhoid fever — *Widal negative*

002.1 Paratyphoid fever A — *serotype paratyphi A*

002.2 Paratyphoid fever B — *serotype schottmulleri*

002.3 Paratyphoid fever C — *serotype hirschfeldii*

002.9 Unspecified paratyphoid fever — *unknown paratyphoid serotype*

Coding Clarification

Report a suspected carrier of typhoid with V02.1 and vaccination against typhoid with V03.1. When typhoid presents with specific manifestations, report those manifestations secondary to the typhoid infection (endocarditis, 421.1; pneumonia, 484.8; perichondritis, 478.71; osteomyelitis, 730.8x; spine, 720.81).

003 Other salmonella infections

This classification is called "other" salmonella infections because typhoid and paratyphoid infections are caused by strains of salmonella. This classification includes all other salmonellas — more than 1,500 serotypes — except congenital salmonella. Salmonella remains a significant health problem in the United States. About 85 percent of salmonella infections present as gastroenteritis. The other 15 percent present as septicemia or as another infectious disease.

Salmonella gastroenteritis, also known as enteritis, is caused by the ingestion of contaminated foods. Meat, poultry, raw milk, and eggs are the most common sources. Other reported sources include infected pet turtles or lizards, infected dyes, or contaminated marijuana. Immunosuppressed patients are most susceptible to localized salmonella infection.

003.0 Salmonella gastroenteritis — *gastrointestinal infection*

003.1 Salmonella septicemia — *bloodstream infection*

003.20 Unspecified localized salmonella infection — *unknown localized site*

003.21 Salmonella meningitis — *infection of membranes of brain/spinal cord*

003.22 Salmonella pneumonia — *infection of lungs*

003.23 Salmonella arthritis — *infection of joint*

003.24 Salmonella osteomyelitis — *infection of bone*

003.29 Other localized salmonella infections — *other localized site*

003.8 Other specified salmonella infections — *other salmonella infection*

003.9 Unspecified salmonella infection

Coding Clarification

Suspected carrier of salmonella is reported with V02.3. Congenital salmonella is reported with 771.81.

004 Shigellosis

Shigellosis is a bacterium that causes an acute infection of the bowel with fever, irritability, drowsiness, anorexia, nausea, vomiting, diarrhea, abdominal pain, and distension. Blood, pus, and mucus are found in the stool. Ingestion of food contaminated by feces of infected individuals is the most common source of infection. Incubation period is one to four days.

There are four species in the *Shigella* genus and they differ according to their biochemical reactions. All cause dysentery in humans and some primates.

004.0 Shigella dysenteriae — *subgroup A, severe dysenteria; type 1 can be fatal in children; Schmitz bacillus, Bacillus dysenteriae or Bacterium dysenteriae*

004.1 Shigella flexneri — *subgroup B; Shigella paradysenteriae and Flexner's bacillus*

004.2 Shigella boydii — *subgroup C; tropical locales, causing severe diarrhea*

004.3 Shigella sonnei — *subgroup D, milder dysentery; Sonne-Duval bacillus or Bacterium sonnei.*

004.8 Other specified shigella infections — *other than A,B,C,D*

004.9 Unspecified shigellosis — *unknown shigella infection*

Coding Clarification

Suspected *Shigella* carrier is reported with V02.3.

005 Other food poisoning (bacterial)

Food poisoning as reported with a code from category 005 reports the ingestion of bacteria that leads to gastrointestinal infection.

Staphylococcal enterotoxin is a common cause of food poisoning that can occur when an infected food handler introduces the staph into egg, milk, or meat products. The infection multiplies in the protein-rich media. An acute bout of diarrhea and vomiting usually occurs within a few hours of ingestion, and resolves within several hours. Hypovolemia poses the greatest risk to the elderly, the young, and the immunosuppressed, but this form of food poisoning rarely is fatal.

Clostridium botulinum is a neurotoxic bacterium and ingestion of contaminated food leads to optic neurology symptoms including diplopia, loss of accommodation, or blepharoptosis. Gastrointestinal symptoms including vomiting and diarrhea may precede neurological symptoms. No fever is present. Improperly canned food is the most common source

 © 2004 Ingenix, Inc.

of botulism. With treatment, the mortality rate of botulism is still significant although at less than 10 percent.

Food poisoning by *V. vulnificus* is the result of eating raw seafood. Resulting gastroenteritis can be severe and may be fatal to persons with liver disease.

Bacillus cereus (005.89) is commonly found in soil, milk, and other dried food, such as cereals, herbs, and spices. Meat pies, fried rice, and puddings are frequently implicated in outbreaks.

Botulism is a muscle-paralyzing disease caused by a toxin made by the bacterium *Clostridium botulinum.*

There are three main types of botulism:

- Foodborne botulism occurs when a person ingests pre-formed toxin that leads to illness within a few hours to days. Foodborne botulism is a public health emergency because the contaminated food may still be available to other persons aside from the patient. Foodborne botulism can occur in all age groups. With foodborne botulism, symptoms begin within six hours to two weeks (most commonly between 12 and 36 hours) after eating toxin-containing food. Symptoms of botulism include double vision, blurred vision, drooping eyelids, slurred speech, difficulty swallowing, dry mouth, muscle weakness that always descends through the body: shoulders are affected, then upper arms, lower arms, thighs, calves, etc. Paralysis of breathing muscles can cause a person to stop breathing and die, unless assistance with breathing (mechanical ventilation) is provided.

- Infant botulism occurs in a small number of susceptible infants each year who harbor *C. botulinum* in their intestinal tract.

- Wound botulism occurs when wounds are infected with *C. botulinum,* which secretes the toxin.

The Centers for Disease Control maintains a supply of antitoxin against botulism. The antitoxin is effective in reducing the severity of symptoms if administered early in the course of the disease. Most patients eventually recover after weeks to months of supportive care.

005.0 Staphylococcal food poisoning — *Staphylococcal toxemia due to food*

005.1 Botulism — *Clostridium botulinum*

005.2 Food poisoning due to Clostridium perfringens (C. welchii) — *enteritis necroticans*

005.3 Food poisoning due to other Clostridia — *other or unknown*

005.4 Food poisoning due to Vibrio parahaemolyticus — *from fish; common to Japan*

005.81 Food poisoning due to Vibrio vulnificus — *severe enteritis from seafood; may progress to septicemia*

005.89 Other bacterial food poisoning — *Bacillus cereus*

005.9 Unspecified food poisoning

Coding Clarification

C. perfringens is commonly found in soil, air, and water. When the bacterium contaminates meat, it forms spores that cause mild gastroenteritis in type A or severe, life-threatening gastroenteritis in type C. Both are reported with 005.2.

Report 005.1 *Botulism for food poisoning by C. botulinum* if botulism was contracted as a result of terrorist acts, E997.1 *Injury due to biological warfare* may be reported in addition to code rubric 005.1. If there is only a suspicion that the patient has been exposed, report V74.8 *Special screening* for other specified bacterial and spirochetal diseases to report the medical necessity of botulism testing.

006 Amebiasis

There are 50 million annual cases of amebiasis worldwide, with 40,000 to 50,000 deaths attributed to amebiasis annually.

Amebiasis is most common in tropical areas where crowded living conditions and poor sanitation exist. Africa, Latin America, Southeast Asia, and India have significant health problems associated with amebiasis. In amebiasis, protozoa can live in the large intestine without causing symptoms or it can invade the colon wall causing colitis, acute dysentery, or chronic diarrhea. The infection may spread through the blood to the liver, and, rarely, to the lungs, brain, or other organs.

Transmission occurs through ingestion of feces in contaminated food or water, use of human feces as fertilizer, or person-to-person contact. Malnutrition and alcoholism predispose a person to more severe disease, as does immunosuppression. Recent travel to a tropical region is a risk factor. In the United States, immunosuppressed populations, people living in institutions, people with disabilities, and male homosexuals are considered higher risk groups, although the infection rate in the United States is low at less than 1 percent.

006.0 Acute amebic dysentery without mention of abscess — *sudden, severe dysentery*

006.1 Chronic intestinal amebiasis without mention of abscess — *persistent dysentery*

006.2 Amebic nondysenteric colitis — *inflamed colon but no dysentery*

006.3 Amebic liver abscess — *liver infection*

006.4 Amebic lung abscess — *lung with or without liver infection*

006.5 Amebic brain abscess — *brain with or without lung and/or liver*

006.6 Amebic skin ulceration — *cutaneous amebiasis*

006.8 Amebic infection of other sites — *including seminal vesicle, bladder, appendix or other site infection, ameboma*

006.9 Unspecified amebiasis — *unknown or unspecified*

Coding Clarification

Codes in the rubric 006 are used to report infection or ulceration due to *Entamoeba histolytica.* If the ameba is other than *E. histolytica,* report 007.8 instead. Meningoencephalitis due to *Naegleria gruber* is reported with 136.2. Suspected carrier of amebic disease is reported with V02.2.

007 Other protozoal intestinal diseases

Giardia lamblia is the most common intestinal parasite in the United States and is classified to this rubric. Giardiasis is an infection of the lumen of the small intestine, spread by contaminated food and water or by direct contact. Commonly, contaminated water from lakes or streams is a source of the disease. Most cases are asymptomatic, but those with symptoms experience diarrhea, nausea, lassitude, anorexia, and weight loss.

Cryptosporidiosis is usually transmitted person-to-person and the symptoms are mild and self-limited in a healthy population. However, cryptosporidiosis is frequently seen as an opportunistic infection in the acquired immune deficiency syndrome (AIDS), causing profound dehydration and electrolyte imbalances. There is no specific antibiotic therapy for cryptosporidiosis. Treatment consists of rehydration and electrolyte management.

007.0 Balantidiasis — *Balantidium coli infection*

007.1 Giardiasis — *Giardia lamblia, lambliasis infection*

007.2 Coccidiosis — *Isospora belli, Isospora hominis infection*

007.3 Intestinal trichomoniasis — *Trichomonas infection*

007.4 Cryptosporidiosis — *Cryptosporidium infection is self-limiting in immunocompetent cattle workers, debilitating in immunosuppressed patients*
AHA: Q4, 1997, 30

007.5 Cyclosporiasis — *dysentery from Cyclospora infection*
AHA: Q4, 2000, 38

007.8 Other specified protozoal intestinal diseases — *including chilomastigiasis, craigiasis*

007.9 Unspecified protozoal intestinal disease — *unknown*

Coding Clarification

In the case of an AIDS patient with cryptosporidiosis and volume depletion, report the AIDS first (042), followed by cryptosporidiosis (007.4) and volume depletion (276.5).

008 Intestinal infections due to other organisms

Intestinal infections caused by *Escherichia* coli are covered in the 008 rubric. The infections are classified by the degree of penetration into intestinal tissue.

008.00 Intestinal infection due to unspecified E. coli — *not otherwise specified*
AHA: Q4, 1992, 17

008.01 Intestinal infection due to enteropathogenic E. coli — *inflammation of intestines*
AHA: Q4, 1992, 17

008.02 Intestinal infection due to enterotoxigenic E. coli — *toxic reaction in intestinal mucosa, causing voluminous watery secretions*
AHA: Q4, 1992, 17

008.03 Intestinal infection due to enteroinvasive E. coli — *infection penetrates intestinal mucosa*
AHA: Q4, 1992, 17

008.04 Intestinal infection due to enterohemorrhagic E. coli — *infection penetrates intestinal mucosa, causing ulceration and bleeding*
AHA: Q4, 1992, 17

008.09 Intestinal infection due to other intestinal E. coli infections

008.1 Intestinal infection due to Arizona group of paracolon bacilli — *Arizona (bacillus)*

008.2 Intestinal infection due to aerobacter aerogenes — *Enterobacter aerogenes*

008.3 Intestinal infections due to proteus (mirabilis) (morganii) — *Morganella morganii, Salmonella morganii*

008.41 Intestinal infections due to staphylococcus

008.42 Intestinal infections due to pseudomonas

008.43 Intestinal infections due to campylobacter

008.44 Intestinal infections due to yersinia enterocolitica

008.45 Intestinal infections due to clostridium difficile

008.46 Intestinal infections due to other anerobes

008.47 Intestinal infections due to other gram-negative bacteria

008.49 Intestinal infection due to other organisms

008.5 Intestinal infection due to unspecified bacterial enteritis

008.61 Intestinal infection, enteritis due to rotavirus

 © 2004 Ingenix, Inc.

008.62 Intestinal infection, enteritis due to adenovirus

008.63 Intestinal infection, enteritis due to Norwalk virus

008.64 Intestinal infection, enteritis due to other small round viruses (SRVs)

008.65 Intestinal infection, enteritis due to calcivirus

008.66 Intestinal infection, enteritis due to astrovirus

008.67 Intestinal infection, enteritis due to enterovirus not elsewhere classified

008.69 Intestinal infection, enteritis due to other viral enteritis

008.8 Intestinal infection due to other organism, NEC

Coding Clarification

Infections or food poisoning caused by other agents are reported with codes in the 005 rubric.

Congenital *E. coli* is coded to 771.81 *Septicemia [Sepsis] of newborn*, 038.42 *Septicemia due to E. coli*, and 041.4 *E. coli in conditions classified elsewhere (code first the disease then the bacterial agent)*.

Gastroenteritis and enteritis due to a specified virus is coded to 008.61-008.69.

Use 008.69 to report a specified virus when it is not elsewhere classified or 008.8 to report the infection when it is not elsewhere classified or otherwise specified.

009 Ill-defined intestinal infections

Colitis is the inflammation of the colon, while enteritis is the inflammation of the intestine, especially small intestine. Gastroenteritis is inflammation of the mucous membranes of the stomach and intestines. Diarrhea describes copious, loose bowels without evidence of infection or inflammation of the gastrointestinal tract.

009.0 Infectious colitis, enteritis, and gastroenteritis — *known to be infectious*
AHA: Q3, 1999, 4

009.1 Colitis, enteritis, and gastroenteritis of presumed infectious origin — *presumed to be infectious*
AHA: Q3, 1999, 6

009.2 Infectious diarrhea — *known to be infectious*

009.3 Diarrhea of presumed infectious origin — *presumed to be infectious*
AHA: Nov-Dec, 1987, 7

Coding Clarification

Use this series of codes only when more specific information in not available. If the source of infection is known, use an infective enteritis code from the 001-008 series. Noninfective colitis, enteritis, or gastroenteritis is reported with codes in the 555-558 series, and diarrhea due to noninfectious causes is reported with 787.91. Allergic diarrhea is reported with 558.3; nervous diarrhea with 306.4.

Coding Scenario

An acute lymphoblastic leukemia patient presents with extreme abdominal pain, having finished his course of chemotherapy the previous week. His laboratory findings are as follows: profound neutropenia- white count of .2, absolute neutrophil count of 20. The hematologist has diagnosed acute neutropenic enterocolitis. Abdominal surgery is not required.

> Code assignment: The physician must be queried as to the nature of the enterocolitis-infectious vs. noninfectious.
>
> If the enteritis is infectious, the codes are as follows: 288.0 *Agranulocytosis;* 009.1 *Colitis, enteritis, and gastroenteritis, of presumed infectious origin;* E933.1 *Adverse effect of antineoplastic drugs;* and 204.00 *Lymphoid leukemia, acute, without mention of remission.*

010–018 Tuberculosis

Tuberculosis (TB) is a bacterial infection that usually attacks the lungs, but which may also affect other organs. The disease is caused by *Mycobacterium tuberculosis.* TB is transmitted by inhaling air droplets exhaled by an infected person, or sometimes, the infection is absorbed through the skin. Medical technicians handling TB specimens may contract the disease through skin wounds. TB has also been reported in people who have received tattoos or circumcisions in nonsterile conditions.

Symptoms of TB include coughing, chest pain, shortness of breath, loss of appetite, weight loss, fever, chills, and fatigue. Children and people with weakened immune systems are the most susceptible to TB.

A person may become infected with TB bacteria and not develop the disease. The immune system may destroy the bacteria completely. Only 5 to 10 percent of people infected with TB actually become sick.

010 Primary tuberculous infection

Primary TB is the stage of the disease absent of any noticeable symptoms. The disease is not contagious in the early stage. Macrophages, immune cells that detect and destroy foreign matter, ingest the TB bacteria and transport them to the lymph nodes where they may be inhibited, destroyed, or may multiply.

The following fifth-digit subclassification is for use with categories 010-018:

0 unspecified
1 bacteriological or histological examination not done
2 bacteriological or histological examination unknown (at present)
3 tubercle bacilli found (in sputum) by microscopy
4 tubercle bacilli not found (in sputum) by microscopy, but found by bacterial culture
5 tubercle bacilli not found by bacteriological examination, but tuberculosis confirmed histologically
6 tubercle bacilli not found by bacteriological or histological examination but tuberculosis confirmed by other methods (inoculation of animals)

010.0 5th Primary tuberculous complex — *first infection, lung*

010.1 5th Tuberculous pleurisy in primary progressive tuberculosis — *first infection, lung and lung lining*

010.8 5th Other primary progressive tuberculosis infection — *primary site other than pulmonary*

010.9 5th Primary tuberculous infection, unspecified — *unknown primary tuberculosis*

011 Pulmonary tuberculosis

If the bacteria multiply, active primary tuberculosis will develop along with typical symptoms of TB: coughing, night sweats, weight loss, and fever. A chest x-ray typically shows shadows or fluid collection between the lung and its lining.

If the bacteria are suppressed but not destroyed, they will be contained in a mass known as a granuloma or tubercle: a wall of immune cells around inactive bacteria to protect the body from infection. As long as the immune system remains strong, the TB bacteria remain walled off and inactive. The tubercle gradually collects calcium deposits to form a Ghon focus.

Initial tubercles in the lung usually heal, leaving permanent scars that appear as shadows in chest x-rays. At this primary stage of TB, the disease does not progress, but bacteria may remain dormant in the body for many years. If the immune system becomes weakened, the tubercle opens, releases the bacteria, and the infection may develop into secondary TB.

011.0 5th Tuberculosis of lung, infiltrative — (Use additional code to identify any associated silicosis, 502) — *clusters of TB bacilli in lung*

011.1 5th Tuberculosis of lung, nodular — (Use additional code to identify any associated silicosis, 502) — *infiltration of TB leads to formation of nodules*

011.2 5th Tuberculosis of lung with cavitation — (Use additional code to identify any associated silicosis, 502) — *further infiltration of TB leads to cavities*

011.3 5th Tuberculosis of bronchus — (Use additional code to identify any associated silicosis, 502) — *clusters of TB bacilli in bronchial tissue*

011.4 5th Tuberculous fibrosis of lung — (Use additional code to identify any associated silicosis, 502) — *TB cells in lungs surrounded by fibrous tissue*

011.5 5th Tuberculous bronchiectasis — (Use additional code to identify any associated silicosis, 502) — *TB causes bronchial dilation and cough*

011.6 5th Tuberculous pneumonia (any form) — (Use additional code to identify any associated silicosis, 502) — *TB causes inflammatory reaction of lung*

011.7 5th Tuberculous pneumothorax — (Use additional code to identify any associated silicosis, 502) — *TB causes spontaneous rupture of lung tissue*

011.8 5th Other specified pulmonary tuberculosis — (Use additional code to identify any associated silicosis, 502) — *not elsewhere classified*

011.9 5th Unspecified pulmonary tuberculosis — (Use additional code to identify any associated silicosis, 502) — *unknown type*

012 Other respiratory tuberculosis

Rubric 012 is used to report tuberculosis of respiratory sites other than the lung without lung involvement, such as the pleura; intrathoracic lymph nodes; trachea or bronchus alone; larynx (including the glottis); and the mediastinum, nasopharynx, nose, or sinus.

Tuberculosis of other respiratory sites, such as the nose, can be due to a primary or secondary infection with *Mycobacterium tuberculosis.*

A pleural effusion occurs after the initial infection. The result of a release of a small amount of tuberculoprotein within the lung into the plural space causing an inflammatory response and a resulting accumlation of fluid.

At the time of the initial infection, hilar and mediastinal lymph nodes become seeded with bacilli, and other lymph nodes may also become involved. The infection may progress to clinical significance, may become active at a late date, or may never become active.

012.0 5th Tuberculous pleurisy — *inflammation of lung lining*

 © 2004 Ingenix, Inc.

012.1 ✓5th Tuberculosis of intrathoracic lymph nodes — *hilar, mediastinal, tracheobronchial lymph infection*

012.2 ✓5th Isolated tracheal or bronchial tuberculosis — *without lung involvement*

012.3 ✓5th Tuberculous laryngitis — *infection of glottis*

012.8 ✓5th Other specified respiratory tuberculosis — *mediastinum, nasopharynx, nose, or sinus infection, other*

013 Tuberculosis of meninges and central nervous system

Nearly all TB in the United States originates as a pulmonary disease, though before pasteurization, infection commonly occurred at other anatomical sites with the ingestion of contaminated milk or milk products. Today in the United States, sites other than the lung are considered secondary to pulmonary infection.

013.0 ✓5th Tuberculous meningitis — *infection of cerebral or spinal meninges*

013.1 ✓5th Tuberculoma of meninges — *enlarged tubercle in lining or brain or spinal cord*

013.2 ✓5th Tuberculoma of brain — *enlarged tubercle in brain*

013.3 ✓5th Tuberculous abscess of brain — *abscess of brain*

013.4 ✓5th Tuberculoma of spinal cord — *enlarged tubercle in spinal cord*

013.5 ✓5th Tuberculous abscess of spinal cord — *abscess of spinal cord*

013.6 ✓5th Tuberculous encephalitis or myelitis — *inflammation of brain or spinal cord*

013.8 ✓5th Other specified tuberculosis of central nervous system — *other CNS site*

013.9 ✓5th Unspecified tuberculosis of central nervous system — *unknown CNS site*

014 Tuberculosis of intestines, peritoneum, and mesenteric glands

Infection of the intestinal tract by the tuberculin bacillus can occur through the blood, through swallowing the organisms from the pulmonary tract, or through penetration of the intestinal layers from granuloma or from other infected sites.

Wide-spread, intra-abdominal infection may result in peritonitis, which may present in an exudative form with ascites, or a fibrotic form with slight to no ascites but with intraperitoneal adhesions. Peritoneal tuberculosis is often associated with a concomitant pleural effusion.

014.0 ✓5th Tuberculous pertonitis — *inflammation of the lining of the abdomen*

014.8 ✓5th Tuberculosis of intestines, peritoneum, and mesentric glands, other

015 Tuberculosis of bones and joints

Tuberculosis of the bone or joints is usually limited to cases in which the primary TB occurs during childhood. Sometimes, the symptoms do not present themselves for years. In joint disease, arthritis is present. In bone infection, bone may be destroyed. In Pott's disease, the patient may be asymptomatic until deformity occurs or vertebrae collapse.

015.0 ✓5th Tuberculosis of vertebral column — (Use additional code to identify manifestation: 711.4, 720.81, 727.01, 730.8, 737.4) — *Pott's disease, sacrum, spine, vertebra, lordosis, scoliosis, intervertebral*

015.1 ✓5th Tuberculosis of hip — (Use additional code to identify manifestation: 711.4, 727.01, 730.8) — *joint or bone infection*

015.2 ✓5th Tuberculosis of knee — (Use additional code to identify manifestation: 711.4, 727.01, 730.8) — *joint or bone infection*

015.5 ✓5th Tuberculosis of limb bones — (Use additional code to identify manifestation: 711.4, 727.01, 730.8) — *long bones, hands, feet, wrist, ankle, dactylitis*

015.6 ✓5th Tuberculosis of mastoid — (Use additional code to identify manifestation: 711.4, 727.01, 730.8) — *mastoiditis*

015.7 ✓5th Tuberculosis of other specified bone — (Use additional code to identify manifestation: 711.4, 727.01, 730.8) — *jaw, bony pelvis, shoulder blade, other bone*

015.8 ✓5th Tuberculosis of other specified joint — (Use additional code to identify manifestation: 711.4, 727.01, 730.8) — *wrist, ankle, sacroiliac, shoulder, other joint*

015.9 ✓5th Tuberculosis of unspecified bones and joints — (Use additional code to identify manifestation: 711.4, 727.01, 730.8) — *cartilage, ganglion, rheumatism, other synovitis or tenosynovitis*

016 Tuberculosis of genitourinary system

Code tuberculosis of the genitourinary system with the appropriate code from the following range, based on the specific organ affected.

016.0 ✓5th Tuberculosis of kidney — (Use additional code to identify manifestation: 583.81, 590.81) — *renal, perinephritic*

016.1 ✓5th Tuberculosis of bladder — *cystitis*

016.2 ✓5th Tuberculosis of ureter — *ureter only*

016.3 ✓5th Tuberculosis of other urinary organs — *urethra*

016.4 ✓5th Tuberculosis of epididymis

016.5 ✓5th Tuberculosis of other male genital organs — (Use additional code to identify manifestation: 601.4, 608.81) — *bulbourethral gland, Cowper's gland, penis, prepuce, prostate, scrotum, spermatic cord, testis*

016.6 ✓5th Tuberculous oophoritis and salpingitis — *fallopian tube, ovary*

016.7 ✓5th Tuberculosis of other female genital organs — *broad ligament, cervix, endometrium, placenta, uterus*

016.9 ✓5th Genitourinary tuberculosis, unspecified — *unknown genitourinary site*

017 Tuberculosis of other organs

Code tuberculosis of other organs with the appropriate code from the following range, based on the specific organ affected.

017.0 ✓5th Tuberculosis of skin and subcutaneous cellular tissue — *cellulitis, colliquativa, cutis, scrofuloderma*

017.1 ✓5th Erythema nodosum with hypersensitivity reaction in tuberculosis — *Bazin's disease, erythema induratum, tuberculosis indurativa*

017.2 ✓5th Tuberculosis of peripheral lymph nodes — *axilla, cervical, neck*

017.3 ✓5th Tuberculosis of eye — (Use additional code to identify manifestation: 363.13, 364.11, 370.31, 370.59, 379.09) — *conjunctiva, globe, iris, lacrimal apparatus, retina*

017.4 ✓5th Tuberculosis of ear — *inner ear, middle ear; excludes mastoid*

017.5 ✓5th Tuberculosis of thyroid gland — *thyroid*

017.6 ✓5th Tuberculosis of adrenal glands — *bronze (Addison's) disease*

017.7 ✓5th Tuberculosis of spleen — *spleen*

017.8 ✓5th Tuberculosis of esophagus — *esophagus*

017.9 ✓5th Tuberculosis of other specified organs — (Use additional code to identify manifestation: 420.0, 422.0, 424.91) — *artery, breast, buccal cavity, endocardium, muscle, palate, parotid, parathyroid, pericardium, perineum, pituitary, thymus, stomach, vein*

018 Miliary tuberculosis

Tuberculosis bacilli may be seeded to distant organs through the lymphatic or vascular system. Miliary tuberculosis is named for the pale, disseminated lesions that resemble millet seeds. Miliary tuberculosis is most commonly seen in bone marrow, eye, lymph nodes, liver, spleen, kidney, adrenal gland, prostate, seminal vesicle, fallopian tube, endometrium, or meninges. Affected organs may eventually develop progressive, isolated organ infection.

018.0 ✓5th Acute miliary tuberculosis — *sudden, severe onset*

018.8 ✓5th Other specified miliary tuberculosis — *other*

018.9 ✓5th Unspecified miliary tuberculosis — *unknown*

Coding Clarification

Some tuberculosis codes are found in other sections of ICD-9-CM. Congenital tuberculosis is reported with 771.2, and the late effects of tuberculosis are reported with codes in the 137 series. If an asymptomatic person tests positive for TB, report 795.5. Report exposure to TB without further information on tests or infection status with V01.1, and report the need for a BCG inoculation against TB with V03.2. Do not report personal history of tuberculosis (V12.01) in patients with active disease.

When coding tuberculosis of bones or joints, report the TB code first (015.xx), followed by codes that best describe the manifestation, such as arthropathy (subclassification 711.4), necrosis or osteitis (730.8x), or synovitis/tenosynovitis (727.01). In Pott's disease, also report any curvature of spine (737.43) or spondylitis (720.81).

When coding tuberculosis of the genitourinary system, report the TB code first (016.xx), followed by codes that best describe the manifestation, such as nephropathy (583.81), prostatitis (601.4), or pyelitis (590.81).

When coding tuberculosis of other organs, report the TB code first (017.xx), followed by codes that best describe the manifestation, such as episcleritis (379.09), myocarditis (422.0), or interstitial keratitis (370.59).

020–027 Zoonotic Bacterial Diseases

020 Plague

Plague, an acute infection caused by the bacillus *Yersinia pestis*, occurs in three forms among people: bubonic plague, pneumonic plague, and septicemic plague. All three varieties have been called "black death" because in untreated cases, respiratory failure precedes death by several hours, and during this time, the hypoxic victim's skin may turn deep purple. Plague responds well to modern antibiotics. In the United States, sporadic infections are seen primarily in the Southwest.

Bubonic plague is transmitted by the bite of insects that are normally rodent parasites. The most important of these insects is the rat flea *Xenopsylla cheopis*. Bubonic plague is characterized by buboes: enlarged, inflamed lymph nodes in the groin, armpit, or neck. Other symptoms include headache, fever, nausea, vomiting, and aching joints. Untreated, bubonic plague's fatality rate is 30 to 75 percent.

Septicemic plague may be initiated by direct contact of contaminated hands, food, or objects with the

© 2004 Ingenix, Inc.

mucous membranes of the nose or throat. Untreated, pneumonic plague's fatality rate is 95 percent; septicemic, nearly 100. In treated cases, the fatality drops to 10 percent or less.

Pneumonic plague is characterized by lung infection and, as a primary infection, is often transmitted by inhaling bacteria-carrying air droplets exhaled by an infected person. Secondary pneumonic plague begins as another form of plague before infecting the lungs.

Pneumonic plague occurs when *Y. pestis* infects the lungs. The first signs of illness in pneumonic plague are fever, headache, weakness, and cough productive of bloody or watery sputum. The pneumonia progresses over two days to five days and may cause septic shock and, without early treatment, death.

Person-to-person transmission of pneumonic plague occurs through respiratory droplets, which can only infect those who have face-to-face contact with the ill patient.

Early treatment of pneumonic plague is essential. Several antibiotics are effective, including streptomycin, tetracycline, and chloramphenicol.

There is no vaccine against plague. Prophylactic antibiotic treatment for seven days will protect persons who have had face-to-face contact with infected patients.

Complications of antibiotics may include nausea, diarrhea, CNS disturbance, local IV site reactions, and abnormalities of hepatic enzymes, eosinophilia, headache, rash, restlessness, vomiting, abdominal pain/discomfort, headache, rash, and restlessness. Code first the symptom of the adverse effect and then the E code for Adverse Effects of a Drug in Therapeutic Use.

020.0	Bubonic plague — *most common, with swollen lymph glands*
020.1	Cellulocutaneous plague — *inflammation and necrosis of the skin*
020.2	Septicemic plague — *infection in bloodstream*
020.3	Primary pneumonic plague — *plague infects lung first*
020.4	Secondary pneumonic plague — *infection spreads to lung*
020.5	Pneumonic plague, unspecified
020.8	Other specified types of plague
020.9	Unspecified plague

Coding Clarification

Rubric 020 is only used for patients with plague. If exposure to plague has been substantiated, report V01.8 *Contact with or exposure to communicable diseases.* If there is only a suspicion that the patient has been exposed, report V74.8 *Special screening for other specified bacterial and spirochetal diseases* to report the medical necessity of plague testing.

Another code that may become appropriate is V03.3 *Prophylactic inoculation against plague.*

If plague was contracted as a result of terrorist acts, E997.1 *Injury due to biological warfare* may be reported in addition to the appropriate code from rubric 020.

If the patient is isolated for contact with plague, report V07.0 Isolation of individual after contact with infectious diseases.

Other coding issues may include reactions to vaccination, such as anaphylatic shock due to serum 999.4, and other serum reaction 999.5. See Complications, vaccination.

021 Tularemia

A sudden fever, chill, headache, myalgia, and fatigue characterize tularemia.

It is a fairly uncommon disease, seen in the United States mostly in Oklahoma, Missouri, and Alaska. The infective agent, *Francisella tularensis,* enters the body through a tick bite or by direct contact with the skin. The bacillus can penetrate unbroken skin, and can therefore be transmitted by handling tainted meat or cleaning wild game, usually rodents such as squirrels or rabbits.

Tularemia responds well to antibiotic treatment and, with treatment, death is rare. Without treatment, mortality of tularemia is about 5 percent. Once infected, the patient develops immunity.

021.0	Ulceroglandular tularemia — *lesion at cutaneous site of bacillus penetration*
021.1	Enteric tularemia — *intestinal infection*
021.2	Pulmonary tularemia — *infection of lung and/or bronchus*
021.3	Oculoglandular tularemia — *conjunctival infection with possible spread to cornea, lacrimal systems*
021.8	Other specified tularemia — *glandular or other*
021.9	Unspecified tularemia — *site unknown*

Coding Clarification

Tularemia codes are selected on the basis of site of initial infection: skin, lung, gastrointestinal system, eye, or other site.

To report prophylactic vaccination against tularemia, see V03.4.

022 Anthrax

AHA: Q4, 2002, 70

Anthrax infection can occur in three forms: cutaneous (skin), inhalation, and gastrointestinal. Symptoms vary according to the form of infection, but usually occur within seven days.

In most cases, the anthrax bacterium enters a cut or abrasion on the skin. This is called cutaneous anthrax. Skin infection begins as a raised itchy bump that resembles an insect bite. The bump develops into a vesicle and, from there, a painless ulcer, usually 1.0 centimeter to 3.0 centimeters in diameter, within 48 hours. Lymph glands in the adjacent area may swell. Not long afterward, the lesions turn black, a hallmark of skin anthrax, as tissue begins to die. About 20 percent of untreated cases of cutaneous anthrax will result in death. However, death is rare with drug therapy.

Pulmonary anthrax is caused by inhalation of the anthrax bacterium. It generally takes two to five days for symptoms to appear, though in some cases, spores lodged in the lungs may take up to 60 days to germinate. Initially, symptoms mimic those of the flu — fever, nausea, muscle aches, and cough — and after several days, as the immune system fails to rid the body of the bacteria, more severe signs appear, including difficulty breathing, high fever, and shock. Fatality is 90 percent if left untreated.

The intestinal form of anthrax is rare, and may follow the consumption of contaminated meat. Intestinal anthrax is characterized by an acute gastroenteritis progressing into septicemia.

Anthrax is caused by the bacterium *B. anthracis,* which once inside the body emerges from the dormant spore phase, begins to reproduce, and in the process of reproduction, produces toxins that can lead to organ failure. DNA analysis can determine the strain of anthrax in an outbreak and whether the strain has been genetically manipulated.

Pulmonary and cutaneous anthrax are the types of anthrax contracted in recent bioterrorism in the United States, with the pulmonary form most likely to result in death because the germs burrow into lung tissue, where they come in close contact with lymph vessels.

There are several types of lab tests that can detect the presence of anthrax, although no single screen can provide a definitive diagnosis. Culturing a sample taken from the mucous membranes, in the case of pulmonary anthrax, is the most conclusive way to confirm anthrax. An antibody-antigen test is another way to confirm anthrax and this test takes less time than the several days for confirmation through culture.

Antibiotics administered early are effective against the disease and, at the time of the bioterrorism, Cipro was the only medication available in the United States approved as an effective drug against anthrax due to the testing (on animals) the Food and Drug Administration (FDA) requires for labeling a product. The FDA has since fast-tracked approval for penicillin and doxycycline. A company manufacturing an anthrax vaccine for the U.S. military stopped its production in 1998, due to quality control standards cited by the FDA. In the wake of the attacks, the company has reapplied for approval, but in the interim, the federal government has been pushing two newer vaccines into clinical trials.

Complications of antibiotics may include nausea, diarrhea, CNS disturbance, local IV site reactions, and abnormalities of hepatic enzymes, eosinophilia, headache, rash, restlessness, vomiting, abdominal pain/discomfort, headache, rash, and restlessness.

022.0 Cutaneous anthrax — *infection through superficial wound*
AHA: Q4, 2002, 70

022.1 Pulmonary anthrax — *infection in lungs*
AHA: Q4, 2002, 70

022.2 Gastrointestinal anthrax — *acute gastrointestinal infection*
AHA: Q4, 2002, 70

022.3 Anthrax septicemia — *infection in bloodstream*
AHA: Q4, 2002, 70

022.8 Other specified manifestations of anthrax — *other site of infection*
AHA: Q4, 2002, 70

022.9 Unspecified anthrax — *unknown site of infection*
AHA: Q4, 2002, 70

Coding Clarification

Rubric 022 is only used in patients testing positive to anthrax exposure. Do not use these codes for false positive tests or for negative tests in cases of exposure.

If septicemia is due to anthrax report 022.3, do not report a code from rubric 038.

In the case of pulmonary anthrax with pneumonia, also report the pneumonia, 484.5.

If there is only a suspicion that the patient has been exposed, report V74.8 *Special screening for other specified bacterial and spirochetal diseases* to report the medical necessity of an anthrax screening test.

Another code that may become appropriate as a result of the recent bioterrorism includes V03.89 *Need for prophylactic vaccination and inoculation against other single bacterial disease.*

If anthrax was contracted as a result of terrorist acts, E997.1 *Injury due to biological warfare* may be reported in addition to the appropriate code from rubric 022.

© 2004 Ingenix, Inc.

Other coding issues may include reactions to vaccination, such as anaphylatic shock due to serum 999.4, and other serum reaction 999.5. See Complications, vaccination.

023 Brucellosis

Brucellosis is also known as "undulant fever" or "Bangs disease" and is a systemic infection caused by exposure to any of several *Brucella* species. The species are specific to the type of animal usually infected: sheep/goats, cattle, swine, or dogs.

The infection enters the body through a break in the skin. Onset of symptoms can be within three days to 30 days. Symptoms of brucellosis infection in humans include fever, night sweats, fatigue, anorexia, weight loss, headache, and arthralgia. In animals, the primary sign of infection is abortion in females and epididymitis in males.

Worldwide, brucellosis remains a major source of disease in humans and domesticated animals. *B. abortus* is the most common form in the United States.

023.0 Brucella melitensis — *contact infected sheep/goats*

023.1 Brucella abortus — *contact infected cattle*

023.2 Brucella suis — *contact infected swine*

023.3 Brucella canis — *contact infected dogs*

023.8 Other brucellosis — *more than one source*

023.9 Burcellosis, unspecified — *unknown animal contact*

024 Glanders OK

Glanders is an equine disease communicable to man and caused by *Burkholderia mallei* (formerly *Pseudomonas mallei*). Nearly all cases of glanders in the United States occur among people who are professionally or recreationally exposed to horses, although glanders can be transmitted from human to human and in the laboratory. Glanders cases have not appeared in the United States since the 1940s. Outbreaks do occur in South America, Asia, Africa, and the Middle East. Symptoms of glanders include headache, chills, fever, and vomiting.

025 Melioidosis OK

Also known as Whitmore's disease or pseudoglanders, melioidosis is a rare infection caused by *Pseudomonas pseudomallei*. Most cases are limited to Asia. The disease is acquired through exposure to contaminated soil or water to a break in the skin. Symptoms range from a skin lesion at the site of infection, to pneumonia or septicemia. Patients with melioidosis may suffer relapses years after the initial infection has resolved.

026 Rat-bite fever

Rat-bite fever begins with a rat bite, scratch, or ingestion of contaminated food or water. While the initial wound may heal promptly, it usually becomes swollen and painful again within a few weeks of the bite. At that time, regional lymph nodes may swell and there may be chills, fever, and a skin rash. Periods of relapse may subside and recur. Code selection is based on the type of infection: *Spirillum minus* or *Streptobacillus moniliformis.*

026.0 Spirillary fever — *Spirillum minus infection, Sodoku*

026.1 Streptobacillary fever — *Streptobacillus moniliformis infection, Haverhill fever*

026.9 Unspecified rat-bite fever — *unknown*

027 Other zoonotic bacterial diseases

Use this rubric to report zoonotic bacterial disease not described earlier in the chapter.

027.0 Listeriosis — (Use additional code to identify manifestation, 320.7) — *infection by Listeria monocytogenes*

027.1 Erysipelothrix infection

027.2 Pasteurellosis — *infection by Pasteurella multocida (P. septica)*

027.8 Other specified zoonotic bacterial diseases — *Yersinia septica, others*

027.9 Unspecified zoonotic bacterial disease — *unknown*

Coding Clarification

In all cases, code the zoonotic bacterial disease first, followed by manifestations of the infection, as in the case of listeriosis with meningitis (320.7). Report congenital listeriosis infection with 771.2.

030–041 Other Bacterial Diseases

030 Leprosy

Mycobacterium leprae causes leprosy. Leprosy, also known as Hansen's disease, can be treated effectively with several drugs. If left untreated, the disease can result in severe disfigurement, especially of the feet, hands, and face. It is rarely fatal.

Ninety percent of the 900,000 leprosy cases worldwide occur in just 16 nations, with India and Brazil having the highest numbers of cases. Only 7,000 registered cases of leprosy currently exist in the United States. Most of these patients are immigrants who acquired the disease in their home countries.

Leprosy has two main forms: tuberculoid and lepromatous. In tuberculoid leprosy, skin lesions are few and small, with few bacteria present. Lepromatous leprosy, is a more severe disease, with symptomatic widespread lesions and significant bacteria.

Leprosy is not easily transmitted, but likely is transmitted person-to-person through nasal droplets released from an infected person. Less than 5 percent of people who are infected with *M. leprae* actually develop leprosy. For most, the immune system fights off infection. Immunosuppressed patients are no more likely to develop leprosy and research has not discovered what, if anything, predisposes a person to the disease.

Treating leprosy using multidrug therapy can halt the progression of the disease, though there are side effects. Inflammation develops in patients when leprosy bacteria are killed and erythema nodosum leprosum (ENL) is a risk in patients during drug therapy. The painful skin sores characteristic of ENL are thought to be a result of abnormal immune reactions to the killed bacteria.

030.0 Lepromatous leprosy (type L) — *widespread lesions and bacteria*

030.1 Tuberculoid leprosy (type T) — *small lesions, few bacteria*

030.2 Indeterminate leprosy (group I) — *uncharacteristic, early manifestation*

030.3 Borderline leprosy (group B) — *transitional; neither tuberculoid or lepromatous; dimorphous*

030.8 Other specified leprosy — *not elsewhere classified*

030.9 Unspecified leprosy — *unknown type*

Coding Clarification

When coding leprosy, report the leprosy code, and identify any manifestations in addition to the leprosy, such as infective and deformity-creating dermatitis of the eyelid (373.4) or corneal lesion (371.89).

Erythema nodosum leprosum (ENL) is reported with 695.2.

031 Diseases due to other mycobacteria

Mycobacteria cause leprosy and tuberculosis. In this rubric, other mycobacterial diseases are classified by site of infection.

Mycobacterium avium-intracellulare (MAC) affects up to 40 percent of human immunodeficiency virus (HIV)-infected people in the United States, while the disseminated form of the disease (DMAC) affects 15 to 24 percent of AIDS patients and other people with severely impaired immune systems. Severe anemia, fever, night sweats, anorexia, and diarrhea characterize DMAC. It is a significant cause of AIDS morbidity.

031.0 Pulmonary diseases due to other mycobacteria — *lung infection; Battey disease, M. avium, M. intracellulare, M. kansasii, M. fortuitum, M. xenopi*

031.1 Cutaneous diseases due to other mycobacteria — *skin infection; Buruli ulcer; M. marinum (M. balnei)*

031.2 Disseminated diseases due to other mycobacteria — *more than one site; DMAC, MAC*
AHA: Q4, 1997, 31

031.8 Other specified diseases due to other mycobacteria — *not elsewhere classified; kasongo, kakerifu*

031.9 Unspecified diseases due to mycobacteria — *unknown or atypical*

Coding Clarification

When coding AIDS related cases, sequence the code for AIDS (042) first, followed by the code for MAC or DMAC (031.2).

032 Diphtheria

An acute, contagious disease, diphtheria is one of the childhood diseases that common immunizations protect against. (The D in DPT is for the diphtheria vaccine). The infective agent is *Corynebacterium diphtheriae.*

Diphtheria usually presents with sore throat, with its hallmark fibrous membrane most commonly seen on the tonsil or nasopharynx. This membrane can combine with pharyngeal edema to obstruct breathing. However, diphtheria can attack other organs rather than presenting as a sore throat, and the codes in this rubric are therefore classified by site of infection.

032.0 Faucial diphtheria — *tonsillar*

032.1 Nasopharyngeal diphtheria — *deep, soft tissue of nose and pharynx*

032.2 Anterior nasal diphtheria — *superficial, soft tissue of the nose*

032.3 Laryngeal diphtheria — *larynx*

032.81 Conjunctival diphtheria — *conjunctiva*

032.82 Diphtheritic myocarditis — *wall of the heart*

032.83 Diphtheritic peritonitis — *abdominal membrane lining*

032.84 Diphtheritic cystitis — *bladder*

032.85 Cutaneous diphtheria — *skin*

032.89 Other specified diphtheria — *neurological or other complication*

032.9 Unspecified diphtheria

Coding Clarification

Report suspected carrier of diphtheria with V02.4 and report prophylactic vaccination against diphtheria with V03.5 (diptheria alone).

Vaccinations for diphtheria in combination with other diseases are in the V06 series of codes.

© 2004 Ingenix, Inc.

033 Whooping cough

An acute, contagious disease, whooping cough is one of the childhood diseases that common immunizations protect against. The P in DPT is for the pertussis (whooping cough) vaccine.

The infective agent in whooping cough is *Bordetella pertussis.* A milder disease clinically indistinguishable from *B. pertussis* is caused by *B. parapertussis. B. bronchiseptica* also creates symptoms of whooping cough.

The course of whooping cough is approximately six weeks and has three stages: catarrhal (nocturnal cough, sneezing, and lacrimation); paroxysmal (thick mucus, choking spells); and convalescence, when the severity of the symptoms diminishes. Mortality for the most severe form of whooping cough, pertussis, is about 2 percent in children younger than 1.

033.0 Whooping cough due to Bordetella pertussis (P. pertussis) — (Use additional code to identify any associated pneumonia, 484.3) — *B. pertussis*

033.1 Whooping cough due to Bordetella parapertussis (B. parapertussis) — (Use additional code to identify any associated pneumonia, 484.3) — *B. parapertussis*

033.8 Whooping cough due to other specified organism — (Use additional code to identify any associated pneumonia, 484.3) — *B. bronchiseptica*

033.9 Whooping cough, unspecified organism — (Use additional code to identify any associated pneumonia, 484.3) — *unknown organism*

Coding Clarification

Report any pneumonia concurrent to whooping cough separately with 484.3. The pneumonia should be coded as a secondary diagnosis.

Prophylactic vaccination is reported with V03.6 (pertussis alone) or with a code from the V06 series for pertussis vaccination in combination with other prophylactic vaccinations.

034 Streptococcal sore throat and scarlet fever

Strep throat is a common pharyngeal infection presenting with a red, sore throat and fever. Strep throat responds readily to antibiotic treatment. Without antibiotics, strep throat can progress into scarlet fever, typified by a red blush to the skin of the chest and abdomen, that blanches under pressure. Streptococcal infections can progress to endocarditis, pneumonias, and septicemias.

034.0 Streptococcal sore throat — *simple strep throat*

034.1 Scarlet fever — *red rash spreading from trunk*

Coding Clarification

Suspected carrier of streptococcus is reported with V02.51 for Group B and V02.52 for other strains of streptococcus.

For streptococcal angina, use code 034.0.

035 Erysipelas OK

Formerly called St. Anthony's fire, erysipelas is a hot, bright red, superficial cellulitis, involving dermal lymphatics that is usually caused by a streptococcal infection.

Coding Clarification

If the erysipelas infection is of the external ear, report the erysipelas first, and the site of infection with 380.13. For erysipelas as a maternal complication of childbirth, see rubric 670.

036 Meningococcal infection

Neisseria meningitidis is a common cause of meningitis. Also called meningococcus, the bacteria may invade the spinal cord, brain, heart, joints, optic nerve, or bloodstream. A pink or petechial rash may accompany the disease. Although the bacterium is found in the nasopharynx of 5 percent of the population, only a fraction of carriers ever develop the disease. It is seen most commonly in infants or in epidemics among persons who live in close quarters (barracks, schools).

036.0 Meningococcal meningitis — *infection of membranes lining brain or spinal cord*

036.1 Meningococcal encephalitis — *infection of brain*

036.2 Meningococcemia — *invasion of bloodstream*

036.3 Waterhouse-Friderichsen syndrome, meningococcal — *vascular collapse and shock*

036.40 Meningococcal carditis, unspecified — *site of heart infection unknown*

036.41 Meningococcal pericarditis — *infection of lining of heart*

036.42 Meningococcal endocarditis — *infection within heart cavities*

036.43 Meningococcal myocarditis — *infection of muscle of heart*

036.81 Meningococcal optic neuritis — *infection of optic nerve*

036.82 Meningococcal arthropathy — *infection of joint*

036.89 Other specified meningococcal infections — *other specific site of infection*

036.9 Unspecified meningococcal infection — *unknown site of infection*

Coding Clarification

Prophylactic meningococcal vaccination is administered during epidemics and is reported with V03.89.

Suspected carrier of meningitis is reported with V02.59.

037 Tetanus OK

Tetanus is an infection by *Clostridium tetani*, and is commonly called "lockjaw" because of the tonic spasms that occur in voluntary muscles. *C. tetani* is found in soil and animal feces, and infection may result from insignificant or deep wounds. The infected patient may have difficulty swallowing, speaking, or respiration as a result of the tonic spasms caused by the infection.

In the United States, the highest number of tetanus cases is seen among intravenous drug abusers and in burn victims or as a complication of abortion or pregnancy. See the index of ICD-9-CM for entries relating to tetanus occurring as a result of abortion or childbirth.

Tetanus has a high mortality rate and is one of the diseases that common childhood immunizations protect against. (The T in DPT is for tetanus vaccine.)

Coding Clarification

Report prophylactic vaccination for tetanus with V03.7. If tetanus immunization occurs in conjunction with other immunizations, see the V06 series of immunization codes.

038 Septicemia

AHA: Q3, 1988, 12; Q4, 1988, 10

Septicemia is the invasion of the bloodstream that results in multisystemic infection. Codes in this series are classified according to the infective bacterial agent.

Septicemia, also called septic syndrome or sepsis, occurs when a localized infection (a urinary tract infection, operative wound infection, or infected tooth) metastasizes and the bacterium is spread throughout the body. The disease is acute, and symptoms may include shaking chills, fever, abdominal pain, vomiting, and diarrhea. Septicemia treatments include antibiotic therapy, drainage of any abscess, or reoperation.

The incidence of septicemia in staphylococcal infection is related to the organism identified. As many as 90 percent of *Staphylococcus aureus* infection cases are true sepsis, while less than 50 percent of non-aureus *Staphylococcus* cases are true sepsis.

Use additional code for systemic inflammatory response syndrome (SIRS), 995.91-995.92.

038.0 Streptococcal septicemia — *other than Streptococcus pneumoniae*
AHA: Q3, 1988, 12; Q4, 1988, 10; Q2, 1996, 5; Q4, 2003, 79

038.10 Unspecified staphylococcal septicemia — *unknown staphylococcus*
AHA: Q3, 1988, 12; Q4, 1988, 10; Q4, 1997, 32

038.11 Staphylococcus aureus septicemia — *also called Staphylococcus pyogenes*
AHA: Q3, 1988, 12; Q4, 1988, 10; Q4, 1997, 32; Q4, 1998, 42; Q2, 2000, 5

038.19 Other staphylococcal septicemia

038.2 Pneumococcal septicemia — *septicemia from bacteria common to pneumonia*
AHA: Q3, 1988, 12; Q4, 1988, 10; Q1, 1991, 13; Q2, 1996, 5

038.3 Septicemia due to anaerobes — *due to bacteroides*
AHA: Q3, 1988, 12; Q4, 1988, 10

038.40 Septicemia due to unspecified gram-negative organism — *not otherwise specified*
AHA: Q3, 1988, 12; Q4, 1988, 10

038.41 Septicemia due to hemophilus influenzae (H. influenzae) — *also called Pfeiffer's bacillus*
AHA: Q3, 1988, 12; Q4, 1988, 10

038.42 Septicemia due to Escherichia coli (E. coli) — *also called colon bacillus and Escherich's bacillus*
AHA: Q3, 1988, 12; Q4, 1988, 10; Q3, 2003, 73

038.43 Septicemia due to pseudomonas — *family Pseudomonadaceae*
AHA: Q3, 1988, 12; Q4, 1988, 10

038.44 Septicemia due to serratia — *family Enterobacteriaceae*
AHA: Q3, 1988, 12; Q4, 1988, 10

038.49 Other septicemia due to gram-negative organism — *including Proteus vulgaris*
AHA: Q3, 1988, 12; Q4, 1988, 10

038.8 Other specified septicemia — *not elsewhere classified*
AHA: Q3, 1988, 12; Q4, 1988, 10

038.9 Unspecified septicemia — *disseminated, unknown cause*
AHA: Q3, 1988, 12; Q4, 1988, 10; Q2, 1996, 6; Q3, 1996, 16; Q1, 1998, 5; Q3, 1999, 5,9; Q2, 2000, 3; Q4, 2003, 79

Documentation Issues

"Sepsis" may be an ambiguous term in the medical record and coding should differentiate generalized sepsis represented in this code rubric from other bacterial infections.

 © 2004 Ingenix, Inc.

When the documentation states the diagnosis of septicemia with shock or general sepsis with septic shock, code and list the septicemia first and use an additional code for the septic shock.

If the documentation has an unclear diagnostic statement as to the site or organ-specific sepsis (e.g., urosepsis), it may require clarification from the physician for accurate code selection.

If the physician has documented urosepsis, verify which of the following the diagnosis is intended to mean:

- Generalized sepsis caused by leakage of urine or toxic urine by-products into the general vascular circulation, code 038.x
- Urine contaminated by bacteria, bacterial by-products, or other toxic material but without other findings, code 599.0

When the physician documents that the sepsis is secondary to a urinary tract infection (UTI) and the blood and urine cultures reveal the presence of the infection, it would be appropriate to code both the septicemia and the UTI.

If the medical record documentation identifies that the septicemia is due to *Candida albicans,* a code would not be selected from the bacterial disease series, categories 030-041. *C. albicans* is one of the mycotic infections and is classified as such. The correct code would be 112.5 *Disseminated candidiasis.*

If the physician documents both pneumococcal pneumonia (481) and pneumococcal septicemia (038.2), both conditions should be coded.

Coding Clarification

Complication of Care: When septicemia is caused by a complication of care (e.g., indwelling urinary catheter, vascular access device), the complication code should be listed as principal/primary diagnosis. Additional codes should be assigned for the septicemia from category 038, and the organism responsible for the sepsis should also be coded if it is not included in the category 038 code descriptor.

Infection Originating in the Perinatal Period: Sepsis of newborn should be coded with two codes: 771.81 *Septicemia [sepsis] of newborn* and a code from category 038 to identify the septicemia.

Negative Blood Cultures: Septicemia is defined as evidence of infection with fever or hypothermia, tachypnea, tachycardia, and impaired organ system perfusion, such as altered mental status, oliguria, and relative hypotension. Metabolic acidosis may also be present secondary to impaired organ perfusion, as evidenced by either an increased lactate level, increased anion gap, or reduced blood pH. So, although the blood culture may be negative, it may still be appropriate to code the septicemia in view of the clinical findings.

Neutropenic/Nadir Sepsis: This is a true sepsis, even though the white cell counts and temperature are at low points, bacteria is still present in the condition. Two codes need to be assigned for this condition: code 038.9 *Unspecified septicemia* and 288.0 *Agranulocytosis, for the neutropenia.*

Noncardiogenic Acute Pulmonary Edema: When acute pulmonary edema is secondary to septicemia it should be coded as an additional code to the septicemia. Use codes 038.9 *Septicemia* and 518.4 *Acute edema of lung, unspecified.*

Sepsis Secondary to Urinary Tract Infection: If a localized urinary infection has entered into the patients blood stream and has developed into a generalized sepsis, use a code from category 038. Code 599.0 *Urinary tract infection, site not specified* would also be reported as an additional code. If the code from category 038 identifies the causative organism (e.g., pseudomonas septicemia 038.43) it would not be necessary to report a code from category 041.

Septicemia with Pneumonia: Septicemia occurring with pneumonia is a true septic infection and should be coded in addition to the pneumonia. Hospital code sequencing is dependent upon the circumstances of the admission.

Streptococcus Pneumoniae: *Streptococcus pneumoniae* is the microbiological term for the germ that causes pneumococcal disease, so only one code is necessary, code 038.2 *Pneumococcal septicemia.*

The following types of septicemia should be coded as follows: Shigella septicemia, 004.9; Salmonella septicemia, 003.1; gonococcal septicemia, 098.89; herpetic septicemia, 054.5; postoperative septicemia, 998.59; septicemia from anthrax, 022.3.

Coding Scenario

A patient is admitted with an infection of the gastrostomy site. The physician documentation confirms the blood culture and gastrostomy site growth of *Staphylococcal aureus.*

> Code assignment: 536.41 *Infection of gastrostomy* and 038.11 *Staphylococcus aureus septicemia*

A patient with chronic renal failure is seen with an infection of their vascular access device. Physician documentation indicates that the patient has septicemia due to the vascular access device.

> Code assignment: 996.62 *Infection and inflammatory reaction due to vascular device, implant and graft,* 038.9 *Unspecified septicemia,* and 585 *Chronic renal failure*

A 2-day-old infant is readmitted to the hospital with a neonatal staphylococcal septicemia.

> Code assignment: 771.81 *Septicemia [sepsis] of newborn* and 038.11 *Staphylococcal septicemia*

A patient is diagnosed with sepsis and septic shock following an abortion performed two days previous.

> Code assignment: 639.0 *Genital and pelvic infection following abortion* and 639.5 *Shock following abortion*

A 3-year-old is admitted via the emergency department with sores on the mouth and fever. The physician documents as the discharge diagnosis Nadir sepsis and neutropenia.

> Code assignment: 038.9 *Unspecified septicemia* and 288.0 *Agranulocytosis*

039 Actinomycotic infections

Infections by *Actinomyces israelii* are classified in this rubric according to site, at which multiple, communicating abscesses often form granulated tissue. The disease is most commonly seen in adult males and is slowly progressive, although it is sometimes seen as a local complication of intrauterine device (IUD) placement in women.

039.0 Cutaneous actinomycotic infection — *superficial skin infection*

039.1 Pulmonary actinomycotic infection — *lung involvement with chest pain, fever, cough*

039.2 Abdominal actinomycotic infection — *intestinal involvement with anorexia, pain, fever, vomiting and irregular bowels*

039.3 Cervicofacial actinomycotic infection — *"lumpy jaw" in oral mucosa or neck*

039.4 Madura foot — *deep foot infection following penetrating injury*

039.8 Actinomycotic infection of other specified sites — *site not elsewhere classified, multiple sites, or generalized*

039.9 Actinomycotic infection of unspecified site — *unknown site*

040 Other bacterial diseases

Gas gangrene is the result of infection by the *Clostridium* bacteria, usually at the site of injury or a recent surgical wound. It is an acute condition, with red, extremely painful tissue swelling in quick progression to surrounding areas. Involved tissue is destroyed. Gas gangrene has a high mortality rate. *Clostridia* species of bacteria produce many toxins that cause tissue death and systemic symptoms, including sweating, fever, and shock. Untreated, gas gangrene can lead to renal failure, coma, and death. Treatments include wound debridement, amputation, antibiotics, and hyperbaric oxygen treatment.

Whipple's disease primarily effects middle-aged men and presents as chronic diarrhea, anemia, arthralgia, and abdominal pain.

040.0 Gas gangrene — *clostridial myonecrosis, malignant edema*
AHA: Q1, 1995, 11

040.1 Rhinoscleroma — *Klebsiella rhinoscleromatis infection of nose, nasopharynx*

040.2 Whipple's disease — *intestinal lipodystrophy*

040.3 Necrobacillosis — *Fusobacterium necrophorum abscess or necrosis*

040.81 Tropical pyomyositis — *including Bungpagga*

040.82 Toxic shock syndrome — (Use additional code to identify the organism) — *Use additional code to identify the organism*
AHA: Q4, 2002, 44

040.89 Other specified bacterial diseases — *not elsewhere classified, including toxic shock syndrome*
AHA: Nov-Dec, 1986, 7

Coding Clarification

Gas gangrene associated with abortion, pregnancy, or labor and delivery should be reported with codes from that section of ICD-9-CM. Check the ICD-9-CM index for more information. Also check the ICD-9-CM index for a complex list of gangrene diagnoses other than gas gangrene.

Arteriosclerosis with gas gangrene is reported with two codes: 440.29 *Other atherosclerosis of native arteries of extremities* and 040.0 *Gas gangrene.* It is inappropriate to use code 440.24 as this code only includes ischemic gangrene.

041 Bacterial infection in conditions classified elsewhere and of unspecified site

AHA: July-Aug, 1984, 19; Q2, 2001, 12

This rubric of ICD-9-CM provides supplemental codes to identify bacterial agents in diseases classified elsewhere. They usually are sequenced after the disease manifestation. Codes in this rubric can also be used to classify bacterial infections of unspecified nature or site.

041.00 Unspecified streptococcus infection in conditions classified elsewhere and of unspecified site — (Note: This code is to be used as an additional code to identify the bacterial agent in diseases classified elsewhere and bacterial infections of unspecified nature or site)

© 2004 Ingenix, Inc.

041.01 Streptococcus infection in conditions classified elsewhere and of unspecified site, group A — (Note: This code is to be used as an additional code to identify the bacterial agent in diseases classified elsewhere and bacterial infections of unspecified nature or site)

041.02 Streptococcus infection in conditions classified elsewhere and of unspecified site, group B — (Note: This code is to be used as an additional code to identify the bacterial agent in diseases classified elsewhere and bacterial infections of unspecified nature or site)

041.03 Streptococcus infection in conditions classified elsewhere and of unspecified site, group C — (Note: This code is to be used as an additional code to identify the bacterial agent in diseases classified elsewhere and bacterial infections of unspecified nature or site)

041.04 Streptococcus infection in conditions classified elsewhere and of unspecified site, group D [Enterococcus] — (Note: This code is to be used as an additional code to identify the bacterial agent in diseases classified elsewhere and bacterial infections of unspecified nature or site)

041.05 Streptococcus infection in conditions classified elsewhere and of unspecified site, group G — (Note: This code is to be used as an additional code to identify the bacterial agent in diseases classified elsewhere and bacterial infections of unspecified nature or site)

041.09 Other streptococcus infection in conditions classified elsewhere and of unspecified site — (Note: This code is to be used as an additional code to identify the bacterial agent in diseases classified elsewhere and bacterial infections of unspecified nature or site)

041.10 Unspecified staphylococcus infection in conditions classified elsewhere and of unspecified site — (Note: This code is to be used as an additional code to identify the bacterial agent in diseases classified elsewhere and bacterial infections of unspecified nature or site)

041.11 Staphylococcus aureus infection in conditions classified elsewhere and of unspecified site — (Note: This code is to be used as an additional code to identify the bacterial agent in diseases classified elsewhere and bacterial infections of unspecified nature or site)

041.19 Other staphylococcus infection in conditions classified elsewhere and of unspecified site — (Note: This code is to be used as an additional code to identify the bacterial agent in diseases classified elsewhere and bacterial infections of unspecified nature or site)

041.2 Pneumococcus infection in conditions classified elsewhere and of unspecified site — (Note: This code is to be used as an additional code to identify the bacterial agent in diseases classified elsewhere and bacterial infections of unspecified nature or site)

041.3 Friedländer's bacillus infection in conditions classified elsewhere and of unspecified site — (Note: This code is to be used as an additional code to identify the bacterial agent in diseases classified elsewhere and bacterial infections of unspecified nature or site) — *Klebsiella pneumoniae infection*
AHA: July-Aug, 1984, 19; Q2, 2001, 12

041.4 Escherichia coli (E. coli) infection in conditions classified elsewhere and of unspecified site — (Note: This code is to be used as an additional code to identify the bacterial agent in diseases classified elsewhere and bacterial infections of unspecified nature or site)

041.5 Hemophilus influenzae (H. influenzae) infection in conditions classified elsewhere and of unspecified site — (Note: This code is to be used as an additional code to identify the bacterial agent in diseases classified elsewhere and bacterial infections of unspecified nature or site)

041.6 Proteus (mirabilis) (morganii) infection in conditions classified elsewhere and of unspecified site — (Note: This code is to be used as an additional code to identify the bacterial agent in diseases classified elsewhere and bacterial infections of unspecified nature or site)

041.7 Pseudomonas infection in conditions classified elsewhere and of unspecified site — (Note: This code is to be used as an additional code to identify the bacterial agent in diseases classified elsewhere and bacterial infections of unspecified nature or site)

041.81 Mycoplasma infection in conditions classified elsewhere and of unspecified site — (Note: This code is to be used as an additional code to identify the bacterial agent in diseases classified elsewhere and bacterial infections of unspecified nature or site)

041.82 Bacterial infection in conditions classified elsewhere, Bacteroides fragilis — (Note: This code is to be used as an additional code to identify the bacterial agent in diseases classified elsewhere and bacterial infections of unspecified nature or site)

041.83 Clostridium perfringens infection in conditions classified elsewhere and of unspecified site — (Note: This code is to be used as an additional code to identify the bacterial agent in diseases classified elsewhere and bacterial infections of unspecified nature or site)

041.84 Infection due to other anaerobes in conditions classified elsewhere and of unspecified site — (Note: This code is to be used as an additional code to identify the bacterial agent in diseases classified elsewhere and bacterial infections of unspecified nature or site) — *gram negative anaerobes, Bacteroides (fragilis)*
AHA: July-Aug, 1984, 19; Q2, 2001, 12

041.85 Infection due to other gram-negative organisms in conditions classified elsewhere and of unspecified site — (Note: This code is to be used as an additional code to identify the bacterial agent in diseases classified elsewhere and bacterial infections of unspecified nature or site) — *Aerobacter aerogenes, Mima polymorpha, Serratia*
AHA: July-Aug, 1984, 19; Q1, 1995, 18; Q2, 2001, 12

041.86 Helicobacter pylori (H. pylori) infection — (Note: This code is to be used as an additional code to identify the bacterial agent in diseases classified elsewhere and bacterial infections of unspecified nature or site) — *associated with peptic ulcers*
AHA: July-Aug, 1984, 19; Q4, 1995, 60; Q2, 2001, 12

041.89 Infection due to other specified bacteria in conditions classified elsewhere and of unspecified site — (Note: This code is to be used as an additional code to identify the bacterial agent in diseases classified elsewhere and bacterial infections of unspecified nature or site) — *not elsewhere classified*
AHA: July-Aug, 1984, 19; Q2, 2001, 12; Q2, 2003, 7

041.9 Bacterial infection, unspecified, in conditions classified elsewhere and of unspecified site — (Note: This code is to be used as an additional code to identify the bacterial agent in diseases classified elsewhere and bacterial infections of unspecified nature or site)

Coding Clarification

Helicobacter pylori with chronic gastritis is reported with two codes: 535.10 *Atrophic gastritis* and 041.86 *Helicobacter pylori (H.pylori).*

When coding a disease caused by an infectious organism, report the disease first, followed by the code that identifies the infectious agent. For example, urinary tract infection due to *E. coli* is sequenced as 599.0, then 041.4.

Coding Scenario

A patient is seen in the clinic for painful urination and fever. A urine culture shows the bacterial agent *Pseudomonas.* The physician's diagnostic statement confirms a urinary tract infection due to *Pseudomonas.*

> Code assignment: 599.0 *Urinary tract infection, site not specified* and 041.7 *Pseudomonas*

042 Human Immunodeficiency Virus (HIV) Infection

HIV is divided into two categories, HIV-1 and HIV-2. HIV-1 is seen worldwide; HIV-2 is limited to Africa and other countries and is seldom seen in the United States. HIV-1 has far-ranging health effects and manifestations. This code is reserved for patients with active HIV-1 infections, or AIDS. HIV-2 cases are reported with 079.53.

HIV-1 is a blood-borne virus in that it is transmitted through body fluids containing blood or plasma. Transmission of HIV-1 can occur sexually or non-sexually through the exchange of body fluids infected with a high concentration of the virus, mainly blood, semen, or vaginal/cervical secretions.

In HIV-1, the body's immune system is attacked, reducing its ability to protect itself against a variety of illnesses. Over time, the infected person becomes more susceptible to opportunistic infections or cancers that attack the body and can cause death. AIDS related complex (ARC) includes general lymphadenopathy, anorexia, fever, malaise, diarrhea, anemia, oral hairy leukoplakia, and oral candidiasis.

042 Human immunodeficiency virus [HIV] OK

AHA: July-Aug, 1987, 8; Q3, 1990, 17; Q2, 1992, 11; Q1, 1993, 21; Q4, 1997, 30,31; Q1, 1999, 14; Q1, 2003, 15

Documentation Issues

In cases where the medical record documentation indicates "possible," "probable," or "questionable" AIDS, not confirmed, without manifestations, that record should be returned to the physician for further clarification. Physicians also need to be aware that unacceptable terminology and abbreviations in the medical record should not be used. These terms only cause confusion in code selection.

 © 2004 Ingenix, Inc.

Do not use 042 in cases of "rule-out" or "suspected" AIDS's; this diagnosis can create a flag in the patient's data files that could interfere with their ability to obtain life or health insurance.

Coding Clarification

If the patient is being treated for AIDS or an AIDS-related illness, the code for HIV-1 infection (042) should be sequenced first, followed by codes for manifestations of HIV-1 infection. If the patient is being treated for an illness unrelated to AIDS, for example, an injury, AIDS would be reported secondarily to the injury.q

Patients with an HIV related illness should be coded to category 042, located in chapter one of the tabular list, Infectious and Parasitic Diseases. Notes in the tabular section advise the coder to use additional codes to identify all manifestations of HIV-1 and to use an additional code (079.53) to identify HIV-2 infection, if present.

Patients with physician-documented asymptomatic HIV infections who have never had an HIV-related illness should be coded to category V08, located in Chapter 18 of the tabular list, which are V Codes. A note is provided under this category that specifically indicates that this code is only to be used when no HIV infection symptoms or conditions are present. If any HIV infection symptoms or conditions are present, the coder is referred to code 042.

Patients (including infants) with inconclusive HIV test results should be classified with code 795.71, located under the Other nonspecific immunological findings subcategory (795.7) in chapter sixteen of the tabular list, Symptoms, Signs and Ill-Defined Conditions. A note is provided that clearly identifies that this code is only to be used when a test finding is reported as nonspecific. Negative findings are not coded.

HIV During Pregnancy: The obstetric code, 647.6x, should be used followed by the appropriate HIV code.

HIV Testing: For asymptomatic patients that solely want testing to identify their HIV status, use code V73.89 *Screening for other specified viral disease.* In addition, use code V69.8 *Other problems related to lifestyle,* if the patient is known to be a high risk individual.

If the patient returns for the results that are negative, use code V65.44 *Human immunodeficiency virus (HIV) counseling.* If the results were positive and the patient is asymptomatic, use code V08 *Asymptomatic HIV infection.* If the results were positive and they are symptomatic, use code 042 *Human Immunodeficiency virus (HIV) disease* with additional codes to identify the HIV-related symptoms or diagnosis. In addition, if counseling is performed, an additional code V65.44 *Human immunodeficiency virus (HIV) counseling* may be used.

AIDS Wasting Syndrome: Assign 042 *Human immunodeficiency virus (HIV) disease* and use the additional code 799.4 *Cachexia.* Also code any associated conditions that are documented.

Positive Newborn Testing: If a newborn has a positive ELISA or Western Blot test for HIV the correct code is 795.71 *Nonspecific serologic evidence of human immunodeficiency virus [HIV].* These tests may reflect the antibodies of the mother and not the baby. If the mother is positive for HIV, the antibody may cross the placenta to the newborn. The antibodies may be carried up to 18 months producing a false-positive result. These false-positive results during the newborns first 18 months are due to the mothers' antibodies that the newborn carries. The newborn may later lose those antibodies, indicating that he or she was actually never infected.

Coding Scenario

A patient is admitted to the hospital with acute bronchitis. Three months prior, the patient tested positive for HIV but has not yet shown any symptoms of the HIV disease.

> Code assignment: 466.0 *Acute bronchitis* and V08 *Asymptomatic HIV infection*

A patient that is six months pregnant is being treated for pneumocystosis secondary to HIV.

> Code assignment: 647.63 *Pregnancy complicated by other viral diseases,* 042 *Human immunodeficiency virus (HIV) disease,* and 136.3 *Pneumocystosis*

A patient with AIDS is admitted to the hospital with severe dehydration and diarrhea. The final diagnosis is Salmonella with dehydration.

> Code assignment: 042 *Human immunodeficiency virus (HIV) disease,* 003.9 *Salmonella infection, unspecified,* and 276.5 *Dehydration*

A 42-year-old white female who has tested positive for HIV is being seen for a follow-up on the status of her condition. She is presently asymptomatic and has shown no signs or symptoms to date.

> Code assignment: V08 *Asymptomatic HIV infection*

An asymptomatic HIV patient is admitted to undergo Interleukin immunotherapy. The documentation implies that the patient has never had an HIV symptomatic illness.

> Code assignment: Code this patient according to the rule for asymptomatic HIV patients-V08. The planned immunotherapy does not interfere with principal/primary diagnosis selection.

045–049 Poliomyelitis and Other Non–arthropod–borne Viral Diseases of Central Nervous System

045 Acute poliomyelitis

Poliomyelitis is an infectious viral disease of the central nervous system that sometimes results in paralysis. The World Health Organization (WHO) declared the Western Hemisphere polio-free in 1994. Today, polio is most prevalent in areas of Africa, the Middle East, and South Asia.

Three types of poliovirus have been identified: the Brunhilde (type I), Lansing (type II), and Leon (type III) strains. Immunity to one strain does not provide protection against the other two. Type I causes 85 percent of paralytic infection, type II causes 5 percent, and type III causes 10 percent.

Polio enters the body through the digestive tract and spreads along nerve cells to affect various parts of the central nervous system. The incubation period ranges from four days to 35 days. Symptoms include fatigue, headache, fever, vomiting, constipation, and stiffness of the neck. Polio infection can cause permanent paralysis. However, nonparalytic cases far outnumber paralytic cases of polio. No drug has proven effective against polio infection, so treatment is symptomatic.

A third of patients who recover from poliomyelitis develop post-polio syndrome (PPS) 30 to 40 years later. PPS causes fatigue, muscle weakness, and muscle and joint pain.

The following fifth-digit subclassification is for use with category 045:

0 poliovirus, unspecified type — unknown

1 poliovirus type I — Brunhilde

2 poliovirus type II — Lansing

3 poliovirus type III — Leon

045.0 ✓5th Acute paralytic poliomyelitis specified as bulbar — *infection at site where brain merges with spinal cord*

045.1 ✓5th Acute poliomyelitis with other paralysis — *infection of peripheral or spinal nerves*

045.2 ✓5th Acute nonparalytic poliomyelitis — *pain, stiffness, or paresthesia without paralysis*

045.9 ✓5th Acute unspecified poliomyelitis — *unknown type*

Coding Clarification

Late effects of polio, including PPS, deformities, or paralysis in non-active disease, are reported with 138. Sequence first the manifestation, for example, progressive muscular atrophy (335.21), then report the late effect.

Congenital polio is reported with 771.2.

Do not report personal history of poliomyelitis (V12.02) in patients with active disease.

Exposure to poliovirus is reported with V01.2, and prophylactic vaccination is reported with V04.0. Routine immunization is largely responsible for the eradication of poliomyelitis in the United States.

046 Slow virus infection of central nervous system

Jakob-Creutzfeldt disease is a progressive, fatal disease causing dementia and seizures in adults. Transmission occurs from contaminated humans or human cadavers, although 10 percent of cases are familial in origin. Jakob-Creutzfeldt disease is related to mad cow disease, another form of spongiform encephalopathy with European outbreaks.

Kuru is limited exclusively to New Guinea natives, where the disease has nearly been eradicated. The disease is linked to cannibalism and Fore tribal rituals.

Subacute sclerosing panencephalitis (SSPE) is a rare, progressive, and grave disorder, occurring months or years following measles or measles vaccination, and usually before age 20. Mental faculties are diminished, seizures occur, and the patient deteriorates until death, usually within three years.

046.0 Kuru — *New Guinea-based neural disease*

046.1 Jakob-Creutzfeldt disease — *spongiform encephalopathy similar to "mad cow" disease*

046.2 Subacute sclerosing panencephalitis — *Dawson's, Van Bogaert's, Bodechtel-Guttmann disease*

046.3 Progressive multifocal leukoencephalopathy — *cerebral cortex infection in immunosuppressed*

046.8 Other specified slow virus infection of central nervous system — *not elsewhere classified*

046.9 Unspecified slow virus infection of central nervous system — *unknown slow virus infection of CNS*

Coding Clarification

All slow virus infections in this rubric may present with manifestations that should be reported in addition to the infection source. Dementia should be reported with 294.11, with behavioral disturbance, or 294.10, without behavioral disturbance.

 © 2004 Ingenix, Inc.

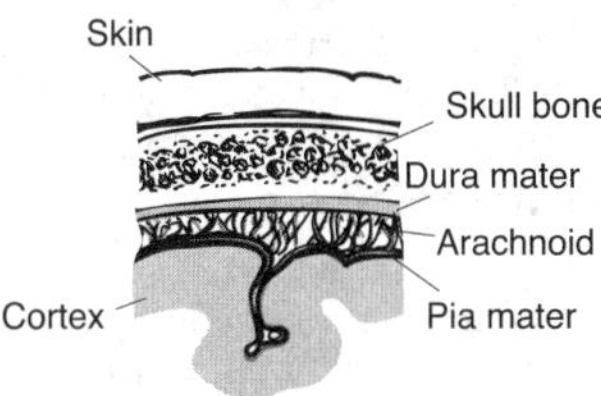

The meninges constitute the three layers that cover the brain and spinal cord: the dura mater, pia mater, and arachnoid

047 Meningitis due to enterovirus

AHA: Jan-Feb, 1987, 6

Meningitis is the inflammation of the membranes surrounding the brain or spinal cord, in this case, due to an aseptic, abacterial, or a viral enterovirus infection not included in other rubrics in this section of ICD-9-CM.

Viral infections must be differentiated from bacterial and other infections. Typically, a viral infection of the central nervous system is suspected by default, when a culture fails to grow bacteria. A virus may be isolated in spinal fluid or other tissues, but viruses causing aseptic meningitis are identified in less than half of all cases.

Coxsackie virus causes symptoms resembling polio, but without paralysis. It is most commonly seen in children during warm months.

ECHO virus is an acronym for enteric cytopathic human orphan virus and is also most prevalent during warm months.

047.0 Meningitis due to coxsackie virus — *coxsackievirus*
AHA: Jan-Feb, 1987, 6

047.1 Meningitis due to ECHO virus — *echovirus*
AHA: Jan-Feb, 1987, 6

047.8 Other specified viral meningitis — *not elsewhere classified*
AHA: Jan-Feb, 1987, 6

047.9 Unspecified viral meningitis — *unknown type*
AHA: Jan-Feb, 1987, 6

048 Other enterovirus diseases of central nervous system OK

This rubric represents all enterovirus disease of the central nervous system not elsewhere classified. Among these is Boston exanthem, a mild illness with a rash and fever caused by echovirus 16. It is named after an epidemic that occurred in Boston, Mass.

049 Other non-arthropod-borne viral diseases of central nervous system

049.0 Lymphocytic choriomeningitis — *arenavirus*

049.1 Meningitis due to adenovirus — *adenovirus*

049.8 Other specified non-arthropod-borne viral diseases of central nervous system — *not elsewhere classified*

049.9 Unspecified non-arthropod-borne viral disease of central nervous system — *unknown type*

Coding Clarification

Late effects of viral encephalitis are reported with 139.0.

050–057 Viral Diseases Accompanied by Exanthem

050 Smallpox

Smallpox is a highly contagious human disease caused by the virus viriolae, of which there are two strains: viriole major, which has severe symptoms and a mortality rate of 20 percent to 40 percent; and viriole minor, which has less severe symptoms and a 1 percent mortality rate. Smallpox can spread from person to person and through infected blankets, linens, and clothing. An infection is usually through the respiratory tract and local lymph nodes from where the virus enters the blood (primary viremia). Internal organs are infected; the virus reenters the blood (secondary viremia) and spreads to the skin. Symptoms appear about 12 days after exposure and mimic a gastrointestinal illness — nausea, vomiting, headache, and backache. Severe abdominal pain and disorientation follows. About two to three days after the onset of illness, the true smallpox rash appears. It begins as macules, which enlarge and become raised papules. By the third day, the papules progress into blisters, 6.0 mm in diameter and deep in the skin. In two more days, the fluid inside becomes turbid; the papules shrink and dry up in the skin. Toxemia may cause death before the rash is fully developed, but more commonly death, if it occurs, is between the 11th and 15th day of the rash. In severe cases the rash may cover the entire body. Secondary infections can include hemorrhaging and gangrene.

Diagnosis is difficult due to variations from the characteristic pattern.

In people exposed to smallpox, the vaccine can lessen the severity of or even prevent illness if given within four days after exposure. There is no proven treatment for smallpox but research to evaluate new antiviral agents is ongoing. Patients with smallpox can benefit from supportive therapy (intravenous fluids, medicine to control fever or pain, etc.) and antibiotics for any secondary bacterial infections that occur.

The vaccine is 100 percent effective if administered before exposure. Unfortunately, considering recent events, the WHO's vaccination campaign ended in 1980 when the disease was officially declared eradicated. No one in the United States has been inoculated since 1972 and since immunity after vaccination lasts up to 10 years, it is unlikely that anyone in the United States is protected against the disease.

Complications of antibiotics may include nausea, diarrhea, CNS disturbance, local IV site reactions, and abnormalities of hepatic enzymes, eosinophilia, headache, rash, restlessness, vomiting, abdominal pain/discomfort, headache, rash, and restlessness.

050.0 Variola major — *severe form*

050.1 Alastrim — *mild form*

050.2 Modified smallpox — *reinfection form*

050.9 Unspecified smallpox — *unknown type*

Coding Clarification

Rubric 050 is only used for patients with smallpox. If exposure to smallpox has been substantiated, report V01.3 *Contact with or exposure to communicable diseases.* If there is only a suspicion that the patient has been exposed, report V73.1 *Special screening for smallpox.*

Another code that may become appropriate as a result of the recent bioterrorism includes V04.1 *Vaccination against smallpox.*

If smallpox was contracted as a result of terrorist acts, E997.1 *Injury due to biological warfare* may be reported in addition to the appropriate code from rubric 050.

If the patient is isolated for contact with smallpox, report V07.0 *Isolation of individual after contact with infectious diseases.*

Code first the symptom of the adverse effect and then the E code for Adverse Effects of a Drug in Therapeutic Use. Other coding issues may include reactions to vaccination, such as anaphylatic shock due to serum 999.4, and other serum reaction 999.5. See Complications, vaccination.

051 Cowpox and paravaccinia

Cowpox is also called vaccinia because it is closely related to variola, the causative virus of smallpox, and infection by cowpox renders the patient immune to smallpox. Cowpox infection is due to Poxvirus bovis infection from milking cattle, and is much milder than smallpox, with hard lesions and low fever.

051.0 Cowpox — *vaccinia from cattle*

051.1 Pseudocowpox — *paravaccinia infection*

051.2 Contagious pustular dermatitis — *Poxvirus from sheep or goats*

051.9 Unspecified paravaccinia — *unknown paravaccinia infection*

Coding Clarification

Vaccinia as a result of inoculation is reported with 999.0, not with 051.1.

052 Chickenpox

Varicella zoster virus causes chickenpox and herpes zoster. Chickenpox is the initial, acute phase of the disease, and herpes zoster is a reactivation of the virus in a latent stage.

Chickenpox is highly contagious and usually mild, but it may be severe in infants, adults, or the immunosuppressed. More than 95 percent of Americans have been infected by chickenpox by the time they reach adulthood. In the United States, four million people are infected with chickenpox each year. Chickenpox has a characteristic itchy rash, which then forms blisters that dry into scabs. An infected person may have anywhere from only a few lesions to more than 500 lesions.

An adult bout of chickenpox is more likely to have complications than a childhood infection. These complications may occur when the varicella zoster virus inflames the brain, lung, or other organ, or when infection is accompanied by manifestations of high fever, or when the patient is immunosuppressed. Secondary infections are also considered complications.

052.0 Postvaricella encephalitis — *with inflammation of brain*

052.1 Varicella (hemorrhagic) pneumonitis — *with lung infection*

052.7 Chickenpox with other specified complications — *complications not listed above*
AHA: Q1, 2002, 3

052.8 Chickenpox with unspecified complication — *unknown complication*

052.9 Varicella without mention of complication — *no complications mentioned*

Coding Clarification

If the complication to chickenpox cannot be described in the codes presented in this rubric, report a code from rubric 052 first, and codes describing the complications or manifestations secondarily, as in the case of myocarditis (422.0) or arthritis (711.50-711.59).

Inoculation against chickenpox is reported with V05.4.

© 2004 Ingenix, Inc.

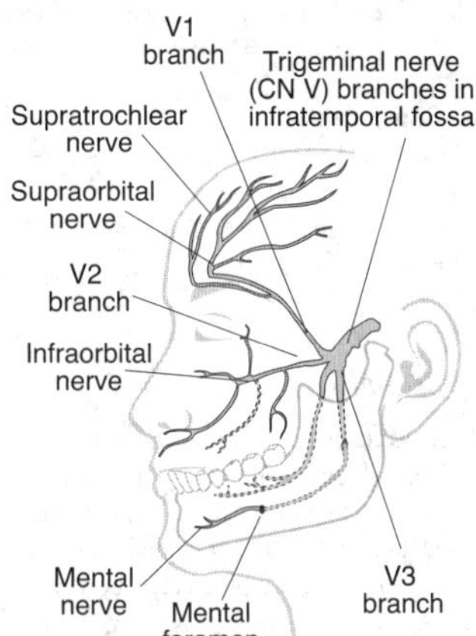

053 Herpes zoster

Varicella zoster virus causes chickenpox and herpes zoster. Chickenpox is the initial, acute phase of the disease, and herpes zoster is a reactivation of the virus in a latent stage. Herpes zoster is often referred to as shingles or zona. In herpes zoster, the virus causes unilateral eruptions and painful neuralgia along a nerve path. The disease is classified according to site.

053.0 Herpes zoster with meningitis — *inflammation of brain and/or spinal cord*

053.10 Herpes zoster with unspecified nervous system complication — *unknown nervous system complication*

053.11 Geniculate herpes zoster — *affecting facial nerve*

053.12 Postherpetic trigeminal neuralgia — *causing oral or nasal pain*

053.13 Postherpetic polyneuropathy — *multiple nerve involvement*

053.19 Other herpes zoster with nervous system complications

053.20 Herpes zoster dermatitis of eyelid — *unilateral, eyelid*

053.21 Herpes zoster keratoconjunctivitis — *unilateral in cornea and conjunctiva*

053.22 Herpes zoster iridocyclitis — *unilateral in iris and ciliary body*

053.29 Other ophthalmic herpes zoster complications — *other eye complication*

053.71 Otitis externa due to herpes zoster

053.79 Other specified herpes zoster complications

053.8 Unspecified herpes zoster complication

053.9 Herpes zoster without mention of complication

054 Herpes simplex

Herpes simplex is an infection of the herpes simplex virus (HSV), including HSV-1 and HSV-2. The infection causes multiple clusters of fluid-filled, inflamed blisters on the skin or mucous membranes and is usually transmitted by direct contact. HSV-1 is commonly seen about the mouth, lips, and conjunctiva. HSV-2 usually affects genitals and is often transmitted through sexual contact. However, either type of HSV can occur in either site.

The virus can remain dormant and be reactivated by emotional stress, fever, or photosensitivity. Typically, the virus is localized, and code selection is based on the anatomy affected. Herpes simplex infections of the lips or mouth are considered the most benign form of the disease and are reported as "uncomplicated," with 054.9. Systemic manifestations can occur, especially in infants and in the immunosuppressed.

054.0 Eczema herpeticum — *invading pre-existing skin inflammation*

054.10 Unspecified genital herpes — *unknown site*
AHA: Jan-Feb, 1987, 15-16

054.11 Herpetic vulvovaginitis — *vulva and vagina*
AHA: Jan-Feb, 1987, 15-16

054.12 Herpetic ulceration of vulva — *vulva*
AHA: Jan-Feb, 1987, 15-16

054.13 Herpetic infection of penis — *penis*
AHA: Jan-Feb, 1987, 15-16

054.19 Other genital herpes — *other specified site*
AHA: Jan-Feb, 1987, 15-16

054.2 Herpetic gingivostomatitis — *oral mucosa*

054.3 Herpetic meningoencephalitis — *inflammation of brain and spinal cord*

054.40 Unspecified ophthalmic complication herpes simplex — *unknown eye complication*

054.41 Herpes simplex dermatitis of eyelid — *inflammation and lesions on lid*

054.42 Dendritic keratitis — *inflammation and ulcers of cornea*

054.43 Herpes simplex disciform keratitis — *inflammation and edema of cornea*

054.44 Herpes simplex iridocyclitis — *inflammation of iris and ciliary body*

054.49 Herpes simplex with other ophthalmic complications — *eye complication not elsewhere classified*

054.5 Herpetic septicemia — *herpes simplex disseminated through bloodstream*
AHA: Q2, 2000, 5

054.6 Herpetic whitlow — *painful herpes lesion on fingertip; "herpetic felon"*

054.71 Visceral herpes simplex — *infection of thoracic or abdominal organ*

054.72 Herpes simplex meningitis — *inflammation of lining of brain or spinal cord*

054.73 Herpes simplex otitis externa — *inflammation and lesions of external ear*

054.79 Other specified herpes simplex complications — *complication not elsewhere classified*

054.8 Unspecified herpes simplex complication — *unknown complications*

054.9 Herpes simplex without mention of complication — *uncomplicated "fever blister"*

Coding Clarification

This rubric excludes congenital herpes simplex, which is reported with 771.2.

055 Measles

Measles is an acute infection caused by paramyxovirus and presents with a hacking cough, rash, and fevers. German measles (rubella) is a different infection, reported with codes from the 056 rubric.

Measles are usually transmitted from person to person via airborne respiratory droplets. Pharyngitis is common. Koplik's spots are white, grainy spots that can occur in the buccal mucosa and are an early symptom of measles.

In the United States, measles outbreaks have been greatly reduced by government immunization programs. Measles has a low mortality rate in healthy individuals, and the disease generally follows a normal course with high fever, Koplik's spots, generalized rash, and cough.

Patients with measles are susceptible to streptococcal infection, worsening of tuberculosis, or reactivation of an inactive mycobacterial infection. Sequence the measles code first, followed by codes for the secondary infection.

Measles are classified according to complication. In most cases, the complication occurs after the symptoms of the measles have diminished. Pneumonia as a complication is most common in infants.

055.0 Postmeasles encephalitis — *brain infection*

055.1 Postmeasles pneumonia — *lung infection*

055.2 Postmeasles otitis media — *middle ear infection*

055.71 Measles keratoconjunctivitis — *inflammation of cornea and conjunctiva*

055.79 Other specified measles complications — *complication not elsewhere classified*

055.8 Unspecified measles complication — *unknown complication*

055.9 Measles without mention of complication — *typical course of rash, fever, and cough*

Coding Clarification

Prophylactic vaccination against measles is reported with V04.2 as a separate inoculation, or V06.4 for measles-mumps-rubella (MMR) inoculation. Measles that follow a normal course should be reported with code 055.9.

056 Rubella

Rubella is also called German measles or three-day measles. It is a highly contagious virus, but the symptoms are mild and short-lived in most people. Symptoms include malaise, arthralgia, rash, headache, and fever. Rubella during pregnancy, however, can result in abortion, stillbirth, or in congenital defects. Because of its highly contagious nature and affect upon the fetus, rubella is considered a serious health threat.

Rubella codes are selected according to complication. Consult the index to report rubella during pregnancy.

056.00 Unspecified rubella neurological complication — *unknown nervous complication*

056.01 Encephalomyelitis due to rubella — *inflammation of brain and spinal cord*

056.09 Other neurological rubella complications — *nervous complication not elsewhere classified*

056.71 Arthritis due to rubella — *inflammation of joint*

056.79 Rubella with other specified complications — *complication not elsewhere classified, not nervous system*

056.8 Unspecified rubella complications — *unknown complication*

056.9 Rubella without mention of complication — *typical course of rash and fever*

Coding Clarification

If the infection runs its normal course, report rubella without complication with 056.9.

This rubric excludes congential rubella, which is reported with 771.0.

Exposure to rubella is reported with V01.4.

Prophylactic vaccination against rubella is reported with V04.3 as a separate inoculation or V06.4 for measles-mumps-rubella (MMR) inoculation.

057 Other viral exanthemata

This rubric captures rash-causing viruses that are not specifically outlined in rubrics 050-056.

© 2004 Ingenix, Inc.

057.0 Erythema infectiosum (fifth disease) — *contagious rash, livid on cheeks*

057.8 Other specified viral exanthemata — *including fourth disease, sixth disease, roseola infantum, monkeypox*

057.9 Unspecified viral exanthem — *unknown viral exanthemata*

Coding Clarification

Report 057.0 for fifth disease, also called Sticker's disease or erythema infectiosum.

Report 057.8 for any of the following: Dukes (-Filatow) disease, exanthema subitum or sixth disease, fourth disease, parascarlatina, pseudoscarlatina, roseola infantum, and Zahorsky's disease.

060–066 Arthropod–borne Viral Diseases

Insects are the carriers that carry the diseases classified to this section of ICD-9-CM. Early attempts to classify these diseases were made along geographic lines and according to the insect believed to be the carrier. An arbovirus is a common shortened name for arthropod-borne virus.

Mosquitoes are the most common carrier, or transmitting agent, for arboviruses. The bite of a mosquito often transmits the disease from bird to mosquito. The bite of a mosquito to man transmits the disease to man. In equine disease, the mosquitoes transmit disease to horses, or from horses to man. Seldom is the disease carried from man to mosquito to man.

060 Yellow fever

Yellow fever is transmitted from mosquito to man. In cities, the bite of an *Aedes aegypti* mosquito causes the infection; in the jungle (sylvan), *Haemagogus* and other forest canopy mosquitoes acquire the virus from jungle primates and transmit the virus to man. In the United States, cases of yellow fever are usually limited to people who have been abroad. Yellow fever is most commonly seen in Central Africa, South America, and Central America.

Yellow fever causes high fever, headache, jaundice, and hemorrhage. The pulse is slow. Mortality rate can be as high as 10 percent.

060.0 Sylvatic yellow fever — (Use additional code to identify any associated meningitis, 321.2) — *origin in jungle or woods; usually transmitted animal to man, by mosquito*

060.1 Urban yellow fever — (Use additional code to identify any associated meningitis, 321.2) — *origin in city or town; usually transmitted man to man, by mosquito*

060.9 Unspecified yellow fever — (Use additional code to identify any associated meningitis, 321.2) — *unknown*

Coding Clarification

Prophylactic inoculation against yellow fever is reported with V04.4.

061 Dengue OK

Dengue is transmitted to man by the bite of the Aedes mosquito. The disease is endemic throughout tropical and subtropical regions, and is usually seen in the United States only when people come to this country already infected with the virus.

Dengue causes chills, headache, backache, and prostration. Joint and leg aches and onset of high fever are rapid.

Coding Clarification

This rubric excludes hemorrhagic fever caused by dengue, which is reported with 065.4.

062 Mosquito-borne viral encephalitis

These diseases cause central nervous system symptoms like tremors, convulsion, coma, confusion, as well as headache, vomiting, and fever. Geographic differences are significant among the varieties. Japanese encephalitis is seen in the Far East. Eastern equine encephalitis (EEE) is most common in the Atlantic and Gulf Coast states, upper New York, and western Michigan. Western equine encephalitis (WEE) is seen in areas west of the Mississippi. St. Louis encephalitis is most common in the United States and Caribbean. Australian encephalitis is usually limited to New Guinea and Australia, and California encephalitis.

062.0 Japanese encephalitis — (Use additional code to identify any associated meningitis, 321.2) — *Flavivirus; Japanese B*

062.1 Western equine encephalitis — (Use additional code to identify any associated meningitis, 321.2) — *Alphavirus; WEE*

062.2 Eastern equine encephalitis — (Use additional code to identify any associated meningitis, 321.2) — *Alphavirus; EEE*

062.3 St. Louis encephalitis — (Use additional code to identify any associated meningitis, 321.2) — *Flavivirus; in United States*

062.4 Australian encephalitis — (Use additional code to identify any associated meningitis, 321.2) — *Flavivirus; in Australia*

062.5 California virus encephalitis — (Use additional code to identify any associated meningitis, 321.2)

062.8 Other specified mosquito-borne viral encephalitis — (Use additional code to identify any associated meningitis, 321.2) — *including Ilheus virus*

062.9 Unspecified mosquito-borne viral encephalitis — (Use additional code to identify any associated meningitis, 321.2) — *unknown*

Coding Clarification

Report Venezuelan equine encephalitis with 066.2.

Report West Nile virus with 066.40-066.49.

063 Tick-borne viral encephalitis

In tick-borne encephalitis, a tick is the carrier instead of a mosquito. Included in this rubric are diseases limited to Russia, Central Europe, and Great Britain. Only Powassan encephalitis is commonly found in North America, both in New York and in Canada. Any other variety is likely to be found among travelers.

063.0 Russian spring-summer (taiga) encephalitis — (Use additional code to identify any associated meningitis, 321.2) — *Russia, central Europe*

063.1 Louping ill — (Use additional code to identify any associated meningitis, 321.2) — *British Isles*

063.2 Central European encephalitis — (Use additional code to identify any associated meningitis, 321.2) — *central Europe*

063.8 Other specified tick-borne viral encephalitis — (Use additional code to identify any associated meningitis, 321.2) — *including Langat and Powassan (New York)*

063.9 Unspecified tick-borne viral encephalitis — (Use additional code to identify any associated meningitis, 321.2)

Coding Clarification

Powassan encephalitis is reported with 063.8

064 Viral encephalitis transmitted by other and unspecified arthropods OK

Report viral encephalitis not otherwise specified, unknown carrier, with 049.9, reserving this code for encephalitis caused by an unidentified arbovirus.

065 Arthropod-borne hemorrhagic fever

This rubric specifies a hemorrhagic fever. If hemorrhage is not a component, seek other codes.

Hemorrhagic fever is not endemic to the United States. Codes in this category may apply to infections obtained while abroad, primarily in Russia and Asia.

065.0 Crimean hemorrhagic fever (CHF Congo virus) — (Use additional code to identify any associated meningitis, 321.2) — *Crimea and Russian Don and Volga river valleys*

065.1 Omsk hemorrhagic fever — (Use additional code to identify any associated meningitis, 321.2) — *Siberia*

065.2 Kyasanur Forest disease — (Use additional code to identify any associated meningitis, 321.2) — *India*

065.3 Other tick-borne hemorrhagic fever — (Use additional code to identify any associated meningitis, 321.2) — *other*

065.4 Mosquito-borne hemorrhagic fever — (Use additional code to identify any associated meningitis, 321.2) — *Dengue hemorrhagic; Chikungunya hemorrhagic*

065.8 Other specified arthropod-borne hemorrhagic fever — (Use additional code to identify any associated meningitis, 321.2) — *including mite-borne hemorrhagic*

065.9 Unspecified arthropod-borne hemorrhagic fever — (Use additional code to identify any associated meningitis, 321.2) — *unknown hemorrhagic arbovirus*

Coding Clarification

Hemorrhagic Dengue fever is reported with 065.4; for dengue fever without mention of hemorrhage, report 061.

Hemorrhagic Chikungunya fever is reported with 065.4; for Chikungunya fever without mention of hemorrhage, report 066.3.

In all cases, with or without hemorrhage, yellow fever is reported with 060.0-060.9.

066 Other arthropod-borne viral diseases

This rubric captures arbovirus infections not classified as hemorrhagic, as causing encephalitis, and not the specific infections of yellow fever or dengue. Colorado tick fever is the arbovirus in this section that would likely be seen in the United States, and causes fever, malaise, headaches, and myalgia. This is a different infection than Rocky Mountain spotted fever, a *Rickettsia* infection that causes a petechial rash in addition to fever, malaise, headache, and myalgia.

West Nile fever is an arbovirus, transmitted to humans by an arthropod, in this case, an infected mosquito. West Nile fever was first isolated 65 years ago in Uganda but was not reported in the continental United States until 1999. It affects humans, birds, and some mammals, including horses, cats, bats, skunks, chipmunks, squirrels, and rabbits. It can cause fatal inflammation of the brain, encephalitis, or of the lining of the brain or spinal cord, meningitis. As a

© 2004 Ingenix, Inc.

result, it is sometimes called West Nile encephalitis or West Nile encephalomyelitis.

066.0	Phlebotomus fever — (Use additional code to identify any associated meningitis, 321.2) — *sandfly-borne; Asia, Mideast, South America*
066.1	Tick-borne fever — (Use additional code to identify any associated meningitis, 321.2) — *American mountain; Colorado*
066.2	Venezuelan equine fever — (Use additional code to identify any associated meningitis, 321.2)
066.3	Other mosquito-borne fever — (Use additional code to identify any associated meningitis, 321.2) — *Bunyamwera; O'nyong-nyong; Rift valley*
066.40	West Nile fever, unspecified
066.41	West Nile fever with encephalitis
066.42	West Nile fever with other neurologic manifestation
066.49	West Nile fever with other complications
066.8	Other specified arthropod-borne viral diseases — (Use additional code to identify any associated meningitis, 321.2) — *including Chandipura and Piry fever*
066.9	Unspecified arthropod-borne viral disease — (Use additional code to identify any associated meningitis, 321.2) — *unknown arbovirus*

Coding Clarification

Colorado tick fever is reported with 066.1.

Rocky Mountain spotted fever is reported with 082.0.

Use an additional code with 066.42 and 066.49 to specify the other conditions.

070–079 Other Diseases Due to Viruses and Chlamydiae

This rubric covers a broad spectrum of infection not elsewhere classified.

070 Viral hepatitis

Hepatitis is an inflammation or infection of the liver. Symptoms of hepatitis range from flu-like illness to liver failure and death. Initially, nausea and malaise are common. Later in the course of the disease, jaundice and an enlarged liver are common.

Hepatitis A (HAV) is spread through fecal contamination or by eating contaminated, raw shellfish and is considered to be a milder form of hepatitis. Exposure to hepatitis B (HBV) is limited to direct contact with contaminated blood or blood products, or through sexual congress. HBV is the source of many chronic liver ailments. The hepatitis C virus (HCV) causes 80 percent of hepatitis cases resulting from blood transfusions, and also is associated with more chronic and severe liver ailments. The hepatitis E virus (HEV) is associated with fecal contamination and is a milder form of the disease.

The following fifth-digit subclassification is for use with categories 070.2 and 070.3:

0 acute or unspecified, without mention of hepatitis delta

1 acute or unspecified, with hepatitis delta

2 chronic, without mention of hepatitis delta

3 chronic, with hepatitis delta

070.0	Viral hepatitis A with hepatic coma
070.1	Viral hepatitis A without mention of hepatic coma
070.2 5th	Viral hepatitis B with hepatic coma
070.3 5th	Viral hepatitis B without mention of hepatic coma
070.41	Acute hepatitis C with hepatic coma
070.42	Hepatitis delta without mention of active hepatitis B disease with hepatic coma
070.43	Hepatitis E with hepatic coma
070.44	Chronic hepatitis C with hepatic coma
070.49	Other specified viral hepatitis with hepatic coma
070.51	Acute hepatitis C without mention of hepatic coma
070.52	Hepatitis delta without mention of active hepatitis B disease or hepatic coma
070.53	Hepatitis E without mention of hepatic coma
070.54	Chronic hepatitis C without mention of hepatic coma
070.59	Other specified viral hepatitis without mention of hepatic coma
070.6	Unspecified viral hepatitis with hepatic coma
070.70	Unspecified viral hepatitis C without hepatic coma
070.71	Unspecified viral hepatitis C with hepatic coma
070.9	Unspecified viral hepatitis without mention of hepatic coma

Documentation Issues

Physician documentation should support answers to the following questions for accurate code selection to be made:

1. Is the hepatitis viral or non-viral?
2. What type of viral hepatitis does the patient have?
3. Is this an acute or chronic phase of the condition?
4. Did the patient experience hepatic coma?

5. Is the patient asymptomatic?

Coding Clarification

Chronic Active Hepatitis: ICD-9-CM classifies hepatitis along two axes, viral and non-viral. Viral forms of the disease are classified to category 070 *Viral hepatitis,* in the Infectious and Parasitic Disease chapter. Non-viral and unspecified hepatitis are classified to category 571 *Chronic liver disease and cirrhosis,* in the digestive system chapter. Further, hepatitis caused by other specific viruses like Epstein-Barr or cytomegaloviruses are considered separately, and do not fall into the general accepted usage of the phrase "viral hepatitis." Viral hepatitis is considered to be hepatitis caused by the hepatitis virus and this rubric covers acute and chronic stages of that disease.

If the diagnostic statement is documented as chronic active hepatitis, a code from category 571 should be selected because the type (viral or non-viral) of hepatitis is unspecified. This category specifically excludes viral forms of hepatitis and an excludes note is provided in the tabular section that references codes 070.0-070.9. If the diagnostic statement specifically indicates chronic active viral hepatitis, it should be assigned one code, 070.30 *Viral hepatitis B, without mention of hepatic coma, acute or unspecified, without mention of hepatitis delta.*

General Guidelines: Code selection is based on serotype, acute or chronic phase, and whether it is documented as with or without hepatic coma (code range: 070.0-070.9).

Viral hepatitis is classified into the following major forms:

- Hepatitis A virus or "infectious hepatitis" is caused by the Hepatitis A Virus and is found to be the generally milder disease transmitted by the fecal oral route. This type of viral hepatitis is less likely to progress to chronic forms of hepatitis or cirrhosis.

- Hepatitis B virus or "serum hepatitis" is the more serious virus. This type is transmitted parenterally (through blood products, injections, and sexual contact) and in a high number of cases progresses into chronic liver disease.

- Hepatitis C virus has been identified as the virus responsible for most cases of parenteral non-A, non-B hepatitis. Although typically associated with blood transfusions, it has been proven to result from other types of exposure (e.g., occupational-health care related, sexual contact). It has been noted that up to 40 percent of cases with this form have no recognized cause for the infection. Patients with hepatitis C are more likely to develop chronic liver disease and chronic manifestations such as chronic active hepatitis and/or cirrhosis.

- Hepatitis D, formally known as "Hepatitis Delta virus," is an incomplete virus and requires the presence of hepatitis B surface antigen (HBSAg) to replicate. Spread mainly by needles and blood, hepatitis delta may present itself as a co-infection during acute infection with hepatitis B, and in these cases is more likely to develop into a fulminant hepatitis than hepatitis B infection alone. Delta hepatitis causes acute and/or chronic liver disease in patients with a concurrent hepatitis B infection. A large number of these patients develop fulminant hepatitis and/or chronic active hepatitis and cirrhosis. Chronic delta infection is a frequent event and manifests as severe forms of chronic hepatitis with accelerated progression to cirrhosis and a high mortality rate.

- Hepatitis E virus or enteric "fecal-oral hepatitis" is serologically different from the other known hepatitis viruses. It is clearly produced by a different type of virus than that causing non-A non-B parenteral hepatitis. This type has been identified during investigations of large epidemics in ill-developing countries. The disease is also a clinically distinct entity as one of the foremost causes of acute viral hepatitis in young to middle aged adults in developing countries and carries a high case-fatality rate among pregnant women. Chronic liver disease has not been reported in these cases.q

Acute and Chronic: Both acute and chronic stages of viral hepatitis are classified to category 070 *Viral hepatitis.* When coding viral hepatitis, keep in mind that the fourth-digit subclassification only provides for identifying serotypes with and without mention of coma. Fifth digits are provided in the viral hepatitis categories to differentiate between acute and chronic viral hepatitis. If the diagnostic statement states that the patient has both, then a code for each should be assigned.

Carrier Status: A carrier is defined as a person who has hepatitis B, C, or D in his/her blood even after all of the symptoms (with the exception of fatigue) have disappeared. If the virus is present in the blood it can be transmitted to others. Codes for carrier or suspected carrier of viral hepatitis would be located in the V Codes chapter, category V02.

Pregnancy and Viral Hepatitis: Use code 647.6x *Other viral diseases,* with an additional code to identify the specific form of viral hepatitis. To identify pregnant women who are carriers, use the code that identifies the carrier state as a secondary diagnosis code with OB code 648.9x *Other current conditions classifiable elsewhere.*

Prophylactic Vaccinations: Currently, prophylactic administration of hepatitis vaccines is being provided to newborns upon parental approval. Since hepatitis B vaccination is recommended for all newborns, V05.3 may be used as an additional code on hospital

 © 2004 Ingenix, Inc.

newborn records. Hospitals assign procedure code 99.55 *Prophylactic administration of vaccine against other diseases.*

Coding Scenario

A 49-year-old female is seen in the office for a pre-employment screening and tested positive for hepatitis B. The patient has shown no symptoms for hepatitis. The patients' past medical history shows a long history of IV drug use.

> Code assignment: V70.5 *Health examination of defined subpopulations* and V02.61 *Hepatitis B carrier*

A 29-year-old male patient is admitted to the hospital with severe hepatic encephalopathy and jaundice. The patient is diagnosed with viral hepatitis B and hepatic encephalopathy.

> Code assignment: 070.21 *Viral hepatitis B with hepatic coma, acute or usnspecified, without hepatitis delta*

A patient is seen in the office for treatment of chronic viral hepatitis, type C.

> Code assignment: 070.54 *Chronic hepatitis C without mention of hepatic coma*

A patient is admitted to the hospital with acute fulminant hepatitis and liver failure due to chronic viral hepatitis type B.

> Code assignment: 070.32 *Viral hepatitis B without mention of hepatic coma, chronic, without mention of hepatitis delta* and 570 *Acute and subacute necrosis of liver*

071 Rabies OK

Rabies, or hydrophobia, is an acute infectious disease caused by a neurotropic virus found in the saliva of rabid mammals. Canine vaccination has nearly eliminated canine rabies in the United States and cases of wild animal bites causing rabies are rare. Rabies causes restlessness, fever, excessive salivation, and painful laryngeal spasms.

Exposure to rabies is usually treated successfully with immediate local wound cleansing and administration of rabies immune globulin.

If the patient develops rabies, the diagnosis is no longer an imminent death sentence. Supportive treatment of respiratory system, circulatory system, and central nervous system complications can result in positive outcome for the symptomatic rabies patient. Rabies is often described as urban or sylvan, depending on the source of infection.

Coding Clarification

This code is used to report active rabies infection, not simple exposure to rabies.

If a person has been exposed to rabies, but infection status is unknown or an infection has not developed, report V01.5.

To report inoculation against rabies, whether following exposure or as a prophylactic measure for high-risk individuals like wildlife handlers, report V04.5.

Whether the carrier is from the city or the wilderness, rabies infection is reported with 071.

072 Mumps

Mumps presents as an acute infection of the salivary glands, usually the parotids, caused by paramyxovirus. Inhaling respiratory droplets from an infected person can spread the disease. Most cases occur in children 2 years of age or older. Mumps causes painful swelling of the salivary glands, pain upon chewing, and high fever. Complications may occur, especially in adults.

072.0 Mumps orchitis — *inflammation of testis*

072.1 Mumps meningitis — *inflammation of lining of brain and/or spinal cord*

072.2 Mumps encephalitis — *inflammation of brain*

072.3 Mumps pancreatitis — *inflammation of pancreas*

072.71 Mumps hepatitis — *inflammation of liver*

072.72 Mumps polyneuropathy — *inflammation of nerves*

072.79 Mumps with other specified complications — *specified inflammation not elsewhere classified*

072.8 Unspecified mumps complication — *complication not elsewhere classified*

072.9 Mumps without mention of complication — *normal course of mumps*

Coding Clarification

Code selection for mumps is determined by complication. In cases that follow the normal uncomplicated course of swollen parotid glands and high fever, report 072.9.

Prophylactic vaccination against mumps is reported with V04.6 as a separate inoculation or V06.4 for measles-mumps-rubella (MMR) inoculation.

073 Ornithosis

Ornithosis is also called psittacosis. The disease is caused by *Chlamydia psittaci* and transmitted most commonly by parrots, parakeets, or lovebirds, but sometimes by domestic birds like pigeons, turkeys, or canaries, or by some seabirds. Infection usually occurs when dust or droppings are inhaled by man or, rarely, by a bird bite. Ornithosis can also be transmitted from man to man, but this is very rare.

Symptoms include fever, malaise, and cough, in the case of lung infection. Ornithosis has a 30 percent mortality rate without treatment, but responds well to antibiotics.

073.0 Ornithosis with pneumonia — *pulmonary infection*

073.7 Ornithosis with other specified complications — *complication not elsewhere classified*

073.8 Ornithosis with unspecified complication — *complication not specified*

073.9 Unspecified ornithosis — *no complications*

Coding Clarification
Code selection for ornithosis is based on type of complication. Report any significant symptoms, like cough or shortness of breath, secondarily.

074 Specific diseases due to Coxsackievirus

Coxsackie virus commonly causes infection in summer and fall and is transmitted man-to-man via oral secretions, feces, or blood. Herpangina is an acute infection of Coxsackie virus, causing throat lesions, fever, and vomiting, generally seen in children during the summer months. Epidemic pleurodynia is a Coxsackie infection causing severe paroxysmal pain in the chest and fever, usually limited to young adults and children. It is also called Bornholm disease or devil's grip.

Coxsackie carditis is infection of the heart. Code selection is based on whether the infection occurs in the outer lining of the heart, the heart cavities, or the heart muscle. In infants, a Coxsackie infection of the heart muscle can be life threatening, but this infection can occur at any age.

Hand, foot, and mouth disease is a Coxsackie infection of the hands, feet, and oral mucosa, most commonly seen in preschool children. It is usually a mild infection.

074.0 Herpangina — *vesicular pharyngitis; typically children in summer*

074.1 Epidemic pleurodynia — *chest pain with fever; typically children and young adults*

074.20 Coxsackie carditis, unspecified — *inflammation of heart unspecified*

074.21 Coxsackie pericarditis — *inflammation of outer lining of heart*

074.22 Coxsackie endocarditis — *inflammation of within the heart cavities*

074.23 Coxsackie myocarditis — *inflammation of muscle of heart*

074.3 Hand, foot, and mouth disease — *lesions on hands, feet, and mouth; typically preschoolers*

074.8 Other specified diseases due to Coxsackievirus — *including acute lymphonodular pharyngitis*

Coding Clarification
Report Coxsackie meningitis with 047.0 and Coxsackie enteritis with 008.67.

Coxsackie virus infection of the nervous system, not elsewhere classified, is reported with 048.

075 Infectious mononucleosis OK

AHA: March-April, 1987, 8; Q3, 2001, 13

Infectious mononucleosis is an active infection by the Epstein-Barr virus, causing fever, sore throat, enlarged lymph glands spleen, and fatigue. It is most commonly seen in teens and young adults, and runs a mild course in most cases.

Coding Clarification
In mononucleosis with hepatitis, report 075 and 573.1.

076 Trachoma

Trachoma is caused by infection with the organism *Chlamydia trachomatis*. It begins slowly as a mild conjunctivitis that develops into a severe onset infection. The initial stage lasts several weeks and is followed by a chronic stage in which the lids remain swollen, and the cornea becomes eroded, scarred, and vascularized. The lids develop contractures and may turn outward, pulling away form the eye. Eventually, the eyelashes turn in, rubbing on the cornea at the front of the eye. The scarring on the cornea leads to severe vision loss and blindness, usually when people are 40 to 50 years of age.

076.0 Initial stage trachoma — *mild inflammation of conjunctiva with pain*

076.1 Active stage trachoma — *acute inflammation of conjunctiva with pain*

076.9 Unspecified trachoma — *stage unknown*

Coding Clarification
Report late effects of trachoma with 139.1. Code the sequelae first, as in vision loss (369.00-369.9), followed by 139.1.

077 Other diseases of conjunctiva due to viruses and Chlamydiae

Codes in this rubric are organized by infective agent and symptoms. Inclusion conjunctivitis is caused by Chlamydia trachomatis and adenovirus type B causes epidemic keratoconjunctivitis and pharyngoconjunctival fever.

077.0 Inclusion conjunctivitis — *due to Chlamydia trachomatis*

 © 2004 Ingenix, Inc.

077.1 Epidemic keratoconjunctivitis — *shipyard eye; due to adenovirus type B*

077.2 Pharyngoconjunctival fever — *due to adenovirus type B*

077.3 Other adenoviral conjunctivitis — *acute adenoviral follicular conjunctivitis*

077.4 Epidemic hemorrhagic conjunctivitis

077.8 Other viral conjunctivitis — *including Newcastle conjunctivitis*

077.98 Unspecified diseases of conjunctiva due to Chlamydiae

077.99 Unspecified diseases of conjunctiva due to viruses — *unknown virus*

Coding Clarification

Other diseases and infections of the conjunctiva can be found in the Nervous System chapter under rubrics 372 and 373, as well as under specific infective agents, for example, herpes zoster keratoconjunctivitis (053.21) or trachoma (076.0-076.9).

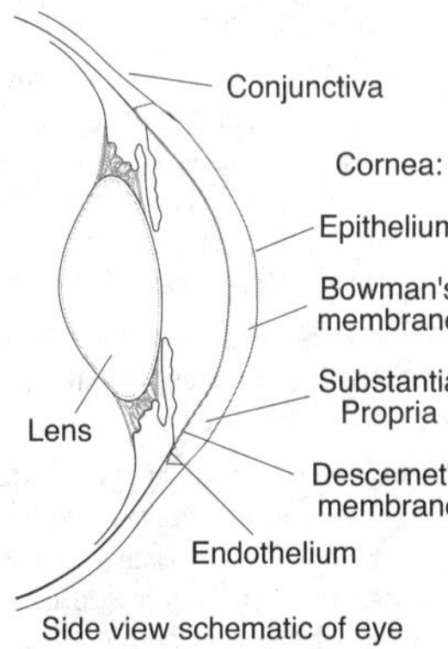

Side view schematic of eye

078 Other diseases due to viruses and Chlamydiae

This rubric addresses specific viral and chlamydial diseases not specified elsewhere.

More than 50 types of human papilloma viruses (HPV) cause plantar and genital warts in humans. These infections may be asymptomatic or produce warts or mucosal lesions.

Commonly, human papilloma virus causes viral warts. They may be documented as condyloma, verruca, or verruca vulgaris. Viral warts caused by condylomata acuminata are sexually transmitted genital warts, distinct from other viral warts in that they are associated with cervical dysplasia and carcinoma of the cervix, penis, and vulva.

Cytomegaloviral disease (CMV) is a human salivary gland virus and member of the herpes group. It affects only humans, and can range in symptoms from being a benign and asymptomatic infection to causing significant impairment or death in infants and the immunosuppressed. In symptomatic cases, fatigue, lymphadenopathy, and low fever may be present.

CMV is a most common and serious organ transplant infection complication.

078.0 Molluscum contagiosum — *poxvirus causing small bumps on skin or conjunctiva*

078.10 Unspecified viral warts — *horny skin wars; human papilloma virus*
AHA: Q4, 1993, 22; Q2, 1997, 9

078.11 Condyloma acuminatum — *clusters of lesions on genitalia; STD*
AHA: Q4, 1993, 22; Q2, 1997, 9

078.19 Other specified viral warts — *including Verruca plantaris, Verruca plana; fig wart*
AHA: Q4, 1993, 22; Q2, 1997, 9

078.2 Sweating fever — *sweating disease; miliary fever*

078.3 Cat-scratch disease — *mild and benign lymphoreticulosis*

078.4 Foot and mouth disease — *aphthous fever; ulcers on mouth, legs and feet*

078.5 Cytomegaloviral disease — (Use additional code to identify manifestation: 484.1, 573.1) — *CMV*
AHA: Q1, 1989, 9; Q2, 1993, 11; Q3, 1998, 4; Q1, 2003, 10

078.6 Hemorrhagic nephrosonephritis — *Russia and Korea*

078.7 Arenaviral hemorrhagic fever — *Argentina and Bolivia*

078.81 Epidemic vertigo — *dizziness*

078.82 Epidemic vomiting syndrome — *winter vomiting disease*

078.88 Other specified diseases due to Chlamydiae — *not elsewhere classified*
AHA: Q4, 1996, 22

078.89 Other specified diseases due to viruses — *including Marburg disease, Lassa fever; green monkey disease, pseudorabies, tanapox, and Aujeszky's disease*

Documentation Issues

Condyloma acuminatum are commonly called genital warts on the patient record, but, unless condyloma acuminatum is specifically noted, the patient record does not substantiate use of code 078.11.

Coding Clarification

Viral warts may be documented as condyloma, verruca, or verruca vulgaris and are reported with 078.10.

Viral warts caused by condylomata acuminata are reported with 078.11.

If CMV infection follows transplant, assign a code from category 996.8 to identify the transplanted organ, and 078.5 to report the infection.

When appropriate, an additional code is used to identify the manifestation of CMV infection, as in hepatitis (573.1) or pneumonia (484.1).

For congenital cytomegaloviral infection, report 771.1.

079 Viral and chlamydial infection in conditions classified elsewhere and of unspecified site

HIV-2, generally not seen in the United States, is on the rise elsewhere in the world.

Respiratory syncytial virus (RSV) is a common cause of respiratory disease in winter in the United States. Infants are most vulnerable to the disease. Each year, RSV causes 4,500 U.S. deaths and 90,000 hospitalizations.

Hantavirus is an arbovirus that causes severe respiratory distress in its victims. The mortality rate for *Hantavirus* is about 50 percent, with treatment. Most commonly transmitted to humans when they inhale dust from feces of infected mice, most cases are seen in the Four Corners area of the United States.

SARS (severe acute respiratory syndrome) is a form of respiratory infection that is spreading rapidly through Southeast Asia and other parts of the world. Patients start out with a fever and often have chills, headache, malaise, body aches, and placid respiratory symptoms. In the early stage, patients have decreased white blood cell counts and some also have diarrhea. After three to seven days, the patient usually develops a dry, non-productive cough that increases in severity. As the disease progresses, chest x-rays show significant congestion in the lungs. Eventually, not enough oxygen gets to the blood and, in 10 to 20 percent of cases, patients will require mechanical ventilation. The severity of illness among patients is variable, ranging from mild symptoms to death. Only patients who have traveled within 10 days of the onset of symptoms to an area with suspected SARS cases, or have had contact with a person suspected of having SARS, are considered possible carriers of the disease.

079.0 Adenovirus infection in conditions classified elsewhere and of unspecified site — (Note: This code is to be used as an additional code to identify the viral agent in diseases classifiable elsewhere and viral infection of unspecified nature or site)

079.1 ECHO virus infection in conditions classified elsewhere and of unspecified site — (Note: This code is to be used as an additional code to identify the viral agent in diseases classifiable elsewhere and viral infection of unspecified nature or site)

079.2 Coxsackievirus infection in conditions classified elsewhere and of unspecified site — (Note: This code is to be used as an additional code to identify the viral agent in diseases classifiable elsewhere and viral infection of unspecified nature or site)

079.3 Rhinovirus infection in conditions classified elsewhere and of unspecified site — (Note: This code is to be used as an additional code to identify the viral agent in diseases classifiable elsewhere and viral infection of unspecified nature or site)

079.4 Human papilloma virus in conditions classified elsewhere and of unspecified site — (Note: This code is to be used as an additional code to identify the viral agent in diseases classifiable elsewhere and viral infection of unspecified nature or site)

079.50 Unspecified retrovirus in conditions classified elsewhere and of unspecified site — (Note: This code is to be used as an additional code to identify the viral agent in diseases classifiable elsewhere and viral infection of unspecified nature or site)

079.52 Human t-cell lymphotrophic virus, type II (HTLV-II), in conditions classified elsewhere and of unspecified site

079.53 Human immunodeficiency virus, type 2 (HIV 2), in conditions classified elsewhere and of unspecified site — (Note: This code is to be used as an additional code to identify the viral agent in diseases classifiable elsewhere and viral infection of unspecified nature or site)

079.59 Other specified retrovirus, in conditions classified elsewhere and of unspecified site — (Note: This code is to be used as an additional code to identify the viral agent in diseases classifiable elsewhere and viral infection of unspecified nature or site)

079.6 Respiratory syncytial virus (RSV) — (Note: This code is to be used as an additional code to identify the viral agent in diseases classifiable elsewhere and viral infection of unspecified nature or site)

079.81 Hantavirus infection — (Note: This code is to be used as an additional code to identify the viral agent in diseases classifiable elsewhere and viral infection of unspecified nature or site)

© 2004 Ingenix, Inc.

079.82 SARS-associated coronavirus — (Note: This code is to be used as an additional code to identify the viral agent in diseases classifiable elsewhere and viral infection of unspecified nature or site) — *severe acute respiratory syndrome*
AHA: Q4, 2003, 46

079.88 Other specified chlamydial infection, in conditions classified elsewhere and of unspecified site — (Note: This code is to be used as an additional code to identify the viral agent in diseases classifiable elsewhere and viral infection of unspecified nature or site)

079.89 Other specified viral infection, in conditions classified elsewhere and of unspecified site — (Note: This code is to be used as an additional code to identify the viral agent in diseases classifiable elsewhere and viral infection of unspecified nature or site)

079.98 Unspecified chlamydial infection, in conditions classified elsewhere and of unspecified site — (Note: This code is to be used as an additional code to identify the viral agent in diseases classifiable elsewhere and viral infection of unspecified nature or site)

079.99 Unspecified viral infection, in conditions classified elsewhere and of unspecified site — (Note: This code is to be used as an additional code to identify the viral agent in diseases classifiable elsewhere and viral infection of unspecified nature or site)

Coding Clarification

For some respiratory infections, report the infection first and RSV as the infective agent secondarily, as in tracheobronchitis due to RSV, with 466.0 and 079.6. If respiratory syncytial virus is noted with acute bronchitis, two codes are required: 466.0 *Acute bronchitis* and 079.6 *Respiratory syncytial virus (RSV)*.

Some respiratory infection codes identify RSV as the infective agent, so only one code is necessary. Bronchiolitis due to RSV is reported with a single code, 466.11, and pneumonia due to RSV is reported with a single code, 480.1.

Report 079.81 secondarily to pneumonia or other infection code from the Respiratory System chapter of ICD-9-CM.

Report HIV-2 with 079.53 and HIV-1 with 042.

080–088 Rickettsioses and Other Arthropod–borne Diseases

Rickettsial diseases are usually perpetuated by a cycle from animal to insect carrier to man. The illnesses are sudden in onset and include fever, myalgia, malaise, headache, and sometimes rash. In some cases, rickettsioses produce a localized ulcer or lesion at the site of the insect bite.

080 Louse-borne (epidemic) typhus OK

Rickettsia prowazekii is transmitted by feces from the human body louse (*Pediculus humanus*), through a break in the skin, often from scratching, or by entry of the louse droppings into mucus membranes. Epidemic typhus causes headache, rash, and high fever, and is most dangerous to people older than 50.

Coding Clarification

Report 080 for primary typhus infection.

081 Other typhus

Other varieties of typhus are classified by infective agent and by carrier.

081.0 Murine (endemic) typhus — *Rickettsia typi (mooseri); rat flea*

081.1 Brill's disease — *R. prowazekii recurrence*

081.2 Scrub typhus — *R. tsutsugamushi; chigger*

081.9 Unspecified typhus — *unknown*

Coding Clarification

Brill's disease is a reoccurrence of epidemic typhus (080) and is reported with 081.1.

082 Tick-borne rickettsioses

These diseases typically begin with a tick bite in which a lesion develops at the site of the bite. This may be called an eschar, or, in boutonneuse fever, a tache noire. Lymphadenopathy, low fever, and a rash usually follow.

Rocky Mountain spotted fever is endemic to the United States. Colorado tick fever is a different infection than Rocky Mountain spotted fever, which causes a petechial rash in addition to fever, malaise, headache, and myalgia.

Boutonneuse fever, caused by *Rickettsia conorii*, occurs in Africa, India, Europe, the Mideast, and near the Caspian, Black, and Mediterranean seas. Normally, boutonneuse fever, Queensland tick typhus, and North Asian tick fever are seen in the United States only among travelers who return with an infection.

Ehrlichiosis is likely caused by various *Ehrlichia* species and code selection is based on the species. Infection resembles Rocky Mountain spotted fever, without a rash, and illness may extend for weeks or months. The infection responds to antibiotics.

082.0 Spotted fevers — *Rocky Mountain spotted fever*

082.1 Boutonneuse fever — *Africa, India, Mediterranean*

082.2 North Asian tick fever — *Siberia*

082.3 Queensland tick typhus — *Australia*

082.40 Ehrlichiosis, unspecified — *unknown type*
AHA: Q4, 2000, 38

082.41 Ehrlichiosis chafeensis [E. chafeensis]

082.49 Other ehrlichiosis — *other than E. chaffeensis*
AHA: Q4, 2000, 38

082.8 Other specified tick-borne rickettsioses

082.9 Unspecified tick-borne rickettsiosis

083 Other rickettsioses

These specific varieties of rickettsioses infection do not fall into the previous rubric classifications.

083.0 Q fever — *Coxiella burnetii*

083.1 Trench fever — *Quintan, Wolhynian, Werner-His fever*

083.2 Rickettsialpox — *Rickettsia akari; mite*

083.8 Other specified rickettsioses — *not elsewhere classified*

083.9 Unspecified rickettsiosis — *unknown*

Coding Clarification

Report 083.9 for an infection known to be rickettsioses, but of unknown type and unknown carrier.

084 Malaria

Malaria is a mosquito-borne protozoan infection endemic to the tropics. It is transmitted man to mosquito to man and has largely been eradicated in the United States through insecticide programs and drugs. Most cases of malaria in the United States are seen in people who have traveled abroad. Sometimes, these infected travelers may even spawn a stateside epidemic of malaria. Rarely, malaria may be transmitted through a blood transfusion or shared needle.

Malaria causes malaise and headache with intermittent fever and chill. Jaundice usually develops. Some varieties, most notably Blackwater fever, can cause more serious complications including hemolysis.

084.0 Falciparum malaria (malignant tertian) — *Plasmodium falciparum*

084.1 Vivax malaria (benign tertian) — *P. vivax*

084.2 Quartan malaria — *P. malariae*

084.3 Ovale malaria — *P. ovale*

084.4 Other malaria — *monkey malaria*

084.5 Mixed malaria — *more than one parasite*

084.6 Unspecified malaria — *unknown*

084.7 Induced malaria — *therapeutically induced*

084.8 Blackwater fever — *P. falciparum; with hemoglobinuria*

084.9 Other pernicious complications of malaria — (Use additional code to identify complication: 573.2, 581.81) — *including algid and cerebral malaria*

Coding Clarification

Malaria is coded according to species of *Plasmodium: P. falciparum, P. malariae, P. ovale, P. vivax,* or mixed species. A code is also provided in this rubric for therapeutically induced malaria (084.7), regardless of species.

Do not report personal history of malaria (V12.03) in patients with active disease.

085 Leishmaniasis

Leishmaniasis is an infection by *Leishmania,* a genus of parasitic protozoa, usually seen in developing nations and rare in the United States, though seen in parts of South America. The focus of infection and the infective agent are variables that create a broad spectrum of disease associated with leishmaniasis.

085.0 Visceral leishmaniasis (kala-azar) — *L. donovani; systemic; in Far East, USSR, Africa, Mediterranean, South and Central America*

085.1 Cutaneous leishmaniasis, urban — *L. tropica minor; dry/ulcerating lesions; boils*

085.2 Cutaneous leishmaniasis, Asian desert — *L. tropica major; wet/necrotizing skin lesions*

085.3 Cutaneous leishmaniasis, Ethiopian — *L. aethiopica; widespread skin lesions*

085.4 Cutaneous leishmaniasis, American — *L. mexicana; L. tegumentaria diffusa; skin lesions*

085.5 Mucocutaneous leishmaniasis, (American) — *L. braziliensis; called espundia, uta, chiclero ulcer*

085.9 Unspecified leishmaniasis — *unknown Leishmania species*

086 Trypanosomiasis

Trypanosomiasis is caused by protozoa *Trypanosoma* and causes chronic disease with symptoms including fever, lymphadenopathy, headache, and edema. Complications can affect the central nervous system and major organs and can be fatal. International travelers may return to the United States with a trypanosomiasis infection, but the protozoa is endemic only in Africa and South America, so it is seldom seen in North America.

086.0 Chagas' disease with heart involvement — *Trypanosoma cruzi; heart involvement*

086.1 Chagas' disease with other organ involvement — *T. cruzi; other organ involvement*

 © 2004 Ingenix, Inc.

086.2 Chagas' disease without mention of organ involvement — *T. cruzi; no organ infection*

086.3 Gambian trypanosomiasis — *T. brucei gambiense*

086.4 Rhodesian trypanosomiasis — *T. brucei rhodesiense*

086.5 African trypanosomiasis, unspecified — *sleeping sickness*

086.9 Unspecified trypanosomiasis — *unknown trypanosomiasis*

Coding Clarification

Report the trypanosomiasis code first, followed by any manifestation codes that may apply, for example, encephalitis (323.2), meningitis (321.3). However, cardiomyopathy from Chagas' disease requires only 086.0, and other specific forms of Chagas' disease are reported with 078.88.

087 Relapsing fever

Relapsing fever is an infection caused by *Borrelia* and the symptoms are episodic and may include fever and arthralgia. Code selection is based on the carrier.

087.0 Louse-borne relapsing fever — *lice as carrier*

087.1 Tick-borne relapsing fever — *tick as carrier*

087.9 Unspecified relapsing fever — *unknown carrier*

Coding Clarification

Report 087.9 if the carrier is unknown.

088 Other arthropod-borne diseases

This category identifies arthropod-borne diseases not elsewhere classified.

Bartonellosis is in infection of *Bartonella bacilliformis*, transmitted by sandflies in the Andes mountains of South America. Cases in the United States are rare.

Babesiosis identifies a group of tick-borne diseases infected with the *Babesia* protozoa. Rare in humans, it causes fever, chills, anemia, splenomegaly, and muscle pain. People with a history of splenectomy have a high mortality rate for babesiosis. In others, it resolves within weeks.

Lyme disease is caused by the bite of a tick infected with *Borrelia burgdorferi* and causes joint disorders, skin lesions, and flu-like symptoms. It is endemic to most parts of the United States as well as in Russia, Australia, and the Far East.

088.0 Bartonellosis — *Bartonella bacilliformis; sandflies; Andes*

088.81 Lyme disease — *Borrelia burgdorferi; ticks, United States*
AHA: Q2, 1989, 10; Q3, 1990, 14; Q4, 1991, 15

088.82 Babesiosis — *Babesia; ticks*
AHA: Q4, 1993, 23

088.89 Other specified arthropod-borne diseases — *not elsewhere classified*

088.9 Unspecified arthropod-borne disease — *unknown*

Coding Scenario

A patient with recently diagnosed Lyme disease is seen in the office for follow-up. She is now complaining of joint pain and swelling of the knees. The physician states that arthritis due to the Lyme disease is now present.

> Code assignment: 088.81 *Lyme disease* and 711.86 *Arthropathy associated with other infectious and parasitic diseases*

090–099 Syphilis and Other Venereal Diseases

It is estimated that 400,000 people seek treatment for syphilis in the United States each year. Syphilis is caused by the spirochete *Treponema pallidum*. The disease is divided into four categories: congenital syphilis and the three stages of acquired syphilis: early syphilis, a contagious stage with mild symptoms; latent syphilis, asymptomatic and infectious; and the late or tertiary stage, with significant symptoms but not contagious. Infection is transmitted by an infected mother to her fetus or by sexual contact. Rare instances of infection from kissing or close bodily contact have been documented, as the spirochete enters the body through the mucous membranes or skin. Syphilis responds to antibiotic treatment.

The disease can manifest itself in any stage, and may be asymptomatic for years. Usually, the first symptoms are lymphadenopathy and a localized chancre. However, the variety of manifestations can make clinical recognition of syphilis difficult.

Syphilis codes are classified as congenital, early, or latent. The disease is further classified according to its manifestations.

090 Congenital syphilis

Up to 80 percent of syphilitic mothers pass the infection to their fetus. Symptoms do not develop in most neonates, so diagnosis in the hospital nursery is usually the result of tests performed on the infant because of the mother's medical history.

Early congenital syphilis may manifest itself within two years of birth with a rash on the patient's palms and soles, swollen lymph glands, an enlarged spleen, and/or characteristic syphilitic chancres near mucous membranes. Other symptoms may include osteochondritis, epiphysitis, periostitis, chronic coryza, or choroiditis. Syphilis is confirmed with serologic tests. Early symptomatic syphilis is sometimes called Wegner's disease.

Latent early congenital syphilis has no clinical manifestations and is diagnosed through serologic testing within the first two years of life. If a test of spinal fluid is positive for syphilis, the disease is not considered latent, even if the patient does not show symptoms. Instead, the condition is reported as congenital syphilitic meningitis (090.42).

090.0 Early congenital syphilis, symptomatic — *from birth to two years old, symptoms*

090.1 Early congenital syphilis, latent — *from birth to two years old, no symptoms*

090.2 Unspecified early congenital syphilis — *from birth to two years, symptoms unknown*

090.3 Syphilitic interstitial keratitis — *congenital corneal infection*

090.40 Unspecified juvenile neurosyphilis — (Use additional code to identify any associated mental disorder) — *unknown site of infection*

090.41 Congenital syphilitic encephalitis — (Use additional code to identify any associated mental disorder) — *infection of brain*

090.42 Congenital syphilitic meningitis — (Use additional code to identify any associated mental disorder) — *infection of the lining of the brain or spinal cord*

090.49 Other juvenile neurosyphilis — (Use additional code to identify any associated mental disorder) — *not elsewhere classified*

090.5 Other late congenital syphilis, symptomatic — *older than two years with symptoms*

090.6 Late congenital syphilis, latent — *older than two years, no symptoms*

090.7 Late congenital syphilis, unspecified — *older than two years, symptoms unknown*

090.9 Congenital syphilis, unspecified — *unknown age in child with unknown symptoms*

Coding Clarification

Report exposure to syphilis with V01.6, and carrier of syphilis with V02.8.

If neurological manifestations are present, use codes from the 090.4 series of codes rather than 090.0.

091 Early syphilis, symptomatic

Generally, early syphilis is the period from initial infection and the first two years of the disease. Early syphilis can be further divided into primary or secondary syphilis. In primary syphilis, a painless chancre appears at the site of infection and regional swelling of lymph nodes occurs as the spirochetes invade the lymphatic system. The lymphadenopathy is sometimes called bubo. In secondary syphilis, the infection spreads to secondary sites. Codes in this section are selected based on whether the infection is primary or secondary and then by anatomic site.

091.0 Genital syphilis (primary) — *genital lesion in new case of syphilis*

091.1 Primary anal syphilis — *anal lesion in new case of syphilis*

091.2 Other primary syphilis — *lesion in new case of syphilis, not genital or anal*

091.3 Secondary syphilis of skin or mucous membranes — *secondary lesions within two years of initial infection*

091.4 Adenopathy due to secondary syphilis — *secondary lymph gland inflammation within two years of initial infection*

091.50 Early syphilis, syphilitic uveitis, unspecified — *secondary inflammation of uvea in eye within two years of initial infection*

091.51 Early syphilis, syphilitic chorioretinitis (secondary) — *secondary inflammation of retina and choroid of eye within two years of initial infection*

091.52 Early syphilis, syphilitic iridocyclitis (secondary) — *secondary inflammation of iris and ciliary body of eye within two years of initial infection*

091.61 Early syphilis, secondary syphilitic periostitis — *secondary inflammation of outer layers of bone within two years of initial infection*

091.62 Early syphilis, secondary syphilitic hepatitis — *secondary inflammation of liver within two years of initial infection*

091.69 Early syphilis, secondary syphilis of other viscera — *secondary inflammation of other abdominal organs within two years of initial infection*

091.7 Early syphilis, secondary syphilis, relapse — *return of symptoms after asymptomatic period within two years of initial infection*

091.81 Early syphilis, acute syphilitic meningitis (secondary) — *sudden, severe inflammation of lining of the brain or spinal cord within two years of initial infection*

091.82 Early syphilis, syphilitic alopecia — *secondary loss of hair of within two years of initial infection*

091.89 Early syphilis, other forms of secondary syphilis — *other secondary manifestation within two years of initial infection*

091.9 Early syphilis, unspecified secondary syphilis

Coding Clarification

Report exposure to syphilis with V01.6, and carrier of syphilis with V02.8.

© 2004 Ingenix, Inc.

If early syphilis has complications involving the heart or nervous system, report codes in the 093 or 094 rubrics instead.

092 Early syphilis, latent

Latent early syphilis has no clinical manifestations and is diagnosed through serologic testing within the first two years of infection. If a test of spinal fluid is positive for syphilis, the disease is not considered latent, even if the patient does not show symptoms. Instead, the condition is reported with a code from the 094 rubric for neurosyphilis.

092.0 Early syphilis, latent, serological relapse after treatment — *other than congenital; results positive-negative-positive within first two years*

092.9 Early syphilis, latent, unspecified — *other than congenital; within first two years, no symptoms*

Coding Clarification

Report exposure to syphilis with V01.6, and carrier of syphilis with V02.8.

093 Cardiovascular syphilis

This rubric is reserved for any syphilitic infection of the cardiovascular system, except congenital infection, which is reported with 090.5 instead. Select the code based on anatomic site of infection. Clinical diagnosis is based on echocardiography (ECG) and serologic test for syphilis. Syphilis infection within the heart may lead to congestive heart failure, which is reported in addition to syphilis with 428.0.

093.0 Aneurysm of aorta, specified as syphilitic — *dilation of syphilitic aorta*

093.1 Syphilitic aortitis — *inflammation of main artery leading from heart*

093.20 Unspecified syphilitic endocarditis of valve — *inflammation of unknown heart valve*

093.21 Syphilitic endocarditis, mitral valve — *inflammation of mitral valve*

093.22 Syphilitic endocarditis, aortic valve — *inflammation of aortic valve*

093.23 Syphilitic endocarditis, tricuspid valve — *inflammation of tricuspid valve*

093.24 Syphilitic endocarditis, pulmonary valve — *inflammation of pulmonary value*

093.81 Syphilitic pericarditis — *inflammation of outer lining of heart*

093.82 Syphilitic myocarditis — *inflammation of muscle of heart*

093.89 Other specified cardiovascular syphilis — *other inflammation of heart, including Babinski-Vaquez syndrome*

093.9 Unspecified cardiovascular syphilis

Coding Clarification

Report exposure to syphilis with V01.6, and carrier of syphilis with V02.8.

Cardiovascular complications occur in tandem with neurosyphilis and, in these cases, report codes from both the 093 and 094 rubrics.

094 Neurosyphilis

In neurosyphilis, spirochetes infect the nerves, spinal cord, or brain. Codes in this rubric are organized by anatomy and severity. Tabes dorsalis is a progressive degeneration of nerves and general paresis describes progressive degeneration of brain. Both conditions are considered the most severe and systemic forms of neurosyphilis.

Most symptomatic neurosyphilis is a form of late syphilis, meaning the patient has been infected for more than two years. Any presence of infection in the spinal fluid is considered a form a neurosyphilis, even if the patient is otherwise asymptomatic.

Disorders including dementia and some forms of arthropathy are associated with some forms of neurosyphilis and should be reported in addition to the neurosyphilis code.

094.0 Tabes dorsalis — (Use additional code to identify any associated mental disorder. Use additional code to identify manifestation, 713.5) — *progressive degeneration of nerves in long-term syphilis*

094.1 General paresis — (Use additional code to identify any associated mental disorder) — *degeneration of brain in long-term syphilis*

094.2 Syphilitic meningitis — (Use additional code to identify any associated mental disorder) — *inflammation of lining of the brain and/or spinal cord*

094.3 Asymptomatic neurosyphilis — (Use additional code to identify any associated mental disorder) — *positive spinal fluid, but no symptoms*

094.81 Syphilitic encephalitis — (Use additional code to identify any associated mental disorder) — *inflammation of the brain in neurosyphilis*

094.82 Syphilitic Parkinsonism — (Use additional code to identify any associated mental disorder) — *tremors, decreased motor function, muscular rigidity*

094.83 Syphilitic disseminated retinochoroiditis — (Use additional code to identify any associated mental disorder) — *inflammation of retina and choroid*

094.84 Syphilitic optic atrophy — (Use additional code to identify any associated mental disorder) — *degeneration of the eye and its nerves*

094.85 Syphilitic retrobulbar neuritis — (Use additional code to identify any associated mental disorder) — *inflammation of the posterior optic nerve*

094.86 Syphilitic acoustic neuritis — (Use additional code to identify any associated mental disorder) — *inflammation of acoustic nerve*

094.87 Syphilitic ruptured cerebral aneurysm — (Use additional code to identify any associated mental disorder) — *rupture of blood vessel in brain*

094.89 Other specified neurosyphilis — (Use additional code to identify any associated mental disorder) — *including Argyll Robertson's syndrome, erosion of spine, Heubner's disease*

094.9 Unspecified neurosyphilis — (Use additional code to identify any associated mental disorder)

Coding Clarification

Report exposure to syphilis with V01.6, and carrier of syphilis with V02.8.

Asymptomatic neurosyphilis can be an early or late form of the disease, and is reported with 094.3.

095 Other forms of late syphilis, with symptoms

This rubric covers symptomatic syphilitic infections of more than two years organized by site of secondary infection. Cardiovascular syphilis (093) and neurosyphilis (094) are excluded from this rubric.

095.0 Syphilitic episcleritis — *inflammation of external surface of sclera*

095.1 Syphilis of lung — *pulmonary infection*

095.2 Syphilitic peritonitis — *inflammation of the abdominal membrane lining*

095.3 Syphilis of liver — *hepatic infection*

095.4 Syphilis of kidney — *inflammation of one or both kidneys*

095.5 Syphilis of bone — *infection of bone*

095.6 Syphilis of muscle — *myositis from syphilis*

095.7 Syphilis of synovium, tendon, and bursa

095.8 Other specified forms of late symptomatic syphilis

095.9 Unspecified late symptomatic syphilis

Coding Clarification

Report exposure to syphilis with V01.6, and carrier of syphilis with V02.8.

096 Late syphilis, latent OK

In latent late syphilis, a positive serologic test has indicated the patient has the disease, but there are no symptoms after an infection of two or more years. The spinal fluid is clear.

Coding Clarification

Report exposure to syphilis with V01.6, and carrier of syphilis with V02.8.

For asymptomatic late syphilis with infected spinal fluid, 094.3 is reported instead.

097 Other and unspecified syphilis

This rubric contains nonspecific codes for use in cases when the timetable of syphilitic infection or the specific site of secondary infection is unknown. These codes are not to be used for patients younger than 2 years of age. See the codes in rubric 090 for congenital and juvenile syphilis.

097.0 Unspecified late syphilis — *after first two years, unknown symptoms*

097.1 Unspecified latent syphilis

097.9 Unspecified syphilis — *unknown acquired syphilis*

Coding Clarification

Report exposure to syphilis with V01.6, and carrier of syphilis with V02.8.

098 Gonococcal infections

Gonorrhea is an acute infection caused by *Neisseria gonorrhoeae*, usually transmitted sexually. Women are often asymptomatic, while men tend to develop urinary symptoms from gonococcus rather quickly. Diagnosis is based on bacteriologic examination of discharge or urine. Gonorrhea responds to antibiotic treatment, though several courses may be required to eradicate the disease.

Gonococcal infection is classified by site. In the most common site of infection, the genitourinary system, a further distinction is made between chronic and acute cases. Report chronic infection codes when the infection has continued for two months or longer.

098.0 Gonococcal infection (acute) of lower genitourinary tract — *sudden onset; bartholinitis, urethritis, vulvovaginitis*

098.10 Gonococcal infection (acute) of upper genitourinary tract, site unspecified — *sudden onset; upper genitourinary tract site unknown*

098.11 Gonococcal cystitis (acute) — *sudden onset; bladder*

098.12 Gonococcal prostatitis (acute) — *sudden onset; prostate*

098.13 Gonococcal epididymo-orchitis (acute) — *sudden onset; epididymis, testis*

098.14 Gonococcal seminal vesiculitis (acute) — *sudden onset; seminal vesicle*

 © 2004 Ingenix, Inc.

098.15 Gonococcal cervicitis (acute) — *sudden onset; cervix*

098.16 Gonococcal endometritis (acute) — *sudden onset; uterus*

098.17 Gonococcal salpingitis, specified as acute — *sudden onset; fallopian tubes*

098.19 Other gonococcal infections (acute) of upper genitourinary tract — *sudden onset; upper genitourinary tract not elsewhere classified*

098.2 Gonococcal infections, chronic, of lower genitourinary tract — *persistent infection; bartholinitis, urethritis, vulvovaginitis*

098.30 Chronic gonococcal infection of upper genitourinary tract, site unspecified — *persistent infection, upper genitourinary tract site unknown*

098.31 Gonococcal cystitis, chronic — *persistent infection; bladder*

098.32 Gonococcal prostatitis, chronic — *persistent infection; prostate*

098.33 Gonococcal epididymo-orchitis, chronic — *persistent infection; epididymis, testis*

098.34 Gonococcal seminal vesiculitis, chronic — *persistent infection; seminal vesicle*

098.35 Gonococcal cervicitis, chronic — *persistent infection; cervix*

098.36 Gonococcal endometritis, chronic — *persistent infection; uterus*

098.37 Gonococcal salpingitis (chronic) — *persistent infection; fallopian tubes*

098.39 Other chronic gonococcal infections of upper genitourinary tract — *persistent infection; upper genitourinary tract not elsewhere classified*

098.40 Gonococcal conjunctivitis (neonatorum) — *infection of conjunctiva at birth*

098.41 Gonococcal iridocyclitis — *inflammation of iris and ciliary body*

098.42 Gonococcal endophthalmia — *inflammation and infection of the contents of the eyeball*

098.43 Gonococcal keratitis — *inflammation and infection of cornea*

098.49 Other gonococcal infection of eye — *other infection of eye due to gonorrhea*

098.50 Gonococcal arthritis — *inflammation of joint*

098.51 Gonococcal synovitis and tenosynovitis — *inflammation of viscid fluid of joint, causing pain and swelling*

098.52 Gonococcal bursitis — *inflammation of sac-like cavities in joint*

098.53 Gonococcal spondylitis — *inflammation of vertebrae*

098.59 Other gonococcal infection of joint — *gonococcal rheumatism; other joint inflammation not elsewhere classified*

098.6 Gonococcal infection of pharynx — *inflammation of pharynx*

098.7 Gonococcal infection of anus and rectum — *proctitis*

098.81 Gonococcal keratosis (blennorrhagica) — *skin lesions*

098.82 Gonococcal meningitis — *inflammation of the lining of the brain or spinal cord*

098.83 Gonococcal pericarditis — *inflammation of the outer lining of the heart*

098.84 Gonococcal endocarditis — *inflammation of the tissues lining the cavities of the heart*

098.85 Other gonococcal heart disease — *heart inflammation, not elsewhere classified*

098.86 Gonococcal peritonitis

098.89 Gonococcal infection of other specified sites — *other infection, not elsewhere classified*

Coding Clarification

If the patient is infected with a penicillin-resistant form of gonorrhea, report V09.0 *Infection with microorganisms resistant to penicillins*, in addition to the code for chronic gonorrhea.

Chlamydial infections frequently occur with gonorrhea and should be reported in addition to the gonorrhea code, with *Chlamydia* codes from the 099 rubric.

Report exposure to gonorrhea with V01.6, and carrier of gonorrhea with V02.7.

Coding Scenario

The patient is seen for UTI. After examination and testing, a diagnosis of acute gonococcal cystitis is confirmed.

> Code assignment: Code 098. 11 *Acute gonococcal cystitis*

099 Other venereal diseases

This category identifies sexually transmitted diseases not elsewhere classified.

Chancroid is a localized infection by *Haemophilus ducreyi*, causing genital ulcers and infecting the inguinal lymph nodes. Care must be taken to distinguish chancroid infection from herpes simplex infection. This diagnosis is made via cultures or microscopic examination.

The most common sexually transmitted disease in the United States is chlamydial infection, and its most common manifestation is urethritis. At least 50 percent of nongonococcal urethritis cases in the United States are due to *Chlamydia*.

099.0 Chancroid — *STD of H. ducreyi; skin lesions*

099.1 Lymphogranuloma venereum — *STD of C. trachomatis; skin lesions*

099.2 Granuloma inguinale — *STD of Calymmatobacterium granulomatis; anogenital skin ulcers*

099.3 Reiter's disease — (Use additional code for associated condition: 372.33, 711.1) — *STD of unknown etiology; urethritis, conjunctivitis*

099.40 Unspecified nongonococcal urethritis (NGU) — *STD, nonspecific NGU*

099.41 Nongonococcal urethritis (NGU) due to Chlamydia trachomatis — *STD, NGU from C. trachomatis*

099.49 Nongonococcal urethritis (NGU) due to other specified organism — *STD, NGU from other specified organism*

099.50 Chlamydia trachomatis infection of unspecified site — *STD, unknown site*

099.51 Chlamydia trachomatis infection of pharynx — *STD, throat*

099.52 Chlamydia trachomatis infection of anus and rectum — *STD, proctitis*

099.53 Chlamydia trachomatis infection of lower genitourinary sites — (Use additional code to specifiy site of infection: 595.4, 616.0, 616.11) — *STD, excluding urethra*

099.54 Chlamydia trachomatis infection of other genitourinary sites — (Use additional code to specifiy site of infection: 604.91, 614.9) — *STD, including pelvic inflammatory disease, testis*

099.55 Chlamydia trachomatis infection of unspecified genitourinary site — *STD, unknown site*

099.56 Chlamydia trachomatis infection of peritoneum — *STD, including perihepatitis*

099.59 Chlamydia trachomatis infection of other specified site — *STD, specified site not elsewhere classified*

099.8 Other specified venereal diseases — *STD, other disease, not elsewhere classified*

099.9 Unspecified venereal disease — *STD, unknown*

Coding Clarification

In the past, chlamydial urethritis was reported generically as NGU. As a result, a specific code for NGU due to chlamydial infection falls under rubric 099.4 *Other nongonococcal urethritis,* rather than under 099.5 *Other veneral diseases due to C. trachomatis.* Codes in the 099.5 rubric exclude urethral infection.

In cases of genitourinary infection, other than urethra and due to *C. trachomatis,* an additional code may be required to specify the site of genitourinary infection. For example, sequence 099.54 *Chlamydia trachomatis infection of other genitourinary site* first and 614.9 *Unspecified inflammatory disease of female pelvic organs and tissues* second to report pelvic inflammatory disease due to *Chlamydia.*

Trachoma, a chlamydial infection of the eye, is not venereal and is reported in the rubric 076.

For Reiter's disease (099.3) use a second code to report manifestations of the infection, such as conjunctivitis (372.33).

100–104 Other Spirochetal Diseases

These spirochetal diseases are not classified as sexually transmitted diseases because they are transmitted from person to person through general body contact.

100 Leptospirosis

Leptospirosis is an infection due to any serotype of *Leptospira.* Dogs and rats are the most common carriers of leptospirosis and, in the United States, the most common source of infection is swimming in contaminated water. The infection usually enters the host through mucous membranes or injured skin. Less than 100 cases are reported in the United States annually.

100.0 Leptospirosis icterohemorrhagica — *Weil's, Mathieu's, Wassilieff's disease*

100.81 Leptospiral meningitis (aseptic) — *inflammation of membranes of brain and spinal cord*

100.89 Other specified leptospiral infections — *including Fort Bragg fever; swamp fever*

100.9 Unspecified leptospirosis — *unknown*

101 Vincent's angina OK

Vincent's angina is an infection of the oral mucosa causing painful bleeding, salivation, edema, and breath odor, caused by fusiform bacillus and a spirochete.

102 Yaws

Yaws is an infection by *Treponema pallidum pertenue* causing lesions of the skin, bone, and soft tissue. Upon infection, a lesion develops at the site and the yaws spirochete enters the body. This lesion is called the "mother yaw." Yaws is endemic to equatorial countries with high humidity, so cases in the United States are limited to travelers.

102.0 Initial lesions of yaws — *initial, mother yaw*

102.1 Multiple papillomata and wet crab yaws due to yaws — *butter, plantar, palmar yaws*

102.2 Other early skin lesions due to yaws — *cutaneous, less than five years since onset*

 © 2004 Ingenix, Inc.

102.3 Hyperkeratosis due to yaws — *overgrowth of skin on palms and bottoms of feet*

102.4 Gummata and ulcers due to yaws — *rubbery lesions and dead skin*

102.5 Gangosa due to yaws — *massive, mutilating lesions of nose and oral cavity*

102.6 Bone and joint lesions due to yaws — *goundou, bone gumma, osteitis*

102.7 Other manifestations due to yaws — *mucosal, juxta-articular nodules*

102.8 Latent yaws — *asymptomatic with positive test*

102.9 Unspecified yaws — *including parangi*

103 Pinta

Pinta is an infection by *Treponema pallidum carateum* confined to the skin and causing progressive lesions. Pinta is confined to the Indians of Mexico, and Central and South America, so cases in the United States are limited to travelers.

103.0 Primary lesions of pinta — *first stage, early disease*

103.1 Intermediate lesions of pinta — *pigmented lesions, mid-disease*

103.2 Late lesions of pinta — *vitiligo, late in disease*

103.3 Mixed lesions of pinta

103.9 Unspecified pinta

104 Other spirochetal infection

Nonvenereal endemic syphilis is an infection of *Treponema pallidum endemicum* found in the eastern Mediterranean region and Africa. It initially causes skin lesions that may progress to soft tissue and bone lesions.

104.0 Nonvenereal endemic syphilis — *lesions on skin and mucosa, not from STD*

104.8 Other specified spirochetal infections — *including bronchospirochetosis, Castellani's bronchitis*

104.9 Unspecified spirochetal infection — *unknown*

110–118 Mycoses

These diseases are usually considered chronic and may be present for years before a diagnosis is made. Seldom are the symptoms acute, except with immunocompromised hosts. In the immunocompromised host, also report the health problem that causes the immune deficiency. Clinical manifestations of mycoses can be fever, anorexia, malaise, and/or depression. Many of the infections are geographically limited; each has a typical clinical course.

110 Dermatophytosis

Dermatophytoses are superficial fungal infections of the skin. Ringworm, though no worm is present, and athlete's foot are common names for the disease. Dermatophytosis is classified according to the site of the lesion. This rubric includes infections by species of *Epidermophyton, Microsporum,* and *Trichophyton tinea.*

110.0 Dermatophytosis of scalp and beard — (Use additional code to identify manifestation: 321.0-321.1, 380.15, 711.6) — *kerion, sycosis, black dot tinea of scalp*

110.1 Dermatophytosis of nail — (Use additional code to identify manifestation: 321.0-321.1, 380.15, 711.6) — *onychomycosis, tinea unguium*

110.2 Dermatophytosis of hand — (Use additional code to identify manifestation: 321.0-321.1, 380.15, 711.6) — *tinea manuum*

110.3 Dermatophytosis of groin and perianal area — (Use additional code to identify manifestation: 321.0-321.1, 380.15, 711.6) — *Dhobie itch, tinea cruris, Baerensprung's disease*

110.4 Dermatophytosis of foot — (Use additional code to identify manifestation: 321.0-321.1, 380.15, 711.6) — *athlete's foot; tinea pedis*

110.5 Dermatophytosis of the body — (Use additional code to identify manifestation: 321.0-321.1, 380.15, 711.6) — *herpes circinatus; tinea imbricata*

110.6 Deep seated dermatophytosis — (Use additional code to identify manifestation: 321.0-321.1, 380.15, 711.6) — *Majocchi's granuloma*

110.8 Dermatophytosis of other specified sites — (Use additional code to identify manifestation: 321.0-321.1, 380.15, 711.6) — *not elsewhere classified*

110.9 Dermatophytosis of unspecified site — (Use additional code to identify manifestation: 321.0-321.1, 380.15, 711.6) — *unknown site*

111 Dermatomycosis, other and unspecified

These superficial fungal infections of the skin are fungal infections other than ringworm, not elsewhere classified, or have an unknown fungal infectious agent.

111.0 Pityriasis versicolor — (Use additional code to identify manifestation: 321.0-321.1, 380.15, 711.6) — *Malassezia (Pityrosporum) furfur; tinea flava, tinea versicolor*

111.1 Tinea nigra — (Use additional code to identify manifestation: 321.0-321.1, 380.15, 711.6) — *Cladosporium infection; pityriasis nigra*

111.2 Tinea blanca — (Use additional code to identify manifestation: 321.0-321.1, 380.15, 711.6) — *Trichosporon (beigelii) (cutaneum); white piedra, Beigel's morbus*

111.3 Black piedra — (Use additional code to identify manifestation: 321.0-321.1, 380.15, 711.6) — *Piedraia hortae infection*

111.8 Other specified dermatomycoses — (Use additional code to identify manifestation: 321.0-321.1, 380.15, 711.6) — *including acladiosis and chromotrichomycosis*

111.9 Unspecified dermatomycosis — (Use additional code to identify manifestation: 321.0-321.1, 380.15, 711.6) — *unknown*

112 Candidiasis

Candidiasis is a yeast infection caused by *Candida* (usually *C. albicans* but also *C. tropicalis, C. parapsilosis*). Topical infections are quite common in the United States and are found in simple cases of diaper rash and vulvovaginal infection. However, *Candida* is an opportunistic illness and significant, systemic infection is seen among the immunosuppressed. Thrush is considered a clinically significant form of *Candida* infection in adults, as it may be an indicator of AIDS. Thrush, an oral infection, is considered benign in children.

112.0 Candidiasis of mouth — (Use additional code to identify manifestation: 321.0-321.1, 380.15, 711.6) — *thrush*

112.1 Candidiasis of vulva and vagina — (Use additional code to identify manifestation: 321.0-321.1, 380.15, 711.6) — *vaginal yeast infection*

112.2 Candidiasis of other urogenital sites — (Use additional code to identify manifestation: 321.0-321.1, 380.15, 711.6) — *other than vulva and vagina*
AHA: Q4, 1996, 33; Q4, 2003, 105

112.3 Candidiasis of skin and nails — (Use additional code to identify manifestation: 321.0-321.1, 380.15, 711.6) — *intertrigo, onychia, perionyxis*

112.4 Candidiasis of lung — (Use additional code to identify manifestation: 321.0-321.1, 380.15, 711.6) — *pneumonia*
AHA: Q2, 1998, 7

112.5 Disseminated candidiasis — (Use additional code to identify manifestation: 321.0-321.1, 380.15, 711.6) — *grave, systemic infection associated with immunosuppression*
AHA: Q2, 1989, 10; Q2, 2000, 5

112.81 Candidal endocarditis — (Use additional code to identify manifestation: 321.0-321.1, 380.15, 711.6) — *infection of lining of cavities of heart*

112.82 Candidal otitis externa — (Use additional code to identify manifestation: 321.0-321.1, 380.15, 711.6) — *infection of outer ear*

112.83 Candidal meningitis — (Use additional code to identify manifestation: 321.0-321.1, 380.15, 711.6) — *infection of lining of brain or spinal cord*

112.84 Candidiasis of the esophagus — (Use additional code to identify manifestation: 321.0-321.1, 380.15, 711.6) — *infection in throat*
AHA: Q4, 1992, 19

112.85 Candidiasis of the intestine — (Use additional code to identify manifestation: 321.0-321.1, 380.15, 711.6) — *infection in intestines*
AHA: Q4, 1992, 19

112.89 Other candidiasis of other specified sites — (Use additional code to identify manifestation: 321.0-321.1, 380.15, 711.6) — *including bronchomoniliasis*
AHA: Q3, 1991, 20; Q1, 1992, 17

112.9 Candidiasis of unspecified site — (Use additional code to identify manifestation: 321.0-321.1, 380.15, 711.6) — *unknown site*

Coding Clarification

Only one code is necessary when reporting a candidal urinary tract infection, 112.2 *Candidiasis of other urogenital sites.*

Candidiasis involving the respiratory system may be considered a clinically defining disease of AIDS. The code for HIV (AIDS) infection (042) should be sequenced first, when it is determined that the patient has AIDS, followed by codes for manifestations of HIV infection.

Candidal Pneumonia is reported with code 112.4 *Candidiasis of lung.*

114 Coccidioidomycosis

AHA: Q4, 1993, 23

Coccidioidomycosis is a fungal disease caused by *Coccidioidomycosis immitis* and common to the Southwestern United States. It is acquired by inhaling contaminated dust. The primary infection is an acute respiratory infection. Progressive disease may infect organs, bones, or nervous system.

Coccidioidomycosis infection is classified by site of infection, and by its primary or progressive form.

114.0 Primary coccidioidomycosis (pulmonary) — (Use additional code to identify manifestation: 321.0-321.1, 380.15, 711.6) — *acute, self-limiting lung infection*
AHA: Q4, 1993, 23

 © 2004 Ingenix, Inc.

114.1 Primary extrapulmonary coccidioidomycosis — (Use additional code to identify manifestation: 321.0-321.1, 380.15, 711.6) — *other acute, self-limited infection*
AHA: Q4, 1993, 23

114.2 Coccidioidal meningitis — (Use additional code to identify manifestation: 321.0-321.1, 380.15, 711.6) — *infection of the lining of the brain or spinal cord*
AHA: Q4, 1993, 23

114.3 Other forms of progressive coccidioidomycosis — (Use additional code to identify manifestation: 321.0-321.1, 380.15, 711.6) — *including disseminated infection*
AHA: Q4, 1993, 23

114.4 Chronic pulmonary coccidioidomycosis — (Use additional code to identify manifestation: 321.0-321.1, 380.15, 711.6) — *persisting infection of lung*
AHA: Q4, 1993, 23

114.5 Unspecified pulmonary coccidioidomycosis — (Use additional code to identify manifestation: 321.0-321.1, 380.15, 711.6) — *lung infection, unknown whether chronic or acute*
AHA: Q4, 1993, 23

114.9 Unspecified coccidioidomycosis — (Use additional code to identify manifestation: 321.0-321.1, 380.15, 711.6) — *unknown infection, or Posada-Wernicke disease*
AHA: Q4, 1993, 23

115 Histoplasmosis

Histoplasmosis is a fungal disease caused by *Histoplasma capsulatum* in the United States or *H. duboisii* in Africa. Pulmonary infection and lesion characterize the disease.

H. capsulatum is common to the eastern and Midwestern United States. It is also called small form histoplasmosis, while the African variety is called large form.

Histoplasmosis is classified according to American (small) or African (large) and by site of infection.

Histoplasmosis can present with significant symptoms, including cough or shortness of breath. Also report any significant symptoms secondarily.

The following fifth-digit subclassification is for use with category 115:

0 without mention of manifestation
1 meningitis
2 retinitis
3 pericarditis
4 endocarditis
5 pneumonia
9 other

115.0 ✓5th Histoplasma capsulatum — (Use additional code to identify manifestation: 321.0-321.1, 380.15, 711.6) — *small form seen in United States*

115.1 ✓5th Histoplasma duboisii — (Use additional code to identify manifestation: 321.0-321.1, 380.15, 711.6) — *large form seen in Africa*

115.9 ✓5th Unspecified Histoplasmosis — (Use additional code to identify manifestation: 321.0-321.1, 380.15, 711.6) — *unknown form*

116 Blastomycotic infection

Blastomycosis is a fungal infection common to North American and Africa. Paracoccidioidomycosis is confined to South America. Lobomycosis is an infection by *Loboa loboi,* uncultured yeast that causes keloidal blastomycosis.

116.0 Blastomycosis — (Use additional code to identify manifestation: 321.0-321.1, 380.15, 711.6) — *Blastomyces (Ajellomyces) dermatitidis; Chicago disease*

116.1 Paracoccidioidomycosis — (Use additional code to identify manifestation: 321.0-321.1, 380.15, 711.6) — *Paracoccidioides (Blastomyces) brasiliensis; South American form*

116.2 Lobomycosis — (Use additional code to identify manifestation: 321.0-321.1, 380.15, 711.6) — *Loboa (Blastomyces) loboi; keloidal form*

117 Other mycoses

The fungus *Aspergillus* is commonly found in decaying leaves, stored grain, or bird droppings. It can cause three types of lung disease: as a colonization or aspergilloma in a healed site of previous lung disease (as in tuberculosis or lung abscess); as an invasive infection of the lung parenchyma that may spread via the blood stream to other parts of the body; or as an allergic reaction in people with asthma, cystic fibrosis, or who are immunosuppressed.

Mycotic mycetomas are infections by various genera and species of Ascomycetes and Deuteromycetes, such as *Acremonium (Cephalosporium) falciforme, Neotestudina rosatii, Madurella grisea, Madurella mycetomi, Pyrenochaeta romeroi, Leptosphaeria senagalensis,* and *Kurtha zopfii.*

Cryptococcosis is an infection by *Cryptococcus neoformans.* The primary infection is respiratory and can be followed by infections in organs, bones, or the nervous system. Cryptococcosis is sometimes called European blastomycosis or torulosis, after its former name, Torula histolytica.

117.0 Rhinosporidiosis — (Use additional code to identify manifestation: 321.0-321.1, 380.15, 711.6) — *Rhinosporidium loboi*

117.1 Sporotrichosis — (Use additional code to identify manifestation: 321.0-321.1, 380.15, 711.6) — *Sporothrix (Sporotrichum) schenckii*

117.2 Chromoblastomycosis — (Use additional code to identify manifestation: 321.0-321.1, 380.15, 711.6) — *Cladosporium carrionii, Fonsecaea compactum, F. pedrosoi, Phialophora verrucosa*

117.3 Aspergillosis — (Use additional code to identify manifestation: 321.0-321.1, 380.15, 711.6) — *Aspergillus fumigatus, A. flavus, A. terreus groups*
AHA: Q4, 1997, 40

117.4 Mycotic mycetomas — (Use additional code to identify manifestation: 321.0-321.1, 380.15, 711.6) — *various Ascomycetes and Deuteromycetes; Madura foot*

117.5 Cryptococcosis — (Use additional code to identify manifestation: 321.0-321.1, 380.15, 711.6) — *Cryptococcus neoformans; Busse-Buschke's disease*

117.6 Allescheriosis (Petriellidosis) — (Use additional code to identify manifestation: 321.0-321.1, 380.15, 711.6) — *Allescheria (Petriellidium) boydii*

117.7 Zygomycosis (Phycomycosis or Mucormycosis) — (Use additional code to identify manifestation: 321.0-321.1, 380.15, 711.6) — *various Absidia, Basidiobolus, Conidiobolus, Cunninghamella, Entomophthora, Mucor, Rhizopus, Saksenaea*

117.8 Infection by dematiacious fungi (Phaehyphomycosis) — (Use additional code to identify manifestation: 321.0-321.1, 380.15, 711.6) — *various fungi including Cladosporium trichoides (bantianum), Dreschlera hawaiiensis, Phialophora gougerotii, Phialophora jeanselmei*

117.9 Other and unspecified mycoses — (Use additional code to identify manifestation: 321.0-321.1, 380.15, 711.6) — *unknown pneumomycosis*

Coding Clarification

In the case of aspergillosis pneumonia, assign codes 117.3 for aspergillosis infection and 484.6 for the pneumonia. For allergic bronchopulmonary aspergillosis (ABA), report 518.6, along with an appropriate asthma code from the 493.9x series.

Report actinomycotic mycetomas with codes from the 039 rubric.

To properly report a urinary tract infection secondary to noncandidal yeast, use two codes: 599.0 *Urinary tract infection, site not specified* and 117.9 *Other and unspecified mycoses.*

118 Opportunistic mycoses OK

Use this code to report infection of skin, subcutaneous tissues, or organs by a wide variety of fungi generally considered to be pathogenic to compromised hosts only. Among the opportunistic mycoses would be the species of *Alternaria, Dreschlera,* and *Fusarium.* These infections are most likely to occur in patients after radiation therapy or during therapy with corticosteroids or immunosuppressants. People with AIDS, Hodgkin's lymphoma, or diabetes are susceptible to opportunistic mycoses.

120–129 Helminthiases

Helminthiases are diseases caused by worms. Worms are soft-bodied invertebrates and the infections can arise in a variety of ways, from person-to-person contact, contact with infested water, or ingestion of larvae in undercooked meat. Most helminthiasis infections occur in underdeveloped countries.

Infection by intestinal parasites is rarely life threatening, especially when the victim is in good health and proper treatment is instituted. Instead, discomfort and inconvenience are the more likely problems caused by intestinal parasites. However, helminthiasis is a significant problem in underdeveloped countries since these infections rob their hosts of essential nutrients. They often cause local irritation throughout the gastrointestinal tract. Diagnosis of intestinal parasites is usually done by analysis of stool specimens.

Worm infestations in ICD-9-CM are initially classified by type of worms: flukes, tapeworms, nematodes, and hookworms.

120 Schistosomiasis (bilharziasis)

Schistosomiasis, also known as bilharzia or blood fluke, is a water-borne parasitic disease carried by water snails. It is the major health risk in the rural areas of Central China and Egypt and continues to rank high in other developing countries. The main forms of schistosomiasis are caused by five species, and classification of infection is based on the species. The disease is contracted through contact with infested water.

The eggs of the schistosomes in the excreta of an infected host open on contact with water and release a parasite, the miracidium, which seeks a fresh water snail. Once it has found its snail host, the miracidium produces thousands of new parasites (cercariae). The snail excretes the cercariae into the surrounding water. They penetrate the skin, continuing the biological cycle once they have made their way to the victim's blood vessels as worms.

 © 2004 Ingenix, Inc.

In intestinal schistosomiasis, the worms reside in the blood vessels lining the intestine. In urinary schistosomiasis, they live in the blood vessels of the bladder. Only about a half of the eggs are excreted in the feces (intestinal schistosomiasis) or in the urine (urinary schistosomiasis). The rest remain in the host, damaging other vital organs. It is the eggs and not the worms that cause damage.

120.0 Schistosomiasis due to schistosoma haematobium — *urinary schistosomiasis; Schistosoma haematobium*

120.1 Schistosomiasis due to schistosoma mansoni — *intestinal schistosomiasis; S. mansoni*

120.2 Schistosomiasis due to schistosoma japonicum — *intestinal schistosomiasis; S. japonicum*

120.3 Cutaneous schistosomiasis

120.8 Other specified schistosomiasis

120.9 Unspecified schistosomiasis — *unknown schistosomiasis*

121 Other trematode infections

Trematodes other than bilharziasis are classified in this rubric. Most are very uncommon in the United States.

121.0 Opisthorchiasis — *Opisthorchis; cat liver fluke*

121.1 Clonorchiasis — *Clonorchis sinensis; oriental liver fluke*

121.2 Paragonimiasis — *Paragonimus; oriental lung fluke*

121.3 Fascioliasis — *Fasciola; sheep liver fluke*

121.4 Fasciolopsiasis — *Fasciolopsis (buski); intestinal fluke*

121.5 Metagonimiasis — *Metagonimus yokogawai*

121.6 Heterophyiasis — *Heterophyes*

121.8 Other specified trematode infections — *other trematode including Dicrocoelium dendriticum, Echinostoma ilocanum; Gastrodiscoides hominis*

121.9 Unspecified trematode infection — *unknown fluke disease*

122 Echinococcosis

Echinococcosis is an infection by the tapeworm *Echinococcus.* Diseases are classified according to serotype — *E. granulosus* or *E. multilocularis* — and by site of infection. Other tapeworm infestations are reported with codes from the 123 rubric.

122.0 Echinococcus granulosus infection of liver — *tapeworm*

122.1 Echinococcus granulosus infection of lung

122.2 Echinococcus granulosus infection of thyroid

122.3 Other echinococcus granulosus infection

122.4 Unspecified echinococcus granulosus infection

122.5 Echinococcus multilocularis infection of liver

122.6 Other echinococcus multilocularis infection

122.7 Unspecified echinococcus multilocularis infection

122.8 Unspecified echinococcus of liver — *unknown type, of liver*

122.9 Other and unspecified echinococcosis

123 Other cestode infection

Tapeworms other than *Echinococcus* are reported under this rubric.

123.0 Taenia solium infection, intestinal form — *adult pork tapeworm*

123.1 Cysticercosis — *larval pork tapeworm*
AHA: Q2, 1997, 8

123.2 Taenia saginata infection — *Taenia saginata; beef tapeworm*

123.3 Taeniasis, unspecified — *unknown Taenia infection*

123.4 Diphyllobothriasis, intestinal — *adult fish tapeworm*

123.5 Sparganosis (larval diphyllobothriasis) — *larval fish tapeworm*

123.6 Hymenolepiasis — *rat tapeworm*

123.8 Other specified cestode infection — *dog tapeworm*

123.9 Unspecified cestode infection — *unknown*

Coding Clarification

Neurocysticercosis is caused by an infestation of the larval form of the parasite *Taenia solium.* Brain involvement of the parasite can result in epilepsy, increased intracranial pressure, and other neurologic conditions. Two codes should be indicated: 123.1 to identify the parasitic infection and code 780.3x indicating the convulsions.

124 Trichinosis OK

Trichinosis is an infection by the roundworm, *Trichinella spiralis,* smallest of the parasitic nematodes. *Trichinella* is found in the muscle of bear and pig and, generally, infection occurs when undercooked meat is eaten. Infection is rare but not unknown in the United States. Patients may be asymptomatic or may have gastrointestinal symptoms, muscle pains, fever, and periorbital edema. Trichinosis is also known as trichinellosis and trichiniasis.

125 Filarial infection and dracontiasis

Worms in the Filaria or Dracunculus family cause diseases in this rubric. Most are uncommon in the United States. Many of the filarial infections cause congestion in the lymphatic system that can lead to other manifestations, including elephantiasis or chyluria.

In dracontiasis, a threadlike worm up to 120 centimeters long inhabits the subcutaneous and muscle tissues of man. Dracontiasis is limited to Africa, India, and Arabia.

125.0 Bancroftian filariasis — *Wuchereria bancrofti*

125.1 Malayan filariasis — *Brugia (Wuchereria) malayi*

125.2 Loiasis — *African eyeworm; Loa loa*

125.3 Onchocerciasis — *Onchocerca volvulus*

125.4 Dipetalonemiasis — *Acanthocheilonema perstans; Caribbean, Central and South America*

125.5 Mansonella ozzardi infection — *Filaria ozzardi*

125.6 Other specified filariasis — *Acanthocheilonema streptocerca, Dipetalonema streptocerca*

125.7 Dracontiasis — *Guinea worm; Africa, India, Asia; subcutaneous worm up to 120 cm*

125.9 Unspecified filariasis — *unknown variety*

126 Ancylostomiasis and necatoriasis

Rubric 126 classifies varieties of hookworm infection. Several infective agents, the most common being *Ancylostoma duodenale* and *Necator americanus,* can cause hookworm. Symptoms include gastrointestinal pain and anemia, though many patients are asymptomatic. *A. duodenale* is common in the Far East and the Mediterranean. N. *americanus* is more common in tropical areas. Currently, incidence of hookworm is very rare in the United States, though the incidence is thought to be as high as one in four people worldwide.

Hookworm is classified according to the infective agent. In symptomatic infection, eggs from the patient's stool can be examined to identify the type of hookworm.

126.0 Ancylostomiasis and necatoriasis due to ancylostoma duodenale — *hookworm*

126.1 Ancylostomiasis and necatoriasis due to necator americanus — *hookworm*

126.2 Ancylostomiasis and necatoriasis due to ancylostoma braziliense — *hookworm*

126.3 Ancylostomiasis and necatoriasis due to ancylostoma ceylanicum — *hookworm*

126.8 Ancylostomiasis and necatoriasis due to other specified ancylostoma — *hookworm not elsewhere classified*

126.9 Unspecified ancylostomiasis and necatoriasis — *unknown hookworm*

127 Other intestinal helminthiases

Ascariasis is infection by *Ascaris lumbricoides* and may cause gastrointestinal or pulmonary symptoms. It is seen worldwide.

Strongyloidiasis is threadworm infection, endemic to the tropics that may cause gastric pain, vomiting, and diarrhea.

127.0 Ascariasis — *Ascaris lumbricoides; roundworm*

127.1 Anisakiasis — *larval infection*

127.2 Strongyloidiasis — *Strongyloides stercoralis*

127.3 Trichuriasis — *Trichuris trichiura; whipworm*

127.4 Enterobiasis — *Enterobius vermicularis; pinworm or threadworm*

127.5 Capillariasis — *Capillaria philippinensis*

127.6 Trichostrongyliasis — *Trichostrongylus species*

127.7 Other specified intestinal helminthiasis — *Oesophagostomum apiostomum*

127.8 Mixed intestinal helminthiasis — *not elsewhere classified*

127.9 Unspecified intestinal helminthiasis — *unknown*

128 Other and unspecified helminthiases

Toxocariasis is an invasion of the viscera by *Toxocara canis* or *Toxocara cati,* which normally cause diseases confined to dogs and cats. Symptoms are fever, cough, or skin rash and some patients experience recurring pneumonias. Most cases are seen in the very young or very old.

128.0 Toxocariasis — *visceral larva migrans syndrome*

128.1 Gnathostomiasis — *Gnathostoma spinigerum*

128.8 Other specified helminthiasis — *not elsewhere classified*

128.9 Unspecified helminth infection — *unknown*

Coding Clarification

Report any significant symptoms or manifestations in addition to the toxocariasis.

129 Unspecified intestinal parasitism OK

Use this code only if the disease is known to be parasitic and the parasite is unknown. If the parasite is known, use the appropriate "not elsewhere classified" code from other rubrics in this section.

 © 2004 Ingenix, Inc.

130–136 Other Infectious and Parasitic Diseases

The diseases in this section of ICD-9-CM are a mixed bag of infections or parasites. Single-cell organisms, amebae, protozoa, mites and lice, fly larvae, or parasites of unknown etiology may cause the infections. As the last subclassification for infectious and parasitic diseases in this chapter, this section provides a hodgepodge of significant diseases.

130 Toxoplasmosis

Toxoplasmosis is caused by a single-celled parasite, *Toxoplasma gondii*. It is found throughout the world. Millions of people in the United States are infected with the *Toxoplasma* parasite, but very few have symptoms because the immune system usually keeps the parasite from causing illness.

Toxoplasmosis is an opportunistic disease and a danger to the unborn and to the immunocompromised patient. Toxoplasmosis is classified according to site or system infected.

130.0 Meningoencephalitis due to toxoplasmosis — *inflammation of brain and its lining*

130.1 Conjunctivitis due to toxoplasmosis — *inflammation of the mucous lining of the eye*

130.2 Chorioretinitis due to toxoplasmosis — *infection of the posterior lining of the eye*

130.3 Myocarditis due to toxoplasmosis — *inflammation of the lining of the heart*

130.4 Pneumonitis due to toxoplasmosis — *inflammation of the lungs*

130.5 Hepatitis due to toxoplasmosis — *inflammation of the liver*

130.7 Toxoplasmosis of other specified sites — *not elsewhere classified*

130.8 Multisystemic disseminated toxoplasmosis — *multiple organ systems; seen in the immunocompromised patient*

130.9 Unspecified toxoplasmosis — *unknown*

Coding Clarification

Congenital toxoplasmosis is classified to the Congenital Anomalies chapter of ICD-9-CM, with 771.2, and toxoplasmosis in pregnancy is classified to the Pregnancy and Childbirth chapter, with a code from the rubric 655.

If multiple sites or systems are infected, report 130.8 *Multisystem disseminated toxoplasmosis.*

In the case of AIDS, the code for HIV infection (042) should be sequenced first, followed by codes for the toxoplasmosis infection. Any functional disturbance (e.g., visual or mental disorder) may be reported secondarily.

131 Trichomoniasis

Trichomonas vaginalis is parasitic flagellated protozoa infestation that is usually sexually transmitted, although transmission by other routes, such as moist, soiled washcloths, has been documented. Most people infected with trichomoniasis are asymptomatic, and most infections are in the genitourinary system. Symptomatic infections are characterized by a white discharge from the genital tract and itching. Complications of infection can be vaginitis, urethritis, enlargement of the prostate, or epididymitis.

131.00 Unspecified urogenital trichomoniasis — *STD with infection of urinary or reproductive organs*

131.01 Trichomonal vulvovaginitis — *STD with infection of vulva or vagina*

131.02 Trichomonal urethritis — *STD with infection of urethra*

131.03 Trichomonal prostatitis — *STD with infection of prostate*

131.09 Other urogenital trichomoniasis — *STD infection at genitourinary site not elsewhere classified*

131.8 Trichomoniasis of other specified sites — *infection, not genitourinary or intestinal, site not elsewhere classified*

131.9 Unspecified trichomoniasis — *unknown*

Coding Clarification

This rubric classifies only trichomoniasis from *T. vaginalis*. Intestinal trichomoniasis may be caused by any of several other forms of *Trichomonas*, and is reported with 007.3.

132 Pediculosis and phthirus infestation

This rubric classifies lice infestations. Lice suck the blood of the host and cause severe itching and loss of sleep. Louse saliva or feces irritate some sensitive hosts, increasing the chance of secondary infection from excessive scratching.

Head lice are *Pediculus capitis*, and they live mainly on the scalp and neck hairs of their human host. Head lice are mainly acquired by direct head-to-head contact with an infested person's hair, but may be transferred with shared combs, hats, and other hair accessories. Infestation is seen most often in children and in whites more frequently than other ethnic groups. Most commonly, epidemics are seen among school children. Head lice do not transmit infectious agents from person to person.

Body lice are Pediculus humanus and are closely related to head lice, but are less frequently encountered in the United States. Body lice feed on the body, though they may be discovered on the scalp and facial hair. They usually remain on clothing near the skin and generally deposit their eggs on or near the seams of garments. Body lice are acquired mainly through direct contact with an infested person or clothing and bedding, and are most commonly found on individuals who infrequently change or wash their clothes. Body lice serve as carriers of certain human pathogens including louse-borne typhus, louse-borne relapsing fever, and trench fever.

Pubic or crab lice are *Phthirus pubis* and have a short crab-like body easily distinguished from that of head and body lice. Pubic lice are most frequently found among the pubic hairs of the infested person, but may also be found elsewhere on the body. The infestation by pubic lice is termed phthiriasis. Pubic lice are acquired mainly through sexual contact or by sharing a bed with an infested person. Public lice do not transmit infectious agents from person to person.

132.0 Pediculus capitis (head louse) — *nits, head lice*

132.1 Pediculus corporis (body louse) — *body lice; may be vector to other disease*

132.2 Phthirus pubis (pubic louse) — *crabs; usually sexually transmitted*

132.3 Mixed pediculosis and phthirus infestation — *infestation of more than one category above*

132.9 Unspecified pediculosis — *unknown infestation by lice*

133 Acariasis

Acariasis is a mite infestation. Acarid infestation is classified according to the type of mite. Scabies causes intense itching and sometimes, secondary infection. Report any significant secondary manifestations.

133.0 Scabies — *Sarcoptes scabiei*

133.8 Other acariasis — *chiggers and other mites, not elsewhere classified*

133.9 Unspecified acariasis — *unknown mite*

Coding Clarification

Scabies (133.0) is caused by *Sarcoptes scabiei;* all other known mites would be classified to 133.8 and unknown infestation would be classified to 133.9.

134 Other infestation

Myiasis is an infestation by fly larvae (maggots), and is most commonly seen in wound or ulcer sites. Myiasis is usually cutaneous, but is also found in nasal mucosa or in the intestines. Hirudiniasis is an infestation of mucous membranes or skin by leeches. While clinical myiasis and hirudiniasis are occasionally pursued as therapeutic interventions, these codes refer to nonclinical infestations.

134.0 Myiasis — *Dermatobia hominis; maggot infestation*

134.1 Other arthropod infestation — *sand fleas or other infestations not elsewhere classified*

134.2 Hirudiniasis — *leech infestation*

134.8 Other specified infestations — *not elsewhere classified*

134.9 Unspecified infestation — *unknown*

135 Sarcoidosis OK

Sarcoidosis is a disease of unknown etiology that has many presentations. It can have an acute onset and rapid resolution, or it can come upon the patient slowly and become an increasingly debilitating chronic condition. Also called sarcoid, the disorder is characterized by epithelioid tubercles in organs and tissues.

Incidence of sarcoid in the United States exceeds that of tuberculosis. Common symptoms include hilar adenopathy, shortness of breath, weight loss, arthralgia, night sweats, and erythema nodosum. The symptoms will vary according to the organs that are affected by sarcoidosis, though nearly all cases show decreased pulmonary function and mediastinal (hilar) adenopathy. Patients with chronic infection frequently have skin lesions. Tissue biopsy is the best method of diagnosing sarcoidosis.

Coding Clarification

Manifestations of sarcoidosis are reported in addition to the infection. These may include cardiac involvement (425.8), pulmonary involvement (517.8), joint involvement (713.7), or erythema nodosum (695.2).

Multiple codes may be required to complete the clinical picture. Report 135 *Sarcoidosis* first, and the manifestations or symptoms of the infection in descending order of severity.

136 Other and unspecified infectious and parasitic diseases

Most of the diseases in this category are "other," not "unspecified." They are listed here by default. There may be no room remaining in the rubric to which they would normally be classified.

Ainhum is an African disease, seen primarily in black males and causing stricture at a distal joint of a digit on the foot or hand. The stricture is progressive, leading to spontaneous amputation. Another name for the disease is dactylolysis spontanea.

Behcet's syndrome is a disease of unknown etiology causing inflammation and lesions of the mucous membrane, joints, and gastrointestinal and nervous systems. It is most common in men in their third decade in Japan and Mediterranean countries.

 © 2004 Ingenix, Inc.

Free-living amoeba, *Naegleria*, can cause a grave form of meningoencephalitis. The infection is acquired by swimming in infected lakes.

Pneumocystosis is an infection of *Pneumocystis carinii* fungus, causing pneumonia in immunocompromised patients. It is the leading cause of death among AIDS patients. Patients with intact immune systems are not affected by pneumocystosis.

Sarcosporidiosis is an infection by *Sarcocystis* causing muscle cysts and intestinal inflammation.

136.0	Ainhum — *African; stricture causes loss of digit*
136.1	Behcet's syndrome — *unknown etiology; inflammation and lesions*
136.2	Specific infections by free-living amebae — *ameba causing meningoencephalitis*
136.3	Pneumocystosis — *Pneumocystis carinii; fungus infection seen in the immunocompromised patient* **AHA:** Nov-Dec, 1987, 5-6; Q1, 2003, 15
136.4	Psorospermiasis — *Psorospermic infection*
136.5	Sarcosporidiosis — *Sarcocystis infection; muscle cysts*
136.8	Other specified infectious and parasitic diseases — *not elsewhere classified, includes candiru infestation, microsporidiosis*
136.9	Unspecified infectious and parasitic diseases — *unknown* **AHA:** Q2, 1991, 8

Coding Clarification

If the source of infection is found no where else in ICD-9-CM and a thorough search of the index does not give better direction, report 136.8 for candiru infestation, microsporidiosis, or an infectious disease not yet classified to ICD-9-CM. If the source of infection remains undiagnosed, report 136.9.

137–139 Late Effects of Infectious and Parasitic Diseases

A late effect is a residual effect of a condition that is no longer acute or an illness that has resolved. There is no time frame associated with a late effect; it can be reported at any time after the condition has resolved. Two codes are required to report late effects: one code for residual condition and the second code for the cause of the late effect. Never report the acute condition that caused the late effect with a late effect code.

137 Late effects of tuberculosis

This category is used to indicate conditions classifiable to 010-018 as the cause of the late effects, which are classified elsewhere. The conditions are reported first, with the late effect code being reported secondarily. Late effects include sequelae, or complications due to old or inactive TB. When using late effect codes from this category, there should be no evidence of active disease.

137.0	Late effects of respiratory or unspecified tuberculosis — *sequelae*
137.1	Late effects of central nervous system tuberculosis
137.2	Late effects of genitourinary tuberculosis
137.3	Late effects of tuberculosis of bones and joints
137.4	Late effects of tuberculosis of other specified organs

138 Late effects of acute poliomyelitis OK

This category is used to indicate conditions classifiable to 045 as the cause of the late effects, which are classified elsewhere. The conditions are reported first, with the late effect code being reported secondarily. Late effects include sequelae or complications due to old or inactive polio. When using late effect codes from this category, there should be no evidence of active disease.

139 Late effects of other infectious and parasitic diseases

This category is to be used to indicate conditions classifiable to 001-009, 020-041, or 046-136 as the cause of the late effects, which are classified elsewhere. The conditions are reported first, with the late effect code being reported secondarily. Late effects include sequelae or complications due to old or inactive infection. When using late effects codes from this category, there should be no evidence of active infection.

139.0	Late effects of viral encephalitis
139.1	Late effects of trachoma
139.8	Late effects of other and unspecified infectious and parasitic diseases

Coding Scenario

A patient who was treated five years ago for Lyme disease is now seen in the office for residual arthritic pain. After examination, the physician's diagnostic statement indicates that the patient has arthritis secondary to Lyme disease. The medical record identifies that the patient is cured of the Lyme disease, but still has the residual arthritis of multiple sites from the disease.

> Code assignment: 139.8 *Late effect of other and unspecified infectious and parasitic diseases* and 711.89 *Arthropathy associated with other infectious and parasitic diseases, multiple sites*

140–239
Neoplasms

Neoplasms in ICD-9-CM are classified as malignant, carcinoma in situ, uncertain, unknown, or benign. In most cases, anatomic location of the neoplasm is specified in code selection.

In malignancy, the neoplasm invades surrounding tissue or sheds cells that seed malignancies in other body sites. Malignant neoplasms are, therefore, classified as primary, for the original site; or secondary, a seeded site. Classifications within malignant neoplasms also specify certain malignancies as leukemias, Kaposi's sarcoma, melanoma, lymphomas, and carcinoma in situ.

A benign neoplasm may grow, but does not invade, and remains a lesion confined to an area. Uncertain behavior is undetermined and unspecified behavior is unknown.

Because of the nature of malignancy, this chapter classifies anatomy differently than other chapters of ICD-9-CM. In this chapter, malignancies are often classified according to contiguous anatomic site rather than by distinct organ system. Therefore, body parts that in other chapters may be classified separately are grouped together here. For example, soft tissue malignancies, whether blood vessels, tendons, or nerves, are classified under a single rubric for connective and soft tissue.

All neoplasms are classified to this chapter, whether or not they are functionally active. A functionally active neoplasm is a growth that performs functions ascribed to surrounding tissue, as in a thyroid tumor that secretes thyroxine and causes hyperthyroidism in the patient.

The index of ICD-9-CM provides a complex and complete table of neoplasms for easy code lookup. The index is organized alphabetically by anatomy. Find the anatomical site, and the table will identify the codes for primary, secondary, and carcinoma in situ, as well as the codes for benign, uncertain, and unspecified behaviors. After looking up the anatomical site and finding the appropriate code, refer to the tabular section of ICD-9-CM to see appropriate includes and excludes notes and instructions for use of that code. Kaposi's sarcoma is excluded from the index and can be found in the alphabetized index under Kaposi's.

ICD-Oncology Classification

The ICD-Oncology identifies the morphology of neoplasms. These are published by the World Health Organization (WHO) and consist of five digits. The first four identify the histological type of neoplasm, and the fifth digit indicates its behavior as benign (/0); uncertain (/1); carcinoma in situ (/2); malignant, primary (/3); malignant, secondary (/6); or malignant, uncertain (/9). These M codes are used in reporting malignancies to the national cancer registry. In many cases, the index to ICD-9-CM can help in M code selections, which are based on morphology and histology rather than anatomic site.

Personal History of Malignant Neoplasm

Codes from the V10 rubric describe personal history of malignant neoplasm, but these codes should never be assigned to patients who have active or recurring disease or are still receiving treatment for their malignancy, except when that disease is secondary. When a previously excised malignant neoplasm recurs at the same site, it is still considered a primary malignancy of that site. If the malignant neoplasm recurs at a different site, it is reported as a secondary malignant neoplasm and an additional code to identify a history of the malignancy of the primary site is reported from the V10 rubric.

Furthermore, when assigning a personal history code, the site should reflect the site of the primary malignant neoplasm, not a metastatic site. Rubric V10 reports only the primary malignancy. There is no method for reporting a history of malignancy in a secondary site.

Sequencing issues

The main rule for sequencing malignancies and their manifestations is to sequence first the reason for the encounter.

In cases of a metastasized malignancy, if a secondary malignancy causes a functional problem, sequence the codes as follows: (1) the functional problem; (2) the secondary malignant neoplasm causing the problem; and (3) the site of the original, metastasized neoplasm (primary site). For example, if a patient with prostate cancer comes to the physician with acute abdominal pain and is found to have a blocked bowel, the result of a secondary malignancy in the ileum, the following codes would be reported in this sequence:

560.89 Other intestinal obstruction without mention of hernia

197.4 Secondary malignant neoplasm of small intestine, including duodenum

185 Malignant neoplasm of the prostate

If the patient is being treated for a condition unrelated to the neoplasm, report the reason for treatment first, followed by the neoplasm only if it could affect the course of care. For example, if a patient with breast cancer fractures her hip, the fracture would be sequenced first, followed by the code for the cancer. However, if the patient's breast neoplasm is known to be benign, only the hip fracture would be reported, since the neoplasm would not affect care, unless the benign neoplasm were discovered in the course of care for the hip fracture. In that case, it would be reported as a secondary diagnosis.

If a patient is seen solely for chemotherapy or radiotherapy, either on an inpatient or outpatient basis, V58.1 *Encounter or admission for chemotherapy* or V58.0 *Encounter or admission for radiotherapy* should be sequenced first, and the code for the malignancy reported secondarily. If the patient receives other care related to the malignancy at the time of the therapy, the therapy would not be sequenced first, but secondary to the malignant neoplasm code.

Codes from the signs and symptoms chapter of ICD-9-CM should never be sequenced first when reporting malignancies. If manifestations cannot be specified with other codes, report the malignancy first, followed by any appropriate signs or symptoms.

140–149 Malignant Neoplasm of Lip, Oral Cavity, and Pharynx

This section of ICD-9-CM classifies malignancies of the mouth and throat. The pharynx (throat) is a tube that begins at the internal nares, behind the nasal cavity, and ends at the larynx. While malignant neoplasms of the pharynx are classified in this subsection of ICD-9-CM, malignant neoplasms of the larynx are found in the respiratory section, under rubric 161.

140 Malignant neoplasm of lip

AHA: Q2, 1990, 7

The lips, or labia, contain skeletal muscles. The primary muscle is the orbicularis oris, the sphincter muscle that encircles the mouth and lies between the outer skin (integument) and the mucous membranes of the lips. The labial glands, which are similar to salivary glands, lie between the muscle and mucous membrane tissues. The lips also have many sensory nerves and abundant capillary vessels that produce the normal reddish color. The external margin of the lips, the vermilion border, marks the boundary between the skin of the face and the mucous membrane that lines the alimentary canal of the digestive system.

Anatomically, the lips are divided into two distinct segments. The vermilion border is the pigmented, fleshy, outer lip, and may be described in the medical record as the lipstick area or external lip. The interior aspect is the second segment. Lined in buccal mucosa, the interior aspect may be described as the mucosa, buccal aspect, or frenulum. The commissure of the lip is the juncture of the upper and lower lips, whether at the vermilion border or interior aspect.

140.0 Malignant neoplasm of upper lip, vermilion border — *pigmented, fleshy margin of upper lip*
AHA: Q2, 1990, 7

140.1 Malignant neoplasm of lower lip, vermilion border — *pigmented, fleshy margin of lower lip*
AHA: Q2, 1990, 7

140.3 Malignant neoplasm of upper lip, inner aspect — *mucous membrane lined, inner margin, upper lip*
AHA: Q2, 1990, 7

140.4 Malignant neoplasm of lower lip, inner aspect — *mucous membrane lined, inner margin, lower lip*
AHA: Q2, 1990, 7

140.5 Malignant neoplasm of lip, inner aspect, unspecified as to upper or lower — *mucous membrane lined inner margin*
AHA: Q2, 1990, 7

140.6 Malignant neoplasm of commissure of lip — *juncture of upper and lower lip*
AHA: Q2, 1990, 7

140.8 Malignant neoplasm of other sites of lip — *contiguous or overlapping sites*
AHA: Q2, 1990, 7

140.9 Malignant neoplasm of lip, vermilion border, unspecified as to upper or lower — *pigmented, fleshy margin*
AHA: Q2, 1990, 7

Coding Clarification

Malignant neoplasms of the lip are classified according to upper, lower, or commissure of lip and whether it is vermilion border or buccal aspect. For overlapping sites, report 140.8 *Other sites of lip.*

141 Malignant neoplasm of tongue

AHA: Q2, 1990, 7

The tongue is a strong muscle that is attached to the floor of the mouth within the curve of the jawbone. It is anchored to muscles at the rear of the mouth, which attach to the base of the skull and to the hyoid bone. The underside of the tongue is attached to the

 © 2004 Ingenix, Inc.

floor of the mouth by membranes. These form a distinct vertical fold in the centerline, called the frenulum linguae. The tongue contains mucous, serous, and lymph glands. The lymph glands at the back of the tongue form the lingual tonsils.

The surface of the tongue is covered with the lingual membrane, a specialized tissue with a variety of papillae protruding from it. These papillae nodules produce the characteristic rough surface of the tongue. Between the papillae are the taste buds, the sensory nerve organs that provide the sensations of flavor. The muscle fibers of the tongue are also heavily supplied with nerves, to provide for manipulation and safe placement of food in the mouth and between the teeth for chewing. The tongue also aids in swallowing and in the formation of sounds of speech.

141.0 Malignant neoplasm of base of tongue — *fixed, dorsal base*
AHA: Q2, 1990, 7

141.1 Malignant neoplasm of dorsal surface of tongue — *dorsal surface, anterior two-thirds*
AHA: Q2, 1990, 7

141.2 Malignant neoplasm of tip and lateral border of tongue — *tip and front edge*
AHA: Q2, 1990, 7

141.3 Malignant neoplasm of ventral surface of tongue — *anterior two-thirds; frenulum linguae*
AHA: Q2, 1990, 7

141.4 Malignant neoplasm of anterior two-thirds of tongue, part unspecified — *mobile part of tongue NOS*
AHA: Q2, 1990, 7

141.5 Malignant neoplasm of junctional zone of tongue — *border of tongue at junction*
AHA: Q2, 1990, 7

141.6 Malignant neoplasm of lingual tonsil — *lymphoid tissue of tongue*
AHA: Q2, 1990, 7

141.8 Malignant neoplasm of other sites of tongue — *contiguous or overlapping sites*
AHA: Q2, 1990, 7

141.9 Malignant neoplasm of tongue, unspecified site

Coding Clarification

Malignant neoplasms of the tongue are classified according to site. If multiple or contiguous sites on the tongue are involved, report 141.8 *Other sites of tongue.* For secondary malignant neoplasm of tongue, report 198.89 and for carcinoma in situ, report 239.0.

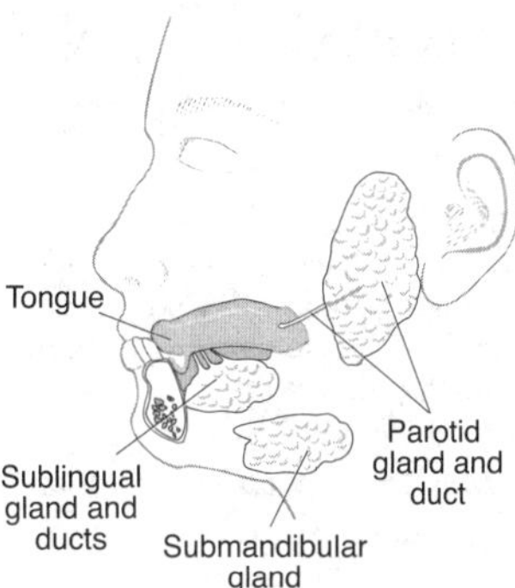

The parotid gland is a common site for malignant lesions. Occurrence is several times the frequency of other major salivary glands

142 *Malignant neoplasm of major salivary glands*

AHA: Q2, 1990, 7

These codes report malignant neoplasms of major salivary glands, but not of surrounding tissues. Salivary glands secrete saliva to aid in mastication and to keep the mouth moist. The major salivary glands are the parotid, sublingual, and submandibular glands.

The parotid is the most common site of salivary gland tumor, and mucoepidermoid carcinoma is the most common type of parotid cancer.

Symptoms of parotid tumor include pain, enlargement of nodule, and sometimes facial nerve paralysis or lymphadenopathy.

Some types of salivary gland tumors classified as malignant are the following carcinomas: mucoepidermoid, adenoid cystic, epithelial-myoepithelial, primary squamous cell, biphasic malignancy, ex-pleomorphic adenoma, malignant onocytoma, clear cell, or acinic cell.

The minor salivary glands are distributed in the lips, palate, uvula, tongue, peritonsillar area, and cheek.

142.0 Malignant neoplasm of parotid gland — *salivary gland in cheek, in front of ear*
AHA: Q2, 1990, 7

142.1 Malignant neoplasm of submandibular gland — *salivary gland at base of mandible*
AHA: Q2, 1990, 7

142.2 Malignant neoplasm of sublingual gland — *salivary gland at base of tongue*
AHA: Q2, 1990, 7

142.8 Malignant neoplasm of other major salivary glands — *contiguous or overlapping sites*
AHA: Q2, 1990, 7

142.9 Malignant neoplasm of salivary gland, unspecified

Coding Clarification

Do not use these codes to report cancers in minor salivary glands. Report malignant neoplasms of minor salivary glands with codes specific to the anatomical site in which they are located.

143 Malignant neoplasm of gum

AHA: Q2, 1990, 7

More than 95 percent of cancers of the oral cavity are squamous cell carcinomas, found most commonly in males, aged 50-70, with a history of tobacco and alcohol use.

143.0 Malignant neoplasm of upper gum — *gingiva, alveolar mucosa, interdental papillae*
AHA: Q2, 1990, 7

143.1 Malignant neoplasm of lower gum — *gingiva, alveolar mucosa, interdental papillae*
AHA: Q2, 1990, 7

143.8 Malignant neoplasm of other sites of gum — *contiguous or overlapping upper and lower sites*
AHA: Q2, 1990, 7

143.9 Malignant neoplasm of gum, unspecified site

Coding Clarification

For malignant neoplasms of contiguous or overlapping sites of the gum, report 143.8 *Other sites of gum.*

144 Malignant neoplasm of floor of mouth

AHA: Q2, 1990, 7

More than 95 percent of cancers of the oral cavity are squamous cell carcinomas, found most commonly in males, aged 50-70, with a history of tobacco and alcohol use. Cancers of the floor of the mouth have a higher incidence of lymph node involvement than do cancers of the lip, palate, or buccal mucosa, which explains their classification separately in ICD-9-CM from other parts of the inside of the mouth.

144.0 Malignant neoplasm of anterior portion of floor of mouth — *anterior to premolar-canine juncture*
AHA: Q2, 1990, 7

144.1 Malignant neoplasm of lateral portion of floor of mouth — *on the side*
AHA: Q2, 1990, 7

144.8 Malignant neoplasm of other sites of floor of mouth — *overlapping site*
AHA: Q2, 1990, 7

144.9 Malignant neoplasm of floor of mouth, part unspecified

Coding Clarification

For malignant neoplasms of contiguous or overlapping sites of the parts of mouth, report 144.8 *Other specified parts of mouth.*

145 Malignant neoplasm of other and unspecified parts of mouth

AHA: Q2, 1990, 7

More than 95 percent of cancers of the oral cavity are squamous cell carcinomas, found most commonly in males, aged 50-70, with a history of tobacco and alcohol use.

The vestibule of the mouth is the part of the oral cavity inside the cheeks and lips and outside the dentoalveolar structures (the teeth and gums). It includes the mucosal and submucosal tissue of the lips and cheeks, and the labial and buccal frenulum, or frenum, the connecting folds of membrane that support and restrain the lips and cheeks. Secretions from the salivary glands lubricate the vestibule.

145.0 Malignant neoplasm of cheek mucosa — *buccal mucosa, inner aspect cheek*
AHA: Q2, 1990, 7

145.1 Malignant neoplasm of vestibule of mouth — *buccal sulcus; labial sulcus*
AHA: Q2, 1990, 7

145.2 Malignant neoplasm of hard palate — *anterior, rigid*
AHA: Q2, 1990, 7

145.3 Malignant neoplasm of soft palate — *posterior, soft*
AHA: Q2, 1990, 7

145.4 Malignant neoplasm of uvula

145.5 Malignant neoplasm of palate, unspecified

145.6 Malignant neoplasm of retromolar area

145.8 Malignant neoplasm of other specified parts of mouth — *overlapping sites*
AHA: Q2, 1990, 7

145.9 Malignant neoplasm of mouth, unspecified site

Coding Clarification

Do not use this rubric for reporting neoplasms of the floor of the mouth (144), lips (140), or nasopharyngeal surface of the soft palate (147).

© 2004 Ingenix, Inc.

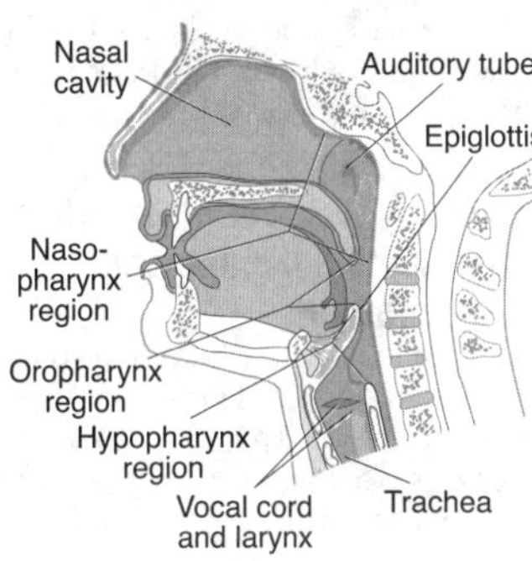

146 Malignant neoplasm of oropharynx

AHA: Q2, 1990, 7

The part of the pharynx that lies posterior to the oral cavity is called the oropharynx. It extends from its upper part at the soft palate down to its lower part that ends at the level of the hyoid bone. The lingual and palatine tonsils are located in the oropharynx. Most oropharyngeal tumors are squamous carcinomas, many with deep infiltrations.

Some tumors of the parapharyngeal space are actually major salivary gland tumors, or carotid body tumors, and should be reported as such. Minor salivary tumors at this site, however, are reported with codes in this rubric.

Oropharyngeal tumors drain bilaterally to lymph nodes, and the incidence of nodal involvement in oropharyngeal malignancy is 70 percent.

146.0 Malignant neoplasm of tonsil — *faucial, palatine*
AHA: Sept-Oct, 1987, 8; Q2, 1990, 7

146.1 Malignant neoplasm of tonsillar fossa — *sinus tonsillaris*
AHA: Q2, 1990, 7

146.2 Malignant neoplasm of tonsillar pillars (anterior) (posterior) — *faucial pillar, palatoglossal arch*
AHA: Q2, 1990, 7

146.3 Malignant neoplasm of vallecula — *Anterior and medial surface of pharyngoepiglottic fold*
AHA: Q2, 1990, 7

146.4 Malignant neoplasm of anterior aspect of epiglottis — *glossoepiglottic fold, epiglottis*
AHA: Q2, 1990, 7

146.5 Malignant neoplasm of junctional region of oropharynx — *junction of free margin of epiglottis, aryepiglottic fold, and pharyngoepiglottic fold*
AHA: Q2, 1990, 7

146.6 Malignant neoplasm of lateral wall of oropharynx — *on the side of the throat*
AHA: Q2, 1990, 7

146.7 Malignant neoplasm of posterior wall of oropharynx — *on the back of the throat*
AHA: Q2, 1990, 7

146.8 Malignant neoplasm of other specified sites of oropharynx — *contiguous or overlapping sites; brachial cleft*
AHA: Q2, 1990, 7

146.9 Malignant neoplasm of oropharynx, unspecified site

147 Malignant neoplasm of nasopharynx

AHA: Q2, 1990, 7

The part of the pharynx that lies behind (posterior) the nasal cavity is called the nasopharynx. The nasopharynx extends from behind the nasal cavity to the soft palate. There are two openings from the nasopharynx to the nose (internal nares) and two openings to the ears (Eustachian tubes). The adenoids (pharyngeal tonsil) are located on the posterior wall of the nasopharynx. The most common tumor of the nasopharynx is squamous cell carcinoma. Lymph node metastases occur in 80 percent of patients with nasopharyngeal cancer.

147.0 Malignant neoplasm of superior wall of nasopharynx — *roof of nasopharynx*
AHA: Q2, 1990, 7

147.1 Malignant neoplasm of posterior wall of nasopharynx — *adenoid; pharyngeal tonsil*
AHA: Q2, 1990, 7

147.2 Malignant neoplasm of lateral wall of nasopharynx — *pharyngeal recess; fossa of Rosenmüller; opening of auditory tube*
AHA: Q2, 1990, 7

147.3 Malignant neoplasm of anterior wall of nasopharynx — *floor of nasopharynx; posterior margin of nasal septum; nasopharyngeal surface of soft palate*
AHA: Q2, 1990, 7

147.8 Malignant neoplasm of other specified sites of nasopharynx — *contiguous or overlapping sites*
AHA: Q2, 1990, 7

147.9 Malignant neoplasm of nasopharynx, unspecified site

140–239

140–239

148 Malignant neoplasm of hypopharynx

AHA: Q2, 1990, 7

The lowest part of the pharynx is called the laryngopharynx or hypopharynx. It extends from the hyoid bone and ends at a point where it breaks into two parts, the esophagus and larynx, by blending in with them. More than 95 percent of hypopharyngeal cancers are squamous carcinoma, and the most common site is the periform sinus, which occur on either side of the larynx. These account for 60 percent of hypopharyngeal cancers. Lymphatic involvement is seen in about 70 percent of hypopharyngeal malignancy.

148.0 Malignant neoplasm of postcricoid region of hypopharynx

148.1 Malignant neoplasm of pyriform sinus — *pyriform fossa*
AHA: Q2, 1990, 7

148.2 Malignant neoplasm of aryepiglottic fold, hypopharyngeal aspect — *aryepiglottic fold NOS*
AHA: Q2, 1990, 7

148.3 Malignant neoplasm of posterior hypopharyngeal wall

148.8 Malignant neoplasm of other specified sites of hypopharynx — *overlapping sites*
AHA: Q2, 1990, 7

148.9 Malignant neoplasm of hypopharynx, unspecified site

149 Malignant neoplasm of other and ill-defined sites within the lip, oral cavity, and pharynx

AHA: Q2, 1990, 7

This rubric captures malignant neoplasms in the pharynx and oral cavity that have less specific anatomic boundaries. Waldeyer's ring includes the lymphatic tissues of the lingual, pharyngeal, and palatine tonsils.

149.0 Malignant neoplasm of pharynx, unspecified — *unknown part*
AHA: Q2, 1990, 7

149.1 Malignant neoplasm of Waldeyer's ring — *lymphatic tissues of the lingual, pharyngeal, and palatine tonsils*
AHA: Q2, 1990, 7

149.8 Malignant neoplasm of other sites within the lip and oral cavity — *point of origin cannot be assigned to any one of the categories 140-148*
AHA: Q2, 1990, 7

149.9 Malignant neoplasm of ill-defined sites of lip and oral cavity

Coding Clarification

Report 149.8 if the malignancy is not limited to one of the specific structures, but has invaded contiguous or overlapping structures.

150–159 Malignant Neoplasm of Digestive Organs and Peritoneum

This subsection of ICD-9-CM classifies malignancies of the body parts that carry food through the digestive system where nutrients are absorbed, to the anus where the waste is excreted. These body parts include the esophagus, stomach, intestines, and anus.

Structures that support the digestive process from outside this continuous tube are also included in this system: gallbladder, pancreas, and liver. These organs provide secretions that are critical to food absorption and use by the body.

The digestive system is a group of organs that breaks down and changes food chemically for absorption as simple, soluble substances by blood, lymph systems, and body tissues. The digestive system begins in the mouth, continues in the pharynx and esophagus, the stomach, the small and large intestines, the rectum, and the anus.

Digestion involves mechanical and chemical processes. Mechanical actions include chewing in the mouth, churning action in the stomach, and intestinal peristaltic action. These mechanical forces move the food through the digestive tract and mix it with secretions containing enzymes, which accomplish three chemical reactions: the conversion of carbohydrates to simple sugars, the breakdown of proteins into amino acids, and the conversion of fats into fatty acids and glycerol.

The stomach churns and mixes the food with hydrochloric acid and enzymes and gradually releases materials into the upper small intestine (the duodenum) through the pyloric sphincter.

The majority of the digestive process occurs in the small intestine where most foods are hydrolysed and absorbed. The products of digestion are actively or passively transported through the wall of the small intestine and assimilated into the body. The stomach and the large intestine (colon) can also absorb water, alcohol, certain salts and crystalloids, and some drugs. Water-soluble digestive products (minerals, amino acids, and carbohydrates) are transferred into the blood system and transported to the liver. Many fats, resynthesized in the intestinal wall, are picked up by the lymphatic system and enter the blood stream through the vena caval system, bypassing the liver.

Remaining undigested matter is passed into the large intestine (the colon) where water is extracted. This solid mass (the stool) is propelled into the rectum, where it is held until excreted through the anus.

© 2004 Ingenix, Inc.

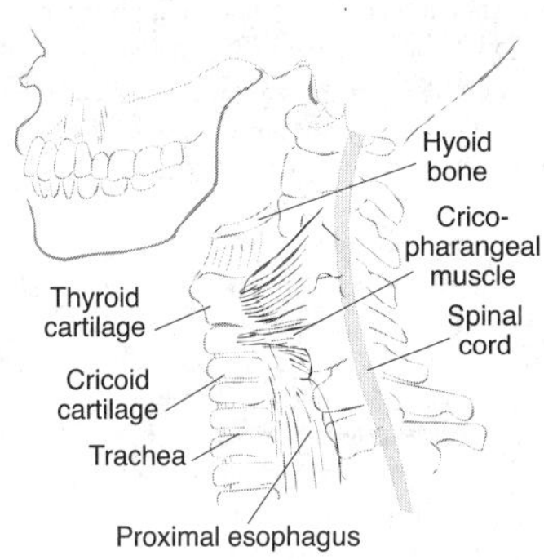

150 Malignant neoplasm of esophagus

AHA: Q2, 1990, 7

The esophagus is the alimentary canal connecting the pharynx to the stomach. Symptoms of carcinoma of the esophagus include difficulty swallowing, weight loss, coughing, and pain. Hoarseness is often seen.

Carcinoma of the esophagus is more common among men and has been linked in the United States to heavy use of alcohol and tobacco. A majority of these cancers are squamous cell or adenocarcinoma. Anatomically, 20 percent occur in the upper third of the esophagus, 30 percent in the mid-esophagus, and 50 percent in the lower esophagus.

Adenocarcinoma is more common in the lower esophagus, while squamous cell carcinoma is common in the mid to the upper esophagus.

150.0 Malignant neoplasm of cervical esophagus — *above the diaphragm*
AHA: Q2, 1990, 7

150.1 Malignant neoplasm of thoracic esophagus — *within the diaphragm*
AHA: Q2, 1990, 7

150.2 Malignant neoplasm of abdominal esophagus — *below the diaphragm*
AHA: Q2, 1990, 7

150.3 Malignant neoplasm of upper third of esophagus — *proximal third*
AHA: Q2, 1990, 7

150.4 Malignant neoplasm of middle third of esophagus — *middle third*
AHA: Q2, 1990, 7

150.5 Malignant neoplasm of lower third of esophagus — *distal third*
AHA: Q2, 1990, 7

150.8 Malignant neoplasm of other specified part of esophagus — *contiguous or overlapping sites of esophagus whose point of origin cannot be determined*
AHA: Q2, 1990, 7

150.9 Malignant neoplasm of esophagus, unspecified site

Coding Clarification

Cancers in this rubric are classified by site, with one exception. According to ICD-9-CM exclusion notes, if squamous cell carcinoma is present at the distal end of the esophagus (the cardia), report 150.5 *Malignant neoplasm of lower third of esophagus.* However, if adenocarcinoma is present in the distal end of the esophagus (the cardia), report 151.0 *Malignant neoplasm of cardia.*

If the malignancy is of contiguous and overlapping sites, report 150.8 *Malignant neoplasm of other specified part of esophagus.*

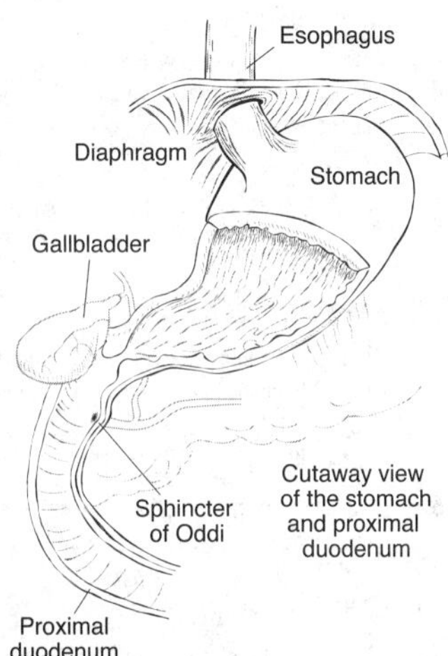

151 Malignant neoplasm of stomach

AHA: Q2, 1990, 7

The stomach has four functions: to act as a reservoir for food, to mix food, to begin the digestive process, and to allow the absorption of some substances.

The stomach begins at the portal between the esophagus and the stomach — the cardia. It ends at the portal to the duodenum — the pylorus. In between is the corpus, or the body of the stomach. The corpus is divided into the upper portion, the fundus, which is served by the oxyntic gland; the lower portion or the antrum, served by the pyloric gland; and the large midportion, the body. There are no clear demarcations between the segments of the corpus. The lesser and greater curvatures of the stomach refer to the short and long walls of the organ.

Stomach cancer is rarely found before age 40 and is twice as common in men as in women. The most common types of stomach cancers are ulcerating carcinomas, polypoid carcinomas, superficial spreading carcinomas, linitis plastica, and advanced carcinoma.

151.0 Malignant neoplasm of cardia — *cardiac orifice; cardio-esophageal junction*
AHA: Q2, 1990, 7

151.1 Malignant neoplasm of pylorus — *pre-pylorus, pyloric canal*
AHA: Q2, 1990, 7

151.2 Malignant neoplasm of pyloric antrum — *lower portion of the stomach preceding the pylorus; antrum of stomach*
AHA: Q2, 1990, 7

151.3 Malignant neoplasm of fundus of stomach — *upper portion of the stomach proceeding from the cardia*
AHA: Q2, 1990, 7

151.4 Malignant neoplasm of body of stomach — *central segment*
AHA: Q2, 1990, 7

151.5 Malignant neoplasm of lesser curvature of stomach, unspecified — *not classifiable to 151.1-151.4*
AHA: Q2, 1990, 7

151.6 Malignant neoplasm of greater curvature of stomach, unspecified — *not classifiable to 151.0-151.4*
AHA: Q2, 1990, 7

151.8 Malignant neoplasm of other specified sites of stomach — *anterior wall, posterior wall, contiguous or overlapping parts*
AHA: Q2, 1990, 7

151.9 Malignant neoplasm of stomach, unspecified site — *carcinoma ventriculi, gastric cancer, Brinton's disease*
AHA: Q2, 1990, 7; Q2, 2001, 17

Coding Clarification

Cancers in this rubric are classified by site, with one exception. According to ICD-9-CM exclusion notes, if squamous cell carcinoma is present at the distal end of the esophagus (the cardia), report 150.5 *Malignant neoplasm of lower third of esophagus.* However, if adenocarcinoma is present in the distal end of the esophagus (the cardia), report 151.0 *Malignant neoplasm of cardia.*

If the malignancy is of contiguous and overlapping sites, report 151.8 *Malignant neoplasm of other specified sites of stomach.*

152 Malignant neoplasm of small intestine, including duodenum

AHA: Q2, 1990, 7

The small intestine, often called the small bowel, is the portion of the alimentary canal from the pylorus to the cecum and is divided into the upper two-fifths, the jejunum, and the balance (the ileum). There is no demarcation between the two portions of small bowel, but, generally, the jejunum resides to the left side of the peritoneum and the ileum resides to the right and into the pelvis. The duodenum lies between the pylorus valve at the exit of the stomach and the jejunum. The most common form of small intestine malignancy is adenocarcinoma in the proximal jejunum.

152.0 Malignant neoplasm of duodenum — *small intestine immediate to the pylorus*
AHA: Q2, 1990, 7

152.1 Malignant neoplasm of jejunum — *middle portion of the small intestine*
AHA: Q2, 1990, 7

152.2 Malignant neoplasm of ileum — *distal small intestine that connects to the large intestine*
AHA: Q2, 1990, 7

152.3 Malignant neoplasm of Meckel's diverticulum — *abnormal pouch near the terminal part of the ilium near the ileocecal juncture*
AHA: Q2, 1990, 7

152.8 Malignant neoplasm of other specified sites of small intestine — *duodenojejunal junction; contiguous or overlapping sites*
AHA: Q2, 1990, 7

152.9 Malignant neoplasm of small intestine, unspecified site

Coding Clarification

The small intestine is a common site for melanoma metastases, and these should be classified as secondary cancers rather than with the 152 rubric.

Cancer of the small bowel is classified by site. If the malignancy is of contiguous or overlapping sites, report 152.8 *Malignant neoplasm of other specified sites of small intestine.* Cancer of the ileocecal valve is reported with 153.4 *Malignant neoplasm of the cecum.*

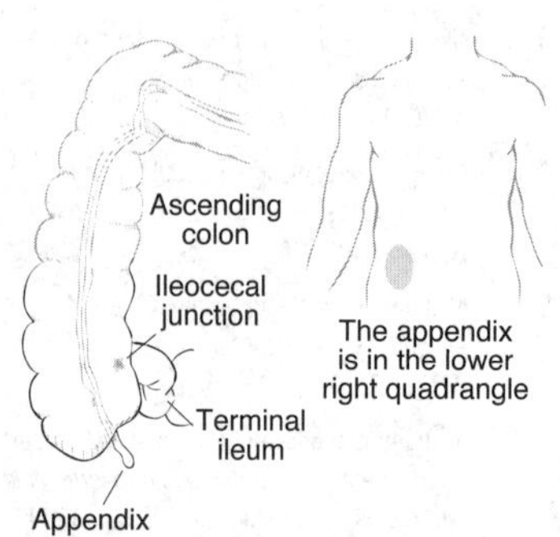

© 2004 Ingenix, Inc.

153 Malignant neoplasm of colon

AHA: Q2, 1990, 7

The large intestine, or colon, extends from the end of the ileum to the rectum. The rectum, however, is excluded from rubric 153 and classified in 154. The right colon consists of the cecum, ascending colon, hepatic flexure, and proximal transverse colon. The left colon consists of the distal transverse colon, the splenic flexure, the descending colon, sigmoid colon, and rectosigmoid colon.

Colon cancer is second to lung cancer as the most common form of cancer in the United States. About 150,000 new cases are diagnosed and 60,000 deaths occur each year. Adenocarcinoma is the most common form of colon cancer.

153.0 Malignant neoplasm of hepatic flexure — *juncture of the ascending and transverse colons*
AHA: Q2, 1990, 7

153.1 Malignant neoplasm of transverse colon — *middle portion of the large intestines, between the hepatic and splenic flexures*
AHA: Q2, 1990, 7

153.2 Malignant neoplasm of descending colon — *between the splenic flexure and the sigmoid colon; left colon*
AHA: Q2, 1990, 7

153.3 Malignant neoplasm of sigmoid colon — *S-shaped colon between the descending colon and the rectum*
AHA: Q2, 1990, 7

153.4 Malignant neoplasm of cecum — *pouch at the beginning of the large intestine, including ileocecal valve*
AHA: Q2, 1990, 7

153.5 Malignant neoplasm of appendix — *attached to the cecum*
AHA: Q2, 1990, 7

153.6 Malignant neoplasm of ascending colon — *first portion of the large intestine between the cecum and the hepatic flexure; right colon*
AHA: Q2, 1990, 7

153.7 Malignant neoplasm of splenic flexure — *bend between the transverse and descending colons*
AHA: Q2, 1990, 7

153.8 Malignant neoplasm of other specified sites of large intestine — *not elsewhere classified or contiguous or overlapping sites*
AHA: Q2, 1990, 7

153.9 Malignant neoplasm of colon, unspecified site

Coding Clarification

If the malignancy is causing obstruction or other manifestation, report the manifestation first, and the neoplasm secondarily.

Coding Scenario

A patient is admitted for blood transfusions for severe anemia. The patient history indicates the patient has colon cancer and chronic obstructive pulmonary disease. The physician documentation specifies the anemia as a chronic simple type.

> Code assignment: 281.9 *Unspecified deficiency anemia*, 153.9 *Malignant neoplasm of colon, unspecified*, and 496 *Chronic airway obstruction, not elsewhere classified*

154 Malignant neoplasm of rectum, rectosigmoid junction, and anus

AHA: Q2, 1990, 7

The rectum begins at the rectosigmoid junction and ends at the anus. The rectum and rectosigmoid junctions are the most common sites for cancer in the colon, accounting for more than 30 percent of cases. In these cancers, the most common symptoms are rectal bleeding with bowel movement and pain upon defecation (tenesmus).

154.0 Malignant neoplasm of rectosigmoid junction — *colon with rectum; rectosigmoid (colon)*
AHA: Q2, 1990, 7

154.1 Malignant neoplasm of rectum — *rectal ampulla*
AHA: Q2, 1990, 7

154.2 Malignant neoplasm of anal canal — *including anal sphincter*
AHA: Q2, 1990, 7; Q1, 2001, 8

154.3 Malignant neoplasm of anus, unspecified site

154.8 Malignant neoplasm of other sites of rectum, rectosigmoid junction, and anus — *anorectum, cloacogenic zone, contiguous or overlapping sites*
AHA: Q2, 1990, 7

Coding Clarification

Diseases in this rubric are classified according to site. Report 154.8 *Malignant neoplasm of other specified sites* if the malignancy is of contiguous or overlapping sites. If the malignancy is causing bleeding, obstruction, or other manifestation, report the manifestation first, and the malignancy secondarily.

155 Malignant neoplasm of liver and intrahepatic bile ducts

AHA: Q2, 1990, 7

140–239

Primary liver cancer is uncommon in the United States; however, the liver is a common site for metastases, and would be reported with 197.7 *Secondary malignant neoplasm of the mediastinum.* About 80 percent of primary liver cancers are hepatomas.

155.0 Malignant neoplasm of liver, primary — *including all lobes; hepatoblastoma, liver carcinoma*
AHA: Q2, 1990, 7

155.1 Malignant neoplasm of intrahepatic bile ducts — *canaliculi biliferi, interlobular bile ducts; intrahepatic biliary passages, gall duct; intrahepatic bile ducts*
AHA: Q2, 1990, 7

155.2 Malignant neoplasm of liver, not specified as primary or secondary — *unknown whether a metastasis*
AHA: Q2, 1990, 7

Coding Clarification

For cancers of the hepatic duct, report 156.1 *Malignant neoplasm of extrahepatic bile ducts.*

156 *Malignant neoplasm of gallbladder and extrahepatic bile ducts*

AHA: Q2, 1990, 7

Gallbladder cancer is uncommon and usually seen only in the elderly. Bile duct tumors are somewhat more common, but still usually limited to older patients. Most of these cancers are adenocarcinomas.

156.0 Malignant neoplasm of gallbladder

156.1 Malignant neoplasm of extrahepatic bile ducts — *biliary, common bile, cystic, hepatic duct; sphincter of Oddi*
AHA: Q2, 1990, 7

156.2 Malignant neoplasm of ampulla of Vater — *area of dilation at the juncture of common bile and pancreatic ducts near their opening into the lumen of the duodenum*
AHA: Q2, 1990, 7

156.8 Malignant neoplasm of other specified sites of gallbladder and extrahepatic bile ducts — *not elsewhere classified or of contiguous or overlapping sites*
AHA: Q2, 1990, 7

156.9 Malignant neoplasm of biliary tract, part unspecified site — *unknown or involving both intrahepatic and extrahepatic bile ducts*
AHA: Q2, 1990, 7

Coding Clarification

Disease is classified according to site. If the malignancy is of contiguous and overlapping sites, report 156.8 *Other specified sites of gallbladder and extrahepatic bile ducts.*

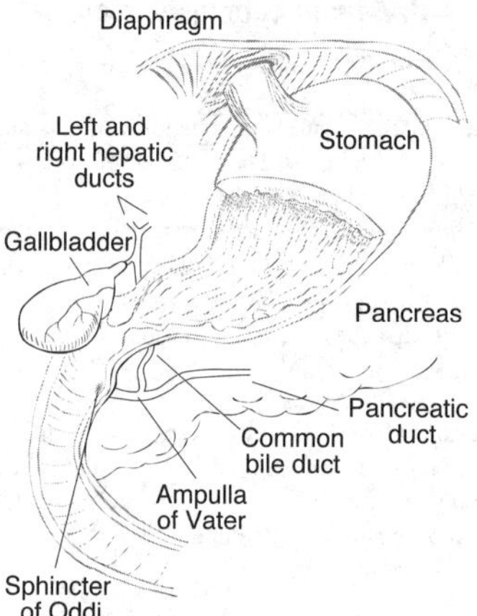

Location of the gallbladder in relation to select surrounding structures

157 *Malignant neoplasm of pancreas*

AHA: Q2, 1990, 7

The pancreas is a slender organ lying behind the stomach in the abdomen. The head of the pancreas is curved near the duodenum; the body is the main portion, and the tail is the portion that abuts the spleen. There are no clear demarcations between the parts of the pancreas.

The pancreas produces pancreatic juice, enzymes that assist in digestion. It also creates insulin, which regulates blood glucose levels.

Pancreatic cancer is one of the most prevalent cancers in the United States, after lung cancer and colon cancer. It is most common in people aged 50-70. Symptoms include weight loss, jaundice, and abdominal or back pain. Pancreatic cancer is most common in the head of the gland, with 66 percent of malignancies occurring there. Ductal adenocarcinoma is the most common type of malignancy in pancreatic cancer.

If the cancer is in the islets of Langerhans, insulin regulation could be affected.

157.0 Malignant neoplasm of head of pancreas — *Bard-Pic's syndrome*
AHA: Q2, 1990, 7; Q4, 2000, 40

157.1 Malignant neoplasm of body of pancreas — *main portion*
AHA: Q2, 1990, 7

157.2 Malignant neoplasm of tail of pancreas

157.3 Malignant neoplasm of pancreatic duct — *Santorini, Wirsung ducts*
AHA: Q2, 1990, 7

© 2004 Ingenix, Inc.

157.4 Malignant neoplasm of islets of Langerhans — (Use additional code to identify any functional activity) — *structures in the pancreas that produce insulin, somatostatin, or glucagon*
AHA: Q2, 1990, 7

157.8 Malignant neoplasm of other specified sites of pancreas — *ectopic tissue, contiguous or overlapping sites*
AHA: Q2, 1990, 7

157.9 Malignant neoplasm of pancreas, part unspecified

Coding Clarification
Any functional activity resulting from the malignancy should be separately reported. If the cancer occurs in overlapping or contiguous portions of the pancreas, report 157.8 *Other specified sites of pancreas.*

158 Malignant neoplasm of retroperitoneum and peritoneum

AHA: Q2, 1990, 7

The retroperitoneum is the space behind the peritoneum and in front of the spine. The peritoneum is the membrane that holds the abdominal organs. A majority of peritoneal malignancies are secondary, with the exception of peritoneal mesothelioma, a rare cancer arising in the mesodermal lining of the peritoneum. Retroperitoneal tumors are usually of mesodermal tissue.

158.0 Malignant neoplasm of retroperitoneum — *periadrenal, perirenal, perinephric, retrocecal tissues*
AHA: Q2, 1990, 7

158.8 Malignant neoplasm of specified parts of peritoneum — *Douglas cul-de-sac, mesentery; mesocolon; omentum; peritoneum; rectouterine pouch; or contiguous or sites*
AHA: Q2, 1990, 7

158.9 Malignant neoplasm of peritoneum, unspecified

Coding Clarification
If the malignancy spans both the peritoneum and retroperitoneum, ICD-9-CM instructs to report this condition with 158.8 *Malignant neoplasm of specified parts of peritoneum.*

159 Malignant neoplasm of other and ill-defined sites within the digestive organs and peritoneum

AHA: Q2, 1990, 7

This rubric is reserved for nonspecific malignancies of digestive sites and the peritoneum.

159.0 Malignant neoplasm of intestinal tract, part unspecified

159.1 Malignant neoplasm of spleen, not elsewhere classified — *angiosarcoma, fibrosarcoma of spleen*
AHA: Q2, 1990, 7

159.8 Malignant neoplasm of other sites of digestive system and intra-abdominal organs — *point of origin cannot be assigned to any one of the categories 150-158*
AHA: Q2, 1990, 7

159.9 Malignant neoplasm of ill-defined sites of digestive organs and peritoneum — *generalized "alimentary canal," "gastrointestinal tract"*
AHA: Q2, 1990, 7

Coding Clarification
When a digestive malignancy has progressed so that the point of origin cannot be assigned to a specific code in rubrics 150-158, report 159.8 *Malignant neoplasm of other sites of digestive system and intra-abdominal organs.*

160–165 Malignant Neoplasm of Respiratory and Intrathoracic Organs

The respiratory system can be divided into two main sections: the upper and the lower respiratory tracts. The upper respiratory tract is located outside the thorax (the chest cavity), and is composed of the nose and the pharynx (nasopharynx, oropharynx, and hypopharynx). Malignant neoplasms of this upper portion of respiratory anatomy are classified in 140-149, as part of the oral cavity. This subsection includes the larynx and the lower respiratory tract contained within the thorax, which consists of the trachea, bronchial tree, lungs, and pleura. Also classified to this subsection because of their anatomic locations are malignant neoplasms of the heart, thymus, and mediastinum. However, great vessels are classified to 171.4.

The respiratory system functions as follows: air enters the body through the nose, where it is warmed, filtered, and humidified as it passes through the nasal cavity. The air passes into the pharynx and from the pharynx into the trachea (the "windpipe"). The epiglottis in the pharynx prevents food from entering the trachea. The upper part of the trachea contains the three parts of the larynx and the vocal chords. At its base, the trachea divides into the left and right primary bronchi. Each bronchus divides into smaller branches known as segmental bronchi. These divide into tiny bronchioles that terminate in the microscopic ducts and alveoli sacs of the lungs where gas exchange takes place.

The lungs are large, paired organs in the thorax. The right lung has three lobes. The left lung cavity

© 2004 Ingenix, Inc.

contains two lobes and encloses the heart. Thin sheets of epithelium (the pleura) separate the inside of the chest cavity from the outer surface of the lungs and the heart.

The respiratory system functions as an air distributor and gas exchanger, to supply oxygen and remove carbon monoxide from the body's cells. All parts of the respiratory system, except the microscopic alveoli of the lungs, function as air distributors. Only the alveoli sacks and ducts serve as gas exchangers. In addition to air distribution and gas exchange, the respiratory system and its structures provide for such functions as yawning, sneezing, coughing, hiccups, sound production (including speech), and the sense of smell (olfaction). The respiratory system also assists in homeostasis (regulation of pH in the body).

Coding Clarification

Malignancies in this section are classified according to anatomic site. If malignancies are found in multiple sites within an anatomic system, a code for "other sites" is in most cases appropriate to report multiple sites. If the malignancy results in functional abnormalities, report the malignancy first, followed by the functional problem. For nonspecific or multiple thoracic or intrathoracic malignancies, report 195.1 *Malignant neoplasm of the thorax.* If the malignancy is carcinoma in situ, report with codes from the 231 rubric instead. If respiratory or thoracic malignancies are secondary, see codes in the 196-199 rubrics.

160 Malignant neoplasm of nasal cavities, middle ear, and accessory sinuses

AHA: Q2, 1990, 7

The nasal cavity opens into the vestibule that is just inside of the nostrils and continues to the respiratory area where bone in three shelves (formed by the nasal cavity) called the superior, middle, and inferior nasal turbinates (nasal conchae) are located. The turbinates come close to the nasal septum and subdivide the nasal cavity into passageways.

160.0 Malignant neoplasm of nasal cavities — *nasal cartilage, septum, conchae, fossa, mucosa, internal nose*
AHA: Q2, 1990, 7

160.1 Malignant neoplasm of auditory tube, middle ear, and mastoid air cells — *eustachian tube, inner ear, middle ear, antrum tympanicum, tympanic cavity*
AHA: Q2, 1990, 7

160.2 Malignant neoplasm of maxillary sinus — *sinus behind cheekbones; maxillary antrum and Highmore antrum*
AHA: Q2, 1990, 7

160.3 Malignant neoplasm of ethmoidal sinus — *sinus between the eyes on either side of the nose*
AHA: Q2, 1990, 7

160.4 Malignant neoplasm of frontal sinus — *sinus above the eyes*
AHA: Q2, 1990, 7

160.5 Malignant neoplasm of sphenoidal sinus — *sinus behind the eyes on either side of the nose*
AHA: Q2, 1990, 7

160.8 Malignant neoplasm of other sites of nasal cavities, middle ear, and accessory sinuses — *contiguous or overlapping sites of nasal cavities, middle ear, and accessory sinuses*
AHA: Q2, 1990, 7

160.9 Malignant neoplasm of site of nasal cavities, middle ear, and accessory sinus, unspecified site

161 Malignant neoplasm of larynx

AHA: Q2, 1990, 7

The larynx has several functions: speech, protection of the airways, respiration, and fixation of the chest. It is commonly called the "voicebox." Most laryngeal malignancies are squamous cell carcinomas and 90 percent of laryngeal cancers occur in males. Hoarseness and throat pain are common symptoms.

161.0 Malignant neoplasm of glottis — *true vocal cord including intrinsic larynx, commissure*
AHA: Q2, 1990, 7

161.1 Malignant neoplasm of supraglottis — *false vocal cord including aryepiglottic fold, epiglottis, extrinsic larynx, ventricular bands*
AHA: Q2, 1990, 7

161.2 Malignant neoplasm of subglottis — *larynx below the vocal cords and above the trachea*
AHA: Q2, 1990, 7

161.3 Malignant neoplasm of laryngeal cartilages — *including arytenoid, cricoid, cuneiform, thyroid cartilage*
AHA: Q2, 1990, 7

161.8 Malignant neoplasm of other specified sites of larynx — *contiguous or overlapping sites of larynx whose point of origin cannot be determined*
AHA: Q2, 1990, 7

161.9 Malignant neoplasm of larynx, unspecified site

Coding Clarification

Malignant neoplasms of the larynx are classified according to site. If the malignancy spans two sites of the larynx, ICD-9-CM instructs to report this condition with 161.8 *Malignant neoplasm of other specified sites of larynx.* Do not use codes in this rubric

© 2004 Ingenix, Inc.

to report malignancies of the epiglottis (146.4) or hypopharynx (rubric 148).

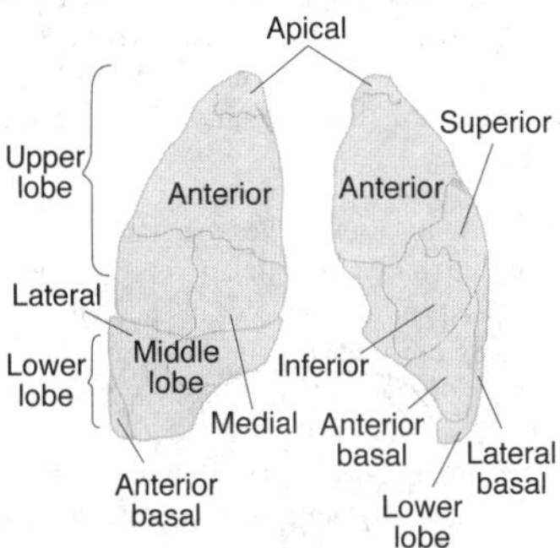

Anterior view of lungs. The left lung is divided into superior and inferior lobes. The right lung has three segments. The subdivisions are defined by the areas served by bronchial divisions

162 Malignant neoplasm of trachea, bronchus, and lung

AHA: Q2, 1990, 7

Lung cancer is the most common cancer in the United States, with more than 150,000 cases diagnosed and more than 100,000 dying from the disease annually. Malignant tumors of the lung may be squamous cell, adenocarcinoma, small cell, large cell, adenosquamous, carcinoid, or bronchial gland carcinoma. Lung cancer is considered one of the most lethal forms of cancer, with only 20 percent of patients surviving one year after diagnosis. Symptoms include wheezing, pneumonia, and pain, as well as symptoms from metastatic sites of disease. The most common site of metastatic lung cancer is the liver; however, brain, kidney, and adrenal gland are also common sites.

162.0 Malignant neoplasm of trachea — *breathing tube anterior to the esophagus and extending from the larynx to the right and left bronchi.*
AHA: Q2, 1990, 7

162.2 Malignant neoplasm of main bronchus — *carina and hilus of lung*
AHA: Q2, 1990, 7

162.3 Malignant neoplasm of upper lobe, bronchus, or lung — *Cuiffini-Pancoase syndrome, Hare's syndrome, Tobias' syndrome*
AHA: Q2, 1990, 7

162.4 Malignant neoplasm of middle lobe, bronchus, or lung — *Middle lobe, bronchus or lung*
AHA: Q2, 1990, 7

162.5 Malignant neoplasm of lower lobe, bronchus, or lung — *Lower lobe, bronchus or lung*
AHA: Q2, 1990, 7

162.8 Malignant neoplasm of other parts of bronchus or lung — *contiguous or overlapping sites of bronchus or lung whose point of origin cannot be determined*
AHA: Q2, 1990, 7

162.9 Malignant neoplasm of bronchus and lung, unspecified site

Coding Clarification

Lung cancer is classified according to the lobe of the lung. Report 162.8 if the cancer invades contiguous or overlapping sites in the lung or bronchus if the point of origin cannot be determined.

Coding Scenario

A patient is admitted with an esophageal obstruction due to esophageal metastasis from the lung.

> Code assignment: 530.3 *Stricture and stenosis of esophagus*, 197.8 *Secondary malignant neoplasm of other respiratory and digestive organs*, and 162.9 *Malignant neoplasm of bronchus, and lung, unspecified*

A 49-year-old female is admitted for severe dehydration. The patient is known to have lung cancer with generalized metastases. The patient is treated with IV fluids for the dehydration. The patient's cancer is not treated during this admission.

> Code assignment: 276.5 *Volume depletion*, 162.9 *Malignant neoplasm of bronchus and lung, unspecified*, and 199.0 *Malignant neoplasm, disseminated*

A patient is admitted for chemotherapy requiring placement of a Hickman catheter for infusion of an anticancer agent for treatment of lung cancer metastases.

> Code assignment: V58.1 *Encounter for chemotherapy*, 162.9 *Malignant neoplasm of bronchus and lung, unspecified*, and 199.1 *Malignant neoplasm without specification of site, other*

A patient develops agranulocytosis associated with the chemotherapy treatment he has been receiving for lung cancer.

> Code assignment: 288.0 *Agranulocytosis*, 162.9 *Malignant neoplasm of bronchus and lung, unspecified*, and E933.1 *Adverse effects in therapeutic use, antineoplastic and immunosuppressive drugs*

163 Malignant neoplasm of pleura

AHA: Q2, 1990, 7

140–239

The pleura line the lung and localized mesothelioma. Diffuse malignant mesothelioma is the most common form of pleural malignancy. Cancers of the pleura are classified according to site. The parietal pleura are the outer lining of the lung, and the visceral pleura are the inner lining.

163.0 Malignant neoplasm of parietal pleura — *outer lining of the lung*
AHA: Q2, 1990, 7

163.1 Malignant neoplasm of visceral pleura — *inner lining of the lung*
AHA: Q2, 1990, 7

163.8 Malignant neoplasm of other specified sites of pleura — *contiguous or overlapping sites of pleura whose point of origin cannot be determined*
AHA: Q2, 1990, 7

163.9 Malignant neoplasm of pleura, unspecified site

Coding Clarification

Report 163.8 if the malignancy is overlapping or in contiguous parts of the pleura.

164 Malignant neoplasm of thymus, heart, and mediastinum

AHA: Q2, 1990, 7

The thymus is a bilateral, lymph-rich organ that produces T lymphocytes that circulate throughout the body to provide an immune function. The organ is anterior to the heart, in the upper mediastinum, and is a common site for neoplasms. The most common type of thymoma is epithelial, accounting for 45 percent of cases. Since some lymphomas and Hodgkin's granulomas arise in thymus tissue, check documentation to be sure of appropriate use of codes from this rubric.

The mediastinum is the compartment between the sternum and lungs/heart (anterior), and the spine and lungs/heart (posterior). Because of the general nature of the mediastinum in anatomical descriptions, care should be taken that a more specific site isn't overlooked when coding malignant neoplasm of the mediastinum. The thymus (164.0) and parathyroid (194.1) reside in the mediastinum, but are reported with more specific codes, as are neurogenic tumors in the mediastinum (classify to nerve).

The heart is the muscle responsible for circulation of blood throughout the body. It is divided into four cavities: the right and left atria and the right and left ventricles. The left atrium receives oxygenated blood from the lung and passes it along to the left ventricle, which pushes the blood through the circulatory system to nourish the body's cells. The right atrium receives the blood that has completed its circuit through the body. From the right atrium, the blood is circulated to the right ventricle, which pumps it back into the lungs for reoxygenation. Four major valves separate the chambers and prevent backflow of blood. The valves consist of flaps called cusps; the ends of the cusps between the atria and ventricles extend into the ventricles where they are connected to the papillary muscles by fibrous cords called the chordae tendineae.

Malignant neoplasms of the heart are rarely seen as primary neoplasms. When primary cancer of the heart occurs, it occurs most commonly in children. The most common cardiac malignancy is cardiac sarcoma, accounting for 30 percent of the cases. Complications from cardiac cancer can be grave and include heart failure, hemorrhagic pericardial effusion with tamponade, and arrhythmia. A primary cancer of the heart is also prone to metastases to the spine and other major organs.

164.0 Malignant neoplasm of thymus — *lymphoid and endocrine organ behind the sternum*
AHA: Q2, 1990, 7

164.1 Malignant neoplasm of heart — *endocardium, epicardium, myocardium and pericardium*
AHA: Q2, 1990, 7

164.2 Malignant neoplasm of anterior mediastinum — *soft and connective tissue between the lungs, in the cavity between the heart and the sternum*
AHA: Q2, 1990, 7

164.3 Malignant neoplasm of posterior mediastinum — *soft and connective tissue between the lungs, in the cavity between the heart and the spinal column*
AHA: Q2, 1990, 7

164.8 Malignant neoplasm of other parts of mediastinum — *contiguous or overlapping sites of thymus, heart, and mediastinum*
AHA: Q2, 1990, 7

164.9 Malignant neoplasm of mediastinum, part unspecified

Coding Clarification

Report malignant neoplasms of the great vessels with 171.4 *Malignant neoplasm of the thorax.* If the malignancy is overlapping or in contiguous parts of the heart and mediastinum, report 164.8 *Malignant neoplasm of other parts of mediastinum.*

165 Malignant neoplasm of other and ill-defined sites within the respiratory system and intrathoracic organs

AHA: Q2, 1990, 7

This rubric is reserved for nonspecific malignancies of respiratory and intrathoracic organs.

 © 2004 Ingenix, Inc.

165.0 Malignant neoplasm of upper respiratory tract, part unspecified — *the respiratory organs above the diaphragm*
AHA: Q2, 1990, 7

165.8 Malignant neoplasm of other sites within the respiratory system and intrathoracic organs — *point of origin cannot be assigned to any one of the categories 160-164*
AHA: Q2, 1990, 7

165.9 Malignant neoplasm of ill-defined sites within the respiratory system — *respiratory tract not otherwise specified*
AHA: Q2, 1990, 7

Coding Clarification

When a respiratory malignancy has progressed to a point that it cannot be assigned to a specific code in rubrics 160-164, report 165.8 *Malignant neoplasm of other sites within the respiratory system and intrathoracic organs.*

170–176 Malignant Neoplasm of Bone, Connective Tissue, Skin, and Breast

Codes in this section of ICD-9-CM refer to malignancies in the bone, connective tissue, skin, and breast.

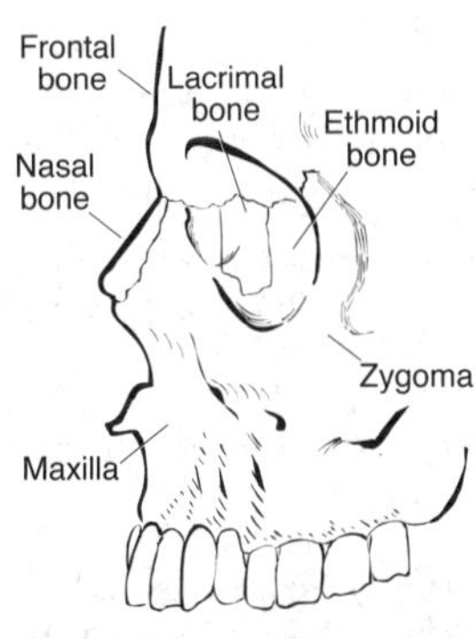

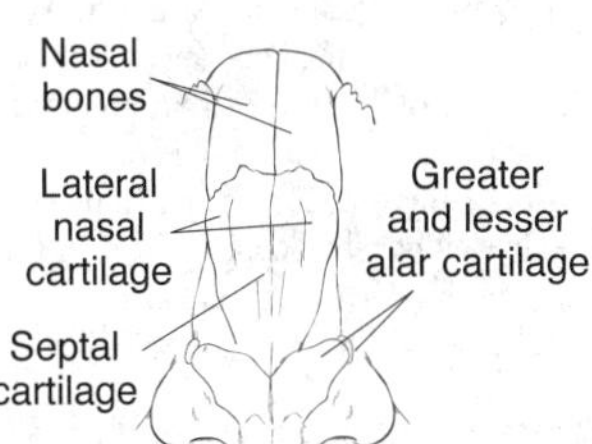

170 *Malignant neoplasm of bone and articular cartilage*

AHA: Q2, 1990, 7

Primary malignancies of the bone are uncommon compared to the incidence of metastases to the bone.

Multiple myeloma is the most common bone malignancy, occurring usually in older adults. Osteosarcoma is most commonly seen in children and young adults. Pain, swelling, limit to range of motion, or pathological fracture are common symptoms.

170.0 Malignant neoplasm of bones of skull and face, except mandible — *ethmoid, frontal, turbinate, malar, occipital, orbital, zygomatic, sphenoid, temporal*
AHA: Q2, 1990, 7

170.1 Malignant neoplasm of mandible — *inferior maxilla, lower jaw bone*
AHA: Q2, 1990, 7

170.2 Malignant neoplasm of vertebral column, excluding sacrum and coccyx — *meaning bony spine, vertebra*
AHA: Q2, 1990, 7

170.3 Malignant neoplasm of ribs, sternum, and clavicle — *costal cartilage, costovertebral joint, xiphoid process*
AHA: Q2, 1990, 7

170.4 Malignant neoplasm of scapula and long bones of upper limb — *acromion, radius, ulna, humerus*
AHA: Q2, 1990, 7; Q2, 1999, 9

170.5 Malignant neoplasm of short bones of upper limb — *bones of hand and wrist; carpal, cuneiform, scaphoid, semilunar of lunate, navicular, phalanges, unciform, trapezoid, pisiform*
AHA: Q2, 1990, 7

170.6 Malignant neoplasm of pelvic bones, sacrum, and coccyx — *coccygeal vertebra, ilium, ischium, pubic bone, sacral vertebra*
AHA: Q2, 1990, 7

170.7 Malignant neoplasm of long bones of lower limb — *femur, fibula, tibia*
AHA: Q2, 1990, 7

170.8 Malignant neoplasm of short bones of lower limb — *bones of knee, foot and ankle; astragalus talus, calcaneus, cuboid, navicular of knee, patella, phalanges, tarsal, metatarsal*
AHA: Q2, 1990, 7

170.9 Malignant neoplasm of bone and articular cartilage, site unspecified

Coding Clarification

For metastasized cancers, see 198.5 *Secondary malignant neoplasm of the bone and bone marrow.* Malignancies of the bone are classified in ICD-9-CM according to anatomic site and type of bone (long or short). Articular cartilage and periosteum malignancies are classified to the appropriate bone

© 2004 Ingenix, Inc.

code. Connective and soft tissue malignancies are classified to the 171 rubric, as connective tissue.

171 Malignant neoplasm of connective and other soft tissue

AHA: Q2, 1990, 7

Malignant neoplasms of the connective tissue and other soft tissue are classified according to site rather than specific type of tissue. These codes can be used to classify malignant neoplasms of blood vessels; bursa; fascia; fat; ligament (except uterine); muscle; peripheral, sympathetic, and parasympathetic nerves; synovia; or tendons.

Cartilage is a type of dense connective tissue (hyaline, elastic, and fibrocartilage) that is found in joints. Hyaline cartilage is located at joints over the ends of long bones; fibrocartilage is found at other body sites, such as the pubic symphysis, intervertebral discs, menisci of the knee, and the point where the hip bones fuse anteriorly.

Soft tissue generally includes the deep fascia, muscles, tendons, and ligaments. Deep fascia lies beneath the second layer of subcutaneous tissue (hypodermis) of the integumentary system. Deep fascia in the musculoskeletal system lines extremities and holds together groups of muscles. There are three types of muscle tissue: skeletal, cardiac, and visceral. Muscle tissue consists of specialized cells that allow contraction to produce voluntary or involuntary movement of body parts.

Tendons are fibrous cords that vary in length. They are found at the ends of muscles and connecting muscles to bones. Ligaments are bands of fibrous tissue that connect two or more bones or cartilage.

171.0 Malignant neoplasm of connective and other soft tissue of head, face, and neck — *blood vessel, fascia, fat, muscle, cartilage of eye and ear, ligament, and peripheral, sympathetic, and parasympathetic nerve and ganglia*
AHA: Q2, 1990, 7; Q2, 1999, 6

171.2 Malignant neoplasm of connective and other soft tissue of upper limb, including shoulder — *blood vessel, fascia, fat, muscle, ligament, and peripheral, sympathetic, and parasympathetic nerve and ganglia*
AHA: Q2, 1990, 7

171.3 Malignant neoplasm of connective and other soft tissue of lower limb, including hip — *blood vessel, fascia, fat, muscle, ligament, and peripheral, sympathetic, and parasympathetic nerve and ganglia*
AHA: Q2, 1990, 7

171.4 Malignant neoplasm of connective and other soft tissue of thorax — *blood vessel, fascia, fat, muscle, ligament, and peripheral, sympathetic, and parasympathetic nerve and ganglia*
AHA: Q2, 1990, 7

171.5 Malignant neoplasm of connective and other soft tissue of abdomen — *blood vessel, fascia, fat, muscle, ligament, and peripheral, sympathetic, and parasympathetic nerve and ganglia*
AHA: Q2, 1990, 7

171.6 Malignant neoplasm of connective and other soft tissue of pelvis — *blood vessel, fascia, fat, muscle, ligament, and peripheral, sympathetic, and parasympathetic nerve and ganglia*
AHA: Q2, 1990, 7

171.7 Malignant neoplasm of connective and other soft tissue of trunk, unspecified site — *blood vessel, fascia, fat, muscle, ligament, and peripheral, sympathetic, and parasympathetic nerve and ganglia*
AHA: Q2, 1990, 7

171.8 Malignant neoplasm of other specified sites of connective and other soft tissue — *contiguous or overlapping sites of connective tissue whose point of origin cannot be determined*
AHA: Q2, 1990, 7

171.9 Malignant neoplasm of connective and other soft tissue, site unspecified

Coding Clarification

If the malignant neoplasm is of contiguous or overlapping soft tissue sites and the point of origin cannot be determined, report 171.8.

172 Malignant melanoma of skin

AHA: Q2, 1990, 7

The integumentary system is a diverse and complex organ forming the boundary and barrier between the internal environment of the body and the outside world. Although quite thin, the skin (or cutaneous membrane) is the largest human organ, usually 12 to 20 square feet in area and composing 12 percent of the total body weight. The depth of the skin varies from 0.5 mm in thin areas such as the eyelids to 5.0 mm or more at its thickest over the back.

There are three integrated layers in the skin: the thinner outer layer (epidermis), the dense connective layer (dermis), and the loose subcutis or subcutaneous layer (also called the hypodermis or superficial fascia), which is composed of fat and areolar tissue.

The epidermis consists of three distinct cell types: keratinocytes that provide structure, melanocytes that

© 2004 Ingenix, Inc.

contribute color and filter ultraviolet light, and Langerhans cells that contribute to the immune response. These cells form up to five strata over the dermal epidermal junction or basement membrane. Beneath the epidermal junction lies the dermis, composed of a papillary and a reticular layer. The dermis is rich in skin receptor nerves, blood vessels, and in sweat glands. It provides attachment for smooth and skeletal muscle fibers and the hair follicles. The lipocyte cells of the subcutis, joined to the bottom of the dermis, produce lipids for the subcutaneous tissue to make the fatty, insulating layer that cushions the body against shocks and provides an energy source.

Melanomas are skin cancers that are usually pigmented but otherwise vary in size and presentation. They are among the most invasive of the cancers. Change is the hallmark of melanoma; adjacent tissue is usually transformed. The most common type of melanoma is superficial spreading melanoma, accounting for 65 percent of all melanomas. They are most common on women's legs, or men's trunks. Other types of melanoma include nodular, with dark papules or plaques, and solar lentigo, arising as a flat tan macule on areas of skin that have had long-term sun exposure, especially on the hands and forehead.

172.0 Malignant melanoma of skin of lip — *skin only, outer aspect only*
AHA: Q2, 1990, 7

172.1 Malignant melanoma of skin of eyelid, including canthus

172.2 Malignant melanoma of skin of ear and external auditory canal — *auricle, external canal, tragus, helix, pinna, concha, pinna*
AHA: Q2, 1990, 7

172.3 Malignant melanoma of skin of other and unspecified parts of face — *external cheek and nose, chin but not neck, forehead, but not scalp*
AHA: Q2, 1990, 7

172.4 Malignant melanoma of skin of scalp and neck — *but not chin or forehead*
AHA: Q2, 1990, 7

172.5 Malignant melanoma of skin of trunk, except scrotum — *axilla, breast, buttock, groin, perianal skin, perineum, umbilicus*
AHA: Q2, 1990, 7

172.6 Malignant melanoma of skin of upper limb, including shoulder — *shoulder, arm, and hand*
AHA: Q2, 1990, 7

172.7 Malignant melanoma of skin of lower limb, including hip — *hip, leg, and foot*
AHA: Q2, 1990, 7

172.8 Malignant melanoma of other specified sites of skin — *contiguous or overlapping sites of skin*
AHA: Q2, 1990, 7

172.9 Melanoma of skin, site unspecified

Coding Clarification

Melanoma begins as a skin cancer, but aggressively metastasizes to other systems or organs. These secondary sites are not classified in ICD-9-CM as melanomas, but as secondary malignant neoplasms, classified by site in rubrics 196-199.

Do not report personal history of malignant melanoma of skin (V10.83) in patients with a recurrence; instead, report the active disease. The personal history code is reserved for patients who have completed treatment and are without recurrence of melanoma.

173 Other malignant neoplasm of skin

AHA: Q2, 1990, 7; Q2, 1996, 12; Q1, 2000, 18

Skin cancers other than melanoma may be basal cell or squamous cell carcinomas. No distinction is made between basal and squamous cells in ICD-9-CM classification. Basal cell carcinoma is usually small, shiny, and firm, but may also be crusty and ulcerous. A squamous cell carcinoma is often more pigmented, but it, too, is highly variable in appearance.

173.0 Other malignant neoplasm of skin of lip — *skin only, outer aspect only*
AHA: Q2, 1990, 7; Q2, 1996, 12; Q1, 2000, 18

173.1 Other malignant neoplasm of skin of eyelid, including canthus

173.2 Other malignant neoplasm of skin of ear and external auditory canal — *auricle, external canal, tragus, helix, pinna, concha, pinna*
AHA: Q2, 1990, 7; Q2, 1996, 12; Q1, 2000, 18

173.3 Other malignant neoplasm of skin of other and unspecified parts of face — *external cheek and nose, chin but not neck, forehead, but not scalp*
AHA: Q2, 1990, 7; Q2, 1996, 12; Q1, 2000, 3; Q1, 2000, 18

173.4 Other malignant neoplasm of scalp and skin of neck — *but not chin or forehead*
AHA: Q2, 1990, 7; Q2, 1996, 12; Q1, 2000, 18

173.5 Other malignant neoplasm of skin of trunk, except scrotum — *axilla, breast, buttock, groin, perianal skin, perineum, umbilicus*
AHA: Q2, 1990, 7; Q2, 1996, 12; Q1, 2000, 18; Q1, 2001, 8

140–239

173.6 Other malignant neoplasm of skin of upper limb, including shoulder — *shoulder, arm and hand*
AHA: Q2, 1990, 7; Q2, 1996, 12; Q1, 2000, 18

173.7 Other malignant neoplasm of skin of lower limb, including hip — *hip, leg and foot*
AHA: Q2, 1990, 7; Q2, 1996, 12; Q1, 2000, 18

173.8 Other malignant neoplasm of other specified sites of skin — *contiguous or overlapping sites of skin*
AHA: Q2, 1990, 7; Q2, 1996, 12; Q1, 2000, 18

173.9 Other malignant neoplasm of skin, site unspecified

Coding Clarification

Skin cancers in this rubric are classified according to location. For melanoma, see codes in rubric 172; for Kaposi's sarcoma, see rubric 176. Cancers of the skin of the genitalia are reported with genitalia codes, 184.0-184.9 and 187.1-187.9.

174 Malignant neoplasm of female breast

AHA: Q4, 1989, 11; Q2, 1990, 7; Q3, 1997, 8

The mammary glands are accessory organs of the female reproductive system. Each breast contains glandular tissue consisting of secreting cells and ducts. The smaller ducts unite into a single milk-carrying duct for each lobe and these converge toward the nipple. The glandular tissue is contained within dense connective tissue that attaches to the pectoral muscle, and with suspensory ligaments that extend from the skin to the pectoral muscle to provide support. Surrounding the nipple is the circular area of pigmented and irregular surfaced skin called the areola.

The function of the mammary gland is lactation — secretion of colostrum and subsequently milk for the nourishment of newborn infants. Successful lactation relies on pre- and postnatal production of hormones including progesterone, estrogen, prolactin, and oxytocin.

Malignant neoplasms of the female breast are classified according to site. The upper, outer quadrant of the breast is the most likely site for a malignancy; a full 50 percent of breast disease occurs in this quadrant. This is followed by 18 percent in the nipple; 15 percent in the upper, inner quadrant; 6 percent in the lower, inner quadrant; and 1 percent in the lower, outer quadrant. The remaining percentage (10 percent) is distributed in the axillary tail and in multiple sites.

174.0 Malignant neoplasm of nipple and areola of female breast

174.1 Malignant neoplasm of central portion of female breast

174.2 Malignant neoplasm of upper-inner quadrant of female breast

174.3 Malignant neoplasm of lower-inner quadrant of female breast

174.4 Malignant neoplasm of upper-outer quadrant of female breast

174.5 Malignant neoplasm of lower-outer quadrant of female breast

174.6 Malignant neoplasm of axillary tail of female breast

174.8 Malignant neoplasm of other specified sites of female breast — *ectopic sites or overlapping sites*
AHA: Q4, 1989, 11; Q2, 1990, 7; Q3, 1997, 8

174.9 Malignant neoplasm of breast (female), unspecified site

Coding Clarification

If a malignancy is found in several sites of the breast, report 174.8 *Malignant neoplasm of other specified sites of female breast,* which includes multiple sites. Do not code each site separately. If the malignancy is in the skin of the breast, report 172.5 (melanoma) or 173.5 (other skin malignancy).

Coding Scenario

A 49-year-old female patient is seen in the hospital ambulatory surgery center for a biopsy of a breast lump at the patient's previous mastectomy site. Pathology report confirms a recurrent breast carcinoma.

> Code assignment: 174.9 *Malignant neoplasm of breast (female), unspecified*

A 63-year-old female is diagnosed with an intraductal comedo carcinoma with focal stromal microinvasion, upper inner quadrant right breast.

> Code assignment: 174.2 *Malignant neoplasm of upper-inner quadrant of female breast*

A 49-year-old female with recent radical mastectomy for breast carcinoma is seen for radiation therapy.

> Code assignment: V58.0 *Encounter for radiotherapy* and 174.9 *Malignant neoplasm of breast (female), unspecified*

175 Malignant neoplasm of male breast

AHA: Q2, 1990, 7

Malignant neoplasms of the male breast are classified by site: both nipple and areola or other.

175.0 Malignant neoplasm of nipple and areola of male breast

 © 2004 Ingenix, Inc.

175.9 Malignant neoplasm of other and unspecified sites of male breast — *ectopic sites*
AHA: Q2, 1990, 7

Coding Clarification

If the malignancy is in the skin of the breast, report 172.5 (melanoma) or 173.5 (other skin malignancy) instead. Breast cancer in men occurs at only 1 percent of the rate it occurs in women.

176 Kaposi's sarcoma

AHA: Q2, 1990, 7; Q4, 1991, 24

Kaposi's sarcoma is a malignancy characterized by numerous vascular skin tumors. Kaposi's sarcoma was once found only rarely, in aging men, usually of Italian or Jewish decent. Today, incidence is common in the United States, as a manifestation of Acquired Immune Deficiency Syndrome (AIDS).

A diagnosis of Kaposi's sarcoma of the skin is significant because it is often the first clinical manifestation of AIDS in a Human Immunodeficiency Virus (HIV) positive patient, though Kaposi's sarcoma itself is rarely a cause of death. Disseminated Kaposi's sarcoma can involve lymph nodes, viscera, and the gastrointestinal tract.

176.0 Kaposi's sarcoma of skin — *any site*
AHA: Q2, 1990, 7; Q4, 1991, 24

176.1 Kaposi's sarcoma of soft tissue — *blood vessel, connective tissue, fat, fascia, ligament, muscle*
AHA: Q2, 1990, 7; Q4, 1991, 24

176.2 Kaposi's sarcoma of palate — *hard or soft*
AHA: Q2, 1990, 7; Q4, 1991, 24

176.3 Kaposi's sarcoma of gastrointestinal sites — *stomach, intestine, anus, liver, spleen, pancreas*
AHA: Q2, 1990, 7; Q4, 1991, 24

176.4 Kaposi's sarcoma of lung — *any site*
AHA: Q2, 1990, 7; Q4, 1991, 24

176.5 Kaposi's sarcoma of lymph nodes — *any site, but excluding lymphatic channels*
AHA: Q2, 1990, 7; Q4, 1991, 24

176.8 Kaposi's sarcoma of other specified sites — *external genitalia, scrotum, vulva, and oral cavity not elsewhere specified*
AHA: Q2, 1990, 7; Q4, 1991, 24

176.9 Kaposi's sarcoma of unspecified site — *viscera not otherwise specified*
AHA: Q2, 1990, 7; Q4, 1991, 24

Coding Clarification

Kaposi's syndrome is classified according to site of lesion. More than one code may be required to describe disseminated sarcoma, and Kaposi's is never reported with secondary neoplasm codes.

Do not reference the table of neoplasms to assign codes for Kaposi's sarcoma; Kaposi's sarcoma codes are omitted from the table. Instead, refer to Kaposi's sarcoma in the index of ICD-9-CM where a complete indexing is provided.

179–189 Malignant Neoplasm of Genitourinary Organs

Codes in this subsection of ICD-9-CM are classified according to site of malignant neoplasm in the female or male reproductive system or in the urinary system.

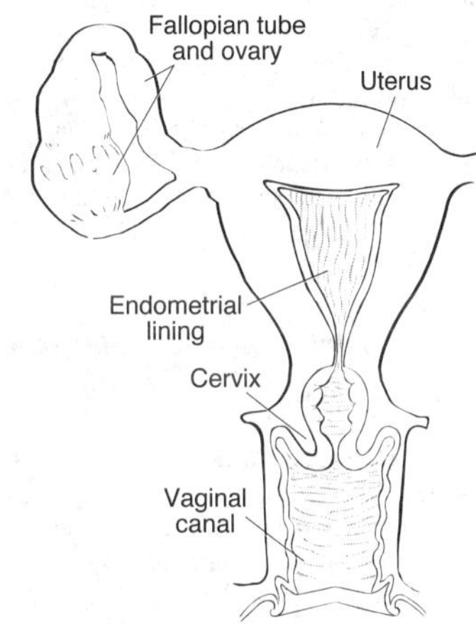

179 Malignant neoplasm of uterus, part unspecified OK

AHA: Q2, 1990, 7

Use this valid three-digit code to report a malignant neoplasm of the uterus when the specific location is unknown. Use a more specific code whenever possible, as this code is nonspecific and its use may cause reimbursement delays.

Coding Clarification

Use 182.8 *Malignant neoplasm of other specified sites of body of uterus* when the neoplasm is of contiguous or overlapping sites of the uterus.

180 Malignant neoplasm of cervix uteri

AHA: Q2, 1990, 7

Cancer of the cervix uteri may be asymptomatic or may cause vaginal discharge, pain, or postcoital bleeding. Most cervical cancers are squamous cell cancers.

Cervical cancer is classified as either of the endocervix, which opens into the uterus, or the exocervix, the part that protrudes into the vagina.

180.0 Malignant neoplasm of endocervix — *cervical canal opening into uterus*
AHA: Q2, 1990, 7

180.1 Malignant neoplasm of exocervix — *cervical canal opening into vagina*
AHA: Q2, 1990, 7

180.8 Malignant neoplasm of other specified sites of cervix — *cervical stump, squamocolumnar junction of cervix, or contiguous or overlapping sites*
AHA: Q2, 1990, 7

180.9 Malignant neoplasm of cervix uteri, unspecified site

Coding Clarification

Report other specified site, 180.8, if the malignancy is of the cervical stump following hysterectomy, of the squamocolumnar junction of the cervix, or if the malignancy is of contiguous or overlapping sites of the endocervix and exocervix.

181 Malignant neoplasm of placenta OK

AHA: Q2, 1990, 7

The placenta is an organ of pregnancy, operating as an exchange point for waste from the fetus and nourishment from the mother. In rare cases, an anomalous placenta may develop when no viable fetus exists, as in the case of hydatidiform mole. Use this valid three-digit code to report choriocarcinoma, also called chorioepithelioma. Hydatidiform mole or pregnancy precedes choriocarcinoma. It is an epithelial malignancy that metastasizes rapidly.

Coding Clarification

Do not use this code to report a hydatidiform mole (630), malignant hydatidiform mole (236.1), or chorioadenoma (236.1).

182 Malignant neoplasm of body of uterus

AHA: Q2, 1990, 7

The uterus is the muscular female organ where the fetus develops until delivery. Normally only three inches long and the shape of a pear, the uterus expands greatly during pregnancy.

Malignant neoplasms of the body of the uterus are classified according to site: the body of the uterus, including the fundus and endometrium; and the isthmus of the uterus, the narrow, distal portion of the uterus between the main body and the cervix. Endometrial carcinoma is a common malignancy that affects primarily postmenopausal women. Symptoms include postmenopausal bleeding, though symptoms may not be present until metastases become symptomatic.

182.0 Malignant neoplasm of corpus uteri, except isthmus — *cornu, endometrium, myometrium, fundus*
AHA: Q2, 1990, 7

182.1 Malignant neoplasm of isthmus — *narrow portion of the uterus between the cervix and the main body of the uterus.*
AHA: Q2, 1990, 7

182.8 Malignant neoplasm of other specified sites of body of uterus — *contiguous or overlapping sites*
AHA: Q2, 1990, 7

Coding Clarification

Endometrial carcinoma is reported with 182.0 *Malignant neoplasm of corpus uteri, except isthmus.*

Report 182.8 *Malignant neoplasm of other specified site of body of uterus* if the malignancy is of contiguous or overlapping sites of the uterus. See codes in the 183 rubric to report cancer of the uterine ligaments.

183 Malignant neoplasm of ovary and other uterine adnexa

AHA: Q2, 1990, 7

The ovary is the female gonad and produces the ova. The organs are situated on either side of the uterus and lie near bilateral fallopian tubes, which carry the ova from the ovary to the uterus. Ligaments secure the female reproductive organs in the abdominal cavity.

Ovarian malignancies often present as an abdominal mass. Common types of ovarian malignancies include mucinous cystadenocarcinoma and endometrioid carcinoma. Other ovarian cancers are hormone producing and include Sertoli-Leydig cell tumors, adrenal cell rest tumors, and granulosa-theca cell tumors. Use an additional code to report any functional activity associated with the ovarian malignancy. If the ovarian malignancy is bilateral, it is usually metastasized disease, rather than a primary malignancy.

183.0 Malignant neoplasm of ovary — (Use additional code to identify any functional activity) — *female gonad*
AHA: Q2, 1990, 7

183.2 Malignant neoplasm of fallopian tube — *oviduct, uterine tube*
AHA: Q2, 1990, 7

183.3 Malignant neoplasm of broad ligament of uterus — *fold of peritoneum extending from the side of the uterus to the wall of the pelvis; mesovarium, parovarian region*
AHA: Q2, 1990, 7

© 2004 Ingenix, Inc.

183.4 Malignant neoplasm of parametrium of uterus — *connective tissue between the uterus and the broad ligament; uterosacral ligament*
AHA: Q2, 1990, 7

183.5 Malignant neoplasm of round ligament of uterus — *ligament between the uterus and the wall of the pelvis*
AHA: Q2, 1990, 7; Q3, 1999, 5

183.8 Malignant neoplasm of other specified sites of uterine adnexa — *tubo-ovarian, utero-ovarian, or contiguous or overlapping sites of ovary and other uterine adnexa*
AHA: Q2, 1990, 7

183.9 Malignant neoplasm of uterine adnexa, unspecified site

Coding Clarification

This rubric excludes Douglas' cul-de-sac, reported with 158.8. If the malignancy is of contiguous or overlapping sites of ovary and uterine adnexa, report 183.8 *Malignant neoplasm of other specified sites of uterine adnexa.*

Coding Scenario

A patient is admitted for treatment of anemia due to the chemotherapy for malignant neoplasm of ovary.

> Code assignment: 285.22 *Anemia in neoplastic disease,* 183.0 *Malignant neoplasm of ovary,* and E933.1 *Adverse reaction to antineoplastic and immunosuppressive drugs*

A patient has a known ovarian cancer currently in the terminal phase. She is admitted at this time to the hospice care facility for palliative care. Treatment is solely for pain management.

> Code assignment: 183.0 *Malignant neoplasm of ovary* and V66.7 *Encounter for palliative care*

184 Malignant neoplasm of other and unspecified female genital organs

AHA: Q2, 1990, 7

Malignancies of external female genitalia and the vagina are classified to this rubric.

184.0 Malignant neoplasm of vagina — *Gartner's duct, vaginal vault*
AHA: Q2, 1990, 7

184.1 Malignant neoplasm of labia majora — *outer fold of skin and fat on either side of the vagina, including Bartholin's gland*
AHA: Q2, 1990, 7

184.2 Malignant neoplasm of labia minora — *inner fold of skin between the labia major and the vagina*
AHA: Q2, 1990, 7

184.3 Malignant neoplasm of clitoris

184.4 Malignant neoplasm of vulva, unspecified site — *specific site in vulva unknown*
AHA: Q2, 1990, 7

184.8 Malignant neoplasm of other specified sites of female genital organs — *Mullerian duct; contiguous or overlapping sites of female genital organs*
AHA: Q2, 1990, 7

184.9 Malignant neoplasm of female genital organ, site unspecified

Coding Clarification

If the malignancy affects both labia majora and labia minor, report 184.8 for contiguous or overlapping sites, rather than 184.4 for unspecified vulva.

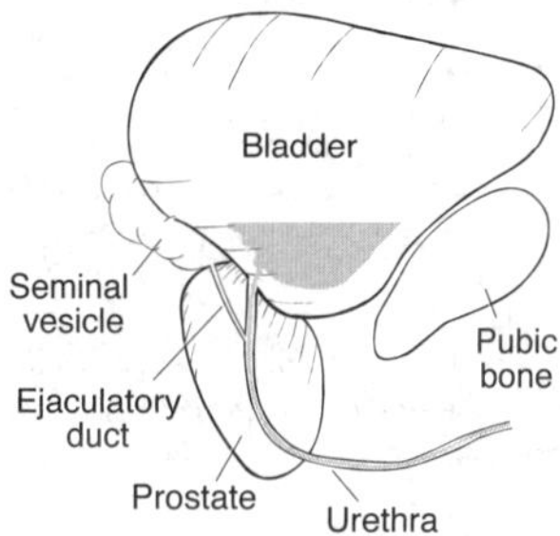

Side view schematic of prostate and related structures

185 Malignant neoplasm of prostate OK

AHA: Q2, 1990, 7; Q3, 1992, 7; Q3, 1999, 5; Q3, 2003, 13

The prostate is a singular, walnut-sized gland in the male. It surrounds the neck of the bladder and its ducts empty into the prostatic portion of the urethra. The prostate contributes fluid that helps to liquefy semen.

Adenocarcinoma of the prostate is the most common form of cancer in males older than 50 in the United States. Symptoms are uncommon until late in the disease course, when ureteral obstruction and hematuria may occur.

Coding Clarification

For cancer of the seminal vesicles, see 187.8 *Malignant neoplasm of other specified sites of male genital organs.*

Coding Scenario

A 69-year-old male is admitted to the facility with urinary retention and undergoes a TURP of the prostate. The final diagnosis is benign prostatic hypertrophy with urinary obstruction. The pathology report identifies microscopic foci of adenocarcinoma and confirms the benign prostatic hyperplasia.

Code assignment: 600.0 *Hypertrophy (benign) of prostate,* 185 *Malignant neoplasm of prostate,* and 788.20 *Retention of urine, unspecified*

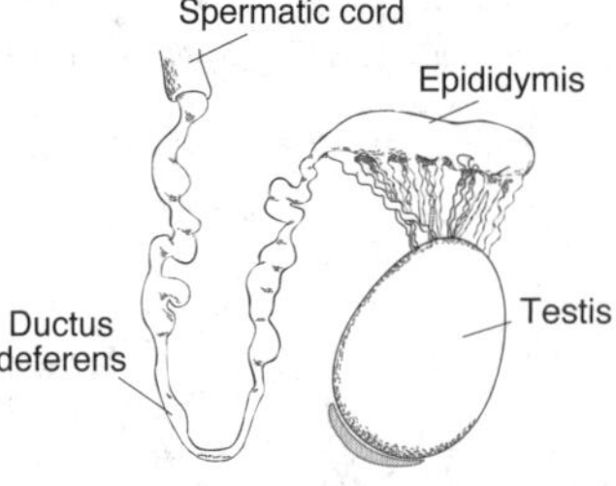

140–239

186 Malignant neoplasm of testis

AHA: Q2, 1990, 7

The testes are a pair of male gonads found in the scrotum and produce spermatozoa for fertilization. Leydig cells in the testes produce testosterone.

Most testicular masses are malignant and testicular cancer is more common among males with a history of undescended testes, even if the condition has been corrected surgically.

186.0 Malignant neoplasm of undescended testis — (Use additional code to identify any functional activity) — *ectopic, retained*
AHA: Q2, 1990, 7

186.9 Malignant neoplasm of other and unspecified testis — (Use additional code to identify any functional activity) — *descended, scrotal*
AHA: Q2, 1990, 7

Coding Clarification

Testicular tumors rarely cause functional problems. If functional problems occur, however, use an additional code to report it.

187 Malignant neoplasm of penis and other male genital organs

AHA: Q2, 1990, 7

The penis has two functions in males: sexual and excretory. The urethra may convey semen or urine. The tip of the penis is called the glans penis, and is covered in mucous membrane. The prepuce, or foreskin, is a fold of skin at the juncture where the body of the penis meets the glans penis; this extra skin is removed in circumcision. The corpora cavernosa are twin cylinders that extend the length of the organ called the body of the penis. Cancer of the penis usually occurs in uncircumcised males and human papillomavirus infection has been linked to penile cancer rates.

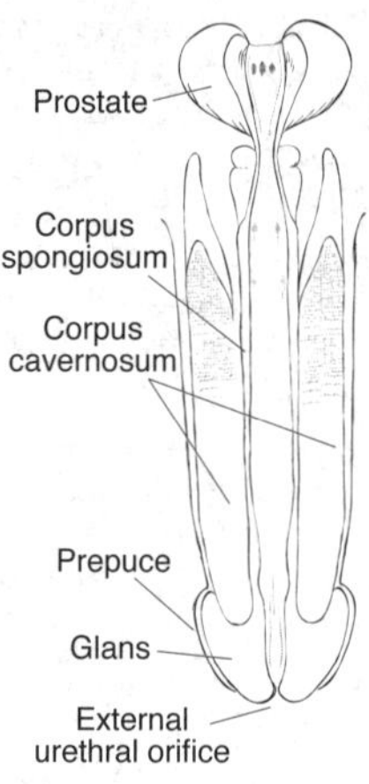

187.1 Malignant neoplasm of prepuce — *foreskin*
AHA: Q2, 1990, 7

187.2 Malignant neoplasm of glans penis — *head, distal end*
AHA: Q2, 1990, 7

187.3 Malignant neoplasm of body of penis — *corpus cavernosum, shaft*
AHA: Q2, 1990, 7

187.4 Malignant neoplasm of penis, part unspecified — *skin of penis not otherwise specified*
AHA: Q2, 1990, 7

187.5 Malignant neoplasm of epididymis — *tube in which sperm is stored*
AHA: Q2, 1990, 7

187.6 Malignant neoplasm of spermatic cord — *tube that carries sperm to the ejaculatory duct; vas deferens*
AHA: Q2, 1990, 7

187.7 Malignant neoplasm of scrotum — *pouch of skin and muscle, but not the contents (testes)*
AHA: Q2, 1990, 7

187.8 Malignant neoplasm of other specified sites of male genital organs — *seminal vesicle, Mullerian duct, tunica vaginalis, and contiguous or overlapping sites of penis and other male genital organs*
AHA: Q2, 1990, 7

187.9 Malignant neoplasm of male genital organ, site unspecified

Coding Clarification

Report 187.8 *Malignant neoplasm of male genital organs* if the malignancy is of contiguous or overlapping sites of the penis or other male reproductive organs.

 © 2004 Ingenix, Inc.

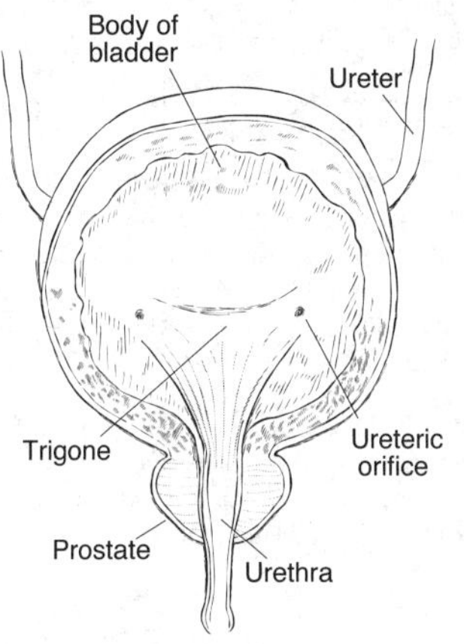

188 Malignant neoplasm of bladder

AHA: Q2, 1990, 7

The bladder lies in front (anterior) of the rectum in men and in front (anterior) of the vagina in women. As the bladder fills with urine, impulses from both voluntary and involuntary nerves signal that the bladder is full. When full, the bladder releases the urine it has stored through urination (voiding) via a tube called the urethra that connects the bladder floor to the outside of the body. Internal and external urinary muscle sphincters control the urine flow and stops the urine.

Malignant neoplasms of the bladder are classified by site. The dome of the bladder is the ceiling and the trigone is the triangular lower portion of the bladder bounded by the ureteral and urethral openings. Symptoms of malignant neoplasm of the bladder include hematuria, urinary urgency or frequency, or secondary infection at the tumor site. Pain or urinary retention may be present.

Males are twice as likely to develop bladder cancers as are females, and more than 90 percent of these cancers are transitional cell carcinomas. The most common site for cancer in the bladder is in the trigone.

188.0 Malignant neoplasm of trigone of urinary bladder — *lower portion of the bladder, bounded by a triangle created by the points at which the urethra and two ureters attach to the bladder*
AHA: Q2, 1990, 7

188.1 Malignant neoplasm of dome of urinary bladder — *top wall of the bladder*
AHA: Q2, 1990, 7

188.2 Malignant neoplasm of lateral wall of urinary bladder — *side wall of the bladder*
AHA: Q2, 1990, 7

188.3 Malignant neoplasm of anterior wall of urinary bladder — *front wall of the bladder*
AHA: Q2, 1990, 7

188.4 Malignant neoplasm of posterior wall of urinary bladder — *back wall of the bladder*
AHA: Q2, 1990, 7

188.5 Malignant neoplasm of bladder neck — *internal urethral orifice*
AHA: Q2, 1990, 7

188.6 Malignant neoplasm of ureteric orifice — *bladder surrounding the ureter's opening*
AHA: Q2, 1990, 7

188.7 Malignant neoplasm of urachus — *remnant of the fetal urinary tract*
AHA: Q2, 1990, 7

188.8 Malignant neoplasm of other specified sites of bladder — *contiguous or overlapping sites of bladder*
AHA: Q2, 1990, 7

188.9 Malignant neoplasm of bladder, part unspecified

Coding Clarification

If the malignancy is of contiguous and overlapping sites and the point of origin cannot be determined, report 188.8 *Malignant neoplasm of other specified sites of bladder.*

189 Malignant neoplasm of kidney and other and unspecified urinary organs

AHA: Q2, 1990, 7

The kidneys are paired organs between the parietal peritoneum and the posterior abdominal wall (retroperitoneal). They are located in the area of the last thoracic vertebrae to the third lumbar vertebrae.

Think of the kidneys as the body's blood filter. Items no longer needed are removed from the blood by the filter (kidneys) and eliminated in the form of urine, and elements needed are put back into the blood to be used by the cells and tissues of the body. Some of the blood the heart outputs with each cardiac cycle is sent to the kidneys to be filtered via two renal arteries (one to each kidney). In the kidneys, the renal arteries drain into other small arteries, then into even smaller arterioles and capillary networks called glomeruli where filtration takes place. Once the blood has been filtered and cleaned in the kidneys, it goes through venous capillaries that change into small veins called venules. Venules drain into larger veins that finally drain into the renal veins. The renal veins return the blood that has been filtered to the heart via the inferior vena cava.

Cup-like projections in each of the kidneys, called the renal calyces, drain the urine. Urine that has collected in the renal pelvis is transported via a process called peristalsis to storage in the bladder. The ureters enter the bladder (one at each side) at its base (top) and deposit the urine they carry into the bladder. Each ureter includes a valve that prevents urine that has been placed into the bladder from backing up into the ureters and the renal pelvis.

189.0 Malignant neoplasm of kidney, except pelvis — *parenchyma, Wilms' tumor*
AHA: Q2, 1990, 7

189.1 Malignant neoplasm of renal pelvis — *portal of the kidney from which the ureters collect urine; renal calyces, ureteropelvic junction*
AHA: Q2, 1990, 7

189.2 Malignant neoplasm of ureter — *one of a pair of tubes that transport urine from the kidneys to the bladder*
AHA: Q2, 1990, 7

189.3 Malignant neoplasm of urethra — *tube that eliminates urine from the bladder, and in males, serves as a genital duct*
AHA: Q2, 1990, 7

189.4 Malignant neoplasm of paraurethral glands — *glands and ducts of the urethra*
AHA: Q2, 1990, 7

189.8 Malignant neoplasm of other specified sites of urinary organs — *contiguous or overlapping sites of kidney and other urinary organs*
AHA: Q2, 1990, 7

189.9 Malignant neoplasm of urinary organ, site unspecified

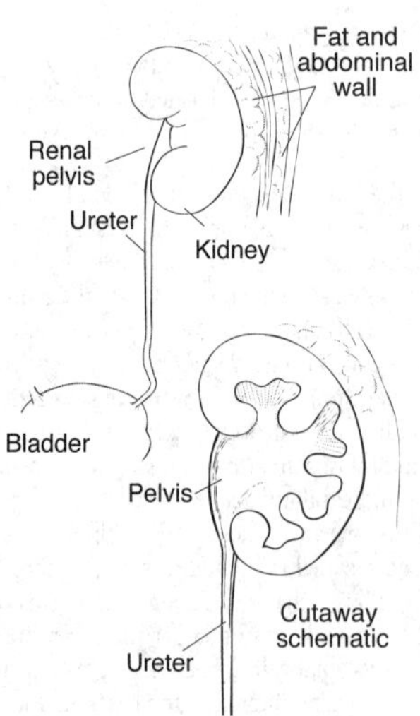

Coding Clarification

Wilms' tumor is nephroblastoma, a childhood malignancy of the kidney and reported with 189.0.

The tumor begins in utero and may be asymptomatic for years, though it is usually diagnosed before age 5.

190–195 Malignant Neoplasm of Other and Unspecified Sites

Anatomical sites that don't fall under other rubrics are classified here for malignant neoplasms. Cancers of the eye, the brain, the central nervous system, and glands, as well as undefined locations are reported in this section of ICD-9-CM.

Secondary malignant neoplasms are also reported in this section. Secondary malignancies are sites to which the primary cancer has spread. They are usually classified by anatomical site.

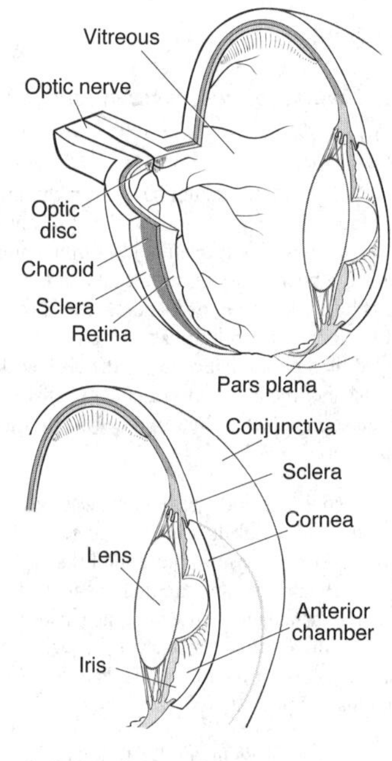

190 Malignant neoplasm of eye

AHA: Q2, 1990, 7

The eye is the organ of sight and has a complex physiology. The eyeball rests in fatty tissue in the bony orbit of the skull where it is protected from jarring actions. A malignant neoplasm of the orbit lies in these fatty and other tissues between the eyeball and the skull. The eyeball can be divided into several segments: the anterior segment, which includes the lens and all tissue anterior to the lens in the eyeball; and the posterior segment, which includes everything in the eyeball that is situated behind the lens. The eye is basically a fluid-filled ball. Intraocular pressure in the anterior segment of the eye is maintained through the flow of aqueous humor, or tears. The lacrimal system provides these tears and is also an agent in

 © 2004 Ingenix, Inc.

their disposal. Tears are produced in the lacrimal glands, located bilaterally behind the eyebrow, and the lacrimal ducts carry the tears to the eye or away from the eye to the nose. Pressure in the posterior segment of the eye is maintained by gel-like vitreous humor.

A thin, vascular, mucous membrane covers the inner eyelids and the white outer shell of the eye (sclera). This membrane is called the conjunctiva. The cornea is the bulging "window" through which we see, and the retina is the light-sensitive "viewing screen" at the back of the eye. The choroid is a vascular layer of the inside of the eyeball.

190.0 Malignant neoplasm of eyeball, except conjunctiva, cornea, retina, and choroid — *ciliary body, sclera, lens, iris, uveal tract*
AHA: Q2, 1990, 7

190.1 Malignant neoplasm of orbit — *tissue between the sclera of the eyeball and the orbital bone; retrobulbar tissue, extraocular muscle*
AHA: Q2, 1990, 7

190.2 Malignant neoplasm of lacrimal gland — *tear-producing gland located behind the eyebrow; excludes lacrimal duct, sac*
AHA: Q2, 1990, 7

190.3 Malignant neoplasm of conjunctiva — *mucous membrane lining the anterior eyeball and the inner aspect of the eyelid*
AHA: Q2, 1990, 7

190.4 Malignant neoplasm of cornea — *clear dome that covers the anterior segment of the eye*
AHA: Q2, 1990, 7

190.5 Malignant neoplasm of retina — *light-sensitive lining of the posterior segment of the eye*
AHA: Q2, 1990, 7

190.6 Malignant neoplasm of choroid — *vascular layer of the globe of the eye*
AHA: Q2, 1990, 7

190.7 Malignant neoplasm of lacrimal duct — *passage that carries tears to the eye and nose; lacrimal sac, nasolacrimal duct.*
AHA: Q2, 1990, 7

190.8 Malignant neoplasm of other specified sites of eye — *contiguous or overlapping sites of eye*
AHA: Q2, 1990, 7

190.9 Malignant neoplasm of eye, part unspecified

Coding Clarification

A congenital cancer that is usually detected before age two, retinoblastoma is reported with 190.5 *Malignant neoplasm of retina.* Retinoblastoma is a malignancy of the retina and occurs bilaterally in 25 percent of patients with the disease.

If the malignant neoplasm is of the skin of the eyelid, it should be reported with codes for malignant neoplasm of the skin (172.1, 173.1). A malignancy of the optic nerve is reported with 192.0 *Malignant neoplasm of cranial nerves,* and of the orbital bone, 170.0 *Malignant neoplasm of skull and face, except mandible.* If the malignant neoplasm is of contiguous or overlapping parts of the eye, report 190.8 *Malignant neoplasm of other specified sites of eye.*

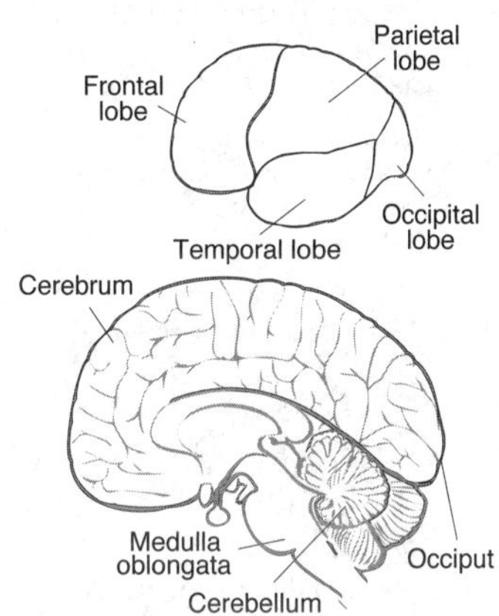

191 Malignant neoplasm of brain

AHA: Q2, 1990, 7

All brain tumors are "malignant" in that they may lead to death as they compromise the circulation of fluids in the brain through compression or obstruction. However, neoplasms classified to this rubric must also be of a metastasizing nature: a true malignancy. The incidences of benign and malignant neoplasms of the brain are about the same at 50 percent.

Symptoms of a neoplasm of the brain include headache, seizures, personality changes, impaired mental or physical functions, or in children, an enlarged head. Use an additional code to report any manifestations associated with the malignancy.

191.0 Malignant neoplasm of cerebrum, except lobes and ventricles — *including basal ganglia, globus pallidus; cerebral cortex; hypothalamus; corpus striatum; thalamus, cerebrum, internal capsule*
AHA: Q2, 1990, 7

191.1 Malignant neoplasm of frontal lobe of brain — *frontal lobe*
AHA: Q2, 1990, 7

191.2 Malignant neoplasm of temporal lobe of brain — *hippocampus, uncus*
AHA: Q2, 1990, 7

140–239

191.3 Malignant neoplasm of parietal lobe of brain — *parietal lobe*
AHA: Q2, 1990, 7

191.4 Malignant neoplasm of occipital lobe of brain — *occipital lobe*
AHA: Q2, 1990, 7

191.5 Malignant neoplasm of ventricles of brain — *choroid plexus, floor of ventricle*
AHA: Q2, 1990, 7

191.6 Malignant neoplasm of cerebellum NOS — *cerebellopontine angle*
AHA: Q2, 1990, 7

191.7 Malignant neoplasm of brain stem — *cerebral peduncle, midbrain, medulla oblongata, pons, stem*
AHA: Q2, 1990, 7

191.8 Malignant neoplasm of other parts of brain — *corpus callosum, tapetum, and contiguous or overlapping sites of brain*
AHA: Q2, 1990, 7

191.9 Malignant neoplasm of brain, unspecified site

Coding Clarification

Malignant neoplasms of the brain are classified according to location. Symptoms usually correspond to site. Malignant neoplasms of contiguous or overlapping sites in the brain are reported with 191.8. Do not use codes in this rubric to report cancers of the cranial nerves (192.0), of the retrobulbar area (190.1), or of the pituitary gland (194.3).

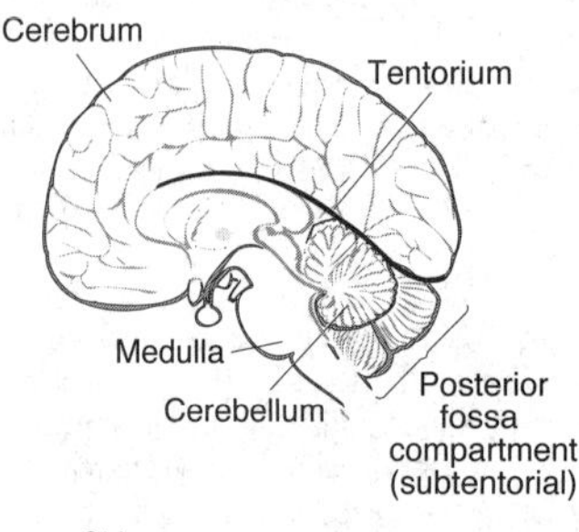

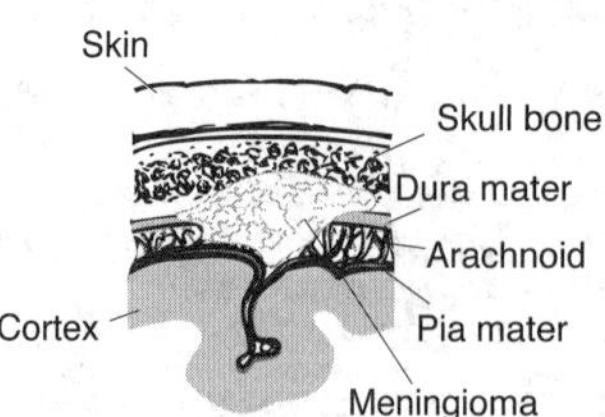

The tentorium is a dural sheath that divides the cranial cavity and supports the occipital lobes

192 Malignant neoplasm of other and unspecified parts of nervous system

AHA: Q2, 1990, 7

Malignant neoplasms of the spine, meninges, cranial nerves, or sites unknown in the nervous system are classified in this rubric. Primary malignancies arising at these sites are much more rare than malignancies of the brain.

192.0 Malignant neoplasm of cranial nerves — *olfactory bulb*
AHA: Q2, 1990, 7

192.1 Malignant neoplasm of cerebral meninges — *dura mater, falx, meninges, tentorium*
AHA: Q2, 1990, 7

192.2 Malignant neoplasm of spinal cord — *cauda equina*
AHA: Q2, 1990, 7

192.3 Malignant neoplasm of spinal meninges — *lining of the spinal cord*
AHA: Q2, 1990, 7

192.8 Malignant neoplasm of other specified sites of nervous system — *contiguous or overlapping sites of other parts of nervous system*
AHA: Q2, 1990, 7

192.9 Malignant neoplasm of nervous system, part unspecified

Coding Clarification

Report 192.8 *Malignant neoplasm of other specified sites of nervous system* if the neoplasm is of overlapping or contiguous sites of the nervous system. Peripheral, sympathetic, or parasympathetic nerve malignancies are classified in rubric 171.

193 Malignant neoplasm of thyroid gland OK

AHA: Q2, 1990, 7

The thyroid gland is located just below the cricoid cartilage near the larynx and its purpose is to secrete thyroxine and triiodothyronine. Thyroxine and triiodothyronine increase the rate of cell metabolism.

Papillary adenocarcinoma accounts for 85 percent of thyroid cancers and usually appears in young adults. Though the only symptom of thyroid cancer may be a palpable node, some patients with thyroid cancer present with symptoms of hyporthyroidism or hyperthyroidism.

Coding Clarification

Use an additional code to report any functional activity associated with the malignancy.

 © 2004 Ingenix, Inc.

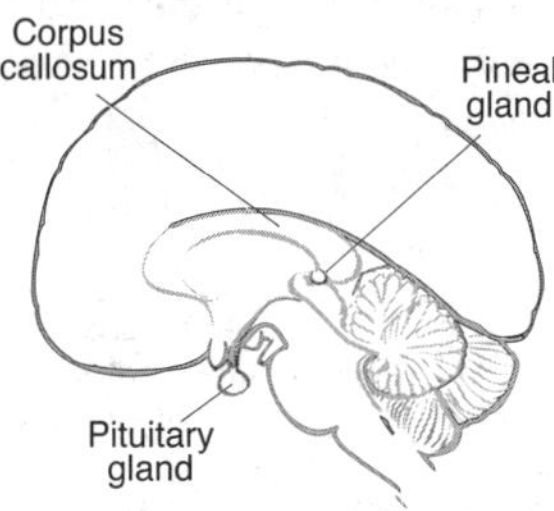

194 Malignant neoplasm of other endocrine glands and related structures

AHA: Q2, 1990, 7

The parathyroid glands come in pairs — the superior and inferior pair — that are embedded in the posterior thyroid. The adrenal glands are situated above each kidney, and the pituitary gland is located in the sella turcica of the sphenoid bone. The pineal gland, located at the base of the corpus callosum, secretes melatonin; the carotid body, located in the fork of the carotid artery, monitors blood oxygen. The aortic body at the aortic arch and right subclavian artery regulates reflex respiration.

Malignancies of the endocrine glands can create functional activities in those glands. For example, adrenal tumors can cause virilizing or feminizing symptoms. Pituitary cancers can cause gigantism, Cushing's disease, amenorrhea or galactorrhea, or acromegaly. Report these functional activities in addition to the cancer.

Neuroblastoma is a common tumor of childhood that may affect the adrenal gland, retroperitoneum, central nervous system, or thoracic cavity. Usually seen in children younger than age 5, neuroblastomas present with a complex of symptoms according to the site of malignancy. A majority of the neuroblastomas arise in the adrenal gland.

194.0 Malignant neoplasm of adrenal gland — (Use additional code to identify any functional activity) — *cortex, medulla, suprarenal gland*
AHA: Q2, 1990, 7

194.1 Malignant neoplasm of parathyroid gland — (Use additional code to identify any functional activity) — *superior and inferior*
AHA: Q2, 1990, 7

194.3 Malignant neoplasm of pituitary gland and craniopharyngeal duct — (Use additional code to identify any functional activity) — *craniobuccal pouch, Rathke's pouch, hypophysis, sella turcica*
AHA: July-Aug, 1985, 9; Q2, 1990, 7

194.4 Malignant neoplasm of pineal gland — (Use additional code to identify any functional activity) — *located at the base of the corpus callosum*
AHA: Q2, 1990, 7

194.5 Malignant neoplasm of carotid body — (Use additional code to identify any functional activity) — *located at the fork in the carotid artery*
AHA: Q2, 1990, 7

194.6 Malignant neoplasm of aortic body and other paraganglia — (Use additional code to identify any functional activity) — *located at aortic arch and right subclavian artery; coccygeal body, para-aortic body, glomus jugulare*
AHA: Q2, 1990, 7

194.8 Malignant neoplasm of other endocrine glands and related structures — (Use additional code to identify any functional activity. Note: If the sites of multiple involvements are known, they should be coded separately.) — *if the sites of multiple involvements are known, they should be coded separately.*
AHA: Q2, 1990, 7

194.9 Malignant neoplasm of endocrine gland, site unspecified — (Use additional code to identify any functional activity)

Coding Clarification

An additional code from Chapter Three may be reported to identify functional activity associated with any neoplasm, for example, catecholamine-producing malignant pheochromocytoma of adrenal, 194.0 for neoplasm and 255.6 for adrenal hypofunction.

The ICD-9-CM index identifies 194.0 *Malignant neoplasm of adrenal gland* as the code for neuroblastoma for unspecified site. However, if a site other than adrenal gland is specified, consult the Neoplasm Table in ICD-9-CM for the correct code as classified by site.

195 Malignant neoplasm of other and ill-defined sites

AHA: Q2, 1990, 7

Use this rubric only as a last resort when the specific site of primary cancer cannot be identified or when the primary cancer has grown to invade two anatomic areas that would normally be reported with two codes and the point of origin cannot be determined.

195.0 Malignant neoplasm of head, face, and neck — *cheek, jaw, nose, supraclavicular region*
AHA: Q2, 1990, 7; Q4, 2003, 107

195.1 Malignant neoplasm of thorax — *axilla, chest wall, or intrathoracic region*
AHA: Q2, 1990, 7

140–239

195.2 Malignant neoplasm of abdomen — *intrabdominal*
AHA: Q2, 1990, 7; Q2, 1997, 3

195.3 Malignant neoplasm of pelvis — *groin; sacrococcygeal, inguinal, or presacral regions; rectovaginal or rectovesical septums; or overlapping sites*
AHA: Q2, 1990, 7

195.4 Malignant neoplasm of upper limb — *shoulder, arm, or hand*
AHA: Q2, 1990, 7

195.5 Malignant neoplasm of lower limb — *hip, leg, or foot*
AHA: Q2, 1990, 7

195.8 Malignant neoplasm of other specified sites — *not elsewhere classified, including back, flank, and trunk*
AHA: Q2, 1990, 7

196–199 Secondary and Unspecified Malignant Neoplasms

All cancers shed cells into the patient's circulation. When these cells adhere to the vascular endothelium and begin to multiply into new tumors, the cancer is said to have metastasized. The new cancers are considered secondary malignancies, the primary malignancy being the "mother" site.

When a cancer recurs at the site of the original malignancy, it is still considered a primary malignancy and should not be reported with secondary malignancy codes. If the cancer recurs at a different site, these codes are appropriate, along with an additional code from the V10 rubric to identify a history of the malignancy of the primary site.

The secondary malignancy is sequenced first in coding if the patient is receiving treatment solely for the secondary malignancy. Otherwise, the code for the secondary site follows the code for the primary malignancy site.

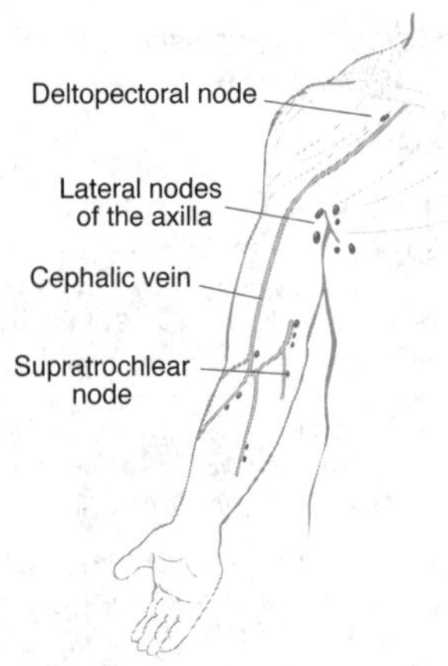

196 Secondary and unspecified malignant neoplasm of lymph nodes

AHA: May-June, 1985, 3; Q2, 1990, 7; Q2, 1992, 3

Secondary malignancies are classified according to site in this rubric. Metastases of cancers to lymphatic sites are fairly common since lymphatic fluid circulates the body and is filtered in the lymph nodes. The primary cancer may be near the affected lymph tissue or distant from it.

196.0 Secondary and unspecified malignant neoplasm of lymph nodes of head, face, and neck — *cervicofacial, supraclavicular*
AHA: May-June, 1985, 3; Q2, 1990, 7; Q2, 1992, 3

196.1 Secondary and unspecified malignant neoplasm of intrathoracic lymph nodes — *bronchopulmonary, mediastinal, intercostal, tracheobronchial, intrathoracic, Virchow's*
AHA: May-June, 1985, 3; Q2, 1990, 7; Q2, 1992, 3

196.2 Secondary and unspecified malignant neoplasm of intra-abdominal lymph nodes — *aortic, intestinal, retroperitoneal, mesenteric,*
AHA: May-June, 1985, 3; Q2, 1990, 7; Q2, 1992, 3; Q4, 2003, 111

196.3 Secondary and unspecified malignant neoplasm of lymph nodes of axilla and upper limb — *axillary, brachial, infraclavicular, epitrochlea, pectoral*
AHA: May-June, 1985, 3; Q2, 1990, 7; Q2, 1992, 3

196.5 Secondary and unspecified malignant neoplasm of lymph nodes of inguinal region and lower limb — *Cloquet, femoral, popliteal, groin, Rosenmueller's, tibial*
AHA: May-June, 1985, 3; Q2, 1990, 7; Q2, 1992, 3

196.6 Secondary and unspecified malignant neoplasm of intrapelvic lymph nodes — *hypogastric, obturator, iliac, parametrial*
AHA: May-June, 1985, 3; Q2, 1990, 7; Q2, 1992, 3

196.8 Secondary and unspecified malignant neoplasm of lymph nodes of multiple sites — *lymphatic channel or vessel not elsewhere classified*
AHA: May-June, 1985, 3; Q2, 1990, 7; Q2, 1992, 3

196.9 Secondary and unspecified malignant neoplasm of lymph nodes, site unspecified

© 2004 Ingenix, Inc.

197 Secondary malignant neoplasm of respiratory and digestive systems

AHA: May-June, 1985, 3; Q2, 1990, 7

Secondary malignancies are classified according to site in this rubric.

197.0 Secondary malignant neoplasm of lung — *bronchus*
AHA: May-June, 1985, 3; Q2, 1990, 7; Q2, 1999, 9

197.1 Secondary malignant neoplasm of mediastinum — *soft tissue between sternum and the spinal column, between the lungs*
AHA: May-June, 1985, 3; Q2, 1990, 7

197.2 Secondary malignant neoplasm of pleura — *lining of the lung*
AHA: May-June, 1985, 3; Q4, 1989, 11; Q2, 1990, 7; Q4, 2003, 110

197.3 Secondary malignant neoplasm of other respiratory organs — *trachea*
AHA: May-June, 1985, 3; Q2, 1990, 7

197.4 Secondary malignant neoplasm of small intestine including duodenum — *duodenum, ilium, jejunum*
AHA: May-June, 1985, 3; Q2, 1990, 7

197.5 Secondary malignant neoplasm of large intestine and rectum — *colon, rectum*
AHA: May-June, 1985, 3; Q2, 1990, 7

197.6 Secondary malignant neoplasm of retroperitoneum and peritoneum — *mesentery, mesocolon, omentum, retroperitoneal tissue*
AHA: May-June, 1985, 3; Q4, 1989, 11; Q2, 1990, 7

197.7 Secondary malignant neoplasm of liver

197.8 Secondary malignant neoplasm of other digestive organs and spleen — *spleen, pancreas, gall bladder/duct, ampulla of Vater, sphincter of Oddi*
AHA: May-June, 1985, 3; Q2, 1990, 7; Q2, 1992, 3; Q2, 1997, 3

Coding Clarification

Report metastases to lymph nodes with codes from the rubric 196.

Coding Scenario

A patient is admitted with an esophageal obstruction due to esophageal metastasis from the lung.

> Code assignment: 197.8 *Secondary malignant neoplasm of other respiratory and digestive organs and spleen,* 162.9 *Malignant neoplasm of bronchus and lung, unspecified,* and 530.3 *Stricture and stenosis of esophagus*

198 Secondary malignant neoplasm of other specified sites

AHA: May-June, 1985, 3; Q2, 1990, 7

Secondary malignancies are classified according to site in this rubric.

198.0 Secondary malignant neoplasm of kidney — *parenchyma, calyx, hilus, pelvis*
AHA: May-June, 1985, 3; Q2, 1990, 7

198.1 Secondary malignant neoplasm of other urinary organs — *bladder, ureter, urethra, prostate utricle*
AHA: May-June, 1985, 3; Q2, 1990, 7

198.2 Secondary malignant neoplasm of skin — *skin of breast and except genital*
AHA: May-June, 1985, 3; Q2, 1990, 7

198.3 Secondary malignant neoplasm of brain and spinal cord — *brain and spinal cord nerve root*
AHA: May-June, 1985, 3; Q2, 1990, 7; Q3, 1999, 7

198.4 Secondary malignant neoplasm of other parts of nervous system — *meninges, parasympathetic, sympathetic, peripheral nerves and ganglia*
AHA: May-June, 1985, 3; Jan-Feb, 1987, 7; Q2, 1990, 7

198.5 Secondary malignant neoplasm of bone and bone marrow — *bone and associated cartilage or marrow*
AHA: May-June, 1985, 3; Q4, 1989, 10; Q2, 1990, 7; Q1, 1991, 16; Q2, 1992, 3; Q3, 1999, 5; Q4, 2003, 110

198.6 Secondary malignant neoplasm of ovary — *female gonad*
AHA: May-June, 1985, 3; Q2, 1990, 7

198.7 Secondary malignant neoplasm of adrenal gland — *suprarenal gland*
AHA: May-June, 1985, 3; Q2, 1990, 7

198.81 Secondary malignant neoplasm of breast — *male or female*
AHA: May-June, 1985, 3; Q2, 1990, 7

198.82 Secondary malignant neoplasm of genital organs — *Mullerian duct, oviduct, cervical stump, endometrial stroma*
AHA: May-June, 1985, 3; Q2, 1990, 7

198.89 Secondary malignant neoplasm of other specified sites — *pharynx, tongue, thyroid, salivary pituitary, connective tissue*
AHA: May-June, 1985, 3; Q2, 1990, 7; Q2, 1997, 4

Coding Clarification

Report metastases to lymph nodes with codes from the rubric 196.

140–239

199 Malignant neoplasm without specification of site

AHA: Q2, 1990, 7

Secondary malignancies in this rubric are general, though they do have some specific uses. Up to 7 percent of cancer patients are diagnosed with a secondary malignancy for which the primary site cannot be found (e.g., UPO [unknown primary origin]).

199.0 Disseminated malignant neoplasm — *carcinomatosis, multiple in unspecified site*
AHA: Q4, 1989, 10; Q2, 1990, 7

199.1 Other malignant neoplasm of unspecified site — *unspecified primary or secondary site; Eaton-Lambert syndrome*
AHA: Q2, 1990, 7

Coding Clarification

In these cases, report the secondary malignancy first, followed by 199.1 *Other malignant neoplasm of unspecified site* to report the unknown primary site. In cases where laboratory results indicate metastases to an unknown site, report the secondary malignancy with the same code, 199.1.

200–208 Malignant Neoplasm of Lymphatic and Hematopoietic Tissue

Malignant neoplasms of the lymphatic and hematopoietic tissues are considered primary neoplasms and do not spread to secondary sites. The malignant cells circulate to other areas through the lymphatic or blood systems.

Cancers of the lymphatic sytem are called lymphomas and they are more common after age 50. They occur most frequently in the groin (inguinal), neck (cervical), and armpit (axillary) nodes.

Some of the types of neoplasms that are included in this section are lymphosarcomas, Hodgkin's disease, lymphomas, malignant histocytosis, multiple myeloma, myeloid leukemia, acute leukemia, and chronic leukemia. These diseases are classified by type, by site, and, in some cases, by status of remission or chronic or acute phase.

Do not use codes in this series to report secondary or unspecified lymph node malignancies, secondary bone marrow malignancies, or spleen cancer.

If the encounter is solely for the purpose of chemotherapy, the V code for chemotherapy (V58.1) should be sequenced first and the malignancy sequenced secondarily.

Behavior Classification: Code categories 200-208 identify neoplastic disorders of the blood-forming tissues and neoplasms arising in the reticuloendothelial and lymphatic systems acknowledged or assumed to be primary malignancies. The difference between lymphohematopoietic system malignancies and other malignancies is that the tumor cells typically circulate in large numbers in the bloodstream.

Malignant neoplasms classified by code categories 200-208 that are identified as metastatic or secondary are still classified within the 200-208 categories and would not be classified to category 196. Do not use codes from code range 200-208 to classify secondary sites or metastatic neoplasms when the primary site is not classified within this code range.

Indications for Transplant: The following are clinical indications for the various forms of bone marrow transplants.

- Autologous-Refractory acute leukemia, Burkitt's lymphoma, undifferentiated lymphoma, diffuse histiocytic lymphoma, refractory acute leukemia, melanoma, central nervous system malignancies, soft tissue sarcomas, central axis Ewing's sarcoma, and carcinomas of breast, ovary, lung, and testes.
- Syngeneic-Acute myelogenous leukemia, acute lymphoblastic leukemia, chronic myelogenous leukemia, non-Hodgkin's lymphoma, Ewing's sarcoma, and hairy cell leukemia.
- Allogeneic-Acute myelogenous leukemia, acute lymphoblastic leukemia, chronic myelogenous leukemia, non-Hodgkin's lymphoma, severe combined immunodeficiency disease, Wiskott-Aldrich syndrome, and aplastic anemia.

Bone marrow transplantation is typically performed on patients whose condition is in the state of remission. Patients in remission are better able to tolerate the bone marrow transplant. They are receiving active treatment for the leukemia during the remission phase; therefore codes in the V10 "History of" category are not appropriate. A code from the 204-208 series would be used to designate the type of leukemia.

200 Lymphosarcoma and reticulosarcoma

AHA: Nov-Dec, 1986, 5; Q2, 1990, 7; Q2, 1992, 3

Lymphosarcoma is a form of non-Hodgkin's lymphoma in which the cells are either a small or large lymphocyte.

Reticulosarcoma (200.1x) along with histiocytic sarcoma is a form of non-Hodgkin's lymphoma derived from the histiocyte, a macrophage present in connective tissue.

Burkitt's tumor or lymphoma is a form of non-Hodgkin's lymphoma characterized by an undifferentiated B-cell tumor. There are two variants:

 © 2004 Ingenix, Inc.

endemic (African) and sporadic. The endemic variant is associated with Epstein-Barr virus infection and has a variable diagnosis. The sporadic variant has a very poor prognosis. Jaw and orbital involvement is typical in endemic Burkitt's lymphoma and abdominal disease predominates in sporadic Burkitt's lymphoma.

The following fifth-digit subclassification is for use with categories 200-202:

0 unspecified site, extranodal and solid organ sites
1 lymph nodes of head, face, and neck
2 intrathoracic lymph nodes
3 intra-abdominal lymph nodes
4 lymph nodes of axilla and upper limb
5 lymph nodes of inguinal region and lower limb
6 intrapelvic lymph nodes
7 spleen
8 lymph nodes of multiple sites

200.0 5th Reticulosarcoma — *reticulum cell sarcoma; pleomorphic cell type*
AHA: Nov-Dec, 1986, 5; Q2, 1990, 7; Q2, 1992, 3

200.1 5th Lymphosarcoma — *lymphoblastoma, prolymphocytic*
AHA: Nov-Dec, 1986, 5; Q2, 1990, 7; Q2, 1992, 3

200.2 5th Burkitt's tumor or lymphoma — *malignant lymphoma*
AHA: Nov-Dec, 1986, 5; Q2, 1990, 7; Q2, 1992, 3

200.8 5th Other named variants of lymphosarcoma and reticulosarcoma — *mixed cell type; reticulolymphosarcoma; lymphoplasmacytoid*
AHA: Nov-Dec, 1986, 5; Q2, 1990, 7; Q2, 1992, 3

201 Hodgkin's disease

AHA: Nov-Dec, 1986, 5; Q2, 1990, 7; Q2, 1992, 3

Hodgkin's disease is the most common type of lymphoma, and most commonly affects young and middle-aged adults. Hodgkin's disease is a painless, progressive replacement of lymph nodes, spleen, and other lymphatic tissue with tumor tissue consisting of atypical histiocytes together with lymphocytes, eosinophils, plasma cells, and fibrous tissue. In Hodgkin's lymphoma, Reed-Sternberg cells are present.

The following fifth-digit subclassification is for use with categories 200-202:

0 unspecified site, extranodal and solid organ sites
1 lymph nodes of head, face, and neck
2 intrathoracic lymph nodes
3 intra-abdominal lymph nodes
4 lymph nodes of axilla and upper limb
5 lymph nodes of inguinal region and lower limb
6 intrapelvic lymph nodes
7 spleen
8 lymph nodes of multiple sites

201.0 5th Hodgkin's paragranuloma

201.1 5th Hodgkin's granuloma

201.2 5th Hodgkin's sarcoma

201.4 5th Hodgkin's disease, lymphocytic-histiocytic predominance

201.5 5th Hodgkin's disease, nodular sclerosis — *cellular phase*
AHA: Nov-Dec, 1986, 5; Q2, 1990, 7; Q2, 1992, 3

201.6 5th Hodgkin's disease, mixed cellularity

201.7 5th Hodgkin's disease, lymphocytic depletion — *lymphocytic depletion; diffuse fibrosis; reticular type*
AHA: Nov-Dec, 1986, 5; Q2, 1990, 7; Q2, 1992, 3

201.9 5th Hodgkin's disease, unspecified type — *Paltauf-Sternberg disease*
AHA: Nov-Dec, 1986, 5; Q2, 1990, 7; Q2, 1992, 3

Coding Scenario

A patient is admitted to the facility with Hodgkin's disease. The final diagnostic statement identifies Hodgkin's disease with lymphocytic depletion (numerous Reed-Sternberg cells) with extensive body involvement.

Code assignment: 201.78 *Hodgkin's disease, lymphocytic depletion, lymph nodes of multiple sites*

202 Other malignant neoplasms of lymphoid and histiocytic tissue

AHA: Nov-Dec, 1986, 5; Q2, 1990, 7; Q2, 1992, 3

Nodular lymphoma is a non-Hodgkin's lymphoma in which lymphoma cells are clustered into identifiable nodules or follicles, and malignant histiocytosis presents with progressive, abnormal histiocytes in the blood. Mycosis fungoides is an uncommon, chronic T-cell lymphoma affecting the skin and sometimes internal organs, usually in patients 50 years or older. T-cell lymphoma often appears as a rash and goes undiagnosed for a period. Sezary disease is an extension of mucosis fungoides that affects the blood. Leukemic reticuloendotheliosis is a chronic leukemia with preponderance of large, mononuclear cells with hairy appearance in the marrow, spleen, liver, and blood. In Letterer-Siwe disease, reticuloendotheliosis occurs in early childhood and presents with skin eruptions, anemia, and enlarged liver, spleen, and lymph nodes.

The following fifth-digit subclassification is for use with categories 200-202:

0 unspecified site, extranodal and solid organ sites
1 lymph nodes of head, face, and neck
2 intrathoracic lymph nodes
3 intra-abdominal lymph nodes
4 lymph nodes of axilla and upper limb
5 lymph nodes of inguinal region and lower limb
6 intrapelvic lymph nodes
7 spleen
8 lymph nodes of multiple sites

202.0 ✓5th Nodular lymphoma — *Brill-Symmers disease; lymphosarcoma; reticulosarcoma*
AHA: Nov-Dec, 1986, 5; Q2, 1990, 7; Q2, 1992, 3

202.1 ✓5th Mycosis fungoides — *cutaneous T-cell lymphoma*
AHA: Nov-Dec, 1986, 5; Q2, 1990, 7; Q2, 1992, 3; Q2, 1992, 4

202.2 ✓5th Sezary's disease — *mycosis fungoides infecting blood*
AHA: Nov-Dec, 1986, 5; Q2, 1990, 7; Q2, 1992, 3; Q2, 1999, 7

202.3 ✓5th Malignant histiocytosis — *histiocytic medullary reticulosis; malignant reticuloendotheliosis/reticulosis*
AHA: Nov-Dec, 1986, 5; Q2, 1990, 7; Q2, 1992, 3

202.4 ✓5th Leukemic reticuloendotheliosis — *hairy cell leukemia*
AHA: Nov-Dec, 1986, 5; Q2, 1990, 7; Q2, 1992, 3

202.5 ✓5th Letterer-Siwe disease — *acute differentiated progressive histiocytosis; histiocytosis X; infantile reticuloendotheliosis*
AHA: Nov-Dec, 1986, 5; Q2, 1990, 7; Q2, 1992, 3

202.6 ✓5th Malignant mast cell tumors — *mast cell sarcoma; mastocytoma; mastocytosis*
AHA: Nov-Dec, 1986, 5; Q2, 1990, 7; Q2, 1992, 3

202.8 ✓5th Other malignant lymphomas — *NOS, diffuse*
AHA: Nov-Dec, 1986, 5; Q2, 1990, 7; Q2, 1992, 3; Q2, 1992, 4

202.9 ✓5th Other and unspecified malignant neoplasms of lymphoid and histiocytic tissue — *Follicular dendritic cell carcinoma, interdigitating dendric cell sarcoma, Langerhans cell sarcoma, malignant neoplasm of bone marrow NOS*
AHA: Nov-Dec, 1986, 5; Q2, 1990, 7; Q2, 1992, 3

Coding Clarification

Cutaneous T-cell Lymphoma with Sezary Syndrome: Cutaneous T-cell lymphoma is synonymous with mycosis fungoides and can be found in the alphabetic index under the main term, Mycosis, fungoides. Use subcategory code 202.1x to report this condition with the appropriate fifth digit. Also code the Sezary disease with 202.2x. When two conditions are present from the same category, as long as the fourth digits are different, it is appropriate to code them both.

Retroperitoneal Follicular Center Cell: Report with code 202.8x *Other malignant lymphomas,* with the fifth digit that identifies the site of the lymphoma.

Coding Scenario

A 59-year-old patient is admitted with intractable bone pain. The patient had been previously diagnosed with malignant lymphoma of the bone. The patient is found to have a lymph node in the chest positive for lymphoma and a biopsy of the bone in the pelvis reveals the same lymphoma cell type.

> Code assignment: 202.88 *Other malignant lymphomas, lymph nodes of multiple sites*

A patient is admitted with Sezary syndrome, diagnosed fairly recently, and with cutaneous T-cell lymphoma, diagnosed four years previous.

> Code assignment: Code both 202.2x *Sezary disease* and 202.1x *Mycosis fungoides, for cutaneous T-cell lymphoma with Sezary syndrome.* It is permissible to code more than one condition from the same three digit-category, so long as the fourth digits are different.

203 Multiple myeloma and immunoproliferative neoplasms

AHA: Q2, 1990, 7; Q4, 1991, 26

Multiple myeloma is an uncontrolled proliferation of plasma cells and results in a number of organ dysfunctions and symptoms of bone pain or fracture, renal failure, infection, anemia, hypercalcemia, as well as clotting and neurologic or vascular abnormalities.

Multiple myeloma is often described as metastatic to the bone, but because this is part of the disease, the bone metastases should not be reported separately as a secondary malignant neoplasm.

 © 2004 Ingenix, Inc.

The following fifth-digit subclassification is for use with categories 203, 204, 205, 206, 207, and 208:

0 without mention of remission

1 in remission

203.0 ✓5th Multiple myeloma — *Kahler's disease; myelomatosis*
AHA: Q4, 1989, 10; Q2, 1990, 7; Q4, 1991, 26; Q1, 1996, 16

203.1 ✓5th Plasma cell leukemia — *plasmacytic leukemia*
AHA: Sept-Oct, 1986, 12; Q2, 1990, 7; Q4, 1990, 26; Q4, 1991, 26

203.8 ✓5th Other immunoproliferative neoplasms

Coding Clarification

When a patient with multiple myelomas develops a complication from the disease, the complication is generally sequenced first, followed by the myeloma. For example, if a patient with multiple myeloma sustains a stress fracture of the femur, the codes would be sequenced:

733.14 Pathologic fracture of the neck of femur

203.00 Multiple myeloma without mention of remission

204 Lymphoid leukemia

AHA: Q2, 1990, 7; Q3, 1993, 4

Lymphoid leukemia is a malignant proliferation of immature lymphocytes called lymphoblasts. The acute condition is common in children and fatal if untreated. The chronic condition is a generalized, progressive form of lymphocytic leukemia predominantly affecting men older than age 50. It is the least malignant form of leukemia.

The following fifth-digit subclassification is for use with categories 203, 204, 205, 206, 207, and 208:

0 without mention of remission

1 in remission

204.0 ✓5th Acute lymphoid leukemia — *lymphoblastic, usually in childhood*
AHA: Q2, 1990, 7; Q3, 1993, 4; Q3, 1999, 6

204.1 ✓5th Chronic lymphoid leukemia — *lymphoblastic, more mature, usually in middle/old age*
AHA: Q2, 1990, 7; Q3, 1993, 4

204.2 ✓5th Subacute lymphoid leukemia

204.8 ✓5th Other lymphoid leukemia — *aleukemic leukemia*
AHA: Q2, 1990, 7; Q3, 1993, 4

204.9 ✓5th Unspecified lymphoid leukemia

Documentation Issues

If the physician documentation specifies that the patient's leukemia has been completely cured, use code V10.6x.

Only when documentation specifically indicates the leukemia is in remission should it be coded as such.

If the physician document[illegible] states the diagnosis of leukemia associated with [illegible]ma, two codes should be used to identify [illegible] as separate entities.

Coding Clarification

Bone Marrow Donor: If the patient has been admitted to donate his/her own marrow for bone marrow transplantation, code V59.3 *Bone marrow donor* would still be appropriate. Use an additional code to identify the specific type of leukemia from code series 204-208. Keep in mind that code V59.3 is only used when the admission is solely for donor purposes.

Coding Scenario

An acute lymphoblastic leukemia patient presents with extreme abdominal pain, having finished his course of chemotherapy the previous week. His laboratory findings are as follows: profound neutropenia-white count of .2, absolute neutrophil count of 20. The hematologist has diagnosed acute neutropenic enterocolitis. Abdominal surgery is not required.

Code Assignment: The physician must be queried as to the nature of the enterocolitis-infectious vs. noninfectious

If the enteritis is infectious, the codes are as follows: 288.0 *Agranulocytosis*, 009.1 *Colitis, enteritis, and gastroenteritis, of presumed infectious origin*, E933.1 *Adverse effect of antineoplastic drugs*, and 204.00 *Acute lymphoid leukemia, without mention of remission.*

If the enteritis is non-infectious, the codes are as follows: 288.0 *Agranulocytosis*, 558.9 *Other and unspecified noninfectious gastroenteritis and colitis*, E933.1 *Adverse effect of antineoplastic and immunosuppressive drugs*, and 204.00 *Acute lymphoid leukemia, without mention of remission.*

205 Myeloid leukemia

AHA: May-June, 1985, 18; Q2, 1990, 7; Q4, 1990, 3; Q4, 1991, 26; Q3, 1993, 3

Myeloid leukemia is a rapid and malignant proliferation of immature myelocytes called myeloblasts. The acute condition is common in children and fatal if untreated. The chronic condition is a fatal disease characterized by abnormal proliferation of premature granulocytes called myeloblasts, promyelocytes, metamyelocytes, and myelocytes, in bone marrow, peripheral blood, and body tissues.

The following fifth-digit subclassification is for use with categories 203, 204, 205, 206, 207, and 208:

0 without mention of remission

1 in remission

205.0 5th Acute myeloid leukemia — *acute promyelocytic; differentiated cell populations*
AHA: May-June, 1985, 18; Q2, 1990, 7; Q4, 1990, 3; Q4, 1991, 26; Q3, 1993, 3

205.1 5th Chronic myeloid leukemia — *more granulocytic cells; usually in young adults, eosinophilic/neutrophilic*
AHA: July-Aug, 1985, 13; May-June, 1985, 18; Q2, 1990, 7; Q4, 1990, 3; Q4, 1991, 26; Q3, 1993, 3; Q1, 2000, 6

205.2 5th Subacute myeloid leukemia

205.3 5th Myeloid sarcoma — *chloroma, granulocytic carcoma, green malignancy airising from bone marrow*
AHA: May-June, 1985, 18; Q2, 1990, 7; Q4, 1990, 3; Q4, 1991, 26; Q3, 1993, 3

205.8 5th Other myeloid leukemia — *aleukemic*
AHA: May-June, 1985, 18; Q2, 1990, 7; Q4, 1990, 3; Q4, 1991, 26; Q3, 1993, 3

205.9 5th Unspecified myeloid leukemia

Documentation Issues

If the physician documentation specifies that the patient's leukemia has been completely cured, use code V10.6x.

Only when documentation specifically indicates the leukemia is in remission should it be coded as such.

If the physician documentation states the diagnosis of leukemia associated with lymphoma, two codes should be used to identify each as separate entities.

Coding Clarification

Blast Crisis: This condition is noted by an abrupt, severe change in the course of chronic myelocytic leukemia that resembles that in acute myelocytic leukemia, with an increase in the proportion of myeloblasts. In some cases, the cells may be lymphoblasts. There is no code to identify the blast crisis as it identifies the progression to chronic myelogenous leukemia. If, for example, the diagnostic statement indicates chronic myelogenous leukemia with blast crisis, it would be coded 205.10 *Chronic myeloid leukemia without mention of remission* and additional codes would be used to identify conditions such as severe anemia due to blood loss (280.0) and thrombocytopenia (287.4). Although a fever may be noted, do not use code 780.6, since it classifies fever of unknown etiology.

Bone Marrow Donor: If the patient has been admitted to donate his/her own marrow for bone marrow transplantation code V59.3 *Bone marrow donor* would still be appropriate. Use an additional code to identify the specific type of leukemia from code series 204-208. Code V59.3 is only used when the admission is solely for donor purposes.

Coding Scenario

A patient is admitted for treatment of chronic myelogenous leukemia with blastic exacerbation.

> Code assignment: 205.10 *Chronic myeloid leukemia, without mention of remission*

A patient with myeloblastic leukemia in the remission stage is admitted for bone marrow transplantation.

> Code assignment: V59.3 *Bone marrow donor* and 205.91 *Unspecified myeloid leukemia, in remission*

206 Monocytic leukemia

AHA: Q2, 1990, 7

The following fifth-digit subclassification is for use with categories 203, 204, 205, 206, 207, and 208:

0 without mention of remission

1 in remission

206.0 5th Acute monocytic leukemia — *uncommon; monocytes as predominant cells*
AHA: Q2, 1990, 7

206.1 5th Chronic monocytic leukemia

206.2 5th Subacute monocytic leukemia

206.8 5th Other monocytic leukemia — *aleukemic*
AHA: Q2, 1990, 7

206.9 5th Unspecified monocytic leukemia — *Schilling-type*
AHA: Q2, 1990, 7

Documentation Issues

If the physician documentation specifies that the patient's leukemia has been completely cured, use code V10.6x.

Only when documentation specifically indicates the leukemia is in remission should it be coded as such.

If the physician documentation states the diagnosis of leukemia associated with lymphoma, two codes should be used to identify each as separate entities.

Coding Clarification

When a patient has an acute exacerbation of chronic monocytic leukemia, assign 206.10 *Chronic monocytic leukemia, without mention of remission* since the acute exacerbation is included in the code for chronic leukemia. The "acute" designation in this rubric is reserved for an uncommon form of myelogenous leukemia with monocytes as predominant cells.

Bone Marrow Donor: If the patient has been admitted to donate his/her own marrow for bone marrow transplantation, code V59.3 *Bone marrow donor*

© 2004 Ingenix, Inc.

would still be appropriate. Use an additional code to identify the specific type of leukemia from code series 204-208. Code V59.3 is only used when the admission is solely for donor purposes.

207 Other specified leukemia

AHA: Q2, 1990, 7

This rubric is reserved for several leukemias that do not classify to the other rubrics.

The following fifth-digit subclassification is for use with categories 203, 204, 205, 206, 207, and 208:

0 without mention of remission

1 in remission

207.0 ✓5th Acute erythremia and erythroleukemia — *acute erythremic myelosis; Di Guglielmo's disease; erythremic myelosis*
AHA: Q2, 1990, 7

207.1 ✓5th Chronic erythremia — *Heilmeyer-Schöner disease*
AHA: Q2, 1990, 7

207.2 ✓5th Megakaryocytic leukemia — *megakaryocytic myelosis; thrombocytic leukemia*
AHA: Q2, 1990, 7

207.8 ✓5th Other specified leukemia — *lymphosarcoma cell leukemia*
AHA: Q2, 1990, 7

Documentation Issues

If the physician documentation specifies that the patient's leukemia has been completely cured, use code V10.6x.

Only when documentation specifically indicates the leukemia is in remission should it be coded as such.

If the physician documentation states the diagnosis of leukemia associated with lymphoma, two codes should be used to identify each as separate entities.

Coding Clarification

Leukemias of unspecified cell types are classified to rubric 208.

Bone Marrow Donor: If the patient has been admitted to donate his/her own marrow for bone marrow transplantation, code V59.3 *Bone marrow donor* would still be appropriate. Use an additional code to identify the specific type of leukemia from code series 204-208. Keep in mind that code V59.3 is only used when the admission is solely for donor purposes.

208 Leukemia of unspecified cell type

AHA: Q2, 1990, 7

Use these leukemia codes when documentation does not provide sufficient information or when the patient's specific diagnosis has not yet been established although leukemia is certain.

The following fifth-digit subclassification is for use with categories 203, 204, 205, 206, 207, and 208:

0 without mention of remission

1 in remission

208.0 ✓5th Acute leukemia of unspecified cell type — *acute leukemia NOS; stem cell leukemia; blast cell leukemia*
AHA: Q2, 1990, 7

208.1 ✓5th Chronic leukemia of unspecified cell type — *not otherwise specified*
AHA: Q2, 1990, 7

208.2 ✓5th Subacute leukemia of unspecified cell type — *not otherwise specified*
AHA: Q2, 1990, 7

208.8 ✓5th Other leukemia of unspecified cell type

208.9 ✓5th Unspecified leukemia — *Bennett's disease*
AHA: Q2, 1990, 7

Documentation Issues

If the physician documentation specifies that the patient's leukemia has been completely cured, use code V10.6x.

Only when documentation specifically indicates the leukemia is in remission should it be coded as such.

If the physician documentation states the diagnosis of leukemia associated with lymphoma, two codes should be used to identify each as separate entities.

Coding Clarification

Bone Marrow Donor: If the patient has been admitted to donate his/her own marrow for bone marrow transplantation, code V59.3 *Bone marrow donor* would still be appropriate. Use an additional code to identify the specific type of leukemia from code series 204-208. Code V59.3 is only used when the admission is solely for donor purposes.

210–212 Benign Neoplasms of Digestive and Respiratory System and Intrathoracic Organs

Benign neoplasms are tumors characterized by dividing cells that adhere to each other, so that the mass remains a circumscribed lesion. Benign neoplasms are classified according to site. Many cysts and embryonic cysts are excluded from this classification.

210 Benign neoplasm of lip, oral cavity, and pharynx

AHA: Q2, 1990, 7

Neoplasms are classified by site in this rubric. Excluded from this rubric are cysts, ranulas, and radicular cysts.

210.0 Benign neoplasm of lip — *frenulum labii, inner aspect, mucosa*
AHA: Q2, 1990, 7

210.1 Benign neoplasm of tongue — *lingual tonsil*
AHA: Q2, 1990, 7

210.2 Benign neoplasm of major salivary glands — *parotid, sublingual, submandibular; Warthin's tumor*
AHA: Q2, 1990, 7

210.3 Benign neoplasm of floor of mouth — *floor of mouth*
AHA: Q2, 1990, 7

210.4 Benign neoplasm of other and unspecified parts of mouth — *gingiva, oral mucosa, palate, uvula, labial commissure*
AHA: Q2, 1990, 7

210.5 Benign neoplasm of tonsil — *faucial, palatine*
AHA: Q2, 1990, 7

210.6 Benign neoplasm of other parts of oropharynx — *mesopharynx, tonsillar fossa/pillars, vallecula, brachial cleft, anterior epiglottis*
AHA: Q2, 1990, 7

210.7 Benign neoplasm of nasopharynx — *adenoid, pharyngeal tonsil, posterior nasal septum, choana*
AHA: Q2, 1990, 7

210.8 Benign neoplasm of hypopharynx — *arytenoid fold, pyriform fossa, postcricoid region, laryngopharynx*
AHA: Q2, 1990, 7

210.9 Benign neoplasm of pharynx, unspecified — *site specified only as "throat"*
AHA: Q2, 1990, 7

211 Benign neoplasm of other parts of digestive system

AHA: Q2, 1990, 7

Neoplasms are classified by site in this rubric.

211.0 Benign neoplasm of esophagus

211.1 Benign neoplasm of stomach — *cardia, body, fundus, pylorus*
AHA: Q2, 1990, 7

211.2 Benign neoplasm of duodenum, jejunum, and ileum — *small intestine*
AHA: Q2, 1990, 7

211.3 Benign neoplasm of colon — *large intestine, appendix, cecum, ileocecal valve, Cronkhite-Canada syndrome*
AHA: Q2, 1990, 7; Q4, 2001, 56

211.4 Benign neoplasm of rectum and anal canal — *sphincter, rectosigmoid junction*
AHA: Q2, 1990, 7

211.5 Benign neoplasm of liver and biliary passages — *ampulla of Vater, gallbladder, sphincter of Oddi, hepatic or cystic or common bile duct*
AHA: Q2, 1990, 7

211.6 Benign neoplasm of pancreas, except islets of Langerhans — *head, tail, or body, except insulin-producing cells*
AHA: Q2, 1990, 7

211.7 Benign neoplasm of islets of Langerhans — (Use additional code to identify any functional activity) — *insulin producing cells*
AHA: Q2, 1990, 7

211.8 Benign neoplasm of retroperitoneum and peritoneum — *mesentery, mesoappendix, mesocolon, omentum, retroperitoneal tissue*
AHA: Q2, 1990, 7

211.9 Benign neoplasm of other and unspecified site of the digestive system — *spleen and generalized sites*
AHA: Q2, 1990, 7

Coding Clarification

Benign neoplasms of the digestive system are classified by site in these rubrics. The margin of the anus is excluded from this rubric and would be reported with 216.5 *Benign neoplasm of skin of trunk, except scrotum.*

Coding Scenario

A patient diagnosed with a nonmalignant gastric lymphoma (pseudolymphoma) returns for a follow up visit.

Code assignment: 211.1 *Benign neoplasm of stomach*

212 Benign neoplasm of respiratory and intrathoracic organs

AHA: Q2, 1990, 7

Neoplasms are classified by site in this rubric.

212.0 Benign neoplasm of nasal cavities, middle ear, and accessory sinuses — *sinus, eustachian tube, septum, nasal cartilage*
AHA: Q2, 1990, 7

212.1 Benign neoplasm of larynx — *vocal cords including laryngeal cartilage, suprahyoid epiglottis, glottis*
AHA: Q2, 1990, 7

212.2 Benign neoplasm of trachea

212.3 Benign neoplasm of bronchus and lung — *carina, hilus*
AHA: Q2, 1990, 7

© 2004 Ingenix, Inc.

212.4 Benign neoplasm of pleura — *membrane surrounding lung*
AHA: Q2, 1990, 7

212.5 Benign neoplasm of mediastinum — *thoracic soft tissue not elsewhere classified*
AHA: Q2, 1990, 7

212.6 Benign neoplasm of thymus — *lymphoid tissue in upper, anterior mediastinum*
AHA: Q2, 1990, 7

212.7 Benign neoplasm of heart — *myocardium, pericardium, endocardium*
AHA: Q2, 1990, 7

212.8 Benign neoplasm of other specified sites of respiratory and intrathoracic organs — *not elsewhere classified*
AHA: Q2, 1990, 7

212.9 Benign neoplasm of respiratory and intrathoracic organs, site unspecified

Coding Clarification

Classify thoracic or intrathoracic benign neoplasms, not otherwise specified to 229.8.

213–215 Benign Neoplasms of Bone, Connective, and Soft Tissues

Neoplasms in this rubric include lipomas and are classified by site.

213 Benign neoplasm of bone and articular cartilage

AHA: Q2, 1990, 7

Bone and cartilage are not differentiated in this rubric. Code selection is based on anatomic site.

213.0 Benign neoplasm of bones of skull and face — *cranial bone, turbinates, orbit, patella*
AHA: Q2, 1990, 7

213.1 Benign neoplasm of lower jaw bone — *mandible*
AHA: Q2, 1990, 7

213.2 Benign neoplasm of vertebral column, excluding sacrum and coccyx — *intervertebral cartilage or disc*
AHA: Q2, 1990, 7

213.3 Benign neoplasm of ribs, sternum, and clavicle — *xiphoid process, costal cartilage*
AHA: Q2, 1990, 7

213.4 Benign neoplasm of scapula and long bones of upper limb — *long bones, upper extremity*
AHA: Q2, 1990, 7

213.5 Benign neoplasm of short bones of upper limb — *short bones, upper extremity*
AHA: Q2, 1990, 7

213.6 Benign neoplasm of pelvic bones, sacrum, and coccyx — *acetabulum, cuboid*
AHA: Q2, 1990, 7

213.7 Benign neoplasm of long bones of lower limb — *long bones, lower extremity*
AHA: Q2, 1990, 7

213.8 Benign neoplasm of short bones of lower limb — *short bones, lower extremity*
AHA: Q2, 1990, 7

213.9 Benign neoplasm of bone and articular cartilage, site unspecified

Coding Clarification

Benign neoplasms for some cartilage sites are classified elsewhere: ear, eyelid, nose (212.0), larynx (212.1), synovia (215.0-215.9), and exostosis NOS (726.91).

214 Lipoma

AHA: Q2, 1990, 7

A lipoma is a soft nodule of fat that can occur subcutaneously or in any organ system. Treatment is not usually required, unless the lipoma is causing discomfort or compression. Other words used to describe lipomas are angiolipoma, fibrolipoma, hibernoma, myelolipoma, and myxolipoma. Lipomas are classified by site.

214.0 Lipoma of skin and subcutaneous tissue of face — *also called angiolipoma, fibrolipoma, hibernoma, or myelolipoma*
AHA: Q2, 1990, 7

214.1 Lipoma of other skin and subcutaneous tissue — *excluding face*
AHA: Q2, 1990, 7

214.2 Lipoma of intrathoracic organs — *intrathoracic, mediastinum, thymus*
AHA: Q2, 1990, 7

214.3 Lipoma of intra-abdominal organs — *peritoneum, retroperitoneum, stomach, kidney*
AHA: Q2, 1990, 7

214.4 Lipoma of spermatic cord — *also called angiolipoma, fibrolipoma, hibernoma, or myelolipoma*
AHA: Q2, 1990, 7

214.8 Lipoma of other specified sites — *not elsewhere classified, including muscle*
AHA: Q2, 1990, 7; Q3, 1994, 7

214.9 Lipoma of unspecified site

215 Other benign neoplasm of connective and other soft tissue

AHA: Q2, 1990, 7

140–239

Soft tissue includes blood vessel; bursa; fascia; ligament; muscle; peripheral, sympathetic, or parasympathetic nerve and ganglia; synovia; and tendon.

215.0 Other benign neoplasm of connective and other soft tissue of head, face, and neck — *blood vessel, bursa, fascia, ligament, muscle, or peripheral, sympathetic, and parasympathetic nerve*
AHA: Q2, 1990, 7

215.2 Other benign neoplasm of connective and other soft tissue of upper limb, including shoulder — *blood vessel, bursa, fascia, ligament, muscle, or peripheral, sympathetic, and parasympathetic nerve*
AHA: Q2, 1990, 7

215.3 Other benign neoplasm of connective and other soft tissue of lower limb, including hip — *blood vessel, bursa, fascia, ligament, muscle, or peripheral, sympathetic, and parasympathetic nerve*
AHA: Q2, 1990, 7

215.4 Other benign neoplasm of connective and other soft tissue of thorax — *blood vessel, bursa, fascia, ligament, muscle, or sympathetic and parasympathetic nerve*
AHA: Q2, 1990, 7

215.5 Other benign neoplasm of connective and other soft tissue of abdomen — *blood vessel, bursa, fascia, ligament, muscle, or sympathetic and parasympathetic nerve*
AHA: Q2, 1990, 7

215.6 Other benign neoplasm of connective and other soft tissue of pelvis — *blood vessel, bursa, fascia, ligament, muscle, or sympathetic and parasympathetic nerve*
AHA: Q2, 1990, 7

215.7 Other benign neoplasm of connective and other soft tissue of trunk, unspecified — *blood vessel, bursa, fascia, ligament, muscle, or sympathetic and parasympathetic nerve*
AHA: Q2, 1990, 7

215.8 Other benign neoplasm of connective and other soft tissue of other specified sites — *not elsewhere classified*
AHA: Q2, 1990, 7

215.9 Other benign neoplasm of connective and other soft tissue of unspecified site

Coding Clarification

Classify benign neoplasm of cartilage to rubric 212 or 213, and of breast to 217. Classify connective tissue of internal organs to the appropriate organ, except for hemangioma or lipoma.

216–217 Benign Neoplasms of Integumentary System

216 Benign neoplasm of skin

AHA: Q2, 1990, 7; Q1, 2000, 21

Codes in this rubric report such benign neoplasms as blue nevus, dermatofibroma, hydrocystoma, pigmented nevus, syringoadenoma, and syringoma.

216.0 Benign neoplasm of skin of lip — *blue nevus, pigmented nevus, dermatofibroma, syringoadenoma, hydrocystoma*
AHA: Q2, 1990, 7; Q1, 2000, 21

216.1 Benign neoplasm of eyelid, including canthus — *blue nevus, pigmented nevus, dermatofibroma, syringoadenoma, hydrocystoma*
AHA: Q2, 1990, 7; Q1, 2000, 21

216.2 Benign neoplasm of ear and external auditory canal — *blue nevus, pigmented nevus, dermatofibroma, syringoadenoma, hydrocystoma*
AHA: Q2, 1990, 7; Q1, 2000, 21

216.3 Benign neoplasm of skin of other and unspecified parts of face — *blue nevus, pigmented nevus, dermatofibroma, syringoadenoma, hydrocystoma*
AHA: Q2, 1990, 7; Q1, 2000, 21

216.4 Benign neoplasm of scalp and skin of neck — *blue nevus, pigmented nevus, dermatofibroma, syringoadenoma, hydrocystoma*
AHA: Q2, 1990, 7; Q3, 1991, 12; Q1, 2000, 21

216.5 Benign neoplasm of skin of trunk, except scrotum — *blue nevus, pigmented nevus, dermatofibroma, syringoadenoma, hydrocystoma*
AHA: Q2, 1990, 7; Q1, 2000, 21

216.6 Benign neoplasm of skin of upper limb, including shoulder — *blue nevus, pigmented nevus, dermatofibroma, syringoadenoma, hydrocystoma*
AHA: Q2, 1990, 7; Q1, 2000, 21

216.7 Benign neoplasm of skin of lower limb, including hip — *blue nevus, pigmented nevus, dermatofibroma, syringoadenoma, hydrocystoma*
AHA: Q2, 1990, 7; Q1, 2000, 21

216.8 Benign neoplasm of other specified sites of skin — *not elsewhere classified*
AHA: Q2, 1990, 7; Q1, 2000, 21

216.9 Benign neoplasm of skin, site unspecified

 © 2004 Ingenix, Inc.

217 Benign neoplasm of breast OK

AHA: Q2, 1990, 7; Q1, 2000, 4

Benign neoplasms of the connective, glandular, or soft parts of the male or female breast are classified to this rubric.

Coding Clarification
Adenofibrosis of the breast is reported with 610.2 *Fibroadenosis of breast.* Benign cyst of the breast is reported with 610.0 *Solitary cyst of breast.* Fibrocystic disease is reported with 610.1 *Diffuse cystic mastopathy* and benign lesion of the skin of the breast with 216.5 *Benign neoplasm of skin of trunk, except scrotum.* Consult the ICD-9-CM index for more information.

218–222 Benign Neoplasms of Genital Organs

218 Uterine leiomyoma

AHA: Q2, 1990, 7

Most leiomyomas are detected during the course of routine pelvic exam; there are often no symptoms. If there are symptoms, they might include abdominal discomfort, urinary frequency, and constipation.

Uterine leiomyomas usually occur in multiples. They are classified according to where they establish within the wall of the uterus. They may be called by alternate names such as uterine fibromyoma or, simply, myoma.

218.0 Submucous leiomyoma of uterus — *Submucous fibroid, fibroma, myoma*
AHA: Q2, 1990, 7

218.1 Intramural leiomyoma of uterus — *interstitial fibroid, fibroma, myoma*
AHA: Q2, 1990, 7

218.2 Subserous leiomyoma of uterus — *fibroid, fibroma, myoma on serous membrane*
AHA: Q2, 1990, 7

218.9 Leiomyoma of uterus, unspecified

219 Other benign neoplasm of uterus

This rubric classifies all benign neoplasms of the uterus, other than leiomyomas, according to site of neoplasm.

219.0 Benign neoplasm of cervix uteri — *cervical stump, internal and external os*

219.1 Benign neoplasm of corpus uteri — *endometrium, fundus, myometrium*

219.8 Benign neoplasm of other specified parts of uterus — *not elsewhere classified*

219.9 Benign neoplasm of uterus, part unspecified

220 Benign neoplasm of ovary OK

AHA: Q2, 1990, 7

The ovary is the female gonad and produces the ova. Some ovarian neoplasms are hormone-producing. Use an additional code to report any functional activity associated with the ovarian neoplasm.

221 Benign neoplasm of other female genital organs

AHA: Q2, 1990, 7

221.0 Benign neoplasm of fallopian tube and uterine ligaments — *oviduct, parametrium, round and broad ligaments*
AHA: Q2, 1990, 7

221.1 Benign neoplasm of vagina

221.2 Benign neoplasm of vulva — *clitoris, Bartholin's gland, labia (majora) (minora), pudendum*
AHA: Q2, 1990, 7

221.8 Benign neoplasm of other specified sites of female genital organs — *not elsewhere classified, including Mullerian duct (female)*
AHA: Q2, 1990, 7

221.9 Benign neoplasm of female genital organ, site unspecified

Coding Clarification
Excluded from this rubric is a cyst of the Bartholin's gland or duct, which is classified to 616.2 *Cyst of Bartholin's gland.*

222 Benign neoplasm of male genital organs

AHA: Q2, 1990, 7

The testes are a pair of male gonads found in the scrotum and produce spermatozoa for fertilization. Leydig cells in the testes produce testosterone. Few testicular masses are malignant. Testicular tumors may cause functional activity problems.

222.0 Benign neoplasm of testis — (Use additional code to identify any functional activity) — *male gonad*
AHA: Q2, 1990, 7

222.1 Benign neoplasm of penis — *corpus cavernosum, foreskin, prepuce, glans penis*
AHA: Q2, 1990, 7

222.2 Benign neoplasm of prostate — *median or lateral lobes*
AHA: Q2, 1990, 7

222.3 Benign neoplasm of epididymis — *parorchis*
AHA: Q2, 1990, 7

© 2004 Ingenix, Inc.

222.4 Benign neoplasm of scrotum — *skin, not contents*
AHA: Q2, 1990, 7

222.8 Benign neoplasm of other specified sites of male genital organs — *not elsewhere classified, including Mullerian duct (male), seminal vesicle, spermatic cord*
AHA: Q2, 1990, 7

222.9 Benign neoplasm of male genital organ, site unspecified

Coding Clarification

If functional activity problems occur, use an additional code to report it.

Benign hyperplasia of the prostate is reported with codes in rubric 600. The codes in rubric 600 describe conditions including adenoma, fibroma, myoma, polyp, cyst, or hyperplasia of prostate.

140–239

223 Benign neoplasm of kidney and other urinary organs

AHA: Q2, 1990, 7

223.0 Benign neoplasm of kidney, except pelvis — *parenchyma*
AHA: Q2, 1990, 7

223.1 Benign neoplasm of renal pelvis — *calyx, hilus*
AHA: Q2, 1990, 7

223.2 Benign neoplasm of ureter — *except orifice of bladder*
AHA: Q2, 1990, 7

223.3 Benign neoplasm of bladder — *dome, neck, orifice, sphincter, trigone, urachus, wall*
AHA: Q2, 1990, 7

223.81 Benign neoplasm of urethra — *except orifice of bladder*
AHA: Q2, 1990, 7

223.89 Benign neoplasm of other specified sites of urinary organs — *paraurethral gland*
AHA: Q2, 1990, 7

223.9 Benign neoplasm of urinary organ, site unspecified

Coding Clarification

Excluded from this rubric are congenital cyst of the kidney (753.11), polycystic kidney (753.12-753.14), and multiple cysts of the kidney (753.19).

224–225 Benign Neoplasms of Nervous System

Benign neoplasms of the brain, eye, spine, meninges, cranial nerves, or sites unknown in the nervous system are classified to rubrics 224 and 225. Peripheral, sympathetic, or parasympathetic nerves are classified to codes in rubric 215.

224 Benign neoplasm of eye

AHA: Q2, 1990, 7

The eye is basically a fluid-filled ball and benign neoplasms can pose two major dangers to sight: neoplasms can disrupt the visual field and cause compression that disrupts the flow of blood or aqueous, leading to permanent tissue damage. In addition, a benign neoplasm can result in significant irritation or pain.

Intraocular pressure in the anterior segment of the eye is maintained through the flow of aqueous humor, or tears. The lacrimal system provides these tears and is also an agent in their disposal. Tears are produced in the lacrimal glands, located bilaterally behind the eyebrow, and the lacrimal ducts carry the tears to the eye, or away from the eye to the nose. Pressure in the posterior segment of the eye is maintained by gel-like vitreous humor.

A thin, vascular, mucous membrane covers the inner eyelids and the white outer shell of the eye (sclera). This membrane is called the conjunctiva. The cornea is the bulging "window" through which we see and the retina is the light-sensitive "viewing screen" at the back of the eye. The choroid is a vascular layer of the inside of the eyeball.

224.0 Benign neoplasm of eyeball, except conjunctiva, cornea, retina, and choroid — *ciliary body, iris, sclera, uveal tract*
AHA: Q2, 1990, 7

224.1 Benign neoplasm of orbit — *soft tissue between eyeball and bony orbit*
AHA: Q2, 1990, 7

224.2 Benign neoplasm of lacrimal gland — *excluding other parts of lacrimal apparatus*
AHA: Q2, 1990, 7

224.3 Benign neoplasm of conjunctiva — *of sclera or inner aspect of eyelid*
AHA: Q2, 1990, 7

224.4 Benign neoplasm of cornea — *limbus*
AHA: Q2, 1990, 7

224.5 Benign neoplasm of retina — *pars optica, pars ciliaris, pars iridica*
AHA: Q2, 1990, 7

224.6 Benign neoplasm of choroid — *choroidea, chorioidea*
AHA: Q2, 1990, 7

224.7 Benign neoplasm of lacrimal duct — *canaliculi, nasal duct, punctum, sac*
AHA: Q2, 1990, 7

224.8 Benign neoplasm of other specified parts of eye

224.9 Benign neoplasm of eye, part unspecified

 © 2004 Ingenix, Inc.

225 Benign neoplasm of brain and other parts of nervous system

AHA: Q2, 1990, 7

All brain tumors are "malignant" in that they may lead to death as they compromise the circulation of fluids in the brain through compression or obstruction. However, neoplasms classified to this rubric are not of a metastasizing nature; they are circumscribed lesions. The incidence of benign and malignant neoplasms of the brain is about the same at 50 percent.

Symptoms of a neoplasm of the brain include headache, seizures, personality changes, impaired mental or physical functions, or in children, an enlarged head. Use an additional code to report any manifestations associated with the neoplasm.

225.0 Benign neoplasm of brain — *cerebrum, cerebellum, hypothalamus, basal ganglia, stem, medulla oblongata*
AHA: Q2, 1990, 7

225.1 Benign neoplasm of cranial nerves — *acoustic neuroma; cranial, trigeminal, trochlear, vagus nerve*
AHA: Q2, 1990, 7

225.2 Benign neoplasm of cerebral meninges — *meninges, meningioma*
AHA: Q2, 1990, 7

225.3 Benign neoplasm of spinal cord — *cauda equina*
AHA: Q2, 1990, 7

225.4 Benign neoplasm of spinal meninges — *meningioma*
AHA: Q2, 1990, 7

225.8 Benign neoplasm of other specified sites of nervous system

225.9 Benign neoplasm of nervous system, part unspecified

Coding Clarification
Acoustic neuroma is a common benign tumor of the acoustic nerve, which can cause hearing interruption, dizziness, and tinnitus. It is classified to 225.1 *Benign neoplasm of cranial nerves.*

226–228 Benign Neoplasms of Other and Unspecified Sites

226 Benign neoplasm of thyroid glands OK

AHA: Q2, 1990, 7

The thyroid gland is located just below the cricoid cartilage near the larynx. Its purpose is to secrete thyroxine and triiodothyronine, which increase the rate of cell metabolism.

Benign thyroid tumors are adenomas, cysts, or involutionary nodules. A majority is follicular.

In many cases, the patient with a benign thyroid growth undergoes surgery because of suspicion of cancer, to improve cosmetic appearance, or to correct a functional activity. Use an additional code to report any functional activity associated with the neoplasm.

227 Benign neoplasm of other endocrine glands and related structures

AHA: Q2, 1990, 7

The parathyroid glands come in pairs — the superior and inferior pair — and they are embedded in the posterior thyroid. The adrenal glands are situated above each kidney, and the pituitary gland is located in the sella turcica of the sphenoid bone. The pineal gland, located at the base of the corpus callosum, secretes melatonin; and the carotid body, located in the fork of the carotid artery, monitors blood oxygen. The aortic body at the aortic arch and right subclavian artery regulates reflex respiration.

Benign neoplasms of the endocrine glands can create functional activities in those glands. For example, adrenal tumors can cause virilizing or feminizing symptoms. Pituitary cancers can cause gigantism, Cushing's disease, amenorrhea or galactorrhea, or acromegaly. Report these functional activities in addition to the neoplasm.

227.0 Benign neoplasm of adrenal gland — (Use additional code to identify any functional activity) — *suprarenal gland*
AHA: Q2, 1990, 7

227.1 Benign neoplasm of parathyroid gland — (Use additional code to identify any functional activity) — *inferior or superior*
AHA: Q2, 1990, 7

227.3 Benign neoplasm of pituitary gland and craniopharyngeal duct (pouch) — (Use additional code to identify any functional activity) — *craniobuccal pouch, Rathke's pouch, hypophysis, sella turcica*
AHA: Q2, 1990, 7

227.4 Benign neoplasm of pineal gland — (Use additional code to identify any functional activity) — *pineal body*
AHA: Q2, 1990, 7

227.5 Benign neoplasm of carotid body — (Use additional code to identify any functional activity) — *glomus caroticum*
AHA: Q2, 1990, 7

227.6 Benign neoplasm of aortic body and other paraganglia — (Use additional code to identify any functional activity) — *coccygeal body, para-aortic body, glomus jugulare*
AHA: Nov-Dec, 1984, 17; Q2, 1990, 7

140–239

227.8 Benign neoplasm of other endocrine glands and related structures — (Use additional code to identify any functional activity) — *not elsewhere specified*
AHA: Q2, 1990, 7

227.9 Benign neoplasm of endocrine gland, site unspecified — (Use additional code to identify any functional activity)

Coding Clarification

An additional code from chapter three may be reported to identify functional activity associated with any neoplasm, for example, basophil adenoma of pituitary with Cushing's syndrome, 227.3 for neoplasm and 255.0 for Cushing's syndrome.

228 Hemangioma and lymphangioma, any site

AHA: Q2, 1990, 7; Q1, 2000, 21

Hemangiomas are neoplasms arising from vascular tissue or malformations of vascular structures. Many are congenital. They can occur topically (on the skin) or within any organ system. Common topical hemangiomas include strawberry nevus, nevus vasculosus, capillary hemangioma, port wine stain, and nevus flammeus. Classify hemangiomas according to site.

A lymphangioma is a benign, congenital malformation in the lymphatic system.

228.00 Hemangioma of unspecified site

228.01 Hemangioma of skin and subcutaneous tissue — *any site*
AHA: Jan-Feb, 1985, 19; Q2, 1990, 7; Q1, 2000, 21

228.02 Hemangioma of intracranial structures — *brain, brain meninges*
AHA: Jan-Feb, 1985, 19; Q2, 1990, 7; Q1, 2000, 21

228.03 Hemangioma of retina

228.04 Hemangioma of intra-abdominal structures — *peritoneum, retroperitoneum*
AHA: Jan-Feb, 1985, 19; Q2, 1990, 7; Q1, 2000, 21

228.09 Hemangioma of other sites — *choroid, heart, iris, spinal meninges, spinal cord; systemic angiomatosis*
AHA: Jan-Feb, 1985, 19; Q2, 1990, 7; Q3, 1991, 20; Q1, 2000, 21

228.1 Lymphangioma, any site — *congenital lymphangioma, lymphatic nevus*
AHA: Q2, 1990, 7; Q1, 2000, 21

Coding Clarification

Lymphangiomas may be superficial or deep and all lymphangiomas classify to 228.1 *Lymphangioma, any site.*

229 Benign neoplasm of other and unspecified sites

AHA: Q2, 1990, 7

Lymphangiomas are excluded from rubric 229.

229.0 Benign neoplasm of lymph nodes — *any site*
AHA: Q2, 1990, 7

229.8 Benign neoplasm of other specified sites — *thoracic or intrathoracic, not otherwise specified*
AHA: Q2, 1990, 7

229.9 Benign neoplasm of unspecified site

Coding Clarification

For intrathoracic or thoracic site not otherwise specified, report 229.8 *Benign neoplasm of other specified sites.*

230–234 Carcinoma In Situ

Carcinoma in situ is defined as a carcinoma that has not invaded neighboring tissue. Once microscopic extension of malignant cells is found in tissue adjacent to carcinoma in situ, it is no longer "in situ," and malignant neoplasm codes should be used.

230 Carcinoma in situ of digestive organs

AHA: Q2, 1990, 7

Carcinoma in situ in this rubric is classified by site within the digestive system.

230.0 Carcinoma in situ of lip, oral cavity, and pharynx — *alveolus, gingiva, palate, pharynx, salivary glands, tongue*
AHA: Q2, 1990, 7

230.1 Carcinoma in situ of esophagus — *distal, proximal, middle*
AHA: Q2, 1990, 7

230.2 Carcinoma in situ of stomach — *body, cardia, fundus, pylorus, cardiac orifice*
AHA: Q2, 1990, 7

230.3 Carcinoma in situ of colon — *appendix, cecum, ileocecal valve, large intestine*
AHA: Q2, 1990, 7

230.4 Carcinoma in situ of rectum — *rectosigmoid junction*
AHA: Q2, 1990, 7

230.5 Carcinoma in situ of anal canal — *anal sphincter*
AHA: Q2, 1990, 7

230.6 Carcinoma in situ of anus, unspecified

230.7 Carcinoma in situ of other and unspecified parts of intestine — *duodenum, jejunum, ileum, small intestine*

 © 2004 Ingenix, Inc.

AHA: Q2, 1990, 7

230.8 Carcinoma in situ of liver and biliary system — *ampulla of Vater, gallbladder, common bile duct, hepatic duct, cystic duct, and sphincter of Oddi*
AHA: Q2, 1990, 7

230.9 Carcinoma in situ of other and unspecified digestive organs — *pancreas, spleen, not elsewhere specified*
AHA: Q2, 1990, 7

231 Carcinoma in situ of respiratory system

AHA: Q2, 1990, 7

Carcinoma in situ in this rubric is classified by site within the respiratory system.

231.0 Carcinoma in situ of larynx — *voice box including cartilage, epiglottis*
AHA: Q2, 1990, 7

231.1 Carcinoma in situ of trachea — *trachea*
AHA: Q2, 1990, 7

231.2 Carcinoma in situ of bronchus and lung — *carina, hilus*
AHA: Q2, 1990, 7

231.8 Carcinoma in situ of other specified parts of respiratory system — *accessory sinus, middle ear, nasal cavities, pleura*
AHA: Q2, 1990, 7

231.9 Carcinoma in situ of respiratory system, part unspecified

232 Carcinoma in situ of skin

AHA: Q2, 1990, 7

Carcinoma in situ in this rubric is classified by site within the skin.

232.0 Carcinoma in situ of skin of lip — *excluding vermilion border, mucosal tissue*
AHA: Q2, 1990, 7

232.1 Carcinoma in situ of eyelid, including canthus

232.2 Carcinoma in situ of skin of ear and external auditory canal — *antitragus, triangular fossa, tragus, lobule, helix, and concha*
AHA: Q2, 1990, 7

232.3 Carcinoma in situ of skin of other and unspecified parts of face — *chin and forehead, but not neck or scalp*
AHA: Q2, 1990, 7

232.4 Carcinoma in situ of scalp and skin of neck — *scalp and neck, but not chin and forehead*
AHA: Q2, 1990, 7

232.5 Carcinoma in situ of skin of trunk, except scrotum — *perianal skin, skin of back, breast, buttock, chest, groin, perineum, umbilicus*
AHA: Q2, 1990, 7

232.6 Carcinoma in situ of skin of upper limb, including shoulder — *arm, hand, shoulder*
AHA: Q2, 1990, 7

232.7 Carcinoma in situ of skin of lower limb, including hip — *leg, foot*
AHA: Q2, 1990, 7

232.8 Carcinoma in situ of other specified sites of skin — *not elsewhere classified*
AHA: Q2, 1990, 7

232.9 Carcinoma in situ of skin, site unspecified

233 Carcinoma in situ of breast and genitourinary system

AHA: Q2, 1990, 7

Carcinoma in situ in this rubric is classified by site within the genitourinary system.

In situ carcinoma of the vulva and vagina are linked to human papilloma virus and occur frequently in premenopausal women.

Dysplasias of the cervix are cellular deviations from the normal structure and function of the cells of the cervix of the uterus. Dysplasias are considered a precursor to carcinoma. Cervical dysplasia is classified to one of three levels of cervical intraepithelial neoplasm.

233.0 Carcinoma in situ of breast — *male or female*
AHA: Q2, 1990, 7

233.1 Carcinoma in situ of cervix uteri — *cervical stump, internal and external os*
AHA: Q2, 1990, 7; Q1, 1991, 11; Q3, 1992, 7; Q3, 1992, 8

233.2 Carcinoma in situ of other and unspecified parts of uterus — *endometrium, fundus, and myometrium*
AHA: Q2, 1990, 7

233.3 Carcinoma in situ of other and unspecified female genital organs — *other and unspecified female genital organs*
AHA: Q2, 1990, 7

233.4 Carcinoma in situ of prostate — *median or lateral lobes*
AHA: Q2, 1990, 7

233.5 Carcinoma in situ of penis — *corpus cavernosum, foreskin, prepuce, glans penis*
AHA: Q2, 1990, 7

233.6 Carcinoma in situ of other and unspecified male genital organs

140–239

233.7 Carcinoma in situ of bladder — *trigone, ureteral orifice, urethral orifice, urachus, sphincter*
AHA: Q2, 1990, 7

233.9 Carcinoma in situ of other and unspecified urinary organs — *not elsewhere classified or unknown*
AHA: Q2, 1990, 7

Coding Clarification

CIN I is reported with 622.11 *Mild dysplasia of cervix.* CIN II is reported with 622.12 *Moderate dysplasia of cervix.* Report low grade squamous intraepithelial lesion (LGSIL) with 795.03. Report high grade squamous intraepithelial lesion (HGSIL) with 795.04, while CIN III is reported with 233.1 *Carcinoma in situ of cervix uteri.* Vulvar intraepithelial neoplasm VIN III is classified to 233.3 *Carcinoma in situ of other and unspecified female genital organs.*

234 Carcinoma in situ of other and unspecified sites

AHA: Q2, 1990, 7

Carcinoma in this rubric is classified by site as the eye, other, or unspecified.

234.0 Carcinoma in situ of eye — *retina, conjunctiva, globe, choroid, iris, ciliary body, cornea*
AHA: Q2, 1990, 7

234.8 Carcinoma in situ of other specified sites — *endocrine glands*
AHA: Q2, 1990, 7

234.9 Carcinoma in situ, site unspecified

Coding Clarification

Classify all parts of the eye to 234.0 *Carcinoma in situ of eye,* except eyelid skin (232.1) and eyelid cartilage, optic nerve, or orbital bone (234.8). Carcinomas in situ of the adrenal, parathyroid, pituitary, pineal glands, and the carotid and pineal bodies are classified to 234.8 *Carcinoma in situ of other specified sites.*

235–238 Neoplasms of Uncertain Behavior

Uncertain behavior is a histomorphological determination, as distinguished from unspecified behavior, which indicates a lack of documentation to support a more specific code assignment. Neoplasms of uncertain behavior are classified by site or organ system. Neurofibromatosis, polycythemia vera, and mast cell tumors are classified in this series of rubics.

235 Neoplasm of uncertain behavior of digestive and respiratory systems

AHA: Q2, 1990, 7

Neoplasms in this rubric are classified by site within the digestive or respiratory systems.

235.0 Neoplasm of uncertain behavior of major salivary glands — *parotid, sublingual, submandibular glands*
AHA: Q2, 1990, 7

235.1 Neoplasm of uncertain behavior of lip, oral cavity, and pharynx — *gingiva, alveolus, pharynx, tongue, minor salivary glands*
AHA: Q2, 1990, 7

235.2 Neoplasm of uncertain behavior of stomach, intestines, and rectum — *ilium, jejunum, cardia, colon, sigmoid, duodenum*
AHA: Q2, 1990, 7

235.3 Neoplasm of uncertain behavior of liver and biliary passages — *ampulla of Vater, gallbladder, bile ducts, liver*
AHA: Q2, 1990, 7

235.4 Neoplasm of uncertain behavior of retroperitoneum and peritoneum — *abdominal soft tissue other than organs*
AHA: Q2, 1990, 7

235.5 Neoplasm of uncertain behavior of other and unspecified digestive organs — *esophagus, pancreas, spleen, anus*
AHA: Q2, 1990, 7

235.6 Neoplasm of uncertain behavior of larynx — *voice box*
AHA: Q2, 1990, 7

235.7 Neoplasm of uncertain behavior of trachea, bronchus, and lung — *all lobes, trachea, bronchi*
AHA: Q2, 1990, 7

235.8 Neoplasm of uncertain behavior of pleura, thymus, and mediastinum — *thoracic soft tissue other than heart, lungs*
AHA: Q2, 1990, 7

235.9 Neoplasm of uncertain behavior of other and unspecified respiratory organs — *accessory sinus, middle ear, nasal cavities*
AHA: Q2, 1990, 7

236 Neoplasm of uncertain behavior of genitourinary organs

AHA: Q2, 1990, 7

Neoplasms in this rubric are classified by site within the genitourinary system. If a neoplasm of the testis or ovary causes functional changes in hormone levels, report the functional activity in addition to the neoplasm of uncertain behavior.

236.0 Neoplasm of uncertain behavior of uterus — *endometrium, fundus, myometrium*
AHA: Q2, 1990, 7

© 2004 Ingenix, Inc.

236.1 Neoplasm of uncertain behavior of placenta — *choriodenoma destruens, malignant hydatidiform mole*
AHA: Q2, 1990, 7

236.2 Neoplasm of uncertain behavior of ovary — (Use additional code to identify any functional activity) — *female gonad*
AHA: Q2, 1990, 7

236.3 Neoplasm of uncertain behavior of other and unspecified female genital organs — *not elsewhere classified or unknown*
AHA: Q2, 1990, 7

236.4 Neoplasm of uncertain behavior of testis — (Use additional code to identify any functional activity) — *male gonad*
AHA: Q2, 1990, 7

236.5 Neoplasm of uncertain behavior of prostate — *median or lateral lobes*
AHA: Q2, 1990, 7

236.6 Neoplasm of uncertain behavior of other and unspecified male genital organs — *not elsewhere classified or unknown*
AHA: Q2, 1990, 7

236.7 Neoplasm of uncertain behavior of bladder — *trigone, ureteral orifice, urethral orifice, urachus, sphincter*
AHA: Q2, 1990, 7

236.90 Neoplasm of uncertain behavior of urinary organ, unspecified

236.91 Neoplasm of uncertain behavior of kidney and ureter — *calyx, hilus, pelvis of kidney*
AHA: Q2, 1990, 7

236.99 Neoplasm of uncertain behavior of other and unspecified urinary organs — *urethra*
AHA: Q2, 1990, 7

237 Neoplasm of uncertain behavior of endocrine glands and nervous system

AHA: Q2, 1990, 7

If a neoplasm causes functional changes in hormone levels or nervous system functions, report the functional activity or manifestation in addition to the neoplasm of uncertain behavior.

237.0 Neoplasm of uncertain behavior of pituitary gland and craniopharyngeal duct — (Use additional code to identify any functional activity) — *pituitary body, fossa, lobe*
AHA: Q2, 1990, 7

237.1 Neoplasm of uncertain behavior of pineal gland — *pineal body*
AHA: Q2, 1990, 7

237.2 Neoplasm of uncertain behavior of adrenal gland — (Use additional code to identify any functional activity) — *suprarenal gland*
AHA: Q2, 1990, 7

237.3 Neoplasm of uncertain behavior of paraganglia — *aortic body, coccygeal body, carotid body, glomus jugulare*
AHA: Nov-Dec, 1984, 17; Q2, 1990, 7

237.4 Neoplasm of uncertain behavior of other and unspecified endocrine glands — *parathyroid gland, thyroid gland*
AHA: Q2, 1990, 7

237.5 Neoplasm of uncertain behavior of brain and spinal cord — *frontal lobe, thalamus, cerebrum, cerebellum, temporal lobe and stem*
AHA: Q2, 1990, 7

237.6 Neoplasm of uncertain behavior of meninges — *cerebral or spinal*
AHA: Q2, 1990, 7

237.70 Neurofibromatosis, unspecified — *type unknown*
AHA: Q2, 1990, 7

237.71 Neurofibromatosis, Type 1 (von Recklinghausen's disease) — *"elephant man" syndrome*
AHA: Q2, 1990, 7

237.72 Neurofibromatosis, Type 2 (acoustic neurofibromatosis) — *bilateral 8th nerve masses*
AHA: Q2, 1990, 7

237.9 Neoplasm of uncertain behavior of other and unspecified parts of nervous system — *cranial, parasympathetic, sympathetic, peripheral nerves or unknown*
AHA: Q2, 1990, 7

238 Neoplasm of uncertain behavior of other and unspecified sites and tissues

AHA: Q2, 1990, 7

238.0 Neoplasm of uncertain behavior of bone and articular cartilage — *long and short ones and associated cartilage*
AHA: Q2, 1990, 7

238.1 Neoplasm of uncertain behavior of connective and other soft tissue — *peripheral, sympathetic, and parasympathetic nerves and ganglia*
AHA: Q2, 1990, 7

238.2 Neoplasm of uncertain behavior of skin — *any site*
AHA: Q2, 1990, 7

238.3 Neoplasm of uncertain behavior of breast — *male or female*
AHA: Q2, 1990, 7

140–239

238.4 Neoplasm of uncertain behavior of polycythemia vera — *Vaquez-Osler disease*
AHA: Q2, 1990, 7

238.5 Neoplasm of uncertain behavior of histiocytic and mast cells — *mastocytoma NOS*
AHA: Q2, 1990, 7

238.6 Neoplasm of uncertain behavior of plasma cells — *plasmacytoma NOS, solitary myeloma*
AHA: Q2, 1990, 7

238.7 Neoplasm of uncertain behavior of other lymphatic and hematopoietic tissues — *idiopathic thrombocythemia; megakaryocytic myelosclerosis; myelodysplastic syndrome; panmyelosis; preleukemic syndrome*
AHA: Q2, 1989, 8; Q2, 1990, 7; Q1, 1997, 5; Q3, 2001, 13

238.8 Neoplasm of uncertain behavior of other specified sites — *eye, heart, nasolacrimal duct, lymph gland, Virchow's gland*
AHA: Q2, 1990, 7

238.9 Neoplasm of uncertain behavior, site unspecified

Coding Clarification

Report pancytopenia, panmyelosis, and myelosclerosis with myeloid metaplasia, myelodysplastic syndrome, megakaryocytic myelosclerosis, and idiopathic thrombocythemia with 238.7.

239 Neoplasms of Unspecified Nature

This rubric classifies neoplasms for unknown or undocumented morphology. Classify the neoplasm according to site in this rubric.

239 Neoplasms of unspecified nature

AHA: Q2, 1990, 7

239.0 Neoplasm of unspecified nature of digestive system — *mouth, esophagus, stomach, intestine, pancreas, gallbladder*
AHA: Q2, 1990, 7

239.1 Neoplasm of unspecified nature of respiratory system — *lungs, pleura, bronchi*
AHA: Q2, 1990, 7

239.2 Neoplasms of unspecified nature of bone, soft tissue, and skin — *bone, blood vessels, muscles*
AHA: Q2, 1990, 7

239.3 Neoplasm of unspecified nature of breast — *male or female*
AHA: Q2, 1990, 7

239.4 Neoplasm of unspecified nature of bladder

239.5 Neoplasm of unspecified nature of other genitourinary organs — *male or female*
AHA: Q2, 1990, 7

239.6 Neoplasm of unspecified nature of brain — *including cerebellum, cerebrum, stem*
AHA: Q2, 1990, 7

239.7 Neoplasm of unspecified nature of endocrine glands and other parts of nervous system — *thyroid, pituitary, pineal gland*
AHA: Q2, 1990, 7

239.8 Neoplasm of unspecified nature of other specified sites — *mediastinum, lymph glands, eye, heart, thymus*
AHA: Q2, 1990, 7

239.9 Neoplasm of unspecified nature, site unspecified

Coding Clarification

Do not use codes from this rubric to classify a "mass." Instead, consult "mass" in the index. Use of any code in this rubric may cause delays in claims processing due to the nonspecific nature of these codes.

 © 2004 Ingenix, Inc.

240–279

Endocrine, Nutritional and Metabolic Diseases, and Immunity Disorders

The endocrine system is a group of specialized organs and body tissues that produces, stores, and secretes chemical substances known as hormones. Hormones provide information and instructions to regulate development, control the function of various tissues, support reproduction, and regulate metabolism.

Hormones from the endocrine system are secreted into the blood, where proteins bind to them to keep them intact as the hormones are disbursed through the body. The proteins also regulate the release of hormones.

Usually, the changes a hormone produces also serve to regulate that hormone's secretion. For example, parathyroid hormone causes the body to increase the level of calcium in the blood. As calcium levels rise, the secretion of parathyroid hormone decreases. Other changes in the body also influence hormone secretions. For example, during illness, the adrenal glands increase the secretions of certain hormones to help the body overcome the stress of illness. The normal regulation of hormone secretion is suspended, allowing for a tolerance of higher levels of hormone in the blood until the illness is resolved.

Nutritional deficiencies in this chapter cover deficiencies in vitamins, minerals, and protein-calorie malnutrition. Deficiencies of anemia are classified to Chapter Four Disease of the Blood and Blood-Forming Organs.

Metabolic diseases in this chapter cover a wide range of diseases, including problems with amino-acid transport, carbohydrate transport, lipoid metabolism, plasma protein metabolism, gout, mineral metabolism, and fluid, electrolyte, and acid-base imbalances. Also covered are cystic fibrosis, porphyrin, purine and pyrimidine metabolism, and obesity.

240–246 Disorders of Thyroid Gland

The thyroid gland is attached to the trachea by loose connective tissue and derives its blood supply from the superior and interior thyroid arteries. The function of the thyroid is to create, store, and secrete thyroxine and triiodothyronine. The thyroid gland secretes hormones in response to stimulation by thyroid stimulating hormone (TSH) from the pituitary gland. The thyroid hormones regulate growth and metabolism and play a role in brain development during childhood.

240 Simple and unspecified goiter

In simple goiter, the thyroid gland is enlarged, but the hormone secretions of the thyroid are still within normal limits. Simple goiter can have several causes. Iodine is essential to thyroid hormone secretion. The thyroid of a person whose diet has insufficient iodine will actually become enlarged so that it can produce more thyroid hormone. Iodine deficiency is the most common cause of simple goiter, but as there is no deficiency in the United States, this cause is rarely seen here. Simple goiter can also occur during puberty, pregnancy, or during menses as a result of hormonal imbalances. If a goiter has enough mass, it may cause compression that may lead to airway restriction, swallowing difficulty, or problems with venous flow.

240.0 Goiter, specified as simple — *not affecting hormone production*

240.9 Goiter, unspecified — *extent unknown*

241 Nontoxic nodular goiter

In nontoxic nodular goiter, the thyroid gland exhibits palpable nodules, though the nodules do not affect thyroid hormone secretion. Goiters in this rubric are classified as having a singular nodule or multiple nodules.

241.0 Nontoxic uninodular goiter — *one node, without clinical hypothyroidism*

241.1 Nontoxic multinodular goiter — *multiple nodes, without clinical hypothyroidism*

241.9 Unspecified nontoxic nodular goiter — *struma nodosa (simplex)*

Coding Clarification

Benign neoplasms of the thyroid are reported with codes in the 226 rubric.

242 Thyrotoxicosis with or without goiter

Thyrotoxicosis is an over-secretion of thyroid hormone, and is also called hyperthyroidism. Symptoms include tachycardia, nervousness, tremor, weight loss, heat intolerance, goiter, and fatigue.

Thyrotoxicosis is eight to 10 times more common in women than in men.

The causes of thyrotoxicosis are varied. Increased hormone secretion can be related to a thyroid nodule or to ectopic thyroid tissue. Thyrotoxicosis can also be the result of a more systemic problem, as in the case of Grave's disease, an autoimmune disorder.

A thyrotoxic storm is a sudden, life-threatening crisis in which symptoms of hyperthyroidism are exacerbated and new symptoms develop. It is most likely to occur at the time of infection, surgical procedure, or trauma in a patient with undertreated hyperthyroidism. The patient may develop a fever, emotional instability or psychosis, heart complications, and an enlarged liver.

Diseases in this rubric are classified first by the cause of hyperthyroidism, and second, by the status of thyrotoxic storm.

The following fifth-digit subclassification is for use with category 242:

0 without mention of thyrotoxic crisis or storm

1 with metnion of thyrotoxic crisis or storm

242.0 5th Toxic diffuse goiter — *Grave's disease, Basedow's disease, Marsh's disease, Parry's syndrome, Parson's disease; exophthalmic goiter*

242.1 5th Toxic uninodular goiter — *single nodule, toxic, or with hyperthyroidism*

242.2 5th Toxic multinodular goiter — *multiple nodules, toxic, or with hyperthyroidism*

242.3 5th Toxic nodular goiter, unspecified type — *nodular, unknown type, with hyperthyroidism or toxic; Plummer's disease*

242.4 5th Thyrotoxicosis from ectopic thyroid nodule — *aberrant thyroid tissue as cause*

242.8 5th Thyrotoxicosis of other specified origin — (Use additional E code to identify cause, if drug-induced) — *overproduction of TSH; thyroid toxicosis factitia*

242.9 5th Thyrotoxicosis without mention of goiter or other cause — *not elsewhere specified; Leopold-Levi's syndrome*

Coding Clarification

If a neoplasm is causing the functional activity, report the appropriate neoplasm code in addition to the hyperthyroidism code. Sequencing varies according to the encounter.

Neonatal thyrotoxicosis is reported with 775.3.

243 Congenital hypothyroidism OK

The most common cause of congenital hypothyroid is absence of a thyroid gland at birth. This requires lifelong hormone therapy since thyroxine regulates metabolism and growth. Untreated, congenital hypothyroidism causes serious problems in the central nervous system, developmental delay, and problems with somatic growth. Screening programs exist in the United States to test newborns for this disorder. By providing replacement thyroid hormones, almost all of the complications of congenital hypothyroidism are avoidable.

Coding Clarification

Congenital goiter with an enzyme defect in synthesis of thyroid hormone is reported with 246.1.

244 Acquired hypothyroidism

Hypothyroidism is a deficiency of thyroid hormone. Primary hypothyroidism usually develops in older adults, usually after age 40, and causes lethargy, fatigue, and mental sluggishness.

244.0 Postsurgical hypothyroidism — *athyroidism or part of thyroid removed*

244.1 Other postablative hypothyroidism — *following irradiation*

244.2 Iodine hypothyroidism — (Use additional E code to identify drug) — *resulting from high iodide intake*

244.3 Other iatrogenic hypothyroidism — (Use additional E code to identify drug) — *resulting from: PAS, phenylbutazone, resorcinol*

244.8 Other specified acquired hypothyroidism — *not elsewhere classified, Gull's disease*
AHA: July-Aug, 1985, 9

244.9 Unspecified hypothyroidism — *Brissaud-Meige syndrome; Strumipriva cachexia; Hoffmann's syndrome*
AHA: Q4, 1996, 29; Q3, 1999, 19

Coding Clarification

For hypothyroidism complicating pregnancy, see rubric 648.

Coding Scenario

A patient in for laboratory testing was recently diagnosed with iron deficiency anemia due to hypothyroidism.

Code assignment: 280.9 *Iron deficiency anemia, unspecified* and 244.9 *Unspecified hypothyroidism*

245 Thyroiditis

Diseases in this rubric are classified as acute, subacute, chronic, and iatrogenic. The most common form of thyroiditis in the United States is Hashimoto's thyroiditis (245.2), a chronic condition that usually leads to chronic hypothyroidism and lifetime treatment with synthetic hormone. Hashimoto's thyroiditis is an autoimmune disorder that often

© 2004 Ingenix, Inc.

240–279

presents with other forms of autoimmune disease, including Type 1 diabetes mellitus, hypoparathyroidism, or Addison's disease. Schmidt's syndrome is Addison's disease with hypothyroidism secondary to Hashimoto's thyroiditis, and is reported with 258.1 *Other combinations of endocrine dysfunction.* In diabetes with hypothyroidism, report both conditions rather than this combination code since, as a significant systemic disease, diabetes should always be coded separately.

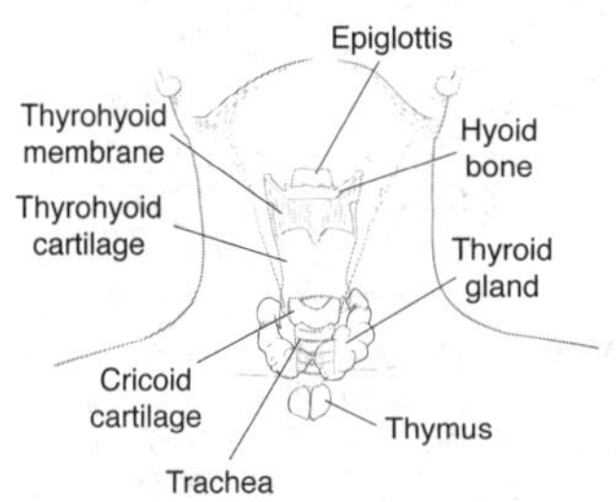

245.0 Acute thyroiditis — (Use additional code to identify organism) — *abscess, pyogenic, suppurative, nonsuppurative*

245.1 Subacute thyroiditis — *de Quervain's, giant cell, granulomatous*

245.2 Chronic lymphocytic thyroiditis — *Hashimoto's disease*

245.3 Chronic fibrous thyroiditis — *Riedel's thyroiditis; struma fibrosa*

245.4 Iatrogenic thyroiditis — (Use additional code to identify cause) — *due to medical treatment other than radiation or excision*

245.8 Other and unspecified chronic thyroiditis — *not elsewhere classified*

245.9 Unspecified thyroiditis

246 Other disorders of thyroid

This rubric captures other disorders of the thyroid, with the exception of neoplasms, which are found in Chapter 2.

246.0 Disorders of thyrocalcitonin secretion — *hypersecretion of calcitonin or thyrocalcitonin*

246.1 Dyshormonogenic goiter — *enzyme defect; congenital dyshormonogenic*

246.2 Cyst of thyroid

246.3 Hemorrhage and infarction of thyroid

246.8 Other specified disorders of thyroid — *atrophy, TBG defect, degeneration*

246.9 Unspecified disorder of thyroid

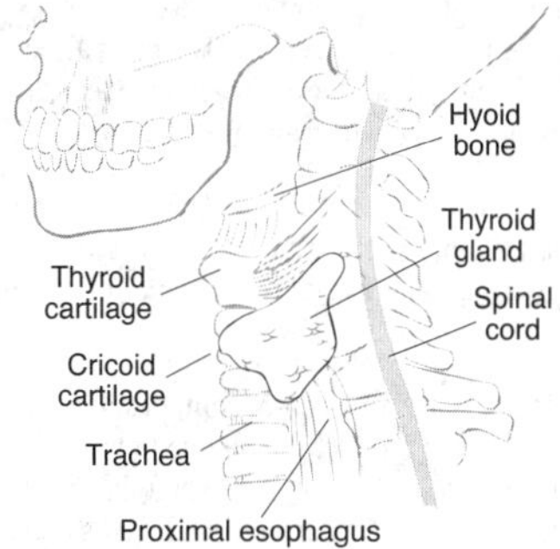

250–259 Diseases of Other Endocrine Glands

Included in this section are diseases associated with insulin-producing cells of the pancreas, the islets of Langerhans, parathyroid, pituitary, hypothalamus, adrenals, ovaries, and testes.

250 Diabetes mellitus

AHA: Nov-Dec, 1985, 11; Q2, 1990, 22; Q3, 1991, 3; Q2, 1992, 5; Q4, 1993, 19; Q3, 1996, 5; Q2, 1997, 14; Q4, 1997, 32; Q2, 1998, 15; Q2, 2001, 16; Q2, 2002, 13

The pancreas is positioned in the upper abdomen, just under the stomach. The major part of the pancreas, called the exocrine pancreas, secretes digestive enzymes into the gastrointestinal tract. Distributed through the pancreas are clusters of endocrine cells that secrete insulin, glucagon, and somatostatin. These hormones all participate in regulating energy and metabolism in the body.

Diabetes is a systemic disease and, as such, should be coded even in the absence of documented, active intervention during the patient encounter.

Diabetes mellitus has two forms. Diabetes mellitus Type I is caused by inadequate secretion of insulin by the pancreas. Diabetes mellitus Type II is caused by the body's inability to respond to insulin. Both have similar symptoms, including excessive thirst, hunger, and urination as well as weight loss. Laboratory tests that detect glucose in the urine and elevated levels of glucose in the blood usually confirm the diagnosis.

Treatment of diabetes mellitus Type I requires regular injections of insulin. Type II can be treated with diet, exercise, oral medication, or injection.

Only about 10 percent of diabetics are juvenile-onset Type I. The primary factor that distinguishes Type I from Type II is the absence of naturally occurring insulin within the body. Type I diabetics require insulin injections to survive. Type II diabetics may improve their health with insulin injections, and may even come to require insulin, but the administration of insulin has no bearing on code selection for diabetes. A patient with Type II diabetes is always coded as having Type II, even when the medical record states the patient requires insulin.

In this rubric, diabetes is classified according to type of complication, as selected by the fourth digit, and by Type I or Type II status and the presence of diabetic control, selected by the fifth digit.

Diabetes can cause a variety of complications, including kidney problems, pain due to nerve damage, blindness, and coronary heart disease. Recent studies have shown that controlling blood sugar levels reduces the risk of developing diabetes complications.

The following fifth-digit subclassification is for use with category 250:

0 type II [non-insulin dependent type] [NIDDM type] [adult-onset type] or unspecified type, not stated as uncontrolled

1 type I [insulin dependent type] [IDDM] [juvenile type], not stated as uncontrolled

2 type II [non-insulin dependent type] [NIDDM type] [adult-onset type] or unspecified type, uncontrolled

3 type I [insulin dependent type] [IDDM] [juvenile type], uncontrolled

250.0 5th Diabetes mellitus without mention of complication — *no complications arising from disease*
AHA: Nov-Dec, 1985, 11; Q2, 1990, 22; Q3, 1991, 3; Q3, 1991, 3,12; Q2, 1992, 5; Q4, 1993, 19; Q3, 1996, 5; Q2, 1997, 14; Q4, 1997, 32; Q2, 1998, 15; Q2, 2001, 16; Q2, 2002, 13

250.1 5th Diabetes with ketoacidosis — *ketosis, acidosis, without coma*
AHA: Nov-Dec, 1985, 11; Q2, 1990, 22; Q3, 1991, 3; Q3, 1991, 6; Q2, 1992, 5; Q4, 1993, 19; Q3, 1996, 5; Q2, 1997, 14; Q4, 1997, 32; Q2, 1998, 15; Q2, 2001, 16; Q2, 2002, 13

250.2 5th Diabetes with hyperosmolarity — *increased osmolarity of the body fluids as a complication of diabetes*
AHA: Nov-Dec, 1985, 11; Q2, 1990, 22; Q3, 1991, 3; Q3, 1991, 7; Q2, 1992, 5; Q4, 1993, 19; Q3, 1996, 5; Q2, 1997, 14; Q4, 1997, 32; Q2, 1998, 15; Q2, 2001, 16; Q2, 2002, 13

250.3 5th Diabetes with other coma — *arising from ketoacidosis or hypoglycemia*
AHA: Nov-Dec, 1985, 11; Q2, 1990, 22; Q3, 1991, 3; Q3, 1991, 7, 12; Q2, 1992, 5; Q4, 1993, 19; Q3, 1996, 5; Q2, 1997, 14; Q4, 1997, 32; Q2, 1998, 15; Q2, 2001, 16; Q2, 2002, 13

250.4 5th Diabetes with renal manifestations — (Use additional code to identify manifestation: 581.81, 583.81) — *kidney disease*
AHA: Sept-Oct, 1984, 3; Nov-Dec, 1985, 11; Sept-Oct, 1987, 9; Q2, 1990, 22; Q3, 1991, 3; Q3, 1991, 8,12; Q2, 1992, 5; Q4, 1993, 19; Q3, 1996, 5; Q2, 1997, 14; Q4, 1997, 32; Q2, 1998, 15; Q2, 2001, 16; Q2, 2002, 13

250.5 5th Diabetes with ophthalmic manifestations — (Use additional code to identify manifestation: 362.01, 362.02, 362.83, 365.44, 366.41, 369.0-369.9) — *ocular disease*
AHA: Sept-Oct, 1985, 11; Nov-Dec, 1985, 11; Q2, 1990, 22; Q3, 1991, 3; Q3, 1991, 8; Q2, 1992, 5; Q4, 1993, 19; Q3, 1996, 5; Q2, 1997, 14; Q4, 1997, 32; Q2, 1998, 15; Q2, 2001, 16; Q2, 2002, 13

250.6 5th Diabetes with neurological manifestations — (Use additional code to identify manifestation: 337.1, 354.0-355.9, 357.2, 358.1, 713.5) — *nerve damage or disease*
AHA: Nov-Dec, 1984, 9; Nov-Dec, 1985, 11; Q2, 1990, 22; Q3, 1991, 3; Q3, 1991, 9; Q2, 1992, 5; Q2, 1992, 15; Q2, 1993, 6; Q4, 1993, 19; Q3, 1996, 5; Q2, 1997, 14; Q4, 1997, 32; Q2, 1998, 15; Q2, 2001, 16; Q2, 2002, 13

250.7 5th Diabetes with peripheral circulatory disorders — (Use additional code to identify manifestation: 443.81, 785.4) — *blood vessel damage or disease*
AHA: Nov-Dec, 1985, 11; Q2, 1990, 22; Q3, 1990, 15; Q3, 1991, 3; Q3, 1991, 10,12; Q2, 1992, 5; Q4, 1993, 19; Q2, 1994, 17; Q3, 1994, 5; Q1, 1996, 10; Q3, 1996, 5; Q2, 1997, 14; Q4, 1997, 32; Q2, 1998, 15; Q2, 2001, 16; Q2, 2002, 13

250.8 5th Diabetes with other specified manifestations — (Use additional code to identify manifestation: 707.10-707.9, 731.8. Use additional E code to identify cause, if drug-induced) — *including hypoglycemic shock*
AHA: Nov-Dec, 1985, 11; Q2, 1990, 22; Q3, 1991, 3; Q3, 1991, 10; Q2, 1992, 5; Q4, 1993, 19; Q4, 1993, 20; Q3, 1996, 5; Q2, 1997, 14; Q2, 1997, 16; Q4, 1997, 32; Q4, 1997, 43; Q2, 1998, 15; Q4, 2000, 44; Q2, 2001, 16; Q2, 2002, 13

250.9 5th Diabetes with unspecified complication

Documentation Issues

The documentation may indicate conditions "with" diabetes, but this does not necessarily mean the condition is due to diabetes. Although diabetic patients are vulnerable to chronic conditions affecting other body systems (e.g., renal, ophthalmologic, vascular), this does not indicate a direct correlation. Clarification must be obtained from the physician as to the cause and effect relationship of the condition. Documentation should identify a direct relation by statements such as "due to," "caused by," or

240–279

 © 2004 Ingenix, Inc.

"secondary to" before diabetic complication codes are assigned.

For example, the documentation states neurogenic bowel in a diabetic patient. Before a code is assigned, consult with the physician on whether the diabetes is the cause of the neurogenic bowel. If the neurogenic bowel is due to the diabetes, use codes 250.6x, 337.1, and 564.81.

When coding inpatient claims, if the documentation indicates that the patient only has diabetes and does not indicate a complication, the admission would be considered questionable. Clarification should be made with the physician for a more complete diagnosis to substantiate the necessity for the admission.

Documentation must specify that the patient is Type I to allow use of the fifth digit 1 or 3. The patient may be receiving insulin but may not be a true insulin dependent diabetic. Verify status with the physician if clarification is needed.

Fifth digits specifying uncontrolled diabetes should not be assigned based on blood glucose levels. These codes should only be used if the physician documents uncontrolled diabetes in the medical record.

If the documentation in the record indicates that the patient has metabolic acidosis and diabetes, clarify with the physician if there is a cause and effect relationship. Note that code 276.2 has an exclusion note for diabetic acidosis and references code 250.1x.

When the patient has had a pancreatic transplant, the diabetes code would apply solely if the physician documents diabetes and/or manifestations of the diabetes.

When the physician documents "pseudodiabetes" of newborn, use code 775.1 *Neonatal diabetes mellitus.* This condition is also known as "transient neonatal diabetes," which occurs in the newborn of a diabetic mother.

If the physician documents that the patient has diabetes with a hyperosmolar coma, it does not necessarily mean the patient is in an unconscious state. This condition involves an altered state of consciousness without notable ketosis, with hyperosmolarity and dehydration. Typically this condition occurs in noninsulin dependent diabetics. Use code 250.2x *Diabetes with hyperosmolarity* to identify this condition.

Diabetes mellitus should not be coded as out of control unless the physician specifically indicates it as such in the final diagnostic statement and/or in the body of the medical record. If the record identifies the uncontrolled state and the final diagnostic statement does not, clarification must be obtained from the physician.

Coding Clarification

For diabetic pregnancy, two codes are required: the pregnancy code from the rubric 648 and also a code from the 250 rubric.

Secondary diabetes should not be reported with this rubric. Instead, the condition causing the diabetes should be reported. For example, in post-pancreatectomy diabetes, assign 251.3 *Postsurgical insulinemia.*

Diabetes is one of a number of the ICD-9-CM classification categories that is used as a primary code to classify both the disease and its major manifestations. Additional codes should be used to provide more specificity in defining the manifestations. When a cause and effect relationship between renal failure and diabetes has been established, the diabetes code 250.4x is listed first and the renal failure code is listed as an additional code. Accordingly, if the diagnosis does not indicate a cause and effect relationship between the diabetes and renal failure, the code for the renal failure may be listed first.

Atherosclerosis: Diabetic atherosclerosis is coded as 250.7x *Diabetes with peripheral circulatory disorders* and 440.2x *Atherosclerosis of native arteries of extremities.* If the diagnosis is diabetes with ischemic heart disease or cerebrovascular disease, code them as separate entities.

Coexisting or Chronic Conditions: Coexisting or chronic conditions that are treated on an ongoing basis should be coded and reported as many times as the patient receives treatment, management, and additional care for the conditions. Conditions such as diabetes that are considered systemic diseases should be coded, even in the absence of documented active intervention.

End Stage Renal Disease: Diabetes is one of the many diseases that may cause end stage renal disease and chronic renal failure due to the progressive nature of the disease. Due to the cause and effect relationship between these conditions, always sequence code 250.4x first and the renal manifestation second. If the documentation does not indicate the cause and effect relationship of the chronic renal disease or failure and the diabetes, the renal condition may be listed as the initial code and the diabetes may be listed as secondary.

Foot Ulcers: Diabetic patients may develop foot ulcers from conditions such as diabetic neuropathy (250.6x), diabetic peripheral vascular disease (250.7x), or superimposed infection. If it is due to the superimposed infection, the foot ulcer would not be coded as a diabetic complication. Use codes 250.0x *Diabetes mellitus* and 707.1x *Ulcer of lower limbs, except decubitus* and an additional code for the causative organism of the infection, if known. If the cause of the diabetic ulcer is not known, use code 250.8x

© 2004 Ingenix, Inc.

Diabetes with other specified manifestations and 707.1x *Ulcer of lower limbs.*

Gangrene: Gangrene noted in the diabetic patient is always coded as a diabetic complication. The exception to this guideline is if there is a history of trauma such as an open wound. If the patient has an open wound that has developed an infection that has progressed to gangrene, use the complicated open wound code with code 785.4 for the gangrene and 250.0x for the diabetes.

Gastroparesis Due to Diabetes: Three codes are required to identify this condition: 250.6x. *Diabetes mellitus with neurological manifestations,* 337.1 *Peripheral autonomic neuropathy in disorders classified elsewhere,* and 536.3 *Gastroparesis.*

Impotence: When coding diabetic impotence, the diabetic condition that caused the impotence would be listed first (e.g., peripheral vascular disease, peripheral neuropathy) followed by the code for the impotence, 607.84. If the cause of the diabetic impotence is not known, use codes 250.8x *Diabetes with other specified manifestations* and 607.84 *Impotence of organic origin.*

Multiple Coding: Multiple coding is required for diabetic complications. Instructions for these conditions appear in the alphabetic index as well as the tabular list of the ICD-9-CM code book. In the alphabetic index, in many cases, both codes are listed with the subentry term. The second code is in brackets. Both codes should be assigned in the same sequence in which they appear in the alphabetic index. In the tabular listing, review instructional terms, such as "Use additional code to identify manifestation" and "Code first the underlying disease." Apply multiple coding instructions throughout the classification where appropriate, whether or not multiple coding directions appear in the alphabetic index. Take steps to avoid indiscriminate multiple coding or irrelevant information, such as symptoms or signs characteristic of the diabetic condition (e.g., acute metabolic complications associated with the diabetes itself).

Ophthalmic Manifestations: Diabetic cataracts, true diabetic cataracts, or those known as "snowflake cataracts" are rare and are found in Type I diabetics. Use codes 250.51 *Diabetes with ophthalmic manifestations* and 366.41 *Diabetic cataract.* Senile cataracts, although commonly seen in diabetics, are not classified as such because they are not caused by the diabetes. Use codes 250.0x *Diabetes mellitus without mention of complication* and 366.10 *Senile cataract, unspecified.*

Codes for diabetic retinopathy (250.5x and 362.0x) include:

- Macular edema in branch retinal vein occlusion
- Macular edema resulting in leakage within the retina
- Background or simple diabetic retinopathy with microaneurysms, hemorrhages, and/or cotton wool spots
- Malignant or proliferative diabetic retinopathy (e.g., retinal neovascularization with or without retinal hemorrhages)

Even though specific codes are available for retinal vein occlusion, macular edema, and retinal hemorrhage, these conditions are included in the codes for diabetic retinopathy and no additional codes are required.

For nondiabetic proliferative retinopathy, assign code 362.29 *Other nondiabetic proliferative retinopathy.*

Osteomyelitis: Diabetic osteomyelitis requires three codes to accurately identify the condition: 250.8x *Diabetes with other specified manifestations,* 731.8 *Other bone involvement in diseases classified elsewhere,* and a code from category 730 *Osteomyelitis, periostitis and other infections involving bone.*

Pregnancy: When coding a condition that is either a complication of pregnancy or that is complicating the pregnancy, always list the code for the obstetric complication first. Additional codes are assigned as needed to provide specificity. Essentially all pregnant diabetics have complications, either with the diabetes or the pregnancy, therefore two codes (648.0x and 250.0x) are always assigned.

Gestational diabetes is not a true diabetes but is often confused as such. Gestational diabetes is a condition that refers to abnormal glucose tolerance during pregnancy. In this condition, the patient may require treatment for control of blood glucose levels, but returns to normal glucose tolerance after childbirth. Use code 648.8x *Abnormal glucose tolerance for gestational diabetes.*

Secondary Diabetes: Secondary diabetes codes should not be selected from category 250. When it has been substantiated that the diabetes is secondary to another condition, code the underlying condition. For example, for postpancreatectomy diabetes, assign code 251.3 *Postsurgical hypoinsulinemia.*

Type I vs Type II: The primary factor that distinguishes between the Type I and Type II is the absence or presence of insulin. The Type I diabetic requires insulin to survive; however, there may be short symptom free periods also known as "honeymoon periods" during which insulin is not required. Type II diabetics can produce sufficient amounts but may receive insulin to assist the body in using the insulin that is present in the body. The Type II diabetic is not dependent on insulin to survive. The administration of insulin has no bearing on code assignment. Only the type (I or II) of diabetes influences the fifth-digit assignment for diabetic codes.

© 2004 Ingenix, Inc.

Diabetic Complication: Diabetic atherosclerosis of the extremities is coded as 250.7x *Diabetes with peripheral circulatory disorders* and 440.2x *Atherosclerosis of native arteries of extremities.* If the diagnosis is diabetes with ischemic heart disease or cerebrovascular disease, they are coded as separate entities.

When the documentation identifies a diabetic patient with cardiomyopathy, these conditions are coded as separate entities. The diabetic complication code 250.7x does not include cardiomyopathy.

Use an additional code to report long term (current) insulin use (V58.67) if applicable.

Coding Scenario

A patient is admitted with chronic renal failure for dialysis. The patient history indicates the patient is a Type II diabetic controlled by oral drugs.

> Code assignment: V56.0 *Encounter for extracorporeal dialysis,* 585 *Chronic renal failure,* and 250.00 *Diabetes mellitus without mention of complication, Type II or unspecified type, not stated as uncontrolled*

A 59-year-old male is seen in the physician's office for episodes of dizziness. He is found to have an elevated blood sugar level. Additional testing is done that shows a minimally elevated blood fasting and glucose tolerance test results within normal range. The physician documentation specifically indicates that diabetes mellitus was ruled out.

> Code assignment: 790.2 *Abnormal glucose tolerance test*

A 48-year-old female is seen in the clinic for her neurogenic bladder disorder secondary to diabetes. Documentation specifically indicates that she is an insulin-requiring Type II diabetic.

> Code assignment: 250.60 *Diabetes with neurological manifestations, Type II or unspecified type, not stated as uncontrolled,* 337.1 *Peripheral autonomic neuropathy in disorders classified elsewhere,* and 596.54 *Syndrome with neurogenic bladder*

A 55-year-old male is admitted with hypertension due to hypervolemia as a direct result of his chronic renal failure. Patient history indicates that the patient is a Type I diabetic with renal failure.

> Code assignment: 250.41 *Diabetes with renal manifestations, Type I, not stated as uncontrolled,* 405.99 *Other secondary hypertension,* 276.6 *Fluid overload,* and 585 *Chronic renal failure*

A 28-year-old male Type II diabetic is seen at a clinic for his chronic pseudo-obstruction of the intestine.

> Code assignment: 250.80 *Diabetes with other specified manifestations, Type II or unspecified, not stated as uncontrolled* and 564.89 *Other functional disorders of intestine*

A patient is admitted with diabetic neuropathy with secondary diabetes. Patient history identifies a previous history of a partial pancreatectomy that has caused the diabetic condition.

> Code assignment: 251.3 *Postsurgical hypoinsulinemia* and 357.4 *Polyneuropathy in other diseases classified elsewhere*

A Type I diabetic female is seen in the emergency department and is diagnosed with hypoglycemia. The physician identifies that the patient has been compliant with her prescribed insulin dosage.

> Code assignment: 250.81 *Diabetes with other specified manifestations, Type I, not stated as uncontrolled* and E932.3 *Adverse effect of insulin and antidiabetic agents*

A Type II diabetic comes into the emergency department after an accidental overdose of insulin. The patient is admitted with hypoglycemic shock.

> Code assignment: 962.3 *Poisonings by hormones and synthetic substitutes, insulin and antidiabetic agents,* 250.80 *Diabetes with other specified manifestations, Type II or unspecified, not stated as uncontrolled,* and E858.0 *Accidental poisoning by drugs, hormones and synthetic substitutes*

A patient is seen in the office for an eye examination that reveals a small snowflake cataract. This patient is a known Type I diabetic since 10 years of age. Verification with the physician confirms this is a diabetic cataract.

> Code assignment: 250.51 *Diabetes with ophthalmic manifestations, Type I, not stated as uncontrolled* and 366.41 *Diabetic cataract*

A Type II diabetic is admitted for a severe chronic left heel ulcer. The patient's history clarifies that the patient's foot ulcer is secondary to diabetic peripheral neuropathy. The final diagnostic statement confirms the diagnosis as diabetic peripheral autonomic neuropathy with chronic left heel ulcer.

> Code assignment: 250.60 *Diabetes with neurological manifestations, Type II or unspecified, not stated as uncontrolled,* 337.1 *Peripheral autonomic neuropathy in disorders classified elsewhere,* and 707.14 *Ulcer of heel and midfoot*

A patient is admitted for gangrene of the left leg secondary to diabetic arteriosclerosis. Record documentation identifies that the patient is a Type I diabetic requiring insulin.

> Code assignment: 250.71 *Diabetes with peripheral circulatory disorders, Type I, not stated as uncontrolled* and 440.24 *Atherosclerosis of the extremities with gangrene*

The physician's final diagnosis states hypertensive renal disease with chronic renal failure due to diabetes, Type II.

> Code assignment: 250.40 *Diabetes with renal manifestations, Type II or unspecified, not stated as uncontrolled* and 403.91 *Hypertensive renal disease with renal failure*

A patient is admitted for hemodialysis. The patient is a true insulin-dependent diabetic, Type I, with progressive nephropathy. The physician also documents chronic renal failure in the medical history.

> Code assignment: 250.41 *Diabetes with renal manifestations, Type I, not stated as uncontrolled,* 583.81 *Nephritis and nephropathy, not specified as acute or chronic, in diseases classified elsewhere,* and 585 *Chronic renal failure*

An elderly patient is transferred from an extended care facility for treatment of a decubitus ulcer. The physician also identifies the patient is a Type II diabetic with related progressive peripheral vascular disease.

> Code assignment: 707.00 *Decubitus ulcer, unspecified site,* 250.70 *Diabetes with peripheral circulatory disorders, Type II or unspecified, not stated as uncontrolled,* and 443.81 *Peripheral angiopathy in diseases classified elsewhere*

240–279

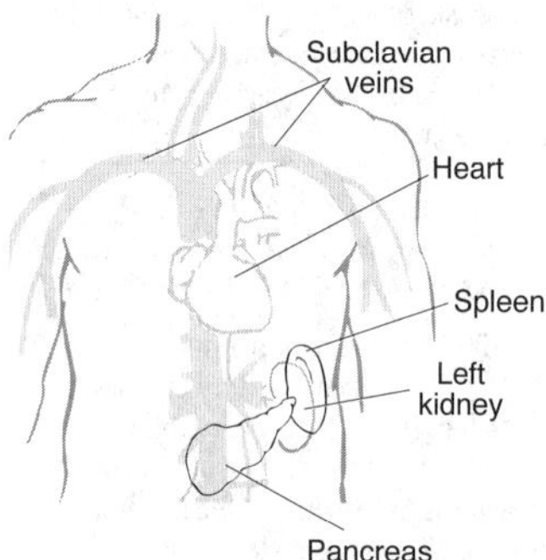

251 Other disorders of pancreatic internal secretion

Diabetes insipidus is caused by a deficiency of vasopressin, one of the antidiuretic hormones (ADH) secreted by the pituitary gland. Symptoms include increased thirst and urination. Treatment is with drugs, such as synthetic vasopressin, that help the body maintain water and electrolyte balance.

251.0 Hypoglycemic coma — (Use additional E code to identify drug, if drug induced) — *Non-diabetic insulin coma*
AHA: March-April, 1985, 8

251.1 Other specified hypoglycemia — (Use additional E code to identify drug, if drug induced) — *including hyperplasia of pancreatic islet beta cells NOS; Harris' syndrome*
AHA: Q1, 2003, 10

251.2 Hypoglycemia, unspecified — *not otherwise specified, including McQuarrie's syndrome*
AHA: March-April, 1985, 8

251.3 Postsurgical hypoinsulinemia — *following complete or partial pancreatectomy*
AHA: Q3, 1991, 6

251.4 Abnormality of secretion of glucagon — *hyperplasia of islet alpha cells with glucagon excess*

251.5 Abnormality of secretion of gastrin — *hyperplasia of alpha cells with gastrin excess; Zollinger-Ellison syndrome*

251.8 Other specified disorders of pancreatic internal secretion — *sclerotic islands of Langerhans*
AHA: Q3, 1991, 6; Q2, 1998, 15

251.9 Unspecified disorder of pancreatic internal secretion — *not elsewhere classified*

252 Disorders of parathyroid gland

The parathyroid glands are four small glands located at the four corners of the thyroid gland. The hormone secreted, parathyroid hormone, regulates the level of calcium in the blood.

Hyperparathyroidism is an excessive secretion of the parathyroid hormone (PTH) from one or more of the parathyroid glands. The parathyroid glands are four pea-sized glands located in the neck on the thyroid. In 85% of cases, a benign tumor, called an adenoma, is found on a gland that causes it be overactive. Most other cases of primary hyperparathyroidism result from enlargement or hyperplasia of two or more glands that also causes overactive hormone production.

Primary hyperparathyroidism is caused by a disorder of the parathyroid glands themselves that results in their secreting too much parathyroid hormone (PTH).

Secondary hyperparathyroidism results from releasing increased levels in response to deconditioning of the body to PTH due to another disease process, such as renal failure. PTH helps regulate the levels of calcium and phosphorus in the body, induces the release of calcium from bone, the amount of calcium taken from food, intestinal absorption of calcium, and the excretion of calcium in the urine. Hypercalcemia, or increased levels of calcium in the blood, is a sign of hyperparathyroidism, when accompanied by a concurrent increase in the level of PTH hormone.

252.00 Hyperparathyroidism, unspecified

252.01 Primary hyperparathyroidism

 © 2004 Ingenix, Inc.

252.02 Secondary hyperparathyroidism, non-renal

252.08 Other hyperparathyroidism

252.1 Hypoparathyroidism — *low secretion of parathyroid hormones causing a severe convulsive disorder known as tetany; parathyroiditis; parathyroid tetany*

252.8 Other specified disorders of parathyroid gland — *cyst, hemorrhage, or infarct*

252.9 Unspecified disorder of parathyroid gland

Coding Clarification

Code 252.02 reports hyperparathyroidism from non-renal causes. Report 588.81 for secondary hyperparathyroidism of renal origin.

Coding Scenario

A 65-year-old woman has come to her physician with fatigue, constipation and increased urination and thirst. The doctor orders urine and blood tests, which come back high for calcium and orders a blood test to check for PTH levels, which also returns high, blood sugar levels are normal. Once the diagnosis is established that she has primary hyperparathyroidism, the doctor has her follow up with a bone density exam and an abdominal radiograph to assess for kidney stones. The condition of an overactive, enlarged gland or benign tumor is discussed with surgical option of removal in the future.

> Code assignment: 252.01 *Primary hyperparathyroidism*

253 Disorders of the pituitary gland and its hypothalamic control

The hypothalamus controls the pituitary gland from deep within the brain. Acting as liaison between the brain and the pituitary gland, the hypothalamus is the primary link between the endocrine and nervous systems.

The pituitary, located in the base of the brain, secretes several hormones that regulate the function of the other endocrine glands. The pituitary gland is divided into two parts, the anterior and posterior lobes, each having separate functions. The anterior lobe regulates the activity of the thyroid, adrenal, and reproductive glands. It also regulates the body's growth and stimulates milk production in women who are breast-feeding. Hormones secreted by the anterior lobe include adrenocorticotropic hormone (ACTH), thyrotropic hormone (TSH), luteinizing hormone (LH), follicle-stimulating hormone (FSH), growth hormone (GH), and prolactin. The anterior lobe also secretes endorphins, chemicals that act on the nervous system to reduce sensitivity to pain.

The posterior lobe of the pituitary gland contains the nerve endings (axons) from the hypothalamus, which stimulate or suppress hormone production. This lobe secretes antidiuretic hormones (ADH), which control water balance in the body, and oxytocin, which controls muscle contractions in the uterus.

253.0 Acromegaly and gigantism — *acromegaly describes unusual growth beginning in middle age; gigantism usually begins in childhood. Both are caused by overproduction of pituitary growth hormone; Erdheim's, Launois', Marie's, syndromes*

253.1 Other and unspecified anterior pituitary hyperfunction — *Forbes-Albright and Argonz-Del Castillo syndromes*
AHA: July-Aug, 1985, 9

253.2 Panhypopituitarism — *organic pituitary dysfunction leading to impaired sexual function, fatigue, bradycardia, depression, and impaired growth in children; including cachexia, necrosis, insufficiency; Sheehan's, hypopituitarism, or postpartum-panhypopituitary syndromes*

253.3 Pituitary dwarfism — *with persistence of infantile physical characteristics due to under-secretion of growth hormone and gonadotropin deficiency; HGH deficiency, Lorain-Levi dwarfism, Burnier's syndrome, Nebecourt's syndrome*

253.4 Other anterior pituitary disorders — *isolated or partial deficiency of an anterior pituitary hormone, other than growth hormone; prolactin deficiency; Kallmann's syndrome*
AHA: July-Aug, 1985, 9

253.5 Diabetes insipidus — *insufficient diuretic hormone release; symptoms include frequent urination, thirst, and weight loss; vasopressin deficiency*

253.6 Other disorders of neurohypophysis — *syndrome of inappropriate secretion of antidiuretic hormone [ADH] and Schwartz-Bartter syndrome*

253.7 Iatrogenic pituitary disorders — (Use additional E code to identify cause) — *drug therapy, radiation therapy, or surgery, causing mild to severe symptoms*

253.8 Other disorders of the pituitary and other syndromes of diencephalohypophyseal origin — *abscess of pituitary; adiposogenital dystrophy; Rathke's pouch, pituitary or intrasellar cyst, empty sella; or hypophyseal, Launois-Cléret syndrome, Fröhlich's syndrome, Rénon-Delille syndrome*

253.9 Unspecified disorder of the pituitary gland and its hypothalamic control

254 Diseases of thymus gland

The thymus gland is comprised of lymphatic and epithelial tissue (Hassall's corpuscles) and is located in the anterior, superior mediastinum. The thymus processes white blood cells (WBC) known as lymphocytes, which kill foreign cells and stimulate

240–279

other immune cells to produce antibodies. The role of the thymus is not entirely understood, though it seems to be most important during infancy and until puberty, when the lymphatic tissue is chiefly replaced by fat. In adults, the thymus can be removed without significant impact on health.

Thymic disease in this rubric is classified as abscess, hyperplasia, or other specified disease.

254.0 Persistent hyperplasia of thymus — *continued, abnormal growth of the twin lymphoid lobes that produce T lymphocytes in the anterior superior mediastinum*

254.1 Abscess of thymus — *pocket of liquid puris caused by infection in the thymus*

254.8 Other specified diseases of thymus gland — *atrophy, cyst, hemorrhage, necrotic tissue, inflammation, thymicolymphaticus shunt, Kopp's asthma, hyperthymism*

254.9 Unspecified disease of thymus gland

Coding Clarification

Excluded from this rubric are aplasia, dysplasia, or hypoplasia of the thymus with immunodeficiency (279.2), myasthenia gravis (358.0), thymoma (212.6), and DiGeorge anomaly (279.11). Congenital absence of the thymus is classified to 759.2 *Anomalies of other endocrine glands.*

255 Disorders of adrenal glands

Located on the kidneys, the adrenal glands have two distinct parts. The outer, called the adrenal cortex, produces a variety of hormones called corticosteroids. Chief among the corticosteroids is cortisol, which regulates salt and water balance in the body, prepares the body for stress, regulates metabolism, interacts with the immune system, and influences sexual function. The inner part, the adrenal medulla, produces catecholamines, such as epinephrine, also called adrenaline, which increases the blood pressure and heart rate during times of stress.

Addison's disease is caused by decreased function of the adrenal cortex. Weakness, fatigue, abdominal pains, nausea, dehydration, fever, and hyperpigmentation (tanning without sun exposure) are among the possible symptoms. Treatment involves providing the body with replacement corticosteroid hormones as well as dietary salt.

Primary Cushing's syndrome is caused by excessive secretion of glucocorticoids, the subgroup of corticosteroid hormones that includes hydrocortisone, by the adrenal glands. Symptoms may develop over many years prior to diagnosis and may include obesity, physical weakness, easily bruised skin, acne, hypertension, and psychological changes. Treatment may include surgery, radiation therapy, chemotherapy, or blockage of hormone production with drugs.

Acromegaly and gigantism both are caused by a pituitary tumor that stimulates production of excessive growth hormone, causing abnormal growth in particular parts of the body. Acromegaly is rare and usually develops over many years in adult subjects. Gigantism occurs when the excess of growth hormone begins in childhood.

255.0 Cushing's syndrome — (Use additional E code to identify cause, if drug-induced) — *over-secretion of adrenal cortisol or use of glucocorticoid medications causing fat deposits in the head and neck and kyphosis; adrenal hyperplasia, ectopic ACTH syndrome*

255.10 Primary aldosteronism — *excessive aldosterone secretion, hypertension, renin suppression, hypokalemia*

255.11 Glucocorticoid-remediable aldosteronism — *inherited as an autosomal dominant trait, with moderate to severe hypertension, moderate hypersecretion of aldosterone, suppressed plasma renin activity , with rapid reversal of these abnormalities with glucocorticoids. Familial type.*

255.12 Conn's syndrome — *an aldosteronoma (benign adrenal tumor), usually less than 2 cm in diameter, benign, golden yellow, causing headaches, nocturia, plyuria, fatigue, hypertension, hypokalemic alkolosis, potassium depletion, hyperfolemia, decreased renin activity*

255.13 Bartter's syndrome — *found in children, hypokalemia alkolosis, elevated rennin, elevated angiotensin, low or normal blood pressure, no edema, retarded growth. Secondary hyperaldosteronism with juxtaglomerular hyperplasia, hyperaldosteronism with hypokalemic alkolosis*

255.14 Other secondary aldosteronism — *due to extra-adrenal disorders, increased renin, increased aldosterone, sodium retention, hypertensive state, secondary reninism due to decreased renal perfusion*

255.2 Adrenogenital disorders — *congenital or acquired disorders of the genitals due to adrenal dysfunction; Achard-Thiers syndrome, Apert-Gallais syndrome, Cooke-Apert-Gallais syndrome, Corticosexual syndrome, and Hercules syndrome*

255.3 Other corticoadrenal overactivity — *acquired benign adrenal androgenic overactivity; Schroeder's syndrome or Slocum's syndrome*

255.4 Corticoadrenal insufficiency — *underproduction of adrenal hormones causing low blood pressure; Addisonian crisis, Bernard-Sergent syndrome*

© 2004 Ingenix, Inc.

255.5 Other adrenal hypofunction — *adrenal medullary insufficiency*

255.6 Medulloadrenal hyperfunction — *catecholamine secretion by pheochromocytoma*

255.8 Other specified disorders of adrenal glands — *abnormality of cortisol-binding globulin, Adrenal collapse; adrenal/suprarenal cyst; adrenal obesity, inflammation, necrosis, sclerosis, swelling*

255.9 Unspecified disorder of adrenal glands

Coding Clarification

A secondary form of the disease can occur as a side effect of drug therapy, and is reported with the same code, 255.0 *Cushing's syndrome.*

Coding Scenario

A 49-year-old patient is seen in the clinic for adrenal-pituitary insufficiency secondary to steroids. The patient is a known steroid-dependent asthmatic.

> Code assignment: 255.4 *Corticoadrenal insufficiency,* 493.90 *Asthma, type unspecified,* and E932.0 *Drug causing adverse effects in therapeutic use, adrenal cortical steroids*

256 Ovarian dysfunction

AHA: Q4, 2000, 51

Female gonads secrete sex hormones in response to stimulation from the pituitary gland. Located in the pelvis, the ovaries produce eggs. They also secrete female sex hormones, estrogen and progesterone, which regulate development of the reproductive organs, female secondary sex characteristics, and menstruation and pregnancy.

256.0 Hyperestrogenism — *over-secretion by the ovary of estrogen*
AHA: Q4, 2000, 51

256.1 Other ovarian hyperfunction — *hypersecretion of ovarian androgens*
AHA: Q3, 1995, 15; Q4, 2000, 51

256.2 Postablative ovarian failure — (Use additional code for states associated with artificial menopause, 627.4) — *iatrogenic, postsurgical, postirradiation*
AHA: Q4, 2000, 51; Q2, 2002, 12

256.31 Premature menopause

256.39 Other ovarian failure — *delayed menarche, ovarian hypofunction, and primary ovarian failure NOS*
AHA: Q4, 2000, 51; Q4, 2001, 41

256.4 Polycystic ovaries — *containing multiple follicular cysts filled with serous fluid; isosexual virilization; Stein-Leventhal syndrome*
AHA: Q4, 2000, 51

256.8 Other ovarian dysfunction — *hyperthecosis, ovary*
AHA: Q4, 2000, 51

256.9 Unspecified ovarian dysfunction

Coding Clarification

The rubric excludes the acquired absence of an ovary (V45.77) and artificial menopause NOS (627.4).

257 Testicular dysfunction

Male gonads produce sperm and secrete androgens. The androgens, the most important of which is testosterone, regulate development of the reproductive organs, male secondary sex characteristics, and muscle.

257.0 Testicular hyperfunction — *over-secretion by the testicles of testosterone*

257.1 Postablative testicular hypofunction — *iatrogenic, postsurgical, postirradiation*

257.2 Other testicular hypofunction — *eunuchoidism; defective biosynthesis of testicular androgen; failure of Leydig's cell, adult; fertile eunuch, Reifenstein's syndrome*

257.8 Other testicular dysfunction — *male pseudohermaphroditism with testicular feminization; Goldberg-Maxwell syndrome, Morris syndrome*

257.9 Unspecified testicular dysfunction

258 Polyglandular dysfunction and related disorders

Autoimmune disorders affecting endocrine glands often occur in multiples. Hashimoto's thyroiditis, for example, often presents with Type I diabetes mellitus, hypoparathyroidism, or Addison's disease.

258.0 Polyglandular activity in multiple endocrine adenomatosis — *abnormal production of hormones by two or more endocrine glands due to hyperplasia; caused by genetic defects; Wermer's syndrome*

258.1 Other combinations of endocrine dysfunction — *Lloyd's syndrome, Schmidt's syndrome, Pierre Mauriac's syndrome*

258.8 Other specified polyglandular dysfunction — *atrophy pluriglandular; polyglandular sclerosis*

258.9 Unspecified polyglandular dysfunction

Coding Clarification

Schmidt's syndrome is Addison's disease with hypothyroidism secondary to Hashimoto's thyroiditis, and is reported with 258.1 *Other combinations of endocrine dysfunction.* In diabetes with hypothyroidism, report both conditions rather than this combination code since, as a significant systemic disease, diabetes should always be codified separately.

259 Other endocrine disorders

The parathyroid glands are four small glands located at the four corners of the thyroid gland. The hormone secreted, parathyroid hormone, regulates the level of calcium in the blood.

259.0 Delay in sexual development and puberty, not elsewhere classified — *delayed puberty*

259.1 Precocious sexual development and puberty, not elsewhere classified — *cryptogenic, constitutional, idiopathic*

259.2 Carcinoid syndrome — *Argentaffin syndrome, Björk (-Thorson) syndrome, Cassidy (-Scholte) syndrome, Hedinger's syndrome*

259.3 Ectopic hormone secretion, not elsewhere classified — *arising from an abnormal site or tissue: antidiuretic hormone secretion [ADH], hyperparathyroidism*
AHA: Nov-Dec, 1985, 4

259.4 Dwarfism, not elsewhere classified — *constitutional*

259.8 Other specified endocrine disorders — *pineal dysfunction, pineal calcification; Werner's syndrome, Donohue's syndrome, Gilford (-Hutchinson) syndrome, Pellizzi's, Progeria trigeminal plate syndrome; progeria, leprechaunism*

259.9 Unspecified endocrine disorder

Coding Clarification

Obesity due to underlying endocrine disease is reported with 259.9 *Unspecified endocrine disorder.*

260–269 Nutritional Deficiencies

In the United States, nutritional and vitamin deficiencies usually are the result of poverty, prolonged parenteral feeding, chronic substance abuse, food fads, or extreme diets. Malnutrition results from insufficiency in the body's total intake of energizing nutrients and proteins, and vitamin or mineral deficiencies are the result of insufficient intake of very specific nutrients. While patients with malnutrition may also commonly have vitamin or mineral deficiencies, it is also possible to develop a vitamin or mineral deficiency without malnutrition.

Coding Clarification

This group of rubrics excludes deficiency anemias, which are reported with 280.0-281.9.

260 Kwashiorkor OK

Kwashiorkor is an African word meaning "first-child, second-child." It refers to the protein-deficit illness that affects the first child when it is weaned to make room for the second child. Instead of protein-rich breast milk, the first child is fed a thin gruel made from sweet potato, banana, or cassava. The gruel is starchy, so there is no energy deficit, but the lack of protein causes edema, lethargy, and impaired growth. Kwashiorkor is considered a third-degree malnutrition disorder.

261 Nutritional marasmus OK

Marasmus results from near starvation with a deficit in protein and nonprotein intake. Typically, marasmus is a childhood disease in underdeveloped countries, and occurs when the mother is unable to breast-feed. The child is very thin, with little muscle or body fat. Marasmus is considered a third-degree malnutrition disorder.

262 Other severe protein-calorie malnutrition OK

AHA: July-Aug, 1985, 12; Q4, 1992, 24

Classify malnutrition to this rubric if there is nutritional edema without mention of dyspigmentation of skin and hair.

263 Other and unspecified protein-calorie malnutrition

AHA: Q4, 1992, 24

Malnutrition results from inadequate intake or malabsorption of nutrients. Infants and children are at highest risk for malnutrition, since there is a high demand for nutrients during the growth years. Pregnancy and old age also pose other significant risks for malnutrition, as does the presence of chronic disease or adherence to some diets. Substance abuse is also a risk factor for malnutrition.

263.0 Malnutrition of moderate degree — *second degree malnutrition characterized by superimposed biochemical changes in electrolytes, lipids, blood plasma.*
AHA: July-Aug, 1985, 1; Q4, 1992, 24

263.1 Malnutrition of mild degree — *first degree malnutrition characterized by tissue wasting in an adult or growth failure in a child, but few or no biochemical changes.*
AHA: July-Aug, 1985, 1; Q4, 1992, 24

263.2 Arrested development following protein-calorie malnutrition — *physical retardation due to malnutrition*
AHA: Q4, 1992, 24

263.8 Other protein-calorie malnutrition — *not elsewhere specified*
AHA: Q4, 1992, 24

263.9 Unspecified protein-calorie malnutrition

264 Vitamin A deficiency

Vitamin A is found in green, leafy vegetables, fish, and dairy products, and serious deficiency can cause growth retardation in children, blindness, and

© 2004 Ingenix, Inc.

increased susceptibility to infection. Vitamin A deficiency is common in kwashiorkor and is endemic in areas in which rice is the staple.

264.0 Vitamin A deficiency with conjunctival xerosis — *conjunctival dryness*

264.1 Vitamin A deficiency with conjunctival xerosis and Bitot's spot — *conjunctival dryness and superficial spots of keratinized epithelium; Bitot's spot in young child*

264.2 Vitamin A deficiency with corneal xerosis — *corneal dryness*

264.3 Vitamin A deficiency with corneal ulceration and xerosis — *corneal dryness and epithelial ulceration*

264.4 Vitamin A deficiency with keratomalacia — *corneal dryness progressing to corneal insensitivity, softness, necrosis; usually bilateral*

264.5 Vitamin A deficiency with night blindness — *failure of vision in dim light*

264.6 Vitamin A deficiency with xerophthalmic scars of cornea — *corneal scars caused by dryness*

264.7 Other ocular manifestations of vitamin A deficiency — *xerophthalmia*

264.8 Other manifestations of vitamin A deficiency — *follicular keratosis, xeroderma, phrynoderma*

264.9 Unspecified vitamin A deficiency

265 Thiamine and niacin deficiency states

Alcoholism is the main cause of thiamine deficiency in the United States. In other countries, it can result from eating a diet of highly polished rice. Infants can develop a thiamine deficiency when breast-fed by thiamine-deficient mothers. Thiamine deficiency causes beriberi, with its manifestations of neuritis, edema, and heart disease.

Niacin deficiency is called pellagra, and is characterized by a light-sensitive rash, diarrhea, glossitis, and psychosis. Pellagra is most common in countries in which corn is the main food source, and is rare in the United States.

265.0 Beriberi — *vitamin B1 deficiency characterized by neuritis, edema, and heart disease*

265.1 Other and unspecified manifestations of thiamine deficiency — *Gayet-Wernicke's syndrome*

265.2 Pellagra — *niacin deficiency causing disturbances in skin, digestion, psyche*

266 Deficiency of B-complex components

Ariboflavinosis is riboflavin, or vitamin B2, deficiency that causes inflammation of the lips, tongue fissures, corneal vascularization, and anemia. Ariboflavinosis is associated with deficiency of milk in the diet, though the disease can also occur secondarily in patients with chronic diseases affecting nutritional absorption.

Vitamin B6 is important in blood, the central nervous system, and skin metabolism. It is uncommon to find a primary deficiency in vitamin B6, but secondary deficiency can result in chronic diseases affecting nutritional absorption, in patients using oral contraceptives, or in alcoholism.

266.0 Ariboflavinosis — *vitamin B2 deficiency causing inflammation of the lips, tongue fissures, corneal vascularization, anemia.*
AHA: Sept-Oct, 1986, 10

266.1 Vitamin B6 deficiency — *skin, lip, and tongue disturbances, peripheral neuropathy, and in infants, convulsions*

266.2 Other B-complex deficiencies — *B12, burning feet syndrome, Gopalan's syndrome*

266.9 Unspecified vitamin B deficiency

Coding Clarification

Report vitamin B6 responsive sideroblastic anemia with 285.0.

267 Ascorbic acid deficiency OK

Vitamin C, or ascorbic acid, is essential for wound healing and connective tissue health and it facilitates absorption of iron. A deficiency in this vitamin is commonly called scurvy or Cheadle-Moller-Barlow syndrome. Vitamin C is common to many fruits and vegetables. Symptoms of scurvy include bleeding gums, weight loss, myalgias, and slowing of the healing process. The symptoms are reversed with ascorbic acid therapy.

Coding Clarification

Anemia related to vitamin C deficiency is reported with 281.8 *Anemia associated with other specified nutritional deficiency.*

268 Vitamin D deficiency

Vitamin D is found in yeast, eggs, and dairy products, fish liver oils, and is also created when skin is exposed to sunlight. Deficiency is commonly called "rickets" in children and osteomalacia in adults. The disease is rare in the United States, though seen occasionally in immigrants from India. Demineralization of bone and bone deformity are the most common side effects of vitamin D deficiency.

Diseases in this rubric are classified as active or late effect, and as rickets or adult osteomalacia.

268.0 Rickets, active — *vitamin D deficiency causing metabolic bone disease in children; rosary, rachitic*

268.1 Rickets, late effect — (Use additional code to identify the nature of late effect) — *distorted or demineralized bones as a result of vitamin D deficiency and stated to be a late effect or sequela of rickets*

268.2 Osteomalacia, unspecified — *vitamin D deficiency causing metabolic bone disease in adults; Looser-Debray syndrome, Milkman-Looser syndrome, Miller's disease*

268.9 Unspecified vitamin D deficiency — *viosterol deficiency*

Coding Clarification

Renal rickets is reported with 588.0 *Renal osteodystrophy* and celiac rickets is reported with 579.0 *Celiac disease.*

Rickets or osteomalacia can also be caused by a metabolic resistance to absorb vitamin D, rather than a deficiency in intake. If this is the case, report the resistance with 275.3 *Disorders of phosphorus metabolism.*

269 Other nutritional deficiencies

269.0 Deficiency of vitamin K

269.1 Deficiency of other vitamins — *including vitamins E and P*

269.2 Unspecified vitamin deficiency — *multiple vitamin deficiency not specified*

269.3 Mineral deficiency, not elsewhere classified — *dietary calcium, iodine*

269.8 Other nutritional deficiency — *not elsewhere classified*

269.9 Unspecified nutritional deficiency

Coding Clarification

Vitamin K deficiencies associated with hypoprothrombinemia and depression of coagulation are reported with 286.7. Vitamin K deficiency of the newborn is reported with 776.0 *Hemorrhagic disease of newborns.*

Do not use codes from this rubric to report failure to thrive or feeding problems. These conditions are classified to rubric 783. Deficiencies of calcium, potassium, and sodium are classified to rubrics 275 or 276.

270–279 Other Metabolic and Immunity Disorders

Use an additional code to identify any associated mental retardation.

270 Disorders of amino-acid transport and metabolism

270.0 Disturbances of amino-acid transport — (Use additional code to identify any associated mental retardation) — *cystinosis, renal glycinuria, cystinuria, Hartnup disease, Fanconi (-de Toni)*

270.1 Phenylketonuria (PKU) — (Use additional code to identify any associated mental retardation) — *inherited error of metabolism affecting phenylalanine; early diagnosis through screening blood test prevents mental retardation; hyperphenylalaninemia*

270.2 Other disturbances of aromatic amino-acid metabolism — (Use additional code to identify any associated mental retardation) — *albinism, hypertyrosinemia, alkaptonuria, Oasthouse urine disease, Mende's syndrome, Smith-Strang disease, van der Hoeve-Halbertsma-Waardenburg syndrome*
AHA: Q3, 1999, 20

270.3 Disturbances of branched-chain amino-acid metabolism — (Use additional code to identify any associated mental retardation) — *of leucine, isoleucine, and valine; hypervalinemia; intermittent branched-chain ketonuria; leucine-induced hypoglycemia; methylmalonic aciduria*
AHA: Q3, 2000, 8

270.4 Disturbances of sulphur-bearing amino-acid metabolism — (Use additional code to identify any associated mental retardation) — *cystathioninuria, cystathioninuria; disturbances of metabolism of methionine, homocystine, and cystathionine, homocystinuria*

270.5 Disturbances of histidine metabolism — (Use additional code to identify any associated mental retardation) — *carnosinemia, histidinemia, hyperhistidinemia, imidazole aminoaciduria*

270.6 Disorders of urea cycle metabolism — (Use additional code to identify any associated mental retardation) — *argininosuccinic aciduria; citrullinemia; disorders of metabolism of ornithine, citrulline, argininosuccinic acid, arginine, and ammonia*

270.7 Other disturbances of straight-chain amino-acid metabolism — (Use additional code to identify any associated mental retardation) — *glucoglycinuria; hyperglycinemia and other disturbances of metabolism of glycine, threonine, serine, glutamine, and lysine; pipecolic acidemia, methylmalonic aciduria with glycinemia*
AHA: Q3, 2000, 8

© 2004 Ingenix, Inc.

270.8 Other specified disorders of amino-acid metabolism — (Use additional code to identify any associated mental retardation) — *alaninemia, aminoacidopathy, ethanolaminuria, prolinemia, glycoprolinuria, prolinuria, hydroxyprolinemia, sarcosinemia familial iminoglycinuria, and Lowe-Terrey-MacLachlan syndrome*

270.9 Unspecified disorder of amino-acid metabolism — (Use additional code to identify any associated mental retardation)

Coding Clarification

Excluded from this rubric are abnormal findings without manifest disease (790.0-796.9), disorders of purine and pyrimidine metabolism (277.1-277.2), and gout (274.0-274.9).

271 Disorders of carbohydrate transport and metabolism

271.0 Glycogenosis — (Use additional code to identify any associated mental retardation) — *excessive storage of glycogen; amylopectinosis, glucose-6-phosphatase deficiency, McArdle's disease, Pompe's disease, von Gierke's disease*
AHA: Q1, 1998, 5

271.1 Galactosemia — (Use additional code to identify any associated mental retardation) — *galactose-1-phosphate uridyl transferase deficiency, galactosuria*

271.2 Hereditary fructose intolerance — (Use additional code to identify any associated mental retardation) — *essential benign fructosuria, fructosemia*

271.3 Intestinal disaccharidase deficiencies and disaccharide malabsorption — (Use additional code to identify any associated mental retardation) — *intolerance or malabsorption: glucose, lactose, or sucrose*

271.4 Renal glycosuria — (Use additional code to identify any associated mental retardation) — *abnormally large amount of sugar in the urine with normal blood sugar, caused by failure of the renal tubules to reabsorb glucose; renal diabetes*

271.8 Other specified disorders of carbohydrate transport and metabolism — (Use additional code to identify any associated mental retardation) — *essential benign pentosuria, mannosidosis, fucosidosis, oxalosis, xylosuria, Bird's disease, glycolic aciduria*

271.9 Unspecified disorder of carbohydrate transport and metabolism — (Use additional code to identify any associated mental retardation)

Coding Clarification

Excluded from this rubric are abnormality of secretion of glucagon (251.4), diabetes mellitus (rubric 250), hypoglycemia not otherwise specified (251.2), and mucopolysaccharidosis (277.5).

272 Disorders of lipoid metabolism

Cholesterol is a waxy fat that is present in the human body. Two sources contribute to the amount of cholesterol in the human body. First, the liver manufactures about 80 percent of it. Second, people consume it by eating animal products such as meat, eggs, and dairy products. Cholesterol is carried through the bloodstream by certain proteins (apolipoproteins). When these proteins wrap around cholesterol and other types of fats (lipids) to transport them through the bloodstream, they combine and are called lipoproteins.

There are three different types of lipoproteins that carry cholesterol through the bloodstream:

- High-density lipoproteins (HDL), which are associated with "good" cholesterol
- Low-density lipoproteins (LDL), which are associated with "bad" cholesterol
- Very low-density lipoproteins (VLDL), which are associated with "very bad" cholesterol

High levels of LDL cholesterol have been associated with arteriosclerosis (hardening of the arteries) and coronary artery disease. In contrast, high levels of HDL cholesterol have been shown to reduce some of the harmful effects of LDL cholesterol.

The following are cholesterol levels (all measurements are in milligrams per deciliter): Total cholesterol levels less than 200 are desirable; total cholesterol levels between 200 and 239 are borderline-high; total cholesterol levels that are 240 or higher are high and considered to be hypercholesterolemia.

272.0 Pure hypercholesterolemia — (Use additional code to identify any associated mental retardation) — *high cholesterol in the blood; familial, Fredrickson Type II A hyperlipoproteinemia; low-density-lipoid-type [LDL] hyperlipoproteinemia*

272.1 Pure hyperglyceridemia — (Use additional code to identify any associated mental retardation) — *elevated level of glyceride, a natural fatty acid, in the blood; endogenous hyperglyceridemia; Fredrickson Type IV hyperlipoproteinemia; very-low-density-lipoid-type [VLDL] hyperlipoproteinemia*

272.2 Mixed hyperlipidemia — (Use additional code to identify any associated mental retardation) — *elevated level of lipoprotein, a complex of fats and proteins, in the blood due to an inherited lipoprotein metabolism disorder; Fredrickson Type IIb or III hyperlipoproteinemia, hypercholesterolemia with endogenous hyperglyceridemia; tubo-eruptive xanthoma*

272.3 Hyperchylomicronemia — (Use additional code to identify any associated mental retardation) — *Bürger-Grütz syndrome; Fredrickson type I or V hyperlipoproteinemia; Hyperlipidemia, Group D*

272.4 Other and unspecified hyperlipidemia — (Use additional code to identify any associated mental retardation) — *elevated level of chylomicrons in the blood. Chylomicrons are a form of lipoproteins which transport dietary cholesterol and triglycerides from the small intestine to the blood; Seeley-Klionsky disease*

272.5 Lipoprotein deficiencies — (Use additional code to identify any associated mental retardation) — *abnormally low level of lipoprotein, a complex of fats and proteins, in the blood; abetalipoproteinemia, hypoalphalipoproteinemia; Bassen-Kornzweig syndrome; high-density lipoid deficiency*

272.6 Lipodystrophy — (Use additional code to identify any associated mental retardation. Use additional E code to identify cause, if iatrogenic) — *disturbance in fat metabolism causing abnormal distribution of the body's fatty tissue; Barraquer-Simons disease, Simons' syndrome*

272.7 Lipidoses — (Use additional code to identify any associated mental retardation) — *chemically-induced; Anderson's disease, Fabry's disease, Gaucher's disease, Niemann-Pick disease, pseudo-Hurler's or mucolipidosis III disease, Wolman's disease; Ruiter-Pompen (-Wyers) syndrome, sea-blue histiocyte syndrome*

272.8 Other disorders of lipoid metabolism — (Use additional code to identify any associated mental retardation) — *Hoffa's, Launois-Bensaude's, Anders' syndrome, Dercum's syndrome, Farber*

272.9 Unspecified disorder of lipoid metabolism — (Use additional code to identify any associated mental retardation)

Coding Clarification

Excluded from this rubric is localized cerebral lipidoses (330.1).

273 Disorders of plasma protein metabolism

Wadenstrom's is a rare chronic form of lymphoma which affects plasma cells. Abnormal plasma cells grow out of control and invade bone marrow, lymph nodes and spleen. The cells cause a thickening of the blood by producing an increased amount of an antibody called IgM. This disease affects men more often than women and may cause few symptoms in the early stages.

Alpha-1 is one of the most common and serious hereditary diseases seen in nearly every population. The cases that have been diagnosed are estimated to be less than 10% of those predicted to have Alpha-1. Millions of people are carriers of the deficient gene that causes Alpha-1 and may pass it on to the next generation.

A person with Alpha-1-antitrypsin deficiency carries a gene that produces an abnormal AAT protein that cannot be secreted by the liver. This results in a severe reduction of the circulating levels of the protein as well as damaging accumulation within the liver. The deficiency also results in lung disease, since the protein is designed to protect the lungs from destructive enzymatic activity.

Since Alpha-1 begins in the liver and is a hereditary problem, liver involvement is often seen in children more than in adults, although chronic liver disease can occur at any time in life. Alpha-1 deficiency is the leading genetic cause of liver transplantation in children. This disease is also a major cause of lung transplantation. Lung disease is usually seen in adults, often striking in the prime of life with debilitating lung damage.

273.0 Polyclonal hypergammaglobulinemia — (Use additional code to identify any associated mental retardation) — *elevated level of gamma globulins in the blood, frequently observed in patients with chronic infectious diseases, including Waldenström's*

273.1 Monoclonal paraproteinemia — (Use additional code to identify any associated mental retardation) — *presence of abnormal proteins in the blood plasma; benign monoclonal hypergammaglobulinemia [BMH], monoclonal gammopathy associated with lymphoplasmacytic dyscrasias, paraproteinemia secondary to malignant or inflammatory disease*

273.2 Other paraproteinemias — (Use additional code to identify any associated mental retardation) — *cryoglobulinemic purpura, vasculitis, mixed cryoglobulinemia*

240–279

© 2004 Ingenix, Inc.

273.3 Macroglobulinemia — (Use additional code to identify any associated mental retardation) — *elevated level of macroglobulins in the blood. Macroglobulins are plasma globulins with an unusually high molecular weight; Waldenström's macroglobulinemia*

273.4 Alpha-1-antitrypsin deficiency

273.8 Other disorders of plasma protein metabolism — (Use additional code to identify any associated mental retardation) — *bisalbuminemia; hyperglobulinemia; hypoalbuminemia; hypoproteinemia; pyroglobulinemia*
AHA: Q2, 1998, 11

273.9 Unspecified disorder of plasma protein metabolism — (Use additional code to identify any associated mental retardation)

Coding Clarification

Excluded from this rubric are agammaglobulinemia and hypogammaglobulinemia (279.0-279.2), coagulation defect (286.0-286.9), and hereditary hemolytic anemias (282.0-282.9).

Coding Scenario

A patient is seen at the clinic for symptoms of peripheral neuropathy. The physician's diagnosis states peripheral neuropathy secondary to POEMS syndrome.

> Code assignment: 273.8 *Other disorders of plasma protein metabolism* and 357.4 *Polyneuropathy in other diseases classified elsewhere*

An adult with a history of untreatable asthma and chronic respiratory infections undergoes pulmonary function testing that indicates decreased lung function. X-rays are taken that show a flattened diaphragm, and gas exchange testing shows that pulmonary emphysema is beginning. The physician orders a blood test for Alpha-1 levels, which return at 11 μ M/L. The levels are phenotyped and the patient is diagnosed with Alpha-1-antitrypsin deficiency emphysema (also known as "genetic" or "inherited" emphysema). Weekly replacement intravenous therapy for protein augmentation of Alpha-1 is initiated.

> Code Assignment: 273.4 *Alpha-1-antitrypsin deficiency*

274 Gout

AHA: Q2, 1995, 4

Deposits of monosodium urate or monohydrate crystals cause gout. The most common site for these deposits is around the joints, especially around the big toe. However, these deposits may be found in organ systems, too. Gout is classified according to site.

274.0 Gouty arthropathy — (Use additional code to identify any associated mental retardation) — *acute inflammatory arthritis caused by deposits of monosodium urate monohydrate crystals in the joints*
AHA: Q2, 1995, 4

274.10 Gouty nephropathy, unspecified — (Use additional code to identify any associated mental retardation) — *any kidney disease characterized by abnormal production and excretion of uric acid*
AHA: Nov-Dec, 1985, 15; Q2, 1995, 4

274.11 Uric acid nephrolithiasis — (Use additional code to identify any associated mental retardation) — *with sodium urate stones in the kidney*
AHA: Q2, 1995, 4

274.19 Other gouty nephropathy — (Use additional code to identify any associated mental retardation) — *not otherwise specified*
AHA: Q2, 1995, 4

274.81 Gouty tophi of ear — (Use additional code to identify any associated mental retardation) — *deposit of sodium urate inflaming external ear*
AHA: Q2, 1995, 4

274.82 Gouty tophi of other sites — (Use additional code to identify any associated mental retardation) — *heart*
AHA: Q2, 1995, 4

274.89 Gout with other specified manifestations — (Use additional code to identify any associated mental retardation. Use additional code to identify manifestations: 357.4, 364.11) — *dermatitis, eczema, episcleritis, iritis, neuritis, phlebitis*
AHA: Q2, 1995, 4

274.9 Gout, unspecified — (Use additional code to identify any associated mental retardation) — *podagra, thesaurismosis urate, uric acid diathesis*
AHA: Q2, 1995, 4

Coding Clarification

Pseudogout is classified to rubric 275. Excluded from this rubric is lead gout, which is classified to 984.0-984.9.

Coding Scenario

A 62-year-old male patient is seen by his physician complaining of pain in the left great toe. An x-ray is negative. Uric acid level is elevated. A diagnosis of gout is made and the patient is prescribed allopurinal.

> Code assignment: 274.0 *Gouty arthropathy*

275 Disorders of mineral metabolism

Hypercalcemia includes symptoms of nausea, vomiting, anorexia, fever, and constipation. Pseudogout is chondrocalcinosis, a disorder of calcium metabolism. Joint disease is due to deposits of dicalcium phosphate or pyrophosphate crystals.

275.0 Disorders of iron metabolism — (Use additional code to identify any associated mental retardation) — *bronzed diabetes, pigmentary cirrhosis, hemochromatosis, Troisier-Hanot-Chauffard syndrome, von Recklinghausen-Applebaum disease*
AHA: Q2, 1997, 11

275.1 Disorders of copper metabolism — (Use additional code to identify any associated mental retardation) — *hepatolenticular degeneration; Wilson's disease; amyostatic syndrome, chorea-athetosis-agitans syndrome, Westphal-Strümpel syndrome*

275.2 Disorders of magnesium metabolism — (Use additional code to identify any associated mental retardation) — *hypermagnesemia, hypomagnesemia*

275.3 Disorders of phosphorus metabolism — (Use additional code to identify any associated mental retardation) — *familial hypophosphatemia, vitamin*

275.40 Unspecified disorder of calcium metabolism — (Use additional code to identify any associated mental retardation)

275.41 Hypocalcemia — (Use additional code to identify any associated mental retardation) — *low level of calcium in the blood with possible symptoms including muscle or abdominal cramps, tendon reflex anomalies, or carpopedal spasms*
AHA: Q4, 1997, 33

275.42 Hypercalcemia — (Use additional code to identify any associated mental retardation) — *elevated level of calcium in the blood with possible symptoms including fatigue, nausea, constipation, depression*
AHA: Q4, 1997, 33; Q4, 2003, 110

275.49 Other disorders of calcium metabolism — (Use additional code to identify any associated mental retardation) — *nephrocalcinosis; pseudohypoparathyroidism; pseudopseudohypoparathyroidism; and Martin-Albright syndrome, Seabright-Bantam syndromes*
AHA: Q4, 1997, 33

275.8 Other specified disorders of mineral metabolism — (Use additional code to identify any associated mental retardation) — *not elsewhere classified*

275.9 Unspecified disorder of mineral metabolism — (Use additional code to identify any associated mental retardation)

Coding Clarification

Iron Overload due to Transfusions: If a sickle cell patient is admitted with an iron overload (hemochromatosis) due to transfusion, three codes would be required: 275.0 *Disorders of iron metabolism for the hemochromatosis*, 282.60 for the sickle cell, and E934.7 *Drugs, medicinal and biological substances causing adverse effects in therapeutic use, natural blood and blood products*, to identify the adverse reaction of the iron overload from the blood.

Patients being treated with chronic transfusions necessitated by their sickle cell anemia are often treated with prophylactic therapy to prevent iron overload. If the patient is noncompliant with this therapy and is admitted for a high dose infusion to prevent an overload, then two codes would be necessary: 282.60 *Sickle-cell disease, unspecified* and V15.81 *Noncompliance with medical treatment.*

276 Disorders of fluid, electrolyte, and acid-base balance

Dehydration is the depletion of total body water and sodium. Dehydration may follow bouts of diarrhea, vomiting, or profuse sweating. It is often a manifestation of the patient's illness (e.g., gastroenteritis), and in such cases, the code for dehydration would not be sequenced first. However, if the patient's dehydration becomes significant enough to warrant separate treatment for rehydration, the dehydration code would be sequenced first.

276.0 Hyperosmolality and/or hypernatremia — (Use additional code to identify any associated mental retardation) — *sodium [Na] excess or overload*

276.1 Hyposmolality and/or hyponatremia — (Use additional code to identify any associated mental retardation) — *sodium [Na] deficiency*

276.2 Acidosis — (Use additional code to identify any associated mental retardation) — *accumulation of acid or depletion of alkali in blood and body tissues; metabolic or respiratory*
AHA: Jan-Feb, 1987, 15

276.3 Alkalosis — (Use additional code to identify any associated mental retardation) — *accumulation of base or loss of acid without relative loss of base in body fluids, caused by increased arterial plasma bicarbonate concentration or by abnormal loss of carbon dioxide due to hyperventilation; metabolic or respiratory*

© 2004 Ingenix, Inc.

276.4 Mixed acid-base balance disorder — (Use additional code to identify any associated mental retardation) — *hypercapnia with mixed acid-base disorder*

276.5 Volume depletion — (Use additional code to identify any associated mental retardation) — *dehydration, hypovolemia, Luetscher's syndrome*
AHA: Q2, 1988, 9; Q4, 1997, 30; Q3, 2002, 21

276.6 Fluid overload — (Use additional code to identify any associated mental retardation) — *fluid retention*

276.7 Hyperpotassemia — (Use additional code to identify any associated mental retardation) — *elevated level of potassium in the blood with symptoms including abnormal EKG readings and weakness; often associated with defective renal excretion; hyperkalemia, potassium [K] intoxication*
AHA: Q2, 2001, 12

276.8 Hypopotassemia — (Use additional code to identify any associated mental retardation) — *decreased level of potassium in the blood with symptoms including neuromuscular disorders; often associated with potassium loss through vomiting and diarrhea; hypokalemia*

276.9 Electrolyte and fluid disorders not elsewhere classified — (Use additional code to identify any associated mental retardation) — *electrolyte imbalance, hypochloremia, hyperchloremia, disequilibrium syndrome*
AHA: Jan-Feb, 1987, 15

Documentation Issues

Sequencing: Because dehydration is often the result of another condition as well as a difficult management issue in itself, it causes confusion for coders when sequencing the codes. The decision of when dehydration is listed first is dependent upon the documented reason for the admission/visit as determined by the physician. If, after study, dehydration is determined to be the condition chiefly responsible for occasioning the admission of the patient to the hospital, or the primary reason for the outpatient visit, then the dehydration should be listed first.

If the physician has documented that the patient was being treated for gastroenteritis on an outpatient basis, and the patient's dehydration became so severe he/she was admitted to the hospital for IV rehydration, the dehydration code (276.5) should be listed first followed by the code for the gastroenteritis (558.9) on the hospital claim.

If the physician indicates in the documentation that the patient was admitted for treatment of severe burns and dehydration secondary to the burns, the burn code would be listed first and the dehydration code would be listed second.

If the documentation in the record indicates that the patient has metabolic acidosis and diabetes, clarify with the physician if there is a direct cause and effect relationship. Note that code 276.2 has an exclusion note for diabetic acidosis and references code 250.1x.

If the documentation does not identify the reason chiefly responsible for the admission/encounter, clarification must be obtained from the physician. Be sure the physician clearly documents the reason for the admission/encounter in the medical record.

Coding Clarification

Etiology: Dehydration is the depletion or deprivation of water, causing an imbalance in homeostasis. Symptoms and signs of dehydration may be a direct result of inadequate intake of fluid, diarrhea, vomiting, sweating, or polyuria. In severe cases, patients may be lethargic, weak, and obtunded. Conditions such as shock and coma may also occur. Many conditions are accompanied by dehydration, such as gastroenteritis, intestinal disorders, burns, renal failure, urinary tract infections, cryptosporidiosis, ascites, and diabetic glycosuria.

When reporting volume depletion due to chemotherapy, also report E933.1 *Drugs, medicinal, and biological substances, causing adverse effects in therapeutic use, antineoplastic and immunosuppresive drugs.*

In ICD-9-CM, the same code, 276.5 *Volume depletion,* reports dehydration and hypovolemia. Dehydration is the depletion of total body water and sodium; hypovolemia speaks specifically to a reduction of volume and concentration of contents of the blood seen as a result of dehydration.

Dialysis Disequilibrium Syndrome: This condition is reported with code 276.9 *Electrolyte and fluid disorder not elsewhere classified.* Code also the underlying disease such as chronic renal failure (585), and also report the renal dialysis status (V45.1).

Coding Scenario

A 19-year-old patient is admitted to the hospital for IV rehydration. The physician documents that the patient is currently being treated with Kaopectate for his diarrhea but his dehydration became so severe that it was necessary to admit for IV therapy. The final diagnosis is documented as dehydration due to viral gastroenteritis.

> Code assignment: 276.5 *Volume depletion* and 008.8 *Intestinal infection due to other organism, not elsewhere classified*

A patient with known HIV is admitted with a diagnosis of diarrhea and dehydration. The physician's final diagnosis was cryptosporidiosis with dehydration secondary to HIV disease.

240–279

Code assignment: 042 *Human immunodeficiency virus [HIV] disease,* 007.4 *Cryptosporidiosis,* and 276.5 *Volume depletion*

A 49-year-old female is admitted for severe dehydration. The patient is known to have lung cancer with generalized metastases. The patient is treated with IV fluids for the dehydration. The patient's cancer is not treated during this admission.

Code assignment: 276.5 *Volume depletion,* 162.9 *Malignant neoplasm of bronchus and lung, unspecified,* and 199.0 *Malignant neoplasm, disseminated*

277 Other and unspecified disorders of metabolism

Cystic fibrosis is a hereditary disorder in which the body secretes thick, sticky mucus that clogs organs and leads to problems with breathing and digestion. About 30,000 children and young adults in the United States have cystic fibrosis. The disease affects one in 2,500 Caucasians and one in 17,000 African-Americans.

Cystic fibrosis is caused by a defect in the manufacture of cystic fibrosis transmembrane conductance regulator (CFTR). Normally, CFTR forms a channel through which chloride ions traverse the cells lining the lungs, pancreas, sweat glands, and small intestine. With cystic fibrosis, malfunctioning CFTR precludes chloride from entering or leaving cells, resulting in production of thick, sticky mucus. In the lungs, this mucus blocks airways. In the digestive system, the mucus prevents enzymes produced in the pancreas from reaching the intestines, impairing digestion. In addition, the malfunctioning CFTR causes excessive amounts of salt to escape in the sweat.

Cystic fibrosis is an autosomal recessive genetic disorder. To have cystic fibrosis, both parents must carry the disease. One in 31 people in the United States carries the gene. With two carriers, there is a 25 percent chance of producing a child with cystic fibrosis.

Cystic fibrosis symptoms may be apparent soon after birth, or the symptoms may go undiagnosed for years. In 20 percent of cases, the first symptom is meconium ileus, intestinal blockage in newborns, which may require surgery.

Disorders of fatty acid oxidation are genetic metabolic disorders that render the body incapable of breaking down fatty acids to make that energy available. Different types of specific enzyme deficiencies, in which one may be missing or improperly functioning, may manifest themselves as the cause. If undiagnosed, fatty acid oxidation disorders can result in serious complications of the liver, heart, eyes, and muscle development, and may lead to coma and possibly death, especially if metabolic crisis arises after a fasting period, such as during an infection or flu. Other signs include chronic bouts of low blood sugar, vomiting, diarrhea, lethargy, and even seizures.

Medium-chain acyl-CoA dehydrogenase deficiency (MCAD) is a disorder of the enzyme involved in mitochondrial fatty acid B-oxidation. This is usually diagnosed when a child is between three and 24 months of age, but may present later. Once the diagnosis is made, the child will require increased feedings to prevent long periods of fasting.

Peroxisomal disorders are problems at the subcellular level involving the improper formation or functioning of peroxisomes. These are special compartments within cells, called organelles, that are bound by their own membrane and contain certain enzymes. These peroxisomes help to do a number of jobs that are needed for digestion, producing certain hormones, and making the nervous system work properly. Peroxisomal disorders occur when a defect in the assembly of the peroxisome happens, such as when needed proteins fail to transport inside the peroxisome membrane, or a defect in a specific, single function of the peroxisome arises.

Mitochondria are another of the subcellular compartment organelles separated from the rest of the cell by its own membrane and containing its own DNA. The mitochondrion is responsible for handling the energy considerations of the cell. Many different clinical problems can present with mitochondrial metabolism disorders, especially involving neurological problems, such as mitochondrial encephalopathies and myoclonus with epilepsy.

277.00 Cystic fibrosis without mention of meconium ileus — (Use additional code to identify any associated mental retardation) — *genetic disorder causing pancreatic and respiratory deficiencies.*
AHA: Q3, 1990, 18; Q4, 1990, 16; Q2, 2003, 12

277.01 Cystic fibrosis with meconium ileus — (Use additional code to identify any associated mental retardation) — *inherited disorder causing pancreatic and respiratory deficiencies; with meconium ileus present at birth*
AHA: Q3, 1990, 18; Q4, 1990, 16

277.02 Cystic fibrosis with pulmonary manifestations — (Use additional code to identify any associated mental retardation. Use additional code to identify any infectious organism present)

277.03 Cystic fibrosis with gastrointestinal manifestations — (Use additional code to identify any associated mental retardation)

277.09 Cystic fibrosis with other manifestations — (Use additional code to identify any associated mental retardation)

© 2004 Ingenix, Inc.

277.1 Disorders of porphyrin metabolism — (Use additional code to identify any associated mental retardation) — *hematoporphyria, hematoporphyrinuria, hereditary coproporphyria, porphyrinuria, protocoproporphyria, Günther's syndrome*

277.2 Other disorders of purine and pyrimidine metabolism — (Use additional code to identify any associated mental retardation) — *hypoxanthine-guanine-phosphoribosyltransferase deficiency [HG-PRT deficiency], Lesch-Nyhan syndrome, xanthinuria*

277.3 Amyloidosis — (Use additional code to identify any associated mental retardation) — *accumulation of insoluble fibrillar proteins compromising organ function; familial Mediterranean fever, hereditary cardiac amyloidosis, Reimann's periodic disease, Siegal-Cattan-Mamou disease*
AHA: Q1, 1996, 16

277.4 Disorders of bilirubin excretion — (Use additional code to identify any associated mental retardation) — *hyperbilirubinemia; Dubin-Johnson syndrome, Gilbert's syndrome, Rotor's syndrome, Crigler-Najjar syndrome*

277.5 Mucopolysaccharidosis — (Use additional code to identify any associated mental retardation) — *gargoylism; osteochondrodystrophy; lipochondrodystrophy; Morquio-Brailsford disease, Hunter's syndrome, Hurler's syndrome, Sanfilippo's syndrome, Scheie's syndrome, Maroteaux-Lamy syndrome*

277.6 Other deficiencies of circulating enzymes — (Use additional code to identify any associated mental retardation) — *alpha 1-antitrypsin deficiency, hereditary angioedema*

277.7 Dysmetabolic Syndrome X — (Use additional code for associated manifestations: 278.00, 278.01, 414.00-414.07. Use additional code to identify any associated mental retardation.)

277.81 Primary carnitine deficiency — (Use additional code to identify any associated mental retardation) — *decreased carnitine, impairs fatty acid oxidation, not associated with another identifiable systemic illness*

277.82 Carnitine deficiency due to inborn errors of metabolism — (Use additional code to identify any associated mental retardation) — *one or more missing enzyme(s) for metabolic process or partial enzyme processing. Cannot break down fats, sugars, proteins for energy. Malaise, cardiomyopathy, seizures, developmental delay, slow growth, slow weight gain, hypoglycemia*

277.83 Iatrogenic carnitine deficiency — (Use additional code to identify any associated mental retardation) — *may be caused by dialysis, ingestion of valproic acid, pivampicillin, emetine, zidovudine, ketogenic diet*

277.84 Other secondary carnitine deficiency — (Use additional code to identify any associated mental retardation) — *Medical conditions decreasing levels of carnitine in plasma or tissues - cirrhosis, chronic renal failure, diabetes mellitus, heart failure, Alzheimer disease*

277.85 Disorders of fatty acid oxidation

277.86 Peroxisomal disorders

277.87 Disorders of mitochondrial metabolism

277.89 Other specified disorders of metabolism — (Use additional code to identify any associated mental retardation) — *Chronic histiosytosis, chronic histiosytosis X, acatalasemia, reticulohistiocytoma, craniohypophyseal xanthomatosis, Christian's syndrome, Hand-Schuller-Christian syndrome*

277.9 Unspecified disorder of metabolism — (Use additional code to identify any associated mental retardation)

Coding Scenario

A 5-year-old patient is admitted with acute bronchitis and possible cystic fibrosis. A chest x-ray is performed, confirming the diagnosis of cystic fibrosis. The diagnosis at discharge is acute bronchitis and cystic fibrosis.

> Code assignment: 466.0 *Acute bronchitis* and 277.00 *Cystic fibrosis without mention of meconium ileus*

A 1-year-old presents to the emergency room for anorexia with vomiting, lethargy, and fever. Initial blood test shows the child to be very hypoglycemic. A complete metabolic profile, CBC with differential, and carnitine level testing is run. The child is immediately started on a glucose IV to raise and maintain blood sugar levels. The physician diagnoses Medium-Chain Acyl-CoA Dehydrogenase Deficiency (MCAD). Diet requirements and eating habits are established and discussed with the patient's parents.

> Code assignment: 277.85 *Disorders of fatty acid oxidation*

278 Obesity and other hyperalimentation

Obesity is defined as a condition in which the body weight of the patient is at least 30 percent above the ideal weight as seen on standardized weight charts. Codes from this rubric are reported to classify obesity when no underlying condition exists, for instance, underlying endocrine disease (259.9).

Obesity is epidemic in the United States. It is more common among women than among men and more common among African-Americans than Caucasians. Obesity occurs when caloric intake chronically outpaces the energy required. Obesity puts patients at risk for diabetes, hypertension, and coronary artery disease.

Obesity is classified in this rubric as morbid obesity or unspecified obesity. Morbid obesity is defined as obesity in which the patient weighs at least double the ideal weight as seen on standardized weight charts.

278.00 Obesity, unspecified — (Use additional code to identify any associated mental retardation) — *not elsewhere classified*
AHA: Q1, 1999, 5,6; Q4, 2001, 42

278.01 Morbid obesity — (Use additional code to identify any associated mental retardation) — *125% or more over normal body weight*
AHA: Q3, 2003, 6-8

278.1 Localized adiposity — (Use additional code to identify any associated mental retardation) — *fat pad*

278.2 Hypervitaminosis A — (Use additional code to identify any associated mental retardation)

278.3 Hypercarotinemia — (Use additional code to identify any associated mental retardation) — *elevated blood carotene levels due to ingestion of excessive amounts of carotenoids or from an inability to convert carotenoids to vitamin A*

278.4 Hypervitaminosis D — (Use additional code to identify any associated mental retardation) — *ingestion of an excessive amount of vitamin D resulting in weakness, fatigue, loss of weight, and other symptoms.*

278.8 Other hyperalimentation — (Use additional code to identify any associated mental retardation) — *cardiopulmonary obesity syndrome, Pickwickian syndrome*

279 Disorders involving the immune mechanism

279.00 Unspecified hypogammaglobulinemia — (Use additional code to identify any associated mental retardation) — *abnormally low levels of immunoglobulins in the blood; agammaglobulinemia or antibody deficiency syndrome*

279.01 Selective IgA immunodeficiency — (Use additional code to identify any associated mental retardation)

279.02 Selective IgM immunodeficiency — (Use additional code to identify any associated mental retardation)

279.03 Other selective immunoglobulin deficiencies — (Use additional code to identify any associated mental retardation) — *selective deficiency of IgG*

279.04 Congenital hypogammaglobulinemia — (Use additional code to identify any associated mental retardation) — *Bruton's type, x-linked agammaglobulinemia, congenital antibody deficiency syndrome*

279.05 Immunodeficiency with increased IgM — (Use additional code to identify any associated mental retardation) — *autosomal recessive and x-linked immunodeficiency with hyper-IgM*

279.06 Common variable immunodeficiency — (Use additional code to identify any associated mental retardation) — *dysgammaglobulinemia and hypogammaglobulinemia*

279.09 Other deficiency of humoral immunity — (Use additional code to identify any associated mental retardation) — *transient hypogammaglobulinemia of infancy*

279.10 Unspecified immunodeficiency with predominant T-cell defect — (Use additional code to identify any associated mental retardation)

279.11 DiGeorge's syndrome — (Use additional code to identify any associated mental retardation) — *pharyngeal pouch syndrome and thymic hypoplasia*

279.12 Wiskott-Aldrich syndrome — (Use additional code to identify any associated mental retardation) — *eczema-thrombocytopenia syndrome*

279.13 Nezelof's syndrome — (Use additional code to identify any associated mental retardation) — *cellular immunodeficiency with abnormal immunoglobulin deficiency*

279.19 Other deficiency of cell-mediated immunity — (Use additional code to identify any associated mental retardation) — *not elsewhere classified*

 © 2004 Ingenix, Inc.

279.2 Combined immunity deficiency — (Use additional code to identify any associated mental retardation) — *agammaglobulinemia; severe combined immunodeficiency [SCID]; thymic alymphoplasia, aplasia or dysplasia with immunodeficiency*

279.3 Unspecified immunity deficiency — (Use additional code to identify any associated mental retardation)

279.4 Autoimmune disease, not elsewhere classified — (Use additional code to identify any associated mental retardation) — *not elsewhere classified*

279.8 Other specified disorders involving the immune mechanism — (Use additional code to identify any associated mental retardation) — *single complement [C1-C9] deficiency or dysfunction, hypocomplementemia*

279.9 Unspecified disorder of immune mechanism — (Use additional code to identify any associated mental retardation)

Coding Clarification

Transplant failure or rejection is classified to the rubric 996 rather than to this rubric.

240–279

280–289
Diseases of the Blood and Blood-Forming Organs

This chapter classifies diseases and disorders of blood and blood-forming (hemopoietic) organs, including anemias, coagulation defects, purpura and other hemorrhagic conditions, diseases of white blood cells, other diseases of blood, and blood-forming organs.

Bone marrow is the principal site for hemopoietic cell proliferation and differentiation. One of the largest organs in the human body, hemopoietic tissue is responsible for producing erythrocytes (red blood cells), neutrophils, eosinophils, basophils, monocytes, platelets, and lymphocytes.

The term "anemia" refers to a lower than normal erythrocyte count or level of hemoglobin in the circulating blood. A clinical sign rather than a diagnostic entity, anemia can be classified by three morphological variations of the erythrocyte: size (volume), hemoglobin content, and shape. These variations give clinicians clues to the specific type of anemia.

In laboratory blood tests, erythrocyte size is gauged by estimating the volume of red cells in the circulating blood. Red cell volume, or mean corpuscular volume, is estimated by dividing the patient's hematocrit (percentage of red blood cells in whole blood) by the red blood cell (count) (RBC). Normal values are normocytic, abnormally low values are microcytic, and abnormally high values are macrocytic.

Hemoglobin content refers to the average amount of hemoglobin in each red blood cell. This value, called the mean cell hemoglobin, is calculated by dividing the patient's hemoglobin by the number of red blood cells. Normal values are normochromic, less than normal values are hypochromic, and greater than normal values are hyperchromic.

Shape is determined by microscopy. Normally, red blood cells have a smooth concave shape. Erythrocytes with irregular shapes are called poikilocytes, a general term meaning abnormally shaped. Terms referring to specific abnormal cell shapes include acanthocytes, leptocytes, nucleated erythrocytes, macro-ovalocytes, schistocytes, helmet cells, teardrop cells, sickle cells, and target cells.

Once the cell morphology is determined, the anemia can be further classified based on certain physiological and pathological criteria. For example, constitutional aplastic anemia (284.0) is classified physiologically as an anemia of hypoproliferation and pathologically as inborn error of heredity.

The term "coagulation defect" refers to deficiencies or disorders of hemostasis. A complicated process involving substances in the injured tissues, formed elements of blood (platelets, monocytes), and the coagulation proteins, coagulation requires the production of thrombin, a substance that stabilizes the platelet plug and forms the fibrin clot. Together, they mechanically block the extravasation of blood from ruptured vessels.

The coagulation process can be interrupted by a genetic or disease-caused protein deficiency, by an increase in the catabolism of coagulation proteins, or by antibodies directed against the coagulation proteins. There are many proteins involved in coagulation, many of which are identified by the term "factor" followed by a Roman numeral. The appropriate Roman numeral followed by the suffix "a" indicates the activated form of a coagulation factor. For example, when the protein Factor II (prothrombin) is activated by the enzyme thrombin, it is designated Factor IIa.

The term "purpura" refers to a condition characterized by hemorrhage, or extravasation of blood, into the tissues, producing bruises and small red patches on the skin. Purpura may be associated with thrombocytopenia or can occur in a nonthrombocytopenic form. Thrombocytopenia is a decrease of the number of platelets in the circulating blood and may be primary (hereditary or idiopathic) or secondary to a known cause.

Diseases of white blood cells refers to increases, decreases, or genetic or idiopathic anomalies of white blood cells not associated with malignant disease classified to categories 200-208.

Excluded from this rubric is anemia complicating pregnancy and the puerperium, classified to category 648.2x.

280 Iron deficiency anemias

Classified to this rubric are chronic hypochromic and microcytic anemias characterized by small, pale erythrocytes and a depletion of iron stores. In adults, iron deficiency anemia is almost always due to blood loss, with loss of as little as 2-4 ml of blood per day enough to deplete iron stores. This condition also is known as hypoferric anemia, hypochromic or microcytic anemia, and chlorosis.

Signs and symptoms of iron deficiency anemias include pallor, lassitude, somnolence, pica, pagophagia, vertigo, headache, tinnitus, behavioral changes, dyspnea, palpitations, anginal chest pains, and brittle hair and nails. Blood work shows hypochromia, microcytosis, and erythrocyte count less reduced than hemoglobin, serum ferritin below 12 ng/ml, low serum iron, and increased total iron-binding capacity. Bone marrow biopsy shows absence of hemosiderin. Associated conditions include Plummer-Vinson syndrome, glossitis, cheilosis, and koilonychia. Therapies include iron supplementation, either dietary (ferrous sulfate, ferrous gluconate) or parenteral (iron dextran, such as Imferon or similar agent), and blood or blood product transfusion in severe cases.

280.0 Iron deficiency anemia secondary to blood loss (chronic) — *normocytic anemia due to blood loss*
AHA: Q4, 1993, 34

Subcategory 280.0 classifies iron deficiency anemia due to prolonged blood loss, usually from a chronically bleeding lesion in the gastrointestinal tract, such as a gastric ulcer or diverticulitis, or a urologic or gynecologic site.

Signs and symptoms of iron deficiency anemias secondary to blood loss (chronic) include history of a chronically bleeding lesion, pallor, lassitude, somnolence, pica, pagophagia, vertigo, headache, tinnitus, behavioral changes, dyspnea, palpitations, anginal chest pains, and brittle hair and nails. Guaiac test reveals occult bleeding. Blood work shows hypochromia, microcytosis, erythrocyte count less reduced than hemoglobin, serum ferritin below 12 ng/ml, low serum iron, and increased total iron-binding capacity. Bone marrow biopsy shows absence of hemosiderin. Therapies include endoscopy to determine the bleeding site, iron supplementation, either dietary (ferrous sulfate, ferrous gluconate) or parenteral (iron dextran, such as Imferon or similar agent), and blood or blood product transfusion in severe cases.

Coding Clarification

Excluded from this rubric is acute posthemorrhagic anemia (285.1).

Excluded from this rubric is familial microcytic anemia (282.4).

280.1 Iron deficiency anemia secondary to inadequate dietary iron intake — *dietary anemia*

Subcategory 280.1 classifies iron deficiency anemia due to excretion of iron that exceeds normal dietary intake. Iron is recycled metabolically so that less than 1 milligram is lost through excretion per day. A normal diet consists of 12-15 mg of iron, of which 0.6-1.5 mg are absorbed. Neonates and young children may develop iron deficiency anemia due to new blood formation and increased iron utilization that exceeds dietary intake.

280.8 Other specified iron deficiency anemias — *Paterson-Kelly syndrome, Plummer-Vinson syndrome, Waldenström-Kjellberg syndrome; sideropenic dysphagia*

Subcategory 280.8 classifies iron deficiency anemias of other specified types and causes, such as gastrectomy, excessive blood donation, and upper small-bowel malabsorption syndromes.

280.9 Unspecified iron deficiency anemia — *achlorhydric, chlorotic, idiopathic hypochromic Witt's anemias; sideropenia, Hayem-Faber syndrome*

Use subcategory 280.9 only when other, more specific codes are not appropriate. Typically classified to 280.9 are microcytic or hypochromic anemias, not otherwise specified and iron deficiency anemia due to impaired iron absorption, not otherwise specified.

281 Other deficiency anemias

281.0 Pernicious anemia — *chronic progressive anemia caused by failure to absorb vitamin B12; Addison's anemia, Biermer's anemia; Dana-Putnam syndrome, Lichtheim's syndrome, Runeberg's disease*
AHA: Nov-Dec, 1984, 1; Sept-Oct, 1984, 16

Use subcategory 281.0 to report chronic, progressive anemia of vitamin B12 deficiency due to an absorption defect. Also known as Addison or Biermer anemia, it rarely occurs before the fourth decade of life. The condition may be due to an inherited genetic defect characterized by a deficiency of intrinsic factor, a substance essential for B12 absorption.

Signs and symptoms of pernicious anemia include anorexia, dyspepsia, pallor with trace of jaundice, weakness, numbness and tingling of extremities, gingival bleeding, and a smooth sore tongue. Blood work reveals oval macrocytes, pancytopenia, hypersegmented neutrophils, elevated serum gastrin, elevated LDH, high serum iron, and absent haptoglobin. Gastric analysis shows no free gastric acid, and reveals a pH above 7. Schilling test measures absorption of vitamin B12. Bone marrow aspiration and analysis shows bone marrow to be megaloblastic. Therapies include parenteral vitamin B12.

281.1 Other vitamin B12 deficiency anemia — *vegan's anemia; selective vitamin B12 malabsorption with proteinuria; Imerslund's syndrome, Imerslund-Gräsbeck syndrome*

Use subcategory 281.1 only when other, more specific codes are not appropriate. Clinical vitamin B12 deficiency may be caused by dietary deficiency, gastrectomy, regional ileitis, diseases of malformation

280–289

© 2004 Ingenix, Inc.

involving the ileum, ileum resection, and fish tapeworm disease.

281.2 Folate-deficiency anemia — (Use additional E code to identify drug) — *congenital, dietary, drug-induced, Zuelzer-Ogden syndrome*

Use subcategory 281.2 to report anemia due to deficient stores of folic acid (pteroylmonoglutamic acid), a water-soluble B complex vitamin essential for cell growth and reproduction. Folate is a salt of folic acid.

Signs and symptoms of folate-deficiency anemia include history of poor nourishment or alcoholism, weight loss, glossitis, and a blunt masklike face. Blood work reveals low serum folate levels, decreased red cell folate levels, and peripheral blood smear shows megaloblastic anemia. Therapies include oral or parenteral folic acid.

Associated conditions include nontropical sprue, malabsorption syndrome, alcoholism, and complicated pregnancy.

Folate deficiency can be the result of drug therapy. If a drug causes the folate deficiency anemia, use an additional E code to identify that drug.

281.3 Other specified megaloblastic anemias not elsewhere classified — *predominance of megaloblasts in bone marrow with few normoblasts; combined B12 and folate-deficiency anemia, refractory megaloblastic anemia*

281.4 Protein-deficiency anemia — *amino-acid-deficiency anemia*

281.8 Anemia associated with other specified nutritional deficiency — *scorbutic anemia and achrestic anemia*

281.9 Unspecified deficiency anemia

282 Hereditary hemolytic anemias

282.0 Hereditary spherocytosis — *genetic hemolytic anemia characterized by jaundice, splenomegaly, and abnormally fragile sphere-shaped erythrocytes; acholuric (familial) jaundice; congenital hemolytic anemia (spherocytic); congenital spherocytosis; Minkowski-Chauffard syndrome; spherocytosis (familial)*

282.1 Hereditary elliptocytosis — *genetic hemolytic anemia characterized by an excessive proportion of abnormally fragile rod-shaped erythrocytes; elliptocytosis, ovalocytosis, Dresbach's syndrome*

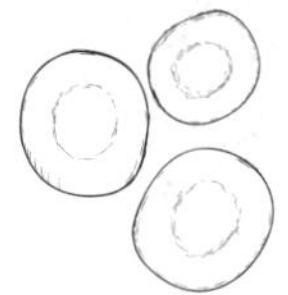
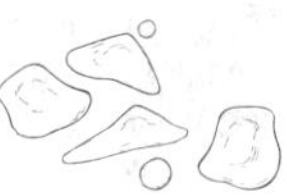

282.2 Anemias due to disorders of glutathione metabolism — *6-phosphogluconic dehydrogenase deficiency; drug-induced enzyme deficiency; erythrocytic glutathione deficiency; glucose-6-phosphate dehydrogenase [G-6-PD] deficiency; disorder of pentose phosphate pathway; favism*

282.3 Other hemolytic anemias due to enzyme deficiency — *hemolytic nonspherocytic (hereditary), type II; hexokinase deficiency; pyruvate kinase [PK] deficiency; triosephosphate isomerase deficiency*

282.4 [5th] Thalassemias — *hereditary anemias characterized by impaired or decreased synthesis of the polypeptide chains of hemoglobin, occurring primarily in Mediterranean or Southeast Asian populations*
AHA: Q4, 2003, 51

282.41 Sickle-cell thalassemia without crisis — *inheritance of a sickle gene from one parent and a gene for either hemoglobin C or beta-thalassemia from the other parent*

282.42 Sickle-cell thalassemia with crisis — (Use additional code for type of crisis: 289.52, 517.3) — *inheritance of a sickle gene from one parent and a gene for either hemoglobin C or beta-thalassemia from the other parent*

Coding Clarification

Sickled cells interfere with oxygen transport, obstructing capillary blood flow. Acidosis, dehydration, and/or decreased prevailing oxygen may bring on a crisis. Crises are attacks of pain that affect any part of the body, without warning, lasting hours or days. Carriers may have frequent infections and high fevers.

282.49 Other thalassemia — *thalassemia minor-one inherited gene thalassemia major - two inherited gene trait. Cooley's anemia, erythroblastic anemia, Dameshek's syndrome, erythorblastic anemia, high fetal gene thalassemia, hemoglobin thalassemia, Mediterranean disease, anemia or syndrome, microdrepanocytosis, mixed hemoglobinopathy, hereditary leptocytosis, Lepore hemoglobin syndrome, Rietti-Greppi-Micheli syndrome, Hb-S disease, silvestroni-Bianco syndrome*

280–289

Coding Clarification

The severity, treatment, and prognosis of thalassemia depend on the globin gene arrangement and deletion type. Thalassemia major, the most severe form, is evident soon after birth and requires lifelong blood transfusions. Life expectancy rarely exceeds the second decade.

282.5 Sickle-cell trait — *Hb-AS genotype*

Coding Clarification

This subcategory reports a heterozygous carrier of both the hemoglobin S and hemoglobin A genes. The condition rarely is associated with a clinical disorder. Couples in which both individuals carry the sickle-cell trait should be counseled about the possibility of having a child with sickle-cell disease.

Excluded from this subcategory is sickle-cell trait with other hemoglobinopathy (282.60-282.69) or that with thalassemia (282.4x).

Sickle-cell anemia is a severe, chronic, and incurable form of anemia occurring in patients who inherit hemoglobin S genes from both their parents. Less severe variations of the disease occur when the patient inherits one hemoglobin S gene from one parent and one hemoglobin C, D, or E gene from the other.

Signs and symptoms of sickle-cell anemia include joint pain, fever, lethargy, weakness, and splenomegaly. Blood work reveals a hematocrit of 20 to 30 percent, a hemoglobin of 6.5-10 g/dl, and a reticulocyte count markedly elevated at 10 to 25 percent. Microscopic exam of erythrocytes reveals characteristic "sickling" deformity. Screening tests, such as sodium metabisulfite test and dithionite solubility test, detect sickle-cell anemia or trait. Hemoglobin electrophoresis or chromatography reveal specific hemoglobin abnormalities such as hemoglobin S. Therapies include IV hydration, analgesics for pain, oxygen for hypoxemia, antibiotics for concomitant infection, blood transfusions, and experimental drugs, such as hydroxyurea, to induce fetal hemoglobin synthesis.

Associated conditions include frequent concomitant infections, dehydration, peripheral vaso-occlusion, and multisystem involvement, e.g., bone (aseptic necrosis), spleen (splenic infarction), pulmonary (pneumonia), neurological (cerebral ischemia), and ophthalmic (retinopathy).

Sickle-cell crisis refers to recurring acute episodes of pain involving any body system, but usually the chest, bones, or abdomen. In children, vaso-occlusive crisis is the most common form, although the term "sickle-cell crisis" may refer to any one of a variety of sudden and potentially serious conditions.

Excluded from this subcategory are sickle-cell thalassemia (282.4x) and sickle-cell trait (282.5).

282.60 Sickle-cell disease, unspecified

282.61 Hb-SS disease without crisis — *Herrick's syndrome*

282.62 Hb-SS disease with crisis — (Use additional code for type of crisis: 289.52, 517.3) — *acute abdominal pain, arthralgia, and leg ulcers in sickle cell anemia; atrophy of the spleen may occur with increased susceptibility to bacterial infection; sickle-cell crisis*
AHA: Q2, 1991, 15; Q2, 1998, 8; Q4, 2003, 56

282.63 Sickle-cell/Hb-C disease without crisis — *Hb-S/Hb-C disease without crisis*

282.64 Sickle-cell/Hb-C disease with crisis — (Use additional code for type of crisis: 289.52, 517.3) — *Sickled cells interfere with oxygen transport, obstructing capillary blood flow, fever, severe pain in joints and abdomen. Acidosis, dehydration and/or decreased prevailing oxygen may bring on a crisis. Hb-S/Hb-C disease with crisis, Sickle-cell/Hb-C disease with vaso-occlusive pain*
AHA: Q4, 2003, 51

282.68 Other sickle-cell disease without crisis — *Hb-S/Hb-D disease without crisis, Hb-S/Hb-E disease without crisis, Sickle-cell/Hb-D disease without crisis, Sickle-cell/Hb-E disease without crisis*
AHA: Q4, 2003, 51

282.69 Other sickle-cell disease with crisis — (Use additional code for type of crisis: 289.52, 517.3) — *Hb-S/Hb-D with crisis; Hb-S/Hb-E with crisis. Other sickle-cell disease with vaso-occlusive pain, sickle-cell/Hb-D disease with crisis, sickle-cell/Hb-E disease with crisis*

282.7 Other hemoglobinopathies — *congenital Heinz-body anemia; hereditary persistence of Hb-Bart's [HPFH], hemoglobin C [Hb-C], hemoglobin D [Hb-D], hemoglobin E [Hb-E], hemoglobin Zurich [Hb-Zurich]*

Coding Clarification

Excluded from this subgroup are familial polycythemia (289.6), hemoglobin M (Hb-M) disease (289.7), and high-oxygen-affinity hemoglobin (289.0).

282.8 Other specified hereditary hemolytic anemias — *stomatocytosis*

282.9 Unspecified hereditary hemolytic anemia

283 Acquired hemolytic anemias

AHA: Nov-Dec, 1984, 1

This rubric reports anemia characterized by the premature destruction of erythrocytes, exclusive of an inherited erythrocyte disorder. Hemolytic anemias may be acquired through infection, injury, drugs, blood transfusions (autoimmune), or other intrinsic

 © 2004 Ingenix, Inc.

or extrinsic causes. Hemolytic uremic syndrome (hemolytic anemia and thrombocytopenia occurring with acute renal failure) is a common manifestation of nonautoimmune hemolytic anemia.

283.0 Autoimmune hemolytic anemias — (Use additional E code to identify cause, if drug-induced) — *hemolytic anemia: cold, warm, or drug-induced*
AHA: Nov-Dec, 1984, 1

283.10 Unspecified non-autoimmune hemolytic anemia — (Use additional E code to identify cause)

283.11 Hemolytic-uremic syndrome — (Use additional E code to identify cause)

283.19 Other non-autoimmune hemolytic anemias — (Use additional E code to identify cause) — *mechanical, microangiopathic, toxic; erythrocyte fragmentation syndrome, Lederer-Brill syndromes*
AHA: Nov-Dec, 1984, 1; Q4, 1993, 25

283.2 Hemoglobinuria due to hemolysis from external causes — (Use additional E code to identify cause) — *acute intravascular hemolysis; hemoglobinuria from exertion or due to hemolysis; Marchiafava-Micheli syndrome, Murri's disease*
AHA: Nov-Dec, 1984, 1

283.9 Acquired hemolytic anemia, unspecified

Coding Clarification

Use an additional E code to identify the cause, as appropriate. Excluded from this rubric are Evan's syndrome (287.3) and hemolytic disease of newborn (773.0-773.5).

284 Aplastic anemia

AHA: Nov-Dec, 1984, 1; Sept-Oct, 1984, 16; Q1, 1991, 14

This rubric reports failure of bone marrow to generate blood cells, resulting in a deficiency of all of the formed elements of the blood (erythrocytes, platelets, and leukocytes).

Signs and symptoms of aplastic anemia include bleeding gums (early), oropharyngeal ulcerations (late), fever, waxy pallor, easily fatigued, weakness, frequent infections, bruising easily, increased menstrual flow, and frequent nosebleeds. Blood work reveals pancytopenia (e.g., thrombocytopenia, neutropenia). Bone marrow biopsy shows aplasia or hypocellularity. Therapies include packed red blood cells and platelet transfusions, bone marrow transplants, splenectomy, and drugs such as androgens and adrenal corticosteroids to stimulate hematopoiesis and marrow regeneration.

Associated conditions include concomitant infections.

284.0 Constitutional aplastic anemia — *Blackfan-Diamond syndrome, Kaznelson's syndrome*
AHA: Nov-Dec, 1984, 1; Sept-Oct, 1984, 16; Q1, 1991, 14

Coding Clarification

Constitutional aplastic anemia is an inherited form of aplastic anemia, both planocellular and unicellular. The etiology is believed to be a fundamental intrinsic abnormality of the stem cells.

284.8 Other specified aplastic anemias — (Use additional E code to identify cause) — *aplastic anemias due to drugs, infection, radiation, toxins, infections, chronic system disease*
AHA: Nov-Dec, 1984, 1; Sept-Oct, 1984, 16; March-April, 1985, 14; Q1, 1991, 14; Q1, 1992, 15; Q1, 1997, 5

Coding Clarification

Subcategory 284.8 reports acquired or secondary forms of aplastic anemia. Etiologies include radiation, chronic systemic disease, infections, drugs, toxic chemicals, and red cell aplasia secondary to thymoma.

284.9 Unspecified aplastic anemia

285 Other and unspecified anemias

AHA: Nov-Dec, 1984, 1; Q1, 1991, 14

285.0 Sideroblastic anemia — (Use additional E code to identify cause, if drug-induced) — *pyridoxine-responsive anemia, sideroblastic anemia, sideroblastic hypochromic with iron loading anemia*
AHA: Nov-Dec, 1984, 1; Q1, 1991, 14

285.1 Acute posthemorrhagic anemia — *secondary to acute blood loss*
AHA: Nov-Dec, 1984, 1; Q1, 1991, 14; Q2, 1992, 15

Coding Clarification

Code 285.1 reports anemia due to frank, rapid blood loss. The etiology may be trauma, spontaneous rupture of a blood vessel, surgical procedures involving major blood vessels, pathology such as bleeding peptic ulcers or neoplasms, or extravasation secondary to a bleeding diathesis such as hemophilia. The anemia is usually normochromic and normocytic in an otherwise healthy patient; blood cells can show morphological changes indicative of other concomitant forms of anemia since the condition can occur with any other form of anemia.

Signs and symptoms of acute posthemorrhagic anemia include faintness, dizziness, thirst, weakness, rapid pulse, rapid respirations, orthostatic changes in blood pressure, and hypovolemic shock. Blood work during and immediately after the hemorrhage may reveal high erythrocyte, hemoglobin, and hematocrit levels due to vasoconstriction. Within a few hours, blood work shows evidence of hemodilution with abnormally low blood indices, polymorphonuclear leukocytosis, and increased thrombocyte production.

Therapies include rapid identification of the bleeding site and establishment of hemostasis, blood transfusions and IV hydration to restore blood volume, iron supplementation, and monitoring for hypovolemic shock.

Associated conditions include angina and hypovolemic shock. Excluded from this rubric is anemia due to chronic blood loss or not specified as acute blood loss (280.0).

Report these codes in conjunction with codes describing the underlying disease as specific end stage renal disease (ESRD), neoplastic disease, or other chronic illness. Sequencing of the codes depends on the presenting patient complaint and clinical circumstances.

285.21 Anemia in end-stage renal disease — *secondary to early stage renal disease [ESRD]*
AHA: Nov-Dec, 1984, 1; Q1, 1991, 14; Q4, 2000, 39

285.22 Anemia in neoplastic disease — *secondary to neoplastic disease*
AHA: Nov-Dec, 1984, 1; Q1, 1991, 14; Q4, 2000, 39

285.29 Anemia of other chronic illness — *secondary to other chronic illness*
AHA: Nov-Dec, 1984, 1; Q1, 1991, 14; Q4, 2000, 39

285.8 Other specified anemias — *not elsewhere classified, von Jaksch's anemia, and Brühl's disease; dyserythropoietic anemia, infantile pseudoleukemia*
AHA: Nov-Dec, 1984, 1; Q1, 1991, 14; Q1, 1991, 16

285.9 Unspecified anemia

Coding Clarification

Use code 285.9 to report normochromic, normocytic anemia of unspecified type, including anemia of chronic disease characterized by shortened red cell survival, suboptimal marrow compensation (sometimes referred to as "relative marrow failure"), defective reutilization of iron, and, occasionally, reduced production of erythropoietin. Such anemias normally do not require treatment unless other characteristics develop, such as iron deficiency anemia (code 280.9) or folic acid deficiency anemia (code 281.2).

Excluded from this rubric are anemias due to chronic blood loss (280.0) or iron deficiency anemia (280.0-280.9).

286 Coagulation defects

Use an additional E code if the coagulation defect is drug induced.

286.0 Congenital factor VIII disorder — *abnormal coagulation characterized by subcutaneous and intramuscular hemorrhage and caused by a mutant gene on the X chromosome; classical, familial, hereditary hemophilia A*

286.1 Congenital factor IX disorder — *abnormality of coagulation characterized by subcutaneous and intramuscular hemorrhage and caused by a mutant gene on the X chromosome; Christmas disease, hemophilia B*

286.2 Congenital factor XI deficiency — *Rosenthal's disease; hemophilia C*

286.3 Congenital deficiency of other clotting factors — *congenital afibrinogenemia; Owren's disease, Stuart-Prower disease; dysfibrinogenemia, parahemophilia*

286.4 Von Willebrand's disease — *angiohemophilia (A) (B); factor VIII deficiency with vascular defect*

286.5 Hemorrhagic disorder due to intrinsic circulating anticoagulants — (Use additional E code to identify cause, if drug-induced) — *acquired abnormality of coagulation caused by presence of tissue factor activity (TFA) which initiates coagulation. Manifestation may be blood clot formation (subacute) or serious bleeding (acute)*
AHA: Q3, 1990, 14; Q3, 1992, 15

286.6 Defibrination syndrome — *consumption coagulopathy; disseminated intravascular coagulation [DIC syndrome], ICF syndrome, IVC syndrome; pathologic fibrinolysis*
AHA: Q4, 1993, 29

286.7 Acquired coagulation factor deficiency — (Use additional E code to identify cause, if drug-induced) — *deficiency of coagulation factor due to liver disease or vitamin K deficiency*
AHA: Q4, 1993, 29

286.9 Other and unspecified coagulation defects — *delay in coagulation or hemostasis disorder*
AHA: Q4, 1993, 29; Q4, 1999, 22

287 Purpura and other hemorrhagic conditions

AHA: Q1, 1991, 14

Excluded from this rubric are hemorrhagic thrombocythemia (238.7) and purpura fulminans (286.6).

© 2004 Ingenix, Inc.

287.0 Allergic purpura — *small hemorrhage into the skin, mucous membrane, or serosal surface caused by sensitization to foods, drugs, insect bites; peliosis rheumatica rheumataica; Schönlein-Henoch purpura*
AHA: Q1, 1991, 14

The definition of allergic purpura is acute and chronic vasculitis. Also known as anaphylactoid purpura and Schönlein-Henoch purpura, allergic purpura affects small vessels of the skin, joints, gastrointestinal tract, and kidneys.

Signs and symptoms of allergic purpura include a rash on the extensor surfaces of the arms, legs, and feet and across the buttocks, fever, polyarthralgia, tenderness and swelling of joints, edema of the hands and feet, colicky abdominal pain, tenderness, melena, hematuria, and proteinuria. Therapies include corticosteroids to control edema and joint and abdominal pain, as well as eliminating the offending drug.

Excluded from this subgroup are hemorrhagic purpura (287.3) and purpura annularis telangiectodes (709.1).

287.1 Qualitative platelet defects — *thrombasthenia; thrombocytasthenia, and Bernard-Soulier thrombopathy*
AHA: Q1, 1991, 14

287.2 Other nonthrombocytopenic purpuras — *Diamond-Gardener syndrome*
AHA: Q1, 1991, 14

287.3 Primary thrombocytopenia — *reduced number of platelets in the circulating blood as the principle disease or condition; Evans' syndrome, Kasabach-Merritt syndrome, thrombopenia-hemangioma syndrome, Werlhof-Wichmann syndrome*
AHA: Q1, 1991, 14

Code 287.3 reports an abnormally small number of platelets in the circulating blood as a result of increased platelet destruction without an identifiable exogenous cause or underlying disease. The condition, also known as Werlhof Wichmann Syndrome and idiopathic thrombocytopenia purpura (ITP), is characterized by the sudden onset of signs and symptoms.

Signs and symptoms of primary thrombocytopenia include petechiae, epistaxis, hematuria or abnormal bleeding of gums, vagina, gastrointestinal tract, and bruising easily. Blood work shows a decreased platelet count, abnormal bleeding time, normal prothrombin time (PT), and partial thromboplastin time (PTT). Bone marrow biopsy and analysis reveal increased megakaryocytes without surrounding platelets. Therapies include drugs such as corticosteroids, immunosuppressive therapy (e.g., vincristine or vinblastine) or IV immunoglobulin, splenectomy, and avoidance of any activity that would expose the patient to bleeding.

Associated conditions include fatal cerebral hemorrhage, hemorrhage of other sites, acute leukemia, macroglobulinemia, and hematoma formation occasionally causing nerve damage. Excluded from this subgroup are thrombotic thrombocytopenic purpura (446.6) and transient thrombocytopenia of newborn (776.1).

287.4 Secondary thrombocytopenia — (Use additional E code to identify cause) — *reduced number of platelets in the circulating blood as a consequence of an underlying disease or condition; posttransfusion purpura, thrombocytopenia due to drugs, extracorporeal circulation of blood, or platelet alloimmunization*
AHA: March-April, 1985, 14; Q1, 1991, 14

This subgroup reports thrombocytopenia due to an identifiable exogenous cause or underlying condition, such as congestive splenomegaly, Felty's syndrome, Gaucher's disease, tuberculosis, sarcoidosis, myelofibrosis, lupus erythematosus, Wiskott-Aldrich syndrome, chronic alcoholism, and scurvy. It also may occur as a result of overhydration, blood transfusions, or drug therapy. Use an additional E code to identify the cause.

Coding Clarification

Transient thrombocytopenia of newborn (776.1) is not classified here.

287.5 Unspecified thrombocytopenia

287.8 Other specified hemorrhagic conditions — *capillary fragility (hereditary) and vascular pseudohemophilia*
AHA: Q1, 1991, 14

287.9 Unspecified hemorrhagic conditions

288 Diseases of white blood cells

AHA: Q1, 1991, 14

Excluded from this rubric is leukemia, reported with codes from the series 204.0-208.9.

288.0 Agranulocytosis — (Use additional E code to identify drug or other cause) — *sudden, severe condition characterized by significant reduction in white blood cells with ulceration of the throat, intestinal tract, and skin; Kostmann's syndrome, Doan-Wiseman syndrome, Werner-Schultz syndrome, Shwachman's syndrome*
AHA: Q1, 1991, 14; Q2, 1996, 6; Q3, 1996, 16; Q2, 1999, 9; Q3, 1999, 6

Agranulocytosis reports an absolute neutrophil count of less than 1,500/cu ml. Also known as neutropenia, agranulocytosis frequently leads to increased susceptibility to bacterial and fungal infections.

Signs and symptoms of agranulocytosis include fever, chills, sore throat, prostration, regional adenopathy, jaundice with liver damage, mucosal ulceration of the throat, vagina, or respiratory tract. Peripheral blood smear reveals absence of granulocytes, reduced monocytes, and lymphocytes. Repeated total and differential white blood cell counts determine if the neutropenia is acute or chronic. Bone marrow aspiration and biopsy typically appear hypoplastic and may reveal bone marrow involvement by leukemia or infiltrative disorders. Serial blood counts and a repeat bone marrow exam at five to seven days typically define the mechanism. Blood and tissue cultures identify infection resulting from agranulocytosis. Therapies include broad-spectrum antibiotics (e.g., penicillin or cephalosporin, as well as aminoglycosides such as gentamicin or tobramycin). If determined to be drug induced, the recommended therapy includes cessation of the causative drug and antipyretics for fever. Associated conditions include sepsis and septicemia, pneumonia, hemorrhagic necrosis of mucous membranes, perirectal abscess, and parenchymal liver damage. Use an additional E code to identify the drug or other cause of agranulocytosis. Transitory neonatal neutropenia (776.7) is not classified here.

288.1 Functional disorders of polymorphonuclear neutrophils — *chronic childhood granulomatous disease, congenital dysphagocytosis, Job's syndrome, lipochrome histiocytosis, and progressive septic granulomatosis*
AHA: Q1, 1991, 14

288.2 Genetic anomalies of leukocytes — *Alder's (-Reilly) syndrome, Chédiak-Steinbrinck (-Higashi) syndrome, Jordan's syndrome, May-Hegglin syndrome, Pelger-Huet syndrome; Döhle body-panmyelopathic syndrome*
AHA: Q1, 1991, 14

288.3 Eosinophilia — *elevated proportion of a type of white blood cell readily stained with eosin; allergic, hereditary, idiopathic, secondary*
AHA: Q1, 1991, 14; Q3, 2000, 11

Subcategory 288.3 reports an absolute eosinophil-count of more than 500/cu ml. Counts of 500-1,000/cu ml are nonspecific and normally are not viewed as a clinical problem. Associated conditions include allergic disorders, parasitic infestation with tissue invasion, skin diseases, tumors, Hodgkin's disease, granulomatous disease, eosinophilic leukemia, fibroplastic endocarditis, systemic vasculitis, and tropical eosinophilia.

Excluded from this rubric are Loffler's syndrome and pulmonary eosinophilia (518.3).

288.8 Other specified disease of white blood cells — *lymphocytopenia, lymphocytosis, monocytosis, leukocytosis, plasmacytosis, hyperleukocytosis, hypoeosinophilia*
AHA: March-April, 1987, 12; Q1, 1991, 14

288.9 Unspecified disease of white blood cells

289 Other diseases of blood and blood-forming organs

289.0 Polycythemia, secondary — *elevated number of red blood cells in the circulating blood occurring as a result to reduced oxygen supply to the tissues; Gaisböck's syndrome*

Polycythemia is an increase in the normal number of red blood cells. Secondary polycythemia is also known as secondary erythrocytosis, spurious polycythemia, and reactive polycythemia. Spurious polycythemia, which is characterized by increased hematocrit and normal or increased erythrocyte total mass, results from a decrease in plasma volume and hemoconcentration. Reactive polycythemia is a condition characterized by excessive production of circulating erythrocytes due to an identifiable secondary condition, such as hypoxia, or an underlying disease, such as a neoplasm.

Excluded from this subcategory are neonatal polycythemia (776.4) and primary polycythemia and polycythemia vera (238.4).

289.1 Chronic lymphadenitis — *persistent inflammation of one or more lymph nodes except mesenteric*

Code 289.1 reports inflammation of the lymph nodes. Any pathogen can cause lymphadenitis. Lymphadenitis may be generalized or restricted to regional lymph nodes and may occur with systemic infections. Acute lymphadenitis (683), mesenteric lymphadenitis (289.2), and enlarged glands not otherwise specified (785.6) are excluded.

289.2 Nonspecific mesenteric lymphadenitis — *inflammation of one or more lymph nodes in the peritoneal fold that encases the abdominal organs; Brennemann's syndrome*

Subcategory 289.2 reports lymphadenitis occurring in a double layer of peritoneum attached to the abdominal wall that encloses a portion or all of one of the mesentery (abdominal viscera).

289.3 Lymphadenitis, unspecified, except mesenteric — *unknown and other than mesenteric*
AHA: Q2, 1992, 8

289.4 Hypersplenism — *cellular components of blood or platelets are removed at an accelerated rate causing deficiency of peripheral blood elements; "big spleen" syndrome; hypoleukemia splenica*

© 2004 Ingenix, Inc.

This subgroup reports a clinical syndrome characterized by splenic hyperactivity and splenomegaly. The condition results in a peripheral blood cell deficiency because the spleen traps and destroys the circulating peripheral blood cells.

Signs and symptoms of hypersplenism include history of frequent infection and bruising easily, and abnormal bleeding from mucous membranes, genitourinary tract, or gastrointestinal tract. There may be ulcers of the mouth, legs, or feet, fever, weakness, and palpitations. Blood work reveals mild, normochromic, and normocytic anemia with elevated reticulocyte count and markedly decreased platelets and granulocytes. A radionuclide scan of chromium-labeled erythrocytes or platelets demonstrates increased splenic activity, while splenic angiography demonstrates portal obstruction or hypertension. A biopsy of the spleen reveals the pathology such as infiltrative disease (e.g., lymphoma, Gaucher's amyloidosis).

Therapies include medical treatment of the underlying etiology or splenectomy, if medical treatment is ineffective.

Associated conditions include recurrent infections such as persistent leg ulcers, Gaucher disease, Niemann-Pick disease, congestive cirrhosis (portal hypertension) or thrombosis, hemolytic anemia, polycythemia vera, Felty's syndrome, subacute bacterial endocarditis, Letterer-Siwe disease, tuberculosis, and cystic or neoplastic disease, such as leukemia, lymphoma, myelofibrosis, or Boeck's sarcoidosis.

Excluded from this rubric is primary splenic neutropenia (288.0).

289.50 Unspecified disease of spleen

289.51 Chronic congestive splenomegaly — *syndrome consisting of anemia, splenic enlargement, hemorrhages, cirrhosis of the liver. Banti's syndrome.*

289.52 Splenic sequestration — (Code first sickle-cell disease in crisis: 282.42, 282.62, 282.64, 282.69)

289.59 Other diseases of spleen — *fibrosis, infarct, rupture, infection, abscess, cyst, atrophy, prolapse, ptosis, torsion, splenocele, wandering spleen*

289.6 Familial polycythemia — *elevation of the number of red blood cells in the blood; benign polycythemia; erythrocytosis*

289.7 Methemoglobinemia — (Use additional E code to identify cause)

Hypercoagulable conditions are inherited and acquired disorders that predispose to venous thromboembolism.

289.81 Primary hypercoagulable state — *activated protein C resistance, antithrombin III deficiency, factor V Leiden mutation, lupus anticoagulant, protein C deficiency, protein S deficiency, prothrombin gene mutation, Antithrombin deficiency hyperhomocystinemia, elevated factor VIII levels dysfibrinogenemia, factor XII deficiency, disorders of plasmin generation*

289.82 Secondary hypercoagulable state — *pregnancy, immobility, trauma, postoperative state, use of oral contraceptives, estrogen, tamoxifen, antiphospholipid syndrome, hyperhomocystinemia, malignancy nephrotic syndrome, myeloproliferative disorders, congestive heart failure, heparin-induced thrombocytopenia with thrombosis, paroxysmal nocturnal hemoglobinuria, Behçet's disease*

289.89 Other specified diseases of blood and blood-forming organs — *hypergammaglobulinemia, myelofibrosis, pseudocholinesterase defiency, osteosclerosis, myelosclerosis, osteomyelosclerosis, osteomyelofibrosis, osteosclerotic anemia, activated protein C resistance*

289.9 Unspecified diseases of blood and blood-forming organs

290–319
Mental Disorders

The World Health Organization (WHO) offers the following guidelines that apply to this chapter: when classifying behavioral disorders, organically based illnesses should get precedence over functional ones, and within the functional group, the order then may be psychoses, neuroses, personality disorders, and others. When coding mental illnesses associated with physical conditions, assign as many codes as necessary to fully describe the clinical picture.

290–299 Psychoses

The term "psychoses" has been applied to many non-psychotic mental disorders historically. For this classification, the definition of psychoses includes only conditions that interfere with activities of daily living and include a gross impairment of reality. Codes in this section represent disorders that exhibit delusions, hallucinations, markedly incoherent speech, disorganized behaviors, and the inability on the part of the patient to comprehend the inappropriateness of this behavior.

290–294 Organic Psychotic Conditions

Included in this section are senile and presenile dementia, arteriosclerotic dementia, dementia and hallucinosis associated with substance abuse, and organic brain syndromes. Assign a code from these rubrics only when the specific organic clinical feature of a confused state, dementia, or delirium is present. Do not use a code from these categories to report the organic etiology of a psychotic mental state that is coded elsewhere in this chapter.

290 Senile and presenile organic psychotic conditions

AHA: Q1, 1988, 3

Arteriosclerotic dementia is attributable to degenerative arterial disease of the brain. Symptoms suggesting a focal lesion in the brain are common. There may be a fluctuating or patchy intellectual defect with insight, and an intermittent course is common. Clinical differentiation from senile or presenile dementia, which may coexist with it, may be very difficult or impossible. Cerebral atherosclerosis should also be reported in addition to the code for the psychosis.

Senile dementia usually occurs after the age of 65 in which any cerebral pathology other than that of senile atrophic change can be reasonably excluded. Presenile dementia occurs before age 65, and is usually associated with diffuse or lobar cerebral atrophy.

In delirium, a superimposed reversible episode of acute confusional state exists; in the delusional type, delusions vary from simple, poorly formed, paranoid delusions to highly formed paranoid delusional states. Hallucinations are also present in a progressive disease of persons in advanced age. Senile dementia, depressed type, is characterized by development in advanced old age, progressive in nature, in which depressive features, ranging from mild to severe forms of manic-depressive affective psychosis, are also present. Disturbance of the sleep-waking cycle and preoccupation with the deceased are often particularly prominent.

In addition to the appropriate code from this rubric, also code first any associated neurological condition such as Pick's disease, Alzheimer's disease, or Jakob-Creutzfeldt disease. Pick's disease, while present in the senile period, may primarily affect the frontal and temporal lobes. Alzheimer's disease is due to a large loss of cells from brain areas such as the cerebral cortex. Jakob-Creutzfeldt disease is a rare, progressive, fatal virus of the central nervous system.

290.0 Senile dementia, uncomplicated — (Code first the associated neurological condition) — *senile dementia, not otherwise specified*
AHA: Q1, 1988, 3; Q4, 1999, 4

290.10 Presenile dementia, uncomplicated — (Code first the associated neurological condition) — *simple type*
AHA: Nov-Dec, 1984, 20; Q1, 1988, 3

290.11 Presenile dementia with delirium — (Code first the associated neurological condition) — *with acute confusional state*
AHA: Nov-Dec, 1984, 20; Q1, 1988, 3

290.12 Presenile dementia with delusional features — (Code first the associated neurological condition) — *paranoid type, including Binswanger's dementia*
AHA: Nov-Dec, 1984, 20; Q1, 1988, 3

290.13 Presenile dementia with depressive features — (Code first the associated neurological condition) — *depressed type*
AHA: Nov-Dec, 1984, 20; Q1, 1988, 3

290.20 Senile dementia with delusional features — (Code first the associated neurological condition) — *paranoid type or senile psychosis not otherwise specified*
AHA: Q1, 1988, 3

290.21 Senile dementia with depressive features — (Code first the associated neurological condition)

290.3 Senile dementia with delirium — (Code first the associated neurological condition) — *with acute confusional state*
AHA: Q1, 1988, 3

290.40 Vascular dementia, uncomplicated — (Code first the associated neurological condition. Use additional code to identify cerebral atherosclerosis, 437.0) — *simple type*
AHA: Q1, 1988, 3

290.41 Vascular dementia, with delirium — (Code first the associated neurological condition. Use additional code to identify cerebral atherosclerosis, 437.0) — *with acute confusional state*
AHA: Q1, 1988, 3

290.42 Vascular dementia, with delusions — (Code first the associated neurological condition. Use additional code to identify cerebral atherosclerosis, 437.0) — *paranoid type*
AHA: Q1, 1988, 3

290.43 Vascular dementia, with depressed mood — (Code first the associated neurological condition. Use additional code to identify cerebral atherosclerosis, 437.0) — *depressed type*
AHA: Q1, 1988, 3

290.8 Other specified senile psychotic conditions — (Code first the associated neurological condition)

290.9 Unspecified senile psychotic condition — (Code first the associated neurological condition)

Documentation Issues

When the physician documents senile dementia with Alzheimer's disease, both conditions should be coded. Report with codes 290.0 *Senile dementia, uncomplicated* and 331.0 *Alzheimer's disease.*

Coding Clarification

Excluded from this rubric are dementias associated with other cerebral conditions (294.10-294.11), psychoses occurring in old age without dementia or delirium (295.0-298.8), senility with mental changes of nonpsychotic severity (310.1), and transient organic psychotic conditions (293.0-293.9).

If mental or behavioral problems are unspecified, report V40.9 *Unspecified mental or behavioral problem.* However, this code is not an acceptable principal diagnosis.

291 Alcohol-induced mental disorders

AHA: Sept-Oct, 1986, 3; Q1, 1988, 3

Alcoholic psychoses are organic psychotic states due mainly to excessive consumption of alcohol. Defects of nutrition are thought to play an important role in alcoholic psychoses. Alcoholic psychoses are classified according to the complex of presenting symptoms.

Alcohol withdrawal delirium is an acute or subacute organic psychotic state in alcoholics characterized by clouded consciousness, disorientation, fear, illusions, delusions, hallucinations of any kind, notably visual and tactile, and restlessness, tremor, and sometimes fever. Alcohol amnestic syndrome is a syndrome of prominent and lasting reduction of memory span, including striking loss of recent memory, disordered time appreciation, and confabulation, occurring in alcoholics as the sequel to an acute alcoholic psychosis (especially delirium tremens) or, more rarely, in the course of chronic alcoholism. It is usually accompanied by peripheral neuritis and may be associated with Wernicke's encephalopathy.

291.0 Alcohol withdrawal delirium — *delirium tremens*
AHA: Sept-Oct, 1986, 3; Q1, 1988, 3; Q2, 1991, 11

291.1 Alcohol-induced persisting amnestic disorder — *Korsakoff's psychosis, alcoholic polyneuritic psychosis*
AHA: Sept-Oct, 1986, 3; Q1, 1988, 3

291.2 Alcohol-induced persisting dementia — *chronic alcoholic brain syndrome*
AHA: Sept-Oct, 1986, 3; Q1, 1988, 3

291.3 Alcohol-induced psychotic disorder with hallucinations — *psychosis with hallucinosis*
AHA: Sept-Oct, 1986, 3; Q1, 1988, 3; Q2, 1991, 11

291.4 Idiosyncratic alcohol intoxication — *pathologic drunkenness*
AHA: Sept-Oct, 1986, 3; Q1, 1988, 3

291.5 Alcohol-induced psychotic disorder with delusions — *psychosis, paranoid type*
AHA: Sept-Oct, 1986, 3; Q1, 1988, 3

291.81 Alcohol withdrawal — *withdrawal symptoms or syndrome*
AHA: July-Aug, 1985, 10; Sept-Oct, 1986, 3; Q1, 1988, 3; Q2, 1991, 11; Q3, 1994, 13; Q4, 1996, 28

291.89 Other specified alcohol-induced mental disorders — *not elsewhere specified*
AHA: July-Aug, 1985, 10; Sept-Oct, 1986, 3; Q1, 1988, 3; Q3, 1994, 13

 © 2004 Ingenix, Inc.

291.9 Unspecified alcohol-induced mental disorders — *chronic alcoholism with psychosis, not otherwise specified*
AHA: Sept-Oct, 1986, 3; Q1, 1988, 3

Documentation Issues

If the documentation references a history of alcohol abuse it should only be reported if it has an impact on the patient treatment or length of stay.

When the medical record indicates that the patient was admitted for a physical complaint related to the alcohol abuse, follow the instructions in the index for the condition described as due to alcohol and sequence the physical condition first, followed by the code for the alcohol abuse.

If the documentation identifies that the patient experienced withdrawal symptoms or syndrome whether prior to, or after admission, report the withdrawal. Use code 291.81 for alcohol withdrawal.

Coding Clarification

Substance Related Mental Conditions: Psychoactive substance-induced organic mental syndromes are identified by physical or psychotic symptoms related to such use. These conditions are classified by category, such as 291 *Alcohol-induced mental disorders.* The alcohol abuse should also be reported as an additional code.

Alcohol Withdrawal: The phenomenon of alcohol withdrawal begins when an individual either greatly reduces or ceases consumption of alcohol after a period of prolonged and heavy use of the substance. Seizures as a result of alcohol withdrawal are coded to 780.39, together with 291.81.

Symptoms are hand tremor, nausea or vomiting, fleeting hallucinations (auditory, tactile, or visual), illusions, grand mal seizures, anxiety, insomnia, autonomic hyperactivity, and psychomotor agitation. These symptoms may cause very noticeable impairment of the sufferer's ability to function at work or in social settings, peaking on the second day, and improving markedly by the fourth day. The symptoms of anxiety, insomnia, and autonomic dysfunction can linger for as long as six months.

Coding Scenario

A patient is admitted in alcohol withdrawal, suffering from delirium tremens.

> Code assignment: 291.0 *Alcohol withdrawal with delirium tremens.* Code 291.81 specifically excludes the use of the code in conjunction with delirium, including delirium tremens.

292 Drug psychoses

AHA: Sept-Oct, 1986, 3; Q1, 1988, 3; Q2, 1991, 11

Drug psychoses are organic mental syndromes that are due to consumption of drugs (notably amphetamines, barbiturates, opiate, and LSD groups) and solvents. Some of the syndromes in this group are not as severe as most conditions labeled "psychotic," but they are included here for practical reasons. Drug psychoses are classified according to the complex of presenting symptoms. In drug withdrawal syndrome, convulsions, tremor, disorientation, and memory disturbances may occur. In hallucinatory/paranoid states, the patient may experience auditory hallucinations and anxiety.

292.0 Drug withdrawal — (Use additional code for any associated drug dependence: 304.00-304.93. Use additional E code to identify drug) — *abstinence syndrome or symptoms*
AHA: Sept-Oct, 1986, 3; Q1, 1988, 3; Q2, 1991, 11; Q1, 1997, 12

292.11 Drug-induced psychotic disorder with delusions — (Use additional code for any associated drug dependence: 304.00-304.93. Use additional E code to identify drug) — *paranoid state induced by drugs*
AHA: Sept-Oct, 1986, 3; Q1, 1988, 3; Q2, 1991, 11

292.12 Drug-induced psychotic disorder with hallucinations — (Use additional code for any associated drug dependence: 304.00-304.93. Use additional E code to identify drug)

292.2 Pathological drug intoxication — (Use additional code for any associated drug dependence: 304.00-304.93. Use additional E code to identify drug) — *reaction resulting in brief psychotic state*
AHA: Sept-Oct, 1986, 3; Q1, 1988, 3; Q2, 1991, 11

292.81 Drug-induced delirium — (Use additional code for any associated drug dependence: 304.00-304.93. Use additional E code to identify drug)

292.82 Drug-induced persisting dementia — (Use additional code for any associated drug dependence: 304.00-304.93. Use additional E code to identify drug)

292.83 Drug-induced persisting amnestic disorder — (Use additional code for any associated drug dependence: 304.00-304.93. Use additional E code to identify drug) — *memory loss*
AHA: Sept-Oct, 1986, 3; Q1, 1988, 3; Q2, 1991, 11

292.84 Drug-induced mood disorder — (Use additional code for any associated drug dependence: 304.00-304.93. Use additional E code to identify drug) — *depressive state induced by drugs*
AHA: Sept-Oct, 1986, 3; Q1, 1988, 3; Q2, 1991, 11

292.89 Other specified drug-induced mental disorder — (Use additional code for any associated drug dependence: 304.00-304.93. Use additional E code to identify drug) — *drug-induced organic personality syndrome, amotivational syndrome, and drug flashback syndrome*
AHA: Sept-Oct, 1986, 3; Q1, 1988, 3; Q2, 1991, 11

292.9 Unspecified drug-induced mental disorder — (Use additional code for any associated drug dependence: 304.00-304.93. Use additional E code to identify drug) — *not otherwise specified*
AHA: Sept-Oct, 1986, 3; Q1, 1988, 3; Q2, 1991, 11

Documentation Issues

If the documentation references a history of drug abuse, it should only be reported if it has an impact on the patient treatment or length of stay.

When the medical record indicates that the patient was admitted for a physical complaint related to the drug abuse, follow the instructions in the index for the condition described as due to drug abuse and sequence the physical condition first, followed by the code for the drug abuse.

If the documentation identifies that the patient experienced withdrawal symptoms or syndrome whether prior to, or after admission, report the withdrawal. Use code 292.0 for drug withdrawal.

Coding Clarification

Use an additional code from rubric 304 to report any associated drug dependence and an E code to identify the drug.

Substance Related Mental Conditions: Psychoactive substance-induced organic mental syndromes are identified by physical or psychotic symptoms related to such use. These conditions are classified by category, such as 292 *Drug-induced mental disorders*. The drug abuse should also be reported as an additional code.

293 Transient organic psychotic conditions

AHA: Q1, 1988, 3

Transient organic psychotic conditions are conditions characterized by clouded consciousness, confusion, disorientation, illusions, and frequently vivid hallucinations. Typically, they are due to some intra- or extracerebral toxic, infectious, metabolic, or other systemic disturbance and generally are reversible.

When using a code from this category, assign an additional code to identify the associated physical or neurological condition.

Acute delirium has an acute or rapid onset and is characterized by extreme disturbances of arousal, attention, orientation, perception, intellectual functions, and affect. These conditions are accompanied commonly by fear and agitation.

Organic affective syndrome is similar to depressive or manic-depressive disorder, but occurs in the presence of specific organic factors such as head trauma, endocranial tumors, exocranial tumors (such as pancreatic carcinoma), steroid overuse, Cushing's syndrome, and other endocrine disorders.

293.0 Delirium due to conditions classified elsewhere — (Code first the associated physical or neurological condition)

293.1 Subacute delirium — (Code first the associated physical or neurological condition) — *organic in origin*
AHA: Q1, 1988, 3

293.81 Psychotic disorder with delusions in conditions classified elsewhere — (Code first the associated physical or neurological condition) — *transient psychotic condition, paranoid type*
AHA: Q1, 1988, 3

293.82 Psychotic disorder with hallucinations in conditions classified elsewhere — (Code first the associated physical or neurological condition) — *transient psychotic condition, hallucinatory type*
AHA: Q1, 1988, 3

293.83 Mood disorder in conditions classified elsewhere — (Code first the associated physical or neurological condition) — *transient psychotic condition, depressive type*
AHA: Q1, 1988, 3

293.84 Anxiety disorder in conditions classified elsewhere — (Code first the associated physical or neurological condition)

293.89 Other specified transient mental disorders due to conditions classified elsewhere, other — (Code first the associated physical or neurological condition) — *Alice in Wonderland syndrome*
AHA: Q1, 1988, 3

293.9 Unspecified transient mental disorder in conditions classified elsewhere — (Code first the associated physical or neurological condition)

294 Persistent mental disorders due to conditions classified elsewhere

AHA: March-April, 1985, 12; Q1, 1988, 3

Amnestic syndrome presents with a prominent and lasting reduction of memory span, including striking loss of recent memory, disordered time appreciation,

© 2004 Ingenix, Inc.

and confabulation. The most common causes are chronic alcoholism (alcohol amnestic syndrome, Korsakoff's alcoholic psychosis), chronic barbiturate dependence, and malnutrition. An amnestic syndrome may be the predominating disturbance in the early states of presenile and senile dementia, arteriosclerotic dementia, and in encephalitis and other inflammatory and degenerative diseases in which there is particular bilateral involvement of the temporal lobes, and certain temporal lobe tumors.

294.0 Amnestic disorder in conditions classified elsewhere — *Korsakoff's psychosis or syndrome (nonalcoholic)*
AHA: March-April, 1985, 12; Q1, 1988, 3

294.10 Dementia in conditions classified elsewhere without behavioral disturbance — (Code first any underlying physical condition: 046.1, 094.1, 275.1, 330.1, 331.0, 331.11, 331.19, 331.82, 333.4, 340, 345.00-345.91, 446.0)

294.11 Dementia in conditions classified elsewhere with behavioral disturbance — (Code first any underlying physical condition: 046.1, 094.1, 275.1, 330.1, 331.0, 331.11, 331.19, 331.82, 333.4, 340, 345.00-345.91, 446.0)

294.8 Other persistent mental disorders due to conditions classified elsewhere — (Use additional code for associated epilepsy: 345.00-345.91) — *mixed paranoid and affective organic psychotic state*
AHA: March-April, 1985, 12; Q1, 1988, 3; Q1, 1988, 5; Q3, 2003, 14

294.9 Unspecified persistent mental disorders due to conditions classified elsewhere — *chronic organic psychosis*
AHA: March-April, 1985, 12; Q1, 1988, 3

Coding Clarification

Other specified chronic organic brain syndromes include conditions that present a clinical picture of organic psychosis but do not take the shape of a confusional state (293), a nonalcoholic Korsakoff's psychosis (294.0), or dementia due to an underlying physical condition (294.1x).

Alzheimer's Dementia: Two codes are required to report this condition. First code the underlying condition 331.0 *Alzheimer's disease,* and then use an additional code to report the dementia, 294.1x *Dementia in conditions classified elsewhere.*

Coding Scenario

A patient is seen for evaluation of Alzheimer's dementia and is referred to a partial hospitalization program for therapy.

Code assignment: 331.0 *Alzheimer's disease* and 294.1x *Dementia in conditions classified elsewhere*

295–299 Other Psychoses

Use an additional code to identify any associated physical disease, injury, or condition affecting the brain with psychoses classifiable to 295-298.

295 Schizophrenic disorders

AHA: Q1, 1988, 3

Schizophrenia is not diagnosed unless there is characteristic disturbance of at least two of these areas: thought, perception, mood, conduct, and personality. Paranoid type schizophrenia includes delusions of persecution or grandeur, thought disorder and hallucinations with less personality disintegration than in other subtypes of schizophrenia. Latent schizophrenia is sometimes called borderline schizophrenia, and is a condition in which there is potential for developing schizophrenia under emotional distress. This term is not recommended for patient diagnosis because a general consensus of its description has not been reached.

Residual schizophrenia presents with symptoms from the acute phase, but the symptoms have lost their prominence or sharpness. Schizoaffective type schizophrenia is a mixture of symptoms from schizophrenia and affective psychoses.

The following fifth-digit subclassification is for use with category 295:

0 unspecified
1 subchronic
2 chronic
3 subchronic with acute exacerbation
4 chronic with acute exacerbation
5 in remission

295.0 [5th] Simple type schizophrenia — (Use additional code to identify any associated physical disease, injury, or condition affecting the brain) — *schizophrenia simplex*
AHA: Q1, 1988, 3

295.1 [5th] Disorganized type schizophrenia — (Use additional code to identify any associated physical disease, injury, or condition affecting the brain) — *hebephrenic type schizophrenia*
AHA: Q1, 1988, 3

295.2 [5th] Catatonic type schizophrenia — (Use additional code to identify any associated physical disease, injury, or condition affecting the brain) — *catatonic schizophrenia*
AHA: Q1, 1988, 3

295.3 ✓5th Paranoid type schizophrenia — (Use additional code to identify any associated physical disease, injury, or condition affecting the brain) — *paraphrenic schizophrenia*
AHA: Q1, 1988, 3

295.4 ✓5th Schizophreniform disorder — (Use additional code to identify any associated physical disease, injury, or condition affecting the brain) — *oneirophrenia, schizophreniform psychosis, confusional*
AHA: Q1, 1988, 3

295.5 ✓5th Latent schizophrenia — (Use additional code to identify any associated physical disease, injury, or condition affecting the brain) — *prodromal, pseudoneurotic, borderline, incipient, prepsychotic*
AHA: Q1, 1988, 3

295.6 ✓5th Residual schizophrenia — (Use additional code to identify any associated physical disease, injury, or condition affecting the brain) — *chronic un-differentiated, Restzustand schizophrenia*
AHA: Q1, 1988, 3

295.7 ✓5th Schizo-affective type schizophrenia — (Use additional code to identify any associated physical disease, injury, or condition affecting the brain) — *cyclic, mixed*
AHA: Q1, 1988, 3

295.8 ✓5th Other specified types of schizophrenia — (Use additional code to identify any associated physical disease, injury, or condition affecting the brain) — *acute, atypical, cenesthopathic*
AHA: Q1, 1988, 3

295.9 ✓5th Unspecified schizophrenia — (Use additional code to identify any associated physical disease, injury, or condition affecting the brain) — *not otherwise specified, including Morel-Kraepelin disease*
AHA: Q1, 1988, 3; Q3, 1995, 6

296 Affective psychoses

AHA: March-April, 1985, 14; Q1, 1988, 3

Affective psychoses are recurrent, severe disturbances of mood accompanied by one or more of the following: delusions, perplexity, disturbed attitude to self, disorder of perception and behavior. Patients with affective psychoses have a strong characteristic inclination toward suicide. This category includes mild disorders of mood if the symptoms closely match the descriptions.

Manic disorder, as a single episode, is characterized by elation, excitement, rapid thought process, increased psychomotor activity, and emotional instability. Diminished interest in activities, fatigue, insomnia or hypersomnia, and change in weight characterize a major depressive disorder as a single episode. In bipolar disorder, the patient cycles between the two states: manic and depressive.

The following fifth-digit subclassification is for use with categories 296.0-296.6:

0 unspecified
1 mild
2 moderate
3 severe, without mention of psychotic behavior
4 severe, specified as with psychotic behavior
5 in partial or unspecified remission
6 in full remission

296.0 ✓5th Bipolar I disorder, single, manic episode — (Use additional code to identify any associated physical disease, injury, or condition affecting the brain) — *hypomania, single episode or unspecified*
AHA: March-April, 1985, 14; Q1, 1988, 3

296.1 ✓5th Manic disorder, recurrent episode — (Use additional code to identify any associated physical disease, injury, or condition affecting the brain) — *hypomania, recurrent*
AHA: March-April, 1985, 14; Q1, 1988, 3

296.2 ✓5th Major depressive disorder, single episode — (Use additional code to identify any associated physical disease, injury, or condition affecting the brain) — *endogenous depression, single episode or unspecified*
AHA: March-April, 1985, 14; Q1, 1988, 3

296.3 ✓5th Major depressive disorder, recurrent episode — (Use additional code to identify any associated physical disease, injury, or condition affecting the brain) — *endogenous depression, recurrent*
AHA: March-April, 1985, 14; Q1, 1988, 3

296.4 ✓5th Bipolar I disorder, most recent episode(or current) manic — (Use additional code to identify any associated physical disease, injury, or condition affecting the brain) — *circular manic depressive psychosis, in manic state*
AHA: March-April, 1985, 14; Q1, 1988, 3

296.5 ✓5th Bipolar I disorder, most recent episode (or current), depressed — (Use additional code to identify any associated physical disease, injury, or condition affecting the brain) — *circular manic depressive psychosis, in depressed state*
AHA: March-April, 1985, 14; Q1, 1988, 3

 © 2004 Ingenix, Inc.

296.6 ✓5th Bipolar I disorder, most recent episode (or current), mixed — (Use additional code to identify any associated physical disease, injury, or condition affecting the brain) — *circular manic depressive psychosis, mixed state*
AHA: March-April, 1985, 14; Q1, 1988, 3

296.7 Bipolar I disorder, most recent episode (or current) unspecified — (Use additional code to identify any associated physical disease, injury, or condition affecting the brain) — *circular manic depressive psychosis, current state unspecified*
AHA: March-April, 1985, 14; Q1, 1988, 3

296.80 Bipolar disorder, unspecified — (Use additional code to identify any associated physical disease, injury, or condition affecting the brain) — *atypical manic depressive psychosis, current state unspecified*
AHA: March-April, 1985, 14; Q1, 1988, 3

296.81 Atypical manic disorder — (Use additional code to identify any associated physical disease, injury, or condition affecting the brain) — *atypical manic only*
AHA: March-April, 1985, 14; Q1, 1988, 3

296.82 Atypical depressive disorder — (Use additional code to identify any associated physical disease, injury, or condition affecting the brain) — *atypical depressive only*
AHA: March-April, 1985, 14; Q1, 1988, 3

296.89 Other and unspecified bipolar disorders, other — (Use additional code to identify any associated physical disease, injury, or condition affecting the brain) — *atypical manic depressive psychosis, mixed status*
AHA: March-April, 1985, 14; Q1, 1988, 3

296.90 Unspecified episodic mood disorder — (Use additional code to identify any associated physical disease, injury, or condition affecting the brain) — *not otherwise specified*
AHA: March-April, 1985, 14; Q1, 1988, 3

296.99 Other specified episodic mood disorder — (Use additional code to identify any associated physical disease, injury, or condition affecting the brain) — *mood swings: brief compensatory, rebound*
AHA: March-April, 1985, 14; Q1, 1988, 3

297 Paranoid states (Delusional disorders)

AHA: Q1, 1988, 3

Paranoia is a condition in which patients show persistent distrust and suspiciousness of others. They typically present with four or more of the following:

- Suspicion that others are exploiting, harming, or deceiving him or her; preoccupied with unjustified doubts about the loyalty or trustworthiness of friends or associates
- Unwillingness to confide in others because of an unwarranted fear that the information will be used maliciously against him or her; reads hidden unbecoming or threatening meanings into benign remarks or events
- Persistently bears grudges, e.g., is unforgiving of insults, injuries, or slights
- Perceives attacks on character or reputation that are not apparent to others and is quick to react angrily or counterattacks
- Has recurrent suspicions, without justification, regarding fidelity of spouse or sexual partner

The disorder must have been present at least one week for this diagnosis.

The illness is not due to organic disease of the brain. This disorder usually occurs in the middle or late in adult life and may be chronic; it often includes resentment and anger that may lead to violence. These patients rarely seek medical attention but are brought for care by associates or relatives.

297.0 Paranoid state, simple — (Use additional code to identify any associated physical disease, injury, or condition affecting the brain) — *simple*
AHA: Q1, 1988, 3

297.1 Delusional disorder — (Use additional code to identify any associated physical disease, injury, or condition affecting the brain) — *chronic, Sander's disease, Cotard's syndrome, systematized delusions*
AHA: Q1, 1988, 3

297.2 Paraphrenia — (Use additional code to identify any associated physical disease, injury, or condition affecting the brain) — *involutional paranoid state, late paraphrenia, paraphrenia (involutional)*
AHA: Q1, 1988, 3

297.3 Shared psychotic disorder — (Use additional code to identify any associated physical disease, injury, or condition affecting the brain) — *folie à deux, induced psychosis or paranoid disorder*
AHA: Q1, 1988, 3

297.8 Other specified paranoid states — (Use additional code to identify any associated physical disease, injury, or condition affecting the brain) — *paranoia querulans, sensitiver Beziehungswahn, psyche passionelle; tarantism*
AHA: Q1, 1988, 3

297.9 Unspecified paranoid state — (Use additional code to identify any associated physical disease, injury, or condition affecting the brain) — *Lasegue's disease*
AHA: July-Aug, 1985, 9; Q1, 1988, 3

Coding Clarification

Excluded from this rubric are acute paranoid reaction (298.3), alcoholic jealousy or paranoid state (291.5), and paranoid schizophrenia (295.3).

Cotard's syndrome, characterized by suicidal tendencies and sensory disturbances, is classified to 297.1.

298 Other nonorganic psychoses

AHA: Q1, 1988, 3

Classified to this rubric are a small group of psychotic conditions that are attributable largely to a recent life experience. They should not be used for the wider range of psychoses in which environmental factors play some, but not a major, part in the etiology.

298.0 Depressive type psychosis — (Use additional code to identify any associated physical disease, injury, or condition affecting the brain) — *psychogenic depressive psychosis*
AHA: Q1, 1988, 3

298.1 Excitative type psychosis — (Use additional code to identify any associated physical disease, injury, or condition affecting the brain) — *acute hysterical psychosis; reactive excitation*
AHA: Q1, 1988, 3

298.2 Reactive confusion — (Use additional code to identify any associated physical disease, injury, or condition affecting the brain) — *psychogenic confusion/twilight state*
AHA: Q1, 1988, 3

298.3 Acute paranoid reaction — (Use additional code to identify any associated physical disease, injury, or condition affecting the brain) — *acute psychogenic paranoid psychosis; Bouffée délirante*
AHA: Q1, 1988, 3

298.4 Psychogenic paranoid psychosis — (Use additional code to identify any associated physical disease, injury, or condition affecting the brain)

298.8 Other and unspecified reactive psychosis — (Use additional code to identify any associated physical disease, injury, or condition affecting the brain) — *hysterical psychosis, psychogenic stupor*
AHA: Q1, 1988, 3

298.9 Unspecified psychosis — (Use additional code to identify any associated physical disease, injury, or condition affecting the brain) — *lycanthropy, nosomania, parergasia, vesania*
AHA: Q1, 1988, 3

Coding Clarification

Lycanthropy, the delusion that the patient believes himself to be a wolf, is classified in the ICD-9-CM index to 298.9, as is nosomania, a delusion of being infected by disease.

299 Pervasive developmental disorders

AHA: Q1, 1988, 3

Infantile autism is a syndrome present from birth or beginning almost invariably in the first 30 months. Responses to auditory and sometimes to visual stimuli are abnormal, and there are usually severe problems in the understanding of spoken language. Speech is delayed and, if it develops, is characterized by echolalia, the reversal of pronouns, immature grammatical structure, and an inability to use abstract terms. There is generally an impaired social use of both verbal and gestural language. Problems in social relationships are most severe before the age of 5 years and include an impaired development of eye-to-eye gaze, social attachments, and cooperative play. Ritualistic behavior is usual and may include abnormal routines, resistance to change, attachment to odd objects, and stereotyped patterns of play. The capacity for abstract or symbolic thought and for imaginative play is diminished. Intelligence ranges from severely subnormal to normal or above. Performance is usually better on tasks involving rote memory or visuospatial skills than on those requiring symbolic or linguistic skills.

The following fifth-digit subclassification is for use with category 299:

0 current or active state

1 residual state

299.0 5th Autistic disorder — *childhood autism; Kanner's syndrome*
AHA: Q1, 1988, 3

299.1 5th Childhood disintegrative disorder — (Use additional code to identify any associated neurological disorder) — *Heller's syndrome*
AHA: Q1, 1988, 3

299.8 5th Other specified pervasive developmental disorders — *atypical childhood psychosis; borderline psychosis of childhood*
AHA: Q1, 1988, 3

299.9 5th Unspecified pervasive developmental disorder

 © 2004 Ingenix, Inc.

Coding Clarification

Excluded from this rubric are adult type psychoses occurring in childhood, as in affective disorders (296.0-296.9), manic-depressive disorders (296.0-296.9), and schizophrenia (295.0-295.9).

300–316 Neurotic Disorders, Personality Disorders, and Other Nonpsychotic Mental Disorders

300 Anxiety, dissociative and somatoform disorders

AHA: Q1, 1988, 3

Neurotic disorders have no obvious evidence of an organic etiology, and there is no lost sense of reality or disorganized personality. Symptoms may include anxiety, hysteria, obsession, compulsion, depression, or phobia. Behavior may be greatly affected although usually remaining within socially acceptable limits.

In psychogenic amnesia, there is a temporary disturbance in the ability to recall important personal information that has already been registered and stored in memory. The sudden onset of this disturbance in the absence of an underlying organic mental disorder, and the extent of the disturbance being too great to be explained by ordinary forgetfulness, are the essential features.

In factitious illness, there are physical or psychological symptoms that are not real, genuine, or natural, which are produced by the individual and are under voluntary control. The presentation of physical symptoms may be fabricated, self-inflicted, an exaggeration or exacerbation of a pre-existing physical condition, or any combination or variation of these.

In phobia, the patient experiences abnormal intense dread of certain objects or specific situations. If the anxiety tends to spread from a specified situation or object to a wider range of circumstances, it becomes akin to or identical with an anxiety state, and should be classified as such.

In obsessive-compulsive behavior, the outstanding symptom is a feeling of subjective compulsion, which must be resisted. The obsessional urge or idea is recognized as alien to the personality but as coming from within the self. Obsessional actions may be quasi-ritual performances designed to relieve anxiety. Attempts to dispel the unwelcome thoughts or urges may lead to a severe inner struggle, with intense anxiety.

300.00 Anxiety state, unspecified — *anxiety neurosis; asphyctic syndrome*
AHA: Q1, 1988, 3; Q1, 2002, 6

300.01 Panic disorder without agoraphobia — *panic attack*
AHA: Q1, 1988, 3

300.02 Generalized anxiety disorder

300.09 Other anxiety states — *not elsewhere classified*
AHA: Q1, 1988, 3

300.10 Hysteria, unspecified

300.11 Conversion disorder — *astasia-abasia; hysterical blindness/deafness; Bergeron's disease*
AHA: Nov-Dec, 1985, 15; Q1, 1988, 3

300.12 Dissociative amnesia — *hysterical amnesia*
AHA: Q1, 1988, 3

300.13 Dissociative fugue — *hysterical fugue*
AHA: Q1, 1988, 3

300.14 Dissociative identity disorder — *dissociative identity disorder*
AHA: Q1, 1988, 3

300.15 Dissociative disorder or reaction, unspecified

300.16 Factitious disorder with predominantly psychological signs and symptoms — *compensation neurosis; Ganser's hysterical syndrome*
AHA: Q1, 1988, 3

300.19 Other and unspecified factitious illness — *factitious illness with physical symptoms, NOS*
AHA: Q1, 1988, 3

300.20 Phobia, unspecified

300.21 Agoraphobia with panic disorder — *fear of open spaces, streets, travel; with panic attacks*
AHA: Q1, 1988, 3

300.22 Agoraphobia without mention of panic attacks — *fear of open spaces, streets, travel; without mention of panic attacks*
AHA: Q1, 1988, 3

300.23 Social phobia — *fear of eating, washing, speaking in public*
AHA: Q1, 1988, 3

300.29 Other isolated or specific phobias — *acrophobia, claustrophobia, animal phobias*
AHA: Q1, 1988, 3

300.3 Obsessive-compulsive disorders — *anancastic neurosis, any obsessional phobia, compulsive neurosis*
AHA: Q1, 1988, 3

300.4 Dysthymic disorder — *anxiety depression, reactive depression*
AHA: Q1, 1988, 3

300.5 Neurasthenia — (Use additional code to identify any associated physical disorder) — *fatigue neurosis, general fatigue, psychogenic asthenia*
AHA: Q1, 1988, 3

300.6 Depersonalization disorder — *neurotic derealization*
AHA: Q1, 1988, 3

300.7 Hypochondriasis — *body dysmorphic disorder*
AHA: Q1, 1988, 3

300.81 Somatization disorder — *Briquet's disorder, severe somatoform disorder*
AHA: Q1, 1988, 3

300.82 Undifferentiated somatoform disorder — *atypical somatoform disorder*
AHA: Q1, 1988, 3; Q4, 1996, 29

300.89 Other somatoform disorders — *occupational neurosis, including writers' cramp, psychasthenia, Janet's disease*
AHA: Q1, 1988, 3

300.9 Unspecified nonpsychotic mental disorder — *neurosis NOS, merergasia, self-mutilation, suicide risk*
AHA: Q1, 1988, 3

Coding Clarification

Excluded from phobic disorders are anxiety states not associated with a specific situation or object (300.00-300.09) and obsessional phobia (300.3).

301 Personality disorders

AHA: Q1, 1988, 3

A dependent personality disorder allows a patient to permit another individual to take control of his/her life. This patient also allows the needs of that person to supersede personal needs. A borderline personality is characterized by instability in interpersonal relationships, behavior, mood, and perception of self-image.

301.0 Paranoid personality disorder — (Use additional code to identify any associated neurosis or psychosis, or physical condition) — *fanatic personality; paranoid traits*
AHA: July-Aug, 1985, 9; Q1, 1988, 3

301.10 Affective personality disorder, unspecified — (Use additional code to identify any associated neurosis or psychosis, or physical condition)

301.11 Chronic hypomanic personality disorder — (Use additional code to identify any associated neurosis or psychosis, or physical condition)

301.12 Chronic depressive personality disorder — (Use additional code to identify any associated neurosis or psychosis, or physical condition)

301.13 Cyclothymic disorder — (Use additional code to identify any associated neurosis or psychosis, or physical condition) — *cycloid personality; cyclothymia*
AHA: Q1, 1988, 3

301.20 Schizoid personality disorder, unspecified — (Use additional code to identify any associated neurosis or psychosis, or physical condition)

301.21 Introverted personality — (Use additional code to identify any associated neurosis or psychosis, or physical condition)

301.22 Schizotypal personality disorder — (Use additional code to identify any associated neurosis or psychosis, or physical condition)

301.3 Explosive personality disorder — (Use additional code to identify any associated neurosis or psychosis, or physical condition) — *excessive emotional instability; pathological emotionality*
AHA: Q1, 1988, 3

301.4 Obsessive-compulsive personality disorder — (Use additional code to identify any associated neurosis or psychosis, or physical condition) — *obsessional personality*
AHA: Q1, 1988, 3

301.50 Histrionic personality disorder, unspecified — (Use additional code to identify any associated neurosis or psychosis, or physical condition) — *not elsewhere classified*
AHA: Q1, 1988, 3

301.51 Chronic factitious illness with physical symptoms — (Use additional code to identify any associated neurosis or psychosis, or physical condition) — *hospital addiction syndrome; Munchausen syndrome*
AHA: Q1, 1988, 3

301.59 Other histrionic personality disorder — (Use additional code to identify any associated neurosis or psychosis, or physical condition) — *emotionally unstable; psychoinfantile; labile*
AHA: Q1, 1988, 3

301.6 Dependent personality disorder — (Use additional code to identify any associated neurosis or psychosis, or physical condition) — *asthenic or passive personality*
AHA: Q1, 1988, 3

301.7 Antisocial personality disorder — (Use additional code to identify any associated neurosis or psychosis, or physical condition) — *amoral or sociopathic personality*
AHA: Sept-Oct, 1984, 16; Q1, 1988, 3

290–319

© 2004 Ingenix, Inc.

301.81 Narcissistic personality disorder — (Use additional code to identify any associated neurosis or psychosis, or physical condition)

301.82 Avoidant personality disorder — (Use additional code to identify any associated neurosis or psychosis, or physical condition)

301.83 Borderline personality disorder — (Use additional code to identify any associated neurosis or psychosis, or physical condition)

301.84 Passive-aggressive personality — (Use additional code to identify any associated neurosis or psychosis, or physical condition)

301.89 Other personality disorder — (Use additional code to identify any associated neurosis or psychosis, or physical condition) — *eccentric, masochistic or psychoneurotic*
AHA: Q1, 1988, 3

301.9 Unspecified personality disorder — (Use additional code to identify any associated neurosis or psychosis, or physical condition) — *Witzelsucht; psychopathic constitutional*
AHA: Q1, 1988, 3

Coding Clarification

Personality disorders include character neuroses, but exclude nonpsychotic personality disorders associated with organic brain syndromes (310.0-310.9). Use an additional code to identify an associated neurosis or psychosis, or physical condition.

302 Sexual and gender identity disorders

AHA: Q1, 1988, 3

The limits and features of normal sexual behavior have not been stated absolutely in different societies and cultures, but applied broadly serve as approved social and biological purposes. The sexual activities of patients with deviant disorders are directed primarily toward sexual acts not associated with coitus normally, or toward coitus performed under abnormal circumstances.

302.0 Ego-dystonic sexual orientation — *ego-dystonic lesbianism; homosexual conflict disorder*
AHA: Q1, 1988, 3

302.1 Zoophilia

302.2 Pedophilia

302.3 Transvestic fetishism

302.4 Exhibitionism

302.50 Trans-sexualism with unspecified sexual history

302.51 Trans-sexualism with asexual history

302.52 Trans-sexualism with homosexual history

302.53 Trans-sexualism with heterosexual history

302.6 Gender identity disorder in children — *feminism in boys; gender identity disorder of childhood*
AHA: Q1, 1988, 3

302.70 Psychosexual dysfunction, unspecified

302.71 Hypoactive sexual desire disorder

302.72 Psychosexual dysfunction with inhibited sexual excitement — *frigidity or impotence*
AHA: Q1, 1988, 3

302.73 Female orgasmic disorder

302.74 Male orgasmic disorder

302.75 Premature ejaculation

302.76 Dyspareunia, psychogenic

302.79 Psychosexual dysfunction with other specified psychosexual dysfunctions — *not elsewhere classified*
AHA: Q1, 1988, 3

302.81 Fetishism

302.82 Voyeurism

302.83 Sexual masochism

302.84 Sexual sadism

302.85 Gender identity disorder in adolescents or adults — *gender identity disorder of adult life*
AHA: Q1, 1988, 3

302.89 Other specified psychosexual disorder — *nymphomania, satyriasis, frotteurism, coprophilia and necrophilia*
AHA: Q1, 1988, 3

302.9 Unspecified psychosexual disorder

Coding Clarification

If the anomalous behavior becomes manifest only during psychosis or other mental illness, the condition should be classified under the major illness. Excluded from psychosexual dysfunction are organic causes of impotence (607.84), occasional or transient failures of erection or sexual excitement, or other dysfunction with organic cause.

303 Alcohol dependence syndrome

AHA: Sept-Oct, 1986, 3; Q1, 1988, 3; Q4, 1988, 8; Q2, 1991, 9; Q3, 1995, 6

Alcohol dependence syndrome is both a psychic and physical state, resulting from excessive alcohol consumption. The syndrome is characterized by behavioral and other responses that always include a compulsion to take alcohol on a continuous or periodic basis in order to experience its psychic effects, and sometimes to avoid the discomfort of its absence; tolerance may or may not be present.

The following fifth-digit subclassification is for use with categories 303, 304, and 305.0, 305.2-305.9:

0 unspecified

1 continuous

2 episodic

3 in remission

303.0 ✓5th Acute alcoholic intoxication — (Use additional code to identify any associated condition: 291.0-291.9, 304.00-304.93, 331.7, 345.00-345.91, 535.3, 571.1, 571.2, 571.3) — *acute drunkenness in alcoholism*
AHA: Sept-Oct, 1986, 3; Q1, 1988, 3; Q4, 1988, 8; Q2, 1991, 9; Q3, 1995, 6

303.9 ✓5th Other and unspecified alcohol dependence — (Use additional code to identify any associated condition: 291.0-291.9, 304.00-304.93, 331.7, 345.00-345.91, 535.3, 571.1, 571.2, 571.3) — *chronic alcoholism; dipsomania*
AHA: Sept-Oct, 1986, 3; Q1, 1988, 3; Q4, 1988, 8; Q2, 1989, 9; Q2, 1991, 9; Q3, 1995, 6; Q2, 2002, 4

Documentation Issues

If the documentation references a history of alcohol dependence, only report it if it has an impact on the current patient treatment or length of stay.

When the diagnostic statement of acute and chronic alcoholism is noted, further review of the documentation should be performed to determine if the patient was acutely intoxicated at the time of the encounter for appropriate code assignment. Verify with the physician if necessary as only one code should be assigned.

When the patient is admitted for detoxification and is currently pregnant, a diagnosis code from Chapter 11 Complications of Pregnancy, Childbirth and Puerperium (630-677) is required unless the physician documents that this condition is not affecting the pregnancy. A code specifying the type of dependence may also be used as an additional diagnosis. If the physician documents that the pregnancy is incidental, use code V22.2 *Pregnant state, incidental* in addition to the dependency code.

If the documentation identifies that the patient experienced withdrawal symptoms or syndrome whether prior to or after admission, report it. Use code 291.81 for alcohol withdrawal.

Coding Clarification

A person may be dependent on alcohol and other drugs; if so, also record the diagnosis of drug dependence to identify the agent. If alcohol dependence is associated with alcoholic psychosis or with physical complications, both diagnoses should be recorded. Use an additional code to identify any associated conditions, as in alcoholic psychosis (291.0-291.9), drug dependence (304.0-304.9), or physical complications of alcohol, including gastritis (535.3), cirrhosis (571.2), hepatitis (571.1), or cerebral degeneration (331.7).

Axes in this rubric classify the alcohol dependence as acute or chronic, and according to the nature of the dependence during the episode of care. When drunkenness is not otherwise specified, report with 305.0x, which reports nondependent abuse of alcohol.

Alcohol Dependence: This chronic condition is identified by the patient who is unable to cease alcohol use even with detriments to health, social interactions, and job performance. These patients generally experience physical signs of withdrawal with any sudden cessation of drinking. Alcohol dependence is classified to category 303. Subcategory code 303.0x is reported for acute alcohol intoxication in chronic alcoholism. Subcategory code 303.9x is reported when the patient is treated when not acutely intoxicated and is alcohol dependent.

Coding Scenario

A 62-year-old male patient is seen in the office for a physical exam. The patient has been alcohol dependent for 32 years. He has quit drinking for the second time and has been dry for a four-month duration.

> Code assignment: 303.93 *Alcohol dependence syndrome, other and unspecified alcohol dependence, in remission*

304 Drug dependence

AHA: Sept-Oct, 1986, 3; Q1, 1988, 3; Q4, 1988, 8; Q2, 1991, 10

Drug dependence is both a mental and physical state, resulting from taking a drug. It is characterized by behavioral and other responses that always include a compulsion to take a drug on a continuous or periodic basis in order to experience its psychic effects, and sometimes to avoid the discomfort of its absence. Tolerance may be present. A person may be dependent on more than one drug.

The following fifth-digit subclassification is for use with categories 303, 304, 305.0, and 305.2-305.9:

0 unspecified

1 continuous

2 episodic

3 in remission

304.0 ✓5th Opioid type dependence — *heroin, opium alkaloids and their derivatives, meperidine, methadone*
AHA: Sept-Oct, 1986, 3; Q1, 1988, 3; Q4, 1988, 8; Q2, 1991, 10

 © 2004 Ingenix, Inc.

304.1 ✓5th Sedative, hypnotic or anxiolytic dependence — *nonbarbiturate sedatives and tranquilizers with similar effect: chlordiazepoxide, meprobamate, diazepam, methaqualone, glutethimide*
AHA: Sept-Oct, 1986, 3; Q1, 1988, 3; Q4, 1988, 8; Q2, 1991, 10

304.2 ✓5th Cocaine dependence — *coca leaves, crack cocaine, coke*
AHA: Sept-Oct, 1986, 3; Q1, 1988, 3; Q4, 1988, 8; Q2, 1991, 10

304.3 ✓5th Cannabis dependence — *hashish, marijuana, pot*
AHA: Sept-Oct, 1986, 3; Q1, 1988, 3; Q4, 1988, 8; Q2, 1991, 10

304.4 ✓5th Amphetamine and other psychostimulant dependence — *methylphenidate, phenmetrazine*
AHA: Sept-Oct, 1986, 3; Q1, 1988, 3; Q4, 1988, 8; Q2, 1991, 10

304.5 ✓5th Hallucinogen dependence — *dimethyltryptamine [DMT], lysergic acid diethylamide [LSD], mescaline, psilocybin*
AHA: Sept-Oct, 1986, 3; Q1, 1988, 3; Q4, 1988, 8; Q2, 1991, 10

304.6 ✓5th Other specified drug dependence — *absinthe; glue sniffing*
AHA: Sept-Oct, 1986, 3; Q1, 1988, 3; Q4, 1988, 8; Q2, 1991, 10

304.7 ✓5th Combinations of opioid type drug with any other drug dependence

304.8 ✓5th Combinations of drug dependence excluding opioid type drug

304.9 ✓5th Unspecified drug dependence — *drug addiction NOS*
AHA: Sept-Oct, 1986, 3; Q1, 1988, 3; Q4, 1988, 8; Q2, 1991, 10

Documentation Issues

If the documentation references a history of drug dependence, only report it if it has an impact on the current patient treatment or length of stay.

When the patient is admitted for detoxification and is currently pregnant, a diagnosis code from chapter 11 Complications of Pregnancy, Childbirth and Puerperium (630-677) is required unless the physician documents this condition as not affecting the pregnancy. A code specifying the type of dependence may also be used as an additional diagnosis. If the physician documents that the pregnancy is incidental, use code V22.2 *Pregnant state, incidental* in addition to the dependency code.

If the documentation identifies that the patient experienced withdrawal symptoms or syndrome whether prior to or after admission, use code 292.0 for drug withdrawal.

Coding Clarification

This rubric excludes nondependent abuse of drugs, which is reported with codes in the 305 rubric.

Drug Dependence: This chronic mental and physical condition is related to the pattern of the patient's drug or drug combination intake and is characterized by behavioral and physiological reactions. These reactions are the obsession to take the drug, the need to have the feeling of its psychic effects, or the attempt to avoid the discomfort of abstinence. Any sudden cessation typically triggers physical signs of withdrawal.

Polydrug Addiction: Report code 304.8x *Combinations of drug dependence excluding opioid type drug* if classifying known combinations not of opium derivatives as well as the polydrug addiction, not otherwise specified. Report code 304.7x *Combinations of opioid type drug with any other drug dependence* when an opioid drug is one of the combinations.

Coding Scenario

A patient is seen for neurogenic bowel disorder secondary to ongoing drug dependence of meperidine and opiates. The physician identifies the neurogenic bowel disorder as constipation in the medical record documentation.

> Code assignment: 304.01 *Drug dependence, Opioid type dependence, continuous* and 564.0 *Constipation*

305 Nondependent abuse of drugs

AHA: Sept-Oct, 1986, 3; Q1, 1988, 3; Q4, 1988, 8; Q2, 1991, 10

Drug abuse includes cases where the individual, for whom no other diagnosis is possible, has come under medical care because of the maladaptive effect of a drug on which the patient is not dependent. In nondependent abuse of drugs, the individual generally has taken the drug on personal initiative to the detriment of health or social functioning. When drug abuse is secondary to a psychiatric disorder, record the disorder as a primary diagnosis.

Codes in this rubric are classified according to the drug being abused, and whether the abuse is continuous, episodic, or in remission.

The following fifth-digit subclassification is for use with categories 303, 304, 305.0, and 305.2-305.9:

0 unspecified
1 continuous
2 episodic
3 in remission

305.0 5th Nondependent alcohol abuse — *drunkenness NOS*
AHA: Sept-Oct, 1986, 3; Q1, 1988, 3; Q4, 1988, 8; Q2, 1991, 10; Q3, 1996, 16

305.1 Nondependent tobacco use disorder — *tobacco dependence*
AHA: Nov-Dec, 1984, 12; Sept-Oct, 1986, 3; Q1, 1988, 3; Q4, 1988, 8; Q2, 1991, 10; Q2, 1996, 10

305.2 5th Nondependent cannabis abuse — *abuse of hashish, marijuana, pot*
AHA: Sept-Oct, 1986, 3; Q1, 1988, 3; Q4, 1988, 8; Q2, 1991, 10

305.3 5th Nondependent hallucinogen abuse — *abuse of dimethyltryptamine [DMT], lysergic acid diethylamide [LSD], mescaline, psilocybin*
AHA: Sept-Oct, 1986, 3; Q1, 1988, 3; Q4, 1988, 8; Q2, 1991, 10

305.4 5th Nondependent barbiturate and similarly acting sedative or hypnotic abuse — *abuse of nonbarbiturate sedatives and tranquilizers with similar effect: chlordiazepoxide, meprobamate, diazepam, methaqualone, glutethimide*
AHA: Sept-Oct, 1986, 3; Q1, 1988, 3; Q4, 1988, 8; Q2, 1991, 10

305.5 5th Nondependent opioid abuse — *abuse of heroin, opium alkaloids, meperidine, methadone*
AHA: Sept-Oct, 1986, 3; Q1, 1988, 3; Q4, 1988, 8; Q2, 1991, 10

305.6 5th Nondependent cocaine abuse — *abuse of coca leaves, crack cocaine, coke*
AHA: Sept-Oct, 1986, 3; Q1, 1988, 3; Q4, 1988, 8; Q2, 1991, 10; Q1, 1993, 25

305.7 5th Nondependent amphetamine or related acting sympathomimetic abuse — *abuse of methylphenidate, phenmetrazine*
AHA: Sept-Oct, 1986, 3; Q1, 1988, 3; Q4, 1988, 8; Q2, 1991, 10

305.8 5th Nondependent antidepressant type abuse

305.9 5th Other, mixed, or unspecified nondependent drug abuse — *laxative habit, nonprescribed drugs or patent medicinals*
AHA: Sept-Oct, 1986, 3; Q1, 1988, 3; Q4, 1988, 8; Q2, 1991, 10; Q3, 1999, 20

Coding Clarification

Cases in which tobacco is used to the detriment of a person's health or social functioning or in which there is tobacco dependence are classified to code 305.1. Dependence is included here rather than under drug dependence because tobacco differs from other drugs of dependence in its psychotoxic effects. Excluded from the code for tobacco dependence is history of tobacco use, V15.82.

Alcohol Abuse: Patients who have been identified as having alcohol abuse represent those who have developed a problem with drinking, including those that drink alcohol in excess but have not arrived at a stage of physical dependency. Symptoms include slurred speech, blackouts, driving difficulty, social dysfunction, and temporary mental disturbance. To report, use subcategory code 305.0x. Simple drunkenness is included in this code.

Drug Abuse: Patients who have been identified as drug abusers have developed a problem with drugs including those that take an excess of drugs but have not arrived at a stage of physical dependency. Representing a maladaptive pattern due to drugs, including social, mental, and physical dysfunction, this condition also includes blackouts, slurred speech, driving difficulty, and temporary mental disturbance. Use code range 305.1x-305.9x for the diagnosis of drug abuse.

Poisoning with Abuse: When the diagnosis of drug and/or alcohol abuse has been noted with a poisoning or reaction to the improper use of the substance, the poisoning code is sequenced first, then the code for the manifestation. Also use an additional code to report the specific form of abuse.

Pregnancy Complication: Report with subcategory code 648.4 with an appropriate fifth digit to denote the current episode of care. A code specifying the type of abuse may also be reported as an additional diagnosis.

Rehabilitation: Do not report code V57.89 as the principal/primary diagnosis when reporting alcohol/drug rehabilitation services. This code is solely used as an additional code to indicate whether rehabilitation and/or detoxification services were furnished.

Tobacco Abuse: Report with code 305.1 *Tobacco use disorder.* If the documentation indicates a past history of smoking, now in remission, code V15.82 *History of tobacco use.* No fifth digit is required for code 305.1.

Coding Scenario

A patient is seen in the emergency department with respiratory failure due to crack overdose. The patient is placed on ventilation and admitted to the intensive care unit for further stabilization.

> Code assignment: 968.5 *Poisoning by other central nervous system depressants and anesthetics, surface [topical] and infiltration anesthetics,* 305.60 *Non-dependent abuse of drugs, cocaine abuse, unspecified,* and 518.81 *Other diseases of lung, respiratory failure*

A patient is seen in the outpatient clinic in an acute drunken state. The patient is complaining of feeling numb. The physician's diagnostic statement confirms acute alcohol intoxication.

> Code assignment: 305.00 *Nondependent abuse of drugs, alcohol abuse*

290–319

© 2004 Ingenix, Inc.

A 17-year-old female is seen in the OB clinic for a prenatal visit. The patient admits to occasional use of cocaine.

> Code assignment: 648.43 *Other current conditions in the mother classifiable elsewhere, but complicating pregnancy, childbirth, or the puerperium, mental disorders, antepartum condition or complication* and 305.60 *Nondependent abuse of drugs, cocaine abuse, unspecified*

A 69-year-old male patient is seen in the physician office for COPD. The patient is currently smoking two packs per day and hasn't had much success with smoking cessation programs.

> Code assignment: 496 *Chronic airway obstruction, not elsewhere classified* and *305.1 Tobacco use disorder*

306 Physiological malfunction arising from mental factors

AHA: Q1, 1988, 3

This rubric includes psychogenic physical and physiological malfunctions that do not include tissue damage.

306.0 Musculoskeletal malfunction arising from mental factors — *psychogenic paralysis or torticollis*
AHA: Q1, 1988, 3

306.1 Respiratory malfunction arising from mental factors — *psychogenic hyperventilation; cough, yawn, or hiccough*
AHA: Q1, 1988, 3

306.2 Cardiovascular malfunction arising from mental factors — *cardiac neurosis*
AHA: July-Aug, 1985, 14; Q1, 1988, 3

306.3 Skin malfunction arising from mental factors — *psychogenic pruritus or hyperhidrosis*
AHA: Q1, 1988, 3

306.4 Gastrointestinal malfunction arising from mental factors — *aerophagy, psychogenic vomiting or diarrhea*
AHA: Q1, 1988, 3; Q2, 1989, 11

306.50 Psychogenic genitourinary malfunction, unspecified

306.51 Psychogenic vaginismus — *vaginal spasm*
AHA: Q1, 1988, 3

306.52 Psychogenic dysmenorrhea — *painful menstruation*
AHA: Q1, 1988, 3

306.53 Psychogenic dysuria — *painful urination*
AHA: Q1, 1988, 3

306.59 Other genitourinary malfunction arising from mental factors — *specified psychogenic pain*
AHA: March-April, 1987, 11; Q1, 1988, 3

306.6 Endocrine malfunction arising from mental factors — *pancreas, thyroid,*
AHA: Q1, 1988, 3

306.7 Malfunction of organs of special sense arising from mental factors — *eyes, ears*
AHA: Q1, 1988, 3

306.8 Other specified psychophysiological malfunction — *bruxism, teeth grinding*
AHA: Q1, 1988, 3

306.9 Unspecified psychophysiological malfunction — *not otherwise specified*
AHA: Q1, 1988, 3

Coding Clarification

If there is tissue damage, see rubric 316. Also excluded are hysteria (300.11-300.19) and specific nonpsychotic mental disorders following organic brain damage (310.0-310.9).

307 Special symptoms or syndromes, not elsewhere classified

AHA: Q1, 1988, 3

This category is intended for psychopathology manifested by a single specific symptom or group of symptoms not part of an organic illness or other mental disorder classified elsewhere.

In anorexia nervosa, the symptoms include persistent active refusal to eat and marked loss of weight. The level of activity and alertness is characteristically high in relation to the degree of emaciation. Typically the disorder begins in teenage girls but it may begin before puberty. It rarely occurs in males. Amenorrhea is usual and, in advanced cases, slowed pulse and respiration, low body temperature, dependent edema, and heart rhythm abnormalities. Manifestations of anorexia nervosa should be reported additionally.

307.0 Stuttering

307.1 Anorexia nervosa — *fear of obesity, usually in females, resulting in emaciation*
AHA: Q1, 1988, 3; Q4, 1989, 11

307.20 Tic disorder, unspecified

307.21 Transient tic disorder

307.22 Chronic motor or vocal tic disorder — *blink, shrug, grimace, cough, jerk*
AHA: Q1, 1988, 3

307.23 Tourette's disorder — *motor-verbal tic disorder; Brissaud's motor-verbal tic*
AHA: Q1, 1988, 3

307.3 Stereotypic movement disorder — *body-rocking; spasmus nutans; head banging*
AHA: Q1, 1988, 3

307.40 Nonorganic sleep disorder, unspecified

307.41 Transient disorder of initiating or maintaining sleep — *associated with intermittent emotional reactions or conflicts*
AHA: Q1, 1988, 3

307.42 Persistent disorder of initiating or maintaining sleep — *associated with anxiety, depression, psychosis*
AHA: Q1, 1988, 3

307.43 Transient disorder of initiating or maintaining wakefulness — *associated with acute or intermittent emotional reactions or conflicts*
AHA: Q1, 1988, 3

307.44 Persistent disorder of initiating or maintaining wakefulness — *associated with depression*
AHA: Q1, 1988, 3

307.45 Circadian rhythm sleep disorder — *jet lag syndrome; shifting sleep-work schedule*
AHA: Q1, 1988, 3

307.46 Sleep arousal disorder — *sleepwalking*
AHA: Q1, 1988, 3

307.47 Other dysfunctions of sleep stages or arousal from sleep — *nightmares*
AHA: Q1, 1988, 3

307.48 Repetitive intrusions of sleep — *environmental disturbances or repeated REM- interruptions*
AHA: Q1, 1988, 3

307.49 Other specific disorder of sleep of nonorganic origin — *subjective "short-sleeper;" pseudoinsomnia*
AHA: Q1, 1988, 3

307.50 Eating disorder, unspecified

307.51 Bulimia nervosa — *binge/purge*
AHA: Q1, 1988, 3

307.52 Pica — *perverted appetite of nonorganic origin*
AHA: Q1, 1988, 3

307.53 Rumination disorder — *regurgitation, of nonorganic origin, of food with reswallowing*
AHA: Q1, 1988, 3

307.54 Psychogenic vomiting — *no physical cause*
AHA: Q1, 1988, 3

307.59 Other disorder of eating — *no physical cause*
AHA: Q1, 1988, 3

307.6 Enuresis — *of nonorganic origin*
AHA: Q1, 1988, 3

307.7 Encopresis — *of nonorganic origin*
AHA: Q1, 1988, 3

307.80 Psychogenic pain, site unspecified

307.81 Tension headache — *stress headache*
AHA: Nov-Dec, 1985, 16; Q1, 1988, 3

307.89 Other pain disorder related to psychological factors — *not elsewhere classified*
AHA: Q1, 1988, 3

307.9 Other and unspecified special symptom or syndrome, not elsewhere classified — *hair plucking, masturbation, lalling, nail-biting, lisping, thumb-sucking*
AHA: Q1, 1988, 3

308 Acute reaction to stress

AHA: Q1, 1988, 3

This rubric is reserved for acute reactions as a response to exceptional physical or mental distress, which usually subside within hours or days. Some examples include catastrophic stress, combat fatigue, or gross stress reaction.

308.0 Predominant disturbance of emotions — *anxiety, emotional crisis, panic*
AHA: Q1, 1988, 3

308.1 Predominant disturbance of consciousness as reaction to stress — *fugues*
AHA: Q1, 1988, 3

308.2 Predominant psychomotor disturbance as reaction to stress — *agitation or stupor*
AHA: Q1, 1988, 3

308.3 Other acute reactions to stress — *brief or acute posttraumatic stress disorder*
AHA: Q1, 1988, 3

308.4 Mixed disorders as reaction to stress — *combination of reactions classified to 308*
AHA: Q1, 1988, 3

308.9 Unspecified acute reaction to stress — *combat fatigue*
AHA: Q1, 1988, 3

Coding Clarification

Excluded from this rubric are adjustment reaction disorders (309.0-309.9) and chronic stress reaction (309.1-309.9).

309 Adjustment reaction

AHA: Q1, 1988, 3

An adjustment or adaptation reaction is a mild or transient disorder lasting longer than acute stress reactions and occurring in individuals of any age without any apparent pre-existing mental disorder. Such disorders are often relatively circumscribed or situation-specific, are generally reversible, and usually last only a few months. They are usually closely related in time and content to stresses such as bereavement, migration, or other experiences. Reactions to major stress that last longer than a few days are also included. In children, such disorders are associated with no significant distortion of development.

 © 2004 Ingenix, Inc.

309.0 Adjustment disorder with depressed mood — *grief reaction*
AHA: Q1, 1988, 3

309.1 Prolonged depressive reaction as adjustment reaction

309.21 Separation anxiety disorder — *abnormal stress upon leaving another person*
AHA: Q1, 1988, 3

309.22 Emancipation disorder of adolescence and early adult life

309.23 Specific academic or work inhibition as adjustment reaction

309.24 Adjustment disorder with anxiety

309.28 Adjustment disorder with mixed anxiety and depressed mood — *adjustment reaction with anxiety and depression*
AHA: Q1, 1988, 3

309.29 Other adjustment reaction with predominant disturbance of other emotions — *culture shock*
AHA: Q1, 1988, 3

309.3 Adjustment disorder with disturbance of conduct — *conduct disturbance or destructiveness as an adjustment reaction*
AHA: Q1, 1988, 3

309.4 Adjustment disorder with mixed disturbance of emotions and conduct

309.81 Posttraumatic stress disorder — *chronic posttraumatic stress disorder; concentration camp syndrome*
AHA: Q1, 1988, 3

309.82 Adjustment reaction with physical symptoms

309.83 Adjustment reaction with withdrawal — *elective mutism, hospitalism*
AHA: Q1, 1988, 3

309.89 Other specified adjustment reaction — *homesickness*
AHA: Q1, 1988, 3

309.9 Unspecified adjustment reaction — *adaptation reaction NOS*
AHA: Q1, 1988, 3

Coding Clarification

Excluded from this rubric are acute reactions to major stress (308.0-308.9) and neurotic disorders (300.1-300.9).

310 Specific nonpsychotic mental disorders due to brain damage

AHA: Q1, 1988, 3

Postconcussion syndrome occurs after generalized contusion of the brain, resembling the overall symptoms found in frontal lobe syndrome or any of the neurotic disorders, but in which headache, giddiness, fatigue, insomnia, and a subjective feeling of impaired intellectual ability are also prominent. Mood may fluctuate, and quite ordinary stress may produce exaggerated fear and apprehension. There may be marked intolerance of mental and physical exertion, undue sensitivity to noise, and hypochondriacal preoccupation. The symptoms are more common in persons who have previously suffered from neurotic or personality disorders. This syndrome is particularly associated with the closed type of head injury when signs of localized brain damage are slight or absent, but it may also occur in other conditions.

Frontal lobe syndrome presents with changes in behavior following damage to the frontal areas of the brain or following interference with the connections of those areas. There is a general diminution of self-control, foresight, creativity, and spontaneity, which may be manifest as increased irritability, selfishness, restlessness, and lack of concern for others. Conscientiousness and powers of concentration are often diminished, but measurable deterioration of intellect or memory is not necessarily present. The overall picture is often one of emotional dullness, lack of drive, and slowness; but, particularly in persons previously with energetic, restless, or aggressive characteristics, there may be a change toward impulsiveness, boastfulness, temper outbursts, silly fatuous humor, and the development of unrealistic ambitions. The direction of change usually depends upon the previous personality. A considerable degree of recovery is possible and may continue over the course of several years.

310.0 Frontal lobe syndrome — *postleucotomy syndrome, Klüver-Bucy (-Terzian) syndrome*
AHA: Q1, 1988, 3

310.1 Personality change due to conditions classified elsewhere — *cognitive or personality change of other type, of nonpsychotic severity; mild memory disturbance; presbyophrenia NOS*
AHA: Q1, 1988, 3

310.2 Postconcussion syndrome — *postconcussion syndrome or encephalopathy*
AHA: Q1, 1988, 3; Q4, 1990, 24

310.8 Other specified nonpsychotic mental disorder following organic brain damage — *postencephalitic syndrome*
AHA: Q1, 1988, 3

310.9 Unspecified nonpsychotic mental disorder following organic brain damage

311 Depressive disorder, not elsewhere classified OK

AHA: Q1, 1988, 3; Q4, 2003, 75

This rubric is reserved for depressive disorders not classified in other sections of this chapter, or depressive orders not assigned a more specific diagnosis.

312 Disturbance of conduct, not elsewhere classified

AHA: Q1, 1988, 3

This rubric is reserved for psychosocial and other conduct disorders not classified in other sections of this chapter, or that cannot be assigned a more specific diagnosis. Conduct disorders mainly involve aggressive and destructive behavior and disorders involving delinquency. Codes in this rubric should be used for abnormal behavior, in individuals of any age, which gives rise to social disapproval although not part of any other psychiatric condition. Minor emotional disturbances may also be present. To be included, the behavior, as judged by its frequency, severity, and type of associations with other symptoms, must be abnormal in its context. Disturbances of conduct are distinguished from an adjustment reaction by a longer duration and by a lack of close relationship in time and content to some stress. They differ from a personality disorder by the absence of deeply ingrained maladaptive patterns of behavior present from adolescence or earlier.

The following fifth-digit subclassification is for use with categories 312.0-312.2:

0 unspecified

1 mild

2 moderate

3 severe

312.0 5th Undersocialized conduct disorder, aggressive type — *aggressive outburst, anger reaction; unsocialized, aggressive disorder*
AHA: Q1, 1988, 3

312.1 5th Undersocialized conduct disorder, unaggressive type — *childhood truancy; tantrums, solitary, stealing; unsocialized*
AHA: Q1, 1988, 3

312.2 5th Socialized conduct disorder — *childhood truancy socialized, group delinquency*
AHA: Q1, 1988, 3

312.30 Impulse control disorder, unspecified

312.31 Pathological gambling

312.32 Kleptomania — *compulsive theft*
AHA: Q1, 1988, 3

312.33 Pyromania — *compulsive fire starting*
AHA: Q1, 1988, 3

312.34 Intermittent explosive disorder

312.35 Isolated explosive disorder

312.39 Other disorder of impulse control — *not elsewhere specified, trichotillomania*
AHA: Q1, 1988, 3

312.4 Mixed disturbance of conduct and emotions — *neurotic delinquency*
AHA: Q1, 1988, 3

312.81 Conduct disorder, childhood onset type

312.82 Conduct disorder, adolescent onset type

312.89 Other specified disturbance of conduct, not elsewhere classified

312.9 Unspecified disturbance of conduct

313 Disturbance of emotions specific to childhood and adolescence

AHA: Q1, 1988, 3

Academic underachievement disorder (313.83) presents as a failure to achieve in most school tasks despite adequate intellectual capacity, a supportive and encouraging social environment, and apparent effort. The failure occurs in the absence of a demonstrable specific learning disability and is caused by emotional conflict not clearly associated with any other mental disorder.

313.0 Overanxious disorder specific to childhood and adolescence — *anxiety and fearfulness in childhood*
AHA: Q1, 1988, 3

313.1 Misery and unhappiness disorder specific to childhood and adolescence

313.21 Shyness disorder of childhood

313.22 Introverted disorder of childhood

313.23 Selective mutism

313.3 Relationship problems specific to childhood and adolescence

313.81 Oppositional defiant disorder

313.82 Identity disorder of childhood or adolescence

313.83 Academic underachievement disorder of childhood or adolescence

313.89 Other emotional disturbance of childhood or adolescence

313.9 Unspecified emotional disturbance of childhood or adolescence

Coding Clarification
This rubric excludes adjustment reactions (309.0-309.9), neurotic emotional disorders (300.0-300.9), and isolated symptoms including masturbation, nail biting, and thumb-sucking (307.0-307.9).

314 Hyperkinetic syndrome of childhood

AHA: Q1, 1988, 3

Hyperkinetic syndromes of childhood are disorders in which the essential features are short attention span and distractibility. In early childhood, the most striking symptom is disinhibited, poorly organized,

© 2004 Ingenix, Inc.

and poorly regulated extreme overactivity but in adolescence this may be replaced by underactivity. Impulsiveness, marked fluctuations in mood, and aggression are also common symptoms. Delays in the development of specific skills are often present and disturbed, poor relationships are common.

314.00 Attention deficit disorder of childhood without mention of hyperactivity

314.01 Attention deficit disorder of childhood with hyperactivity

314.1 Hyperkinesis of childhood with developmental delay — (Use additional code to identify any associated neurological disorder)

314.2 Hyperkinetic conduct disorder of childhood — *without developmental delay*
AHA: Q1, 1988, 3

314.8 Other specified manifestations of hyperkinetic syndrome of childhood

314.9 Unspecified hyperkinetic syndrome of childhood

Coding Clarification
If the hyperkinesis is symptomatic of an underlying disorder, the diagnosis of the underlying disorder is recorded instead. This rubric excludes hyperkinesis as a symptom of an underlying disorder.

315 Specific delays in development

AHA: Q1, 1988, 3

This rubric classifies a group of disorders in which a specific delay in development is the main feature. For many, the delay is not explicable in terms of general intellectual delay or of inadequate schooling. In each case, development is related to biological maturation, but it is also influenced by nonbiological factors. A diagnosis of a specific developmental delay carries no etiological implications. A diagnosis of specific delay in development should not be made if it is due to a known neurological disorder.

315.00 Developmental reading disorder, unspecified

315.01 Alexia — *inability to comprehend words*
AHA: Q1, 1988, 3

315.02 Developmental dyslexia — *impaired reading ability*
AHA: Q1, 1988, 3

315.09 Other specific developmental reading disorder

315.1 Mathematics disorder — *dyscalculia*
AHA: Q1, 1988, 3

315.2 Other specific developmental learning difficulties — *spelling difficulty*
AHA: Q1, 1988, 3

315.31 Expressive language disorder — *expressive language disorder*
AHA: Q1, 1988, 3

315.32 Mixed receptive-expressive language disorder — *receptive, expressive language disorder*
AHA: Q1, 1988, 3; Q4, 1996, 30

315.39 Other developmental speech or language disorder — *dyslalia*
AHA: Q1, 1988, 3

315.4 Developmental coordination disorder — *clumsiness/dyspraxia syndrome*
AHA: Q1, 1988, 3

315.5 Mixed development disorder

315.8 Other specified delay in development

315.9 Unspecified delay in development

Coding Clarification
Excluded from this rubric are delays in development that are due to neurological disorders (320.0-389.9).

316 Psychic factors associated with diseases classified elsewhere OK

AHA: Q1, 1988, 3

This rubric is used to report psychological factors in physical conditions classified elsewhere.

Coding Clarification
Use an additional code to report the associated physical condition, as in psychogenic ulcerative colitis (556.x), eczema (691.8, 692.9), paroxysmal tachycardia (427.2), or psychosocial dwarfism (259.4). Do not use this rubric to report physical symptoms and physiological malfunctions not involving tissue damage or mental origin. For those cases, see 306.0-306.9.

317–319 Mental Retardation

Mental retardation is defined as general intellectual functioning at least two standard deviations below the norm as measured in a standardized intelligence test, when it is accompanied by significant limitation in communication, self-care, home living, interpersonal skills, self-direction, work, leisure, health, or safety. The onset must occur before adulthood.

Use additional codes to identify any associated psychiatric or physical conditions.

317 Mild mental retardation OK

AHA: Q1, 1988, 3

In mild mental retardation, the patient has an IQ of 50-70. Individuals with this level of retardation are usually educable. During the preschool period, they can develop social and communication skills, have minimal delay in sensorimotor areas, and often are not distinguished from normal children until a later age. During the school age period they can learn academic skills up to approximately the sixth-grade level. During the adult years, they can usually achieve social and vocational skills adequate for minimum self-support, but may need guidance and assistance when under social or economic stress.

318 Other specified mental retardation

AHA: Q1, 1988, 3

In moderate mental retardation, the patient has an IQ of 35-49. Individuals with this level of retardation are usually trainable. During the preschool period they can talk or learn to communicate. They have poor social awareness and fair motor development. During the school age period they can profit from training in social and occupational skills, but they are unlikely to progress beyond the second-grade level in academic subjects. During their adult years they may achieve self-maintenance in unskilled or semi-skilled work under sheltered conditions. They need supervision and guidance when under mild social or economic stress.

In severe mental retardation, the patient has an IQ of 20-34. Individuals with this level of retardation evidence poor motor development, minimal speech, and are generally unable to profit from training and self-help during the preschool period. During the school age period they can talk or learn to communicate, can be trained in elementary health habits, and may profit from systematic habit training. During the adult years they may contribute partially to self-maintenance under complete supervision.

In profound mental retardation, the patient has an IQ under 20. Individuals with this level of retardation evidence minimal capacity for sensorimotor functioning and need nursing care during the preschool period. During the school age period some further motor development may occur, and they may respond to minimal or limited training in self-help.

During the adult years some motor and speech development may occur, and they may achieve very limited self-care and need nursing care.

318.0 Moderate mental retardation — (Use additional code(s) to identify any associated psychiatric or physical condition) — *IQ 35-49*
AHA: Q1, 1988, 3

318.1 Severe mental retardation — (Use additional code(s) to identify any associated psychiatric or physical condition) — *IQ 20-34*
AHA: Q1, 1988, 3

318.2 Profound mental retardation — (Use additional code(s) to identify any associated psychiatric or physical condition) — *IQ under 20*
AHA: Q1, 1988, 3

319 Unspecified mental retardation OK

AHA: Q1, 1988, 3

This rubric is reserved for patients who evidence obvious mental retardation, but the severity of the condition has not been measured with standardized testing.

© 2004 Ingenix, Inc.

320–389 Diseases of the Nervous System and Sense Organs

This chapter classifies diseases and disorders of the nervous system including meninges (the covering of the brain and spinal cord), central nervous system, and peripheral nervous system (the nerves that relay signals between the central nervous system and the organs of the body). This chapter also classifies conditions affecting the eye and ear.

320–326 Inflammatory Diseases of the Central Nervous System

The central nervous system (CNS) comprises the brain, the spinal cord, and associated membranes. The brain can be subdivided into several regions:

- The cerebral hemispheres form the largest part of the brain, occupying the anterior and middle cranial fossae in the skull.
- The diencephalon includes the thalamus, hypothalamus, epithalamus and subthalamus, and forms the central core of the brain.
- The midbrain is located at the junction of the middle and posterior cranial fossae.
- The pons is in the anterior part of the posterior cranial fossa; fibers within the pons connect one cerebral hemisphere with its opposite cerebellar hemisphere.
- The medulla oblongata is continuous with the spinal cord and controls the respiratory and cardiovascular systems.
- The cerebellum overlies the pons and medulla and controls motor functions that regulate muscle tone, coordination, and posture.

The spinal column, which encloses the spinal cord, consists of vertebrae linked by intervertebral disks and held together by ligaments. The spinal cord extends from the first lumbar vertebra to the medulla at the base of the brain. The outer layer of the spinal cord consists of myelin-sheathed nerve fibers bundled that conduct impulses triggered by pressure, pain, heat, and other sensory stimuli or conduct motor impulses activating muscles and glands. The inner layer, or gray matter, is primarily composed of nerve cell bodies. The central canal, within the gray matter, circulates the cerebrospinal fluid. The three meninges wrap around the spinal cord and cover the brain; the pia mater is the innermost layer, the arachnoid lies in the middle, and the dura mater is the outside layer, to which the spinal nerves are attached. The 31 pairs of spinal nerves deliver impulses into the spinal cord, which in turn relays them to the brain. Conversely, motor impulses generated in the brain are relayed by the spinal cord to the spinal nerves, which pass the impulses to muscles and glands. Nerve fibers in the spinal cord usually do not regenerate if injured by accident or disease.

Diseases in this rubric are often the result of bacterial invasion spreading from a nearby infection (i.e., a chronic sinus or middle ear infection). The bloodstream may carry bacteria from other sites to the CNS and, in rare cases, head trauma or surgical procedures may introduce bacteria directly into the CNS.

Bacterial infection of the CNS can result in abscesses and empyemas. CNS infections are classified according to the location where they occur. For example, a spinal epidural abscess is located above the dura mater, and a cranial subdural empyema occurs between the dura mater and the arachnoid. As pus and other material from an infection accumulate, pressure is exerted on the brain or spinal cord. This pressure can damage the nervous system tissue and, without treatment, the infection can be fatal. Specific symptoms of CNS infections depend on location, but may include severe headache or back pain, weakness, sensory loss, and a fever. An individual may complain of a stiff neck, nausea or vomiting, and tiredness or disorientation. There is a potential for seizures, paralysis, or coma. The fatality rate associated with CNS infections ranges from 10 to 40 percent, and those surviving an infection may experience permanent damage, resulting in partial paralysis, speech problems, or seizures.

These categories include meningitis, encephalitis, cerebral abscesses, late effects of infections of the central nervous system, and other types of inflammations such as meningitis due to sarcoidosis and lead poisoning (toxic) encephalitis. However, many infections of the central nervous system are excluded.

320 Bacterial meningitis

AHA: Jan-Feb, 1987, 6

Bacterial meningitis is inflammation of the CNS covering of meninges due to a bacterial organism. Bacterial meningitis can be caused by a variety of pyogenic bacterial organisms, most commonly *Haemophilus influenzae (type B), Streptococcus pneumoniae,* Pneumococcus, Neisseria meningitis, *Staphylococcus aureus,* Klebsiella, *Pseudomonas,* and *Escherichia coli.* Code selection is based upon the infective agent.

Anaerobic bacteria are organisms that thrive only in the absence of free oxygen and can be either gram-negative or gram-positive. *Clostridium tetani* is an example of a gram-positive anaerobe, and *Proteus vulgaris* is an example of a gram-negative anaerobe.

The terms "gram-negative" and "gram-positive" refer to a method of differential staining of bacteria for bacterial taxonomy and identification. Gram-positive bacteria retain the basic dye crystal violet, and gram-negative bacteria lose the crystal violet dye to become colorless. Counterstains color gram-negative bacteria pink to red and leave gram-positive bacteria dark purple.

Signs and symptoms of bacterial meningitis include fever and chills, headache, stiff neck, nausea and vomiting, alterations in sensorium, seizure, positive Kernig's and Brudzinski's signs, and rash. These signs and symptoms, in addition to chronically draining ear, are associated with pneumococcal meningitis.

Diagnostic tests include lumbar puncture to obtain cerebrospinal fluid for verifying elevated fluid pressure. Culture of cerebrospinal fluid is performed to identify the organism and a gram stain of cerebrospinal fluid reveals polymorphonuclear leukocytes, elevated white blood cell count, decreased glucose level, and elevated protein content. In addition, a limulus lysate assay test may be performed to detect endotoxins due to gram-negative bacteria and a cranial CT scan may indicate cerebral edema early and subdural effusion or empyema later. Therapies include isolation, avoidance of temperature extremes, antimicrobials administered intravenously in large doses, IV hydration, medication such as Dilantin to control seizures, diuretics or withdrawal of cerebrospinal fluid through an intraventricular catheter to reduce intracranial pressure, oxygen therapy for hypoxia, and intubation and ventilation for hypoventilation with hypercapnia.

Associated conditions include seizures due to increased intracranial pressure, respiratory distress or failure, altered state of consciousness, vasomotor collapse or shock, intravascular coagulation, syndrome of inappropriate antidiuretic hormone secretion (SIADH), dehydration, or various electrolyte imbalances.

320.0 Hemophilus meningitis — *meningitis due to Hemophilus influenzae (H. influenzae)*
AHA: Jan-Feb, 1987, 6

320.1 Pneumococcal meningitis — *pneumococcal infection causing inflammation of the membranes enveloping the brain and/or spinal cord*
AHA: Jan-Feb, 1987, 6

320.2 Streptococcal meningitis — *streptococcal infection causing inflammation of the membranes enveloping the brain and/or spinal cord*
AHA: Jan-Feb, 1987, 6

320.3 Staphylococcal meningitis — *staphylococcal infection causing inflammation of the membranes enveloping the brain and/or spinal cord*
AHA: Jan-Feb, 1987, 6

320.7 Meningitis in other bacterial diseases classified elsewhere — (Code first underlying disease: 002.0, 027.0, 033.0-033.9, 039.8) — *actinomycosis, listeriosis, typhoid fever, and whooping cough*
AHA: Jan-Feb, 1987, 6

320.81 Anaerobic meningitis — *bacteroides (fragilis); gram-negative anaerobes*
AHA: Jan-Feb, 1987, 6

320.82 Meningitis due to gram-negative bacteria, not elsewhere classified — *Aerobacter aerogenes; Klebsiella pneumoniae; Proteus morganii; Pseudomonas*
AHA: Jan-Feb, 1987, 6

320.89 Meningitis due to other specified bacteria — *Bacillus pyocyaneus*
AHA: Jan-Feb, 1987, 6

320.9 Meningitis due to unspecified bacterium

Documentation Issues

If the medical documentation indicates aseptic, viral, or nonbacterial meningitis without further specification, see category 047 *Meningitis due to enterovirus.* When meningitis is a manifestation of another disease process (320.7), code the underlying disease first.

321 Meningitis due to other organisms

AHA: Jan-Feb, 1987, 6

Meningitis due to other organisms is inflammation of the CNS covering of meninges due to organisms other than bacteria. These can be fungal organisms, viruses not classified elsewhere, or other nonbacterial organisms.

Signs and symptoms of meningitis due to other organisms vary according to infectious agent. Therapies include specific treatment depending on the infectious agent (e.g., antifungal agents such as

© 2004 Ingenix, Inc.

amphotericin B for fungal meningitis and corticosteroids for sarcoid meningitis).

321.0 Cryptococcal meningitis — (Code first underlying disease, 117.5) — *cryptococcus infection causing inflammation of the membranes enveloping the brain and/or spinal cord*
AHA: Jan-Feb, 1987, 6

321.1 Meningitis in other fungal diseases — (Code first underlying disease: 110.0-118)

321.2 Meningitis due to viruses not elsewhere classified — (Code first underlying disease: 060.0-066.9)

321.3 Meningitis due to trypanosomiasis — (Code first underlying disease: 086.0-086.9) — *trypanosomiasis infection causing inflammation of the membranes enveloping the brain and/or spinal cord*
AHA: Jan-Feb, 1987, 6

321.4 Meningitis in sarcoidosis — (Code first underlying disease, 135) — *sarcoidosis causing inflammation of the membranes enveloping the brain and/or spinal cord*
AHA: Jan-Feb, 1987, 6

321.8 Meningitis due to other nonbacterial organisms classified elsewhere — (Code first underlying disease)

Documentation Issues

If the medical documentation indicates aseptic, viral, or nonbacterial meningitis without further specification, see category 047 *Meningitis due to enterovirus.* When meningitis is a manifestation of another disease process (320.7), code the underlying disease first.

322 Meningitis of unspecified cause

AHA: Jan-Feb, 1987, 6

322.0 Nonpyogenic meningitis — *meningitis with clear cerebrospinal fluid*
AHA: Jan-Feb, 1987, 6

322.1 Eosinophilic meningitis — *presence of cells readily stained with eosin causing inflammation of the membranes enveloping the brain and/or spinal cord*
AHA: Jan-Feb, 1987, 6

322.2 Chronic meningitis — *persistent inflammation of the membranes enveloping the brain and/or spinal cord*
AHA: Jan-Feb, 1987, 6

322.9 Unspecified meningitis — *leptomeningopathy; ventriculitis, cerebral*
AHA: Jan-Feb, 1987, 6

323 Encephalitis, myelitis, and encephalomyelitis

Encephalitis, myelitis, and encephalomyelitis are inflammations of the central nervous system that alter the function of various portions of the brain (encephalitis), spinal cord (myelitis), or both (encephalomyelitis). The inflammation usually results from either a direct invasion of the central nervous system by a virus or postinfection involvement of the central nervous system after a viral disease. Bacteria, medications, toxic substances, and parasites also may cause it. Arthropod-borne viruses as seen in mosquitoes most often cause encephalitis. Myelitis infection results from direct invasion or tick bites classified to categories 062 and 063.

Signs and symptoms of encephalitis, myelitis, and encephalomyelitis, with mild benign forms, are malaise, fever, headache, dizziness, apathy, neck stiffness, nausea and vomiting, ataxia, tremors, hyperactivity, and speech difficulties. With severe central nervous system involvement, there is high fever, stupor, seizures, disorientation, ocular palsies, paralysis, spasticity, and coma that may proceed to death.

Diagnostic tests include lumbar puncture with analysis of cerebrospinal fluid to show lymphocytes, moderate rises in protein, and markedly elevated specific viral antibody titers with acute encephalitis. Cultures (i.e., cerebrospinal fluid, blood, and saliva) may identify the specific virus (except arboviruses that rarely are detected in the blood or spinal fluid). A brain biopsy may rule out herpes simplex.

Therapies include IV hydration and control of temperature. Specific treatment depends on the etiology (e.g., chelation therapy for lead poisoning encephalitis and chloroquine for malarial encephalitis).

323.0 Encephalitis in viral diseases classified elsewhere — (Code first underlying disease: 073.7, 075, 078.3) — *cat-scratch disease, infectious mononucleosis, and ornithosis*

323.1 Encephalitis in rickettsial diseases classified elsewhere — (Code first underlying disease: 080-083.9) — *inflammation of the brain caused by rickettsial disease carried by louse, tick or mite*

323.2 Encephalitis in protozoal diseases classified elsewhere — (Code first underlying disease: 084.0-084.9, 086.0-086.9) — *malaria and trypanosomiasis*

323.4 Other encephalitis due to infection classified elsewhere — (Code first underlying disease)

323.5 Encephalitis following immunization procedures — (Use additional E code to identify vaccine)

323.6 Postinfectious encephalitis — (Code first underlying disease) — *infection and inflammation of the brain several weeks following outbreak of a systemic infection*

323.7 Toxic encephalitis — (Code first underlying cause: 961.3, 982.1, 984.0-984.9, 985.0, 985.8) — *inflammation of the brain due to toxic effect of exposure to a chemical*
AHA: Q2, 1997, 8

323.8 Other causes of encephalitis

323.9 Unspecified cause of encephalitis — *syringomyelitis*

Coding Clarification

Diseases in this rubric are classified according to causative organism. Sequence the underlying disease first. If the organism is unspecified or the encephalitis has a noninfectious or toxic etiology, see codes 323.5, 323.8, and 323.9.

324 Intracranial and intraspinal abscess

Intracranial and intraspinal abscess is the localized collection of pus in a cavity involving the brain or spinal column, respectively.

Intracranial abscess is the localized collection of purulent material and liquified brain tissue involving the many layers of the brain, including the epidural or subdural spaces, or within the substance of the brain itself. The etiology is usually bacterial and occurs through direct extension from a contiguous focus, blood-borne metastases, or by penetrating injury. The most common cause of direct extension in a brain abscess is a contiguous infection such as in the middle ear, mastoid, or sinuses. The most common site of origin for blood-borne metastasis is the lung (empyema, bronchiectasis). When the abscess is due to trauma, a skull fracture or penetrating injury is usually involved. The most common organisms are streptococci, pneumococci, and staphylococci.

Signs and symptoms of intracranial abscess, with brain abscess, include headache, altered sensorium (lethargy, irritability, confusion, or coma), nausea and vomiting, fever, seizures, multiple alternation nerve palsies, and other neurologic deficits. Signs and symptoms of intracranial abscess, with subdural abscess, include headache, sinusitis, altered sensorium (lethargy, obtundation, or coma), seizures, fever and chills, hemiparesis, and aphasia. Signs and symptoms of intracranial abscess, with cerebral epidural abscess, involve limited localized symptoms.

Diagnostic tests include MRI and radionuclide or CT scans to identify the location and size of abscess. With subdural abscess, plain skull x-rays reveal underlying sinus or mastoid disease, while cerebral arteriography shows space between cerebral vessels and the inner surface of the cranium. Therapies include antimicrobials for early abscess, incision and drainage, or excision of abscess.

The definition of intraspinal abscess is the localized collection of pus in a cavity involving the layers of the spinal cord, including the epidura, extradura, and subdura. It is usually bacterial, and the most common organisms are streptococci, pneumococci, and staphylococci. The etiology is usually due to blood-borne spread, direct extension from contiguous sites, or as a consequence of an invasive procedure. Most spinal abscesses are epidural.

Signs and symptoms of intraspinal abscess include spinal ache, root pain, weakness, paresthesias, and eventually paralysis. Diagnostic tests include lumbar puncture with analysis of cerebrospinal fluid to show elevated protein, xanthochromia, and normal glucose. Culture identifies the bacterial agent. Myelography, CT scan, and MRI visualize the abscess. Therapies include antimicrobials for early abscess, incision and drainage, or excision for fully established intraspinal abscess.

324.0 Intracranial abscess — *cerebellar (embolic) abscess; abscess (embolic) of brain (any part)*

324.1 Intraspinal abscess — *abscess (embolic) of spinal cord (any part); epidural, extradural or subdural*

324.9 Intracranial and intraspinal abscess of unspecified site — *extradural or subdural abscess NOS*

325 Phlebitis and thrombophlebitis of intracranial venous sinuses OK

This rubric identifies the inflammation and formation of a blood clot in a vein within the brain or its lining. The principal veins in the cranial cavity are incorporated into the dura mater, which is closely bound to the inner bone of the cavity. The venous sinuses (e.g., the sagittal, cavernous, petrosal, sphenoparietal, sigmoid, and transverse sinuses) are held in an open position and generally occur where there is a wide separation between major anatomical entities. The sinuses contain an endothelial lining continuous into the veins connected to them. There are no valves in the sinuses or in the veins and the majority of the venous blood in the sinus drains from the cranium via the internal jugular vein.

Intracranial venous thrombosis occurs as a complication of intracranial infections and can result in symptoms such as headaches, focal seizures, and focal neurologic signs affecting the legs more than the arm. Massive venous infarction, due to thrombosis, may be fatal. The thrombus can be identified by its signal intensity on MRI and the flow void in the affected sinus is clearly documented on MR angiography.

 © 2004 Ingenix, Inc.

Septic intracranial thrombophlebitis is an extremely serious complication that even with appropriate therapy is fatal in more that one-third of cases. Deep or superficial septic phlebitis can occur by direct invasion from adjacent non-vascular infections associated with a long-term intravenous cannula being used for chronic administration of fluids or medications. The etiologic agent usually can be cultured both from blood and from any metastatic sites of infection and the organism responsible often can be predicted from the site of infection. The worst complications are in patients with phlebitis due to *Staphylococcus aureus*, often the cause of septic intracranial venous sinus thrombophlebitis.

The injection of contrast material into a central catheter often permits visualization of a catheter-associated thrombus or of an extensive fibrin sheath that extends, cloud-like, away from the catheter. Contrast enhanced CT or magnetic resonance imaging (MRI) can identify the extent of the thrombus, the local anatomy of the affected tissues, and any pockets of purulent material that may require drainage.

Extended high-dose anti-microbial therapy is recommended because of the high risk of septic emboli. Heparin halts the progression of septic thrombophlebitis and eliminates an ongoing source of septic emboli. Because septic phlebitis is associated with a high incidence of secondary infection, high-dose antibiotics are continued for at least six weeks after blood cultures become negative.

Coding Clarification

Excluded from this rubric is phlebitis and thrombophlebitis of intracranial venous sinuses associated with pregnancy (671.5) or of nonpyogenic origin (437.6).

326 Late effects of intracranial abscess or pyogenic infection OK

Late effects of intracranial abscess or pyogenic infection are the late effects of meningitis, encephalitis, myelitis, encephalomyelitis, intracranial and intraspinal abscess, and phlebitis or thrombophlebitis of the intracranial sinuses except when these conditions are manifestations of another disease process identified by italics in the ICD-9-CM tabular list.

Coding Clarification

Use an additional code to describe the condition, as in hydrocephalus (331.4) or paralysis (rubrics 342 and 344).

330–337 Hereditary and Degenerative Diseases of the Central Nervous System

Excluded from this section are hepatolenticular degeneration (275.1), multiple sclerosis (340), and other demyelinating diseases of the central nervous system (rubric 341).

330 Cerebral degenerations usually manifest in childhood

330.0 Leukodystrophy — (Use additional code to identify associated mental retardation) — *Krabbe's disease; globoid cell or metachromatic leukodystrophy; sulfatide lipidosis*

330.1 Cerebral lipidoses — (Use additional code to identify associated mental retardation) — *amaurotic (familial) idiocy; Batten disease; gangliosidosis; Tay-Sachs disease*

330.2 Cerebral degeneration in generalized lipidoses — (Code first underlying disease, 272.7. Use additional code to identify associated mental retardation) — *Fabry's disease, Gaucher's disease, Niemann-Pick disease*

330.3 Cerebral degeneration of childhood in other diseases classified elsewhere — (Code first underlying disease, 272.7. Use additional code to identify associated mental retardation) — *Hunter's disease, mucopolysaccharidosis*

330.8 Other specified cerebral degenerations in childhood — (Use additional code to identify associated mental retardation)

330.9 Unspecified cerebral degeneration in childhood — (Use additional code to identify associated mental retardation) — *childhood cerebral degeneration NOS*

Coding Clarification

Report Rett's syndrome with 330.8. For 330.2 and 330.3, sequence first the underlying disease, as in Fabry's, Gaucher's, Niemann-Pick, or sphingolipidosis (272.7), or Hunter's disease or mucopolysaccharidosis (277.5).

331 Other cerebral degenerations

Alzheimer's disease is a form of presenile dementia caused by the destruction of the subcortical white matter of the brain and characterized by increasing loss of intellectual functioning beginning with minor memory loss and eventually resulting in total loss of ability to function.

Signs and symptoms of Alzheimer's disease include loss of interest in usual pursuits and marked changes of habits. CT scan of the brain shows shrinkage of white matter and an increase in the size of the ventricles. A microscopic exam of brain tissue shows neuronal loss with neurofibrillar and granulovacuolar degeneration and may also show amyloid plaques in the cerebral cortex tissue. Neurochemical studies show changes in the cholinergic system (reduced acetylcholine and choline acetyltransferase) and noradrenergic system (decreased norepinephrine) and may reveal low serotonin levels in caudate and hippocampus nuclei.

Therapies include sedatives, such as chloral hydrate or phenhydramine, for sleep disorders; benzodiazapines, such as lorazepam or oxazepam, for aggressive or assaultive behavior or neuroleptics, such as chlorpromazine or haloperidol, for extreme aggressiveness.

331.0 Alzheimer's disease — *chronic, progressive form of dementia, characterized by plaque formations in the brain, eventually leading to total dependence on others*
AHA: Nov-Dec, 1984, 20; Q4, 1999, 7; Q4, 2000, 41

331.11 Pick's disease — (Use additional code for associated behavioral disturbance: 294.10-294.11) — *presenile dementia due to atrophy of frontal and temporal lobes of the brain*

331.19 Other frontotemporal dementia — (Use additional code for associated behavioral disturbance: 294.10-294.11) — *frontal dementia*

331.2 Senile degeneration of brain — *decline in intellectual function due to brain deterioration*

331.3 Communicating hydrocephalus

331.4 Obstructive hydrocephalus — *acquired hydrocephalus NOS*
AHA: Q1, 1999, 9; Q4, 2003, 106

331.7 Cerebral degeneration in diseases classified elsewhere — (Code first underlying disease: 140.0-239.9, 244.0-244.9, 265.0, 266.2, 303.00-303.93, 430-438, 741.0, 742.3)

331.81 Reye's syndrome — *occurs in children under age 15, and is marked by acute encephalopathy and fatty infiltrates of multiple organs*

331.82 Dementia with Lewy bodies — (Use additional code for associated behavioral disturbance: 294.10-294.11)

331.89 Other cerebral degeneration — *cerebral ataxia*

331.9 Unspecified cerebral degeneration

Documentation Issues

When the physician documents senile dementia with Alzheimer's disease, both conditions should be coded. Report with codes 290.0 *Senile dementia, uncomplicated* and 331.0 *Alzheimer's disease.*

Coding Clarification

Assign an additional code to identify any mental condition, such as presenile dementia in rubric 290, associated with the current condition.

Alzheimer's Dementia: Two codes are required to report this condition. First code the underlying condition 331.0 *Alzheimer's disease,* and then use an additional code to report the dementia 294.1 *Dementia in conditions classified elsewhere.*

Feeding Difficulty: As this disease progresses many patients require a feeding tube due to feeding difficulties. When the Alzheimer's patient is admitted for a feeding tube because of the feeding difficulty, report code 331.0 for the Alzheimer's disease and an additional code, 783.3, for the feeding difficulty.

Coding Scenario

A patient is seen in the clinic with progressive memory loss and disorientation. The physician's diagnostic statement indicates progressive Alzheimer's disease.

> Code assignment: 331.0 *Alzheimer's disease*

A patient is seen for evaluation of Alzheimer's dementia and referred to partial hospitalization program for therapy.

> Code assignment: 331.0 *Alzheimer's disease* and 294.1x *Dementia in conditions classified elsewhere*

332 Parkinson's disease

Paralysis agitans is an idiopathic neurological disease causing degeneration and dysfunction of the basal ganglia. This disease, also known as Parkinsonism or Parkinson's disease, is due to a toxic degeneration of the nigral neurons, a group of specialized cells in the midbrain that contain neuromelanin and manufacture the neurotransmitter substance dopamine. When 75 to 80 percent of the dopamine innervation is destroyed, signs and symptoms of Parkinsonism appear.

Signs and symptoms of paralysis agitans include tremor, rigidity, difficulty starting movement or slowness in movement, "pill-rolling" movement of fingers, shuffling gait with short steps and dragging feet, drooling, and problems of articulation.

Therapies include Levodopa or anticholinergic agents, transplantation of catecholamine tissue (autologous adrenal medulla) into brain adjacent to striatum, and surgery to destroy areas controlling specific functions to control severe tremor.

This disease is associated with mental disorders such as dementia, depression, and delirium. True dementia affects 20 to 30 percent of patients.

Secondary Parkinsonism is a neurologic disease similar to paralysis agitans that affects the central

© 2004 Ingenix, Inc.

nervous system. It is caused by a number of other diseases or by the adverse affect of certain drugs and chemicals.

Associated conditions include Wilson's disease, postencephalic Parkinsonism, midbrain injury or trauma (dementia pugalistica), neoplasms, vascular malformations, Binswanger's disease, etat lacunaire, and hypertensive cerebrovascular disease with normal pressure hydrocephalus. Use the appropriate E code to identify the causative drug or chemical such as carbon monoxide, manganese, methylphenyltetra-hydropyridine (MPTP), or reserpine.

332.0 Paralysis agitans — *Parkinson's disease; NOS, idiopathic, primary*
AHA: March-April, 1987, 7

332.1 Secondary Parkinsonism — (Use additional E code to identify drug, if drug-induced) — *Parkinsonism due to drugs*

Coding Clarification
If the medical record documentation indicates Huntington's disease, see 333.4. For progressive supranuclear palsy, striatonigral degeneration, corticodentationigral degeneration with neuronal achromasia, olivopontocerebellar atrophy, Shy-Drager syndrome, or multiple system atrophy, see 333.0. If the Parkinsonism is secondary to syphilis, see 094.82.

333 Other extrapyramidal disease and abnormal movement disorders

333.0 Other degenerative diseases of the basal ganglia — *progressive supranuclear ophthalmoplegia; Parkinsonian syndrome associated with idiopathic orthostatic hypotension or symptomatic orthostatic hypotension*
AHA: Q3, 1996, 8

333.1 Essential and other specified forms of tremor — (Use additional E code to identify drug, if drug-induced) — *benign essential tremor; familial tremor*

333.2 Myoclonus — (Use additional E code to identify drug, if drug-induced) — *familial essential myoclonus; progressive myoclonic epilepsy*
AHA: March-April, 1987, 12; Q3, 1997, 4

333.3 Tics of organic origin — (Use additional E code to identify drug, if drug-induced)

333.4 Huntington's chorea — *inherited, progressive disease involving CNS, leading to involuntary movements and deterioration of mental faculties ending in dementia*

Coding Clarification
Huntington's chorea is a fatal hereditary disease affecting the basal ganglia and cerebral cortex. The onset varies but usually begins in the fourth decade of life. Death usually follows within 15 years. Signs and symptoms of Huntington's chorea include family history of Huntington's chorea; weight loss; facial grimacing; ceaseless rapid, complex, jerky movements; personality changes, including irritability and indifference; mental deterioration until dementia is reached; and, in children, rigid rather than choreic movements and seizures.

Diagnostic tests include MRI or CT scan of the head to reveal gross atrophy and caudate neuronal loss in with lesser changes elsewhere in the brain. Microscopic exam of tissue identifies gliosis and loss of intrinsic neurons. Neurochemical studies reveal loss of gamma-aminobutyric acid (GABA), acetylcholine, substance P (a tachykinin of 11 amino acids), and enkephalin.

333.5 Other choreas — (Use additional E code to identify drug, if drug-induced) — *hemiballism; paroxysmal choreo-athetosis*

333.6 Idiopathic torsion dystonia — *deformans progressiva or musculorum deformans dystonia*

333.7 Symptomatic torsion dystonia — (Use additional E code to identify drug, if drug-induced) — *athetoid cerebral palsy (Vogt's disease); double athetosis syndrome*

333.81 Blepharospasm — (Use additional E code to identify drug, if drug-induced) — *spasmodic contraction of orbicularis oculi muscle caused by a number of conditions*

333.82 Orofacial dyskinesia — (Use additional E code to identify drug, if drug-induced) — *defect in voluntary movement of orofacial muscles*

333.83 Spasmodic torticollis — (Use additional E code to identify drug, if drug-induced) — *impermanent condition in which head tilts to one side*

333.84 Organic writers' cramp — (Use additional E code to identify drug, if drug-induced) — *cramp affecting thumb, index finger and third finger due to prolonged writing*

333.89 Other fragments of torsion dystonia — (Use additional E code to identify drug, if drug-induced)

333.90 Unspecified extrapyramidal disease and abnormal movement disorder — *extrapyramidal disorder NOS*

333.91 Stiff-man syndrome — *disease of the CNS marked by progressive muscle rigidity and spasms*

333.92 Neuroleptic malignant syndrome — (Use additional E code to identify drug)

333.93 Benign shuddering attacks — *protracted period of convulsive tremors*
AHA: Q4, 1994, 37

333.99 Other extrapyramidal disease and abnormal movement disorder — *restless legs*
AHA: Q4, 1994, 37

Coding Clarification

Benign Shuddering Attacks: This movement disorder is not coded as an epileptic condition; it is a nonepileptic disorder. Use code 333.93 to classify this condition.

334 Spinocerebellar disease

334.0 Friedreich's ataxia — *inherited disease marked by dorsal and lateral columnar sclerosis of the spinal cord*

334.1 Hereditary spastic paraplegia — *paralysis of lower half of body marked by increased muscle tone and heightened tendon reflexes*

334.2 Primary cerebellar degeneration — *Sanger-Brown cerebellar ataxia; dyssynergia cerebellaris myoclonica; primary cerebellar degeneration NOS*
AHA: March-April, 1987, 9

334.3 Other cerebellar ataxia — (Use additional E code to identify drug, if drug-induced) — *cerebellar ataxia NOS*

334.4 Cerebellar ataxia in diseases classified elsewhere — (Code first underlying disease: 140.0-239.9, 244.0-244.9, 303.00-303.93)

334.8 Other spinocerebellar diseases — *ataxia-teleangiectasis (Louis-Bar syndrome); corticostriatal-spinal degeneration*

334.9 Unspecified spinocerebellar disease

335 Anterior horn cell disease

335.0 Werdnig-Hoffmann disease — *infantile spinal muscular atrophy; progressive muscular atrophy of infancy*

335.10 Unspecified spinal muscular atrophy — *muscular atrophy of the spine NOS*

335.11 Kugelberg-Welander disease — *familial spinal muscular atrophy*

335.19 Other spinal muscular atrophy — *adult spinal muscular atrophy*

335.20 Amyotrophic lateral sclerosis — *motor neuron disease (bulbar) (mixed type); Lou Gehrig's disease*
AHA: Q4, 1995, 81

335.21 Progressive muscular atrophy — *Duchenne-Aran muscular atrophy; progressive muscular atrophy (pure)*

335.22 Progressive bulbar palsy — *degeneration of the nuclear cells of lower cranial nerves leading to paralysis*

335.23 Pseudobulbar palsy — *condition in which balance and walking are affected by arteriosclerosis-mediated mini-strokes that damage the pertinent areas of the brain*

335.24 Primary lateral sclerosis — *sclerosis of lateral column of spinal cord*

335.29 Other motor neuron diseases

335.8 Other anterior horn cell diseases

335.9 Unspecified anterior horn cell disease

Coding Scenario

A patient is admitted for chemotherapy treatment for amyotrophic lateral sclerosis.

> Code assignment: 335.20 *Amyotrophic lateral sclerosis*

336 Other diseases of spinal cord

336.0 Syringomyelia and syringobulbia — *progressive spinal cord disease marked by cavitation and gliosis of surrounding tissues*
AHA: Q1, 1989, 10

336.1 Vascular myelopathies — *acute infarction of spinal cord (embolic) (nonembolic); arterial thrombosis of spinal cord; hematomyelia*

336.2 Subacute combined degeneration of spinal cord in diseases classified elsewhere — (Code first underlying disease: 266.2, 281.0, 281.1)

336.3 Myelopathy in other diseases classified elsewhere — (Code first underlying disease: 140.0-239.9)

336.8 Other myelopathy — (Use additional E code to identify cause) — *drug-induced myelopathy; radiation-induced myelopathy*

336.9 Unspecified disease of spinal cord — *cord compression NOS; myelopathy NOS*

337 Disorders of the autonomic nervous system

The nervous system consists of the central nervous system (the brain and the spinal cord) and the peripheral nervous system (the sense organs and the nerves linking the sense organs, muscles, and glands to the central nervous system). The structures of the peripheral nervous system are subdivided into the autonomic nervous system (automatic bodily processes — parasympathetic and sympathetic) and the somatic nervous system. The autonomic nervous system conveys sensory impulses from the blood vessels, the heart, and all of the organs in the chest, abdomen, and pelvis through nerves to other parts of the brain (mainly the medulla, pons, and hypothalamus). These impulses are largely automatic or reflex responses through the efferent autonomic nerves, and cause reactions of the heart, the vascular system, and all the organs of the body to variations in environmental temperature, posture, food intake, stressful experiences, and other changes to which all individuals are exposed.

There are two major components of the autonomic nervous system, the sympathetic and the

© 2004 Ingenix, Inc.

parasympathetic systems. The parasympathetic division of the autonomic nervous system controls anabolism (energy storage); an anabolic activity occurs in normal, nonstressful situations, such as initiating digestion after eating. In general, sympathetic processes reverse parasympathetic responses. The sympathetic division operates for defense or in response to stress. In defensive situations, catabolism (energy use) produces an increased heart rate, an expansion of the lungs to hold more energy, dilated pupils, and blood flow to the muscles.

Abnormalities of the autonomic nervous system include anxiety disorders, such as muscular tension, hyperventilation, increased heart rate, and high blood pressure that can lead to physiological illnesses such as headaches and digestive problems. At times, parasympathetic responses occur simultaneously, such as involuntary discharge of the bladder and bowels in extremely stressful situations.

Damage to the sympathetic nerve to the eye may result in Horner's syndrome (337.9), which causes a small, regular pupil, ptosis (drooping) of the eyelid on the same side, and occasionally loss of sweat formation on the forehead of the affected eye. The pupil will still react to light stimulus and accommodate to distant vision, but will not enlarge in the dark. The diagnosis of Horner's syndrome is by topical application of liquid cocaine. In many cases there is no treatment that improves or reverses the condition. Treatment in acquired cases is directed toward eradicating the disease that is producing the syndrome.

337.0 Idiopathic peripheral autonomic neuropathy — *carotid sinus syncope or syndrome; cervical sympathetic dystrophy or paralysis*

337.1 Peripheral autonomic neuropathy in disorders classified elsewhere — (Code first underlying disease: 250.6, 277.3)

Coding Clarification

Peripheral autonomic neuropathy in disorders classified elsewhere are the chronic and progressive disorders of the peripheral autonomic nerves most often associated with diabetes mellitus, usually insulin dependent or of long-standing duration. Other common etiologies include amyloidosis, botulism, porphyria, and multiple endocrine adenomas.

Signs and symptoms of peripheral autonomic neuropathy in disorders classified elsewhere include impotence, bladder atony, nocturnal diarrhea, orthostatic hypotension, hypersensitivity to cold, and gustatory sweating.

Diagnostic tests include voiding cystometrogram to study urinary neuropathy and motility studies for the esophagus, stomach, and duodenum. Therapies include rigorous control of blood glucose for diabetic autonomic polyneuropathy and symptomatic therapies such as stool bulking agents for diabetic diarrhea, bladder neck resection for urinary bladder dysfunction, and penile implants for impotence.

Associated conditions include foot ulcers, gangrene, other diabetic complications such as diabetic nephropathy, Charcot's joint, or diabetic gastroparesis.

Use codes 250.6x and 337.1 to report diabetic peripheral/cranial neuropathy. For more specific diagnosis identification, more specific codes should be used. For example, orthostatic hypotension secondary to diabetes should be reported with codes 250.6x *Diabetes with neurological manifestations,* 337.1 *Peripheral autonomic neuropathy in disorders classified elsewhere,* and 458.0 *Orthostatic hypotension.*

Gastroparesis, also known as gastroparalysis, requires three codes for accurate reporting: 250.6x *Diabetes mellitus with neurological manifestations,* 337.1 *Peripheral autonomic neuropathy in disorders classified elsewhere,* and 536.3 *Gastroparesis.*

337.20 Unspecified reflex sympathetic dystrophy

337.21 Reflex sympathetic dystrophy of the upper limb

337.22 Reflex sympathetic dystrophy of the lower limb

337.29 Reflex sympathetic dystrophy of other specified site

337.3 Autonomic dysreflexia — (Use additional code to identify the underlying cause: 560.39, 599.0, 707.0)

337.9 Unspecified disorder of autonomic nervous system

340–349 Other Disorders of the Central Nervous System

340 Multiple sclerosis OK

Multiple sclerosis is chronic demyelinating disease affecting the white matter of the spinal cord and brain. Multiple sclerosis is characterized by the breaking down of the myelin fibers of the nervous system; patches of scarred nervous fibers develop at these sites. The etiology is unknown, but recent studies suggest the condition may be a cell-mediated autoimmune disease due to an inherited disorder of immune regulation. The disease affects adults between ages 20 and 40 and occurs more often in women.

Signs and symptoms of multiple sclerosis include acute optic neuritis, diplopia, internuclear ophthalmoplegia, frequent dropping of articles, stumbling or falling for no reason, Lhermitte's phenomenon (flexion of the neck producing tingling and paresthesias of legs), and mental changes.

Lab work shows cerebrospinal fluid with five to 100 lymphocytes per cubic millimeter, elevated gamma globulin level (IgG), and abnormal gold curve.

Evoked-potential testing of the visual evoked response, brainstem auditory evoked response, and somatosensory evoked response is abnormally delayed. Therapies include corticosteroids to lessen the intensity and duration of acute exacerbations, physical and occupational therapy to preserve muscle strength and maintain motor function, and muscle relaxant and transcutaneous electrical nerve stimulation (TENS) units to treat spasm and pain. Immunosuppressive therapy with agents such as oral azathioprine and high dose IV cyclophosphamide is in the experimental phase.

Associated conditions include poor bladder tone (atonic and neurogenic) and urinary incontinence.

341 Other demyelinating diseases of central nervous system

341.0 Neuromyelitis optica — *syndrome involving demyelination of spinal cord, optic nerves and optic chiasma*

341.1 Schilder's disease — *Balo's concentric sclerosis; encephalitis periaxialis diffusa*

341.8 Other demyelinating diseases of central nervous system — *central demyelination of corpus callosum; central pontine myelinosis*
AHA: Nov-Dec, 1987, 6

341.9 Unspecified demyelinating disease of central nervous system

342 Hemiplegia and hemiparesis

AHA: Q4, 1994, 38

Flaccid hemiplegia is the loss of muscle tone in paralyzed body parts with absence of tendon reflex. It may be caused by disease or trauma affecting the nerves associated with the involved muscles.

Spastic hemiplegia is muscle spasm within paralyzed parts of the body with increased tendon reflexes. It may be caused by disease or trauma affecting the nerves associated with the involved muscles.

The following fifth-digit subclassification is for use with codes 342.0-342.9:

0 affecting unspecified side

1 affecting dominant side

2 affecting nondominant side

342.0 5th Flaccid hemiplegia — *hemiplegia (paralysis of half the body) with absent or defective muscle tone*
AHA: Q4, 1994, 38

342.1 5th Spastic hemiplegia — *hemiplegia (paralysis of half the body) with increased muscular tone*
AHA: Q4, 1994, 38

342.8 5th Other specified hemiplegia — *hemiplegia (paralysis of half the body) NEC*
AHA: Q4, 1994, 38

342.9 5th Unspecified hemiplegia — *hemiplegia (paralysis of half the body NOS*
AHA: Q4, 1994, 38; Q4, 1998, 87

343 Infantile cerebral palsy

Infantile cerebral palsy is chronic nonprogressive disorders, present from birth, due to damage to the motor function of the brain. The functional impairment may range from disorders of movement or coordination to paresis.

The term "congenital diplegia" is used to include a group of cases characterized by bilateral and symmetrical disturbances of motility present from birth and that remain stationary or tend to improve. Traditionally, the term "diplegia" is used when all four limbs are affected, but weakness and spasticity are more severe in the lower limbs. Quadriplegia or tetraplegia is the term used when all four limbs are affected to an equal extent.

Congenital hemiplegia refers to conditions demonstrated at birth while infantile hemiplegia is the term applied to hemiplegia that develops during the first few years of life. Clinically, the distinction between congenital and infantile hemiplegia is academic.

343.0 Diplegic infantile cerebral palsy — *congenital paraplegia; stiffness is greater in legs than in arms*

343.1 Hemiplegic infantile cerebral palsy — *congenital hemiplegia*

343.2 Quadriplegic infantile cerebral palsy

343.3 Monoplegic infantile cerebral palsy — *infantile cerebral palsy which affects a single limb or a single group of muscles*

343.4 Infantile hemiplegia — *infantile hemiplegia (postnatal) NOS*

343.8 Other specified infantile cerebral palsy — *congenital or infantile triplegia*

343.9 Unspecified infantile cerebral palsy — *cerebral palsy NOS*

344 Other paralytic syndromes

344.00 Unspecified quadriplegia — *quadriplegia NOS*
AHA: Q4, 1998, 38; Q4, 2003, 103

344.01 Quadriplegia and quadriparesis, C1-C4, complete — *paralysis at least below the level of C4 and lesion transects cord*

344.02 Quadriplegia and quadriparesis, C1-C4, incomplete — *paralysis at least below the level of C4 and does not completely transect the cord*

 © 2004 Ingenix, Inc.

344.03 Quadriplegia and quadriparesis, C5-C7, complete — *paralysis at least below the level of C7 and lesion transects cord*

344.04 C5-C7, incomplete — *incomplete; paralysis at least below the level of C7 and does not completely transect the cord*

344.09 Other quadriplegia and quadriparesis

344.1 Paraplegia — *paralysis of both lower limbs; paraplegia (lower)*
AHA: March-April, 1987, 10; Q4, 2003, 110

344.2 Diplegia of upper limbs — *diplegia (upper); paralysis of both upper limbs*

344.30 Monoplegia of lower limb affecting unspecified side — *paralysis of lower limb NOS*

344.31 Monoplegia of lower limb affecting dominant side

344.32 Monoplegia of lower limb affecting nondominant side

344.40 Monoplegia of upper limb affecting unspecified side — *monoplegia of upper limb NOS*

344.41 Monoplegia of upper limb affecting dominant side

344.42 Monoplegia of upper limb affecting nondominant side

344.5 Unspecified monoplegia

344.60 Cauda equina syndrome without mention of neurogenic bladder

344.61 Cauda equina syndrome with neurogenic bladder — *acontractile bladder; autonomic hyperreflexia of bladder; cord bladder*
AHA: March-April, 1987, 10; May-June, 1987, 12

344.81 Locked-in state — *victim cannot communicate except sometimes through eye-blinking, that he is fully conscious*
AHA: Q4, 1993, 24

344.89 Other specified paralytic syndrome — *alternating oculomotor paralysis, Avellis' syndrome, Babinski-Nageotte syndrome, Benedikt's paralysis, Brown-Sequard syndrome, Cestan-Chenais syndrome, tegmental syndrome, triplegia, Weber-Leyden syndrome*
AHA: Q2, 1999, 4

344.9 Unspecified paralysis

Coding Clarification

Neurogenic Bladder: Many conditions may result in neurogenic bladder including cauda equina syndrome, injury to the spine and spinal cord, spondylitis, neoplasms, fractures, and congenital defects. When the neurogenic bladder is not due to a spinal condition, it is classified to one of the bladder dysfunction categories.

Cauda Equina Syndrome: This condition is due to a compression of the lumbosacral nerve roots. Symptoms include a dull aching pain in the sacral region and/or pain in the legs. There is weakness or paralysis of the muscles. These symptoms slowly progress and a loss of bladder control may eventually occur. When a neurogenic bladder is caused by cauda equina syndrome, code 344.61 is assigned.

Posterior Midline Disk Prolapse: A compression of the nerve roots at the level of L2-3 may result in acute cauda equina syndrome. In these instances, code 722.73 should be reported as well as code 344.61 to indicate both the prolapsed disc and the cauda equina syndrome with neurogenic bladder.

Spondylosis is a compression of any or all of the nerve roots of the cauda equina and causes a variety of sensory and motor deficits. Spondylosis with myelopathy indicates deficits due to nerve compression and would include neurogenic bladder. However, it is appropriate to code lumbar or sacral spondylosis with neurogenic bladder by reporting both codes 721.42 and 344.61.

345 Epilepsy

AHA: Q2, 1992, 8; Q4, 1992, 23; Q1, 1993, 24

Epilepsy is a disorder characterized by recurrent transient disturbances of the cerebral function. An abnormal paroxysmal neuronal discharge in the brain usually results in convulsive seizures, but may result in loss of consciousness, abnormal behavior, and sensory disturbances in any combination. Epilepsy may be secondary to prior trauma, hemorrhage, intoxication (toxins), chemical imbalances, anoxia, infections, neoplasms, or congenital defects.

Signs and symptoms of epilepsy include momentary interruption of activity, staring, and mental blankness. More severe symptoms include complete loss of consciousness, sudden momentary loss or contracture of muscle tone, rolling of the eyes, stiffness, violent jerking movements, and incontinence of urine and feces.

Diagnostic tests include lab work such as CBC for signs of infection and serum lead levels for signs of lead poisoning. Lumbar puncture may rule out suspected cerebrospinal infection or trauma, while a CT scan of the brain may rule out intracranial lesions, and an EEG may detect abnormal electrical activity in the brain.

Therapies include anticonvulsives such as phenobarbital, Tegretol, phenytoin (Dilantin), and surgery (temporal lobectomy, extratemporal cortical resections, hemispherectomy, and CT- or MRI-based stereotactic resections of epileptogenic lesions) for severe, intractable, or life-threatening disease.

The following fifth-digit subclassification is for use with categories 345.0, 345.1, and 345.4-345.9:

0 without mention of intractable epilepsy

1 with intractable epilepsy

345.0 ✔5th Generalized nonconvulsive epilepsy — *atonic absences; minor epilepsy; petit mal; atonic seizures*
AHA: Q2, 1992, 8; Q4, 1992, 23; Q1, 1993, 24

345.1 ✔5th Generalized convulsive epilepsy — *clonic, tonic, myoclonic epileptic seizures; grand mal; major epilepsy*
AHA: Q2, 1992, 8; Q4, 1992, 23; Q1, 1993, 24; Q3, 1997, 4

345.2 Epileptic petit mal status — *epileptic absence status*
AHA: Q2, 1992, 8; Q4, 1992, 23; Q1, 1993, 24

345.3 Epileptic grand mal status — *status epilepticus NOS*
AHA: Q2, 1992, 8; Q4, 1992, 23; Q1, 1993, 24

345.4 ✔5th Partial epilepsy with impairment of consciousness — *limbic system epilepsy; partial secondarily graded epilepsy; psychomotor epilepsy; epileptic automatism*
AHA: Q2, 1992, 8; Q4, 1992, 23; Q1, 1993, 24

345.5 ✔5th Partial epilepsy without mention of impairment of consciousness — *Bravais-Jacksonian epilepsy NOS; motor partial epilepsy; sensory-induced epilepsy; visceral epilepsy; temporal lobe epilepsy*
AHA: Q2, 1992, 8; Q4, 1992, 23; Q1, 1993, 24

345.6 ✔5th Infantile spasms — *hypsarrhythmia; lightning spasms*
AHA: Nov-Dec, 1984, 12; Q2, 1992, 8; Q4, 1992, 23; Q1, 1993, 24

345.7 ✔5th Epilepsia partialis continua — *Kojevnikov's epilepsy*
AHA: Q2, 1992, 8; Q4, 1992, 23; Q1, 1993, 24

345.8 ✔5th Other forms of epilepsy — *cursive or gelastic epilepsy*
AHA: Q2, 1992, 8; Q4, 1992, 23; Q1, 1993, 24

345.9 ✔5th Unspecified epilepsy — *epileptic convulsions, fits or seizures NOS*
AHA: Nov-Dec, 1987, 12; Q2, 1992, 8; Q4, 1992, 23; Q1, 1993, 24

Documentation Issues

Only if the diagnosis specifically indicates epilepsy should it be coded as such. Assign code 780.3x, unless the documentation states epilepsy.

The terms grand mal and tonic-clonic seizures in the documentation do not establish the diagnosis of epilepsy.

In cases where repeated admissions for seizures have occurred during the first three years after birth, verify with the physician if the patient's diagnosis of "convulsions" or "seizures" should be classified as infantile spasms, code 345.6x. If the physician does not verify that the condition is infantile spasms and no underlying pathology is found, use code 780.39 for convulsions of unknown etiology.

When the documentation only indicates the diagnosis of posttraumatic seizure disorder, clarify with the physician if the seizure disorder is to be coded seizure (780.39) or epilepsy (345.9x).

Only if the documentation specifically indicates intractable epilepsy should it be coded as such. Documentation of recurrence does not substantiate an intractable epilepsy because all seizures in an epileptic patient are recurrent.

Coding Clarification

Assign a fourth digit to indicate the type of epilepsy. If the physician does not indicate the type of epilepsy in the medical record, report 345.9x with the appropriate fifth digit.

A series of seizures at intervals too brief to allow consciousness between attacks is known as status epilepticus and can result in death. Status epilepticus not otherwise specified is classified to code 345.3x, grand mal status, but status epilepticus can occur in other specified forms of epilepsy.

Benign Shuddering Attacks: This movement disorder is not coded as an epileptic condition; it is a nonepileptic disorder. Use code 333.93 to classify this condition.

Posttraumatic Epilepsy: Posttraumatic epilepsy is classified with a late effect code, 907.0 *Late effect intracranial injury without mention of skull fracture.* When using a code from the late effect categories (905-909), code first the residual condition, then list the late effect code. The late effects include those specified as such, or as sequelae, which may occur at any time after the acute injury.

Recurrent Seizures: Recurrent seizures are not epilepsy although all seizures in an epileptic patient are recurrent.

Seizure Disorder vs. Epilepsy: Other conditions may cause recurrent seizures such as central nervous system neoplasms, cerebral infarction, and metabolic disorders. Only if the diagnosis specifically indicates epilepsy should it be coded as such.

 © 2004 Ingenix, Inc.

Coding Scenario

A 4-year-old female is admitted for introduction of a ketogenic diet therapy for myoclonic seizure disorder. The patient's history states the patient has generalized epilepsy. The patient has had multiple admissions for recurrent seizures.

> Code assignment: 345.10 *Generalized convulsive epilepsy, without mention of intractable epilepsy*

A patient is admitted via the emergency department with grand mal seizures. The history indicates the patient is known to have intractable epilepsy.

> Code assignment: 345.31 *Epileptic, grand mal status, with intractable epilepsy*

A patient with known epilepsy is admitted after having experienced a grand mal seizure.

> Code assignment: 345.30 *Epileptic, grand mal status, without mention of intractable epilepsy*

346 Migraine

The most common type of vascular headache is migraine. The precise cause of a migraine is unclear; however, people who get migraine headaches appear to have blood vessels that overreact to various triggers. According to current thinking, blood flow changes in the vessels may be a nervous system response to a trigger such as stress or an allergic reaction to food in susceptible people by creating a spasm in the arteries at the base of the brain. The spasm constricts several arteries supplying blood to the brain, which reduces blood flow to the brain. Reduced blood flow decreases the brain's supply of oxygen. The arteries within the brain dilate in response to the reduced oxygen supply that, in turn, triggers the release of pain-producing substances called prostaglandins. The result is a throbbing pain in the head.

No medical test exists for migraine, so the diagnosis is based on having some or all of the following symptoms:

- Moderate to severe throbbing pain for up to 72 hours that is frequently on one side of the head (the word migraine comes from the Greek hemicranios, meaning half a head)
- Nausea, with or without vomiting
- Sensitivity to light and sound

About 20 percent of migraine sufferers experience visual and other disturbances about 15 minutes before the head pain. These symptoms, collectively known as "aura," may include flashing lights, bright spots, loss of part of one's field of vision, or numbness or tingling in the hand, tongue, or side of the face. Migraines preceded by an aura are called classic migraines; others are referred to as common migraines of which symptoms beforehand include mental fuzziness, mood changes, fatigue, and unusual retention of fluids. Common migraine pain can last three to four days. In addition to classic and common, migraine headache can take several other forms:

- Patients with hemiplegic migraine have temporary paralysis on one side of the body.
- In ophthalmoplegic migraine, the pain is around the eye and is associated with a droopy eyelid, double vision, and other sight problems.
- Basilar artery migraine involves a disturbance of a major brain artery and occurs primarily in adolescent and young adult women and is often associated with the menstrual cycle.
- Status migrainosus is a rare and severe type of migraine that can last 72 hours or longer, with pain and nausea so intense that people must be hospitalized.

Migraines affect both males and females, and most often the disorder begins between the ages of 5 and 35. The condition is more common in adult women.

Drug therapy, biofeedback training, stress reduction, and cutting certain foods from the diet are the most common methods of preventing and controlling migraine headaches. For infrequent migraines, drugs can be taken at the first sign of a headache, but for most migraine sufferers who get moderate to severe headaches, and for all cluster patients, stronger drugs may be necessary to control the pain.

The following fifth-digit subclassification is for use with category 346:

0 without mention of intractable migraine

1 with intractable migraine, so stated

346.0 ✓5th Classical migraine — *migraine preceded or accompanied by transient focal neurological symptoms; migraine with aura*

346.1 ✓5th Common migraine — *atypical migraine; sick headache*

346.2 ✓5th Variants of migraine — *cluster headache; histamine cephalgia; abdominal migraine; migrainous or ciliary neuralgia*

346.8 ✓5th Other forms of migraine — *hemiplegic or ophthalmoplegic migraine*

346.9 ✓5th Unspecified migraine

347 Cataplexy and narcolepsy

Cataplexy is a neurologic condition, often confused with epilepsy. Patients with cataplexy experience sudden loss of muscle tone and fall to the floor because of laughter, stress, or frightening experiences. The cataplectic patient does not lose consciousness but lies without moving for a few minutes until normal body tone returns. Cataplexy can exist by itself, or more commonly, as a feature of narcolepsy.

Narcolepsy is a disorder characterized by sudden attacks of irrepressible REM sleep. It is sometimes associated with the following:

- Cataplexy
- Frightening and recurring visual hallucinations when falling to or arousing from sleep
- Paralysis of voluntary musculature while falling asleep

Narcolepsy rarely begins before adolescence. Patients with narcolepsy are easily aroused and become spontaneously alert and are often treated by stimulants such as caffeine, amphetamines, and methylphenidate. These same stimulants are not useful in treating cataplexy, which can be controlled with imipramine or desipramine, given in gradually increasing doses.

347.00 Narcolepsy, without cataplexy

347.01 Narcolepsy, with cataplexy

347.10 Narcolepsy in conditions classified elsewhere, without cataplexy

347.11 Narcolepsy in conditions classified elsewhere, with cataplexy

348 Other conditions of brain

348.0 Cerebral cysts — *arachnoid cyst; pseudoporencephaly*

348.1 Anoxic brain damage — (Use additional E code to identify cause)

348.2 Benign intracranial hypertension — *pseudotumor cerebri*

348.30 Encephalopathy, unspecified — *cerebral or cortical dysrhythmia*

348.31 Metabolic encephalopathy — *organic brain dysfunction from metabolic causes; septic encephalopathy, HIV-1-associated dementia (HAD)*

348.39 Other encephalopathy

348.4 Compression of brain — *brain (stem) compression or herniation*
AHA: Q4, 1994, 37

348.5 Cerebral edema — *swelling of the brain*

348.8 Other conditions of brain — *cerebral fungus or calcification*
AHA: Sept-Oct, 1987, 9

348.9 Unspecified condition of brain

349 Other and unspecified disorders of the nervous system

349.0 Reaction to spinal or lumbar puncture — *headache following lumbar puncture*
AHA: Q3, 1990, 18; Q2, 1999, 9

349.1 Nervous system complications from surgically implanted device

349.2 Disorders of meninges, not elsewhere classified — *meningeal adhesions, (cerebral), (spinal); acquired meningocele; acquired pseudomeningocele*
AHA: Q3, 1994, 4; Q2, 1998, 18

349.81 Cerebrospinal fluid rhinorrhea — *escape of CSF through nose*

349.82 Toxic encephalopathy — (Use additional E code to identify cause)

349.89 Other specified disorder of nervous system — *nervous system disorders NEC*

349.9 Unspecified disorders of nervous system — *disorder of nervous system (central) NOS*

350–359 Disorders of the Peripheral Nervous System

The Cranial Nerves

Ten of the 12 pairs of cranial nerves originate from the brain stem, but all leave the skull through the foramina of the skull. The nerves are designated by Roman numerals that indicate the order in which the nerves arise from the brain (anterior to posterior), while the name of each pair indicates the function — sensory, motor, or mixed motor/sensory. The name and order of each cranial nerve are as follows: olfactory (I) nerve, optic (II) nerve, oculomotor (III) nerve, trochlear (IV) nerve, trigeminal (V) nerve, abducens (VI) nerve, facial (VII) nerve, vestibulocochlear (VIII) nerve, glossopharyngeal (IX) nerve, vagus (X) nerve, accessory (XI) nerve, and hypoglossal (XII) nerve.

350 Trigeminal nerve disorders

This rubric identifies disorders of the trigeminal (V) nerve, which is a mixed (motor/sensory) cranial nerve and the largest of the cranial nerves. The trigeminal nerve has three branches: ophthalmic, maxillary, and mandibular. Trigeminal neuralgia (350.1) is characterized by intermittent, shooting pain in the gums, teeth, and lower face initiated by shaving, chewing, or a particular jaw motion. The pain may present for weeks or months and then cease spontaneously for a variable period of time. Diagnosis is based on medical history and an exam that rules out other conditions. An enlarged looping artery or vein pressing the trigeminal nerve is the most common cause. A brain tumor identified by magnetic resonance imaging (MRI) may also cause the disorder. Trigeminal neuralgia can occur at any age, though onset is generally 50 years of age or older. Treatment includes medication and surgery (i.e., microvascular decompression, glycerol injections, gamma knife radiation, electrocoagulation, and balloon compression).

350.1 Trigeminal neuralgia — *tic douloureux; trifacial neuralgia*

350.2 Atypical face pain

© 2004 Ingenix, Inc.

350.8 Other specified trigeminal nerve disorders — *auriculotemporal syndrome; compression fifth cranial nerve; Frey's syndrome; gustatory sweating syndrome; lesion of gasserian ganglion*

350.9 Unspecified trigeminal nerve disorder

Coding Clarification

A disorder of any of the cranial nerves can produce severe loss of function of which the most common are trigeminal neuralgia (350.1) and Bell's palsy (351.0).

351 Facial nerve disorders

This rubric identifies disorders of the facial (VII) nerve, which is a mixed (motor/sensory) cranial nerve. Its motor fibers originate from the pons and are distributed to facial, scalp, and neck muscles. The sensory fibers convey sensations from the face and scalp and taste buds of the tongue. Bell's palsy (351.0) describes paralysis of muscles on one side of the face that results from temporary damage to the facial nerve. Abnormal tearing from the eye may result when the weakened eyelid can no longer funnel tears into the lacrimal ducts. Severity depends on the extent of nerve damage and although the cause is unknown, a viral infection is suspected. The disorder occurs at all ages, but is most frequent between ages 30 and 60. Ninety percent of patients with Bell's palsy recover without treatment. A cortisone substance may be prescribed to reduce inflammation if the diagnosis is made within the first 48 hours. If eyelid function is compromised, the eye must be covered to prevent drying or injury. Electrophysiologic testing of facial nerve function, though not diagnostic of Bell's palsy, may locate a lesion.

351.0 Bell's palsy — *facial palsy*

351.1 Geniculate ganglionitis — *geniculate ganglionitis NOS*

351.8 Other facial nerve disorders — *facial myokymia; Melkersson's syndrome*
AHA: Q3, 2002, 13

351.9 Unspecified facial nerve disorder — *facial nerve disorder NOS*

352 Disorders of other cranial nerves

352.0 Disorders of olfactory (1st) nerve — *disorders of olfactory (1st) nerve*

352.1 Glossopharyngeal neuralgia — *pain between the throat and the ear along the petrosal and jugular ganglia*
AHA: Q2, 2002, 8

352.2 Other disorders of glossopharyngeal (9th) nerve

352.3 Disorders of pneumogastric (10th) nerve — *disorders of vagal nerve*

352.4 Disorders of accessory (11th) nerve — *disorder in the nerves affecting the palate, pharynx, larynx, thoracic viscera, and sternocleidomastoid and trapezius muscles*

352.5 Disorders of hypoglossal (12th) nerve — *disorder in the nerves affecting the muscles of the tongue*

352.6 Multiple cranial nerve palsies — *Collet-Sicard syndrome; polyneuritis cranialis*

352.9 Unspecified disorder of cranial nerves

353 Nerve root and plexus disorders

This rubric identifies disorders arising from the nerve networks of the peripheral nervous system. Thoracic outlet syndrome (353.0) is a group of symptoms arising from the upper extremity, the chest, neck, shoulders, and head. The Selmonosky Triad test (e.g., tenderness in the supra clavicular area, tingling and burning sensations in the hand on elevation, and adduction and abduction weakness of fingers) during physical examination may be used for diagnosis. The brachial plexus is a network of nerves formed by fibers located between the shoulder and the neck. Severe shoulder and upper arm pain followed by marked upper arm weakness characterizes Parsonage-Turner Syndrome, also known as brachial plexus neuritis or neuralgic amyotrophy (353.5). Magnetic resonance imaging (MRI) of the shoulder and upper arm musculature may reveal denervation, allowing prompt diagnosis. Electromyography three to four weeks after the onset of symptoms can localize the lesion and confirm the diagnosis. Treatment includes analgesics and physical therapy. Phantom limb syndrome (353.6) is a side effect of the brain's attempt to reorganize following a serious disruption in the sensory information processed in the cerebral cortex, thalamus, and brainstem. Those who have lost limbs through amputation are not the only people who have phantom sensations; those with spinal cord injuries, peripheral nerve injury, diabetic neuropathy, and stroke survivors all report similar feelings.

353.0 Brachial plexus lesions — *cervical rib syndrome; thoracic outlet syndrome; scalenus anticus syndrome*

353.1 Lumbosacral plexus lesions — *acquired defect in tissue along the network of nerves in the lower back, causing corresponding motor and sensory dysfunction*

353.2 Cervical root lesions, not elsewhere classified — *cervicodorsal outlet syndrome*

353.3 Thoracic root lesions, not elsewhere classified

353.4 Lumbosacral root lesions, not elsewhere classified

353.5 Neuralgic amyotrophy — *Parsonage-Aldren-Turner syndrome*

353.6 Phantom limb (syndrome) — *postamputation neural disorder causing itch, ache, or pain as if in the nerves of the amputated limb*

353.8 Other nerve root and plexus disorders

353.9 Unspecified nerve root and plexus disorder

354 Mononeuritis of upper limb and mononeuritis multiplex

Carpal tunnel syndrome is a common disorder that is inflammation of the tendons in the carpal tunnel, which can normally be attributed to repetitive use of the hand and/or wrist.

At the base of the palm is a tight canal or "tunnel" (carpal tunnel) through which tendons and nerves must pass on their way from the forearm to the hand and fingers. The median nerve passes through this narrow tunnel to reach the hand. If anything takes extra room in the canal, things become too tight and the nerve in the canal becomes constricted or "pinched." This pinching of the nerve causes numbness and tingling in the area of the hand that the nerve travels to.

The most common cause of carpal tunnel syndrome is repetitive strain injuries (RSIs). This is caused by long periods of steady hand movement. RSIs tend to come with work that demands repeated grasping, turning, and twisting; they are especially likely to get carpal tunnel syndrome if the work requires repeated twisting or involves repetitive vibration, as in hammering nails or operating a power tool.

A number of sports can bring on repetitive stress injuries: rowing, golf, tennis, downhill skiing, archery, competitive shooting, and rock climbing are examples of activities that stress the hand and wrist joints. Injuries and ailments that cause swelling or compression of soft tissue on nerves, such as sprains, leukemia, and rheumatoid arthritis, can lead to stress injuries. Diabetes, thyroid problems, and other systemic disorders are also associated with discomfort from stressed nerves, as is the fluid accumulation that sometimes accompanies pregnancy. Some clinicians believe that a pyridoxine (vitamin B6) deficiency can also induce the symptoms.

354.0 Carpal tunnel syndrome — *median nerve entrapment; partial thenar atrophy*

354.1 Other lesion of median nerve — *acquired defect in tissue in the ulnar nerve, causing corresponding motor and sensory dysfunction in the forearm and hand; cubital tunnel syndrome; tardy ulnar nerve palsy*

354.2 Lesion of ulnar nerve

354.3 Lesion of radial nerve — *acquired defect in tissue in the radial nerve, causing corresponding motor and sensory dysfunction in the forearm and hand; acute radial nerve palsy*
AHA: Nov-Dec, 1987, 6

354.4 Causalgia of upper limb — *dysfunction of peripheral nerve of upper limb, usually due to injury, causing burning pain and trophic skin changes*

354.5 Mononeuritis multiplex — *combinations of single conditions classifiable to 354 or 355*

354.8 Other mononeuritis of upper limb — *paralysis nerve phrenic (acquired); paralysis subscapularis; subcostal nerve compression syndrome*

354.9 Unspecified mononeuritis of upper limb

355 Mononeuritis of lower limb and unspecified site

355.0 Lesion of sciatic nerve — *acquired defect in tissue in the sciatic nerve, causing corresponding motor and sensory dysfunction in the back, buttock, and leg; pyriformis syndrome*
AHA: Q2, 1989, 12

355.1 Meralgia paresthetica — *lateral cutaneous femoral nerve of thigh compression or syndrome*

355.2 Other lesion of femoral nerve

355.3 Lesion of lateral popliteal nerve — *lesion of common peroneal nerve*

355.4 Lesion of medial popliteal nerve

355.5 Tarsal tunnel syndrome — *neuropathy of distal tibial nerve*

355.6 Lesion of plantar nerve — *Morton's metatarsalgia, neuralgia or neuroma*

355.71 Causalgia of lower limb

355.79 Other mononeuritis of lower limb

355.8 Unspecified mononeuritis of lower limb

355.9 Mononeuritis of unspecified site — *causalgia NOS*

356 Hereditary and idiopathic peripheral neuropathy

356.0 Hereditary peripheral neuropathy — *Dejerine-Sottas disease*

356.1 Peroneal muscular atrophy — *Charcot-Marie-Tooth disease; neuropathic muscular atrophy*

356.2 Hereditary sensory neuropathy — *inherited defect in dorsal root ganglia, optic nerve, and cerebellum causing sensory losses, shooting pains, foot ulcers*

356.3 Refsum's disease — *heredopathia atactica polyneuritiformis*

356.4 Idiopathic progressive polyneuropathy — *advancing disease or dysfunction of multiple nerves; cause unknown*

356.8 Other specified idiopathic peripheral neuropathy — *supranuclear paralysis*

© 2004 Ingenix, Inc.

356.9 Unspecified hereditary and idiopathic peripheral neuropathy

357 Inflammatory and toxic neuropathy

Inflammatory and toxic neuropathy is pain, swelling, and loss of function of the peripheral nerves in response to another disease process, injury, or unknown etiology (inflammatory neuropathy), or in response to a toxic substance (toxic neuropathy).

357.0 Acute infective polyneuritis — *Guillain-Barré syndrome; postinfectious polyneuritis*
AHA: Q2, 1998, 12

Acute infective polyneuritis is polyneuropathy due to an infective organism, usually viral or bacterial. The most common infective organism causing polyneuritis is herpes zoster, which is classified to code 053.13. Guillain-Barré syndrome, the most common diagnosis classified here, is characterized by rapid development of symmetrical weakness or flaccid paralysis affecting the lower extremities. The upper extremities and face are less often affected.

Signs and symptoms of acute infective polyneuritis include history of recent herpesvirus (cytomegalovirus, Epstein-Barr virus) infection or immunization, paresthesia and tingling, depressed respirations in severe disease, weakness of hands and feet, and inability to perform fine movements.

Diagnostic tests include lumbar puncture with analysis of cerebrospinal fluid to show elevated protein level, often in normal cell counts. Therapies include plasmapheresis (plasma exchange), immunoglobulins in high doses, IV corticosteroids, and respiratory assistance.

Use an additional code to identify the organism causing the infection. Human immunodeficiency virus (HIV) is becoming a common cause of acute or infective polyneuropathy and is coded 042, along with code 357.0 or 079.53.

357.1 Polyneuropathy in collagen vascular disease — (Code first underlying disease: 446.0, 710.0, 714.0)

357.2 Polyneuropathy in diabetes — (Code first underlying disease: 250.6)

Polyneuropathy in diabetes is neuropathy involving the long sensory nerves supplying the hands and feet. The axons of the sensory nerves degenerate from the most distal sites and gradually spread more proximally.

Signs and symptoms of polyneuropathy in diabetes include loss of sensation to body part involved, thin and shiny skin, hair loss, "stocking and glove" effect, decreased sensation, and paresthesias.

Therapies include strict control of blood glucose levels, vitamin B and thiamine, drugs such as phenytoin, carbamazepine, amitriptyline, and fluphenazine.

Associated conditions include complications of diabetes mellitus such as diabetic nephropathy, ulcers, gangrene, and frequent infections of hands and feet.

Use codes 250.6x and 357.2 to report diabetic polyneuropathy.

357.3 Polyneuropathy in malignant disease — (Code first underlying disease: 140.0-208.9)

357.4 Polyneuropathy in other diseases classified elsewhere — (Code first underlying disease: 032.0-032.9, 135, 251.2, 265.0, 265.2, 266.0-266.9, 277.1, 277.3, 585)

357.5 Alcoholic polyneuropathy

Alcoholic polyneuropathy, also called polyneuritis potatorum, is due to thiamine and other vitamin deficiency caused by chronic alcohol abuse. In addition, alcohol is believed to be neurotoxic.

Signs and symptoms of alcoholic polyneuropathy are pain, particularly in the midcalf and soles of the feet, tingling, loss of sensation, weakness of hands and feet, inability to perform fine movements, diminished tendon reflexes, excessive perspiration, and atrophy of lower limbs.

Diagnostic tests include EMG to show axonal sensorimotor neuropathy. Lab work reveals low vitamin B levels, anemia (chronic alcoholism interferes with eating balanced meals), and elevated liver enzymes (SGOT, SGPT, and bilirubin). Therapies include control of alcohol intake, correction of nutritional deficiencies, and physiotherapy in severe cases.

Associated conditions include cirrhosis of the liver, foot drop and wrist drop, and Korsakoff's psychosis.

357.6 Polyneuropathy due to drugs — (Use additional E code to identify drug)

357.7 Polyneuropathy due to other toxic agents — (Use additional E code to identify toxic agent)

357.81 Chronic inflammatory demyelinating polyneuritis

357.82 Critical illness polyneuropathy — *acute motor neuropathy*
AHA: Q4, 203, 111; Q2, 1998, 12; Q4, 2002, 47

357.89 Other inflammatory and toxic neuropathy

357.9 Unspecified inflammatory and toxic neuropathy

Coding Clarification

Toxic Neuropathy: A common toxic effect of anticancer drugs is peripheral neuropathy. To accurately report this condition, use codes 357.6 *Polyneuropathy due to drugs* and E933.1 *Drugs, medicinal*

and biological substances causing adverse effects in therapeutic use, antineoplastic and immunosuppressive drugs.

Coding Scenario

A patient is admitted with diabetic neuropathy with secondary diabetes. Patient history identifies the patient has a previous history of a partial pancreatectomy that has caused the diabetic condition.

> Code assignment: 251.3 *Postsurgical hypoinsulinemia* and 357.4 *Polyneuropathy in other diseases classified elsewhere*

358 Myoneural disorders

Myasthenia gravis is a disorder of neuromuscular transmission due to the presence of autoimmune antibodies at the neuromuscular junction.

Signs and symptoms of myasthenia gravis include skeletal muscle weakness and fatigability, dysarthria, chewing fatigue, dysphagia, fever, respiratory distress, ptosis, and ocular muscle weakness.

Diagnostic tests include blood serum with AChR-ab (gamma globulin antibody found in 90 percent of patients). CT scan of mediastinum or chest x-ray may show thymoma or prominent thymus gland, while an EMG shows abnormalities in muscle fiber performance. Therapies include drugs such as anticholinesterase, adrenal corticosteroids, and immunosuppressants such as azathioprine, thymectomy, plasmapheresis, and leukoplasmapheresis.

Associated conditions include thymus gland abnormalities, osteoporosis, cataracts, frequent infections, and cholinergic crisis (primarily respiratory depression and paroxysmal atrial tachycardia) due to anticholinesterase medications.

358.00 Myasthenia gravis without (acute) exacerbation — *Goldflam-Erb disease or syndrome, Hoppe-Goldflam disease or syndrome, pseudoparalytica, asthenic bulbar, bulbopsinal paralysis*

358.01 Myasthenia gravis with (acute) exacerbation — *crisis includes life-threatening inability to use respiratory muscles*

358.1 Myasthenic syndromes in diseases classified elsewhere — (Code first underlying disease: 005.1, 140.0-208.9, 242.00-242.91, 244.0-244.9, 250.6, 281.0) — *amyotrophy or Eaton-Lambert syndrome from stated cause classified elsewhere*

358.2 Toxic myoneural disorders — (Use additional E code to identify toxic agent)

358.8 Other specified myoneural disorders — *amyotonia congenita; Oppenheim's disease*

358.9 Unspecified myoneural disorders

Coding Clarification

If the documentation states that the patient's myasthenic symptoms are due to another underlying condition, see subcategory 358.1.

359 Muscular dystrophies and other myopathies

Muscular dystrophies and other myopathies are disease processes that are genetic in origin and cause the degeneration of muscle and nerve fibers.

359.0 Congenital hereditary muscular dystrophy — *benign congenital myopathy; central core disease; centronuclear myopathy*

359.1 Hereditary progressive muscular dystrophy — *Gower's or Duchenne's muscular dystrophy*

Hereditary progressive muscular dystrophy is a disease process that is genetic in origin and causes the degeneration of muscle and nerve fibers. This condition usually has an early onset, primarily affects males, and has a relentless progression until death. In the final stages, wasting of the muscles of the diaphragm and respiratory system causes respiratory failure. Classified here are any of the X-linked recessive types of dystrophy such as Duchenne's, Erb's dystrophy, Landouzy-Dejerine disease, or Gower's dystrophy.

Signs and symptoms of hereditary progressive muscular dystrophy include wasting of muscles and deformities of small and large joints.

Diagnostic tests include serum enzyme measurements that may reveal extremely high levels of serum creatine phosphokinase, aldolase, and glutamic-oxaloacetic transaminase in the first two years, diminishing (but not returning to normal) as the disease progresses. A muscle biopsy shows degeneration of muscle fibers, and an EMG reveals a decrease in amplitude and duration of motor unit potentials. Therapies include physical and occupational therapy to maintain muscle function and treatment of complications such as heart failure or concomitant infection.

Associated conditions include atrophy of the liver, frequent infections, contracture deformities, heart failure, and respiratory failure.

359.2 Myotonic disorders — *dystrophia myotonica; Thomsen's disease*

359.3 Familial periodic paralysis — *hypokalemic familial periodic paralysis*

359.4 Toxic myopathy — (Use additional E code to identify toxic agent) — *muscle disorder caused by toxic agent*
AHA: Q1, 1988, 5

© 2004 Ingenix, Inc.

359.5 Myopathy in endocrine diseases classified elsewhere — (Code first underlying disease: 242.00-242.91, 244.0-244.9, 253.2, 255.0, 255.4)

359.6 Symptomatic inflammatory myopathy in diseases classified elsewhere — (Code first underlying disease: 135, 140.0-208.9, 277.3, 446.0, 710.0, 710.1, 710.2, 714.0)

359.81 Critical illness myopathy

359.89 Other myopathies

359.9 Unspecified myopathy

360–379 Disorders of the Eye and Adnexa

Endophthalmitis is inflammation of the eye that may affect either the anterior or posterior chamber or both, caused by an infection. Noninfectious or sterile endophthalmitis may be a result or retained lens material and/or toxic agents. There are two types of endophthalmitis: endogenous, with results from the hematogenous spread of organisms from a distant source of infection (e.g., endocarditis); and exogenous, which is the result from a direct inoculation, such as a complication of ocular surgery, foreign bodies, or blunt or penetrating ocular trauma. These may also be fungal or candidial in nature.

Endophthalmitis may include white nodules on the lens capsule, iris, retina, or choroid, or inflammation of all of the ocular tissues, which leads to a globe of full, purulent exudates. Inflammation may spread to the orbital soft tissue. Symptoms usually present as acute pain, redness, lid swelling, decreased visual acuity, headache, photophobia, and ocular discharge.

360 Disorders of the globe

360.00 Unspecified purulent endophthalmitis

360.01 Acute endophthalmitis — *sudden, severe infection of the eyeball, with pus*

360.02 Panophthalmitis — *sudden, severe infection throughout the eyeball*

360.03 Chronic endophthalmitis — *persistent infection and inflammation of the eyeball*

360.04 Vitreous abscess — *a pocket of pus in the gel-like fluid that fills the eyeball*

360.11 Sympathetic uveitis — *inflammation of the vascular layer of the uninjured eye following an injury to the patient's other eye*

360.12 Panuveitis — *inflammation of the entire vascular layer of the eye, including the choroid, iris and ciliary body*

360.13 Parasitic endophthalmitis NOS — *inflammation of the entire eye in a parasitic infection*

360.14 Ophthalmia nodosa — *inflammation of the conjunctiva of the eye caused by embedded caterpillar hairs*

360.19 Other endophthalmitis — *not elsewhere classified*

360.20 Unspecified degenerative disorder of globe

360.21 Progressive high (degenerative) myopia — *malignant myopia*
AHA: Q3, 1991, 3

360.23 Siderosis of globe — *deposits of iron pigment within the tissues of the eyeball, caused by high iron content of blood*
AHA: Q3, 1991, 3

360.24 Other metallosis of globe — *chalcosis*
AHA: Q3, 1991, 3

360.29 Other degenerative disorders of globe — *not elsewhere classified*
AHA: Q3, 1991, 3

360.30 Unspecified hypotony of eye

360.31 Primary hypotony of eye — *low intraocular pressure without apparent cause*

360.32 Ocular fistula causing hypotony — *low intraocular pressure due to leak through abnormal passage*

360.33 Hypotony associated with other ocular disorders — *associated with other ocular disorders*

360.34 Flat anterior chamber of eye — *obliteration of the eye, anterior chamber*

360.40 Unspecified degenerated globe or eye

360.41 Blind hypotensive eye — *atrophy of globe; phthisis bulbi*

360.42 Blind hypertensive eye — *absolute glaucoma*

360.43 Hemophthalmos, except current injury — *pool of blood within the eyeball, not from current injury*

360.44 Leucocoria — *reflection from mass behind lens, so that the pupil may look white, often indicative of retinoblastoma*

360.50 Foreign body, magnetic, intraocular, unspecified

360.51 Foreign body, magnetic, in anterior chamber of eye

360.52 Foreign body, magnetic, in iris or ciliary body

360.53 Foreign body, magnetic, in lens

360.54 Foreign body, magnetic, in vitreous

360.55 Foreign body, magnetic, in posterior wall

360.59 Intraocular foreign body, magnetic, in other or multiple sites

360.60 Foreign body, intraocular, unspecified

360.61 Foreign body in anterior chamber

360.62 Foreign body in iris or ciliary body

360.63 Foreign body in lens

360.64 Foreign body in vitreous

360.65 Foreign body in posterior wall of eye

360.69 Foreign body in other or multiple sites of eye

360.81 Luxation of globe — *double whammy syndrome*

360.89 Other disorders of globe — *acquired deformity of globe; adhesion of globe*

360.9 Unspecified disorder of globe

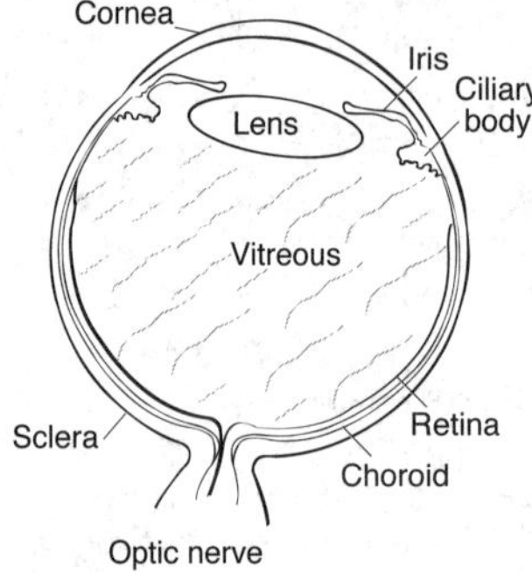

361 Retinal detachments and defects

The retina is sensitive nervous tissue that sends messages via the optic nerve to the brain and one of three layers of the eyeball. The outer, white layer is the sclera, which is the true wall of the eyeball. Lining the sclera is the choroid, a thin membrane that supplies nutrients to part of the retina. The retina, the innermost layer, begins just posterior to the iris, just behind the area called the pars plana, and lines the inner wall of the eye. The central portion of the retina is the macula, which is roughly the area inside of the arcade vessels that extend from the optic nerve and around the macula. The macula is the area of the retina where central vision is the clearest for color and reading vision. The true focal point of the eye is the foveal avascular zone (FAZ), which is only 400 microns wide (0.4mm). The single-layer retinal pigment epithelium (RPE) outside the retina provides nutrients to the photoreceptors; it is also dark with melanin, which decreases light scatter within the eye. The rod and cone are photoreceptors; the cone system dominates vision in daytime, whereas the rod system dominates night vision. Below the RPE is a multi-layered membrane called Bruch's membrane, which separates the RPE and retina from the choroid. The choroid is a vascular layer that provides most of the oxygen to the photoreceptors and RPE. The vitreous is a clear gel-like substance that fills up most of the inner space of the eyeball. It lies behind the lens and is in contact with the retina.

361.00 Retinal detachment with retinal defect, unspecified

361.01 Recent retinal detachment, partial, with single defect

361.02 Recent retinal detachment, partial, with multiple defects

361.03 Recent retinal detachment, partial, with giant tear

361.04 Recent retinal detachment, partial, with retinal dialysis — *dialysis (juvenile) of retina (with detachment)*

361.05 Recent retinal detachment, total or subtotal

361.06 Old retinal detachment, partial — *delimited old retinal detachment*

361.07 Old retinal detachment, total or subtotal

Retinoschisis and retinal cysts involve the splitting of the retina due to microcystoid degeneration (retinoschisis) and development of fluid-filled sacs on the retina (retinal cysts). Retinoschisis often is bilateral and is seen in older persons. Retinal detachment is an occasional complication.

This subcategory excludes juvenile retinoschisis (362.73) and cystic or cytoid degeneration of the retina (362.62).

361.10 Unspecified retinoschisis

361.11 Flat retinoschisis — *slowly progressive split of retinal sensory layers*

361.12 Bullous retinoschisis — *fluid retention between split retinal sensory layers*

361.13 Primary retinal cysts — *abnormal fluid-filled cavities or sacs within the retina*

361.14 Secondary retinal cysts — *abnormal fluid-filled cavities or sacs within the retina, caused by another condition or disease*

361.19 Other retinoschisis and retinal cysts — *cyst of ora serrata*

361.2 Serous retinal detachment

Coding Clarification

Serous retinal detachment is separation of the retina from the choroid. Usually spontaneous, although it may be due to a trauma, this condition usually occurs in patients 50 years of age or older. Aging may cause the vitreous to shrink, which causes the retina to tear.

Signs and symptoms of serous retinal detachment include reduced vision, flashing lights (photopsia), vitreous floaters, with total detachment, and no light perception.

Diagnostic tests include exam with an ophthalmoscope and a scleral depressor, which allows visualization of the tear. Therapies include scleral buckling.

Retinal defects that predispose a patient to retinal detachment classified elsewhere include peripheral cystoid degeneration, senile retinoschisis, peripheral chorioretinal degeneration, lattice degeneration, and dialysis of retina.

 © 2004 Ingenix, Inc.

361.30 Unspecified retinal defect

361.31 Round hole of retina without detachment — *hole of retina*

361.32 Horseshoe tear of retina without detachment — *operculum of retina*

361.33 Multiple defects of retina without detachment

361.81 Traction detachment of retina — *traction detachment with vitreoretinal organization*

361.89 Other forms of retinal detachment — *not elsewhere classified*
AHA: Q3, 1999, 12

361.9 Unspecified retinal detachment

362 Other retinal disorders

362.01 Background diabetic retinopathy — (Code first diabetes, 250.5) — *diabetic macular edema; diabetic retina microaneurysm*
AHA: Q3, 1991, 8

362.02 Proliferative diabetic retinopathy — (Code first diabetes, 250.5) — *neovascularization, vitreous hemorrhage and detachment in a diabetic retina*
AHA: Q3, 1991, 8; Q3, 1996, 5

362.10 Unspecified background retinopathy

362.11 Hypertensive retinopathy — *retinal irregularities caused by systemic hypertension*
AHA: Q3, 1990, 3

362.12 Exudative retinopathy — *Coat's syndrome*
AHA: Q3, 1999, 12

362.13 Changes in vascular appearance of retina — (Use additional code for any associated atherosclerosis, 440.8) — *vascular sheathing of retina*

362.14 Retinal microaneurysms NOS — *microscopic dilation of retinal vessels in nondiabetic*

362.15 Retinal telangiectasia — *permanent dilation of blood vessels of the retina*

362.16 Retinal neovascularization NOS — *choroidal or subretinal revascularization*

362.17 Other intraretinal microvascular abnormalities — *retinal varices*

362.18 Retinal vasculitis — *Eales' disease; retinal arteritis or endarteritis*

362.21 Retrolental fibroplasia — *Terry's syndrome*

362.29 Other nondiabetic proliferative retinopathy

362.30 Unspecified retinal vascular occlusion

362.31 Central artery occlusion of retina

362.32 Arterial branch occlusion of retina

362.33 Partial arterial occlusion of retina — *Hollenhorst plaque; retinal microembolism*

362.34 Transient arterial occlusion of retina — *amaurosis fugax*
AHA: Q1, 2000, 16

362.35 Central vein occlusion of retina

362.36 Venous tributary (branch) occlusion of retina

362.37 Venous engorgement of retina — *incipient or partial occlusion of retinal vein*

362.40 Unspecified retinal layer separation

362.41 Central serous retinopathy — *serous-filled blister causing localized detachment of retina from pigment epithelium*

362.42 Serous detachment of retinal pigment epithelium — *exudative detachment of retinal pigment epithelium*

362.43 Hemorrhagic detachment of retinal pigment epithelium — *blood-filled blister causing localized detachment of retina from pigment epithelium*

362.50 Macular degeneration (senile) of retina, unspecified — *Behr's disease*

362.51 Nonexudative senile macular degeneration of retina — *atrophic or dry senile macular degeneration*

362.52 Exudative senile macular degeneration of retina — *Kuhnt-Junius degeneration; disciform or wet senile macular degeneration*

362.53 Cystoid macular degeneration of retina — *cystoid macular edema*

362.54 Macular cyst, hole, or pseudohole of retina — *break or tear in macula*

362.55 Toxic maculopathy of retina — (Use additional E code to identify drug, if drug-induced) — *macular disease caused by toxic substance*

362.56 Macular puckering of retina — *preretinal fibrosis*

362.57 Drusen (degenerative) of retina — *white hyaline deposits on the retinal pigment epithelium*

362.60 Unspecified peripheral retinal degeneration

362.61 Paving stone degeneration of peripheral retina — *spots of retinal thinning through which the choroid can be seen*

362.62 Microcystoid degeneration of peripheral retina — *Blessig's or Iwanoff's cysts*

362.63 Lattice degeneration of peripheral retina — *palisade degeneration of retina*

362.64 Senile reticular degeneration of peripheral retina — *net-like appearance of retina; a sign of degeneration*

362.65 Secondary pigmentary degeneration of peripheral retina — *pseudoretinitis pigmentosa*

362.66 Secondary vitreoretinal degenerations peripheral retina — *non-ocular disease causing vitreoretinal change*

362.70 Unspecified hereditary retinal dystrophy

362.71 Retinal dystrophy in systemic or cerebroretinal lipidoses — (Code first underlying disease: 272.7, 330.1) — *cerebroretinal lipidoses, systemic lipidoses*

362.72 Retinal dystrophy in other systemic disorders and syndromes — (Code first underlying disease: 272.5, 356.3) — *Bassen-Kornzweig syndrome, Refsum's disease*

362.73 Vitreoretinal dystrophies — *juvenile retinoschisis*

362.74 Pigmentary retinal dystrophy — *retinal dystrophy, albipunctate; retinitis pigmentosa*

362.75 Other dystrophies primarily involving the sensory retina — *progressive cone (-rod) dystrophy; Stargardt's disease*

362.76 Dystrophies primarily involving the retinal pigment epithelium — *fundus flavimaculatus; vitelliform dystrophy*

362.77 Retinal dystrophies primarily involving Bruch's membrane — *hyaline or pseudoinflammatory foveal dystrophy; hereditary drusen*

362.81 Retinal hemorrhage — *preretinal, retinal (deep) (superficial) or subretinal hemorrhage*
AHA: Q4, 1996, 43

362.82 Retinal exudates and deposits — *fatty fluids or denser deposits leaking into the retina*

362.83 Retinal edema — *cotton wool retinal spots; retinal edema (localized) (macular) (peripheral)*

362.84 Retinal ischemia — *abnormal reduction of retinal blood supply*

362.85 Retinal nerve fiber bundle defects — *anomalies within the retinal nerves*

362.89 Other retinal disorders — *hyperemian of retina; phakoma; tessellated fundus, retina (tigroid)*

362.9 Unspecified retinal disorder

Coding Clarification

Hypertensive Retinopathy: To report this condition accurately, two codes are required, code 362.11 *Hypertensive retinopathy;* and an appropriate code from categories 401-405 to identify the specific type of hypertension.

363 Chorioretinal inflammations, scars, and other disorders of choroid

The choroid is the layer of blood vessels and connective tissue between the sclera and the retina. Blood vessels first appear in the choroid during the 15th week of development, and arteries and veins can be recognized by the 22nd week. Part of the choroid develops into the cores of the ciliary processes. At the posterior end of the optic cup, the choroid forms a sheath around the optic nerve. The choroid, iris, and ciliary body are also referred to as the uvea. The choroid is heavily pigmented, which prevents stray light from reaching the retina. It supplies nutrients to the inner parts of the eye and acts to exchange heat generated by retinal metabolism. The outer layer, which surrounds the choroid, is the sclera. Diseases of the choroid include choroidal melanoma, which is a common form of cancer that primarily affects the adult's eye, and choroiditis, which is the inflammation of the choroid. Melanoma of the uveal tract is the most common primary ocular cancer in adults.

363.00 Unspecified focal chorioretinitis

363.01 Focal choroiditis and chorioretinitis, juxtapapillary

363.03 Focal choroiditis and chorioretinitis of other posterior pole

363.04 Focal choroiditis and chorioretinitis, peripheral

363.05 Focal retinitis and retinochoroiditis, juxtapapillary — *neuroretinitis*

363.06 Focal retinitis and retinochoroiditis, macular or paramacular

363.07 Focal retinitis and retinochoroiditis of other posterior pole

363.08 Focal retinitis and retinochoroiditis, peripheral

363.10 Unspecified disseminated chorioretinitis

363.11 Disseminated choroiditis and chorioretinitis, posterior pole

363.12 Disseminated choroiditis and chorioretinitis, peripheral

363.13 Disseminated choroiditis and chorioretinitis, generalized — (Code first any underlying disease, 017.3)

363.14 Disseminated retinitis and retinochoroiditis, metastatic — *metastatic*

363.15 Disseminated retinitis and retinochoroiditis, pigment epitheliopathy — *acute posterior multifocal placoid pigment epitheliopathy*

363.20 Unspecified chorioretinitis

363.21 Pars planitis — *posterior cyclitis*

363.22 Harada's disease — *uveomeningeal syndrome*

363.30 Unspecified chorioretinal scar

363.31 Solar retinopathy — *macular damage from staring at the sun*

363.32 Other macular scars of chorioretina — *not elsewhere classified*

363.33 Other scars of posterior pole of chorioretina

© 2004 Ingenix, Inc.

363.34 Peripheral scars of the chorioretina

363.35 Disseminated scars of the chorioretina

363.40 Unspecified choroidal degeneration

363.41 Senile atrophy of choroid — *wasting away of choroid due to advanced age*

363.42 Diffuse secondary atrophy of choroid — *wasting away of choroid in systemic disease*

363.43 Angioid streaks of choroid — *cracks radiating from the optic disk in the layer separating the choriocapillaris from retinal epithelium*

363.50 Unspecified hereditary choroidal dystrophy or atrophy

363.51 Circumpapillary dystrophy of choroid, partial

363.52 Circumpapillary dystrophy of choroid, total — *helicoid dystrophy of choroid*

363.53 Central dystrophy of choroid, partial — *central areolar choroidal dystrophy; circinate choroidal dystrophy*

363.54 Central choroidal atrophy, total — *central gyrate choroidal dystrophy; serpiginous choroidal dystrophy*

363.55 Choroideremia — *degeneration of choroid, affecting both sexes, leading to blindness in males*

363.56 Other diffuse or generalized dystrophy of choroid, partial — *diffuse choroidal sclerosis*

363.57 Other diffuse or generalized dystrophy of choroid, total — *generalized gyrate atrophy, choroid*

363.61 Unspecified choroidal hemorrhage

363.62 Expulsive choroidal hemorrhage

363.63 Choroidal rupture

363.70 Unspecified choroidal detachment

363.71 Serous choroidal detachment — *blister of serous fluid causing localized detachment of choroid from the sclera*

363.72 Hemorrhagic choroidal detachment — *blood-filled blister causing localized detachment of choroid from the sclera*

363.8 Other disorders of choroid — *not elsewhere classified*

363.9 Unspecified disorder of choroid

364 Disorders of iris and ciliary body

The ciliary body is formed from the two layers composing the rim of the optic cup, which undergo folding to form the ciliary processes. The ciliary body produces the clear fluid into the eye that goes through the pupil and drains back into the blood stream through a tissue in front of the periphery of the iris. The ciliary body also contains the muscle that attaches to the outside of the lens of the eye and alters the focus of the eye. In turn, the ciliary body is continuous with a pigmented layer, the choroid, which lines the back of the eye outside the light sensitive retina. The iris, which extends partly over the lens, is composed of the two layers forming the edge of the optic cup and a layer of vascularized connective tissue containing the pupillary muscle. The iris muscles can make the pupil larger or smaller and the pigmented layer is responsible for eye color. The iris is continuous with the ring shaped ciliary body behind it. The iris, ciliary body, and choroid ensure that light only enters the eye through the pupil, and blood vessels in the choroid help to nourish the retina.

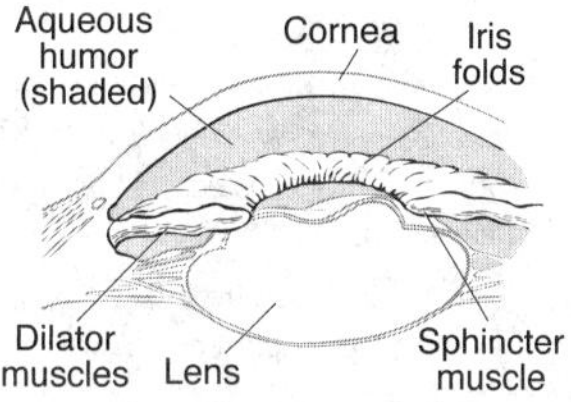

Sideview of iris and lens

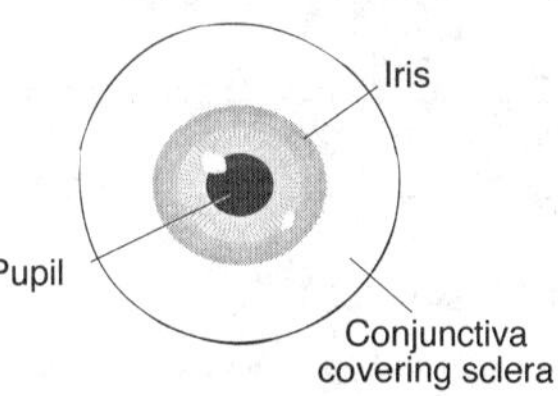

Iridocyclitis is a combination of inflammation of the iris and inflammation of the ciliary body. When the iris is inflamed, its blood vessels dilate and the blood vessels of the white of the eye make it reddened. The dilated vessels leak proteins and blood cells into the clear eye fluid, which tends to prevent fluid from going through the pupil. The iris tissue and the ciliary body are richly supplied with sensory nerves so that the inflamed tissue causes pain especially when it moves in bright light or when focusing for near objects.

364.00 Unspecified acute and subacute iridocyclitis

364.01 Primary iridocyclitis — *inflammation of the iris and ciliary body*

364.02 Recurrent iridocyclitis — *repeated bouts of inflammation of the iris and ciliary body*

364.03 Secondary iridocyclitis, infectious — *inflammation of the iris and ciliary body as a result of a primary infection elsewhere*

364.04 Secondary iridocyclitis, noninfectious — *inflammation of the iris and ciliary body as a result of a other systemic disease or disorder; aqueous fibrin or flare*

364.05 Hypopyon — *accumulation of pus between the cornea and the lens*

© 2004 Ingenix, Inc.

364.10 Unspecified chronic iridocyclitis — *persistent inflammation of the iris and ciliary body as a result of an underlying disease or condition*

364.11 Chronic iridocyclitis in diseases classified elsewhere — (Code first underlying disease: 017.3, 135)

364.21 Fuchs' heterochromic cyclitis — *unilateral inflammation of the ciliary body and iris, making the eyes appear to be different colors*

364.22 Glaucomatocyclitic crises — *uveal inflammation causing acute rise in intraocular pressure*

364.23 Lens-induced iridocyclitis — *immune reaction to proteins in the lens; follows lens trauma or extraction and causes inflammation of the iris*

364.24 Vogt-Koyanagi syndrome — *oculocutaneous syndrome; uveocutaneous syndrome*

364.3 Unspecified iridocyclitis

364.41 Hyphema — *hemorrhage of iris or ciliary body*

364.42 Rubeosis iridis — *neovascularization of iris or ciliary body*

364.51 Essential or progressive iris atrophy — *weakened and defective iris of unknown cause*

364.52 Iridoschisis — *splitting of the iris into two layers*

364.53 Pigmentary iris degeneration — *acquired heterochromia of iris; translucency of iris*

364.54 Degeneration of pupillary margin — *atrophy of sphincter of iris; ectropion of pigment epithelium of iris*

364.55 Miotic cysts of pupillary margin

364.56 Degenerative changes of chamber angle

364.57 Degenerative changes of ciliary body

364.59 Other iris atrophy — *iris atrophy (generalized) (sector shaped)*

364.60 Idiopathic cysts of iris, ciliary body, and anterior chamber — *fluid-filled sacs of the iris or ciliary body of unknown etiology*

364.61 Implantation cysts of iris, ciliary body, and anterior chamber — *epithelial down-growth, anterior chamber; implantation cysts (surgical) (traumatic)*

364.62 Exudative cysts of iris or anterior chamber — *protein or fatty fluid-filled sacs of the iris or ciliary body caused by leak of fluid from blood vessels*

364.63 Primary cyst of pars plana — *fluid-filled sacs of the outermost ciliary ring*

364.64 Exudative cyst of pars plana — *protein or fatty fluid-filled sacs of the outermost ciliary ring, caused by leak of fluid from blood vessels*

364.70 Unspecified adhesions of iris

364.71 Posterior synechiae — *adhesions binding iris to the lens*

364.72 Anterior synechiae — *adhesions binding iris to cornea*

364.73 Goniosynechiae — *peripheral anterior synechiae*

364.74 Adhesions and disruptions of pupillary membranes — *iris bombe; pupillary occlusion or seclusion*

364.75 Pupillary abnormalities — *deformed pupil; rupture of pupillary sphincter; ectopic pupil*

364.76 Iridodialysis — *tear at the base of the iris, separating it from the ciliary body*

364.77 Recession of chamber angle of eye

364.8 Other disorders of iris and ciliary body — *hernia of ciliary body; hernia of iris; iridodonesis*

364.9 Unspecified disorder of iris and ciliary body

365 Glaucoma

Glaucoma is an increase in intraocular pressure due to an abnormal aqueous humor outflow from the anterior chamber or, rarely, from an above normal rate of aqueous humor production by the ciliary body. If untreated, glaucoma ultimately leads to optic nerve damage and loss of vision.

365.00 Unspecified preglaucoma

365.01 Borderline glaucoma, open angle with borderline findings — *open angle with cupping of optic discs*
AHA: Q1, 1990, 8

365.02 Borderline glaucoma with anatomical narrow angle — *defect restricting aqueous flow in the anterior segment, possibly resulting in high intraocular pressure*
AHA: Q1, 1990, 8

365.03 Borderline glaucoma with steroid responders

365.04 Borderline glaucoma with ocular hypertension — *high fluid pressure within the eye due to no apparent cause*
AHA: Q1, 1990, 8

Open-angle glaucoma is an increase in intraocular pressure due to the free access of aqueous humor to the trabecular network in the angle of the anterior chamber. Heredity may play a factor in patients developing primary open-angle glaucoma as well as trauma.

Signs and symptoms of open-angle glaucoma include progressive loss of peripheral vision over a span of

© 2004 Ingenix, Inc.

years, blurred or foggy vision, seeing halos around lights, reduced night vision, and aching in the eyes.

Diagnostic tests include tonometry using an applanation such as a Schiotz or pneumatic tonometer to measure intraocular pressure. An exam (ophthalmoscope, slit lamp) shows the fundus, optic disk, and anterior structure of the eyes, while a gonioscopy differentiates between chronic open-angle glaucoma and acute closed-angle glaucoma. Perimetry and visual field tests determine the extent of peripheral vision loss and fundus photography records and monitors changes in the optic disk.

Therapies include topical miotic drugs (Pilocarpine, Carcholin), carbonic anhydrase inhibitors (acetazolamide), surgery (iridectomy, trephine procedures, trabeculectomy, posterior lip sclerectomy, thermal sclerotomy) to reduce intraocular pressure, Argon laser trabeculoplasty or iridectomy, and cyclodialysis or cyclocryotherapy.

365.10 Unspecified open-angle glaucoma

365.11 Primary open-angle glaucoma — *chronic simple glaucoma*

365.12 Low tension open-angle glaucoma — *comparatively low rise in intraocular pressure*

365.13 Pigmentary open-angle glaucoma — *high intraocular pressure due to iris pigment granules breaking free and blocking aqueous flow*

365.14 Open-angle glaucoma of childhood — *infantile or juvenile glaucoma*

365.15 Residual stage of open angle glaucoma

Primary angle-closure glaucoma is an increase in intraocular pressure due to the iris occluding the anterior chamber structures and preventing the aqueous humor from reaching its usual outflow channel. Acute angle-closure glaucoma is a medical emergency and requires immediate, definitive treatment.

Signs and symptoms of primary angle-closure glaucoma include progressive loss of peripheral vision over a span of years, blurred or foggy vision, seeing colored halos around lights, severe eye pain and headache, corneal epithelial edema, and nausea and vomiting.

Diagnostic tests include exam (flashlight, slit lamp, or ophthalmoscope) to reveal corneal epithelial edema as a fine rough haziness in light and to allow visualization of the fundus and optic disk. Gonioscopy confirms angle closure and tonometry, using an applanation such as a Schiotz or pneumatic tonometer, measures intraocular pressure. Perimetry and visual field tests determine the extent of peripheral vision loss, and fundus photography records and monitors changes in the optic disk.

Therapies include systemic osmotics (glycerol, mannitol, and acetazolamide) to lower intraocular pressure, topical miotic drugs (Pilocarpine, Carcholin), carbonic anhydrase inhibitors (acetazolamide), argon laser iridotomy, and surgical peripheral iridectomy.

365.20 Unspecified primary angle-closure glaucoma — *interval or subacute angle-closure glaucoma*

365.21 Intermittent angle-closure glaucoma

365.22 Acute angle-closure glaucoma — *sudden, severe rise in intraocular pressure due to blockage in aqueous drainage*

365.23 Chronic angle-closure glaucoma — *persistent elevation of intraocular pressure due to continued blockage in aqueous drainage*
AHA: Q2, 1998, 16

365.24 Residual stage of angle-closure glaucoma

365.31 Corticosteroid-induced glaucoma, glaucomatous stage

365.32 Corticosteroid-induced glaucoma, residual stage

365.41 Glaucoma associated with chamber angle anomalies — (Code first associated disorder, 743.44)

365.42 Glaucoma associated with anomalies of iris — (Code first associated disorder: 364.51, 743.45)

365.43 Glaucoma associated with other anterior segment anomalies — (Code first associated disorder, 743.41)

365.44 Glaucoma associated with systemic syndromes — (Code first associated disease: 237.7, 759.6)

365.51 Phacolytic glaucoma — (Use additional code for associated hypermature cataract, 366.18)

365.52 Pseudoexfoliation glaucoma — (Use additional code for associated pseudoexfoliation of capsule, 366.11)

365.59 Glaucoma associated with other lens disorders — (Use additional code for associated disorder: 379.33, 379.34, 743.36)

365.60 Glaucoma associated with unspecified ocular disorder

365.61 Glaucoma associated with pupillary block — (Use additional code for associated disorder, 364.74)

365.62 Glaucoma associated with ocular inflammations — (Use additional code for associated disorder: 364.00-364.3, 364.22)

365.63 Glaucoma associated with vascular disorders of eye — (Use additional code for associated disorder: 362.35, 364.41)

365.64 Glaucoma associated with tumors or cysts — (Use additional code for associated disorder: 190.0-190.9, 224.0-224.9, 364.61)

365.65 Glaucoma associated with ocular trauma — (Use additional code for associated condition: 364.77, 921.3)

365.81 Hypersecretion glaucoma

365.82 Glaucoma with increased episcleral venous pressure

365.83 Aqueous misdirection — *malignant glaucoma*
AHA: Q4, 2002, 48

365.89 Other specified glaucoma

365.9 Unspecified glaucoma

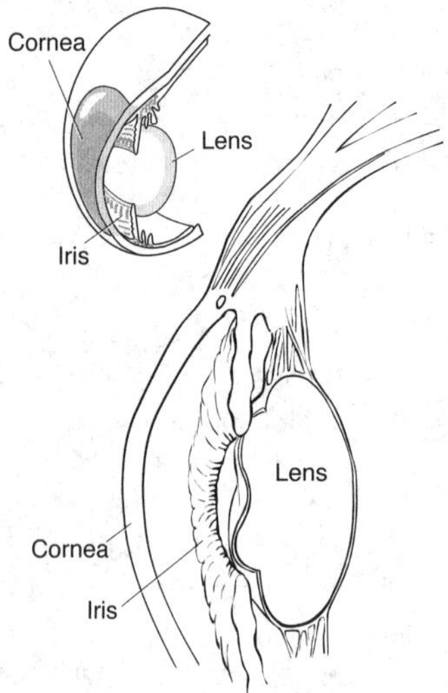

Sideview schematic of anterior chamber

366 Cataract

Cataract is the partial or total opacity of the crystalline lens or lens capsule. Cataracts form gradually and occur bilaterally usually in patients older than 70 years of age, with the exception of traumatic and congenital cataracts. Cataracts are classified by the zones of the lens involved in the opacity: anterior and posterior cortical, equatorial cortical, and supranuclear and nuclear. They are further subdivided into congenital, degenerative, traumatic, secondary, or complicated (due to ocular or systemic disease, radiation, or other external influences), toxic, and after-cataracts (meaning one remaining in the lens or capsule following cataract extraction).

The definition of infantile, juvenile, and presenile cataract is the partial or total opacity of the lens occurring in an infant, a young child, or a young adult. This type of cataract usually is the result of an injury or associated with conditions such as nutritional deficiencies (e.g., galactosemia), previous inflammation, or convulsions.

Signs and symptoms of infantile, juvenile, and presenile cataract include slowly progressing and painless loss of vision, leukocoria, behavioral problems indicative of vision problems, and strabismus.

Senile cataract is partial or total opacity of the lens due to degenerative changes in the lens in patients older than 55 years of age.

Signs and symptoms of senile cataract include slowly progressing and painless loss of vision, leukocoria, difficulty in night driving, altered color perception, and strabismus.

Diagnostic tests include tests of visual acuity to detect any loss of vision sharpness or clarity. An exam (flashlight, slit lamp, or ophthalmoscope) reveals opacity of the lens and pupil, shows the anterior portion of the eye, and detects nuclear cataracts. Refraction and retinoscopy detect nuclear myopia and lenticonus. A-scan and B-scan ultrasound measure thickness and location of the cataract.

Therapies include cataract extraction, intra- or extracapsular, phacoemulsification and aspiration, lensectomy and phacofragmentation, intraocular lens implantation, and cataract glasses postoperatively.

Associated conditions include galactosemia and galactokinase deficiency, hypoglycemia (neonatal), Lowe's syndrome (oculocerebrorenal syndrome), myotonic dystrophy, congenital ichthyosis, Rothmund-Thomson syndrome, rubella, Werner's syndrome, and Hallermann-Streiff-Francois syndrome.

366.00 Unspecified nonsenile cataract

366.01 Anterior subcapsular polar cataract, nonsenile

366.02 Posterior subcapsular polar cataract, nonsenile

366.03 Cortical, lamellar, or zonular cataract, nonsenile

366.04 Nuclear cataract, nonsenile

366.09 Other and combined forms of nonsenile cataract

366.10 Unspecified senile cataract

366.11 Pseudoexfoliation of lens capsule

366.12 Incipient cataract

366.13 Anterior subcapsular polar senile cataract

366.14 Posterior subcapsular polar senile cataract

366.15 Cortical senile cataract

366.16 Nuclear sclerosis

366.17 Total or mature senile cataract

© 2004 Ingenix, Inc.

366.18 Hypermature senile cataract

366.19 Other and combined forms of senile cataract

366.20 Unspecified traumatic cataract

366.21 Localized traumatic opacities of cataract

366.22 Total traumatic cataract

366.23 Partially resolved traumatic cataract

366.30 Unspecified cataracta complicata

366.31 Cataract secondary to glaucomatous flecks (subcapsular) — (Code first underlying glaucoma: 365.00-365.9)

366.32 Cataract in inflammatory ocular disorders — (Code first underlying condition: 363.00-363.22)

366.33 Cataract with ocular neovascularization — (Code first underlying condition, 364.10)

366.34 Cataract in degenerative ocular disorders — (Code first underlying condition: 360.21, 360.24, 362.74)

366.41 Diabetic cataract — (Code first diabetes, 250.5)

366.42 Tetanic cataract — (Code first underlying disease: 252.1, 275.4)

366.43 Myotonic cataract — (Code first underlying disorder, 359.2)

366.44 Cataract associated with other syndromes — (Code first underlying condition: 271.1, 756.0)

366.45 Toxic cataract — (Use additional E code to identify drug or other toxic substance)

366.46 Cataract associated with radiation and other physical influences — (Use additional E code to identify cause)

366.50 Unspecified after-cataract

366.51 Soemmering's ring

366.52 Other after-cataract, not obscuring vision

366.53 After-cataract, obscuring vision

366.8 Other cataract

366.9 Unspecified cataract

Documentation Issues

When the documentation states the patient is being seen for an eye examination for cataracts based on long-term use of a high risk medication, and the exam is normal, use codes V58.69 *Long-term (current) use of other medications* and the code for the condition for which the prescribed medication was being taken (e.g., rheumatoid arthritis).

When the documentation identifies a cataract in a diabetic patient, then clarification should be obtained from the physician as to the cause and effect relationship of the cataract and the diabetes. Senile cataracts are commonly seen in diabetics but are not always associated with the diabetes.

Coding Clarification

Diabetic Complication: True diabetic cataracts, or those known as "snowflake cataracts," are rare and are found in Type I diabetics. Use codes 250.51 *Diabetes with ophthalmic manifestations* and 366.41 *Diabetic cataract.* Senile cataracts, although commonly seen in diabetics, are not classified as such because they are not caused by the diabetes. Use codes 250.0x *Diabetes mellitus, without mention of complication* and 366.10 *Senile cataract, unspecified.*

Drug-Induced: Also known as "toxic" cataracts, drug-induced cataracts are noted in patients who have been taking prescribed medications (e.g., steroids) for conditions such as asthma and rheumatoid arthritis. Use code 366.45 *Toxic cataract,* along with a code to identify the condition for which the prescribed medication was being taken (e.g., asthma). In addition, code V58.69 *Long term (current) use of other medications,* should be used. An E-code may also be used to identify the specific drug or other toxic substance that caused the cataract.

Coding Scenario

A patient is seen for steroid-induced cataracts. The patient has a long-standing history of chronic obstructive asthma.

> Code assignment: 366.45 *Toxic cataract,* 493.20 *Chronic obstructive asthma,* and E932.0 *Adverse effect, therapeutic use, adrenal cortical steroids*

A patient who has completed a high-risk medication regimen for rheumatoid arthritis is given an eye exam. A cataract is noted on the eye exam.

> Code assignment: V67.51 *Follow-up examination following completed treatment with high-risk medications, not elsewhere classified,* 366.45 *Toxic cataract,* and 714.0 *Rheumatoid arthritis*

A patient is seen in the office for an eye examination that reveals a small snowflake cataract. This patient is a known insulin-dependent Type I diabetic. Verification with the physician confirms that this is a diabetic cataract.

> Code assignment: 250.51 *Diabetes with ophthalmic manifestations, Type I* and 366.41 *Diabetic cataract*

367 Disorders of refraction and accommodation

A refractive error occurs due to a disorder among the optical components of the eye (i.e., the curvatures, refractive indices, and distances between the cornea, aqueous, crystalline lens, and vitreous) and the overall axial length of the eye. There are four kinds of refractive types: normal eyesight, myopia (nearsightedness), hyperopia (farsightedness), and astigmatism.

In myopia, parallel light rays from an object are focused in front of the retina, with accommodation relaxed. The term nearsightedness comes from the manifestation, which is blurred distance vision. Correction includes concave spectacle or contact lenses or corneal modification to decrease refractive power. In some cases of pseudomyopia, unaided distance vision can be improved with vision therapy.

Myopia can increase the risk for more severe conditions such as retinal breaks or detachment and glaucoma.

In hyperopia, parallel rays of light entering the eye reach a focal point behind the plane of the retina, while accommodation is maintained in a state of relaxation. The additional dioptic power of the converging lenses required to advance the focusing of light rays onto the retina determines the degree of impairment. Corrective lenses may be spherical or spherocylindrical, depending on the nature of the hyperopia and the amount of astigmatic refractive error present.

Astigmatism is due to an elliptically shaped cornea, rather than the normal spherical shape. A point of light, going through an astigmatic cornea, has two points of focus, instead of one sharp image on the retina, resulting in blurred vision. The degree of impairment depends upon the amount and the direction of the astigmatism. A person with myopia or hyperopia may see a dot as a blurred circle, while a person with astigmatism may see the same dot as a blurred oval-shape.

Accommodation is the ability of both eyes to adjust to change in the printed word at various distances and to different print sizes. Tests to check accommodation include negative relative accommodation (NRA) and positive relative accommodation (PRA). In NRA, the patient looks through a phoropter and plus lenses are added binocularly as the patient fixates at 40 centimeters. The PRA is performed immediately after the NRA. In this test, minus lenses are added in front of the eyes until the patient reports a blurred image. The endpoint of both tests is reached when the lenses in front of the eyes provide the first sustained blur.

367.0 Hypermetropia — *far-sightedness; hyperopia*

367.1 Myopia — *near-sightedness*

367.20 Unspecified astigmatism — *light rays are refracted over a diffuse area, rather than over a focus on the retina*

367.21 Regular astigmatism — *refers to a state of mutual perpendicularity of the sharp (maximum curvatures) and flat (minimum curvatures) of the meridians of the lens and cornea*

367.22 Irregular astigmatism — *axes are irregular, not usually correctable with spherocylinder lens*

367.31 Anisometropia — *refractive errors differing by at least one diopter when eyes are compared*

367.32 Aniseikonia — *unequal retinal image sizes in eyes, usually caused by differing refractive errors*

367.4 Presbyopia — *loss of elasticity of the elderly lens causing errors of accommodation*

367.51 Paresis of accommodation — *cycloplegia*

367.52 Total or complete internal ophthalmoplegia — *large pupil incapable of focus due to total paralysis of ciliary muscle*

367.53 Spasm of accommodation — *focus dysfunction due to abnormal contraction of ciliary muscle*

367.81 Transient refractive change — *temporary change in refractive error*

367.89 Other disorders of refraction and accommodation — *drug-induced disorders of refraction and accommodation*

367.9 Unspecified disorder of refraction and accommodation

368 Visual disturbances

Amblyopia (368.0), also referred to by the public as "lazy eye," is a unilateral, rarely a bilateral, condition in which the best corrected visual acuity is less than normal (20/20) in the absence of any obvious structural anomalies or ocular disease. Functional amblyopia develops in children up to the age of 6 to 8 years, although it may persist for life once established.

Diplopia (368.2) may be the result of a refractive error, light splitting objects into two images by a defect in the eye's optical system, or it may result from failure of both eyes to point at the object being viewed, a condition referred to as ocular misalignment. If the eyes do not point at the same object, the image seen by each eye is different and cannot be fused. This results in double vision.

Color blindness (368.5) is a lack of perceptual sensitivity to certain colors. There are three types of color receptors in our eyes — red, green, and blue — in addition to black and white receptors. Color blindness is due to a lack of one or more color receptors. Red-green color blindness (368.51) is due to a lack of red receptors. Yellow-blue (368.53) is the second most common form. Lack of all three receptors results in black and white only vision (368.54).

Night blindness (368.6) is an eye disorder in which vision is abnormally impaired in dim light or at night due to a deficiency in rhodopsin (visual purple) in the rods, which is responsible for light sensitivity and the degree of dark adaptation. Night blindness most commonly occurs as a result of retinitis pigmentosa, a degenerative condition of the retina. Visual purple

 © 2004 Ingenix, Inc.

may also decrease if there is a dietary deficiency of its principal component vitamin A.

368.00 Unspecified amblyopia

368.01 Strabismic amblyopia — *suppression amblyopia*

368.02 Deprivation amblyopia — *decreased vision associated with suppression of retinal image of one eye*

368.03 Refractive amblyopia — *decreased vision in one eye associated with uncorrected refractive error*

368.10 Unspecified subjective visual disturbance

368.11 Sudden visual loss

368.12 Transient visual loss — *concentric fading; scintillating scotoma*

368.13 Visual discomfort — *asthenopia; eye strain*

368.14 Visual distortions of shape and size — *distortions of shape and size, including macropsia; micropsia*

368.15 Other visual distortions and entoptic phenomena — *photopsia; refractive diplopia; visual halos*

368.16 Psychophysical visual disturbances — *visual agnosia; visual hallucinations; disorientation syndrome; Riddoch's syndrome*

368.2 Diplopia — *double vision*

368.30 Unspecified binocular vision disorder

368.31 Suppression of binocular vision

368.32 Simultaneous visual perception without fusion

368.33 Fusion with defective stereopsis

368.34 Abnormal retinal correspondence

368.40 Unspecified visual field defect

368.41 Scotoma involving central area in visual field — *centrocecal scotoma; chiasmatic syndrome*

368.42 Scotoma of blind spot area in visual field — *enlarged angioscotoma; paracecal scotoma*

368.43 Sector or arcuate defects in visual field — *Bjerrum scotoma*

368.44 Other localized visual field defect — *scotoma NOS; nasal step visual field defect*

368.45 Generalized contraction or constriction in visual field

368.46 Homonymous bilateral field defects in visual field — *hemianopsia (altitudinal) (homonymous); quadrant anopia*

368.47 Heteronymous bilateral field defects in visual field — *binasal hemianopsia; bitemporal hemianopsia*

368.51 Protan defect in color vision — *protanomaly; protanopia*

368.52 Deutan defect in color vision — *deuteranomaly; deuteranopia*

368.53 Tritan defect in color vision — *tritanomaly; tritanopia*

368.54 Achromatopsia — *monochromatism (cone) (rod)*

368.55 Acquired color vision deficiencies

368.59 Other color vision deficiencies — *anomalous trichromatopsia (congenital)*

368.60 Unspecified night blindness

368.61 Congenital night blindness — *hereditary night blindness; Oguchi's disease*

368.62 Acquired night blindness

368.63 Abnormal dark adaptation curve — *abnormal threshold of cones or rods; delayed adaptation of cones or rods*

368.69 Other night blindness

368.8 Other specified visual disturbances

368.9 Unspecified visual disturbance

369 Blindness and low vision

Blindness typically refers to vision loss that is not correctable with eyeglasses or contact lenses, and some people who are considered blind may perceive slowly moving lights or colors. Low vision refers to moderately impaired vision. People with low vision may have a visual impairment that affects only central vision or peripheral vision. Visual acuity and visual field are the two measurements used to assess vision. Visual acuity is the ability to see details (normal vision is 20/20) and visual field refers to peripheral vision (normal visual field is 180 degrees in diameter). Cataract, trachoma, macular degeneration, and glaucoma account for more than 70 percent of all blindness and low vision. Cataracts are not a disease, but a condition affecting the eye. Cataracts usually start as a slight cloudiness that grows more opaque. Light that does reach the retina becomes increasingly blurred and distorted. If left untreated, cataracts can cause blindness. Trachoma is caused by the bacterium Chlamydia trachomatis. It begins in childhood and repeated infections into adulthood irritate and scar the inside of the eyelid and, eventually, the cornea. Scarring on the cornea leads to vision loss. Macular degeneration is a disturbance of the retina and the leading cause of legal blindness in people older than 55 years of age. Glaucoma is a group of conditions related by optic nerve damage, predominantly as a result of elevated intraocular pressure (IOP). The pressure on the optic nerve affects peripheral vision and with glaucoma, central vision is affected as the disease progresses.

Classification		Levels of Visual Impairment	Additional descriptors which may be encountered
"Legal"	WHO	Visual acuity and/or visual field limitation (whichever is worse)	
	(Near-) Normal Vision	Range of Normal Vision 20/10 20/13 20/16 20/20 20/25 2.0 1.6 1.25 1.0 0.8	
		Near-Normal Vision 20/30 20/40 20/50 20/60 0.7 0.6 0.5 0.4 0.3	
	Low Vision	Moderate Visual Impairment 20/70 20/80 20/100 20/125 20/160 0.25 0.20 0.16 0.12	Moderate low vision
Legal Blindness (U.S.A.) Both Eyes		Severe Visual Impairment 20/200 20/250 20/320 20/400 0.10 0.08 0.06 0.05 Visual field: 20 degrees or less	Severe low vision, "Legal" blindness
	Blindness (WHO) One or Both Eyes	Profound Visual Impairment 20/500 20/630 20/800 20/1000 0.04 0.03 0.025 0.02 Count fingers at: less than 3m (10 ft.) Visual field: 10 degrees or less	Profound low vision, Moderate blindness
		Near-Total Visual Impairment Visual acuity: less than 0.02 (20/1000) Count fingers at: 1m (3 ft.) or less Hand movements: 5m (15 ft.) or less Light projection, light perception Visual field: 5 degrees or less	Severe blindness, Near-total blindness
		Total Visual Impairment No light perception (NLP)	Total blindness

Visual acuity refers to best achievable acuity with correction.
Non-listed Snellen fractions may be classified by converting to the nearest decimal equivalent, e.g., 10/200 = 0.05, 6/30 = 0.20.
CF (count fingers) without designation of distance, may be classified to profound impairment.
HM (hand motion) without designation of distance, may be classified to near-total impairment.
Visual field measurements refer to the largest field diameter for a 1/100 white test object.

369.00 Blindness of both eyes, impairment level not further specified — *blindness, both eyes*

369.01 Better eye: total vision impairment; lesser eye: total vision impairment

369.02 Better eye: near-total vision impairment; lesser eye: not further specified

369.03 Better eye: near-total vision impairment; lesser eye: total vision impairment

369.04 Better eye: near-total vision impairment; lesser eye: near-total vision impairment

369.05 Better eye: profound vision impairment; lesser eye: not further specified

369.06 Better eye: profound vision impairment; lesser eye: total vision impairment

369.07 Better eye: profound vision impairment; lesser eye: near-total vision impairment

369.08 Better eye: profound vision impairment; lesser eye: profound vision impairment

369.08 Better eye: profound vision impairment; lesser eye: profound vision impairment

369.10 Profound, moderate or severe vision impairment, not further specified — *blindness, one eye, low vision other eye*

369.11 Better eye: severe vision impairment; lesser eye: blind, not further specified

369.12 Better eye: severe vision impairment; lesser eye: total vision impairment

369.13 Better eye: severe vision impairment; lesser eye: near-total vision impairment

369.14 Better eye: severe vision impairment; lesser eye: profound vision impairment

369.15 Better eye: moderate vision impairment; lesser eye: blind, not further specified

369.16 Better eye: moderate vision impairment; lesser eye: total vision impairment

369.17 Better eye: moderate vision impairment; lesser eye: near-total vision impairment

369.18 Better eye: moderate vision impairment; lesser eye: profound vision impairment

369.20 Vision impairment, both eyes, impairment level not further specified

369.21 Better eye: severe vision impairment; lesser eye; impairment not further specified

369.22 Better eye: severe vision impairment; lesser eye: severe vision impairment

369.23 Better eye: moderate vision impairment; lesser eye: impairment not further specified

369.24 Better eye: moderate vision impairment; lesser eye: severe vision impairment

369.25 Better eye: moderate vision impairment; lesser eye: moderate vision impairment

369.3 Unqualified visual loss, both eyes

369.4 Legal blindness, as defined in USA — *blindness according to U.S.A. definition*

369.60 Impairment level not further specified — *including blindness one eye*

369.61 One eye: total vision impairment; other eye: not specified

369.62 One eye: total vision impairment; other eye: near-normal vision

369.63 One eye: total vision impairment; other eye: normal vision

 © 2004 Ingenix, Inc.

369.64 One eye: near-total vision impairment; other eye: vision not specified

369.65 One eye: near-total vision impairment; other eye: near-normal vision

369.66 One eye: near-total vision impairment; other eye: normal vision

369.67 One eye: profound vision impairment; other eye: vision not specified

369.69 One eye: profound vision impairment; other eye: normal vision

369.70 Low vision, one eye, not otherwise specified

369.71 One eye: severe vision impairment; other eye: vision not specified

369.72 One eye: severe vision impairment; other eye: near-normal vision

369.73 One eye: severe vision impairment; other eye: normal vision

369.74 One eye: moderate vision impairment; other eye: vision not specified

369.75 One eye: moderate vision impairment; other eye: near-normal vision

369.76 One eye: moderate vision impairment; other eye: normal vision

369.8 Unqualified visual loss, one eye

369.9 Unspecified visual loss

370 Keratitis

Keratitis is inflammation of the cornea, the transparent membrane at the front of the eye, with or without associated conjunctivitis (keratoconjunctivitis). Keratitis usually is due to Type 1 herpes simplex virus (dendritic keratitis, code 054.42), but may be due to bacteria, fungus, amoeba, radiation, trauma, or another source of inflammatory reaction.

Signs and symptoms of keratitis include impaired vision (early) or blindness (late), opacity of the cornea, irritation and tearing, and photophobia.

Diagnostic tests include exam (flashlight, slit lamp) to reveal exudate and hypopyon, which are typical of corneal ulcer, and to confirm keratitis. Instillation of fluorescein dye outlines corneal ulcers. Culture and sensitivity of corneal exudate or hypopyon identify the causative organism. For corneal ulcer, superficial keratectomy may provide culture material.

Therapies include antimicrobials for infection, eye lubricants, plastic bubble eye shield or eye patch, and replacement of cornea from a cadaver (keratoplasty) for corneal scarring.

370.00 Unspecified corneal ulcer

370.01 Marginal corneal ulcer — *tissue loss and inflammation in the margins of the cornea*

370.02 Ring corneal ulcer — *continuous, peripheral tissue loss ringing the cornea*

370.03 Central corneal ulcer — *corneal tissue loss in the center of the cornea*

370.04 Hypopyon ulcer — *serpiginous ulcer*

370.05 Mycotic corneal ulcer — *fungal infection causing corneal tissue loss*

370.06 Perforated corneal ulcer — *tissue loss through all layers of the cornea*

370.07 Mooren's ulcer — *painful chronic inflammation and tissue loss at the junction of the cornea and sclera; seen in elderly*

370.20 Unspecified superficial keratitis

370.21 Punctate keratitis — *Thygeson's superficial punctate keratitis*

370.22 Macular keratitis — *nummular or areolar keratitis*

370.23 Filamentary keratitis — *painful and inflamed cornea due to flaking of corneal cells*

370.24 Photokeratitis — *snow blindness; welders' keratitis*
AHA: Q3, 1996, 6

370.31 Phlyctenular keratoconjunctivitis — (Use additional code for any associated tuberculosis, 017.3)

370.32 Limbar and corneal involvement in vernal conjunctivitis — (Use additional code for vernal conjunctivitis, 372.13)

370.33 Keratoconjunctivitis sicca, not specified as Sjögren's — *inadequate tear production causing dry, burning eye*

370.34 Exposure keratoconjunctivitis — *incomplete closure of eyelid causing dry, inflamed eye*
AHA: Q3, 1996, 6

370.35 Neurotrophic keratoconjunctivitis — *corneal and conjunctival inflammation, insensitivity, and nerve damage following injury*

370.40 Unspecified keratoconjunctivitis — *superficial keratitis with conjunctivitis*

370.44 Keratitis or keratoconjunctivitis in exanthema — (Code first underlying condition: 050.0-052.9) — *corneal inflammation accompanying infection and rash*

370.49 Other unspecified keratoconjunctivitis

370.50 Unspecified interstitial keratitis

370.52 Diffuse interstitial keratitis — *Cogan's syndrome*

370.54 Sclerosing keratitis — *chronic corneal inflammation leading to opaque scarring*

370.55 Corneal abscess — *pocket of pus and inflammation on the cornea*

370.59 Other interstitial and deep keratitis — *other interstitial and deep keratitis*

370.60 Unspecified corneal neovascularization

370.61 Localized vascularization of cornea — *limited infiltration of the cornea by new blood vessels*

370.62 Pannus (corneal) — *shallow infiltration of the cornea by new blood vessels*
AHA: Q3, 2002, 20

370.63 Deep vascularization of cornea — *deep infiltration of the cornea by new blood vessels*

370.64 Ghost vessels (corneal) in corneal neovascularization — *transparent, empty blood vessels remaining in cornea after the inflammation that created them has resolved*

370.8 Other forms of keratitis

370.9 Unspecified keratitis

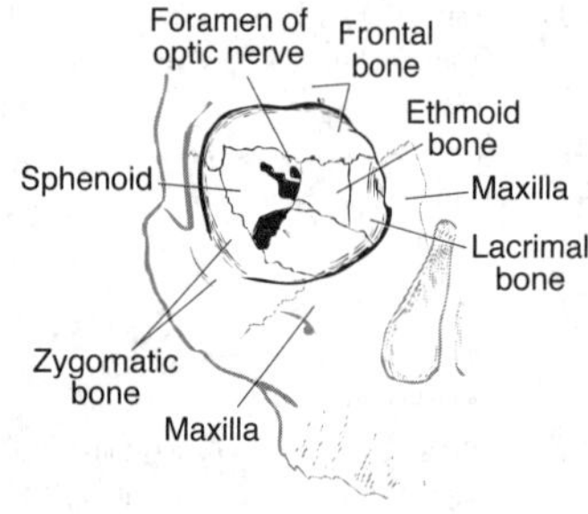

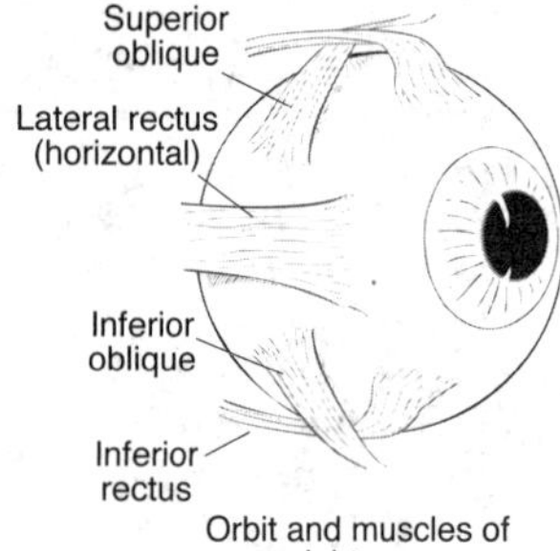

Orbit and muscles of right eye

371 Corneal opacity and other disorders of cornea

The cornea is the transparent tissue that covers the front of the eye. It has three layers:

1. The epithelium blocks the passage of foreign material and provides a smooth surface that absorbs oxygen and other needed cell nutrients that are contained in tears.
2. The stroma gives the cornea its strength and elasticity, and the protein fibers of the stroma produce the cornea's light-conducting transparency.
3. The endothelium pumps excess water out of the stroma.

Unlike most tissues in the body, the cornea contains no blood vessels to protect it against infection. The cornea serves as a physical barrier that shields the inside of the eye from germs, dust, and other foreign objects. It also acts as the eye's outermost lens. When light strikes the cornea, it refracts the incoming light onto the crystalline lens. The lens focuses the light onto the retina. Although much thinner than the lens, the cornea provides about 65 percent of the eye's power to bend light. Most of this power resides in the center of the cornea, which is rounder and thinner than the outer part of the tissue and is better suited to bend light waves.

371.00 Unspecified corneal opacity — *corneal sear*

371.01 Minor opacity of cornea — *corneal nebula*

371.02 Peripheral opacity of cornea — *corneal macula not interfering with central vision*

371.03 Central opacity of cornea — *corneal leucoma or macula interfering with central vision*

371.04 Adherent leucoma — *dense, opaque corneal growth adhering to the iris*

371.05 Phthisical cornea — (Code first underlying tuberculosis, 017.3)

371.10 Unspecified corneal deposit

371.11 Anterior pigmentations of cornea — *Stähli's lines*

371.12 Stromal pigmentations of cornea — *hematocornea*

371.13 Posterior pigmentations of cornea — *Krukenberg spindle*

371.14 Kayser-Fleischer ring — *copper deposits forming ring at outer edge of cornea*

371.15 Other deposits of cornea associated with metabolic disorders

371.16 Argentous deposits of cornea — *silver deposits in cornea*

371.20 Unspecified corneal edema

371.21 Idiopathic corneal edema — *corneal swelling and fluid retention of unknown cause*

371.22 Secondary corneal edema — *corneal swelling and fluid retention caused by underlying disease, injury or condition*

371.23 Bullous keratopathy — *small blisters formed on swollen corneal epithelium*

371.24 Corneal edema due to wearing of contact lenses

371.30 Unspecified corneal membrane change

371.31 Folds and rupture of Bowman's membrane — *folds and rupture in the second outermost layer of the cornea*

371.32 Folds in Descemet's membrane — *folds in the second innermost layer of the cornea*

© 2004 Ingenix, Inc.

371.33 Rupture in Descemet's membrane — *rupture in the second innermost layer of the cornea*

371.40 Unspecified corneal degeneration

371.41 Senile corneal changes — *arcus senilis; Hassall-Henle bodies*

371.42 Recurrent erosion of cornea

371.43 Band-shaped keratopathy — *horizontal bands of superficial corneal calcium deposits*

371.44 Other calcerous degenerations of cornea

371.45 Keratomalacia NOS — *corneal softening with the development of opacities*

371.46 Nodular degeneration of cornea — *Salzmann's nodular dystrophy*

371.48 Peripheral degenerations of cornea — *marginal degeneration of cornea (Terrien's)*

371.49 Other corneal degenerations — *discrete colliquative keratopathy*

371.50 Unspecified hereditary corneal dystrophy — *unspecified corneal dystrophy*

371.51 Juvenile epithelial corneal dystrophy

371.52 Other anterior corneal dystrophies — *microscopic, cystic corneal dystrophy*

371.53 Granular corneal dystrophy

371.54 Lattice corneal dystrophy

371.55 Macular corneal dystrophy

371.56 Other stromal corneal dystrophies — *crystalline corneal dystrophy*

371.57 Endothelial corneal dystrophy — *combined corneal dystrophy; cornea guttata; Fuchs' endothelial dystrophy*

371.58 Other posterior corneal dystrophies — *polymorphous corneal dystrophy*

371.60 Unspecified keratoconus

371.61 Keratoconus, stable condition

371.62 Keratoconus, acute hydrops

371.70 Unspecified corneal deformity

371.71 Corneal ectasia — *bulging protrusion of a thinned, scarred cornea*

371.72 Descemetocele — *protrusion of Descemet's membrane into the cornea*

371.73 Corneal staphyloma — *protrusion of the cornea into surrounding tissue*

371.81 Corneal anesthesia and hypoesthesia — *decreased or absent sensitivity of the cornea*

371.82 Corneal disorder due to contact lens

Coding Clarification

Corneal disorders can arise due to contact lens use. Complications associated with contact lens use include, but are not limited to, foreign body sensation and irritation, infectious and noninfectious infiltrates, anterior chamber reaction, peripheral vascularization, corneal distortion, corneal perforations, and giant papillary conjunctivitis.

371.89 Other corneal disorder — *hypertrophic cornea*
AHA: Q3, 1999, 12

371.9 Unspecified corneal disorder

372 Disorders of conjunctiva

Acute conjunctivitis is an inflammation of the mucous membrane covering the anterior surface of the eyeball and the lining of the eyelids. Acute conjunctivitis usually is due to bacteria such as *Staphylococcus aureus, Staphylococcus epidermidis, Streptococcus pneumoniae, Streptococcus pyogenes, Moraxella lacunata,* and *Neisseria gonorrhoeae* (098.40). Acute conjunctivitis also may be due to viruses and chlamydiae (rubric 077), and to allergies (atopic).

Signs and symptoms of acute conjunctivitis include hyperemia of conjunctiva, pain and itching, tearing, sticky mucopurulent discharge, injection of bulbar conjunctival vessels, and history of contact lens wear.

Diagnostic tests include culture and sensitivity of discharge to identify the infective organism. Stain may show predominant eosinophils if allergy related, neutrophils if bacterial, and monocytes if caused by a virus (category 077).

Therapies include topical antibiotics for bacterial conjunctivitis, corticosteroid drops, antihistamines and cold compresses for allergic conjunctivitis, and eye lubricants.

372.00 Unspecified acute conjunctivitis — *unspecified acute conjunctivitis*

372.01 Serous conjunctivitis, except viral — *severe conjunctival inflammation with watery discharge*

372.02 Acute follicular conjunctivitis — *conjunctival folliculitis NOS; Parinaud's oculoglandular syndrome*

372.03 Other mucopurulent conjunctivitis — *catarrhal conjunctivitis*

372.04 Pseudomembranous conjunctivitis — *membranous conjunctivitis*

372.05 Acute atopic conjunctivitis — *sudden severe conjunctivitis due to allergies*

Chronic conjunctivitis is chronic inflammation of the conjunctiva characterized by acute exacerbations and remissions occurring over months or years. Degenerative changes or damage may occur from repeated acute attacks. The clinical presentation is similar in most respects to acute conjunctivitis except that it is more innocuous at the onset and runs a more protracted course.

372.10 Unspecified chronic conjunctivitis

372.11 Simple chronic conjunctivitis — *persistent conjunctival inflammation*

372.12 Chronic follicular conjunctivitis — *persistent conjunctival inflammation with dense, localized infiltrations of lymphoid tissues of inner eyelids*

372.13 Vernal conjunctivitis — *persistent seasonal conjunctival inflammation in childhood*
AHA: Q3, 1996, 8

372.14 Other chronic allergic conjunctivitis

372.15 Parasitic conjunctivitis — (Code first underlying disease: 085.5, 125.0-125.9)

372.20 Unspecified blepharoconjunctivitis

372.21 Angular blepharoconjunctivitis — *inflammation at the junction where the upper and lower eyelids meet; usually blocks lacrimal secretions*

372.22 Contact blepharoconjunctivitis — *inflammation of the eyelid margin and conjunctiva due to an allergic reaction*

372.30 Unspecified conjunctivitis

372.31 Rosacea conjunctivitis — (Code first underlying rosacea dermatitis, 695.3)

372.33 Conjunctivitis in mucocutaneous disease — (Code first underlying disease: 099.3, 695.1)

372.39 Other and unspecified conjunctivitis

372.40 Unspecified pterygium

372.41 Peripheral ptergium, stationary

372.42 Peripheral pterygium, progressive

372.43 Central pterygium

372.44 Double pterygium

372.45 Recurrent pterygium

372.50 Unspecified conjunctival degeneration

372.51 Pinguecula — *benign subconjunctival elevation on either side of the cornea*

372.52 Pseudopterygium

372.53 Conjunctival xerosis — *conjunctival dryness due to insufficient secretions*

372.54 Conjunctival concretions — *hard masses in the conjunctiva*

372.55 Conjunctival pigmentations — *conjunctival argyrosis*

372.56 Conjunctival deposits

372.61 Granuloma of conjunctiva — *abnormal dense collection of cells in the conjunctiva*

372.62 Localized adhesions and strands of conjunctiva — *abnormal fibrous connections in conjunctiva*

372.63 Symblepharon — *extensive adhesions of conjunctiva*

372.64 Scarring of conjunctiva — *contraction of eye socket (after enucleation)*

372.71 Hyperemia of conjunctiva — *conjunctival blood vessel congestion causing eye redness*

372.72 Conjunctival hemorrhage — *hyposphagma; subconjunctival hemorrhage*

372.73 Conjunctival edema — *subconjunctival edema*

372.74 Vascular abnormalities of conjunctiva — *aneurysm (ata) of conjunctiva*

372.75 Conjunctival cysts — *abnormal thin-walled sacs of fluid in the conjunctiva*

372.81 Conjunctivochalasis

372.89 Other disorders of conjunctiva

372.9 Unspecified disorder of conjunctiva

373 Inflammation of eyelids

The patient presenting with a chalazion differs from the patient presenting with a hordeolum (stye) in that the chalazion is usually painless after a few days, while discomfort from a hordeolum usually escalates. A chalazion will usually resolve within a few months and can be treated with hot compresses to hasten resolution. Intrachalazion administration of corticosteroid is another method of treatment.

373.00 Blepharitis, unspecified

373.01 Ulcerative blepharitis — *inflammation of the eyelid with erosion of tissue*

373.02 Squamous blepharitis — *inflammation of eyelid margin with scaling of tissue*

373.11 Hordeolum externum — *hordeolum NOS; stye*

373.12 Hordeolum internum — *infection of meibomian gland; stye*

373.13 Abscess of eyelid — *furuncle of eyelid*

373.2 Chalazion — *meibomian (gland) cyst*

373.31 Eczematous dermatitis of eyelid — *itchy inflammation of eyelid*

373.32 Contact and allergic dermatitis of eyelid — *inflammation of the eyelid due to allergic reaction*

373.33 Xeroderma of eyelid — *rough, dry, and scaly skin of the eyelid*

373.34 Discoid lupus erythematosus of eyelid — *swollen eyelids from discoid lupus erythematosus*

373.4 Infective dermatitis of eyelid of types resulting in deformity — (Code first underlying disease: 017.0, 030.0-030.9, 102.0-102.9)

373.5 Other infective dermatitis of eyelid — (Code first underlying disease: 039.3, 051.0, 110.0-111.9, 684, 999.0)

373.6 Parasitic infestation of eyelid — (Code first underlying disease: 085.0-085.9, 125.2, 125.3, 132.0)

© 2004 Ingenix, Inc.

373.8 Other inflammations of eyelids — *inflammations of eyelids NEC*

373.9 Unspecified inflammation of eyelid

374 Other disorders of eyelids

374.00 Unspecified entropion — *entropion NOS*

374.01 Senile entropion — *eyelid margin curves inward in an elderly eye*

374.02 Mechanical entropion — *eyelid margin curves inward due to external forces*

374.03 Spastic entropion — *eyelid margin curves inward intermittently and involuntarily*

374.04 Cicatricial entropion — *eyelid margin curves inward due to scarring*

374.05 Trichiasis of eyelid without entropion — *eyelashes curve inward, without eyelid margin defect*

374.10 Unspecified ectropion — *ectropion NOS*

374.11 Senile ectropion — *lower eyelid droops away from the elderly eye*

374.12 Mechanical ectropion — *lower eyelid droops away from eye due to external forces*

374.13 Spastic ectropion — *lower eyelid droops away from eye intermittently and involuntarily*

374.14 Cicatricial ectropion — *cicatricial*

374.20 Unspecified lagophthalmos — *lagophthalmos NOS*

374.21 Paralytic lagophthalmos — *full closure of eyelid prevented by nerve defect*

374.22 Mechanical lagophthalmos — *outside force prevents full closure of eyelids*

374.23 Cicatricial lagophthalmos — *scar tissue prevents full closure of eyelids*

374.30 Unspecified ptosis of eyelid

374.31 Paralytic ptosis — *drooping of upper eyelid due to nerve defect*

374.32 Myogenic ptosis — *drooping of upper eyelid due to muscular defect*

374.33 Mechanical ptosis — *outside force causes drooping of upper eyelid*

374.34 Blepharochalasis — *drooping or relaxation of upper eyelid due to atrophy of intercellular tissue*

374.41 Eyelid retraction or lag

374.43 Abnormal innervation syndrome of eyelid — *jaw-blinking; paradoxical facial movements*

374.44 Sensory disorders of eyelid

374.45 Other sensorimotor disorders of eyelid — *deficient blink reflex*

374.46 Blepharophimosis — *ankyloblepharon*

374.50 Unspecified degenerative disorder of eyelid

374.51 Xanthelasma of eyelid — (Code first underlying condition: 272.0-272.9)

374.52 Hyperpigmentation of eyelid — *chloasma; dyspigmentation*

374.53 Hypopigmentation of eyelid — *vitiligo of eyelid*

374.54 Hypertrichosis of eyelid — *excessive eyelash growth*

374.55 Hypotrichosis of eyelid — *less than normal amount, or absence of, eyelashes; madarosis of eyelid*

374.56 Other degenerative disorders of skin affecting eyelid — *other degenerative skin disorders affecting eyelid NEC*

374.81 Hemorrhage of eyelid — *bleeding eyelid*

374.82 Edema of eyelid — *hyperemia of eyelid*

374.83 Elephantiasis of eyelid — *filarial disease causing dermatitis and enlargement of eyelid*

374.84 Cysts of eyelids — *sebaceous cyst of eyelid*

374.85 Vascular anomalies of eyelid

374.86 Retained foreign body of eyelid

374.87 Dermatochalasis — *loss of elasticity causing skin under eye to sag*

374.89 Other disorders of eyelid — *blepharoplegia; granuloma of eyelid*

374.9 Unspecified disorder of eyelid

375 Disorders of lacrimal system

The lacrimal system produces and distributes the tears that lubricate and clean the eye and keep nasal tissues moist. Excluded from this rubric are congenital disorders of the lacrimal system.

375.00 Unspecified dacryoadenitis

375.01 Acute dacryoadenitis — *severe, sudden inflammation of the lacrimal gland*

375.02 Chronic dacryoadenitis — *persistent inflammation of the lacrimal gland*

375.03 Chronic enlargement of lacrimal gland

375.11 Dacryops — *overproduction and constant flow of tears*

375.12 Other lacrimal cysts and cystic degeneration

375.13 Primary lacrimal atrophy — *wasting away of the lacrimal gland*

375.14 Secondary lacrimal atrophy — *wasting away of the lacrimal gland due to other disease process*

375.15 Unspecified tear film insufficiency — *dry eye syndrome*
AHA: Q3, 1996, 6

375.16 Dislocation of lacrimal gland

375.20 Epiphora, unspecified as to cause

375.21 Epiphora due to excess lacrimation — *overflow of tears due to overproduction*

375.22 Epiphora due to insufficient drainage — *overflow of tears due to blocked drainage*

375.30 Unspecified dacryocystitis

375.31 Acute canaliculitis, lacrimal — *sudden, severe inflammation of the tear drainage system*

375.32 Acute dacryocystitis — *acute peridacryocystitis*

375.33 Phlegmonous dacryocystitis — *infection of the tear sac with pockets of pus*

375.41 Chronic canaliculitis — *persistent inflammation of the tear drainage system*

375.42 Chronic dacryocystitis — *persistent inflammation of the tear sac*

375.43 Lacrimal mucocele — *enlarged pocket of mucus in lacrimal system*

375.51 Eversion of lacrimal punctum — *abnormal turning outward of the tear duct*

375.52 Stenosis of lacrimal punctum — *abnormal narrowing of tear duct*

375.53 Stenosis of lacrimal canaliculi — *abnormal narrowing of the tear drainage system*

375.54 Stenosis of lacrimal sac — *abnormal narrowing of tear sac*

375.55 Obstruction of nasolacrimal duct, neonatal — *acquired narrowing of the tear drainage system from the eye to the nose*

375.56 Stenosis of nasolacrimal duct, acquired

375.57 Dacryolith — *concretion of stone anywhere in lacrimal system*

375.61 Lacrimal fistula — *abnormal communication from the lacrimal system*

375.69 Other change of lacrimal passages — *changes of lacrimal passage NOS*

375.81 Granuloma of lacrimal passages — *abnormal nodules within the tear drainage system*

375.89 Other disorder of lacrimal system — *disorders of lacrimal system NOS*

375.9 Unspecified disorder of lacrimal system

376 Disorders of the orbit

This rubric identifies disorders of the orbit, which is the bony housing for the eyeball that expands for the first two years of life as the eye grows. Between the bony housing and the eyeball are other structures such as fat, muscle, blood vessels, and glands. The orbital fat cushioning each globe is divided into central and peripheral compartments. The central space contains the optic, oculomotor, abducent, and nasociliary nerves. The peripheral space contains the trochlear, lacrimal, frontal, and infraorbital nerves.

Codes in subclassification 376.0 are selected by site. In orbital cellulitis, the infection is between the orbital bone and the eyeball. In orbital periostitis, the infection is in the connective tissue covering the orbital bone. In orbital osteomyelitis, the bone is infected; and in tenonitis, the infection is in the Tenon's capsule, the thin membrane that envelops the eyeball.

376.00 Unspecified acute inflammation of orbit — *acute orbital inflammation NOS*

376.01 Orbital cellulitis — *abscess of orbit*

376.02 Orbital periostitis — *inflammation of connective tissue covering the orbital bone*

376.03 Orbital osteomyelitis — *inflammation of the orbital bone*

376.04 Orbital tenonitis — *inflammation of Tenon's capsule, the thin membrane that envelops the eyeball*

376.10 Unspecified chronic inflammation of orbit — *chronic orbital inflammation NOS*

376.11 Orbital granuloma — *pseudotumor (inflammatory) of orbit*

376.12 Orbital myositis — *painful inflammation of the muscles of the eye*

376.13 Parasitic infestation of orbit — (Code first underlying disease: 122.3, 122.6, 122.9, 134.0)

376.21 Thyrotoxic exophthalmos — *bulging eyes as a result of hyperthyroidism*

376.22 Exophthalmic ophthalmoplegia — *inability to rotate eyes as a result of bulging eyes*

376.30 Unspecified exophthalmos

376.31 Constant exophthalmos — *continuous, abnormal protrusion or bulging of eyeball*

376.32 Orbital hemorrhage — *bleeding behind the eyeball, causing it to bulge forward*

376.33 Orbital edema or congestion — *fluid retention behind eyeball, causing it to bulge forward*

376.34 Intermittent exophthalmos — *separate incidences of abnormal bulging of the eyeball*

376.35 Pulsating exophthalmos — *throbbing bulge or protrusion of the eyeball, usually associated with a carotid-cavernous fistula*

376.36 Lateral displacement of globe of eye — *abnormal displacement of the eyeball away from the nose, toward the temple*

376.40 Unspecified deformity of orbit

376.41 Hypertelorism of orbit — *congenital anomaly in which the eyes are widely placed*

376.42 Exostosis of orbit — *abnormal bony growth of orbit*

 © 2004 Ingenix, Inc.

376.43 Local deformities of orbit due to bone disease — *acquired abnormalities of the orbit due to bone disease*

376.44 Orbital deformities associated with craniofacial deformities — *congenital malformation of the orbital bone*

376.45 Atrophy of orbit — *wasting away of bone tissue of orbit*

376.46 Enlargement of orbit

376.47 Deformity of orbit due to trauma or surgery

376.50 Enophthalmos, unspecified as to cause — *recession of eyeball deep into eye socket*

376.51 Enophthalmos due to atrophy of orbital tissue — *recession of eyeball deep into eye socket due to atrophy of orbital tissue*

376.52 Enophthalmos due to trauma or surgery

376.6 Retained (old) foreign body following penetrating wound of orbit — *retrobulbar foreign body*

376.81 Orbital cysts — *encephalocele of orbit; mucocele of orbit*
AHA: Q3, 1999, 13

376.82 Myopathy of extraocular muscles — *disease in one or more of the six muscles that control eyeball movement*

376.89 Other orbital disorder — *emphysema of eye; retrobulbar hemorrhage*

376.9 Unspecified disorder of orbit

Coding Clarification

A second code from Infectious and Parasitic Diseases (001-139) can be reported to identify the infective agent.

Orbital cellulitis (376.01) is the inflammation of the orbital tissues caused by infection that extends from the nasal sinuses or teeth, by metastatic spread from infections elsewhere, or by bacteria introduced via orbital trauma. Exophthalmos (376.30, 376.31) describes the protrusion of one eyeball or both that results from orbital inflammation, edema, tumors, injuries, cavernous sinus thrombosis, or enlargement of the eyeball (as in congenital glaucoma and unilateral high myopia). When an infection or tumor develops, the tissues swell, causing the eye to protrude. Aggressive therapy, including surgical intervention, may be necessary to save the eye and retain functional sight. Hypertelorism (376.41) describes increased space between the eyes and is often associated with other skeletal abnormalities such as an encephalocele or syndromes such as Apert syndrome. Craniofacial surgery is often required for orbital deformities associated with craniofacial deformity (376.44). In congenital or trauma-induced enophthalmos (376.50, 376.51, 376.52), the eyeballs are displaced far back into the orbit.

When an underlying disease causes the orbital disorder, sequence the underlying disease code first and a code from this rubric secondarily.

377 Disorders of optic nerve and visual pathways

The optic nerve is the extent of the visual system pathway from the back of the eyeball up to the optic chiasm. It contains axons of ganglion cells in the retina of the ipsilateral (i.e., same side) eye. Each optic nerve splits and half of its fibers cross over to the other side at the optic chiasm. If the optic nerve is damaged between an eyeball and the optic chiasm, the person may become blind in that eye. If the problem lies farther back in the optic nerve pathway, both eyes may lose half of the visual fields, a condition called hemianopia. If both eyes lose peripheral vision, the cause may be damage at the optic chiasm. If both eyes lose half of the visual field on the same side, the cause is usually damage to the optic nerve pathway on the opposite side of the brain caused by a stroke, hemorrhage, or tumor. Dysfunction of the optic nerve may be congenital or acquired. If congenital, it is usually hereditary. The acquired type may be due to vascular disturbances, secondary to degenerative retinal disease (e.g., papilledema or optic neuritis), a result of pressure against the optic nerve, or related to metabolic diseases (e.g., diabetes), trauma, glaucoma, or toxicity (to alcohol, tobacco, or other poisons).

377.00 Unspecified papilledema

377.01 Papilledema associated with increased intracranial pressure — *pressure within the brain causes swelling and engorgement of the optic disc and its blood vessels*

377.02 Papilledema associated with decreased ocular pressure — *reduced pressure within the eyeball causes swelling and engorgement of the optic disc and its blood vessels*

377.03 Papilledema associated with retinal disorder — *retinal disease or dysfunction causes swelling and engorgement of optic disc and its blood vessels*

377.04 Foster-Kennedy syndrome — *basofrontal syndrome*

377.10 Unspecified optic atrophy

377.11 Primary optic atrophy — *disc is grayish white with sharp edges*

377.12 Postinflammatory optic atrophy — *eye wastes away due to inflammation*

377.13 Optic atrophy associated with retinal dystrophies — *wasting away of eye due to progressive changes in retinal tissue due to metabolic defects*

377.14 Glaucomatous atrophy (cupping) of optic disc — *wasting away of eye as a result of high intraocular pressure*

377.15 Partial optic atrophy — *temporal pallor of optical disc*

377.16 Hereditary optic atrophy — *Leber's optic atrophy*

377.21 Drusen of optic disc — *glistening white nodules within optic nerve head*

377.22 Crater-like holes of optic disc — *crater-like holes*

377.23 Coloboma of optic disc — *congenital cleft, or defect in continuity of the optic disc*

377.24 Pseudopapilledema — *optic nerve head deformity resembling a choked optic disc*

377.30 Unspecified optic neuritis

377.31 Optic papillitis — *swelling and inflammation of the optic disc*

377.32 Retrobulbar neuritis (acute) — *inflammation of optic nerve in the orbit behind the eye*

377.33 Nutritional optic neuropathy — *optic nerve disorder caused by malnutrition*

377.34 Toxic optic neuropathy — *toxic amblyopia*

377.39 Other optic neuritis — *optic neuritis NEC*

377.41 Ischemic optic neuropathy — *optic nerve disorder due to decreased blood flow*

377.42 Hemorrhage in optic nerve sheaths — *bleeding in optic nerve sheaths*

377.49 Other disorder of optic nerve — *compression of optic nerve*

377.51 Disorders of optic chiasm associated with pituitary neoplasms and disorders — *disruption in nerve chain from retina to brain, caused by abnormal pituitary growth*

377.52 Disorders of optic chiasm associated with other neoplasms — *disruption in nerve chain from retina to brain, caused by abnormal growth, other than pituitary*

377.53 Disorders of optic chiasm associated with vascular disorders — *disruption in nerve chain from retina to brain, caused by a vascular disorder*

377.54 Disorders of optic chiasm associated with inflammatory disorders — *disruption in nerve chain from retina to brain, caused by inflammatory disease*

377.61 Disorders of other visual pathways associated with neoplasms

377.62 Disorders of other visual pathways associated with vascular disorders

377.63 Disorders of other visual pathways associated with inflammatory disorders

377.71 Disorders of visual cortex associated with neoplasms

377.72 Disorders of visual cortex associated with vascular disorders

377.73 Disorders of visual cortex associated with inflammatory disorders

377.75 Disorders of visual cortex associated with cortical blindness — *blindness due to brain disorder, not eye disorder*

377.9 Unspecified disorder of optic nerve and visual pathways

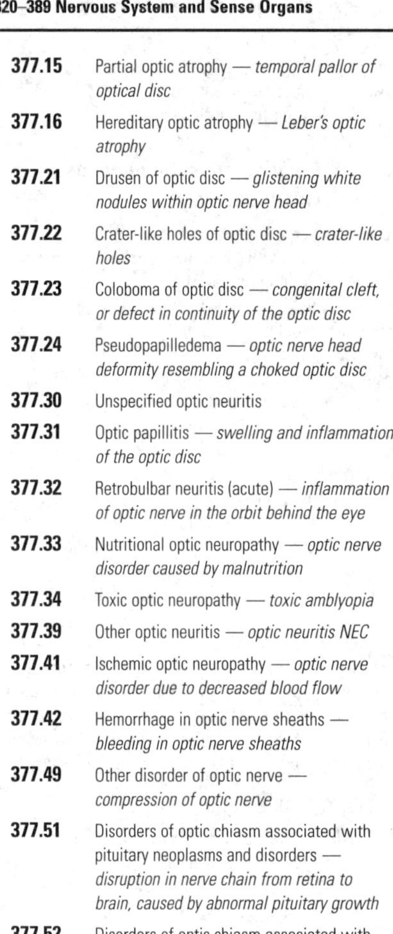

The various heterophorias present when the visual axis fails upon removal of the fusioning stimuli. The eye then wanders in the indicated direction

378 Strabismus and other disorders of binocular eye movements

Binocular fixation is necessary to see three-dimensionally and to aid in depth perception. A visual defect in which the two eyes fail to work together results in a partial or total loss of binocular depth perception and stereoscopic vision. At least 12 percent of the population has some type of binocular vision disability, of which amblyopia and strabismus are the most common types.

Strabismus is a condition in which the eyes do not point in the same direction. It can also be referred to as a tropia or squint. The disorder occurs in 2 to 5 percent of all children. About half are born with the condition, which causes one or both eyes to turn:

- Esotropia — inward turning of the eye
- Exotropia — outward turning of the eye
- Hypertropia — upward turning of the eye
- Hypotropia — downward turning of the eye

A baby's eyes should be straight and parallel by three or four months of age. A child who develops strabismus after the age of 8 or 9 years is said to have adult-onset strabismus. Most children with strabismus have comitant strabismus, in which the degree of deviation does not change. In incomitant strabismus,

© 2004 Ingenix, Inc.

the amount of misalignment depends upon which direction the eyes are pointed.

To determine misalignment, the ophthalmologist looks at a flashlight reflection on the cornea when the patient looks in all directions. The light should be reflected on the same portion of the cornea bilaterally or the diagnosis may be made with the cover test, in which each eye is covered in turn as the child looks at an object about 20 feet away. When the eye is covered, the uncovered eye should not move in a normal individual. In those with strabismus, the uncovered eye will move to focus properly on the object. Treatment may be surgical for muscle imbalance, use of refractive lenses, or patching the normal eye to allow the affected eye to regain strength and vision.

There is a genetic basis for several types of inherited strabismus, including those associated with genetic multisystem disorders such as Moebius syndrome, Prader-Willi syndrome, craniofacial dysostoses, and mitochondrial myopathies. It is especially common in children who have brain tumors, hydrocephalus, or genetic disorders (i.e., Down syndrome). In adults, diabetes, head trauma, stroke, or brain tumor may cause strabismus. Untreated strabismus can damage vision in the unused eye and possibly result in amblyopia (lazy eye). Amblyopia involves lowered visual acuity and poor muscle control in one eye. The result is often a loss of stereoscopic vision and binocular depth perception. Other binocular disorders include visual fine motor difficulties, eye movement inefficiencies, and visual perceptual lags that can result in eye strain, headache, double vision, blurred vision, learning related vision problems, and poor eye-hand coordination.

378.00 Unspecified esotropia

378.01 Monocular esotropia — *one eye turns inward*

378.02 Monocular esotropia with A pattern — *one eye turns inward with A pattern*

378.03 Monocular esotropia with V pattern — *one eye turns inward with V pattern*

378.04 Monocular esotropia with other noncomitancies — *monocular esotropia with X or Y pattern*

378.05 Alternating esotropia — *each eye takes turns deviating toward inner eye*

378.06 Alternating esotropia with A pattern — *each eye takes turns deviating toward inner eye with A pattern*

378.07 Alternating esotropia with V pattern — *each eye takes turns deviating toward inner eye with V pattern*

378.08 Alternating esotropia with other noncomitancies — *each eye takes turns deviating toward inner eye with X or Y pattern*

378.10 Unspecified exotropia

378.11 Monocular exotropia — *one eye turns outward*

378.12 Monocular exotropia with A pattern — *one eye turns outward with A pattern*

378.13 Monocular exotropia with V pattern — *one eye turns outward with V pattern*

378.14 Monocular exotropia with other noncomitancies — *monocular exotropia with X or Y pattern*

378.15 Alternating exotropia — *each eye takes turns deviating outward*

378.16 Alternating exotropia with A pattern — *each eye takes turns deviating outward with A pattern*

378.17 Alternating exotropia with V pattern — *each eye takes turns deviating outward with V pattern*

378.18 Alternating exotropia with other noncomitancies — *each eye takes turns deviating outward with X or Y pattern*

378.20 Unspecified intermittent heterotropia — *intermittent esotropia NOS or intermittent exotropia NOS*

378.21 Intermittent esotropia, monocular — *monocular*

378.22 Intermittent esotropia, alternating — *alternating*

378.23 Intermittent exotropia, monocular — *monocular*

378.24 Intermittent exotropia, alternating — *alternating*

378.30 Unspecified heterotropia

378.31 Hypertropia — *vertical heterotropia (constant) (intermittent)*

378.32 Hypotropia

378.33 Cyclotropia

378.34 Monofixation syndrome — *microtropia*

378.35 Accommodative component in esotropia

378.40 Unspecified heterophoria

378.41 Esophoria

378.42 Exophoria

378.43 Vertical heterophoria

378.44 Cyclophoria

378.45 Alternating hyperphoria

378.50 Unspecified paralytic strabismus

378.51 Paralytic strabismus, third or oculomotor nerve palsy, partial

378.52 Paralytic strabismus, third or oculomotor nerve palsy, total — *Nothnagel's syndrome; ophthalmoplegia-cerebellar ataxia syndrome*
AHA: Q2, 1989, 12

378.53 Paralytic strabismus, fourth or trochlear nerve palsy

378.54 Paralytic strabismus, sixth or abducens nerve palsy

378.55 Paralytic strabismus, external ophthalmoplegia — *Tolosa-Hunt syndrome*

378.56 Paralytic strabismus, total ophthalmoplegia

378.60 Unspecified mechanical strabismus

378.61 Mechanical strabismus from Brown's (tendon) sheath syndrome — *unilateral defect in sheath of superior oblique muscle, mimicking palsy*

378.62 Mechanical strabismus from other musculofascial disorders

378.63 Mechanical strabismus from limited duction associated with other conditions

378.71 Duane's syndrome — *eye retraction syndrome*

378.72 Progressive external ophthalmoplegia — *von Graefe's syndrome*

378.73 Strabismus in other neuromuscular disorders

378.81 Palsy of conjugate gaze — *oculomotor syndrome' Parinaud's syndrome*

378.82 Spasm of conjugate gaze — *muscle contractions impairing parallel movement of eyes*

378.83 Convergence insufficiency or palsy in binocular eye movement

378.84 Convergence excess or spasm in binocular eye movement — *overcompensation in parallel movement of eye*

378.85 Anomalies of divergence in binocular eye movement

378.86 Internuclear ophthalmoplegia — *eye movement anomaly attributed to brainstem lesion*

378.87 Other dissociated deviation of eye movements — *skew deviation*

378.9 Unspecified disorder of eye movements

379 Other disorders of eye

Aphakia is classified to this rubric.

Scleritis is the inflammation of the sclera (the white, outer wall of the eye) that can be superficial or deep. It is usually associated with autoimmune diseases such as rheumatoid arthritis, lupus erythematosis, infections, or chemical injuries, but sometimes the cause is unknown. It occurs most often in people between the ages of 30 and 60 and is rare in children. Symptoms include severe eye pain, blurred vision, sensitivity to light, and tearing of the eyes.

Staphyloma is a protrusion of the cornea or sclera, consisting of uveal tissue, caused by thinning of the sclera. No treatment has shown its effectiveness and evisceration is usually indicated.

379.00 Unspecified scleritis — *episcleritis NOS*

379.01 Episcleritis periodica fugax — *inflammation of outermost layer of the sclera, with blood engorgement*

379.02 Nodular episcleritis — *inflammation of outermost layer of the sclera, with nodular formations*

379.03 Anterior scleritis — *scleritis adjacent to corneal limbus*

379.04 Scleromalacia perforans — *softening and thinning of sclera*

379.05 Scleritis with corneal involvement — *scleroperikeratitis*

379.06 Brawny scleritis — *severe scleral inflammation with thickening corneal margins*

379.07 Posterior scleritis — *sclerotenonitis*

379.09 Other scleritis and episcleritis — *scleral abscess; scleral ulcer*

379.11 Scleral ectasia — *scleral staphyloma NOS*

379.12 Staphyloma posticum — *stretched, bulging sclera and uveal tissue at the posterior pole of eye*

379.13 Equatorial staphyloma — *stretched, bulging sclera and uveal tissue midway between anterior and posterior portions of eye*

379.14 Anterior staphyloma, localized — *stretched, bulging sclera and uveal tissue at the anterior pole of eye*

379.15 Ring staphyloma — *stretched, bulging sclera and uveal tissue in ring shape*

379.16 Other degenerative disorders of sclera

379.19 Other scleral disorder

379.21 Vitreous degeneration — *vitreous cavitation, detachment or liquefaction*

379.22 Crystalline deposits in vitreous — *asteroid hyalitis; synchysis scintillans*

379.23 Vitreous hemorrhage — *bleeding into the vitreous*
AHA: Q3, 1991, 15

379.24 Other vitreous opacities — *vitreous floaters*

379.25 Vitreous membranes and strands — *membranes and strands*

379.26 Vitreous prolapse — *vitreous slippage from normal position*

379.29 Other disorders of vitreous

379.31 Aphakia — *condition of being without natural optical lens*

379.32 Subluxation of lens — *partial dislocation of natural lens*

 © 2004 Ingenix, Inc.

379.33	Anterior dislocation of lens — *anterior displacement of natural lens toward iris*
379.34	Posterior dislocation of lens — *backward displacement of natural lens toward vitreous*
379.39	Other disorders of lens
379.40	Unspecified abnormal pupillary function
379.41	Anisocoria — *unequal pupils, differing by 1mm or more*
379.42	Miosis (persistent), not due to miotics — *sustained, abnormal contraction of pupil*
379.43	Mydriasis (persistent), not due to mydriatics — *sustained, abnormal dilation of pupil*
379.45	Argyll Robertson pupil, atypical — *Argyll Robertson phenomenon or pupil, nonsyphilitic*
379.46	Tonic pupillary reaction — *Adie's pupil or syndrome; Saenger's syndrome*
379.49	Other anomaly of pupillary function — *pupillary paralysis*
379.50	Unspecified nystagmus
379.51	Congenital nystagmus — *oscillating eye movements, congenital*
379.52	Latent nystagmus
379.53	Visual deprivation nystagmus — *oscillating eye movements caused by darkness*
379.54	Nystagmus associated with disorders of the vestibular system — *oscillating eye movements due to inner ear disease*
379.55	Dissociated nystagmus — *oscillating eye movements independent of each other*
379.56	Other forms of nystagmus
379.57	Nystagmus with deficiencies of saccadic eye movements — *abnormal optokinetic response*
379.58	Nystagmus with deficiencies of smooth pursuit movements — *dysfunction in normal tracking focus and movement of eyes*
379.59	Other irregularities of eye movements — *opsoclonus*
379.8	Other specified disorders of eye and adnexa
379.90	Unspecified disorder of eye
379.91	Pain in or around eye
379.92	Swelling or mass of eye
379.93	Redness or discharge of eye
379.99	Other ill-defined disorder of eye

Coding Clarification

Report aphakia as a condition warranting treatment with 379.31, while aphakia (pseudophakia) as a post-cataract extraction status is reported with V45.61. Congenital aphakia is reported with 743.35.

380–389 Diseases of the Ear and Mastoid Process

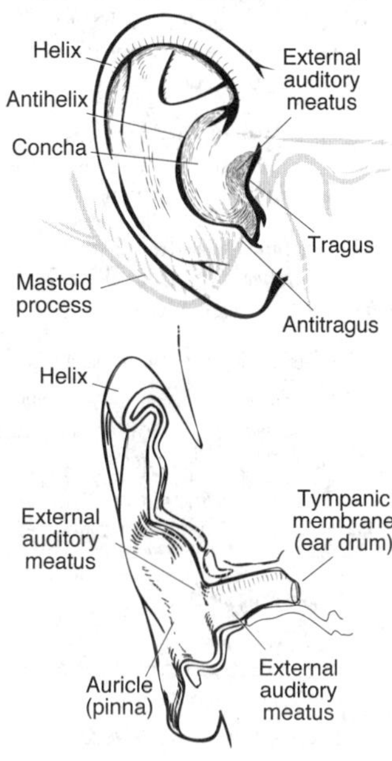

380 Disorders of external ear

Disorders of the external ear include those of the auricle (pinna) and external auditory meatus. The auricle consists of the helix, anthelix, scapha, concha, tragus, antitragus, intertragic notch, and lobule. The auricle is a single, elastic cartilage covered in skin and normal adnexal features (hair follicles, sweat glands, and sebaceous glands). The ridged nature of the auricle is to channel sounds into the acoustic meatus. The semicircular depression leading to the ear is named the concha, Latin for shell. The external auditory meatus consists of cartilaginous and osseous portions with the canal lined with epidermis, hair, and ceruminous glands that extend to the tympanic membrane.

Perichondritis is infection of the skin and tissue layer surrounding the cartilage of the ear and often happens after trauma or another infection has occurred. Chondritis is infection that has progressed into the cartilage itself. Though not a common infection, the recent increase in ear piercing through the cartilage around the outside of the ear has increased this risk. It is also a serious complication following surgery or injury as the damage can be severe, progressing to necrosis, requiring removal and reconstruction of the pinna.

Infective otitis externa is inflammation and infection of the auricle and external meatus. Bacteria, such as Pseudomonas, *Proteus vulgaris, Streptococci,* and

Staphylococcus aureus, or fungal infections such as Candida albicans can cause this condition.

Signs and symptoms of infective otitis externa include redness and swelling that can obstruct the meatus, serous or purulent drainage, external ear tenderness, and enlarged regional lymph nodes.

Diagnostic tests include culture and sensitivity to identify the infective organism. An otoscopy reveals inflammation and ceruminous impaction.

Therapies include antimicrobials (topically, systemically, or both), heat therapy to relieve pain, and gentle ear cleansing.

380.00 Unspecified perichondritis of pinna

380.01 Acute perichondritis of pinna — *sudden, severe inflammation of the connective tissue of the cartilage of the outer ear*

380.02 Chronic perichondritis of pinna — *persistent inflammation of the connective tissue of outer ear*

380.03 Chondritis of pinna

380.10 Unspecified infective otitis externa — *otitis externa (acute), circumscribed; otitis externa (acute), hemorrhagica*

380.11 Acute infection of pinna — *sudden, severe infection of outer ear canal*

380.12 Acute swimmers' ear — *beach ear; tank ear*

380.13 Other acute infections of external ear — (Code first underlying disease: 035, 684, 690.10-690.18)

380.14 Malignant otitis externa — *severe infection of outer ear canal with some tissue destruction*

380.15 Chronic mycotic otitis externa — (Code first underlying disease: 111.9, 117.3)

380.16 Other chronic infective otitis externa — *chronic infective otitis externa NOS*

380.21 Cholesteatoma of external ear — *keratosis obturans of external ear (canal)*

380.22 Other acute otitis externa — *actinic, chemical, contact, eczematoid, reactive*

380.23 Other chronic otitis externa — *chronic otitis externa NOS*

380.30 Unspecified disorder of pinna

380.31 Hematoma of auricle or pinna — *collection of blood in the tissue of the fleshy external ear*

380.32 Acquired deformities of auricle or pinna

380.39 Other noninfectious disorder of pinna — *ossification ear*

380.4 Impacted cerumen — *wax in ear*

380.50 Acquired stenosis of external ear canal unspecified as to cause

380.51 Acquired stenosis of external ear canal secondary to trauma — *narrowing of the external ear canal due to trauma*

380.52 Acquired stenosis of external ear canal secondary to surgery — *postsurgical narrowing of external ear canal*

380.53 Acquired stenosis of external ear canal secondary to inflammation — *narrowing of the external ear canal due to inflammation*

380.81 Exostosis of external ear canal

380.89 Other disorder of external ear — *auricular calcification; cicatrix of auricle; fistula of ear canal*

380.9 Unspecified disorder of external ear

Coding Clarification

Assign a fifth digit to indicate the exact nature and/or location of the inflammation.

Coding Scenario

A 16-year-old girl presented to her physician's office with her outer ear severely abscessed and the surrounding tissue beginning to show signs of vascular compromise, following multiple ear piercings. When the physician asked her why she waited so long to come in, she told him her mother had forbidden her to get multiple ear piercings around her ear and she had hoped it would heal with topical antiseptic. A culture was taken which revealed a *Pseudomonas aeruginosa* infection. The physician had her hospitalized where drains were inserted, some wound debridement was done, and she was placed on intravenous antibiotic therapy to stop the approach of gangrene.

> Code assignment: 380.03 *Chondritis of pinna*
> 041.7 *Pseudomonas infection*

381 Nonsuppurative otitis media and Eustachian tube disorders

Suppurative and unspecified otitis media are infections of the middle ear due to pyogenic organisms such as *staphylococci, pneumococci, Haemophilus influenzae, beta-hemolytic streptococci,* and gram-negative bacteria.

Signs and symptoms of suppurative and unspecified otitis media include chills and fever, malaise, deep throbbing ear pain, nausea and vomiting, dulled or impaired hearing, ear drainage, bulging of tympanic membrane, signs of upper respiratory infection, and a tender and swollen mastoid process.

Diagnostic tests include otoscopy to reveal obscured or distorted bony landmarks of the tympanic membrane, with scarring and thickening in chronic otitis media. A pneumatoscope shows decreased tympanic membrane motility. Culture and sensitivity of purulent material identify the infective organism.

© 2004 Ingenix, Inc.

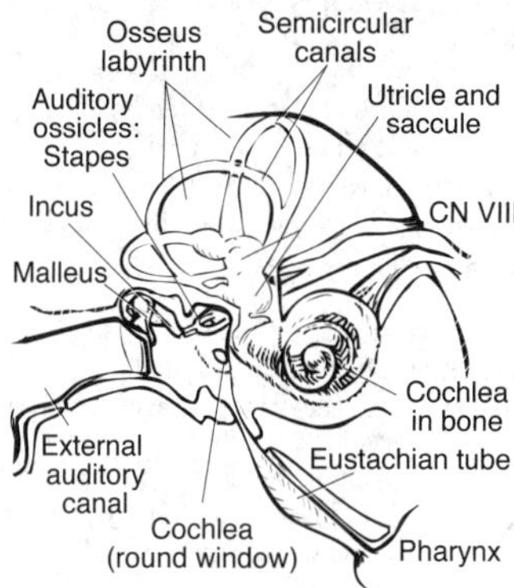

Exposed view of middle and inner ear

Therapies include systemic antibiotics, nasal decongestants, and analgesics such as aspirin to control pain and fever, and myringotomy with aspiration of the middle ear fluid if the tympanic membrane is in danger of rupture. Surgery may be performed (tympanoplasty, myringoplasty, mastoidectomy, excision of cholesteatomas) for chronic otitis media.

Associated conditions include adenoiditis or tonsillitis, colds or sinusitis, cholesteatoma, adhesions or scarring of middle ear structures, conductive hearing loss, abscesses, meningitis, mastoiditis, suppurative labyrinthitis, facial paralysis, otitis externa, sigmoid sinus, and jugular vein thrombosis.

381.00 Unspecified acute nonsuppurative otitis media

381.01 Acute serous otitis media — *acute or subacute secretory otitis media*

381.02 Acute mucoid otitis media — *acute or subacute seromucinous otitis media; blue drum syndrome*

381.03 Acute sanguinous otitis media — *sudden, severe infection of the middle ear, with blood*

381.04 Acute allergic serous otitis media — *allergic serous*

381.05 Acute allergic mucoid otitis media — *allergic mucoid*

381.06 Acute allergic sanguinous otitis media — *allergic sanguinous*

381.10 Simple or unspecified chronic serous otitis media — *persistent infection of the middle ear, without pus*

381.19 Other chronic serous otitis media — *serosanguinous chronic otitis media*

381.20 Simple or unspecified chronic mucoid otitis media

381.29 Other chronic mucoid otitis media — *mucosanguineous chronic otitis media*

381.3 Other and unspecified chronic nonsuppurative otitis media — *otitis media, chronic - allergic, exudative, secretory, transudative, with effusion*

381.4 Nonsuppurative otitis media, not specified as acute or chronic — *allergic, catarrhal, exudative, secretory, serous, transudative, with effusion, otitis media*

381.50 Unspecified Eustachian salpingitis

381.51 Acute Eustachian salpingitis — *sudden, severe inflammation of the Eustachian tube*

381.52 Chronic Eustachian salpingitis — *persistent inflammation of the Eustachian tube*

381.60 Unspecified obstruction of Eustachian tube — *obstruction of Eustachian tube NOS*

381.61 Osseous obstruction of Eustachian tube — *obstruction of Eustachian tube from cholesteatoma, polyp, or other osseous lesion*

381.62 Intrinsic cartilagenous obstruction of Eustachian tube — *Eustachian tube blockage caused by Eustachian cartilage overgrowth*

381.63 Extrinsic cartilagenous obstruction of Eustachian tube — *compression of Eustachian tube; Eustachian tube blockage caused by other cartilage overgrowth*

381.7 Patulous Eustachian tube — *distended, oversized*

381.81 Dysfunction of Eustachian tube

381.89 Other disorders of Eustachian tube — *adhesion of Eustachian tube; diverticula of Eustachian tube*

381.9 Unspecified Eustachian tube disorder

Coding Scenario

A 5-year-old male is seen in the emergency department. His mother states that he suffered a seizure. Upon examination the child is found to have acute nonsuppurative otitis media and a temperature of 104.2.

> Code assignment: 780.31 *Febrile convulsions* and 381.00 *Acute nonsuppurative otitis media, unspecified*

382 Suppurative and unspecified otitis media

The middle ear cleft extends from the nasopharyngeal orifice of the eustachian tube to the mastoid air cells. The three main segments are the eustachian tube, middle ear (tympanum), and the air cells of the mastoid, petrosa, and related areas. Suppurative otitis media is a serious bacterial infection of the middle ear that can follow untreated acute otitis media.

Infections with *Streptococcus pneumoniae, Haemophilus influenza,* and *Moraxella catarrhalis* are the most common causes of acute suppurative otitis media (382.0). Most complications of otitis media are associated with chronic or subacute disease. Acute and chronic otitis media infection may spread beyond the temporal bone and cause intratemporal (i.e., mastoiditis, petrositis, labyrinthitis, and facial nerve paralysis) and intracranial (i.e., extradural abscess, brain abscess, subdural abscess, sigmoid sinus thrombophlebitis, otic hydrocephalus, and meningitis) complications. The classic signs of acute otitis media are redness and bulging of the tympanic membrane. If the process continues to worsen, necrosis of the tympanic membrane occurs and the effusion passes into the ear canal through a perforation (suppurative otitis media). Diagnosis includes use of a pneumotoscopy when the presence of fluid behind the eardrum is not clear or an otomicroscopy using the operating microscope to visualize depth and three-dimensional structure. Antibiotics are usually prescribed for infection. Once osteitis is diagnosed, mastoidectomy is generally warranted to remove the infected, often necrotic bone. If an abscess is present, surgery is performed for drainage of pus and removal of the infected bone.

382.00 Acute suppurative otitis media without spontaneous rupture of eardrum — *severe inflammation of middle ear, with pus*

382.01 Acute suppurative otitis media with spontaneous rupture of eardrum — *sudden, severe inflammation of middle ear, with pressure tearing ear drum tissue, with pus*

382.02 Acute suppurative otitis media in diseases classified elsewhere — (Code first underlying disease: 034.1, 487.8)

382.1 Chronic tubotympanic suppurative otitis media — *benign chronic suppurative otitis media or chronic tubotympanic disease with anterior perforation of ear drum*

382.2 Chronic atticoantral suppurative otitis media — *chronic atticoantral disease or persistent mucosal disease with posterior or superior marginal perforation of ear drum*

382.3 Unspecified chronic suppurative otitis media — *chronic purulent otitis media*

382.4 Unspecified suppurative otitis media — *purulent otitis media NOS*

382.9 Unspecified otitis media — *otitis media NOS, acute otitis media NOS; chronic otitis media NOS*
AHA: Nov-Dec, 1984, 16

383 Mastoiditis and related conditions

Mastoiditis and related conditions describe inflammation and/or infection of the mastoid bone or an abscess in the mastoid antrum. The infections usually are due to Pneumococcus, *Haemophilus influenzae, beta-hemolytic Streptococci,* and gram-negative organisms.

Signs and symptoms of mastoiditis and related conditions include dull ache and tenderness over the mastoid process, low-grade fever, thick and purulent discharge, postauricular edema, erythema, and conductive hearing loss.

Diagnostic tests include x-rays of the mastoid area to reveal hazy signs of infection and an otoscopy to reveal dull and thick edematous tympanic membrane.

Therapies include antibiotics, myringotomy and drainage of purulent fluid, mastoidectomy (simple or radical), sequestrectomy, or debridement of necrotic bone.

Associated conditions include meningitis, facial paralysis, brain abscess, suppurative labyrinthitis, chronic otitis media, and conductive hearing loss.

383.00 Acute mastoiditis without complications — *sudden, severe inflammation of the mastoid air cells*

383.01 Subperiosteal abscess of mastoid — *von Bezold's abscess*

383.02 Acute mastoiditis with other complications — *Gradenigo's syndrome*

383.1 Chronic mastoiditis — *caries of mastoid; fistula of mastoid*

383.20 Unspecified petrositis

383.21 Acute petrositis — *sudden, severe inflammation of the dense bone behind the ear*

383.22 Chronic petrositis — *persistent inflammation of the dense bone behind the ear*

383.30 Unspecified postmastoidectomy complication — *postmastoidectomy complication NOS*

383.31 Mucosal cyst of postmastoidectomy cavity — *mucous-lined cyst cavity following removal of mastoid bone*

383.32 Recurrent cholesteatoma of postmastoidectomy cavity — *cystlike mass of cell debris in cavity following removal of mastoid bone*

383.33 Granulations of postmastoidectomy cavity — *chronic inflammation of postmastoidectomy cavity*

383.81 Postauricular fistula — *abnormal passage behind mastoid cavity*

383.89 Other disorder of mastoid — *perforation of mastoid (antrum) (cell)*

383.9 Unspecified mastoiditis

 © 2004 Ingenix, Inc.

384 Other disorders of tympanic membrane

The tympanic membrane (eardrum), which separates the outer ear from the middle ear, is a three-layer structure. The outer layer and inner layer are squamous and respiratory epithelia, which attempt to bridge defects in the middle ear. If there is a poor blood supply, or if there is an infection during the healing process, the squamous and respiratory epithelial layers may interfere with the process of spontaneous repair. A perforated eardrum (384.2x) is a hole or rupture in the eardrum, of which there are several causes, such as a skull fracture, infection, or from pushing a foreign object too far into the ear. Middle ear infections may cause pain, hearing loss, and spontaneous rupture of the eardrum resulting in a perforation. Most eardrum perforations heal spontaneously within weeks after rupture, during which time the ear must be protected from water and trauma. The location of the perforation affects the degree of hearing loss. If severe trauma (e.g., skull fracture) disrupts the bones in the middle ear or causes injury to the inner ear structures, the loss of hearing may be quite severe. Permanent hearing loss occurs in 3 percent of patients operated on for chronic otitis media and is associated with excessive ossicular mobilization, fracture of stapedial foot plate, direct trauma, or introduction of toxic materials.

384.00 Unspecified acute myringitis

384.01 Bullous myringitis — *myringitis bullosa hemorrhagica*

384.09 Other acute myringitis without mention of otitis media

384.1 Chronic myringitis without mention of otitis media — *chronic tympanitis*

384.20 Unspecified perforation of tympanic membrane

384.21 Central perforation of tympanic membrane

384.22 Attic perforation of tympanic membrane — *attic perforation including pars flaccida*

384.23 Other marginal perforation of tympanic membrane

384.24 Multiple perforations of tympanic membrane

384.25 Total perforation of tympanic membrane

384.81 Atrophic flaccid tympanic membrane — *healed perforation of ear drum*

384.82 Atrophic nonflaccid tympanic membrane

384.9 Unspecified disorder of tympanic membrane

Coding Clarification

Myringitis (384.0x) is always associated with otitis media. Bullous myringitis (384.01) is an inflammatory and contagious disorder of the eardrum or tympanum (caused by infection) resulting in painful blisters on the eardrum.

385 Other disorders of middle ear and mastoid

The mastoid is a part of the temporal bone of the skull (e.g., bony bump just behind and slightly above the level of the external ear) that is connected with the middle ear. In the adult, the mastoid portion of the temporal bone contains mastoid air cells that are separated from the brain by thin bony partitions. When there is a collection of fluid in the middle ear, there is usually also a slight collection of fluid within the airspaces of the mastoid. Attached to the eardrum (tympanic membrane) are three ear bones known as the malleus, incus, and stapes. The malleus pushes the incus; the incus pushes the stapes. When sound waves strike the eardrum, it vibrates and sets the bones into a motion that is transmitted to the inner ear, which generates nerve impulses that are sent to the brain. The muscles of the middle ear modify the performance of the middle ear bones and act as safety devices to protect the ear against excessively large vibrations from loud noises. As the noise level rises, one set of muscles tightens to restrict the movement of the malleus thus weakening the vibrations transmitted within the middle ear. At the same time, the stapes muscle contracts to pull the stapes away from the oval window so that less vibration is passed along to the very sensitive inner ear. The middle ear is connected to the nose by the Eustachian tube, which equalizes pressure in the middle ear. A healthy middle ear must contain air at the same atmospheric pressure as outside of the ear, so all these structures can vibrate freely. Tympanosclerosis is a common sequela after acute and chronic otitis media; the pathological calcified plaques are found in the tympanic membrane and the middle ear ossicles, leading to hearing impairment. Treatment is surgery but recurrencies are common and there is also a risk for iatrogenic sensorineural hearing loss.

385.00 Tympanosclerosis, unspecified as to involvement

385.01 Tympanosclerosis involving tympanic membrane only — *tough fibrous tissue impeding functions of the ear drum*

385.02 Tympanosclerosis involving tympanic membrane and ear ossicles — *tough fibrous tissue impeding functions of the eardrum and middle ear bones (stapes, malleus, and incus)*

385.03 Tympanosclerosis involving tympanic membrane, ear ossicles, and middle ear — *tough fibrous tissue impeding functions of the ear drum, middle ear bones, and middle ear canal*

385.09 Tympanosclerosis involving other combination of structures

385.10 Adhesive middle ear disease, unspecified as to involvement

385.11 Adhesions of drum head to incus

385.12 Adhesions of drum head to stapes

385.13 Adhesions of drum head to promontorium

385.19 Other middle ear adhesions and combinations

385.21 Impaired mobility of malleus — *ankylosis of malleus*

385.22 Impaired mobility of other ear ossicles — *ankylosis of ear ossicles, except malleus*

385.23 Discontinuity or dislocation of ear ossicles — *disruption in the auditory chain created by the malleus, incus, and stapes*

385.24 Partial loss or necrosis of ear ossicles — *loss of tissue in the malleus, incus, or stapes*

Coding Clarification

Cholesteatoma of the middle ear and mastoid is an abnormal growth of squamous epithelial cells within the middle ear extending from the external meatus. The dead epithelial tissue, which usually is forced to the exterior of the ear with the movement of the earwax, forms a sac, and produces keratin.

Signs and symptoms of cholesteatoma of the middle ear and mastoid include hearing loss and history of acute or chronic otitis media.

Otoscopy reveals white debris in the middle ear and destruction of the external auditory canal bone; x-rays of the middle ear and mastoid show tumor formation.

Therapies include control of concomitant infection, excision of cholesteatoma in extreme cases, tympanoplasty (reconstruction of ossicles), and myringoplasty.

Associated conditions include acute or chronic otitis media, hearing loss due to bony destruction of the ossicles, middle ear hemorrhage, attic and marginal perforations of the tympanic membrane, aural polyps, purulent labyrinthitis, facial paralysis, and intracranial abscess.

385.30 Unspecified cholesteatoma

385.32 Cholesteatoma of middle ear — *cystlike mass of cell debris in middle ear*

385.33 Cholesteatoma of middle ear and mastoid — *cystlike mass of cell debris in middle ear and mastoid air cells behind ear*
AHA: Q3, 2000, 10

385.35 Diffuse cholesteatosis of middle ear and mastoid — *cystlike masses of cell debris throughout middle ear*

385.82 Cholesterin granuloma of middle ear — *fatty granulations in the middle ear*

385.83 Retained foreign body of middle ear

385.89 Other disorders of middle ear and mastoid — *caries of middle ear; cicatrix of middle ear; hemotympanum; neuralgic mastoid; fistula of middle ear*

385.9 Unspecified disorder of middle ear and mastoid — *disorder of middle ear or mastoid NOS*

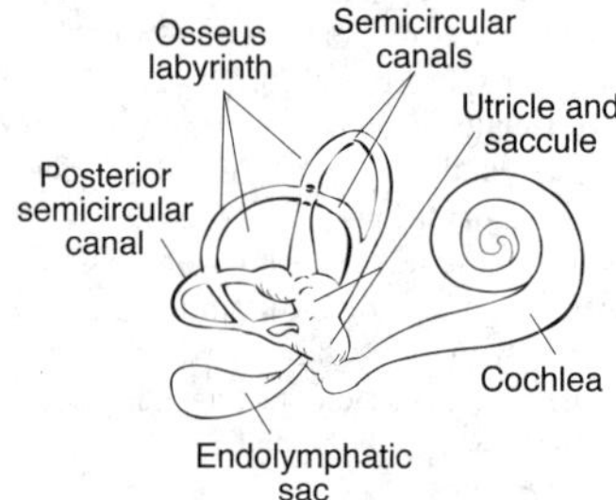

Schematic of labyrinth and semicircular ducts

386 Vertiginous syndromes and other disorders of vestibular system

AHA: March-April, 1985, 12

The inner ear consists of a system of fluid-filled tubes and sacs called the labyrinth, as well as the nerves that connect the labyrinth to the brain. The labyrinth, which rests inside the bone of the skull, contains the cochlea, and other organs, called the vestibular system, which control balance and eye movements. The first part of the vestibular system is made up of three semicircular canals that respond to angular acceleration of the head. The second part consists of the utricle and the saccule, which contain otoliths, or macular organs that respond to linear acceleration of the head as well as gravity.

Labyrinthitis and neuronitis are bacterial or viral inflammations of the inner ear or the nerves connecting the inner ear to the brain. Inflammation of the cochlea can cause disturbances in hearing, such as tinnitus. Dizziness, unsteadiness or imbalance when walking, and nausea are the most common symptoms of vestibular disorders. Because the vestibular system interacts with other parts of the nervous system, there may be problems with vision, muscles, thinking, and memory. Patients with vestibular disorders often report fatigue and loss of stamina and an inability to concentrate. Diagnosis depends on a variety of tests, including a physical exam to rule out other causes (i.e., cardiovascular disorders), vestibular testing, electronystagmography to record eye movements, and balance testing. Treatment consists of drug therapy, physical therapy, or, in severe cases, surgery.

In many cases, the underlying cause cannot be determined, though head trauma is a frequent cause in individuals younger than age 50. Ear infections such as otitis media and labyrinthitis and conditions that reduce blood flow to the inner ear (i.e., stroke) may damage the vestibular and hearing structures of the inner ear. High doses or long-term use of certain

 © 2004 Ingenix, Inc.

antibiotics can also cause permanent damage to the inner ear. Other drugs, such as aspirin, caffeine, alcohol, nicotine, sedatives, and tranquilizers can cause temporary dizziness but do not result in permanent damage to the vestibular system.

Menierè's disease is a disorder of the inner ear that causes episodes of vertigo, tinnitus, a feeling of fullness or pressure in the ear, and fluctuating hearing loss, and which can last two to four hours. Menierè's episodes may occur in clusters, or weeks, months, or years may pass between episodes. Between the acute attacks, most people are free of symptoms or note only mild imbalance and tinnitus. Between attacks, medication may be prescribed to help regulate the fluid pressure in the inner ear, reducing the severity and frequency of episodes. A hydrops diet regimen results in significant improvement in most patients. Surgery (possibly including instillation of gentamicin or other substances) may be performed to relieve the pressure on the inner ear or to block the transmission of information from the affected ear to the brain.

Benign paroxysmal positional vertigo (386.11) is a type of vertigo often induced when a patient turns over in bed, or gets in and out of bed. It is a benign disorder due to calcium impacted inner ear canals and treated with removal of the impaction. Diagnosis is through the Dix Halpike maneuver, which involves moving the patient rapidly from a sitting position, to the head hanging position, below horizontal, such as with a head hanging off the end of an examining table.

Vestibular neuronitis (386.12) is characterized by a sudden loss of balance that can be so severe that the patient may not be able to walk for several days or weeks. Viral neuronitis or a blood clot in the arterial system may precipitate the disorder. Diagnosis is based on symptoms, a physical exam, and tests, including audiometry, electronystagmography, and magnetic resonance imaging of the head. Treatment depends on the extent of balance loss (e.g., partial or total) and the onset of the disease in relation to treatment. Anticoagulants may be prescribed in conjunction with vasodilators to expand the blood vessels and allow the clot to pass. Corticosteroids may be used to treat a viral infection.

Labyrinthitis is a bacterial or viral infection secondary to acute otitis media or to purulent meningitis. When bacterial, there is a total loss of hearing on the affected side; if tuberculosis or syphilis is the cause, the hearing loss may be only partial. Diagnosis is by clinical exam of the ear and the patient's description of symptoms. Treatment of bacteria-caused labyrinthitis consists of heavy doses of antibiotics. The viral form is usually self-limiting, and the only treatment is bed rest, tranquilizers, and a medication to combat the dizziness.

386.00 Unspecified Meniere's disease — *Menierè's disease (active); Lermoyez' syndrome*
AHA: March-April, 1985, 12

386.01 Active Meniere's disease, cochleovestibular

386.02 Active Meniere's disease, cochlear

386.03 Active Meniere's disease, vestibular

386.04 Inactive Meniere's disease — *Menierè's disease in remission*
AHA: March-April, 1985, 12

386.10 Unspecified peripheral vertigo

386.11 Benign paroxysmal positional vertigo

386.12 Vestibular neuronitis — *Pedersen's (epidemic) vertigo*
AHA: March-April, 1985, 12

386.19 Other and unspecified peripheral vertigo — *aural vertigo; otogenic vertigo; otolith syndrome*
AHA: March-April, 1985, 12

386.2 Vertigo of central origin — *central positional nystagmus; malignant positional vertigo*
AHA: March-April, 1985, 12

386.30 Unspecified labyrinthitis

386.31 Serous labyrinthitis — *Serous labyrinthitis; diffuse labyrinthitis; inflammation with fluid buildup*
AHA: March-April, 1985, 12

386.32 Circumscribed labyrinthitis — *focal labyrinthitis; localized inflammation*
AHA: March-April, 1985, 12

386.33 Suppurative labyrinthitis — *purulent labyrinthitis; inflammation with pus*
AHA: March-April, 1985, 12

386.34 Toxic labyrinthitis — *inflammation caused by toxic reaction*
AHA: March-April, 1985, 12

386.35 Viral labyrinthitis — *inflammation caused by virus*
AHA: March-April, 1985, 12

386.40 Unspecified labyrinthine fistula

386.41 Round window fistula

386.42 Oval window fistula

386.43 Semicircular canal fistula

386.48 Labyrinthine fistula of combined sites

386.50 Unspecified labyrinthine dysfunction

386.51 Hyperactive labyrinth, unilateral — *oversensitivity of labyrinth, one ear*
AHA: March-April, 1985, 12

386.52 Hyperactive labyrinth, bilateral — *bilateral; oversensitivity of labyrinth, both ears*
AHA: March-April, 1985, 12

386.53 Hypoactive labyrinth, unilateral — *reduced sensitivity of labyrinth, one ear*
AHA: March-April, 1985, 12

386.54 Hypoactive labyrinth, bilateral — *reduced sensitivity of labyrinth, both ears*
AHA: March-April, 1985, 12

386.55 Loss of labyrinthine reactivity, unilateral — *reduced reaction of labyrinth, one ear*
AHA: March-April, 1985, 12

386.56 Loss of labyrinthine reactivity, bilateral — *bilateral; reduced reaction of labyrinth, both ears*
AHA: March-April, 1985, 12

386.58 Other forms and combinations of labyrinthine dysfunction

386.8 Other disorders of labyrinth — *caries of labyrinth; hemorrhage of cochlea; otoconia*
AHA: March-April, 1985, 12

386.9 Unspecified vertiginous syndromes and labyrinthine disorders — *vertiginous syndrome or labyrinthine disorder NOS*
AHA: March-April, 1985, 12

387 Otosclerosis

Otosclerosis is an inherited disorder involving the growth of abnormal spongy bone in the middle ear, which prevents the stapes from vibrating in response to sound waves. The condition leads to progressive hearing loss and is the most frequent cause of middle ear hearing loss in young adults, most commonly in women, 15 to 30 years old. Risks include a family history of hearing loss in pregnancy, which may trigger the onset. Diagnosis depends on a physical exam to rule out other causes of hearing loss and an audiometry exam to determine the extent of hearing loss. A computed tomography scan or x-ray of the head may be used to distinguish otosclerosis from other causes of hearing loss. Treatment includes medications such as oral fluoride, calcium, or vitamin D to stabilize the hearing loss. Surgery involves removal of the stapes and replacement with a prosthesis; this may be a total replacement (stapedectomy) or a laser may be used to make a hole in the stapes to allow placement of the prosthesis.

387.0 Otosclerosis involving oval window, nonobliterative — *tough, fibrous tissue impeding functions of the oval window*

387.1 Otosclerosis involving oval window, obliterative — *tough, fibrous tissue blocking the oval window*

387.2 Cochlear otosclerosis — *otosclerosis involving otic capsule or round window*

387.8 Other otosclerosis

387.9 Unspecified otosclerosis — *ossification of middle ear; otoporosis; otospongiosis*

388 Other disorders of ear

388.00 Unspecified degenerative and vascular disorders — *degenerative and vascular disorders NOS*

388.01 Presbyacusis — *loss of hearing associated with aging process*

388.02 Transient ischemic deafness — *temporary loss of hearing due to restricted blood flow to auditory organs*

388.10 Unspecified noise effects on inner ear — *effects on inner ear NOS*

388.11 Acoustic trauma (explosive) to ear — *otitic blast injury*

388.12 Noise-induced hearing loss — *noise-induced loss*

388.2 Unspecified sudden hearing loss — *sudden hearing loss NOS*

388.30 Unspecified tinnitus

388.31 Subjective tinnitus — *noises heard only by patient; usually biochemical in nature*

388.32 Objective tinnitus — *noises originating within patient and audible to others*

388.40 Unspecified abnormal auditory perception — *abnormal auditory perception NOS*

388.41 Diplacusis — *cochlear dysfunction causing patient to hear a single auditory stimulus as two sounds*

388.42 Hyperacusis — *acute hearing sensitivity; not necessarily painful*

388.43 Impairment of auditory discrimination — *impairment in ability to distinguish sound*

388.44 Other abnormal auditory perception, recruitment — *impairment in ability to distinguish volume of sound*

388.5 Disorders of acoustic nerve — *acoustic neuritis; degeneration or disorder of acoustic or eighth nerve*
AHA: March-April, 1987, 8

388.60 Unspecified otorrhea — *discharging ear NOS*

388.61 Cerebrospinal fluid otorrhea — *spinal fluid leakage from ear*

388.69 Other otorrhea — *otorrhagia*

388.70 Unspecified otalgia — *earache NOS*

388.71 Otogenic pain — *ear pain caused by a condition within the ear*

388.72 Referred otogenic pain — *ear pain caused by a condition outside the ear*

388.8 Other disorders of ear — *swelling ear*

388.9 Unspecified disorder of ear — *atrophic ear*

 © 2004 Ingenix, Inc.

389 Hearing loss

The ear consists of three parts: the outer ear, middle ear, and inner ear. The outer ear is the visible part plus the canals. The canals lead to the eardrum (middle ear), which is attached to the ossicles that amplify and conduct sound to the inner ear. The inner ear consists of the cochlea, which contains hair cells that vibrate when a sound is conducted to them by the eardrum and ossicles. The movement of the hair cells transmits electrical impulses down the auditory nerve to the brain, which is the sound heard.

Conductive hearing loss results from external or middle ear problems, which are often mechanical in nature. There are various causes for conductive hearing loss, including otitis media and otosclerosis. The most common cause of conductive hearing loss in children is otitis media infection in the middle ear cavity. The most common cause of conductive hearing loss in adults is otosclerosis. The loss results from fixation of the stapes (the third bone in the middle ear) so that sounds cannot be transported to the inner ear. Conductive hearing loss can be either temporary or permanent, and is treatable with medication and/or surgery.

Sensory hearing losses are due to disorders in the inner ear, specifically, the cochlea. This type of loss may be congenital, resulting from abnormal cochlea development or inherited conditions, or the loss may be the result of an acquired condition, such as meningitis, an infection of the fluid around the brain often extending into the inner ear.

Neural hearing loss results from a problem with the auditory nerve, often caused by an acoustic neuroma, which is a benign tumor that grows on the vestibular nerve and presses upon the auditory nerve. Early detection and prompt removal of the tumor is curative and may prevent future hearing loss. The acoustic reflex is a way of testing for neural hearing loss. The stapedius is a small muscle attached to the stapes that contracts in response to any loud sound, thus protecting the ear. The level of sound required to elicit this acoustic reflex can be used as a rough measure of hearing sensitivity. If the middle ear is normal, absence of the acoustic reflex may indicate a neural type of hearing loss. Neural hearing loss is also characterized by a greater loss of speech discrimination than experienced with sensory loss.

Sensorineural hearing loss is usually permanent loss of hearing sensitivity, usually more in the high frequencies than the lower frequencies and may affect the ability to understand conversations, especially in difficult listening situations and is best treated with the use of hearing aids. Malformations of the semicircular canal of the inner ear can be the cause of conductive and sensorineural hearing loss. If a sensorineural cause is suspected, an electrocochleography and auditory brainstem response tests are performed to measure the activity of the cochlea, auditory nerve, and brain.

Central auditory dysfunction refers to auditory impairment resulting from problems in the brain. Fortunately, central problems are uncommon. While they cause communication difficulties, they do not cause deafness because they usually affect only one side of the brain: both sides of the brain are involved in hearing. Central auditory dysfunction can result from aging, from Alzheimer's disease, and from other uncommon problems.

389.00	Unspecified conductive hearing loss
389.01	Conductive hearing loss, external ear
389.02	Conductive hearing loss, tympanic membrane
389.03	Conductive hearing loss, middle ear
389.04	Conductive hearing loss, inner ear
389.08	Conductive hearing loss of combined types
389.10	Unspecified sensorineural hearing loss
389.11	Sensory hearing loss
389.12	Neural hearing loss
389.14	Central hearing loss
389.18	Sensorineural hearing loss of combined types
389.2	Mixed conductive and sensorineural hearing loss — *deafness or hearing loss of type classifiable to 389.0 with 389.1*
389.7	Deaf mutism, not elsewhere classifiable — *deaf, nonspeaking*
389.8	Other specified forms of hearing loss
389.9	Unspecified hearing loss — *deafness NOS*

390–459
Diseases of the Circulatory System

Coding diseases of the circulatory system can be complex for several reasons, some of which are among the following:

- Interrelationship of conditions
- Specificity of coding guidelines
- Varied medical lexicon used to describe circulatory conditions

390–392 Acute Rheumatic Fever

Acute rheumatic fever is defined as a systemic disease/nonsuppurative acute complication, generally affecting joints (arthritis), subcutaneous tissue (nodules), skin (erythema marginatum), heart (carditis), and brain (chorea). The fever usually follows a throat infection by Group A Streptococci. Therapies include medications such as antibiotics (including subsequent antistreptococcal prophylaxis), analgesics, and anti-inflammatory agents.

Rheumatic fever is classified according to the site of inflammation. In acute rheumatic fever, the infection is active. Excluded from these rubrics are chronic heart conditions caused by rheumatic fever (393.0-398.9).

390 Rheumatic fever without mention of heart involvement OK

This rubric is limited to rheumatic fever that may have acute or subacute arthritis, but no heart involvement.

391 Rheumatic fever with heart involvement

Acute rheumatic pericarditis is an acute rheumatic fever with fibrinous involvement of the pericardium without mention of other cardiac involvement. It is uncommon in adults.

Acute rheumatic endocarditis is an acute rheumatic fever with involvement of the endocardium. This form of acute rheumatic fever principally involves one or more of the heart valves. Echocardiography of a patient with acute rheumatic endocarditis reveals large, friable "vegetations" on the heart valves or chordae tendineae.

Acute rheumatic myocarditis is an acute rheumatic fever with involvement of the heart muscle. Signs and symptoms may include tachycardia out of proportion to fever, cardiac manifestations such as heart blocks and arrhythmias, or a history of recent upper respiratory infection, pharyngitis, or tonsillitis. Diagnostic tests, such as stool and throat cultures, may identify the bacteria present, while endomyocardial biopsy provides a definite diagnosis. Disorders associated with acute rheumatic myocarditis may include cardiac arrhythmias, congestive heart failure, thromboembolism, or pericarditis. Therapies include antibiotics for bacterial infection, anti-arrhythmics for cardiac arrhythmias, and/or anticoagulants for possible thromboembolism.

391.0 Acute rheumatic pericarditis — *sudden, severe inflammation of the lining of the heart*

391.1 Acute rheumatic endocarditis — *sudden, severe inflammation of the heart cavities*

391.2 Acute rheumatic myocarditis — *sudden, severe inflammation of the heart muscle*

391.8 Other acute rheumatic heart disease — *sudden, severe inflammation of multiple sites in heart*

391.9 Unspecified acute rheumatic heart disease — *sudden, severe inflammation of unknown site of heart*

392 Rheumatic chorea

Rheumatic chorea is an inflammatory complication of Group A streptococcal infection involving the central nervous system. It is also known as chorea minor, chorea dance, Sydenham's chorea, and Saint Vitus dance. It generally affects children and young adults. Signs and symptoms may include involuntary, irregular, jerky movements of the face (excluding eyes), neck, or limbs.

392.0 Rheumatic chorea with heart involvement — *involuntary muscle movement and weakness*

392.9 Rheumatic chorea without mention of heart involvement — *involuntary muscle movement and weakness*

390–459

393–398 Chronic Rheumatic Heart Disease

Chronic rheumatic heart disease is a chronic disease resulting from single or repeated attacks of acute rheumatic fever that produce late effects in the structure of the heart, usually the endocardium. Sequelae include rigidity and deformity of the valvular cusps, fusion of the commissures, or shortening and fusion of the chordae tendinea. Damage also may occur in the myocardium following severe bouts of acute rheumatic myocarditis affecting cardiac performance. Associated conditions may include valvular stenosis and/or insufficiency and, usually, mitral and myocardial damage.

393 Chronic rheumatic pericarditis OK

Chronic rheumatic pericarditis is a set of conditions such as adhesive pericarditis and constrictive pericarditis when specified as a manifestation following an acute rheumatic infection. Adhesive pericarditis (chronic) occurs when adhesions develop between the two-pericardial layers, or between the pericardium and the heart or other neighboring structures. Constrictive pericarditis (chronic) is a thickening of the pericardial membrane with constriction of the cardiac chambers.

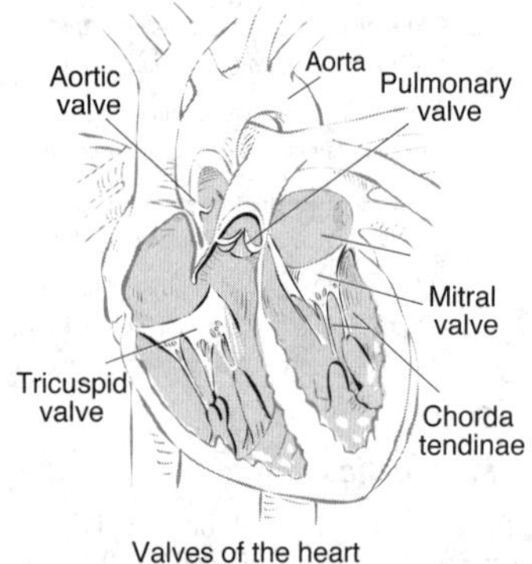

Valves of the heart

394 Diseases of mitral valve

Mitral stenosis, mitral valve disease (unspecified), and mitral valve failure are presumed to be rheumatic in origin for classification purposes and need not be stated as rheumatic. Other manifestations, such as insufficiency, incompetence, or regurgitation (without stenosis) must be specified as due to rheumatic heart disease for classification under rubric 394.

Mitral stenosis is a narrowing of the orifice of the mitral valve due to (presumed) rheumatic heart disease that impedes left ventricular filling. Signs and symptoms include left or combined left and right heart failure, hemoptysis, systematic embolism, hoarseness, atrial fibrillation, or pulmonary rales and increased S1/S2 heart sounds.

Rheumatic mitral insufficiency is a reflux of a portion of blood back into the left atrium instead of forward into the aorta, resulting in increased atrial pressure and decreased forward cardiac output. Signs and symptoms may include dyspnea due to left ventricular failure (which may be combined with right heart failure in severe cases), pulmonary hypertension, holosystolic apical murmur, S3 heart sound, or brisk carotid upstroke. An EKG may show left ventricular hypertrophy and left atrial enlargement in cases of rheumatic mitral insufficiency, and a chest x-ray usually shows heart enlargement and vascular congestion when the insufficiency has resulted in heart failure. Echocardiography may visualize scarring and retraction of the mitral leaflets. Cardiac catheterization with a pulmonary capillary wedge monitor (Swan-Ganz) may reveal systolic volume overload, which is characterized by a large V wave on right heart catheterization, and left ventriculography demonstrates systolic regurgitation of contrast material into the left atrium. Therapies for rheumatic mitral insufficiency may include medications (digitalis, diuretics, or vasodilators) to increase forward cardiac output and reduce pulmonary venous hypertension. Anticoagulants may be prescribed for patients with atrial fibrillation or surgery, such as annuloplasty or replacement of the mitral valve, for chronic mitral valve insufficiency and sometimes in cases demonstrating relatively mild symptoms to forestall significant ventricular muscle dysfunction. Conditions associated with rheumatic mitral insufficiency include atrial fibrillation, pulmonary hypertension, left or congestive heart failure, and systemic embolism.

394.0	Mitral stenosis — *obstruction*
394.1	Rheumatic mitral insufficiency — *incompetence, regurgitation*
394.2	Mitral stenosis with insufficiency — *obstruction with incompetence or regurgitation*
394.9	Other and unspecified mitral valve diseases — *unknown or not otherwise specified*

395 Diseases of aortic valve

Rheumatic aortic stenosis is a pathological narrowing of the aortic valve orifice due to fibrosis of the commissures and/or degenerative distortion of the aortic valve cusps. Commissural fusion and scarring may be present early in the progression of the disease, and calcification of the valve is often a late complication. The resulting stenosis produces a pressure overload on the left ventricle due to the increased pressure needed to force the blood through the narrowed aortic valve orifice. Signs and symptoms of rheumatic aortic stenosis include angina, syncope, heart failure, delayed carotid upstroke, and/or a sustained forceful apex beat, systolic ejection murmur,

 © 2004 Ingenix, Inc.

or softened singular S2 heart sound with S4 heart sound. An EKG normally shows left ventricular hypertrophy in cases of rheumatic aortic stenosis, and cardiac catheterization provides definitive diagnosis and evaluation of the condition. Echocardiography and fluoroscopy may be of limited value in assessing the severity of the stenosis. Therapies include medications (digitalis, diuretics, and antiarrhythmics) as temporary symptomatic measures, or aortic valve replacement. Associated conditions include left heart failure, mitral valve disease, angina (exertional), heart blocks due to calcification of the conduction system, and atrial and ventricular arrhythmias.

Rheumatic aortic insufficiency is the reflux of blood into the left ventricle during diastole due to an incompetent aortic valve. Chronic aortic insufficiency eventually leads to left ventricular dysfunction and failure. The condition is also known as rheumatic aortic regurgitation and rheumatic aortic incompetence. Signs and symptoms include left ventricular failure, syncope, angina, diastolic murmur along the left sternal border or an Austin Fling murmur, and/or stroke volume increase. An EKG normally shows left ventricular hypertrophy in cases of rheumatic aortic insufficiency. Chest x-rays show cardiac enlargement in severe chronic cases. Echocardiography demonstrates an enlarged left ventricular cavity and frequently reveals diastolic vibration of the mitral valve. Cardiac catheterization and arteriography demonstrate regurgitation of contrast material back into the left ventricle. Therapies include medications (digitalis, diuretics, and vasodilators) for symptomatic relief, and aortic valve replacement in severe cases. Associated conditions include angina and left heart failure, and congestive heart failure.

395.0 Rheumatic aortic stenosis — *obstruction*
AHA: Q4, 1988, 8

395.1 Rheumatic aortic insufficiency — *incompetence or regurgitation*

395.2 Rheumatic aortic stenosis with insufficiency — *obstruction with incompetence or regurgitation*

395.9 Other and unspecified rheumatic aortic diseases — *unknown or not otherwise specified*

396 Diseases of mitral and aortic valves

AHA: Nov-Dec, 1987, 8

For more information about the subcategories of this rubric, refer to the detailed descriptions of the individual components of combined aortic and mitral valve disease.

396.0 Mitral valve stenosis and aortic valve stenosis — *narrowing of both valves*
AHA: Nov-Dec, 1987, 8

396.1 Mitral valve stenosis and aortic valve insufficiency — *narrowing of mitral valve with incompetence or regurgitation of aortic valve*
AHA: Nov-Dec, 1987, 8

396.2 Mitral valve insufficiency and aortic valve stenosis — *incompetence or regurgitation of mitral valve with narrowing of aortic valve*
AHA: Nov-Dec, 1987, 8; Q2, 2000, 16

396.3 Mitral valve insufficiency and aortic valve insufficiency — *incompetence or regurgitation of both valves*
AHA: Nov-Dec, 1987, 8

396.8 Multiple involvement of mitral and aortic valves — *stenosis and insufficiency of mitral or aortic valve with stenosis or insufficiency, or both, of the other valve*
AHA: Nov-Dec, 1987, 8

396.9 Unspecified mitral and aortic valve diseases

Coding Clarification

When both the mitral and aortic valves are involved, ICD-9-CM presumes an etiology of rheumatic heart disease for classification purposes. In all cases, when both the aortic and mitral valves are diseased, the ICD-9-CM index will lead to rubric 396.

397 Diseases of other endocardial structures

This rubric includes chronic rheumatic heart diseases of the tricuspid, pulmonary, and unspecified heart valves. Note that diseases of the tricuspid valve are presumed to be of rheumatic etiology, but diseases of the pulmonary or unspecified heart valves must be stated as due to a late effect of rheumatic heart disease.

Diseases of the tricuspid valve are classified to codes in the 397.0 subclassification and report insufficiency, obstruction, regurgitation, and stenosis of the tricuspid valve. Tricuspid regurgitation may occur secondary to right ventricular pressure overload from left-sided lesions. It also may occur as a result of primary rheumatic heart disease of the tricuspid valve itself. Tricuspid stenosis serves as a mechanical obstruction blocking the return of blood to the right ventricle of the heart.

Rheumatic diseases of pulmonary valves (397.1) include valve insufficiency and stenosis. Pulmonary valve insufficiency is a reflux of blood back into the right ventricle through an incompetent pulmonary valve and may be associated with pulmonary hypertension. Pulmonary valve stenosis is an obstruction of the blood through the pulmonary valve.

397.0 Diseases of tricuspid valve — *insufficiency, obstruction, regurgitation, stenosis*
AHA: Q2, 2000, 16

397.1 Rheumatic diseases of pulmonary valve — *insufficiency, obstruction, regurgitation, stenosis*

397.9 Rheumatic diseases of endocardium, valve unspecified — *unknown valve*

Coding Clarification

All diseases of the tricuspid valve not specifically directed to other code categories in the ICD-9-CM index are included in 397.0.

Code 397.1 includes all diseases of the pulmonary valve specified as due to a late effect of rheumatic heart disease not directed to other code categories in the ICD-9-CM index.

398 Other rheumatic heart disease

This rubric includes rare occurrences of chronic rheumatic heart disease not involving the heart valves.

398.0 Rheumatic myocarditis — *myocardium*

398.90 Unspecified rheumatic heart disease

398.91 Rheumatic heart failure (congestive) — *left ventricular failure*
AHA: Q3, 1988, 3; Q1, 1995, 6

398.99 Other and unspecified rheumatic heart diseases — *not otherwise specified, inactive pancarditis with rheumatic fever*

Coding Clarification

Chronic inflammation of the muscular walls of the heart (myocarditis) specified as due to or a late effect of rheumatic heart disease is reported with 398.0. Code this condition in addition to rheumatic valve disease when indicated. Congestive rheumatic heart failure is reported with 398.91 and includes left heart failure and congestive heart failure due to rheumatic heart disease. Left and congestive heart failure, common in the rheumatic valvular diseases described in rubrics 394-396, may be coded in addition to rheumatic valvular disease when indicated.

401–405 Hypertensive Disease

Hypertensive disease is a condition in which the diastolic pressure exceeds 100 mm Hg in persons 60 years of age or older or 90 mm Hg in persons younger than 60 years of age. The World Health Organization (WHO) defines hypertension as pressures exceeding 160/90 mm Hg, but studies have shown that increased morbidity and mortality are associated with diastolic pressures of just 85 mm Hg. It is generally asymptomatic until complications develop. Complications may include retinal changes, loud aortic sounds and early systolic ejection click heard on auscultation, headache, tinnitus, and palpitations.

Rubrics 401-404 include primary (essential) hypertension of no known cause and account for approximately 90 percent of the population. The remaining 10 percent of the population have secondary hypertension classifiable to 405, due to definitive and diagnosable disease such as Cushing's syndrome. Use the hypertension table in the ICD-9-CM index to distinguish between primary and secondary hypertension and assign the correct code.

Use the fourth digits in categories 401-405 to specify the course of hypertensive disease as malignant, benign, or unspecified. Do not try to make the distinction between benign and malignant without first obtaining physician verification for coding and classification purposes.

401 Essential hypertension

AHA: July-Aug, 1984, 11; Sept-Oct, 1987, 9; Q2, 1989, 12; Q3, 1990, 3; Q2, 1992, 5

High blood pressure, also called hypertension, occurs when the arterioles narrow, causing the blood to exert excessive pressure against the vessel wall and the heart must work harder to maintain the higher pressure. Over time, damage to the brain, eye, and kidney can result ("target organ damage"). Essential or primary hypertension means that there is no underlying condition that is causing the blood pressure to increase. Up to 95 percent of hypertension is the essential type and, unless blood pressure readings are very high, efforts to control blood pressure are usually based on changes in lifestyle (weight loss, exercise, dietary changes, and reducing stress). Use rubric 401 to report all primary forms of hypertension without mention of heart or renal disease, including arterial, idiopathic, systemic, and vascular hypertension.

401.0 Essential hypertension, malignant — *severe high arterial blood pressure without apparent organic cause*
AHA: July-Aug, 1984, 11; May-June, 1985, 19; Sept-Oct, 1987, 9; Q2, 1989, 12; Q3, 1990, 3; Q2, 1992, 5

401.1 Essential hypertension, benign — *mild elevation in arterial blood pressure without apparent organic cause*
AHA: July-Aug, 1984, 11; Sept-Oct, 1987, 9; Q2, 1989, 12; Q3, 1990, 3; Q2, 1992, 5

401.9 Unspecified essential hypertension

Documentation Issues

Unless documentation identifies a cause and effect relationship between hypertension and congestive heart failure they should be coded as separate entities, 428.0 and 401.x. However, if the documentation indicates the congestive heart failure is due to the hypertension, only one code is necessary, 402.91.

The physician must document the type and nature (e.g., malignant, benign) of the hypertension for accurate classification of the condition.

When the documentation identifies a postoperative hypertension, the physician needs to document

 © 2004 Ingenix, Inc.

whether it was caused by inadequate control of pain or patient agitation, and if the hypertension was merely an elevation in blood pressure without mention of hypertension (796.2), or a benign hypertension (401.1).

Documentation indicates the patient has congestive heart failure and hypertension. If the documentation does not identify a cause and effect relationship, verify with the physician. Ask the physician if this was hypertensive heart disease with congestive heart failure (402.91). If no clarification as to the cause and effect relationship is obtained, use codes 428.0 and 401.9.

If the patient is diagnosed as having hypertension and renal failure, request that documentation clarify if the hypertension is malignant or accelerated for accurate code selection.

When documentation identifies hypertension in a patient who is status post-renal transplant for chronic renal failure, more information is required for accurate code selection. Review the medical record or obtain the information necessary from the physician, such as:

- If the hypertension is caused by a complication of the transplant, use codes 996.81 and 405.99.
- If the hypertension is a side effect of the postoperative immunotherapy given after the transplantation, use codes 405.99, E933.1, and V42.0.
- If the hypertension existed prior to the transplant and is still present, use a code from the hypertension code series 401-404.

If the physician documents the diagnosis of hypertensive cardiovascular disease, review the medical record for any reference to coronary arteriosclerosis, angina, or chronic myocardial ischemia. If these conditions are noted, code them in addition to the hypertensive heart disease. If the documentation also notes any myocardial ischemic conditions, they need to be coded separately.

Coding Clarification

Coexisting or Chronic Conditions: Coexisting or chronic conditions that are treated on an ongoing basis should be coded and reported as many times as the patient receives treatment, management, and additional care for the conditions. Conditions such as hypertension that are considered systemic diseases should be coded even in the absence of documented active intervention.

Elevated Blood Pressure: Also known as transient hypertension, this is an elevated blood pressure reading without a diagnosis of hypertension and may be characteristic of older age groups or due to emotional stress. For these cases, report code 796.2 *Elevated blood pressure reading without diagnosis of hypertension.*

Hypertensive Cerebrovascular Disease: Cerebral symptoms resulting in an abrupt elevation in blood pressure, such as confusion, agitation, headaches, obtundation, stupor, and convulsions, are known as cerebral encephalopathy (437.2 and an additional code from categories 401-405). An extended exposure to arterial benign hypertension may cause intracerebral hemorrhage, which may result from a rupture of an arteriosclerotic vessel (431 and an additional code from categories 401-405). Malignant hypertension could result in a cerebral infarction; use codes 434.0 and 401.0.

Malignant Hypertension: Interchangeable terms also identifying malignant hypertension are necrotizing or accelerating hypertension. This condition is distinguished by symptoms of progressive heart failure, impairment of vision, ocular hemorrhage, exudates, and papilledema. By definition, papilledema is always associated with malignant hypertension. More serious outcomes are uremia, cerebral hemorrhage, or heart failure. To report, use code 401.0 *Essential hypertension, malignant.*

Postoperative Hypertension: It is appropriate to use complication code 997.91 *Complications affecting specified body systems, NEC, hypertension* and an additional code to identify the specific type of hypertension. Sequence the complication code first and the hypertension code second. If the physician documents hypertension sometime after the operative episode, but does not indicate it as postoperative or as a complication of surgery, use a code from categories 401-405 only.

Pregnancy Complication: If the hypertension is noted as a mild pre-eclampsia, hypertension in pregnancy with mild proteinuria and edema, use code 642.4x. If the diagnosis states pregnancy with severe proteinuria or severe pre-eclampsia (HELLP syndrome), use code 642.5x. Hypertension that develops in the second half of pregnancy through the last trimester should be reported with code 642.4x and, if stated as severe, code 642.5x. For pregnancy with hypertension secondary to renal disease, use code 642.1x and, if pre-eclampsia or eclampsia is also present, use code 642.7x. If the diagnosis is stated as transient hypertension of pregnancy, use code 642.3x.

Questionable Admission Diagnosis: CMS issued a list of codes to the medical review entities that usually do not warrant inpatient admissions. When these diagnoses appear as the principal diagnoses, the justification for admission is considered questionable. Benign essential hypertension code 401.1 is on this questionable diagnosis list.

Retinopathy: To accurately report this condition, two codes are required: code 362.11 *Hypertensive*

390–459

retinopathy and an appropriate code from categories 401-405 to identify the specific type of hypertension.

Secondary Hypertension: This condition may be due to a number of underlying causes. Always code the underlying cause first, if indicated as a current condition, and then the secondary hypertension.

Systolic Hypertension: This is typically defined as a systolic pressure higher that 160 mm Hg and a diastolic pressure of less than 95 mm Hg. It is also known as arteriosclerotic hypertension because patients have a tendency to develop arteriosclerosis of the central aorta and its branches. Code 401.1 *Benign hypertension* should be used to identify this condition as there appears to be no reference to it as a malignant hypertension.

Uncontrolled Hypertension: This does not indicate the hypertension is malignant, only that the condition is in an uncontrolled state. It typically indicates the need for diuretics or other antihypertensive drugs, such as beta-blockers. There is no code to identify this condition so classification would be to its type and nature.

Coding Scenario

A patient previously diagnosed with atherosclerotic hypertension is now seen in the clinic for follow up. Medical record indicates coronary atherosclerosis and benign hypertension.

> Code assignment: 414.00 *Coronary atherosclerosis of unspecified type of vessel, native or graft* and 401.1 *Essential hypertension, benign*

A patient is admitted with a diagnosis of hypertension. The physician's final diagnosis at discharge is atherosclerosis of the aorta and generalized arteriosclerosis.

> Code assignment: 440.0 *Atherosclerosis of aorta,* and 440.9 *Generalized and unspecified atherosclerosis*

A patient is seen in the emergency department with uncontrolled hypertension. The patient was previously treated with diuretics. The physician's documentation identifies the hypertension as benign. The patient is discharged to follow up with attending the next day.

> Code assignment: 401.1 *Essential hypertension, benign*

A patient is seen in the outpatient clinic for a follow-up visit for hypertension and angina. The physician prescribes nitroglycerin for the angina and a diuretic for the hypertension. The patient history also identifies the patient had pneumonia six months ago.

> Code assignment: 401.9 *Essential hypertension, unspecified* and 413.9 *Angina pectoris, unspecified*

A patient is admitted and treated for acute renal failure and essential hypertension.

> Code assignment: 584.9 *Acute renal failure, unspecified* and 401.9 *Essential hypertension, unspecified*

402 Hypertensive heart disease

AHA: July-Aug, 1984, 11; Nov-Dec, 1984, 18; Sept-Oct, 1987, 9; Q2, 1989, 12; Q3, 1990, 3; Q2, 1993, 9; Q4, 2002, 49

Use rubric 402 to report heart disease due to the effects of systemic hypertension. It is characterized by concentric hypertrophy of the left ventricle that in time can lead to left ventricular failure.

402.00 Malignant hypertensive heart disease without heart failure — *severe high blood pressure causing heart complications*
AHA: July-Aug, 1984, 11; Nov-Dec, 1984, 18; Sept-Oct, 1987, 9; Q2, 1989, 12; Q3, 1990, 3; Q2, 1993, 9; Q4, 2002, 49

402.01 Malignant hypertensive heart disease with heart failure — *severe high blood pressure causing heart complications*
AHA: July-Aug, 1984, 11; Nov-Dec, 1984, 18; Sept-Oct, 1987, 9; Q2, 1989, 12; Q3, 1990, 3; Q2, 1993, 9; Q4, 2002, 49

402.10 Benign hypertensive heart disease without heart failure — *mild elevation in blood pressure causing heart complications*
AHA: July-Aug, 1984, 11; Nov-Dec, 1984, 18; Sept-Oct, 1987, 9; Q2, 1989, 12; Q3, 1990, 3; Q2, 1993, 9; Q4, 2002, 49

402.11 Benign hypertensive heart disease with heart failure — *mild elevation in blood pressure causing heart complications*
AHA: July-Aug, 1984, 11; Nov-Dec, 1984, 18; Sept-Oct, 1987, 9; Q2, 1989, 12; Q3, 1990, 3; Q2, 1993, 9; Q4, 2002, 49

402.90 Unspecified hypertensive heart disease without heart failure — *high blood pressure of unknown degree causing heart complications*
AHA: July-Aug, 1984, 11; Nov-Dec, 1984, 18; Sept-Oct, 1987, 9; Q2, 1989, 12; Q3, 1990, 3; Q2, 1993, 9; Q4, 2002, 49

402.91 Unspecified hypertensive heart disease with heart failure — *high blood pressure of unknown degree causing heart complications*
AHA: July-Aug, 1984, 11; Nov-Dec, 1984, 18; Sept-Oct, 1987, 9; Q2, 1989, 12; Q3, 1990, 3; Q1, 1993, 19; Q2, 1993, 9; Q4, 2002, 49; Q4, 2002, 52

Documentation Issues

If the documentation indicates that the patient has heart failure, review the record for any hypertensive heart or hypertensive heart and renal disease. If documentation identifies these conditions, a

 © 2004 Ingenix, Inc.

combination code may be used from categories 402 and 404.

Even if the patient is being seen for another condition, if the heart failure is noted in the record and the patient is still under treatment, the heart failure should be coded as a secondary condition.

Note that there must be a stated or implied cause and effect relationship between the heart disease and the hypertension. For example, the statement "benign hypertension with congestive heart failure" is coded to 401.1 and 428.0; but the statement "benign hypertensive heart disease with heart failure" is reported with 402.11.

Coding Clarification

Hypertension and Atherosclerosis: Hypertension frequently accelerates atherosclerosis and if both are documented, code both conditions. Systolic hypertension may be referenced as "arteriosclerotic hypertension" of the elderly. In younger patients, systolic hypertension may be associated with an arteriovenous fistula or thyrotoxicosis, and would be classified as a secondary hypertension.

Hypertensive cardiovascular arteriosclerotic disease with heart failure is coded 402.91. Use an additional code of 414.0x to identify the coronary arteriosclerosis.

Coding Scenario

A patient is admitted with hypertensive cardiovascular disease. Documentation identifies that the patient was having chest pain due to angina. The physician's final diagnosis is hypertensive cardiovascular disease, benign, with angina pectoris.

> Code assignment: 402.10 *Benign hypertensive heart disease, without heart failure* and 413.9 *Other and unspecified angina pectoris*

A patient is seen in the clinic for evaluation of treatment for hypertensive cardiomyopathy. Record documentation identifies that the cardiomyopathy was secondary to hypertensive heart disease.

> Code assignment: 402.90 *Unspecified hypertensive heart disease, without heart failure* and 425.8 *Cardiomyopathy in other diseases classified elsewhere*

Cardiology consultation identifies a benign hypertensive heart disease with left ventricular failure.

> Code assignment: 402.11 *Benign hypertensive heart disease, with heart failure*

A patient is admitted with fluid overload. Final diagnosis indicates that the patient has heart failure due to hypertensive cardiovascular disease. Documentation also reveals the patient has arteriosclerotic heart disease without previous surgical intervention.

> Code assignment: 402.91 *Unspecified hypertensive heart disease, with heart failure* and 414.01 *Coronary atherosclerosis of native coronary artery*

A 57-year-old male is admitted to the facility with left ventricular failure and benign hypertensive heart disease.

> Code assignment: 402.11 *Benign hypertensive heart disease, with heart failure*

403 Hypertensive renal disease

AHA: July-Aug, 1984, 11; Sept-Oct, 1987, 9; Q2, 1989, 12; Q3, 1990, 3; Q2, 1992, 5; Q4, 1992, 22

Hypertensive renal disease is a condition also known as arteriolar nephrosclerosis, and is reported with codes from rubric 403. It is characterized by intimal thickening of the afferent arteriole of the glomerulus and due to long-standing or poorly controlled hypertension. In severe nephrosclerosis, the nephron is deprived of its blood supply, and areas of infarction occur with subsequent scar formation. Renal insufficiency occurs when the kidney is scarred and contracted. In most cases, the patient will eventually develop renal failure.

This rubric reports chronic renal failure associated with hypertensive renal disease due to progressive and irreversible destruction of the nephrons and should not be confused with acute renal failure. Acute renal failure is classified to rubric 584 and describes failure of the kidneys to perform their essential function due to trauma, impaired blood flow, toxic substances, bacterial infection, or obstruction of the urinary tract.

Both diabetes mellitus and hypertension have associated renal manifestations such as renal failure.

The following fifth-digit subclassification is for use with category 403:

0 without mention of renal failure

1 with renal failure

403.0 5th Hypertensive renal disease, malignant — *severe high blood pressure causing kidney malfunctions*

AHA: July-Aug, 1984, 11; Sept-Oct, 1987, 9; Q2, 1989, 12; Q3, 1990, 3; Q2, 1992, 5; Q4, 1992, 22

403.1 5th Hypertensive renal disease, benign — *mild high blood pressure causing kidney malfunctions*

AHA: July-Aug, 1984, 11; Sept-Oct, 1987, 9; Q2, 1989, 12; Q3, 1990, 3; Q2, 1992, 5; Q4, 1992, 22

403.9 5th Unspecified hypertensive renal disease — *high blood pressure of unknown degree causing kidney malfunctions*

AHA: July-Aug, 1984, 11; Sept-Oct, 1987, 9; Q2, 1989, 12; Q3, 1990, 3; Q2, 1992, 5; Q4, 1992, 22; Q1, 2003, 20

390–459

Documentation Issues

In cases where the diagnostic statement indicates hypertensive renal failure due to diabetes mellitus, report the diabetes with renal manifestations from the series 250.4x and 403.91 to indicate the hypertensive renal failure. If the diagnostic statement indicates diabetes with chronic renal failure and hypertension secondary to hypervolemia, report codes from the series 250.4x and rubrics 405 and 585.

For coding and classification purposes, any condition classifiable to categories 585-587 with hypertension is presumed due to hypertension, so no cause and effect relationship need be stated or implied in the diagnostic statement.

Coding Clarification

Hypertensive Renal Disease: Category 403 identifies hypertensive renal disease with renal failure with the fifth-digit assignment of "1." For example, in many cases renal failure is seen in hypertensive renal disease only when the hypertension becomes malignant or accelerated. In these cases, only one code is necessary, 403.01 *Hypertensive renal disease, malignant, with renal failure.* Category 403 excludes acute renal failure; when this is noted, an additional code will be required from category 584 *Acute renal failure.*

Nephrosclerosis: This condition is presumed to be a secondary process of hypertensive renal disease. When chronic renal failure is documented as secondary to nephrosclerosis, only one code is necessary. The code is selected from category 403 *Hypertensive renal disease,* with the fifth-digit subclassification of "1" to identify the renal failure.

Coding Scenario

The physician's final diagnosis states hypertensive renal disease with chronic renal failure due to diabetes, Type II.

> Code assignment: 250.40 *Diabetes with renal manifestations, Type II* and 403.91 *Hypertensive renal disease, unspecified, with renal failure*

A patient is seen for acute renal failure that has an established hypertensive renal nephrosclerosis.

> Code assignment: 584.9 *Acute renal failure, unspecified* and 403.91 *Hypertensive renal disease, unspecified, with renal failure*

404 Hypertensive heart and renal disease

AHA: July-Aug, 1984, 11; July-Aug, 1984, 14; Sept-Oct, 1987, 9; Q2, 1989, 12; Q3, 1990, 3; Q4, 2002, 49

This category is used for combined forms of heart and renal disease as classified in categories 402 and 403.

The following fifth-digit subclassification is for use with category 404:

- 0 without mention of congestive heart failure or renal failure
- 1 with congestive heart failure
- 2 with renal failure
- 3 with congestive heart failure and renal failure

404.0 ✓5th Hypertensive heart and renal disease, malignant

404.1 ✓5th Hypertensive heart and renal disease, benign

404.9 ✓5th Unspecified hypertensive heart and renal disease

Documentation Issues

For coding and classification purposes, the heart disease must be stated or implied as due to hypertension, but the renal disease may be presumed. For example, the statement "hypertensive heart failure and chronic renal failure" would be coded 404.93 even though hypertension is not the stated cause of the chronic renal failure.

Coding Clarification

Hypertensive Heart and Renal Disease: Category 404 identifies hypertensive heart and renal disease and has a fifth-digit subclassification to identify renal failure. For example, in many cases renal failure is only seen in hypertensive heart and renal disease when the hypertension becomes malignant or accelerated. In these cases, only one code is necessary, 404.02 *Hypertensive heart and renal disease, malignant, with renal failure.* Category 404 excludes acute renal failure; when this is noted, an additional code is required from category 584 *Acute renal failure.*

Coding Scenario

A patient is admitted with a diagnosis of heart failure. Record documentation identifies that the patient has benign hypertensive heart and renal disease with chronic renal failure in addition to the heart failure.

> Code assignment: 404.13 *Hypertensive heart and renal disease, benign, with heart failure and renal failure*

405 Secondary hypertension

AHA: July-Aug, 1984, 11; July-Aug, 1984, 14; Sept-Oct, 1987, 9,11; Q2, 1989, 12; Q3, 1990, 3

Secondary hypertension is a condition caused by renovascular or other diseases. Renovascular hypertension is the obstruction of renal blood flow at the level of the renal artery. The obstruction stimulates the renin-angiotensin system causing an increase in systemic angiotensin, which in turn causes the retention of sodium and water resulting in hypertension. Surgical reconstruction of the renal artery or percutaneous transluminal angioplasty may be performed to relieve the obstruction. Other causes

 © 2004 Ingenix, Inc.

of secondary hypertension include renal parenchymal diseases, oral contraceptives, primary aldosteronism, Cushing's syndrome, pheochromocytoma, hyperparathyroidism, hyperthyroidism, and acromegaly.

405.01 Secondary renovascular hypertension, malignant — *severe high blood pressure as a result of an underlying disease or condition*
AHA: July-Aug, 1984, 11; July-Aug, 1984, 14; Sept-Oct, 1987, 9,11; Q2, 1989, 12; Q3, 1990, 3

405.09 Other secondary hypertension, malignant — *severe high blood pressure as a result of an underlying disease or condition*
AHA: July-Aug, 1984, 11; July-Aug, 1984, 14; Sept-Oct, 1987, 9,11; Q2, 1989, 12; Q3, 1990, 3

405.11 Secondary renovascular hypertension, benign — *mild high blood pressure as a result of an underlying disease or condition*
AHA: July-Aug, 1984, 11; July-Aug, 1984, 14; Sept-Oct, 1987, 9,11; Q2, 1989, 12; Q3, 1990, 3

405.19 Other secondary hypertension, benign — *mild high blood pressure as a result of an underlying disease or condition*
AHA: July-Aug, 1984, 11; July-Aug, 1984, 14; Sept-Oct, 1987, 9,11; Q2, 1989, 12; Q3, 1990, 3

405.91 Secondary renovascular hypertension, unspecified — *high blood pressure of unknown degree as a result of an underlying disease or condition*
AHA: July-Aug, 1984, 11; July-Aug, 1984, 14; Sept-Oct, 1987, 9,11; Q2, 1989, 12; Q3, 1990, 3; Q3, 2000, 4

405.99 Other secondary hypertension, unspecified — *high blood pressure of unknown degree as a result of an underlying disease or condition*
AHA: July-Aug, 1984, 11; July-Aug, 1984, 14; Sept-Oct, 1987, 9,11; Q2, 1989, 12; Q3, 1990, 3; Q3, 2000, 4

Coding Clarification

ICD-9-CM separates only renovascular hypertension from all other etiologies at the fifth-digit level. Renal parenchymal diseases are conditions that reduce kidney function by affecting the kidney's ability to excrete water and sodium and are not the same as renovascular hypertension. Do not code renal parenchymal disease to the neovascular fifth-digit "1."

Secondary Hypertension: Category 405 *Secondary hypertension* does not include renal failure, so two codes are necessary to identify cases of renal failure with secondary hypertension.

Coding Scenario

A 55-year-old male is admitted with hypertension due to hypervolemia as a direct result of his chronic renal failure. Patient history indicates that the patient is an adult onset insulin-dependent diabetic with renal failure.

> Code assignment: 250.40 *Diabetes with renal manifestations, adult-onset Type II*, 405.99 *Other secondary hypertension, unspecified*, 276.6 *Fluid overload*, and 585 *Chronic renal failure*

410–414 Ischemic Heart Disease

Ischemic heart disease is an inadequate flow of blood through the coronary arteries to the tissue of the heart. The predominant etiology of the ischemia is arteriosclerosis. Partially obstructed coronary artery blood flow can manifest in angina pectoris; complete obstruction results in an infarction of the myocardium.

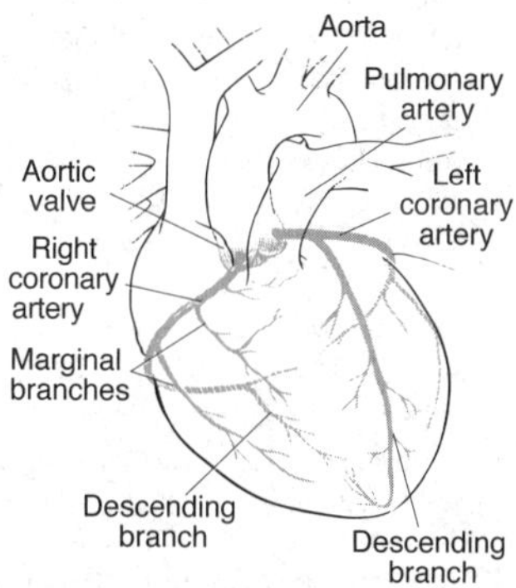

410 Acute myocardial infarction

AHA: July-Aug, 1984, 5; Q3, 1989, 3; Q1, 1991, 14; Q3, 1991, 10,18; Q1, 1992, 10; Q4, 1992, 24; Q3, 1995, 9; Q4, 1997, 37; Q3, 1998, 15; Q3, 2001, 21

Rubric 410 reports sudden partial or total reduction in the supply of blood to the heart, which results in necrosis of the myocardium. Occlusion of one of the coronary arteries due to thrombosis is believed to be the most common etiology. Other possible precipitating conditions include prolonged coronary artery spasm, subintimal hemorrhage at the site of atheromatous narrowing, and nonocclusive etiologies such as postoperative or traumatic shock, gastrointestinal bleeding with acute blood loss anemia, hypotension, and dehydration.

The following fifth-digit subclassification is for use with category 410:

0 episode of care unspecified

Use when the source document does not contain sufficient information for the assignment of fifth digit 1 or 2.

1 initial episode of care

Use fifth digit 1 to designate the first episode of care (regardless of facility site) for a newly diagnosed myocardial infarction. The fifth digit 1 is assigned regardless of the number of times a patient may be transferred during the initial episode of care.

2 subsequent episode of care

Use fifth-digit 2 to designate an episode of care following the initial episode when the patient is admitted for further observation, evaluation, or treatment for a myocardial infarction that has received initial treatment, but is still less than eight weeks old.

410.0 ✓5th Acute myocardial infarction of anterolateral wall — (Use additional code to identify presence of hypertension: 401.0-405.9) — *coronary artery embolism, occlusion, rupture, thrombosis*
AHA: July-Aug, 1984, 5; Q3, 1989, 3; Q1, 1991, 14; Q3, 1991, 10,18; Q1, 1992, 10; Q4, 1992, 24; Q3, 1995, 9; Q4, 1997, 37; Q3, 1998, 15; Q3, 2001, 21

410.1 ✓5th Acute myocardial infarction of other anterior wall — (Use additional code to identify presence of hypertension: 401.0-405.9)

410.2 ✓5th Acute myocardial infarction of inferolateral wall — (Use additional code to identify presence of hypertension: 401.0-405.9) — *coronary artery embolism, occlusion, rupture, thrombosis*
AHA: July-Aug, 1984, 5; Q3, 1989, 3; Q1, 1991, 14; Q3, 1991, 10,18; Q1, 1992, 10; Q4, 1992, 24; Q3, 1995, 9; Q4, 1997, 37; Q3, 1998, 15; Q3, 2001, 21

410.3 ✓5th Acute myocardial infarction of inferoposterior wall — (Use additional code to identify presence of hypertension: 401.0-405.9) — *coronary artery embolism, occlusion, rupture, thrombosis*
AHA: July-Aug, 1984, 5; Q3, 1989, 3; Q1, 1991, 14; Q3, 1991, 10,18; Q1, 1992, 10; Q4, 1992, 24; Q3, 1995, 9; Q4, 1997, 37; Q3, 1998, 15; Q3, 2001, 21

410.4 ✓5th Acute myocardial infarction of other inferior wall — (Use additional code to identify presence of hypertension: 401.0-405.9) — *diaphragmatic wall or inferior wall, not otherwise specified; coronary artery embolism, occlusion, rupture, thrombosis*
AHA: July-Aug, 1984, 5; Q3, 1989, 3; Q1, 1991, 14; Q3, 1991, 10,18; Q1, 1992, 10; Q4, 1992, 24; Q3, 1995, 9; Q3, 1997, 10; Q4, 1997, 37; Q3, 1998, 15; Q4, 1999, 9; Q1, 2000, 7,26; Q3, 2001, 21

410.5 ✓5th Acute myocardial infarction of other lateral wall — (Use additional code to identify presence of hypertension: 401.0-405.9) — *apical-lateral, basal-lateral, high lateral, posterolateral; including coronary artery embolism, occlusion, rupture, thrombosis*
AHA: July-Aug, 1984, 5; Q3, 1989, 3; Q1, 1991, 14; Q3, 1991, 10,18; Q1, 1992, 10; Q4, 1992, 24; Q3, 1995, 9; Q4, 1997, 37; Q3, 1998, 15; Q3, 2001, 21

410.6 ✓5th Acute myocardial infarction, true posterior wall infarction — (Use additional code to identify presence of hypertension: 401.0-405.9) — *posterobasal, strictly posterior; including coronary artery embolism, occlusion, rupture, thrombosis*
AHA: July-Aug, 1984, 5; Q3, 1989, 3; Q1, 1991, 14; Q3, 1991, 10,18; Q1, 1992, 10; Q4, 1992, 24; Q3, 1995, 9; Q4, 1997, 37; Q3, 1998, 15; Q3, 2001, 21

410.7 ✓5th Acute myocardial infarction, subendocardial infarction — (Use additional code to identify presence of hypertension: 401.0-405.9) — *nontransmural; including coronary artery embolism, occlusion, rupture, thrombosis*
AHA: July-Aug, 1984, 5; Q3, 1989, 3; Q1, 1991, 14; Q3, 1991, 10,18; Q1, 1992, 10; Q4, 1992, 24; Q3, 1995, 9; Q4, 1997, 37; Q3, 1998, 15; Q1, 2000, 7; Q3, 2001, 21

410.8 ✓5th Acute myocardial infarction of other specified sites — (Use additional code to identify presence of hypertension: 401.0-405.9) — *not otherwise specified, including atrium, papillary muscle, septum alone; including coronary artery embolism, occlusion, rupture, thrombosis*
AHA: July-Aug, 1984, 5; Q3, 1989, 3; Q1, 1991, 14; Q3, 1991, 10,18; Q1, 1992, 10; Q4, 1992, 24; Q3, 1995, 9; Q4, 1997, 37; Q3, 1998, 15; Q3, 2001, 21

410.9 ✓5th Acute myocardial infarction, unspecified site — (Use additional code to identify presence of hypertension: 401.0-405.9) — *unknown site; including coronary artery embolism, occlusion, rupture, thrombosis*
AHA: July-Aug, 1984, 5; Q3, 1989, 3; Q1, 1991, 14; Q3, 1991, 10,18; Q1, 1992, 9; Q1, 1992, 10; Q4, 1992, 24; Q3, 1995, 9; Q1, 1996, 17; Q4, 1997, 37; Q3, 1998, 15; Q3, 2001, 21

Documentation Issues

A common documentation problem for myocardial infarctions is that the physician does not identify the site of the infarction. The site of the infarction must be documented in the medical record for accurate code selection. Contact the physician for identification and be sure the documentation is updated to identify the site.

 © 2004 Ingenix, Inc.

Coding Clarification

Use an additional code to identify presence of hypertension (401.0-405.9) with ischemic heart disease.

The fourth digits for rubric 410 identify the site of the acute myocardial infarction as identified on an EKG. One exception to this is the fourth digit 7, which is for subendocardial and nontransmural infarctions regardless of site. A subendocardial infarction is one that involves the pericardium and not the endocardium; a nontransmural infarction is one that fails to extend from the endocardium to the epicardium. "Non-Q-wave" infarctions also are classified here. In some instances, the diagnostic statement will include the term "subendocardial" or "nontransmural" along with a specific site for the infarction.

Acute myocardial infarction is classified as an initial episode of care when the history does not mention a previous infarction. A myocardial infarction of greater than eight weeks duration with persistent symptoms is classified to 414.8.

Duration: When a myocardial infarction is identified as occurring within an eight-week time frame, a code may be selected from category 410 and the appropriate fifth digit would identify the episode of care (e.g., initial, subsequent). If a myocardial infarction is noted of greater than eight weeks duration with persistent symptoms, use code 414.8.

Impending Myocardial Infarction: If the final diagnostic statement indicates an impending myocardial infarction, documentation should be reviewed to ensure that the myocardial infarction did not occur. If not, use code 411.1 *Intermediate coronary syndrome* to identify the condition.

Infarction of the Inferior Wall-Acute, Subsequent Episode: This is coded as 410.42. This is a correction for advice given in *Coding Clinic for ICD-9-CM* Fourth Quarter, 1999, page 9.

Multiple Myocardial Infarctions: The key to correct coding of multiple myocardial infarctions is to code all of the events as long as they occurred at different sites. Do not use two codes in an attempt to describe various sites if the patient had only one infarction. A reinfarction in the same episode occurring at the same site is considered an extension of the original MI and is not coded.

Reinfarction: If a reinfarction occurs at the same site of the myocardial infarction (an extension), it is only coded once. If the reinfarction or extension occurs at a different site of the heart, assign two codes from category 410.

Coding Scenario

A patient is admitted with congestive heart failure directly from the physician's office. Final diagnosis states acute anterior myocardial infarction with benign hypertensive cardiovascular disease and coronary atherosclerosis of native artery.

> Code assignment: 410.11 *Acute myocardial infarction of other anterior wall, initial episode of care*, 402.11 *Benign hypertensive heart disease, with congestive heart failure*, and 414.01 *Coronary atherosclerosis of nati[illegible]nary artery*

A patient is admitted for [illegible] catheterization. History identifies an acute [illegible]nterior wall infarction three weeks prior. The cardiac catheterization is performed, followed by a percutaneous transluminal coronary angioplasty.

> Code assignment: 410.42 *Acute myocardial infarction of other inferior wall, subsequent episode of care*

A 59-year-old male patient presents to the hospital as an emergency admission. The admitting diagnosis is severe cresendo angina. In an effort to avert an impending myocardial infarction, single vessel PTCA with thrombolic agent administration is performed. Despite these measures, the patient's condition evolves to an inferolateral wall myocardial infarction.

> Code assignment: 410.21 *Acute myocardial infarction of inferolateral wall, initial episode of care*

A 72-year-old female is admitted to observation with chest pain. Later in the day, she is admitted to the coronary care unit with a diagnosis of impending myocardial infarction. Discharge diagnosis states acute diaphragmatic wall myocardial infarction.

> Code assignment: 410.41 *Acute myocardial infarction of other inferior wall, initial episode of care*

A 65-year old male is admitted through the emergency department with an acute MI, initial episode beginning one hour prior to arrival. At discharge, the diagnosis listing is as follows: Subendocardial myocardial infarction, inferior wall 10/1/03, and infarction, inferolateral wall, 10/1/03.

> Code assignment: The patient has suffered two infarctions, so both are coded: 410.71 *Acute myocardial infarction, subendocardial infarction* and 410.21 *Acute myocardial infarction of inferolateral wall*

A patient is admitted to the facility via the emergency department with severe chest pain and shortness of breath. The final diagnosis is an acute nontransmural infarction complicated by acute respiratory failure.

> Code assignment: 410.71 *Acute myocardial infarction, subendocardial infarction* and 518.81 *Acute respiratory failure*

411 *Other acute and subacute forms of ischemic heart disease*

AHA: July-Aug, 1984, 5; Q3, 1991, 10,24; Q4, 1994, 55

This rubric includes all acute and subacute forms of ischemic heart disease excluding acute myocardial infarction. Acute forms of ischemia include conditions with a relatively short and severe course, and subacute forms of ischemia denote a course of ischemic disease that falls in between acute and chronic disease.

411.0 Postmyocardial infarction syndrome — (Use additional code to identify presence of hypertension: 401.0-405.9) — *fever, pain, and inflammation within six weeks of MI; Dressler's syndrome*
AHA: July-Aug, 1984, 5; Q3, 1991, 10,24; Q4, 1994, 55

411.1 Intermediate coronary syndrome — (Use additional code to identify presence of hypertension: 401.0-405.9) — *impending infarction, preinfarction angina, unstable angina*
AHA: July-Aug, 1984, 5; Q4, 1989, 10; Q3, 1990, 6; Q1, 1991, 14; Q3, 1991, 24; Q3, 1991, 10,24; Q4, 1994, 55; Q2, 1996, 10; Q4, 1998, 86; Q2, 2001, 7,9; Q3, 2001, 15; Q1, 2003, 12

411.81 Acute coronary occlusion without myocardial infarction — (Use additional code to identify presence of hypertension: 401.0-405.9) — *interruption of blood flow without death of heart tissue*
AHA: July-Aug, 1984, 5; Q3, 1989, 4; Q1, 1991, 14; Q3, 1991, 18; Q3, 1991, 24; Q3, 1991, 10,24; Q4, 1994, 55

411.89 Other acute and subacute form of ischemic heart disease — (Use additional code to identify presence of hypertension: 401.0-405.9) — *coronary insufficiency, subendocardial ischemia*
AHA: July-Aug, 1984, 5; Q3, 1989, 4; Q3, 1991, 18; Q3, 1991, 10,24; Q1, 1992, 9; Q4, 1994, 55; Q3, 2001, 14

Documentation Issues

Often, the diagnosis of "angina" is documented without further details. Clarification should be obtained from the physician as to the specific type of angina, because a patient who is admitted to the hospital would usually be treated for preinfarctional or unstable angina (411.1). If further specification cannot be obtained, the diagnosis of "angina" would be assigned code 413.9 *Other and unspecified angina pectoris.*

Angina identified in the documentation by terms such as preinfarction, crescendo, initial onset, or unstable should be reported with code 411.1 *Intermediate coronary syndrome.*

When documentation indicates "acute ischemic (coronary) heart disease" or "acute myocardial ischemia" and the diagnostic tests reveal no evidence of myocardial infarction and this is verified with the physician, it may be appropriate to use a code from category 411 *Other acute and subacute forms of ischemic heart disease.* Clarification must be obtained from the physician as to whether code 411.1 or 411.8x should be used or if it should be classified to ischemic anginal pain from the 413 category.

Coding Clarification

Postmyocardial infarction syndrome is reported with 411.0 and is a complication occurring several days to several weeks following an acute myocardial infarction. Also known as Dressler's syndrome, this condition is believed to be due to an antibody antigen reaction that takes place in the myocardial tissue during the healing phase of an infarction. Some patients will continue to experience unstable angina pectoris after their recent myocardial infarction because of persistent coronary artery disease. Do not confuse angina due to ischemic heart disease (coronary artery disease) following a myocardial infarction with postmyocardial infarction syndrome. Code postmyocardial angina due to myocardial ischemia to 413.9 or 411.1. Code Dressler's syndrome and postmyocardial angina due to postmyocardial infarction syndrome to 411.0.

Intermediate coronary syndrome is reported with 411.1 and is an intermediate state between angina pectoris of effort and acute myocardial infarction. Since the mortality rate for myocardial infarction is greatest within the first few hours, unstable angina, with its increased likelihood of impeding myocardial infarction, is a medical emergency and requires acute care hospitalization. The term "class III' and "class IV" describing the functional classification of patients with heart disease may be used in conjunction with unstable angina. However, do not assume every patient with class III or class IV angina or heart disease has unstable angina. Code 411.1 cannot be assigned when the condition evolves into a myocardial infarction for which a code from rubric 410 will be assigned.

Coronary occlusion without myocardial infarction is reported with 411.81. This code classifies patients with an acute or subacute, complete or incomplete, occlusion of the coronary artery, not associated with acute myocardial infarction. The occlusion may be embolic, thrombotic, other, or unspecified and will usually be associated with some form of angina. This code may be used in conjunction with a diagnosis of stable or unstable angina.

 © 2004 Ingenix, Inc.

Coding Scenario

A patient is admitted with a severe anginal episode. A cardiac catheterization is performed and a diagnosis of an incomplete coronary artery occlusion is established. Documentation in the record indicates that an infarction did not occur. Final diagnosis is an incomplete coronary artery occlusion with severe angina.

> Code assignment: 411.81 *Acute coronary occlusion without myocardial infarction* and 413.9 *Other and unspecified angina pectoris*

A 63-year-old female is admitted with unstable angina. After successful treatment with IV thrombolytic agents, the patient is discharged.

> Code assignment: 411.1 *Intermediate coronary syndrome*

A patient is admitted with severe chest pain resembling an acute myocardial infarction and TPA is administered. After the TPA administration, the physician documents aborted myocardial infarction and subsequently transfers the patient to another facility for further diagnostic testing.

> Code assignment: 411.1 *Intermediate coronary syndrome*

412 Old myocardial infarction OK

AHA: July-Aug, 1984, 5; Q3, 1990, 7; Q2, 1991, 22; Q3, 1991, 10; Q3, 1998, 15; Q2, 2001, 9; Q2, 2003, 10

This rubric includes diagnoses with a history of myocardial infarction. These patients usually demonstrate EKG changes but currently present no symptoms and warrant no clinical intervention.

Coding Clarification

Patients can have both an acute myocardial infarction and an old myocardial infarction in different sites during the same episode of care. Code both conditions. Also, it is possible that an old myocardial infarction may "reinfarct," extending the degree of necrosis at the site of the old myocardial infarction. In this case, code only the acute myocardial infarction.

Coding Scenario

A patient is admitted for treatment of impending myocardial infarction with a known history of coronary atherosclerosis, status post myocardial infarction several years ago. After the patient is treated with intravenous thrombolytic agents, the acute myocardial infarction is averted.

> Code assignment: 414.01 *Coronary atherosclerosis of native coronary artery,* 411.1 *Intermediate coronary syndrome,* and 412 *Old myocardial infarction*

413 Angina pectoris

AHA: July-Aug, 1984, 5; Q3, 1991, 10

Angina pectoris is a clinical syndrome due to myocardial ischemia caused by atherosclerotic heart disease, but may be due to coronary artery spasm, severe aortic stenosis or insufficiency, syphilitic aortitis, vasculitis, marked anemia, paroxysmal tachycardia with rapid ventricular rates, or any disease or disorder that markedly increases metabolic demands. Angina decubitus is a form of angina occurring at night or when the patient is resting quietly. Prinzmetal angina is a variant characterized by chest pain at rest and by sinus tachycardia (ST) segment elevation, rather than depression, during the attack.

413.0 Angina decubitus — (Use additional code to identify presence of hypertension: 401.0-405.9) — *nocturnal angina; occurs only when lying down*
AHA: July-Aug, 1984, 5; Q3, 1991, 10

413.1 Prinzmetal angina — (Use additional code to identify presence of hypertension: 401.0-405.9) — *occurs when lying down; associated with ST-segment elevations; variant angina pectoris*
AHA: July-Aug, 1984, 5; Q3, 1991, 10

413.9 Other and unspecified angina pectoris — (Use additional code to identify presence of hypertension: 401.0-405.9) — *Herberden's, Likoff's, X syndromes; syncope anginosa, stenocardia*
AHA: July-Aug, 1984, 5; Q3, 1990, 6; Q3, 1991, 10; Q3, 1991, 16; Q3, 2002, 4

Documentation Issues

Often, the diagnosis of "angina" is documented without further details. Clarification should be obtained from the physician as to the specific type of angina, because a patient who is admitted to the hospital would usually be treated for preinfarctional or unstable angina (411.1). If further specification cannot be obtained, the diagnosis of "angina" would be assigned code 413.9 *Other and unspecified angina pectoris.*

Angina identified in the documentation by terms such as preinfarction, crescendo, initial onset, or unstable, should be reported with code 411.1 *Intermediate coronary syndrome.*

When documentation indicates "acute ischemic (coronary) heart disease" or "acute myocardial ischemia" and the diagnostic tests reveal no evidence of myocardial infarction and this is verified with the physician, it may be appropriate to use a code from category 411 *Other acute and subacute forms of ischemic heart disease.* Clarification must be obtained from the physician as to whether code 411.1 or 411.8x should be used or if it should be classified to ischemic anginal pain from the 413 category.

If the physician documents a diagnosis of hypertensive cardiovascular disease, review the documentation in the record for any mention of angina pectoris, arteriosclerosis, or chronic myocardial ischemia. If any of these are present, code them in addition.

Only if documentation identifies that angina was a complication of a procedure should it be coded as such.

If the patient is admitted with unstable angina but the documentation states that the condition progressed to a myocardial infarction, only code the infarction.

Angina due to coronary atherosclerosis or coronary artery disease must be documented as such. If the etiology of the angina is not documented, the code for the angina is listed first. When the etiology (e.g., atherosclerosis) is documented, the code for that condition should be listed first.

When a patient is admitted with unstable angina and then has a cardiac catheterization that identifies coronary atherosclerosis as the cause of the angina, the atherosclerosis would be listed as the principal/primary diagnosis and the unstable angina as secondary.

If the diagnosis is documented as atherosclerosis, verify the site of the disease with the physician.

Coding Clarification

Report 413.9 for angina not specified or classified elsewhere, including stable angina pectoris. Angina described with class I or class II heart disease is often classified to 413.9; do not equate these functional classifications of heart disease as synonymous for stable angina.

Assignment of a code from rubric 413 cannot be made in addition to a code from rubric 410 for the same episode of care.

Coexisting Conditions: These conditions should not be coded unless they require or affect patient care treatment or management. In many cases angina may be asymptomatic, but if still being treated it would qualify as a reportable condition and should be coded. Do not code conditions that were previously treated and no longer exist.

Intermediate Coronary Syndrome: This condition is also known as unstable angina, preinfarction angina, or crescendo angina. This condition represents an intermediate stage between angina of effort and acute myocardial infarction. The patient's pain is more acute, longer lasting and more frequent then angina, and more resistant to anti-anginal treatment. This type of angina often results in an acute myocardial infarction. Initial onset of angina is also classified to code 411.1. Code 413.9 excludes preinfarctional angina.

Myocardial Infarction with Angina: Angina is a symptom of the myocardial infarction and should not be coded in addition.

Other and Unspecified: Code 413.9 encompasses the commonly and uncommonly used descriptors that are not specific to codes 413.0 and 413.1 (e.g., anginal syndrome, status anginosus, stenocardia), typically stable forms of angina. Make sure you use the following guidelines:

- Code the significant sign or symptom that prompted the admission if no actual clinical diagnosis is documented
- Code the condition that was concluded after study
- Use a code from category V71 if no other diagnosis was made

Postinfarctional Angina: Code selection is based on the type of angina indicated. If unstable, assign code 411.1 *Intermediate coronary syndrome.* If stable, use code 413.9 *Other and unspecified angina pectoris.*

Coding Scenario

A patient is admitted with hypertensive cardiovascular disease. Documentation identifies that the patient was having chest pain due to angina. The physician's final diagnosis is hypertensive cardiovascular disease, benign, with angina pectoris.

> Code assignment: 402.10 *Benign hypertensive heart disease, without heart failure* and 413.9 *Other and unspecified angina pectoris*

A 59-year-old male is admitted to the facility with chest pain and possible myocardial infarction. After study the patient is diagnosed with an acute anginal attack. The physician indicates in his final diagnosis that the myocardial infarction was ruled out.

> Code assignment: 413.9 *Other and unspecified angina pectoris*

A patient is admitted with a severe anginal episode. A cardiac catheterization is performed and a diagnosis of an incomplete coronary artery occlusion is established. Documentation in the record indicates that an infarction did not occur. Final diagnosis is an incomplete coronary artery occlusion with severe angina.

> Code assignment: 411.81 *Acute coronary occlusion without myocardial infarcation* and 413.9 *Other and unspecified angina pectoris*

A patient is admitted via the emergency department with chest pain. The physician's final diagnosis is chest pain, due to either angina or esophageal spasm.

 © 2004 Ingenix, Inc.

Code assignment: 786.50 *Chest pain, unspecified,* 413.9 *Other and unspecified angina pectoris,* and 530.5 *Dyskinesia of esophagus*

A 67-year-old male is admitted to the facility with stable angina. After performing a combined left and right cardiac catheterization, the physician determines that the patient has severe atherosclerotic heart disease. The patient has no previous history of bypass grafting.

Code assignment: 414.01 *Coronary atherosclerosis of native coronary artery* and 413.9 *Other and unspecified angina pectoris*

A patient is seen in the outpatient clinic for a follow-up visit for hypertension and angina. The physician prescribes nitroglycerin for the angina and a diuretic for the hypertension. The patient history also identifies the patient had pneumonia six months ago.

Code assignment: 401.9 *Essential hypertension, unspecified* and 413.9 *Angina pectoris, unspecified*

414 Other forms of chronic ischemic heart disease

AHA: July-Aug, 1984, 5; Q3, 1991, 10

This rubric classifies obstruction of blood flow to the heart, usually due to a mechanical obstruction of one or more of the coronary arteries. Obliterative atherosclerosis of the coronary arteries is by far the most common form of ischemic heart disease. In time, the accumulations may calcify throughout the cardiovascular system, leading to the condition known as "hardening of the arteries."

Coronary atherosclerosis is localized, subintimal accumulations of fatty and fibrous tissue caused by proliferation of smooth muscle cells in combination with a disorder of lipid metabolism. Atherosclerotic heart disease eventually leads to acute and subacute forms of ischemic heart disease such as unstable angina and myocardial infarction.

Aneurysm of the heart is a dilatation, stretching, weakening, or bulging of the tissue of the heart or of the coronary arteries. An aneurysm of the heart wall is an aneurysm of heart muscle, known as a cardiac, mural, or ventricular wall aneurysm, which is usually a consequence of myocardial infarction. Aneurysm of the coronary vessels is a circumscribed dilation of a coronary artery or a blood-containing tumor connecting directly with the lumen of a coronary artery.

414.00 Coronary atherosclerosis of unspecified type of vessel, native or graft — (Use additional code to identify presence of hypertension: 401.0-405.9)

414.01 Coronary atherosclerosis of native coronary artery — (Use additional code to identify presence of hypertension: 401.0-405.9) — *ASHD, arteriosclerosis, arteritis, atheroma, sclerosis, stricture in natural heart vessels*
AHA: July-Aug, 1984, 5; Q3, 1990, 7; Q3, 1991, 10; Q1, 1994, 6; Q2, 1994, 13; Q4, 1994, 49; Q2, 1995, 17; Q2, 1996, 10; Q4, 1996, 31; Q2, 1997, 13; Q3, 1997, 15; Q2, 2001, 8,9; Q3, 2001, 15; Q3, 2002, 4-9; Q3, 2003, 9, 14; Q4, 2003, 105, 108

414.02 Coronary atherosclerosis of autologous vein bypass graft — (Use additional code to identify presence of hypertension: 401.0-405.9) — *plaque deposit in grafted vein originating within patient*
AHA: July-Aug, 1984, 5; Q3, 1990, 7; Q3, 1991, 10; Q1, 1994, 6; Q2, 1994, 13; Q4, 1994, 49; Q2, 1995, 17; Q2, 1997, 13

414.03 Coronary atherosclerosis of nonautologous biological bypass graft — (Use additional code to identify presence of hypertension: 401.0-405.9) — *plaque deposit in grafted vessel originating outside patient*
AHA: July-Aug, 1984, 5; Q3, 1990, 7; Q3, 1991, 10; Q1, 1994, 6; Q2, 1994, 13; Q4, 1994, 49; Q2, 1995, 17; Q2, 1997, 13

414.04 Coronary atherosclerosis of artery bypass graft — (Use additional code to identify presence of hypertension: 401.0-405.9) — *plaque deposit in grafted artery originating within patient*
AHA: July-Aug, 1984, 5; Q3, 1990, 7; Q3, 1991, 10; Q1, 1994, 6; Q2, 1994, 13; Q4, 1994, 49; Q2, 1995, 17; Q4, 1996, 31; Q2, 1997, 13

414.05 Coronary atherosclerosis of unspecified type of bypass graft — (Use additional code to identify presence of hypertension: 401.0-405.9) — *plaque deposit in grafted vessel of unknown origin*
AHA: July-Aug, 1984, 5; Q3, 1990, 7; Q3, 1991, 10; Q1, 1994, 6; Q2, 1994, 13; Q4, 1994, 49; Q2, 1995, 17; Q4, 1996, 31; Q2, 1997, 13; Q3, 1997, 15

414.06 Coronary atherosclerosis, of native coronary artery of transplanted heart — (Use additional code to identify presence of hypertension: 401.0-405.9)

414.07 Coronary atherosclerosis, Of bypass graft (artery) (vein) of transplanted heart — (Use additional code to identify presence of hypertension: 401.0-405.9)

414.10 Aneurysm of heart — (Use additional code to identify presence of hypertension: 401.0-405.9) — *dilation of a wall in the heart*
AHA: July-Aug, 1984, 5; Q3, 1991, 10; Q4, 2002, 54

390–459

414.11 Aneurysm of coronary vessels — (Use additional code to identify presence of hypertension: 401.0-405.9) — *dilation of a wall of a coronary vessel*
AHA: July-Aug, 1984, 5; Q3, 1991, 10; Q1, 1999, 17; Q4, 2002, 54; Q3, 2003, 10

414.12 Dissection of coronary artery — (Use additional code to identify presence of hypertension: 401.0-405.9)

414.19 Other aneurysm of heart — (Use additional code to identify presence of hypertension: 401.0-405.9) — *acquired arteriovenous fistula*
AHA: July-Aug, 1984, 5; Q3, 1991, 10; Q4, 2002, 54

AHA: July-Aug, 1984, 5; Q3, 1991, 10; Q4, 2002, 54

414.8 Other specified forms of chronic ischemic heart disease — (Use additional code to identify presence of hypertension: 401.0-405.9) — *chronic coronary insufficiency, chronic myocardial ischemia*
AHA: July-Aug, 1984, 5; Q2, 1990, 19; Q3, 1990, 7,15; Q3, 1991, 10; Q1, 1992, 10; Q3, 2001, 15

414.9 Unspecified chronic ischemic heart disease — (Use additional code to identify presence of hypertension: 401.0-405.9) — *unknown or not otherwise specified*
AHA: July-Aug, 1984, 5; Q3, 1991, 10

Documentation Issues

If the physician documents both ischemic congestive cardiomyopathy and idiopathic ischemic cardiomyopathy, only one code is necessary as all ischemic cardiomyopathies are classified with code 414.8 *Other specified forms of chronic ischemic heart disease.*

When the documentation identifies a diabetic patient with cardiomyopathy, these conditions are coded as separate entities. The diabetic complication code 250.7x does not include cardiomyopathy.

Coding Clarification

Report 414.11 for abnormal communication between a coronary artery and vein resulting in the formation of an arteriovenous aneurysm, usually resulting from myocardial infarction. Report 414.19 for an arteriovenous fistula of the coronary vessels.

Myocardial Bridge: This condition has been identified as a congenital disorder that develops when the heart muscle wraps around the coronary artery causing constriction. This bridge typically builds over the middle component of the left anterior descending artery. There is increasing evidence that this condition causes conditions such as myocardial infarction, ischemia, ventricular fibrillation, conduction disturbances, and even sudden death. For reporting, use code 746.85 *Myocardial bridge, congenital* and a code that identifies chronic ischemic disease, 414.8.

Hypertension and Atherosclerosis: Hypertension frequently accelerates atherosclerosis and if both are documented, code both conditions. Systolic hypertension may be referenced as "arteriosclerotic hypertension" of the elderly. In younger patients, systolic hypertension may be associated with an arteriovenous fistula or thyrotoxicosis, and would be classified as a secondary hypertension.

Hypertensive cardiovascular arteriosclerotic disease with heart failure is coded 402.91. Use an additional code of 414.0x to identify the coronary arteriosclerosis.

Occlusion of Bypass Grafts: Coronary artery bypass graft occlusions are reported with codes 414.02 (autologous), 414.03 (nonautologous), 414.04 (of artery), 414.05 (unspecified type), and 414.07 (of transplanted heart). If the graft type is unknown, use code 414.05 *Coronary atherosclerosis of unspecified type of bypass graft.*

Post-Coronary Artery Bypass Graft: Although a coronary artery bypass was done, coronary artery disease (CAD) is still present. When a patient is admitted with unstable angina post coronary artery bypass graft, assign code 414.00 *Coronary atherosclerosis of unspecified type of vessel, native or graft* as the principal diagnosis and code 411.1 *Intermediate coronary syndrome.* Use code V45.81 as an additional code to identify the aortocoronary bypass status.

Re-occlusion Post PTCA: A PTCA leaves the coronary artery intact and no grafting is performed. When a PTCA is performed, a balloon device is used to apply pressure inside the vessel, which compresses the arteriosclerotic plaque against the wall of the artery. Re-occlusion is typically caused by progression of the disease or re-expansion of the plaque within the vessel. Assign code 414.0x *Coronary atherosclerosis,* unless the physician specifically indicates that re-occlusion was due to a complication of the procedure. Use code V45.82 as an additional code to identify the angioplasty status.

Peripheral: Arteriosclerosis (occlusive) of the extremities is reported with code 440.2x.

If the documentation indicates the patient has coronary artery disease with diastolic dysfunction, use code 414.9 *Chronic ischemic heart disease, unspecified.*

Ischemic Cardiomyopathy: The term "ischemic" cardiomyopathy is used to specify the condition in which ischemic heart disease causes diffuse fibrosis or multiple infarctions, resulting in heart failure with left ventricular dilation. All ischemic heart diseases are classified to the code series 410-414. Unless more specific documentation is obtained from the physician, ischemic cardiomyopathy is reported with

 © 2004 Ingenix, Inc.

code 414.8 *Other specified forms of chronic ischemic heart disease.*

Coding Scenario

A 56-year-old male is admitted for stent placement and vein allograft of a left anterior descending (LAD) aneurysm. Final diagnostic statement verifies the LAD aneurysm.

> Code assignment: 414.11 *Aneurysm of coronary vessels*

A patient previously diagnosed with atherosclerotic hypertension is now seen in the clinic for follow up. Medical record indicates coronary atherosclerosis and benign hypertension.

> Code assignment: 414.00 *Coronary atherosclerosis of unspecified type of vessel, native or graft* and 401.1 *Benign essential hypertension*

A 67-year-old male is admitted to the facility with stable angina. After performing a combined left and right cardiac catheterization, the physician determines that the patient has severe atherosclerotic heart disease. The patient has no previous history of bypass grafting.

> Code assignment: 414.01 *Coronary atherosclerosis of native coronary artery* and 413.9 *Other and unspecified angina pectoris*

A 63-year-old patient is seen in the office for progression of his coronary atherosclerosis. The patient has a history of a heart transplant five years ago.

> Code assignment: 414.06 *Coronary atherosclerosis of coronary artery of transplanted heart* and V42.1 *Organ or tissue replaced by transplant, heart*

A patient is admitted for treatment of impending myocardial infarction with a known history of coronary atherosclerosis, status post myocardial infarction several years ago. After the patient is treated with intravenous thrombolytic agents, the acute myocardial infarction is averted.

> Code assignment: 411.1 *Intermediate coronary syndrome,* 414.00 *Coronary atherosclerosis of unspecified type of vessel, native or graft,* and 412 *Old myocardial infarction*

415–417 Diseases of Pulmonary Circulation

Diseases of the pulmonary circulation include acute pulmonary heart disease (415), chronic pulmonary heart disease (416), and other diseases of the pulmonary circulation (417).

415 Acute pulmonary heart disease

Acute cor pulmonale is a dilation and failure of the right side of the heart due to pulmonary embolism. The condition is usually reversible. Pulmonary embolism and infarction is a condition that occurs when a thrombus, usually forming in the veins of the lower extremities or pelvis but may be secondary to atrial fibrillation or flutter, travels through the right-sided circulation, and becomes lodged in the pulmonary artery. Pulmonary infarction is the consequential hemorrhagic consolidation and necrosis of the lung parenchyma.

415.0 Acute cor pulmonale

415.11 Iatrogenic pulmonary embolism and infarction — *death of lung tissue due to blocked vessels from medical treatment*
AHA: Q4, 1990, 25; Q4, 1995, 58

415.19 Other pulmonary embolism and infarction — *not otherwise specified*
AHA: Q4, 1990, 25

416 Chronic pulmonary heart disease

Chronic pulmonary heart disease is a rare increase in pulmonary circulation, often resulting in right ventricular failure or fatal syncope.

Primary pulmonary hypertension is a condition characterized by pulmonary hypertension and raised pulmonary vascular resistance in the lungs in the absence of any other disease of the lungs or heart. It is marked by diffuse narrowing of the pulmonary arterioles and, in moderate to severe cases, formation of pulmonary thrombi and emboli. The clinical picture is similar to pulmonary hypertension from any other cause, and has a poor prognosis with patients developing severe right heart failure within two to three years.

Kyphoscoliotic heart disease arises from a forward and lateral deformity of the spine. It is characterized by difficult breathing, respiratory alkalosis, pulmonary hypertension, and, in severe cases, congestive heart failure. It is a form of chronic secondary pulmonary hypertension.

416.0 Primary pulmonary hypertension — *idiopathic pulmonary arteriosclerosis, pulmonary hyptertension, Arrillaga-Ayerza and Cardiacos negros syndromes*

416.1 Kyphoscoliotic heart disease — *high blood pressure within the lungs as a result of curvature of the spine*

416.8 Other chronic pulmonary heart diseases — *pulmonary hypertension, secondary*

416.9 Unspecified chronic pulmonary heart disease

Coding Clarification

Report 416.8 in cases of pulmonary hypertension secondary to a known etiology (excluding kyphoscoliosis), such as chronic bronchitis, chronic obstructive pulmonary disease, obesity-hypoventilation syndrome, chronic mountain

390–459

sickness, obstructive sleep apnea, and neuromuscular disease.

417 Other diseases of pulmonary circulation

Arteriovenous fistula of the pulmonary vessels is an abnormal communication between a pulmonary artery and vein that may result in embolization or ischemia. It may occur as a result of previous pulmonary infarction. An aneurysm of the pulmonary artery is a dilation of the pulmonary artery or a blood-containing tumor within the lumen of the pulmonary artery.

417.0 Arteriovenous fistula of pulmonary vessels — *abnormal communication between blood vessels within the lung*

417.1 Aneurysm of pulmonary artery — *dilation of the wall of the main artery in the lung*

417.8 Other specified disease of pulmonary circulation — *arteritis; rupture or stricture of pulmonary vessel, endarteritis*

417.9 Unspecified disease of pulmonary circulation

Coding Clarification

Both true and false (pseudo-) aneurysms are reported with 417.1

420–429 Other Forms of Heart Disease

This section covers inflammatory conditions of the pericardium, endocardium, and myocardium, as well as heart valve disorders, cardiomyopathies, and nerve conduction disorders of the heart.

420 Acute pericarditis

Acute pericarditis is inflammation of the fibroserous membrane that surrounds the heart. The inflammation may be described as fibrinous, serous, sanguineous, hemorrhagic, or purulent. Etiologies for acute pericarditis include myocardial infarction, Dressler's syndrome, viral and bacterial infections, collagen vascular disease, adverse reaction to drugs (such as procainamide, hydralazine, and isoniazid), metastatic disease, and uremia.

420.0 Acute pericarditis in diseases classified elsewhere — (Code first underlying disease: 017.9, 039.8, 066.8, 585) — *secondary to disease*

420.90 Unspecified acute pericarditis

420.91 Acute idiopathic pericarditis — *inflammation of heart lining, cause unknown*

420.99 Other acute pericarditis — *pneumococcal, purulent, staphylococcal, streptococcal, pneumopyopericardium, pyopericardium*

Coding Clarification

Subclassification 420.0 reports acute pericarditis in diseases classified elsewhere. Report the etiology first, then the manifestation.

Unspecified acute pericarditis, including cases in which the specific infective organism is unknown, or in which the etiology is unknown, is reported with 420.90. This code may also be used to report acute pericarditis due to a malignant neoplasm. Acute idiopathic pericarditis, a benign, nonspecific, or viral pericarditis that often follows upper respiratory infections, is reported with 420.91. Use this code only when other etiologies have been ruled out.

Report 420.99 for acute pericarditis caused by bacterial infection or when the acute pericarditis has no known etiology.

421 Acute and subacute endocarditis

Use this rubric for diseases in which the endocardium is inflamed, usually due to bacterial infection. A variety of organisms may cause endocarditis, but *Staphylococcus aureus* is the most common pathogen. Infection of previously damaged valves is due to *Viridans streptococci* or other organisms comprising normal oral flora and may be secondary to a dental procedure. Infection of a prosthetic valve usually is due to Staphylococci within the first two months of surgery, and Streptococci more than two months after surgery. Infection of normal valves is rare and usually associated with intravenous drug abuse.

421.0 Acute and subacute bacterial endocarditis — (Use additional code to identify infectious organism) — *bacterial, infective, lenta, malignant, purulent, septic, ulcerative, vegetative, SBE*
AHA: Q1, 1991, 15; Q1, 1999, 12

421.1 Acute and subacute infective endocarditis in diseases classified elsewhere — (Code first underlying disease: 002.0, 083.0, 116.0) — *sudden, severe inflammation of lining of the heart secondary to other disease*

421.9 Unspecified acute endocarditis

Coding Clarification

Acute endocarditis due to fungal infection is excluded from this rubric, and classified to rubrics 112 and 115.

422 Acute myocarditis

This rubric reports focal or diffuse inflammation of the myocardium that may be due to toxins, adverse reactions to drugs, or viral, bacterial, rickettsial, fungal, or parasitic disease.

In myocarditis in disease classified elsewhere, code first the underlying disease, as in influenza (487.8) or tuberculosis (017.9).

© 2004 Ingenix, Inc.

For acute myocarditis secondary to metastatic disease, report 422.99.

422.0 Acute myocarditis in diseases classified elsewhere — (Code first underlying disease: 017.9, 487.8) — *sudden severe inflammation of muscle of the heart secondary to other disease*

422.90 Unspecified acute myocarditis

422.91 Idiopathic myocarditis — *giant cell, isolated, nonspecific, Fiedler's myocarditis*

422.92 Septic myocarditis — (Use additional code to identify infectious organism) — *caused by bacteria, including pneumococcal and staphylococcal*

422.93 Toxic myocarditis — *as a reaction to a toxic substance*

422.99 Other acute myocarditis — *not otherwise specified*

Coding Clarification

Excluded from this rubric are myocarditis due rheumatic fever (391.2), to Coxsackie virus (074.23), diphtheritic infection (032.82), meningococcal infection (036.43), syphilis (093.82), and toxoplasmosis (130.3).

423 Other diseases of pericardium

Hemopericardium is the presence of blood in the pericardial sac. It includes cardiac tamponade due to hemoperitoneum. Emergency pericardiocentesis is usually performed.

Report adhesive pericarditis for adhesions between the two pericardial layers, between the heart and the pericardium, or between the pericardium and other contiguous structures in the chest.

Constrictive pericarditis is a diffuse thickening of the pericardium as a late effect of inflammation. Cardiac output is limited due to the reduced distensibility of the cardiac chambers, and filling pressures are increased in response to the external constrictive force placed on the heart by the pericardium. This condition may be associated with congestive heart failure.

423.0 Hemopericardium — *escape of blood into the lining of the heart*

423.1 Adhesive pericarditis — *adherent, fibrosis, milk spots, obliterative*

423.2 Constrictive pericarditis — *loss of elasticity; Concato's or Pick's disease, Gouley's syndrome*

423.8 Other specified diseases of pericardium — *not elsewhere specified; calcification, fistula, acquired diverticula, cholesterol pericarditis, cyst*
AHA: Q2, 1989, 12

423.9 Unspecified disease of pericardium

Coding Clarification

Excluded from this rubric is hemopericardium due to trauma, classified as an internal injury of the chest in rubric 860.

Report 423.8 for diseases of the pericardium not reported elsewhere in this rubric, including calcified pericardium, diverticula of pericardium, cyst of pericardium, and fistula of pericardium. Code 423.9 is usually reserved for cardiac tamponade due to nontraumatic pericardial effusion, not specified as hemorrhagic or due to hemopericardium, pericardial compression scarring, and pneumohemopericardium.

424 Other diseases of endocardium

This rubric includes diseases of the heart valves that are specified or presumed to be non-rheumatic in origin, classified to categories 394-397.

424.0 Mitral valve disorders — *incompetence, insufficiency, regurgitation, prolapse; ballooning posterior leaflet syndrome, Barlow's syndrome*
AHA: Nov-Dec, 1984, 8; Nov-Dec, 1987, 8; Q3, 1998, 11; Q2, 2000, 16

424.1 Aortic valve disorders — *incompetence, insufficiency, regurgitation, stenosis, nonrheumatic*
AHA: Nov-Dec, 1987, 8; Q4, 1988, 8

424.2 Tricuspid valve disorders, specified as nonrheumatic — *incompetence, insufficiency, regurgitation, stenosis, nonrheumatic*

424.3 Pulmonary valve disorders — *incompetence, insufficiency, regurgitation, stenosis, nonrheumatic*

424.90 Endocarditis, valve unspecified, unspecified cause — *incompetence, insufficiency, regurgitation, stenosis, endocardial tag, nonrheumatic, unknown cause*

424.91 Endocarditis in diseases classified elsewhere — (Code first underlying disease: 017.9, 710.0) — *secondary to underlying disease*

424.99 Other endocarditis, valve unspecified — *incompetence, insufficiency, regurgitation, stenosis, nonrheumatic, with specified cause*

Coding Clarification

Syphilitic endocarditis is excluded from 424.91 *Endocarditis in diseases classified elsewhere*. For this code, sequence first the underlying disease, for example, tuberculosis (017.9) or disseminated lupus erythematosus (710.0).

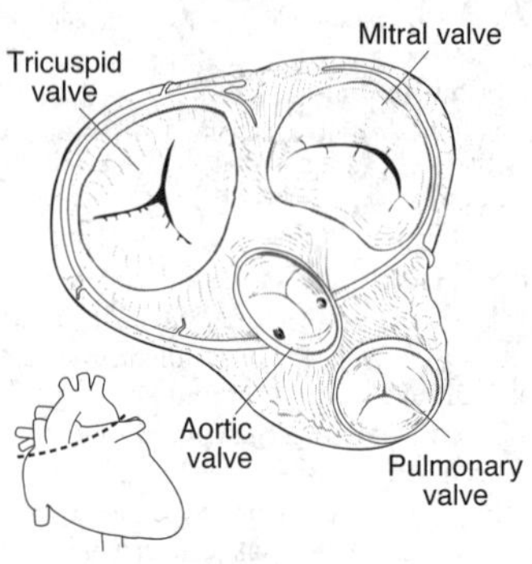

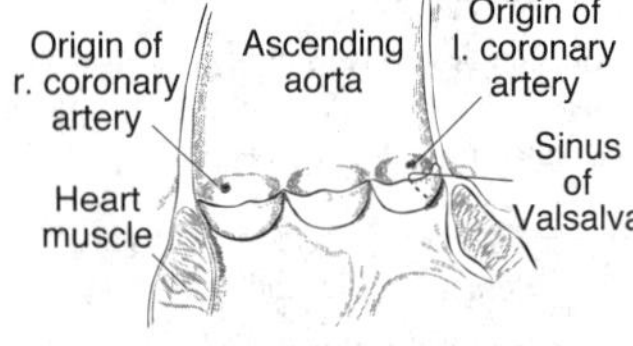

Depiction of opened aortic root showing semilunar cusps

425 Cardiomyopathy

AHA: July-Aug, 1985, 15

Cardiomyopathy is a complex and heterogenous group of diseases of the heart muscle. Rubric 425 includes diseases of the heart muscle itself that are classified to specific etiologies.

Endomyocardial fibrosis is a thickening of the ventricular endocardium due to fibrosis. Occasionally, the tricuspid and mitral valves may be involved and there is thrombus formation.

Hypertrophic obstructive cardiomyopathy, idiopathic hypertrophic subaortic stenosis, and asymmetrical septal hypertrophy are reported with 425.1. The etiology is believed to be an autosomal dominant genetic disorder and is characterized by an excessively hypertrophied interventricular septum. Left ventricular outflow obstruction results when the septum mechanically obstructs the anterior leaflet of the mitral valve.

425.0 Endomyocardial fibrosis — *fibrous tissue invading the muscle of the heart*
AHA: July-Aug, 1985, 15

425.1 Hypertrophic obstructive cardiomyopathy — *abnormal growth of the left ventricle wall causing obstructed blood flow; idiopathic hypertrophic subaortic stenosis*
AHA: July-Aug, 1985, 15

425.2 Obscure cardiomyopathy of Africa — *Becker's disease, South African cardiomyopathy syndrome, idiopathic mural endomyocardial disease*
AHA: July-Aug, 1985, 15

425.3 Endocardial fibroelastosis — *increased elastic tissue production with enlarged left ventricle wall; elastomyofibrosis*
AHA: July-Aug, 1985, 15

425.4 Other primary cardiomyopathies — *congestive, restrictive, familial, hypertrophic, idiopathic, nonobstructive, obstructive, restrictive, cardiovascular collagenosis*
AHA: July-Aug, 1985, 15; Q2, 1990, 19; Q4, 1997, 55; Q1, 2000, 22

425.5 Alcoholic cardiomyopathy — *heart disease resulting from excessive alcohol consumption*
AHA: Sept-Oct, 1985, 15; July-Aug, 1985, 15

425.7 Nutritional and metabolic cardiomyopathy — (Code first underlying disease: 242.00-242.91, 265.0, 271.0, 277.3, 277.5) — *secondary to specific underlying disease*
AHA: July-Aug, 1985, 15

425.8 Cardiomyopathy in other diseases classified elsewhere — (Code first underlying disease: 135, 334.0, 359.1, 359.2) — *secondary to specific underlying disease*
AHA: July-Aug, 1985, 15; Q2, 1993, 9

425.9 Unspecified secondary cardiomyopathy

Coding Clarification

Note that the term "cardiomyopathy" often is used for a disease or disorder that should be classified elsewhere. For example, the term, "ischemic cardiomyopathy" should be interpreted as ischemic heart disease and classified to the series 414.8.

Endomyocardial fibrosis is reported with 425.0.

Idiopathic cardiomegaly, idiopathic mural endomyocardial disease, Becker's disease, and South African cardiomyopathy are all types of obscure cardiomyopathy of Africa, reported with 425.2. These conditions are thought to be late effects of an infectious myocarditis, and are rarely encountered in the United States.

Endocardial fibroelastosis (425.3) is a congenital condition characterized by thickening of the endocardium and subendocardium, with malformation of the cardiac valves, hypertrophy of the heart, and proliferation of elastic tissue in the myocardium. It is also called elastomyofibrosis. Many patients with this condition do not survive infancy.

Report 425.4 for unspecified cardiomyopathy and cardiomyopathy of unknown or obscure etiology. Both obstructive cardiomyopathy and hypertrophic cardiomyopathy may be classified to 425.4, but the

© 2004 Ingenix, Inc.

combined form of hypertrophic obstructive cardiomyopathy is reported with 425.1.

For cardiomyopathy due to underlying disease, code first the underlying disease, then the myopathy with 435.7 or 435.8. Some examples of underlying disease include amyloidosis (277.3), beriberi (265.0), cardiac glycogenesis (271.0), mucopolysaccharidosis (277.5), thyrotoxicosis (242.0-242.9), Friedreich's ataxia (334.0), myotonia atrophica (359.1), and sarcoidosis (135). Subclassification 435.7 excludes gouty tophi of the heart, reported with 274.82, and subclassification 437.8 excludes cardiomyopathy in Chagas' disease (086.0).

Holiday Heart Syndrome: This condition is noted in patients with no known heart disease who develop cardiac arrhythmias due to acute alcohol consumption. The condition may appear in patients who are alcohol dependent (303.00) or nondependent (305.00). Two codes are necessary to identify this condition — one for the specific type of arrhythmia (e.g., atrial fibrillation, atrial flutter) and the other for the acute ingestion of alcohol. If the specific arrhythmia is not known, use code 427.9 *Cardiac dysrhythmia, unspecified.*

This syndrome may also be noted in patients with a diagnosis of chronic alcohol consumption with associated congestive cardiomyopathy. In this situation, three codes are required to accurately report the patient's diagnoses. Code the type of arrhythmia from category 427, the alcoholic cardiomyopathy with code 425.5, and the acute alcoholic intoxication in alcoholism, dependent with 303.00.

Congestive Cardiomyopathy: This condition, also known as congestive dilated cardiomyopathy (425.4), is a heart muscle disease of unknown etiology or a heart muscle disorder secondary to a disease elsewhere in the body. The symptoms are basically the same as those noted in congestive heart failure (CHF). It is possible to have a diagnosis of both congestive cardiomyopathy and congestive heart failure, and both conditions would be reported. In the majority of cases of CHF and cardiomyopathy, patient care revolves around the treatment of the CHF, and in those instances the CHF is listed first.

Diastolic Dysfunction: Cardiomyopathy can result in diastolic dysfunction. If documentation identifies that the diastolic dysfunction is due to cardiomyopathy, use code 425.4 *Other primary cardiomyopathies.*

Hypertensive Cardiomyopathy: If the physician documentation identifies that the hypertensive heart disease is the cause of the cardiomyopathy, use codes 402.9x *Unspecified hypertensive heart disease* and 425.8 *Cardiomyopathy in other diseases classified elsewhere.*

Coding Scenario

A patient is admitted with congestive heart failure and congestive cardiomyopathy.

> Code assignment: 428.0 *Congestive heart failure* and 425.4 *Other primary cardiomyopathies*

A patient is seen in the clinic for evaluation of treatment for hypertensive cardiomyopathy. Record documentation identifies that the cardiomyopathy was secondary to hypertensive heart disease.

> Code assignment: 402.90 *Unspecified hypertensive heart disease without mention of congestive heart failure* and 425.8 *Cardiomyopathy in other diseases classified elsewhere*

A patient's diagnostic condition is documented as idiopathic dilated cardiomyopathy.

> Code assignment: 425.4 *Other primary cardiomyopathies*

A patient is admitted in decompensated congestive failure resulting from end-stage cardiomyopathy. Laboratory findings are metabolic acidosis, elevated BUN/creatine, and elevated liver enzymes. The physician diagnoses both renal and heart failure and liver shock.

> Code assignment: 428.0 *Congestive heart failure, unspecified,* is the principal diagnosis. Assign 570 Subacute necrosis of the liver for the liver shock. Assign code 584.9 *Acute renal failure, unspecified* and 425.4 *Other primary cardiomyopathies*

426 Conduction disorders

Nerve conduction disorders include a group of conditions in which the transmission of cardiac electrical impulses controlling heart rhythm is abnormal, slowed, or interrupted.

Complete atrioventricular block is the most advanced form of heart block. Usually, there is a lesion distal to the bundle of His and is associated with bilateral bundle branch block. Some patients may go through periods of transition between partial and complete heart block.

426.0 Atrioventricular block, complete — *third degree atrioventricular block, Lev's and Rytand-Lipsitch syndrome*

426.10 Unspecified atrioventricular block — *AV block, incomplete or partial*

426.11 First degree atrioventricular block — *first degree incomplete AV block; prolonged P-R interval not specified elsewhere*

426.12 Mobitz (type) II atrioventricular block — *incomplete AV block, Mobitz Type II, second degree*

426.13 Other second degree atrioventricular block — *incomplete AV block, Mobitz, Type I, second degree; Wenckebach's phenomenon*

426.2 Left bundle branch hemiblock — *left anterior or posterior fascicular block*

390–459

390–459

426.3 Other left bundle branch block — *complete, main stem, anterior fascicular with posterior fascicular, not otherwise specified*

426.4 Right bundle branch block

426.50 Unspecified bundle branch block

426.51 Right bundle branch block and left posterior fascicular block

426.52 Right bundle branch block and left anterior fascicular block

426.53 Other bilateral bundle branch block — *bifascicular block not otherwise specified; right bundle ranch with left bundle brand block*

426.54 Trifascicular block

426.6 Other heart block — *intraventricular, diffuse, myofibrillar, sinoatrial, sinoauricular block*

426.7 Anomalous atrioventricular excitation — *accelerated, accessory, pre-excitation; including bundle of Kent syndrome, Wolff-Parkinson-White syndrome*

426.81 Lown-Ganong-Levine syndrome — *short P-R interval, normal QRS complexes, and supraventricular tachycardias*

426.89 Other specified conduction disorder — *AV, interference, isorhythmic dissociation, nonparoxysmal AV nodal tachycardia*

426.9 Unspecified conduction disorder

427 Cardiac dysrhythmias

AHA: July-Aug, 1985, 15

Cardiac dysrhythmias are disturbances in cardiac rate and rhythm, including abnormalities in the rate, regularity, and sequence of atrial and/or ventricular contractions. Cardiac dysrhythmias can take many forms; the clinical significance of each depends on the extent to which they lower blood pressure and reduce cardiac output with resulting hypoperfusion of vital organs such as the brain, kidneys, and the heart. Cardiac dysrhythmias may be benign or malignant, depending on the severity of the dysrhythmia and the patient's ability to tolerate it.

The etiology of cardiac dysrhythmia may be idiopathic, due to heart disease such as arteriosclerosis and rheumatic heart disease or due to other noncardiac etiologies such as thyrotoxicosis, alcoholism, trauma, and intravenous drug abuse. Many cardiac dysrhythmias are chronic, but acute dysrhythmias also can occur in cases of acute infection or digitalis toxicity. Symptoms may include fatigue, light-headedness, decreased exercise tolerance, or syncope, but often, there are no symptoms.

427.0 Paroxysmal supraventricular tachycardia — *very rapid atrial rhythm; including PAT, AV, junctional, nodal*
AHA: July-Aug, 1985, 15

427.1 Paroxysmal ventricular tachycardia — *very rapid ventricular rhythm*
AHA: July-Aug, 1985, 15; March-April, 1986, 11; Q3, 1995, 9

427.2 Unspecified paroxysmal tachycardia — *Bouveret-Hoffmann syndrome, essential paroxysmal tachycardia*
AHA: July-Aug, 1985, 15

427.31 Atrial fibrillation — *irregular, rapid atrial contractions*
AHA: July-Aug, 1985, 15; Q3, 1995, 9; Q2, 1999, 17; Q1, 2003, 8; Q4, 2003, 95, 105

427.32 Atrial flutter — *regular, rapid atrial contractions*
AHA: July-Aug, 1985, 15; Q4, 2003, 94

427.41 Ventricular fibrillation — *irregular, rapid ventricular contractions*
AHA: July-Aug, 1985, 15; Q3, 2002, 5

427.42 Ventricular flutter — *regular, rapid ventricular contractions*
AHA: July-Aug, 1985, 15

427.5 Cardiac arrest — *heart stops and atrial blood pressure flattens*
AHA: July-Aug, 1985, 15; Q2, 1988, 8; Q3, 1995, 8; Q2, 2000, 12; Q3, 2002, 5

427.60 Unspecified premature beats — *ectopic beats, extrasystolic arrhythmia, premature contractions; unknown site*
AHA: July-Aug, 1985, 15

427.61 Supraventricular premature beats — *ectopic beats, extrasystolic arrhythmia, premature contractions; atrial*
AHA: July-Aug, 1985, 15

427.69 Other premature beats — *ectopic beats, extrasystolic arrhythmia, premature contractions, site not otherwise specified*
AHA: July-Aug, 1985, 15; Q4, 1993, 42

427.81 Sinoatrial node dysfunction — *persistent or severe sinus bradycardia; including sick sinus syndrome*
AHA: July-Aug, 1985, 15; Q3, 2000, 8

427.89 Other specified cardiac dysrhythmias — *not otherwise specified, including bigeminy, trigeminy, split heart sounds, wandering pacemaker, gallop rhythm*
AHA: July-Aug, 1985, 15

427.9 Unspecified cardiac dysrhythmia

Coding Clarification

Congenital Long QT Syndrome: This condition is classified as a congenital anomaly of the heart, code 746.89. If torsade de pointe (ventricular arrhythmia with long QT interval) is noted, assign code 427.1 *Paroxysmal ventricular tachycardia* in addition to the congenital anomaly code.

© 2004 Ingenix, Inc.

Holiday Heart Syndrome: This condition is noted in patients with no known heart disease who develop cardiac arrhythmias due to acute alcohol consumption. The condition may appear in patients who are alcohol dependent (303.00) or nondependent (305.00). Two codes are necessary to identify this condition — one for the specific type of arrhythmia (e.g., atrial fibrillation, atrial flutter) and the other for the acute ingestion of alcohol. If the specific arrhythmia is not known use code 427.9 *Cardiac dysrhythmia, unspecified.*

This syndrome may also be noted in patients with a diagnosis of chronic alcohol consumption with associated congestive cardiomyopathy. In this situation, three codes are required to accurately report the patient's diagnoses. Code the type of arrhythmia from category 427, the alcoholic cardiomyopathy with code 425.5, and the acute alcoholic intoxication in alcoholism, dependent with 303.00.

Postural Orthostatic Tachycardia Syndrome (POTS): This condition is classified as a specified cardiac dysrhythmia, other, code 427.89. If orthostatic hypotension is noted, assign code 458.0. If the documentation identifies that any neurological factors are present, they should be coded also.

Ventricular Dysfunction: This condition is not a cardiac arrhythmia. The alphabetic index entry, Dysfunction, heart, 427.9, refers to dysrhythmia. The appropriate code for ventricular dysfunction, if a more definitive diagnosis cannot be established, is 428.9 *Unspecified heart failure.*

Coding Scenario

A patient receives ambulatory cardiac monitoring. The patient is being treated with antiarrhythmic drug therapy for paroxysmal tachycardia. Monitoring is being performed for effectiveness of drug therapy.

> Code assignment: 427.2 *Unspecified paroxysmal tachycardia*

A 59-year-old male is seen in the emergency department after passing out at an office party. The patient is extremely intoxicated but states that his heart is racing. The patient has a known alcohol dependency. EKG findings indicate atrial fibrillation. The physician's diagnosis states holiday heart syndrome with atrial fibrillation and acute alcoholic intoxication in alcoholism.

> Code assignment: 427.31 *Atrial fibrillation* and 303.00 *Acute alcoholic intoxication in alcoholism, dependent*

The diagnosis is documented as ventricular tachycardia secondary to holiday heart syndrome secondary to acute alcohol intoxication. The final diagnosis also indicates chronic alcoholism with alcoholic cardiomyopathy.

> Code assignment: 427.0 *Paroxysmal supraventricular tachycardia,* 425.5 *Alcoholic cardiomyopathy,* and 303.00 *Acute alcoholic intoxication in alcoholism, dependent*

428 Heart failure

AHA: Q3, 1988, 3; Q2, 1989, 10; Q2, 1990, 16, 19; Q3, 1998, 5; Q4, 2002, 49

Congestive heart failure is a mechanical inability of the heart to pump blood efficiently, thus compromising circulation and causing systemic complications due to congestion and edema of fluids in the tissues. Etiologies fall into three groups: disorders that decrease contractile function, disorders than increase myocardial overload, and abnormalities in myocardial preload.

Contractile function of the heart decreases when the myocardium has been damaged as in myocardial infarction, thus reducing the ventricles' ability to contract forcefully.

Increased myocardial afterload refers to the increased force that the myocardium must generate to contract the ventricles. For example, in acute and severe systemic hypertension, the force exerted upon the ventricle by increased blood pressure exceeds the force the ventricle must generate to contract, leading to pulmonary congestion.

Myocardial preload refers to the stretching of the myocardial fibers prior to myocardial contraction. Although this stretching increases the force-generating capabilities of the ventricles, eventually pulmonary congestion occurs when the ventricular filling pressure concomitantly increases.

In ICD-9-CM, congestive heart failure also is defined as right ventricular failure or right ventricular failure due to left ventricular failure. Right ventricular failure is most frequently due to failure of the left ventricle, but may occur independently of left ventricular failure. Chronic obstructive pulmonary disease can produce a pressure overload in the right ventricle independent of any failure on the left side.

428.0 Congestive heart failure, unspecified — *right heart failure; decreased efficiency of heart output causing fluid collection in lungs, hypertension, and congestion of the vessels*
AHA: Q3, 1988, 3; Q2, 1989, 10; Q2, 1989, 12; Q2, 1990, 16, 19; Q3, 1991, 18, 19; Q3, 1996, 9; Q3, 1997, 10; Q4, 1997, 55; Q3, 1998, 5; Q1, 1999, 11; Q4, 1999, 4; Q1, 2000, 22; Q2, 2000, 16; Q4, 2000, 48; Q2, 2001, 13; Q4, 2002, 49; Q4, 2002, 52; Q1, 2003, 9; Q4, 2003, 109

428.1 Left heart failure — *decreased efficiency of the left ventricle of the heart causing fluid in lungs*
AHA: Q3, 1988, 3; Q2, 1989, 10; Q2, 1990, 16, 19; Q3, 1998, 5; Q4, 2002, 49

390–459

428.20 Unspecified systolic heart failure

428.21 Acute systolic heart failure

428.22 Chronic systolic heart failure

428.23 Acute on chronic systolic heart failure

428.30 Unspecified diastolic heart failure

428.31 Acute diastolic heart failure

428.32 Chronic diastolic heart failure

428.33 Acute on chronic diastolic heart failure

428.40 Unspecified combined systolic and diastolic heart failure

428.41 Acute combined systolic and diastolic heart failure

428.42 Chronic combined systolic and diastolic heart failure

428.43 Acute on chronic combined systolic and diastolic heart failure

428.9 Unspecified heart failure — *unknown whether right or left*

AHA: Nov-Dec, 1985, 14; Q3, 1988, 3; Q2, 1989, 10; Q2, 1990, 16, 19; Q3, 1998, 5; Q4, 2002, 49

Documentation Issues

If the documentation indicates that the patient has congestive heart failure, review the record for any hypertensive heart or hypertensive heart and renal disease. If documentation identifies these conditions, a combination code may be used from categories 402 and 404.

Even if the patient is being seen for another condition, if the heart failure is noted in the record and the patient is still under treatment, the heart failure should be coded as a secondary condition.

Unless documentation identifies a cause and effect relationship between hypertension and congestive heart failure, they should be coded as separate entities, 428.0 and 401.x. However, if the documentation indicates the heart failure is due to the hypertension, only one code is necessary, 402.91.

If fluid overload is identified in conjunction with congestive heart failure, it is not coded separately because it is a component of the congestive heart failure.

When the documentation states an acute and chronic heart failure, check with the physician to see if the diagnosis refers to congestive heart failure, such as a congestive heart failure that has become decompensated. If so, use code 428.0. If no clarification can be obtained, use code 428.9 *Unspecified heart failure.*

Coding Clarification

Documentation of an impaired heart muscle or left ventricular dysfunction does not indicate heart failure unless symptoms of fatigue, shortness of breath, and fluid retention are documented. Documentation indicating impaired heart muscle implies definitive causes, such as virus or drug abuse. Documentation of idiopathic or dilated congested cardiomyopathy indicates only that there is four-chamber enlargement of the heart, which may occur without heart failure. Classify compensated and decompensated heart failure to 428.0.

Ventricular Dysfunction: This condition is not a cardiac arrhythmia. The alphabetic index entry, Dysfunction, heart 427.9, refers to dysrhythmia. The appropriate code for ventricular dysfunction, if a more definitive diagnosis cannot be established, is 428.9 *Unspecified heart failure.*

If the congestive heart failure occurs as a result of the patient noncompliance to diet, medication, or dialysis treatment, code the congestive heart failure (428.0) and use an additional code to identify the noncompliance (V15.81).

Etiology: In general, heart failure is defined as an abnormality of heart function and is accountable for the inability of the heart to pump blood at a rate adequate for tissue metabolism or can do so only from an abnormal filling pressure.

Congestive heart failure (CHF) is a typical manifestation of an underlying organic heart condition (e.g., arteriosclerotic, rheumatic, congenital) defined as the inability of the heart to supply adequate output relative to the body's requirement. Uncompensated congestive heart failure results in pulmonary edema.

Heart Transplant Complications: If the patient develops an illness that affects the transplanted organ it is coded as a complication of the transplanted organ (e.g., 996.83 *Complications of transplanted organ, heart*), and an additional diagnosis code is used to identify the illness that affected the organ (e.g., 428.0 *Congestive heart failure, unspecified*).

Myocardial Infarction with CHF: Congestive heart failure is a typical manifestation of a myocardial infarction and would be sequenced as a secondary diagnosis if an infarction is detected.

Pleural Effusion: Pleural effusion is typically noted in cases of heart failure because there is usually some collection of fluid in the pleural space. If pleural effusion is identified with heart failure, it should only be coded if it is specifically evaluated and treated.

Rheumatic: When heart failure is present with rheumatic aortic and mitral valve insufficiency, the heart failure is always classified as rheumatic.

 © 2004 Ingenix, Inc.

Types of Heart Failure

Right vs. Left-sided Heart Failure

- Right-sided heart failure is caused by liver hypertrophy, systemic venous congestion, pitting edema, or ascites due to congestion of fluid behind the left ventricle.
- Left-sided heart failure is demonstrated by paroxysmal nocturnal dyspnea, cardiac asthma, dyspnea, orthopnea, and/or acute pulmonary edema caused by the collection of excess fluid behind the left ventricle.

Low Output vs. High Output Heart Failure

- Low output can be defined as either left or right-sided heart failure. It may be due to ischemic heart disease, cardiomyopathy, hypertension, or valvular or pericardial disease.
- High output can develop with anemia, hyperthyroidism, arteriovenous fistulas, or beriberi and Paget's disease.

Compensated vs. Decompensated Heart Failure

- Compensated heart failure describes the state achieved when the heart develops compensatory mechanisms on a chronic basis such as increased force of contraction, elevated atrial pressures, hypertrophy, and ventricular dilation.
- Decompensated heart failure occurs when these measures are unable to handle the additional workload.

Coding Scenario

A patient is admitted with congestive heart failure and congestive cardiomyopathy.

> Code assignment: 428.0 *Congestive heart failure, unspecified* and 425.4 *Other primary cardiomyopathies*

A patient is admitted in decompensated congestive failure resulting from end-stage cardiomyopathy. Laboratory findings are: metabolic acidosis, elevated BUN/creatine, and elevated liver enzymes. The physician diagnosis both renal and heart failure and liver shock.

> Code assignment: 428.0 *Congestive heart failure, unspecified,* is the principal diagnosis. Assign 570 *Subacute necrosis of the liver* for the liver shock. Assign code 584.9 *Acute renal failure, unspecified* and 425.4 *Other primary cardiomyopathies*

A patient arrives in the emergency department with severe respiratory distress. The patient is found to have cardiogenic pulmonary edema and respiratory failure. Subsequently the patient is intubated in the emergency department and then admitted for treatment of the congestive heart failure.

> Code assignment: 428.0 *Congestive heart failure, unspecified* and 518.81 *Acute respiratory failure*

429 Ill-defined descriptions and complications of heart disease

429.0 Unspecified myocarditis — (Use additional code to identify presence of arteriosclerosis) — *inflammation, cause unknown, but not rheumatic*

429.1 Myocardial degeneration — (Use additional code to identify presence of arteriosclerosis) — *Beau's syndrome, softening, fatty, mural, muscular disease*

429.2 Unspecified cardiovascular disease — (Use additional code to identify presence of arteriosclerosis) — *ASCVD, specifics unknown*

429.3 Cardiomegaly — *enlargement of the heart; dilation, hypertrophy, dilatation*

429.4 Functional disturbances following cardiac surgery — *or due to prosthesis*
AHA: Nov-Dec, 1985, 6; Q2, 2002, 12

429.5 Rupture of chordae tendineae — *torn tissue between heart valves and papillary muscles*

429.6 Rupture of papillary muscle — *torn muscle between chordae tendineae and heart wall*

429.71 Acquired cardiac septal defect — (Use additional code to identify the associated myocardial infarction: with onset of 8 weeks of less, 410.00-410.92; with onset of more than 8 weeks, 414.8)

429.79 Other certain sequelae of myocardial infarction, not elsewhere classified — (Use additional code to identify the associated myocardial infarction: with onset of 8 weeks of less, 410.00-410.92; with onset of more than 8 weeks, 414.8) — *mural thrombus following MI, not otherwise specified*
AHA: Q3, 1989, 5; Q1, 1992, 10

429.81 Other disorders of papillary muscle — *atrophy, degeneration, dysfunction, incompetence, incoordination, scarring*

429.82 Hyperkinetic heart disease — *abnormally increased motor function of the heart*

429.89 Other ill-defined heart disease — *not specified elsewhere, including carditis, hemorrhage of heart, ventricular asynergy, ventricular dyssnergia*
AHA: Q1, 1992, 10

429.9 Unspecified heart disease — *unknown type or site*
AHA: Q1, 1993, 19

430–438 Cerebrovascular Disease

This section of ICD-9-CM classifies the acute, organic conditions of the cerebrovascular system. Conditions coded to this section are nontraumatic in origin and include hemorrhages, thromboses, embolisms, transient cerebral ischemia, other ill-defined cerebrovascular diseases, and the late effects of cerebrovascular disease.

430 Subarachnoid hemorrhage OK

AHA: March-April, 1985, 6; Q2, 1989, 8; Q3, 1990, 3; Q3, 1991, 10; Q1, 1993, 27

A subarachnoid hemorrhage is an extravasation of blood into the subarachnoid space. The episodes usually are sudden in nature and account for 5 to 10 percent of all cerebrovascular accidents. The etiology may be secondary to head trauma and classified to the injury chapter, or due to primary disease such as arteriosclerotic aneurysm, arteriovenous malformation, or hemorrhagic diathesis.

Coding Clarification

This rubric excludes syphilitic ruptured cerebral aneurysm (094.87).

431 Intracerebral hemorrhage OK

AHA: March-April, 1985, 6; Q2, 1989, 8; Q3, 1990, 3; Q3, 1991, 10; Q1, 1993, 27

An intracerebral hemorrhage is a spontaneous extravasation of blood within the brain. Etiologies include hypertension with microaneurysmal formation, bleeding diathesis (leukemia, thrombocytopenia, hemophilia), disseminated intravascular coagulation, anticoagulant therapy, liver disease, cerebral amyloid angiopathy, AV malformation, and brain neoplasms.

432 Other and unspecified intracranial hemorrhage

AHA: March-April, 1985, 6; Q2, 1989, 8; Q3, 1990, 3; Q3, 1991, 10; Q1, 1993, 27

This rubric classifies nontraumatic extradural (epidural) and subdural hemorrhage of the cerebrovascular system.

432.0 Nontraumatic extradural hemorrhage — (Use additional code to identify presence of hypertension) — *bleeding between the skull and the lining of the brain*
AHA: March-April, 1985, 6; Q2, 1989, 8; Q3, 1990, 3; Q3, 1991, 10; Q1, 1993, 27

432.1 Subdural hemorrhage — (Use additional code to identify presence of hypertension) — *bleeding between the outermost and other layers of the lining of the brain*
AHA: March-April, 1985, 6; Q2, 1989, 8; Q3, 1990, 3; Q3, 1991, 10; Q1, 1993, 27

432.9 Unspecified intracranial hemorrhage — (Use additional code to identify presence of hypertension) — *unknown site*
AHA: March-April, 1985, 6; Q2, 1989, 8; Q3, 1990, 3; Q3, 1991, 10; Q1, 1993, 27

Coding Clarification

Excluded from this rubric is extradural and subdural hemorrhage as a spinal cord vascular disease.

433 Occlusion and stenosis of precerebral arteries

AHA: March-April, 1985, 6; Q2, 1989, 8; Q3, 1990, 3,16; Q3, 1991, 10; Q1, 1993, 27; Q2, 1995, 14

The precerebral arteries — basilar, carotid, and vertebral — extend from the aortic arch. Blood is supplied to the brain by the internal carotid arteries and vertebral arteries. The right and left vertebral arteries come together at the base of the brain to form the basilar artery. The right common carotid originates in the innominate artery and the left common carotid is normally the second branch from the aortic arch. The common carotids have no branches until their terminal bifurcation. The internal carotid artery ascends through the base of the skull to give rise to the anterior and middle cerebral arteries. The external carotid artery supplies blood to the face and scalp. The vertebral arteries arise from the subclavian arteries and emerge from the posterior base of the skull to form the basilar artery. Occasionally, the basilar splits into two vessels that reunite. The vertebral artery takes blood to the basilar artery, and from there the blood goes to the circle of Willis, which controls blood pressure in the brain and allows a continued supply of oxygenated blood to the brain in the event that a vessel becomes occluded.

Syndromes of the aortic arch, also referred to as vertebral-basilar artery disease, carotid artery occlusive syndrome, and subclavian steal syndrome, are associated with structural defects resulting from athereosclerosis, trauma, blood clots, or congenital abnormalities of vessel structure. Atherosclerotic occlusive disease of the external portion of the carotid artery is the most common cause of a stroke. Strokes can result from a blocked blood vessel due to an embolism or a constriction or narrowing of an artery in the head or neck (stenosis). Bleeding of a blood vessel is called hemorrhagic stroke. Symptoms include neurologic changes (i.e., dizziness, blurred vision, or weakness), blood pressure changes, and reduced pulse. An embolism can obstruct the vessels causing damage from the lack of blood supply reaching the brain and can occur as a result of surgery if multiple punctures are required or if an atherosclerotic plaque becomes dislodged by the catheter or guidewire. Occlusion of the posterior cerebral arteries can result in loss of pain information from the face and vertigo.

 © 2004 Ingenix, Inc.

Occlusion of the superior cerebellar arteries interferes with the major output of the cerebellum.

The following fifth-digit subclassification is for use with categories 433 and 434:

0 without mention of cerebral infarction

1 with cerebral infarction

433.0 ✓5th Occlusion and stenosis of basilar artery — (Use additional code to identify presence of hypertension) — *embolism, narrowing, obstruction, thrombosis*
AHA: March-April, 1985, 6; Q2, 1989, 8; Q3, 1990, 3,16; Q3, 1991, 10; Q1, 1993, 27; Q2, 1995, 14

433.1 ✓5th Occlusion and stenosis of carotid artery — (Use additional code to identify presence of hypertension) — *embolism, narrowing, obstruction, thrombosis*
AHA: March-April, 1985, 6; Q2, 1989, 8; Q3, 1990, 3,16; Q3, 1991, 10; Q1, 1993, 27; Q2, 1995, 14; Q1, 2000, 16

433.2 ✓5th Occlusion and stenosis of vertebral artery — (Use additional code to identify presence of hypertension) — *embolism, narrowing, obstruction, thrombosis*
AHA: March-April, 1985, 6; Q2, 1989, 8; Q3, 1990, 3,16; Q3, 1991, 10; Q1, 1993, 27; Q2, 1995, 14

433.3 ✓5th Occlusion and stenosis of multiple and bilateral precerebral arteries — (Use additional code to identify presence of hypertension) — *embolism, narrowing, obstruction, thrombosis*
AHA: March-April, 1985, 6; Q2, 1989, 8; Q3, 1990, 3,16; Q3, 1991, 10; Q1, 1993, 27; Q2, 1995, 14; Q2, 2002, 19

433.8 ✓5th Occlusion and stenosis of other specified precerebral artery — (Use additional code to identify presence of hypertension) — *pontine, meningeal, hypophyseal, communicating posterior, choroidal, cerebellar, internal auditory, anterior spinal artery; embolism, narrowing, obstruction, thrombosis*
AHA: March-April, 1985, 6; Q2, 1989, 8; Q3, 1990, 3,16; Q3, 1991, 10; Q1, 1993, 27; Q2, 1995, 14

433.9 ✓5th Occlusion and stenosis of unspecified precerebral artery — (Use additional code to identify presence of hypertension) — *embolism, narrowing, obstruction, thrombosis; unknown site*
AHA: March-April, 1985, 6; Q2, 1989, 8; Q3, 1990, 3,16; Q3, 1991, 10; Q1, 1993, 27; Q2, 1995, 14

Coding Scenario

A patient is admitted via the emergency department with episodes of syncope, possible CVA. A bilateral cerebral arteriogram identifies bilateral carotid occlusions. The left carotid artery identifies a 75 percent occlusion and the right carotid at 95 percent occlusion. The patient undergoes a bilateral endarterectomy and is discharged in good condition. The final diagnosis is bilateral carotid occlusion.

Code assignment: 433.30 *Occlusion and stenosis of multiple and bilateral precerebral arteries, without mention of cerebral infarction*

434 Occlusion of cerebral arteries

AHA: March-April, 1985, 6; Q2, 1989, 8; Q3, 1990, 3; Q3, 1991, 10; Q1, 1993, 27; Q2, 1995, 14

Cerebrovascular accident (CVA) is a vague term often used to describe a condition best classified to this category.

The following fifth-digit subclassification is for use with categories 433 and 434:

0 without mention of cerebral infarction

1 with cerebral infarction

434.0 ✓5th Cerebral thrombosis — (Use additional code to identify presence of hypertension) — *blood clot*
AHA: March-April, 1985, 6; Q2, 1989, 8; Q3, 1990, 3; Q3, 1991, 10; Q1, 1993, 27; Q2, 1995, 14

434.1 ✓5th Cerebral embolism — (Use additional code to identify presence of hypertension) — *complete blockage*
AHA: March-April, 1985, 6; Q2, 1989, 8; Q3, 1990, 3; Q3, 1991, 10; Q1, 1993, 27; Q2, 1995, 14; Q3, 1997, 11

434.9 ✓5th Unspecified cerebral artery occlusion — (Use additional code to identify presence of hypertension) — *extent unknown*
AHA: March-April, 1985, 6; Q2, 1989, 8; Q3, 1990, 3; Q3, 1991, 10; Q1, 1993, 27; Q2, 1995, 14; Q4, 1998, 87

Documentation Issues

Do not classify CVA to this category without obtaining physician verification, since the term can also describe other acute cerebrovascular conditions that would be properly classified elsewhere.

When the physician documentation states that the patient had a lacunar infarction, use code 434.91 *Cerebral artery occlusion, unspecified, with cerebral infarction*. Lacunar infarctions occur in small vessels that are due to occlusion of branches of the middle cerebral, posterior cerebral, and basilar arteries.

Coding Clarification

Cerebral Artery: Occlusion of cerebral arteries is classified with a code from category 434 *Occlusion of cerebral arteries*. Review the medical record for information identifying if the occlusion is due to thrombosis (434.0x) or embolism (434.1x). If unspecified, use code 434.9x. Fifth digits are required with category 434 to identify if the event occurred with or without a cerebral infarction during the current admission.

435 *Transient cerebral ischemia*

AHA: March-April, 1985, 6; Q2, 1989, 8; Q3, 1990, 3; Q3, 1991, 10; Q1, 1993, 27

Transient cerebral ischemia describes episodes of focal neurological symptoms. Its most common form is known as a transient ischemic attack (TIA). A typical TIA lasts between two and 15 minutes and always resolves within 24 hours. Commonly, the etiology of the TIA is embolization due to cardiac causes such as rheumatic heart disease, cardiac dysrhythmias, mitral valve disease, infective endocarditis, mural thrombi complicating myocardial infarction, and myxoma.

This rubric includes reversible ischemic neurological deficits (RIND), if the patient's neurological deficits are associated with TIA and abate within 24 hours.

435.0 Basilar artery syndrome — (Use additional code to identify presence of hypertension)

435.1 Vertebral artery syndrome — (Use additional code to identify presence of hypertension) — *Verbiest's syndrome*
AHA: March-April, 1985, 6; Q2, 1989, 8; Q3, 1990, 3; Q3, 1991, 10; Q1, 1993, 27

435.2 Subclavian steal syndrome — (Use additional code to identify presence of hypertension)

435.3 Vertebrobasilar artery syndrome — (Use additional code to identify presence of hypertension)

435.8 Other specified transient cerebral ischemias — (Use additional code to identify presence of hypertension) — *carotid artery insufficiency*
AHA: March-April, 1985, 6; Q2, 1989, 8; Q3, 1990, 3; Q3, 1991, 10; Q1, 1993, 27

435.9 Unspecified transient cerebral ischemia — (Use additional code to identify presence of hypertension) — *TIA, Alvarez syndrome, impending cerebrovascular accident*
AHA: March-April, 1985, 6; Nov-Dec, 1985, 12; Q2, 1989, 8; Q3, 1990, 3; Q3, 1991, 10; Q1, 1993, 27

Coding Clarification

RIND also may be associated with other conditions in rubrics 430-437 and should be coded to the underlying condition causing the deficits. RIND may require a second code to classify the specific neurological deficit and the appropriate code from categories 430-437.

Coding Scenario

A patient is admitted with left leg weakness and facial numbness. The physician's final diagnosis indicates transient ischemic attack with RIND. The discharge summary identifies that the neurological deficits have subsided with the exception of minimal weakness.

> Code assignment: 435.9 *Unspecified transient cerebral ischemia*

436 *Acute, but ill-defined, cerebrovascular disease* OK

AHA: March-April, 1985, 6; Q2, 1989, 8; Q3, 1990, 3; Q3, 1991, 10; Q1, 1993, 27; Q4, 1999, 3

Wallenberg syndrome is characterized by difficulty in swallowing and hoarseness due to paralysis of the ipsilateral vocal cord and, in some cases, partial loss of the sense of taste due to associated affects on the tongue. The glossopharyngeal (IX) & vagus (X) are the primary cranial nerves involved in this syndrome. Occlusion of the posterior inferior cerebellar artery (PICA) leads to damage to the posterior region of the medulla, which explains the name "lateral medullary plate syndrome" often used to refer to this disorder.

Documentation Issues

If the documentation is limited to "stroke" or "cerebrovascular accident," review the medical record for additional information as to the cause. Code 436 *Acute, but ill-defined, cerebrovascular disease* should only be used when no further information is available and should never be used when the etiology of the CVA has been specified. Code 436 should never be used with a code from category 430-435.

437 *Other and ill-defined cerebrovascular disease*

AHA: March-April, 1985, 6; Q2, 1989, 8; Q3, 1990, 3; Q3, 1991, 10; Q1, 1993, 27

437.0 Cerebral atherosclerosis — (Use additional code to identify presence of hypertension) — *deposits narrowing arteries that branch into the brain*
AHA: March-April, 1985, 6; Q2, 1989, 8; Q3, 1990, 3; Q3, 1991, 10; Q1, 1993, 27

437.1 Other generalized ischemic cerebrovascular disease — (Use additional code to identify presence of hypertension) — *chronic cerebral ischemia, acute cerebrovascular insufficiency not otherwise specified*
AHA: March-April, 1985, 6; Q2, 1989, 8; Q3, 1990, 3; Q3, 1991, 10; Q1, 1993, 27

© 2004 Ingenix, Inc.

437.2 Hypertensive encephalopathy — (Use additional code to identify presence of hypertension) — *brain disease caused by high blood pressure*
AHA: July-Aug, 1984, 14; March-April, 1985, 6; Q2, 1989, 8; Q3, 1990, 3; Q3, 1991, 10; Q1, 1993, 27

437.3 Cerebral aneurysm, nonruptured — (Use additional code to identify presence of hypertension) — *dilation of artery in the brain*
AHA: March-April, 1985, 6; Q2, 1989, 8; Q3, 1990, 3; Q3, 1991, 10; Q1, 1993, 27

437.4 Cerebral arteritis — (Use additional code to identify presence of hypertension) — *inflammation of artery within the brain*
AHA: March-April, 1985, 6; Q2, 1989, 8; Q3, 1990, 3; Q3, 1991, 10; Q1, 1993, 27; Q4, 1999, 21

437.5 Moyamoya disease — (Use additional code to identify presence of hypertension) — *tiny neovacularizations in patients with ischemia*
AHA: March-April, 1985, 6; Q2, 1989, 8; Q3, 1990, 3; Q3, 1991, 10; Q1, 1993, 27

437.6 Nonpyogenic thrombosis of intracranial venous sinus — (Use additional code to identify presence of hypertension)

437.7 Transient global amnesia — (Use additional code to identify presence of hypertension) — *temporary memory loss not due to psychological factors*
AHA: March-April, 1985, 6; Q2, 1989, 8; Q3, 1990, 3; Q3, 1991, 10; Q4, 1992, 20; Q1, 1993, 27

437.8 Other ill-defined cerebrovascular disease — (Use additional code to identify presence of hypertension) — *cerebral hyperemia, hypertensive paralysis, necrotic brain, mollities, cortical or cerebral quadriplegia*
AHA: March-April, 1985, 6; Q2, 1989, 8; Q3, 1990, 3; Q3, 1991, 10; Q1, 1993, 27

437.9 Unspecified cerebrovascular disease — (Use additional code to identify presence of hypertension)

438 Late effects of cerebrovascular disease

AHA: March-April, 1985, 6; March-April, 1986, 7; Nov-Dec, 1986, 12; Q2, 1989, 8; Q3, 1990, 3; Q3, 1991, 10; Q4, 1992, 21; Q1, 1993, 27; Q4, 1997, 35,37; Q4, 1998, 39,88; Q4, 1999, 4,6,7

This rubric classifies conditions in categories 430-437 as the cause of a late effect. ICD-9-CM classifies late effects of cerebrovascular disease according to the neurological deficit.

438.0 Cognitive deficits due to cerebrovascular disease — (Use additional code to identify presence of hypertension) — *thought, memory, perception*
AHA: March-April, 1985, 6; March-April, 1986, 7; Nov-Dec, 1986, 12; Q2, 1989, 8; Q3, 1990, 3; Q3, 1991, 10; Q4, 1992, 21; Q1, 1993, 27; Q4, 1997, 35,37; Q4, 1998, 39,88; Q4, 1999, 4,6,7

438.10 Unspecified speech and language deficit due to cerebrovascular disease — (Use additional code to identify presence of hypertension)

438.11 Aphasia due to cerebrovascular disease — (Use additional code to identify presence of hypertension) — *speech loss or deficit*
AHA: March-April, 1985, 6; March-April, 1986, 7; Nov-Dec, 1986, 12; Q2, 1989, 8; Q3, 1990, 3; Q3, 1991, 10; Q4, 1992, 21; Q1, 1993, 27; Q4, 1997, 36; Q4, 1997, 35,37; Q4, 1998, 39,88; Q4, 1999, 4,6,7; Q4, 2003, 105

438.12 Dysphasia due to cerebrovascular disease — (Use additional code to identify presence of hypertension) — *inability to organize words in their appropriate order*
AHA: March-April, 1985, 6; March-April, 1986, 7; Nov-Dec, 1986, 12; Q2, 1989, 8; Q3, 1990, 3; Q3, 1991, 10; Q4, 1992, 21; Q1, 1993, 27; Q4, 1997, 35,37; Q4, 1998, 39,88; Q4, 1999, 3,9; Q4, 1999, 4,6,7

438.19 Other speech and language deficits due to cerebrovascular disease — (Use additional code to identify presence of hypertension) — *not otherwise specified*
AHA: March-April, 1985, 6; March-April, 1986, 7; Nov-Dec, 1986, 12; Q2, 1989, 8; Q3, 1990, 3; Q3, 1991, 10; Q4, 1992, 21; Q1, 1993, 27; Q4, 1997, 35,37; Q4, 1998, 39,88; Q4, 1999, 4,6,7

438.20 Hemiplegia affecting unspecified side due to cerebrovascular disease — (Use additional code to identify presence of hypertension)

438.21 Hemiplegia affecting dominant side due to cerebrovascular disease — (Use additional code to identify presence of hypertension)

438.22 Hemiplegia affecting nondominant side due to cerebrovascular disease — (Use additional code to identify presence of hypertension)

438.30 Monoplegia of upper limb affecting unspecified side due to cerebrovascular disease — (Use additional code to identify presence of hypertension)

438.31 Monoplegia of upper limb affecting dominant side due to cerebrovascular disease — (Use additional code to identify presence of hypertension)

390–459

438.32 Monoplegia of upper limb affecting nondominant side due to cerebrovascular disease — (Use additional code to identify presence of hypertension)

438.40 Monoplegia of lower limb affecting unspecified side due to cerebrovascular disease — (Use additional code to identify presence of hypertension)

438.41 Monoplegia of lower limb affecting dominant side due to cerebrovascular disease — (Use additional code to identify presence of hypertension)

438.42 Monoplegia of lower limb affecting nondominant side due to cerebrovascular disease — (Use additional code to identify presence of hypertension)

438.50 Other paralytic syndrome affecting unspecified side due to cerebrovascular disease — (Use additional code to identify type of paralytic syndrome: 344.81, 344.00-344.09. Use additional code to identify presence of hypertension)

438.51 Other paralytic syndrome affecting dominant side due to cerebrovascular disease — (Use additional code to identify type of paralytic syndrome: 344.81, 344.00-344.09. Use additional code to identify presence of hypertension)

438.52 Other paralytic syndrome affecting nondominant side due to cerebrovascular disease — (Use additional code to identify type of paralytic syndrome: 344.81, 344.00-344.09. Use additional code to identify presence of hypertension)

438.53 Other paralytic syndrome, bilateral — (Use additional code to identify type of paralytic syndrome: 344.81, 344.00-344.09. Use additional code to identify presence of hypertension)

438.6 Alteration of sensations as late effect of cerebrovascular disease — (Use additional code to identify the altered sensation. Use additional code to identify presence of hypertension)

438.7 Disturbance of vision as late effect of cerebrovascular disease — (Use additional code to identify the visual disturbance. Use additional code to identify presence of hypertension)

438.81 Apraxia due to cerebrovascular disease — (Use additional code to identify presence of hypertension) — *inability to properly use an object or carry out normal tasks*
AHA: March-April, 1985, 6; March-April, 1986, 7; Nov-Dec, 1986, 12; Q2, 1989, 8; Q3, 1990, 3; Q3, 1991, 10; Q4, 1992, 21; Q1, 1993, 27; Q4, 1997, 35,37; Q4, 1998, 39,88; Q4, 1999, 4,6,7

438.82 Dysphagia due to cerebrovascular disease — (Use additional code to identify presence of hypertension) — *difficulty in swallowing*
AHA: March-April, 1985, 6; March-April, 1986, 7; Nov-Dec, 1986, 12; Q2, 1989, 8; Q3, 1990, 3; Q3, 1991, 10; Q4, 1992, 21; Q1, 1993, 27; Q4, 1997, 35,37; Q4, 1998, 39,88; Q4, 1999, 4,6,7

438.83 Facial weakness as late effect of cerebrovascular disease — (Use additional code to identify presence of hypertension) — *facial droop*
AHA: March-April, 1985, 6; March-April, 1986, 7; Nov-Dec, 1986, 12; Q2, 1989, 8; Q3, 1990, 3; Q3, 1991, 10; Q4, 1992, 21; Q1, 1993, 27; Q4, 1997, 35,37; Q4, 1998, 39,88; Q4, 1999, 4,6,7

438.84 Ataxia as late effect of cerebrovascular disease — (Use additional code to identify presence of hypertension)

438.85 Vertigo as late effect of cerebrovascular disease — (Use additional code to identify presence of hypertension)

438.89 Other late effects of cerebrovascular disease — (Use additional code to identify the late effect. Use additional code to identify presence of hypertension) — *not specified elsewhere*
AHA: March-April, 1985, 6; March-April, 1986, 7; Nov-Dec, 1986, 12; Q2, 1989, 8; Q3, 1990, 3; Q3, 1991, 10; Q4, 1992, 21; Q1, 1993, 27; Q4, 1997, 35,37; Q4, 1998, 39; Q4, 1998, 39,88; Q4, 1999, 4,6,7

438.9 Unspecified late effects of cerebrovascular disease due to cerebrovascular disease — (Use additional code to identify presence of hypertension)

Documentation Issues

If documentation only identifies a previous cerebrovascular accident but no residual neurological deficits are noted, use code V12.59 *Personal history of other diseases of the circulatory system.* Codes from category 438 are not appropriate if no residual neurologic deficit remains.

Coding Clarification

Excluded from this rubric is history of cerebrovascular disease when no neurological deficit is present as a late effect. The appropriate code in that case would be V12.59 *Personal history of other disease of the circulatory system.*

Assign a code from rubric 438 in addition to a code from 430-437 if the patient has a current CVA in addition to deficits from an old CVA.

Neurogenic Bladder: When neurogenic bladder occurs as a result of a cerebrovascular hemorrhage, thrombosis, infarction, or obstruction, it is reported with codes 438.89 *Other late effects of cerebrovascular*

 © 2004 Ingenix, Inc.

disease and 596.54 *Neurogenic bladder NOS.* Two codes are necessary since there is no specific combination code for this condition.

Official Inpatient Coding Guidelines: The residual condition or nature of the late effect is sequenced first, followed by the cause of the late effect, except in those few instances where the code for the late effect is followed by a manifestation code identified in the tabular list and the title of the late effect code has been expanded (at the fourth- and fifth-digit levels) to include the manifestation. Unlike other late effect codes, codes from category 438 should be assigned as principal/primary diagnosis when there is a late effect of CVA:

- Late Effect of Cerebrovascular Disease — Category 438 is used to indicate conditions classifiable to categories 430-437. The neurologic deficits caused by cerebrovascular disease may be present from the onset or may arise at any time after the onset of the condition classifiable to 430-437.
- Codes from category 438 may be assigned along with codes from 430-437, if the patient has a recurrent CVA and deficits from an old CVA. Assign code V12.59 (not a code from category 438) as an additional code for history of cerebrovascular disease when no neurologic deficits are present.

Do not assign a code from category 438 when a current diagnosis classifiable to the 430-437 series is present.

Coding Scenario

A 62-year-old male is seen for speech therapy of his aphasia. This patient has a history of a CVA five months ago.

> Code assignment: V57.3 *Care involving use of rehabilitation procedures, speech therapy* and 438.11 *Late effect of cerebrovascular disease, speech and language deficits, aphasia*

440–448 Diseases of Arteries, Arterioles, and Capillaries

This section includes conditions affecting the arteries, arterioles, and capillaries, including atherosclerosis, aneurysm, peripheral vascular disease, embolism and thrombosis, arteritis, and stricture.

440 *Atherosclerosis*

Atherosclerosis is a form of arteriosclerosis characterized by irregularly distributed atheromas accumulating within the tunica intima of arteries. The deposits are associated with calcification and fibrosis, reducing the size of the arterial lumen and resulting in obstructive ischemia.

440.0 Atherosclerosis of aorta — *atheroma, degeneration, endarteritis*
AHA: Q4, 1988, 8; Q2, 1993, 7; Q2, 1993, 8

440.1 Atherosclerosis of renal artery — *atheroma, degeneration, endarteritis*

440.20 Atherosclerosis of native arteries of the extremities, unspecified — *unknown manifestations*
AHA: March-April, 1987, 6; Q3, 1990, 15; Q4, 1992, 25; Q4, 1993, 27; Q4, 1994, 49

440.21 Atherosclerosis of native arteries of the extremities with intermittent claudication — *Charcot's due to atherosclerosis*
AHA: March-April, 1987, 6; Q3, 1990, 15; Q4, 1992, 25; Q4, 1993, 27; Q4, 1994, 49

440.22 Atherosclerosis of native arteries of the extremities with rest pain

440.23 Atherosclerosis of native arteries of the extremities with ulceration — (Use additional code for any associated ulceration: 707.10-707.9)

440.24 Atherosclerosis of native arteries of the extremities with gangrene

440.29 Other atherosclerosis of native arteries of the extremities — *not otherwise specified*
AHA: March-April, 1987, 6; Q3, 1990, 15; Q4, 1992, 25; Q4, 1993, 27; Q4, 1994, 49

440.30 Atheroslerosis of unspecified bypass graft of extremities — *graft origin unknown*
AHA: Q4, 1994, 49

440.31 Atheroslerosis of autologous vein bypass graft of extremities — *graft from patient*
AHA: Q4, 1994, 49

440.32 Atheroslerosis of nonautologous biological bypass graft of extremities — *graft other than from patient*
AHA: Q4, 1994, 49

440.8 Atherosclerosis of other specified arteries — *not otherwise specified; arteriosclerotic retinitis*

440.9 Generalized and unspecified atherosclerosis — *unknown or disseminated*

Documentation Issues

When documentation identifies that a patient with aortic atherosclerosis has an occlusion of the aortoiliac artery due to an embolus, two codes should be used: 444.0 *Arterial embolism and thrombosis of abdominal aorta* and 440.0 *Atherosclerosis of aorta.* Even though the index assumes aortic occlusions are thromboembolic, if the etiology is specified (e.g., atherosclerosis), then that condition should be coded.

If the documentation states that the patient has an aortoiliac artery occlusion due to a stricture in conjunction with aortic arteriosclerosis, two codes are required: 447.1 *Other disorders of arteries and arterioles, stricture of artery* and 440.0 *Atherosclerosis of aorta.*

When the documentation states gangrene of amputation stump and the patient has diabetic arteriosclerosis, obtain clarification from the physician as to the cause of the gangrene. If it is an actual complication of the amputation, use codes 997.62 *Amputation stump infection* and 785.4 *Gangrene.* If it is due to a natural progression of the diabetic arteriosclerotic disease, use codes 250.7x *Diabetes with peripheral circulatory diseases* and 440.24 *Atherosclerosis of native arteries of the extremities with gangrene.*

Coding Clarification

Peripheral: Arteriosclerosis (occlusive) of the extremities is reported with code 440.2x.

Combination Code Hierarchy: Fifth digits used with subcategory code 440.2 identify additional manifestations of the atherosclerotic peripheral vascular disease. These codes are listed by order of increasing priority. All patients classified to this subcategory who have gangrene (regardless whether they have rest pain, ulceration, and/or intermittent claudication) are coded to 440.24. Patients without gangrene but with ulceration (regardless of whether they have rest pain and/or intermittent claudication) are coded to 440.23. Patients without gangrene or ulceration, with rest pain (with or without intermittent claudication) are assigned code 440.22, and those with only intermittent claudication use code 440.21.

Diabetic Complication: Diabetic atherosclerosis of extremities is coded as 250.7x *Diabetes with peripheral circulatory disorders* and 440.2x *Atherosclerosis of native arteries of extremities.* If the diagnosis is diabetes with ischemic heart disease or cerebrovascular disease, they are coded as separate entities.

Gas Gangrene: Arteriosclerosis with gas gangrene is reported with two codes: 440.29 *Other atherosclerosis of native arteries of extremities* and 040.0 *Gas gangrene.* It is inappropriate to use code 440.24; this code only includes ischemic gangrene.

Coding Scenario

A patient is admitted for gangrene of the left leg secondary to diabetic arteriosclerosis. Record documentation identifies that the patient is Type I insulin dependent.

> Code assignment: 250.71 *Diabetes with peripheral circulatory disorders, Type I, not stated as uncontrolled* and 440.24 *Atherosclerosis of native arteries of the extremities with gangrene*

A patient is admitted to the hospital with leg pain and weakness. The final diagnosis indicates peripheral arteriosclerosis with rest pain and intermittent claudication.

> Code assignment: 440.22 *Atherosclerosis of native arteries of the extremities with rest pain*

A 49-year-old female is admitted for occlusion of peripheral artery bypass graft. Her history and physical report indicates that a nonautologous biological bypass graft was performed one year ago. The physician's documentation identifies the occlusion as a progression of the artherosclerotic disease.

> Code assignment: 440.32 *Atherosclerosis of nonautologous biological bypass graft of extremities*

A patient is admitted with a diagnosis of hypertension. The physician's final diagnosis at discharge is atherosclerosis of the aorta and generalized arteriosclerosis.

> Code assignment: 440.0 *Atherosclerosis of aorta,* and 440.9 *Generalized and unspecified atherosclerosis*

Inpatient consultation is provided for a 69-year-old female with pain and weakness in both legs. The patient undergoes a peripheral vascular plethysmography for confirmation of arterial occlusion. The physician's diagnosis states atherosclerosis of bilateral extremities with intermittent claudication.

> Code assignment: 440.21 *Atherosclerosis of native arteries of the extremities with intermittent claudication*

A 53-year-old male is admitted for atherosclerosis. The discharge summary states the final diagnosis as aortoiliac artery occlusion secondary to stricture and aortic atherosclerosis.

> Code assignment: 447.1 *Other disorders of arteries and arterioles, stricture of artery* and 440.0 *Atherosclerosis of aorta*

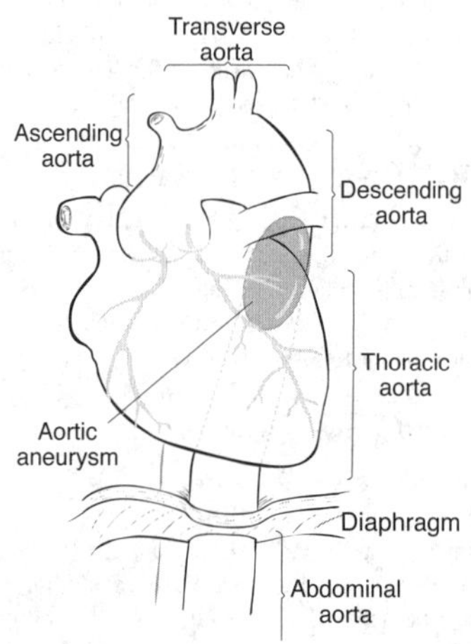

 © 2004 Ingenix, Inc.

441 Aortic aneurysm and dissection

Aortic aneurysms are circumscribed dilations of the aorta or a blood-containing tumor connecting directly within the lumen of the aorta. Generally, an aneurysm is considered clinically significant if its diameter is twice that of the normal artery. A dissecting aneurysm is characterized by blood entering through a split or tear in the intima of the artery wall or by interstitial hemorrhage. Dissecting aortic aneurysms may rupture, constituting a medical emergency. This condition is most frequently seen in men between 40 and 60 years of age.

441.00 Dissecting aortic aneurysm (any part), unspecified site — *dilation and split of aorta lining, site unknown*
AHA: Q4, 1989, 10

441.01 Dissecting aortic aneurysm (any part), thoracic — *dilation and split of aorta lining in the chest cavity*
AHA: Q4, 1989, 10

441.02 Dissecting aortic aneurysm (any part), abdominal — *dilation and split of aorta lining in the abdomen*
AHA: Q4, 1989, 10

441.03 Dissecting aortic aneurysm (any part), thoracoabdominal — *dilation and split of aorta lining in chest and abdomen*
AHA: Q4, 1989, 10

441.1 Thoracic aneurysm, ruptured — *dilation and tear in aorta in chest*

441.2 Thoracic aneurysm without mention of rupture — *dilation in aorta in chest*
AHA: Q3, 1992, 10

441.3 Abdominal aneurysm, ruptured — *dilation and tear of aorta in abdomen*

441.4 Abdominal aneurysm without mention of rupture — *dilation of aorta in abdomen*
AHA: Q3, 1992, 10; Q1, 1999, 15,16,17; Q4, 2000, 64

441.5 Aortic aneurysm of unspecified site, ruptured — *dilation and tear of aorta in unknown site*

441.6 Thoracoabdominal aneurysm, ruptured — *dilation and tear of aorta in abdomen and chest*

441.7 Thoracoabdominal aneurysm without mention of rupture — *dilation of aorta in abdomen and chest*

441.9 Aortic aneurysm of unspecified site without mention of rupture — *dilation of aorta, site and rupture status unknown*

Documentation Issues

If the documentation states Type I, Type II, Type III abdominal aortic aneurysm, the condition is still classified to 441.0x *Dissection of aorta.* The fifth-digit for this category identifies the site of the aneurysm (e.g., abdominal, thoracic, thoracoabdominal).

Coding Clarification

Aneurysms of Adjoining Sites: When an aneurysm develops at an adjoining site, code each site separately unless a code is provided that identifies the adjoining site. For example, aortoiliac aneurysm requires two codes: 441.4 and 442.2; for a dissecting thoracoabdominal aneurysm one code is required: 441.03.

Coding Scenario

A 68-year-old female patient was admitted with a possible myocardial infarction. After study, the patient was diagnosed with a dissecting thoracoabdominal aortic aneurysm.

> Code assignment: 441.03 *Dissection of aorta, thoracoabdominal*

A 43-year-old patient is admitted with thoracic aneurysm and hypertension. The physician documents the final diagnosis as a dissecting aneurysm of the thoracic aorta with nonmalignant systemic hypertension.

> Code assignment: 441.01 *Dissection of aorta, thoracic* and 401.1 *Essential hypertension, benign*

442 Other aneurysm

442.0 Aneurysm of artery of upper extremity — *dilation; brachial, radial, interosseous, ulnar, superficial palmar arch*

442.1 Aneurysm of renal artery — *dilation*

442.2 Aneurysm of iliac artery — *dilation*
AHA: Q1, 1999, 16,17

442.3 Aneurysm of artery of lower extremity — *dilation; femoral, popliteal artery, medial plantar, posterior tibial, anterior tibial*
AHA: Q1, 1999, 16; Q3, 2002, 24-26

442.81 Aneurysm of artery of neck — *dilation; internal, external, common carotid*

442.82 Aneurysm of subclavian artery — *dilation*

442.83 Aneurysm of splenic artery — *dilation*

442.84 Aneurysm of other visceral artery — *dilation; celiac, gastroduodenal, hepatic, pancreaticoduodenal, superior mesenteric, gastroepiploic*

442.89 Aneurysm of other specified artery — *dilation; mediastinal, spinal artery*

442.9 Other aneurysm of unspecified site

443 Other peripheral vascular disease

443.0 Raynaud's syndrome — (Use additional code to identify gangrene, 785.4) — *construction of arteries of the digits caused by cold or stress*

390–459

443.1 Thromboangiitis obliterans (Buerger's disease) — *inflammation and swelling in distal arteries, causing occlusions*

443.21 Dissection of carotid artery

443.22 Dissection of iliac artery

443.23 Dissection of renal artery

443.24 Dissection of vertebral artery

443.29 Dissection of other artery

443.81 Peripheral angiopathy in diseases classified elsewhere — (Code first underlying disease, 250.7) — *secondary to underlying disease*
AHA: Q3, 1991, 10

443.89 Other peripheral vascular disease — *not otherwise specified, Crocq's, Gerhardt's, Weir Mitchell's disease, acrocyanosis, erythrocyanosis, Schultz's acroparesthesia, Nothnagel's vasomotor acroparesthesia, erythromelalgia*

443.9 Unspecified peripheral vascular disease

Coding Scenario

An elderly patient is transferred from an extended care facility for treatment of a decubitus ulcer. The physician also identifies the patient as a Type I insulin dependent diabetic with related progressive peripheral vascular disease.

> Code assignment: 707.0 *Decubitus ulcer,* 250.71 *Diabetes with peripheral circulatory disorders, Type I [insulin dependent type], not stated as uncontrolled,* and 443.81 *Peripheral angiopathy in diseases classified elsewhere*

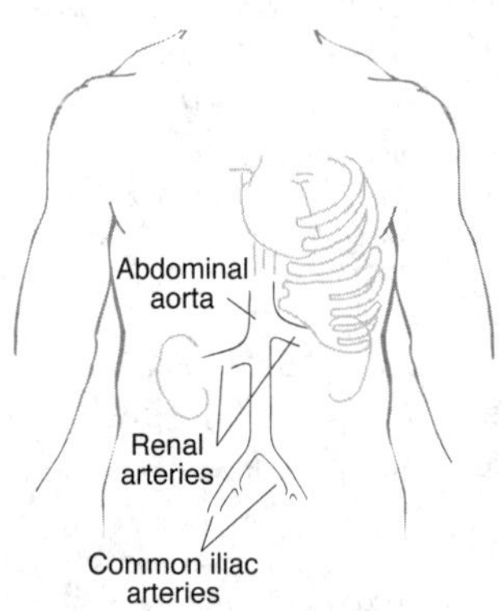

444 *Arterial embolism and thrombosis*

AHA: Q4, 1990, 27; Q2, 1992, 11

An arterial embolism is a partial or complete obstruction of an artery due to the migration of a blood clot or other foreign material. An arterial thrombosis is the formation of a blood clot within the lumen of an artery. In each case, infarction of the tissues perfused by the artery is a potential complication.

444.0 Embolism and thrombosis of abdominal aorta — *aortic bifurcation and Leriche's syndromes, saddle embolus, aortoiliac obstruction*
AHA: Q4, 1990, 27; Q2, 1992, 11; Q2, 1993, 7

444.1 Embolism and thrombosis of thoracic aorta — *embolism of thrombosis of thoracic aorta*
AHA: Q4, 1990, 27; Q2, 1992, 11

444.21 Embolism and thrombosis of arteries of upper extremity — *brachial, radial, interosseous, ulnar, superficial palmar arch*
AHA: March-April, 1987, 6; Q4, 1990, 27; Q2, 1992, 11

444.22 Embolism and thrombosis of arteries of lower extremity — *femoral, popliteal artery, medial plantar, posterior tibial, anterior tibial*
AHA: March-April, 1987, 6; Q3, 1990, 16; Q4, 1990, 27; Q2, 1992, 11; Q1, 2003, 17; Q3, 2003, 10

444.81 Embolism and thrombosis of iliac artery

444.89 Embolism and thrombosis of other specified artery — *hepatic and splenic arteries*
AHA: Q4, 1990, 27; Q2, 1992, 11

444.9 Embolism and thrombosis of unspecified artery

Documentation Issues

When documentation identifies that a patient with aortic atherosclerosis has an occlusion of the aortoiliac artery due to an embolus, two codes should be used: 444.0 *Arterial embolism and thrombosis of abdominal aorta* and 440.0 *Atherosclerosis of aorta.* Even though the index assumes aortic occlusions are thromboembolic, if the etiology is specified (e.g., atherosclerosis), then that condition should be coded.

445 *Atheroembolism*

AHA: Q4, 2002, 57

Atheroembolism occurs when fragments of atherosclerotic plaques break off from their location in an artery and travel to another site, such as the kidney, where the embolus then gets lodged. This may occur spontaneously but often happens as a result of manipulation in the aorta, such as during cardiac catheterization.

445.01 Atheroembolism of upper extremity

445.02 Atheroembolism of lower extremity

445.81 Atheroembolism of kidney — (Use additional code for any associated kidney failure: 584, 585)

445.89 Atheroembolism of other site

 © 2004 Ingenix, Inc.

446 Polyarteritis nodosa and allied conditions

446.0 Polyarteritis nodosa — *inflammation of small and medium size arteries causing tissue death; disseminated necrotizing periarteritis, necrotizing angiitis, Harkavy's syndrome*

446.1 Acute febrile mucocutaneous lymph node syndrome (MCLS) — *inflammatory disease causing fever, skin eruptions, and edema; including Kawasaki disease*

446.20 Unspecified hypersensitivity angiitis — *unknown inflammatory disease of vessels caused by antigen sensitivity*

446.21 Goodpasture's syndrome — (Use additional code to identify renal disease, 583.81) — *antiglomerular basement membrane antibody-mediated nephritis with pulmonary hemorrhage*

446.29 Other specified hypersensitivity angiitis — *not otherwise specified*
AHA: Q1, 1995, 3

446.3 Lethal midline granuloma — *tumor that begins midface and leads to death; malignant granuloma of face*

446.4 Wegener's granulomatosis — *necrotizing granulomatous inflammation of vessels of respiratory tract; Churg-Strauss syndrome*
AHA: Q3, 2000, 11

446.5 Giant cell arteritis — *giant cells and inflammation in large artery, leading to occlusion; including cranial arteritis, Horton's disease, Bagratuni's syndrome*

446.6 Thrombotic microangiopathy — *blockages in the smallest arteries and arterioles; including Moschcowitz's syndrome, Baehr-Schiffrin disease*

446.7 Takayasu's disease — *progressive inflammation of brachiocephalic truck and left common carotid arteries above source in aortic arch; including Martorell-Fabre, Raeder-Harbitz, young female syndromes, pulseless disease*

Coding Clarification

Polyarteritis nodosa is a systemic disease characterized by segmental inflammation with infiltration and necrosis of medium-sized or small arteries. It is most common in males and produces symptoms related to involvement of arteries in the kidneys, muscles, gastrointestinal tract, and heart, and is reported with 446.0.

Septic Leukocytoclastic Vasculitis: Two codes are required to report this condition: 446.29 *Other specified hypersensitivity angiitis* and a code from category 682 *Other cellulitis and abscess.*

447 Other disorders of arteries and arterioles

447.0 Arteriovenous fistula, acquired — *communication between an artery and vein caused by error in healing*

447.1 Stricture of artery — *structurally narrow section of an artery*
AHA: March-April, 1987, 6; Q2, 1993, 8

447.2 Rupture of artery — *tearing of artery with bleeding, not associated with aneurysm, but caused by erosion, (not arteriovenous) fistula or ulcer*

447.3 Hyperplasia of renal artery — *overgrowth of cells in the muscular lining of the renal artery*

447.4 Celiac artery compression syndrome — *compression of the celiac artery by the median arcuate ligament; celiac axis, Marable's, medial arcuate ligament syndromes*

447.5 Necrosis of artery — *death of arterial tissue*

447.6 Unspecified arteritis

447.8 Other specified disorders of arteries and arterioles — *not otherwise specified; fibromuscular hyperplasia of nonrenal artery; Dego's, Wright's, or popliteal artery entrapment syndromes; dilation, hyperabduction, hypertrophy, papulosis*

447.9 Unspecified disorders of arteries and arterioles

Documentation Issues

If the documentation states that the patient has an aortoiliac artery occlusion due to a stricture in conjunction with aortic arteriosclerosis, two codes are required: 447.1 *Stricture of artery* and 440.0 *Atherosclerosis of aorta.*

Coding Scenario

A 53-year-old male is admitted for atherosclerosis. The discharge summary states the final diagnosis as aortoiliac artery occlusion secondary to stricture and aortic atherosclerosis.

> Code assignment: 447.1 *Stricture of artery* and 440.0 *Atherosclerosis of aorta*

448 Disease of capillaries

Arterioles entering tissue that branch into vessels are called capillaries. Nutrients and wastes are exchanged between the blood and body through the walls of the capillaries, which, before leaving the tissues, reunite to form the venules. Although found near almost every cell in the body, their distribution is regulated by the activity of the tissue (i.e., capillary supplies are dense in the liver, kidneys, lungs, muscles, and nervous system and less extensive in tendons and ligaments). Telangiectasia is the permanent dilatation

© 2004 Ingenix, Inc.

of groups of superficial capillaries and venules that can be caused by dermatoses, rosacea, and collagen vascular diseases. A nevus flammeus is a flat capillary hemangioma that is present at birth and varies from pale red to deep reddish purple. It rarely causes any problems.

448.0 Hereditary hemorrhagic telangiectasia

448.1 Nevus, non-neoplastic — *araneus, senile, spider, stellar*

448.9 Other and unspecified capillary diseases — *not otherwise specified, or unknown; thrombosis, rupture, hemorrhage, hyperpermeability, telangiectasia*

451–459 Diseases of Veins and Lymphatics, and Other Diseases of Circulatory System

451 Phlebitis and thrombophlebitis

AHA: Q1, 1992, 16

Phlebitis is inflammation of a vein. Thrombophlebitis is a partial or complete obstruction of a vein with secondary inflammatory reaction in the wall of the vein.

451.0 Phlebitis and thrombophlebitis of superficial vessels of lower extremities — (Use additional E code to identify drug, if drug-induced) — *inflammation and formation of a blood clot in the superficial veins of the legs and feet; including greater and lesser saphenous veins*
AHA: Q3, 1991, 16; Q1, 1992, 16

451.11 Phlebitis and thrombophlebitis of femoral vein (deep) (superficial) — (Use additional E code to identify drug, if drug-induced) — *inflammation and formation of a femoral blood clot*
AHA: Q3, 1991, 16; Q1, 1992, 16

451.19 Phlebitis and thrombophlebitis of other deep vessels of lower extremities — (Use additional E code to identify drug, if drug-induced) — *inflammation and formation of a blood clot in the femoropopliteal, tibia, popliteal veins; blue phlebitis*
AHA: Q3, 1991, 16; Q1, 1992, 16

451.2 Phlebitis and thrombophlebitis of lower extremities, unspecified — (Use additional E code to identify drug, if drug-induced)

451.81 Phlebitis and thrombophlebitis of iliac vein — (Use additional E code to identify drug, if drug-induced) — *inflammation and formation of a blood clot*
AHA: Q1, 1992, 16

451.82 Phlebitis and thrombophlebitis of superficial veins of upper extremities — (Use additional E code to identify drug, if drug-induced) — *inflammation and formation of a blood clot in the antecubital, basilic, cephalic veins*
AHA: Q1, 1992, 16

451.83 Phlebitis and thrombophlebitis of deep veins of upper extremities — (Use additional E code to identify drug, if drug-induced) — *inflammation and formation of a blood clot in the brachial, radial, ulnar veins*
AHA: Q1, 1992, 16

451.84 Phlebitis and thrombophlebitis of upper extremities, unspecified — (Use additional E code to identify drug, if drug-induced)

451.89 Phlebitis and thrombophlebitis of other site — (Use additional E code to identify drug, if drug-induced) — *not otherwise specified, axillary, jugular, subclavian, hepatic, umbilical veins*
AHA: Q1, 1992, 16

451.9 Phlebitis and thrombophlebitis of unspecified site — (Use additional E code to identify drug, if drug-induced)

Coding Clarification

This rubric excludes thrombophlebitis that is due to or following an implant or a catheter device (996.61-996.62) or infusion, perfusion, or transfusion (999.2).

Classify phlebitis and thrombophlebitis according to the vessel. Use an additional E code to identify the drug, if the condition is drug induced.

Deep Venous Thrombosis and Thrombophlebitis: The correct way to code a diagnosis of thrombosis and thrombophlebitis is to report only the thrombophlebitis. Thrombosis is the formation of a clot within a blood vessel. Thrombophlebitis is inflammation of a vein associated with thrombus formation. Thrombophlebitis has the characteristic signs of swelling, pain, induration, and redness.

Often the term "DVT," or deep venous thrombosis, is used as a synonym for thrombophlebitis. If the signs and symptoms described above are seen in the documentation, query the physician and obtain an addendum to the record if the physician states that the patient has thrombophlebitis. It will then be appropriate to code the thrombophlebitis as the only code. An excludes note gives direction to assign only a code from category 451 if both conditions are present.

Deep Vein Category: The femoropopliteal vein, the tibial vein, and the popliteal vein belong to the "deep" category.

Codes in category 451 distinguish between the superficial, deep, and unspecified veins of the upper and lower extremities. The need for this specificity

 © 2004 Ingenix, Inc.

arose with the increasing use of catheters and cannulas, which are often placed in the arm. Included in the deep vessels of the upper extremities are the following veins: branchial vein, radial vein, and ulner vein.

Coding Scenario

The patient is diagnosed with DVT and thrombophlebitis of the superficial femoral vein.

> Code assignment: 451.11 *Phlebitis and thrombophlebitis of femoral vein (deep) (superficial)*

A 24-year-old female is discharged with a diagnostic statement of "DVT of the basilic vein." The nursing notes state that the arm is reddened, indurated, painful, and swollen.

> Code assignment: Code the case as 453.8 *Embolism and thrombosis of other specified veins.* Documentation from the physician must determine thrombophlebitis in order to assign a code from 451

452 Portal vein thrombosis OK

This type of thrombosis describes inflammation and blood clot in the main vein of the liver.

Coding Clarification

The classification excludes hepatic vein thrombosis (453.0) and phlebitis of portal vein (572.1).

453 Other venous embolism and thrombosis

AHA: Q1, 1992, 16

Budd-Chiari syndrome is a thrombus in the main vein that leaves the liver. Symptoms of this syndrome include ascites, jaundice and abnormal liver function tests.

The formation of a blood clot, or thrombus, in the deep veins of the leg not only impedes blood circulation, but also may become life-threatening if the clot or pieces of the blood clot break loose and travel to the lungs where they lodge in an artery, causing pulmonary embolism. The American Heart Association estimates that up to 2 million people a year are affected by DVT, and up to 200,000 die from developing pulmonary embolism—that is more that breast cancer and AIDS combined, and accounts for one of the nation's leading, but preventable causes of death.

People develop deep vein thrombosis from prolonged sitting, immobility, or bed rest that may be occasioned by long distance traveling, major injuries, paralysis, surgery, or pregnancy. Surgery that involves the legs or pelvis, existing heart or circulation problems, hormone replacement therapy, obesity, age, and certain genetic conditions that make blood clotting more likely than usual increase the risk. When a thrombus forms, blood flow back to the heart is impeded, causing redness, swelling, and pain in the leg below the clot that may be perceived as aching or tightness.

Deep vein thrombosis may be associated with inflammation, phlebitis, and thrombophlebitis.

453.0 Budd-Chiari syndrome — *hepatic vein thrombosis with liver enlargement and severe hypertension*
AHA: Q1, 1992, 16

453.1 Thrombophlebitis migrans — *spontaneous, recurring inflammation of veins with blood clots; including Trousseau's and carcinogenic thrombophlebitis syndromes*
AHA: Q1, 1992, 16

453.2 Embolism and thrombosis of vena cava — *blockage and clotting of vena cava*
AHA: Q1, 1992, 16

453.3 Embolism and thrombosis of renal vein — *blockage and clotting of major kidney vein*
AHA: Q1, 1992, 16

453.40 Venous embolism and thrombosis of unspecified deep vessels of lower extremity

453.41 Venous embolism and thrombosis of deep vessels of proximal lower extremity

453.42 Venous embolism and thrombosis of deep vessels of distal lower extremity

453.8 Embolism and thrombosis of other specified veins — *not otherwise specified; iliac, femoral axillary veins; Paget-Schroetter syndrome*
AHA: March-April, 1987, 6; Q3, 1991, 16; Q1, 1992, 16

453.9 Embolism and thrombosis of unspecified site

Documentation Issues

If the documentation states that the thrombus is not associated with inflammation, assign the appropriate code from rubric 453. If the signs and symptoms associated with inflammation (swelling, erythema, pain, induration) are documented, query the physician as to whether the condition is thrombophlebitis and, if it is, assign a code from rubric 451 instead.

Coding Clarification

Report code from rubric 451 for thrombosis with thrombophlebitis.

Coding Scenario

A 56-year-old female, who has recently undergone back surgery, presents to her physician's office complaining of pain and tenderness in her right leg. The physician notes swelling and redness developing in the lower half of her upper leg. As a deep vein thrombosis is suspected, with a greater risk of

390–459

developing pulmonary embolism from its location, she is taken to the hospital where doppler ultrasound and venography are done that confirm a thrombus in the femoral vein. She is admitted, the leg is held in elevated position, and she is monitored closely as intravenous heparin is administered.

> Code assignment: 453.41 *Venous embolism and thrombosis of deep vessels of proximal lower extremity*

454 Varicose veins of lower extremities

AHA: Q2, 1991, 20

Varicose veins are dilated, elongated, and tortuous networks in the subcutaneous venous system resulting from valvular incompetence. Other etiologies include congenital or acquired arteriovenous fistulas and valve damage following deep venous thrombophlebitis. The condition develops predominantly in the lower extremities. Most commonly, the long saphenous vein and its tributaries are involved, but the short saphenous vein also may be affected. Symptoms include night cramps, localized pain, edema, inflammation, or hemorrhage and a dull aching or fatigue exacerbated by standing in place.

454.0 Varicose veins of lower extremities with ulcer — *incompetent vein valves allow reversed blood flow and erosion of tissue*
AHA: Q2, 1991, 20; Q4, 1999, 18

454.1 Varicose veins of lower extremities with inflammation — *incompetent vein valves allow reversed blood flow and inflammation*
AHA: Q2, 1991, 20

454.2 Varicose veins of lower extremities with ulcer and inflammation — *incompetent vein valves allow reversed blood flow, erosion of tissue, and inflammation*
AHA: Q2, 1991, 20

454.8 Varicose veins of the lower extremities with other complications — *Edema, pain, swelling*
AHA: Q2, 1991, 20; Q4, 2002, 58

454.9 Asymptomatic varicose veins

Coding Clarification

Stasis Dermatitis: Determine which of the following diagnoses is appropriate: stasis dermatitis with varicosity, with or without ulceration; stasis dermatitis with venous peripheral insufficiency, and previous deep venous thrombosis. While stasis dermatitis often occurs with varicosity, it also appears after a deep venous thrombosis and may appear as a singular entity (venous peripheral insufficiency).

When consulting the index, a basic coding rule is the requirement for further research if the code title suggested by the index is in contradiction to the condition. In the example for chronic venous insufficiency and previous deep vein thrombosis, the user must reject the suggestion of the index (varicose veins) because they are not the clinical entity at issue.

The codes that may be used to describe stasis dermatitis are: 454.1 *Varicose veins of lower extremity with inflammation*, 454.2 *Varicose veins of lower extremity with ulcer and inflammation*, 459.1x *Post phlebitic syndrome*, and 459.81 *Venous insufficiency, unspecified.*

Varicose vein with ulceration and hemorrhage: When coding ulcerated varicose veins that have ruptured and are hemorrhaging, the coder does not need to code the hemorrhage as a separate clinical entity. Also, the term "ruptured" is a non-essential modifier. Typically after rupture of a varicose vein, bleeding will occur.

Coding Scenario

An 80-year-old presents to the emergency department with stasis dermatitis on the right lower extremity. The physical examination reveals varicosities on the same extremity that have ulcerated.

> Code assignment: 454.2 *Varicose veins of lower extremities with ulcer and inflammation*

A patients presents to the emergency department for control of bleeding from an ulcerated varicose vein of the right lower extremity. The diagnostic statement reads "Varicose veins with ulceration and hemorrhage."

> Code assignment: 454.0 *Varicose veins of lower extremities with ulcer.* Do not assign a separate code for the hemorrhage.

455 Hemorrhoids

Hemorrhoids are dilated veins of the hemorrhoidal plexus in the lower rectum. External hemorrhoids are on the outer side of the external sphincter, covered by skin of the anal canal. Internal hemorrhoids are within the external sphincter, covered with rectal mucosa.

Internal hemorrhoids may be classified as first, second, third, or fourth degree. Fourth-degree hemorrhoids are the most severe and are characterized as both incarcerated and prolapsed; third-degree hemorrhoids are prolapsed. Both third- and fourth-degree hemorrhoids should be classified as complicated.

455.0 Internal hemorrhoids without mention of complication — *reversed blow flow and dilation of vein; contained within rectum*

455.1 Internal thrombosed hemorrhoids — *reversed blow flow and clotted blood in vein; contained within rectum*

© 2004 Ingenix, Inc.

455.2 Internal hemorrhoids with other complication — *reversed blow flow with strangulation, ulcer, prolapse, or bleeding; contained within rectum*
AHA: Q1, 2003, 8

455.3 External hemorrhoids without mention of complication — *reversed blow flow and dilation of vein; extending beyond anus*

455.4 External thrombosed hemorrhoids — *reversed blow flow and clotted blood in vein; extending beyond anus*

455.5 External hemorrhoids with other complication — *reversed blow flow with strangulation, ulcer, prolapse, or bleeding; extending beyond anus*
AHA: Q1, 2003, 8

455.6 Unspecified hemorrhoids without mention of complication — *reversed blow flow and dilation of vein; unknown site*

455.7 Unspecified thrombosed hemorrhoids — *reversed blow flow and clotted blood in vein; unknown site*

455.8 Unspecified hemorrhoids with other complication — *reversed blow flow with strangulation, ulcer, prolapse, or bleeding; unknown site*

455.9 Residual hemorrhoidal skin tags — *redundant tissue remains in anus or rectum following treatment of hemorrhoids*

456 Varicose veins of other sites

Varicose veins may occur at sites other than the lower extremities. Esophageal varices are the most clinically significant and comprise longitudinal venous varices located in the distal end of the esophagus.

456.0 Esophageal varices with bleeding — *distended, tortuous veins of the esophagus, with leaking of blood*

456.1 Esophageal varices without mention of bleeding — *distended, tortuous veins of the esophagus, without bleeding*

456.20 Esophageal varices with bleeding in diseases classified elsewhere — (Code first underlying disease: 571.0-571.9, 572.3) — *secondary to underlying disease*
AHA: Nov-Dec, 1985, 14

456.21 Esophageal varices without mention of bleeding in diseases classified elsewhere — (Code first underlying disease: 571.0-571.9, 572.3) — *secondary to underlying disease*
AHA: Q2, 2002, 4

456.3 Sublingual varices — *distended, tortuous veins beneath the tongue*

456.4 Scrotal varices — *distended, tortuous veins of the scrotum*

456.5 Pelvic varices — *distended, tortuous veins within the pelvic region*

456.6 Vulval varices — *distended, tortuous veins of the external female genitalia*

456.8 Varices of other sites — *distended, tortuous veins of sites not otherwise specified, including orbit, pharynx, renal papilla, spine, spleen, urethra, vocal cord, nasal septum*
AHA: Q2, 2002, 4

Coding Clarification

Varicose veins are almost always due to portal hypertension (456.2). Code the portal hypertension first, followed by 456.20, if bleeding is present, or 456.21, without bleeding.

390–459

457 Noninfectious disorders of lymphatic channels

Lymphatic vessels originate in spaces between cells called lymph capillaries, which originate throughout the body (excluding avascular tissue, the central nervous system, splenic pulp, and bone marrow). The vessels contain lymph nodes at various intervals. The lymphatics of the skin converge with the lymphatics of the viscera to form the lymphatic channels (the thoracic duct and the right lymphatic duct). The thoracic duct receives lymph from the left side of the head, neck, and chest, the left upper extremity, and the entire body below the ribs. The right lymphatic duct collects lymph from the right jugular trunk, which drains the right side of the head and neck; from the right subclavian trunk, which drains the right upper extremity; and from the right bronchomediastinal trunk, which drains the right side of the thorax, right lung, right side of the heart, and part of the convex surface of the liver. Skeletal muscle contractions and respiratory movements are factors maintaining lymph flow.

Postmastectomy syndrome is a form of lymphedema due to excision of the axillary lymphatic structures during mastectomy.

457.0 Postmastectomy lymphedema syndrome — *edema in arms and hands caused by pooling in interstitial fluids, due to reduced lymphatic circulation*
AHA: Q2, 2002, 12

457.1 Other noninfectious lymphedema — *other retention of fluids due to reduced lymphatic circulation; including elephantiasis, lymphedema*

457.2 Lymphangitis — *subacute or chronic inflammation of the lymph glands*

457.8 Other noninfectious disorders of lymphatic channels — *not otherwise specified, including sclerotic lymph gland, chylocele, or lymph node fistula, cyst infarction, or rupture*
AHA: Q3, 2003, 17

457.9 Unspecified noninfectious disorder of lymphatic channels

458 Hypotension

458.0 Orthostatic hypotension — *abnormally low blood pressure worsened when the seated patient stands*
AHA: Q3, 1991, 9; Q3, 2000, 8

458.1 Chronic hypotension — *persistent abnormally low blood pressure*

458.2 ✓5th Iatrogenic hypotension — *abnormally low blood pressure as a result of medical treatment*
AHA: Q4, 1995, 57; Q3, 2002, 12; Q4, 2003, 60

458.21 Hypotension of hemodialysis — *intra-dialytic hypotension*
AHA: Q4, 2003, 61

458.29 Other iatrogenic hypotension — *postoperative hypotension*

458.8 Other specified hypotension — *not otherwise specified*
AHA: Q4, 1997, 37

458.9 Unspecified hypotension

Coding Clarification

Orthostatic hypotension is an excessive fall in blood pressure when assuming an erect position. Severe orthostatic hypotension can be associated with a neuropathic disorder known as Shy-Drager syndrome or idiopathic orthostatic hypotension, classified to 333.0. It may also be due to volume depletion.

Iatrogenic hypotension or postoperative hypotension is classified to 458.29. This code fully describes postoperative hypotension and does not require an additional code to indicate complication of surgical or medical care.

Use code 458.8 to code postmyocardial infarction hypotension. Sequence the myocardial infarction code first.

459 Other disorders of circulatory system

Postphlebitic syndrome is a complex of symptoms due to venous hypertension as a consequence of postphlebitic incompetence of communicating veins.

459.0 Unspecified hemorrhage — *spontaneous rupture of blood vessel, not otherwise specified*
AHA: Q4, 1990, 26

459.10 Postphlebitic syndrome without complications

459.11 Postphlebitic syndrome with ulcer

459.12 Postphlebitic syndrome with inflammation

459.13 Postphlebitic syndrome with ulcer and inflammation

459.19 Postphlebitic syndrome with other complication

459.2 Compression of vein — *stricture of vein; vena cava syndrome*

459.3 ✓5th Chronic venous hypertension — *stasis edema*
AHA: Q4, 2002, 59

459.30 Chronic venous hypertension without complications

459.31 Chronic venous hypertension with ulcer

459.32 Chronic venous hypertension with inflammation

459.33 Chronic venous hypertension with ulcer and inflammation

459.39 Chronic venous hypertension with other complication

459.81 Unspecified venous (peripheral) insufficiency — (Use additional code for any associated ulceration: 707.10-707.9)

459.89 Other specified circulatory system disorders — *not otherwise specified*

459.9 Unspecified circulatory system disorder — *unknown site and unknown disorder*

Coding Clarification

Excluded from this rubric are cases of hemorrhage due to trauma.

Coding Scenario

A 45-year-old female, a data entry clerk by occupation, presents with a stasis dermatitis of the left lower extremity. The history reveals that three weeks previously, she suffered a deep venous thrombosis of the same leg. The physician has not documented any varicosity of the extremity.

Code assignment: 459.1x *Postphlebitic syndrome*

© 2004 Ingenix, Inc.

460–519
Diseases of the Respiratory System

This chapter classifies diseases and disorders of the nose (external, nasal cavity), sinuses (frontal, ethmoid, sphenoid, maxillary), pharynx (nasopharynx, oropharynx), larynx (true and false vocal cords, glottis), trachea, bronchi (left, right, main, carina), and lungs (intrapulmonary bronchi, bronchioli, lobes, alveoli, pleura).

This complex of organs is responsible for pulmonary ventilation and the exchange of oxygen and carbon dioxide between the lungs and ambient air. The organs of the respiratory system also perform nonrespiratory functions such as warming and moisturizing the air passing into the lungs, providing airflow for the larynx and vocal cords for speech, and releasing excess body heat in the process of thermoregulation for homeostasis. The lungs also perform important metabolic and embolic filtering functions.

460–466 Acute Respiratory Infections

Pneumonia and influenza are excluded from this section and can be found in rubrics 480-487.8.

460 Acute nasopharyngitis (common cold) OK

AHA: Q1, 1988, 12

This rubric classifies nasopharyngitis, rhinitis, coryza, or nasal catarrh of an acute nature. Acute nasopharyngitis is the most common of the upper respiratory infections, and is characterized by edema of the nasal mucous membrane, discharge, and obstruction.

Coding Clarification

Chronic nasopharyngitis is reported with 472.2.

461 Acute sinusitis

This rubric classifies sinusitis that is sudden and severe, according to the site of infection: frontal, maxillary, ethmoidal, sphenoidal, or multiple sites. Included in the definition of acute sinusitis are abscess, empyema, and suppuration. Acute sinusitis is usually preceded by an acute respiratory infection. A second code from Chapter 1 Infectious and Parasitic Diseases can be reported to identify the infectious agent, which most commonly is streptococci, pneumococci, *H. influenzae,* or staphylococci. In the case of immuno-compromised patients, the infectious agents are more likely to be aspergillosis, candidiasis, or fungal infections of the order Mucorales.

461.0 Acute maxillary sinusitis — *behind cheekbones*

461.1 Acute frontal sinusitis — *above the eyes*

461.2 Acute ethmoidal sinusitis — *between the eyes on either side of the nose*

461.3 Acute sphenoidal sinusitis — *behind the eyes on either side of the nose*

461.8 Other acute sinusitis — *pansinusitis*

461.9 Acute sinusitis, unspecified

Coding Clarification

Chronic sinusitis is excluded from this rubric and is reported with 473.0-473.9.

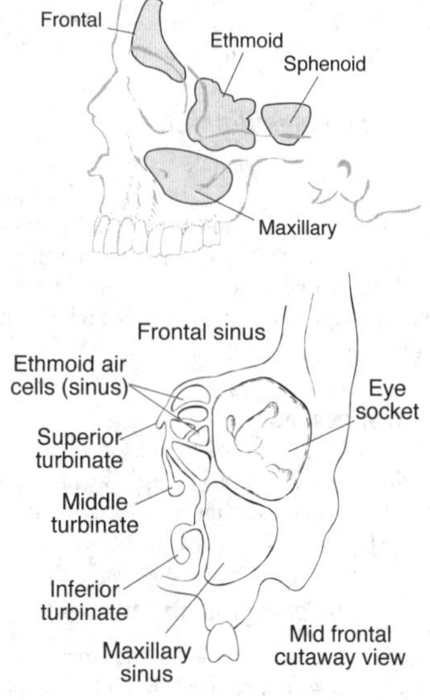

460–519

462 Acute pharyngitis OK

AHA: Sept-Oct, 1985, 8; Q4, 1999, 26

Acute pharyngitis is an acute inflammatory disorder of the throat, which may be caused by a virus or bacteria. Frequently, coryza or other communicable disease precedes acute pharyngitis.

Signs and symptoms of acute pharyngitis include history of tobacco or alcohol abuse, sore throat, dysphagia, fever, headache, and muscle and joint pain.

Therapies include warm saline gargles and analgesics such as aspirin to relieve throat discomfort, bed rest, IV hydration in severe cases, and antibiotics for suspected bacterial acute pharyngitis. Associated conditions include dehydration, sinusitis, and allergies.

Coding Clarification

A code from Chapter 1 Infectious and Parasitic Diseases can be reported secondarily to identify the infective agent in pharyngitis. The most common causes are the infectious agents streptococci, *Mycoplasma pneumoniae, Chlamydia pneumoniae,* or a virus.

Do not use this code to report chronic pharyngitis (472.1) or an abscess of the peritonsillar region (475), pharynx (478.29), or retropharynx (478.24). Also excluded is acute pharyngitis due to Coxsackie virus (074.0), gonococcus (098.6), herpes simplex (054.79), flu (487.1), or streptococcus (034.0). Septic pharyngitis is reported with 034.0.

463 Acute tonsillitis OK

AHA: Nov-Dec, 1984, 16

A sudden severe inflammation of the palatine tonsil is classified to this rubric. The infective agent is most commonly streptococcal or viral. Tonsillitis may be accompanied by throat pain, high fever, and, in some cases, vomiting.

Coding Clarification

Excluded from this rubric are chronic tonsillitis (474.0), hypertrophy of tonsil (474.1), streptococcal tonsillitis (034.0), and sore throat, not otherwise specified (462).

464 Acute laryngitis and tracheitis

Sudden and severe inflammation of the larynx, trachea, and epiglottis associated with infection are classified to this rubric, with obstruction of the airway being an axis for code choice. Laryngitis and tracheitis usually follow an upper respiratory infection, but may occur during the course of pneumonia, bronchitis, flu, or measles.

Acute epiglottitis usually is due to an infection by *Haemophilus influenzae,* pneumococci, or group A streptococci and can develop into a laryngeal airway obstruction. Signs and symptoms of acute epiglottitis include history of upper respiratory infection or chronic lung disease, high fever, sore throat, dysphagia, stridor, and respiratory distress.

Diagnostic tests/reports/findings include a throat exam to reveal an enlarged, edematous epiglottis. Laryngoscopy or lateral neck x-rays reveal inflammatory changes and signs of obstruction. Therapies include endotracheal intubation for obstruction, IV hydration to prevent dehydration, antibiotics (parenteral), oxygen therapy, and blood gas monitoring for hypoxia and hypercapnia.

Croup is an acute laryngotracheobronchitis usually seen in early childhood and characterized by stridor, respiratory distress, and swelling. Parainfluenza virus is usually the infective agent, although respiratory syncytial virus can also cause croup.

464.00 Acute laryngitis, without mention of obstruction

464.01 Acute laryngitis, with obstruction

464.10 Acute tracheitis without mention of obstruction — *sudden, severe inflammation of vocal cords*

464.11 Acute tracheitis with obstruction — *sudden, severe inflammation of vocal cords w/ obstruction*

464.20 Acute laryngotracheitis without mention of obstruction — *sudden, severe inflammation of trachea and vocal cords*

464.21 Acute laryngotracheitis with obstruction — *sudden, severe inflammation of trachea and vocal cords w/ obstruction*

464.30 Acute epiglottitis without mention of obstruction — *sudden, severe inflammation of epiglottis*

464.31 Acute epiglottitis with obstruction — *sudden, severe inflammation of epiglottis w/ obstruction*

464.4 Croup — *barking cough with inflammation of larynx*

464.50 Unspecified supraglottis, without mention of obstruction

464.51 Unspecified supraglottis, with obstruction

Coding Clarification

Excluded from this rubric are cases associated with the flu (487.1) or strep infection (034.0). For chronic laryngitis, see rubric 476; for chronic tracheitis, report 491.8.

If inflammation of the larynx is combined with inflammation of the trachea, report codes from subclassification 464.2 *Acute laryngotracheitis.*

© 2004 Ingenix, Inc.

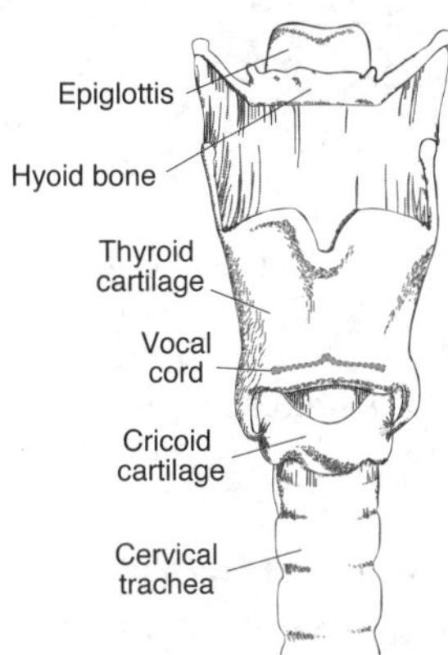

465 Acute upper respiratory infections of multiple or unspecified sites

This rubric is reserved for acute infections of multiple sites or when the site is not otherwise specified.

465.0 Acute laryngopharyngitis — *sudden, severe inflammation of vocal cords and pharynx*

465.8 Acute upper respiratory infections of other multiple sites — *multiple URI*

465.9 Acute upper respiratory infections of unspecified site — *unknown site, URI*

Coding Clarification

Excluded from this rubric are upper respiratory infections due to flu (487.1) or strep (034.0).

466 Acute bronchitis and bronchiolitis

Acute bronchitis is sudden and severe inflammation of the tracheobronchial tree. Acute bronchitis may have an infectious or irritative etiology.

Signs and symptoms of acute bronchitis include a history of upper respiratory infection or exposure to irritants such as dust or fumes, cough, malaise, fever, and pain in the back and chest. Therapies include bed rest and antibiotics such as oral tetracycline when purulent sputum is present. For patients with chronic respiratory disease, therapy includes antipyretics for fever, bronchodilators for bronchial asthma, and monitoring of arterial blood gases (ABGs) in cases of significant underlying chronic respiratory disease.

466.0 Acute bronchitis — *sudden, severe inflammation of bronchial tree main branches*
AHA: Q1, 1988, 12; Q4, 1991, 24; Q4, 1996, 28; Q4, 2002, 46

466.11 Acute bronchiolitis due to respiratory syncytial virus (RSV) — *bronchiolitis, capillary pneumonia due to RSV*
AHA: Q4, 1996, 27

466.19 Acute bronchiolitis due to other infectious organisms — (Use additional code to identify infectious organism) — *bronchiolitis, capillary pneumonia, other infectious agent*

Documentation Issues

When the documentation identifies acute and chronic bronchitis, report 491.22. If the documentation states chronic bronchitis, with or without mention of centrilobular emphysema (blue bloater), use code 491.2x.

If the physician documentation indicates COPD with asthmatic bronchitis, often the physician is referring to chronic obstructive pulmonary emphysema (492.8) with chronic pulmonary heart disease (416.8). Verify with the physician if this is the appropriate classification to identify the condition.

Coding Clarification

Acute and Chronic Bronchitis: Use two codes (466.0 and 491.9) when reporting acute and chronic bronchitis. This will correspond with the following coding guideline: If the same condition is described as both acute (subacute) and chronic and separate subentries exist in the Alphabetic Index at the same level, code both and list the acute (subacute) code first.

Acute Bronchitis and Emphysema: Two codes are required (466.0 *Acute bronchitis* and 492.8 *Other emphysema*) to accurately report this condition as per the National Center for Health Statistics.

Respiratory Syncytial Virus (RSV): If respiratory syncytial virus is noted with acute bronchitis, two codes are required: 466.0 *Acute bronchitis* and 079.6 *Respiratory syncytial virus (RSV)*. If the RSV is noted with acute bronchiolitis, use only code 466.11 *Acute bronchiolitis due to respiratory syncytial virus (RSV)*.

Associated conditions include underlying chronic lung disease such as chronic obstructive bronchitis or COPD, pneumonia or bronchopneumonia, or allergies. Excluded from this rubric are acute bronchitis with asthma (493), bronchiectasis (494.1), and COPD (491.21).

Coding Scenario

A 5-year-old patient is admitted with acute bronchitis and possible cystic fibrosis. A chest x-ray is performed, confirming the diagnosis of cystic fibrosis. The diagnosis at discharge is acute bronchitis and cystic fibrosis.

> Code assignment: 466.0 *Acute bronchitis* and 277.00 *Cystic fibrosis without mention of meconium ileus*

470–478 Other Diseases of the Upper Respiratory Tract

Included in this rubric are many chronic inflammatory diseases of the upper respiratory tract.

The upper respiratory tract includes the nasal cavity and the pharynx and any structure connecting to or associated with them (the paranasal sinus cavities, lacrimal apparatus and conjunctival sac, auditory tube, and middle ear). Though these accessory structures are associated with functions other than breathing or gas exchange, they are all lined with mucous membrane that is continuous with the nasal cavity and pharynx, and infections beginning anywhere in that mucous membrane can readily spread to adjacent structures. The larynx, which can be considered with either upper or lower respiratory structures, is the voice box and connects the pharynx with the tracheo-bronchial tree. It is lined with mucous membrane.

The nasal cavity has a mucociliary lining similar to that of the lower respiratory tract. The inside of the nose is lined with hair that filters inhaled particles. Mucous covering the turbinate bones, or baffle plates, captures particles not filtered by nasal hairs. The change in direction of the airway from the sinuses to the pharynx causes a large number of larger particles to impinge on the back of the throat. The adenoids and tonsils are lymphoid organs in the upper respiratory tract that are vital to an immune response to pathogens. A layer of mucous and ciliated cells covers the lower portion of the lower respiratory tract. Single and subepithelial cells secrete mucous. Particles or respiratory pathogens that reach the lower respiratory tract are first trapped in the mucous layer and are driven upwards by ciliary action to the back of the throat. There are two main obstacles a bacterium or virus must overcome in order to initiate an infection in the respiratory tract: the microorganism must avoid the mucous layers of the upper respiratory tract; however, if the microorganism gets past the mucous layers, it can travel to the lower respiratory tract or lung, where it either is destroyed by phagocytosis or multiplies in the phagocytic cell.

Most of the surfaces of the upper respiratory tract (including nasal and oral passages, nasopharynx, oropharynx, and trachea) are colonized by normal flora. These organisms rarely cause disease, but compete with pathogenic organisms for attachment sites.

Normal flora found in the nose, nasopharynx, and sinuses is as follows:

- Staphylococcus epidermidis
- Staph. aureus (especially in hospital staff)
- Streptococci (including *S. pyogenes* and *S. pneumoniae*)
- Haemophilus sp.
- Neisseria sp.

Normal flora found in the mouth and throat is as follows:

- Streptococci (mainly *S. mitis* and *S. salivarius*)
- Diphtheroids
- Anaerobes (e.g., Fusobacterium sp.)
- Staph. epidermidis

470 Deviated nasal septum OK

Deviated nasal septum is a common disorder that often requires no treatment. However, in some cases, the deviation in the septum, the result of past trauma, causes obstructions in the nasal passages that lead to chronic conditions like sinusitis or epistaxis. If the deviation predisposes the patient to chronic problems, the condition may be treated surgically. When coding, sequence the code for sinusitis or epistaxis first and the deviation secondarily.

Coding Clarification
Excluded from this rubric is congenital deviated septum, which is reported with 754.0.

471 Nasal polyps

Nasal polyps are a natural reaction to chronic sinusitis due to infection or allergy. Polyps most commonly form around the ostia of the maxillary sinus, and are classified according to site. Polyps may be asymptomatic or they may block the nasal airways or promote chronic sinus infection.

471.0 Polyp of nasal cavity — *choanal, nasopharyngeal*

471.1 Polypoid sinus degeneration — *Woakes' syndrome or ethmoiditis*

471.8 Other polyp of sinus — *accessory, ethmoidal, maxillary, sphenoidal, frontal, turbinate, mucous membrane*

471.9 Unspecified nasal polyp

Coding Clarification
Excluded from this rubric is adenomatous polyps (212.0).

472 Chronic pharyngitis and nasopharyngitis

Persistent inflammation of the pharynx and nasopharynx can be the result of an infective agent or due to an allergy or exposure to an irritant.

472.0 Chronic rhinitis — *persistent ozena, atrophic, granulomatous, purulent, ulcerative*

 © 2004 Ingenix, Inc.

472.1 Chronic pharyngitis — *persistent sore throat, atrophic, hypertrophic*

472.2 Chronic nasopharyngitis — *persistent inflammation from the nares to the pharynx*

Coding Clarification

Allergic rhinitis (477) is excluded from this rubric, as are all acute forms of pharyngitis or nasopharyngitis.q

473 Chronic sinusitis

Chronic sinusitis includes any persistent abscess, empyema, or infection of the nasal sinuses. It can be caused by an infective agent or by exposure to an allergic agent or irritant. Code selection is based on site: maxillary, frontal, ethmoidal, sphenoidal, or multiple sites.

473.0 Chronic maxillary sinusitis — *persistent inflammation of the sinus cavities behind the cheekbone; cloudy antrum*

473.1 Chronic frontal sinusitis — *persistent inflammation of the sinus cavities above the eyes*

473.2 Chronic ethmoidal sinusitis — *persistent inflammation of the sinus cavities between the eyes on either side of the nose*

473.3 Chronic sphenoidal sinusitis — *persistent inflammation of the sinus cavities behind the eyes on either side of the nose*

473.8 Other chronic sinusitis — *persistent pansinusitis*

473.9 Unspecified sinusitis (chronic) — *persistent sinusitis, unknown site*

Coding Clarification

Excluded from this rubric is acute sinusitis, which is classified to rubric 461.

474 Chronic disease of tonsils and adenoids

474.00 Chronic tonsillitis — *persistent inflammation, tonsil*
AHA: Q4, 1997, 38

474.01 Chronic adenoiditis — *persistent inflammation, adenoid*
AHA: Q4, 1997, 38

474.02 Chronic tonsillitis and adenoiditis — *persistent inflammation tonsil and adenoid*
AHA: Q4, 1997, 38

474.10 Hypertrophy of tonsil with adenoids — *enlargement, tonsil and adenoid*

474.11 Hypertrophy of tonsils alone — *enlargement, tonsil*

474.12 Hypertrophy of adenoids alone — *enlargement, adenoid*

474.2 Adenoid vegetations — *fungus-like growth*

474.8 Other chronic disease of tonsils and adenoids — *amygdalolith, calculus, cicatrix, tag, ulcer, cyst, plica, necrosis*

474.9 Unspecified chronic disease of tonsils and adenoids

Coding Clarification

Excluded from this rubric is acute or unspecified tonsillitis, which is classified to 463.

475 Peritonsillar abscess OK

Use this code to report an abscess of the tonsil, peritonsillar cellulitis, or Quinsy. In peritonsillar abscess, tonsillitis extends beyond tonsillar tissue to include the soft palate or the space between the tonsillar pillars.

Coding Clarification

Excluded from this rubric are chronic tonsillitis (474.0) and acute tonsillitis (463).

476 Chronic laryngitis and laryngotracheitis

Chronic laryngitis and laryngotracheitis are related to allergic reactions, inhalation of irritants, gastroesophageal reflux, or voice overuse. The voice is compromised, hoarse, or absent.

476.0 Chronic laryngitis — *persistent inflammation, vocal cords*

476.1 Chronic laryngotracheitis — *persistent inflammation, vocal cords and trachea*

Coding Clarification

Excluded from this rubric are chronic inflammations of the trachea (491.8) and acute laryngitis or tracheitis, classified to 464.00-464.51.

477 Allergic rhinitis

Allergic rhinitis, more commonly referred to as hay fever, is an inflammation of the nasal passages caused by allergic reaction to airborne substances. There are two types of allergic rhinitis: seasonal and perennial. The seasonal type occurs when airborne plant pollens are at highest levels. Home or workplace airborne pollutants are usually the cause of the perennial type. Both types of allergies can develop at any age, although childhood through early adulthood onset is most common. Common allergens include pollen, mold, fungi, animal dander, and dust mites. Oftentimes, the animal need not be present to cause the reaction to animal dander; it can occur upon exposure to the allergens left in a room where the animal has previously been. Common symptoms include inflammation of the nose, or rhinitis, accompanied by sneezing, runny nose, redness, and tenderness. Sinus swelling can constrict the eustachian tube, causing a congested feeling. Allergy tests, including skin testing and provocation testing, can help identify the allergen. When it is not possible to avoid one or more allergens, there are two major forms of medical treatment; drugs and immunotherapy.

477.0 Allergic rhinitis due to pollen — *pollinosis*

477.1 Allergic rhinitis, due to food

477.2 Allergic rhinitis, due to animal (cat) (dog) hair and dander

477.8 Allergic rhinitis due to other allergen

477.9 Allergic rhinitis, cause unspecified — *unknown cause*
AHA: Q2, 1997, 9

Coding Scenario

A 9-year-old girl is brought to see her pediatrician because she has been suffering nasal congestion, runny nose, and itchy eyes that have not subsided and now she appears to be having breathing trouble. The family just adopted a new pet, a cat, and that seems to be when the sneezing started. The doctor recommends finding the cat a new home and doing a thorough cleaning to remove the allergens left behind and diagnoses her with acute allergic rhinitis from cat hair.

Code assignment: 477.2 *Allergic rhinitis due to animal (cat) (dog) dander*

460–519

478 Other diseases of upper respiratory tract

Tornwaldt's cyst is a superficial nasopharyngeal cyst that causes purulent exudate and drainage, sore throat, and eustachian tube complications. It is reported with 478.26.

478.0 Hypertrophy of nasal turbinates — *overgrowth of nasal cavity bones*

478.1 Other diseases of nasal cavity and sinuses — *abscess, necrosis, ulcer, cyst, mucocele, rhinolith*

478.20 Unspecified disease of pharynx

478.21 Cellulitis of pharynx or nasopharynx — *inflammation of deep, soft tissues*

478.22 Parapharyngeal abscess — *pocket of pus*

478.24 Retropharyngeal abscess — *pocket of pus*

478.25 Edema of pharynx or nasopharynx — *fluid retention*

478.26 Cyst of pharynx or nasopharynx — *fluid-filled sac*

478.29 Other disease of pharynx or nasopharynx — *including abscess, hyperactive gag reflex, polyp, Tornwaldt's bursitis, ulcer, perforation, spontaneous rupture*

478.30 Unspecified paralysis of vocal cords or larynx — *unknown side*

478.31 Unilateral partial paralysis of vocal cords or larynx — *one side*

478.32 Unilateral complete paralysis of vocal cords or larynx — *one side*

478.33 Bilateral partial paralysis of vocal cords or larynx — *both sides*

478.34 Bilateral complete paralysis of vocal cords or larynx — *both sides*

478.4 Polyp of vocal cord or larynx — *growth of benign tissue*

478.5 Other diseases of vocal cords — *abscess, cellulitis, granuloma, leukoplakia, chorditis, singer's nodes*

478.6 Edema of larynx — *fluid retention*

478.70 Unspecified disease of larynx

478.71 Cellulitis and perichondritis of larynx — *inflammation of deep soft tissue*

478.74 Stenosis of larynx — *narrowing of the diameter of larynx*

478.75 Laryngeal spasm — *involuntary muscle contraction; laryngismus, Millar's asthma*

478.79 Other diseases of larynx — *abscess, necrosis, obstruction, pachyderma, ulcer, nodule, ossification, sclerosis*
AHA: Q3, 1991, 20

478.8 Upper respiratory tract hypersensitivity reaction, site unspecified — *site unknown*

478.9 Other and unspecified diseases of upper respiratory tract — *abscess and cicatrix of trachea, not otherwise specified*

Coding Clarification

Excluded from this rubric is ulcerative laryngitis, classified to 464.00-464.01.

480–487 Pneumonia and Influenza

Pneumonia and influenza are inflammations in the alveolar parenchyma of the lung caused by microbial infection, irradiation, or physicochemical agents. Microbial agents include viral, bacterial, fungal, protozoal, mycobacterial, mycoplasmal, or rickettsial pathogens. Physicochemical agents may be inhaled or reach the lung via the bloodstream. Inhaled agents include toxic gases, irritant particles, or irritant fluids such as gastric juice. Bleomycin is an example of a blood-borne anticancer agent that can cause pneumonia.

The terms "pneumonia" and "pneumonitis" describe two clinical patterns of inflammatory reaction in the lung. The unqualified term "pneumonia" generally refers to pneumonia with exudation in the air spaces. Inflammatory exudate fills the lung alveoli, which are then rendered airless and solid, in a process called consolidation. The terms "pneumonitis" and "interstitial pneumonia" commonly refer to pneumonia with interstitial exudate.

Signs and symptoms of pneumonia vary according to etiology (e.g., with bacterial pneumonia: coughing,

© 2004 Ingenix, Inc.

sputum production, pleuritic chest pain, shaking chills, fever; with aspiration pneumonia: chest rales, dyspnea, cyanosis, hypotension, and tachycardia).

In pneumonia, chest x-ray shows infiltration or consolidation. Blood work may show normal, slightly elevated or markedly elevated white blood cell count (WBC), depending on etiology. Smears, cultures, and gram stains of sputum and/or pleural fluid isolate and identify bacteria. Percutaneous aspiration of lung tissue, endoscopic or open lung biopsy identifies difficult nonbacterial agents such as cytomegalovirus.

Therapies include antibiotics for confirmed and suspected bacterial pneumonia, oxygen therapy, complete bed rest, and intubation and ventilatory support for critically ill patients developing respiratory failure. In addition, there is respiratory therapy, which involves suctioning, coughing, and deep breathing exercises.

Associated conditions include pleural effusion, respiratory failure, empyema, atelectasis, and underlying chronic lung disease such as COPD.

To ensure proper code assignment, first refer to the ICD-9-CM index under the main terms "Pneumonia" and "Pneumonitis." Many forms of pneumonia are classified to other chapters of ICD-9-CM because of etiology. For example, candidal pneumonia is classified to code 112.4 and congenital toxoplasmosis pneumonitis is classified to codes 771.2 and 484.8.

480 Viral pneumonia

480.0 Pneumonia due to adenovirus — *viral infection of lung*

480.1 Pneumonia due to respiratory syncytial virus — *viral infection of lung*
AHA: Q1, 1988, 12; Q4, 1996, 28

480.2 Pneumonia due to parainfluenza virus — *viral infection of lung*

480.3 Pneumonia due to SARS-associated coronavirus — *due to severe acute respiratory syndrome; symptoms include fever, dry cough, dyspnea, headache, hypoxemia (low blood oxygen concentration); usual laboratory findings include lymphopenia (reduced lymphocyte numbers), mildly elevated aminotransferase levels, possible respiratory failure and death due to alveolar damage*
AHA: Q4, 2003, 46-47

480.8 Pneumonia due to other virus not elsewhere classified — *viral infection*

480.9 Unspecified viral pneumonia — *viral infection of lung, unknown virus*
AHA: Q3, 1998, 5

481 Pneumococcal pneumonia (streptococcus pneumoniae pneumonia) OK

AHA: March-April, 1985, 6; Q1, 1988, 13; Q1, 1991, 13; Q1, 1992, 18; Q4, 1992, 19; Q2, 1998, 7

482 Other bacterial pneumonia

AHA: Q4, 1993, 39

482.0 Pneumonia due to Klebsiella pneumoniae — *bacterial infection*
AHA: Q4, 1993, 39

482.1 Pneumonia due to Pseudomonas — *bacterial infection of lung*
AHA: Q4, 1993, 39

482.2 Pneumonia due to Hemophilus influenzae (H. influenzae) — *bacterial infection of lung*
AHA: Q4, 1993, 39

This rubric excludes pneumonia due to *Streptococcus pneumoniae* (481).

482.30 Pneumonia due to unspecified Streptococcus — *strep infection of lung, unknown variety*
AHA: Q1, 1988, 13; Q4, 1993, 39

482.31 Pneumonia due to Streptococcus, group A — *strep infection of lung*
AHA: Q1, 1988, 13; Q4, 1993, 39

482.32 Pneumonia due to Streptococcus, group B — *strep infection of lung*
AHA: Q1, 1988, 13; Q4, 1993, 39

482.39 Pneumonia due to other Streptococcus — *strep infection of lung, not otherwise specified*
AHA: Q1, 1988, 13; Q4, 1993, 39

482.40 Pneumonia due to Staphylococcus, unspecified — *staph infection of lung, unknown variety*
AHA: Q3, 1991, 16; Q4, 1993, 39

482.41 Pneumonia due to Staphylococcus aureus — *staph infection of lung*
AHA: Q3, 1991, 16; Q4, 1993, 39

482.49 Other Staphylococcus pneumonia — *staph infection of lung, unknown variety*
AHA: Q3, 1991, 16; Q4, 1993, 39

482.81 Pneumonia due to anaerobes — *bacteroides, gram-negative anaerobes*
AHA: Q3, 1988, 11; Q4, 1993, 39

482.82 Pneumonia due to escherichia coli (E. coli)

482.83 Pneumonia due to other gram-negative bacteria — *proteus, Serratia marcescens, gram-negative not otherwise specified*
AHA: Q3, 1988, 11; Q4, 1993, 39; Q3, 1994, 9; Q2, 1998, 5

482.84 Legionnaires' disease

460–519

© 2004 Ingenix, Inc.

482.89 Pneumonia due to other specified bacteria — *not elsewhere classified*
AHA: Q3, 1988, 11; Q4, 1993, 39; Q2, 1997, 6

482.9 Unspecified bacterial pneumonia — *bacterial pneumonia, unknown*
AHA: Q4, 1993, 39; Q1, 1994, 17; Q2, 1997, 6; Q2, 1998, 6

483 Pneumonia due to other specified organism

AHA: Nov-Dec, 1987, 5

Mycoplasma pneumoniae is also known as Eaton agent pneumonia.

Signs and symptoms of pneumonia due to *Mycoplasma pneumoniae* include history of recent upper respiratory infection or bronchitis, headache, fever, severe and minimally productive cough, harsh or diminished breath sounds, earache, and cervical lymphadenopathy.

Diagnostic tests include gram stain and culture of sputum or throat washing to reveal polymorphonuclear leukocytes with no dominant organism. Other lab work demonstrates fourfold or greater rise in complement-fixing antibodies and elevated cold agglutinins (IgM antibodies binding to the erythrocyte I antigen). Chest x-ray shows pulmonary infiltrates resembling bacterial or viral pneumonia.

Therapies include antibiotics such as erythromycin or tetracycline, bed rest, and high protein diet.

Associated conditions include cold agglutinin induced hemolytic anemia, arthralgia and polyarthritis, skin rashes, Stevens-Johnson syndrome, transverse myelitis, meningoencephalitis, and myocarditis.

483.0 Pneumonia due to Mycoplasma pneumoniae — *Eaton's agent, pleuropneumonia-like organism [PPLO]*
AHA: Nov-Dec, 1987, 5

483.1 Pneumonia due to Chlamydia

483.8 Pneumonia due to other specified organism — *not elsewhere classified*
AHA: Nov-Dec, 1987, 5

484 Pneumonia in infectious diseases classified elsewhere

484.1 Pneumonia in cytomegalic inclusion disease — (Code first underlying disease, 078.5) — *infection of lung*

484.3 Pneumonia in whooping cough — (Code first underlying disease: 033.0-033.9) — *infection of lung*

484.5 Pneumonia in anthrax — (Code first underlying disease, 022.1) — *infection of lung*

484.6 Pneumonia in aspergillosis — (Code first underlying disease, 117.3) — *infection of lung*
AHA: Q4, 1997, 40

484.7 Pneumonia in other systemic mycoses — (Code first underlying disease) — *infection of lung*

484.8 Pneumonia in other infectious diseases classified elsewhere — (Code first underlying disease: 002.0, 083.0) — *infection of lung*

485 Bronchopneumonia, organism unspecified OK

486 Pneumonia, organism unspecified OK

AHA: Q3, 1988, 11; Q3, 1994, 10; Q3, 1997, 9; Q1, 1998, 8; Q2, 1998, 4,5; Q3, 1998, 7; Q3, 1999, 9; Q4, 1999, 6

487 Influenza

Influenza is an acute respiratory infection due to orthomyxoviruses characterized by the abrupt onset of acute tracheobronchitis. The severity of the disease varies from a mild upper respiratory infection to an extensive pneumonia that can be fatal.

Influenza virus type A is the most common and causes epidemics of varying severity. Influenza virus type B is associated with more limited epidemics and has been linked to Reye's syndrome. Influenza virus type C is an uncommon strain that causes very mild upper respiratory symptoms.

Signs and symptoms of influenza include fever, chills, malaise, cough, muscle aches, and excessive catarrh.

Diagnostic tests/reports/findings include blood work that may show leukopenia and proteinuria. Inoculation of embryonated eggs or cell cultures of throat washing isolate the virus. Chest x-ray may show pneumonia, commonly due to secondary pneumococcal or staphylococcal pneumonia.

Therapies include bed rest, antibiotics for secondary bacterial pneumonia, antipyretics for fever, and aerosol ribavirin for influenza type A or B.

Associated conditions include Reye's syndrome, secondary pneumococcal or staphylococcal pneumonia, acute sinusitis, otitis media, and, rarely, circulatory system complications such as pericarditis, myocarditis, and thrombophlebitis.

487.0 Influenza with pneumonia — *flu with any form of pneumonia or bronchopneumonia*

460–519

© 2004 Ingenix, Inc.

487.1 Influenza with other respiratory manifestations — *flu with upper respiratory infection [URI], except pneumonia or bronchopneumonia*
AHA: Q4, 1999, 26

487.8 Influenza with other manifestations — *encephalopathy*

490–496 Chronic Obstructive Pulmonary Disease and Allied Conditions

490 Bronchitis, not specified as acute or chronic OK

AHA: Q3, 1988, 5

Coding Clarification

Excluded from this rubric is bronchitis due to allergy (493.9), fumes and vapors (506.0), or with asthma (493.9).

491 Chronic bronchitis

AHA: Q3, 1988, 5

Obstructive chronic bronchitis is chronic bronchitis combined with obstructive lung disease. Chronic bronchitis is defined as a persistent cough with sputum production occurring on most days for at least three months of the year for at least two years. Obstructive lung disease is defined as a chronic or recurrent reduction in expiratory airflow within the lungs. Obstructive chronic bronchitis is characterized by an increased mass of mucous glands in the lungs, resulting in an increase in the thickness of the bronchial mucosa. Its most common etiology is cigarette smoking, but it also may be caused by environmental pollution or inhalation of irritant chemicals.

Signs and symptoms of obstructive chronic bronchitis include history of cigarette smoking or other respiratory irritants, sputum productive cough, exertional dyspnea, weight gain due to edema, cyanosis, tachypnea, rhonchi, wheezing with prolonged expiratory time, use of accessory muscles for respiration, jugular or neck vein distention, and pedal edema.

Diagnostic tests include chest x-ray that may show hyperinflation with increased bronchovascular markings. Pulmonary function tests show increased residual volume, decreased vital capacity, and forced expiratory volumes, normal static compliance, and diffusing capacity; ABGs reveal decreased pO2 and normal or increased pCO2. Culture of sputum reveals many neutrophils and varied organisms.

Therapies include oxygen therapy for hypoxia, antibiotics for concomitant respiratory infections, bronchodilators such as aminophylline to control bronchospasm and promote mucociliary expectoration, diuretics for edema, and ultrasonic or mechanical nebulizer treatments to loosen and help mobilize secretions.

Associated conditions include respiratory failure, atrial arrhythmias, and acute respiratory infections.

Acute bronchitis is sudden and severe inflammation of the tracheobronchial tree. Acute bronchitis may have an infectious or irritative etiology.

Signs and symptoms of acute bronchitis include a history of upper respiratory infection or exposure to irritants such as dust or fumes, cough, malaise, fever, and pain in the back and chest. Therapies include bed rest and antibiotics such as oral tetracycline when purulent sputum is present.

491.0 Simple chronic bronchitis — *persistent, catarrhal, smoker's cough*
AHA: Q3, 1988, 5

491.1 Mucopurulent chronic bronchitis — *persistent, purulent, recurrent*
AHA: Q3, 1988, 5; Q3, 1988, 12

491.20 Obstructive chronic bronchitis, without exacerbation

491.21 Obstructive chronic bronchitis, with (acute) exacerbation

491.22 Obstructive chronic bronchitis with acute bronchitis

491.8 Other chronic bronchitis — *tracheitis or tracheobronchitis*
AHA: Q3, 1988, 5

491.9 Unspecified chronic bronchitis — *unknown type*
AHA: Q3, 1988, 5

Documentation Issues

If the documentation states chronic bronchitis, with or without mention of centrilobular emphysema (blue bloater), use code 491.2x.

If the physician documentation indicates COPD with asthmatic bronchitis, often the physician is referring to chronic obstructive pulmonary emphysema (492.8) with chronic pulmonary heart disease (416.8). Verify with the physician if this is the appropriate classification to identify the condition.

Assign a fifth digit 0 to indicate obstructive chronic bronchitis without mention of acute exacerbation and fifth digit 1 for obstructive chronic bronchitis with acute exacerbation. Acute exacerbation of chronic obstructive bronchitis is not the same as acute bronchitis.

Coding Clarification

Excluded from this rubric is chronic obstructive asthma with acute exacerbation, classified to 493.22.

460–519

492 Emphysema

AHA: Q3, 1988, 5; Q2, 1991, 21

Emphysema refers to any condition in which air is present in a small area of an organ or tissue, for example, in the interstices of the conjunctival tissue. Emphysema classified to category 492 refers to pulmonary emphysema only.

The definition of emphysematous bleb is a disease characterized by the formation of subpleural, air-filled cystlike structures that are greater than 1.0 centimeter in diameter. Also known as emphysematous bullae, they can be found in association with other forms of pulmonary emphysema or can occur alone, especially in younger patients. Apical bullae are the most common cause of spontaneous pneumothorax in young patients.

492.0 Emphysematous bleb — *tension pneumatocele, vanishing lung, giant bullous emphysema*
AHA: Q3, 1988, 5; Q2, 1991, 21; Q2, 1993, 3

492.8 Other emphysema — *pink puffer, MacLeod's syndrome, Swyer-James syndrome*
AHA: July-Aug, 1984, 17; Q3, 1988, 5; Q2, 1991, 21; Q4, 1993, 41

Coding Clarification

Other emphysema is abnormal irreversible enlargement of the air spaces distal to the terminal bronchioli accompanied by destruction of alveolar walls. The condition results in a reduction of the alveolar surface necessary for gas exchange. There are two major types of pulmonary emphysema: centroacinar and panacinar.

Centroacinar or centrilobar, emphysema affects the central parts of the lung acini and destroys the respiratory bronchioli. It often is associated with chronic bronchitis and smoking.

Panacinar, or pan lobar, emphysema destroys the alveolar walls and is distributed uniformly among the lung acini. The disease is more diffuse than centroacinar emphysema. Like centroacinar emphysema, panacinar emphysema occurs in cigarette smokers, but is also found in young adults with a familial history of emphysema.

Signs and symptoms of other emphysema include history of cigarette smoking, barrel-chested appearance, shortness of breath, anorexia, weight loss, breathing abnormalities such as the use of accessory muscles, prolonged expiration, grunting, pursed lip breathing, tachypnea, peripheral cyanosis, and digital clubbing.

Associated conditions include recurrent respiratory infections, cor pulmonale, and respiratory failure.

Other forms of pulmonary emphysema classified to this subcategory are distal acinar or paraseptal emphysema, irregular or paracicatricial emphysema, mixed emphysema, and unclassified forms of emphysema.

493 Asthma

AHA: Nov-Dec, 1984, 17; July-Aug, 1985, 8; Q3, 1988, 5,9; Q1, 1991, 13; Q4, 2000, 42; Q4, 2001, 43; Q4, 2003, 62

Asthma is the narrowing of the airways due to increased responsiveness of the trachea and bronchi to various stimuli. Asthma is reversible, changing in severity either spontaneously or as a result of treatment. Asthma is associated with bronchospasm and pathologic features such as increased mucous secretion, mucosal edema and hyperemia, hypertrophy of bronchial smooth muscle, and acute inflammation.

Signs and symptoms of asthma include recurrent or chronic episodes of wheezing, dyspnea, cough, chest tightness, chest pain, tachycardia, tachypnea, increased accessory muscle respiration, and history of familial allergy.

Diagnostic tests include blood work that may show increased WBC during acute attack and eosinophilia. ABGs may show hypoxemia and respiratory alkalosis. Gross exam of sputum demonstrates viscidity, while microscopic exam of sputum reveals mucous casts, eosinophils, and elongated rhomboid crystals. Pulmonary function tests show typical abnormalities of obstructive dysfunction. Chest x-ray may show hyperinflated lungs and skin tests and inhalation bronchial challenge tests identify and evaluate the clinical significance of allergens.

Therapies include bronchodilators such as epinephrine, aminophylline, albuterol; other medications such as cromolyn sodium, anticholinergics, corticosteroids, hyposensitization or "allergy" shots; oxygen therapy; and intubation and ventilation therapy for severe attacks of asthma.

Associated conditions include respiratory failure, eosinophilia, pneumothorax, acute cor pulmonale, and atelectasis.

Triad asthma is a syndrome that occurs in patients with three conditions that can be coded: intrinsic asthma (subclassification 493.0), aspirin sensitivity (apply codes according to ICD-9-CM coding rules regarding adverse reaction), and nasal polyposis (rubric 471).

In ICD-9-CM, asthma is classified as extrinsic, intrinsic, chronic obstructive, or unspecified. Extrinsic asthma is asthma due to allergenic exposure to substances such as pollen, house dust, animal dander, molds, food or beverages, vapors, or drugs. Most prevalent in children, this condition is associated with abnormally high levels of IgE immunoglobulins, indicating an allergic reaction.

 © 2004 Ingenix, Inc.

Intrinsic asthma is asthma due to nonallergenic factors such as emotional stresses, fatigue, endocrine changes, irritants (nonallergenic) such as dust and chemicals, and acute respiratory infection. More prevalent in adults, intrinsic asthma is associated with normal IgE immunoglobulin levels, indicating a nonallergic reaction.

This differentiation between extrinsic or intrinsic is considered archaic by many clinicians because manifestations of both extrinsic and intrinsic diseases commonly occur in the same patient. It is recommended that hospitals and physician offices develop coding policies for patients diagnosed with both intrinsic and extrinsic asthmatic conditions.

Chronic obstructive asthma is used to identify obstructive forms of asthma (in obstructive lung disease). Patients with chronic obstructive pulmonary disease with asthma have a continuous obstruction to airflow on expiration, which is different than patients with nonobstructive asthma, who wheeze during an asthma attack, but return to normal breathing once the attack subsides. Respiratory insufficiency is included in subcategory 493.2x because it is integral to COPD; do not code separately.

Status asthmaticus refers to a prolonged, severe asthmatic attack or airway obstruction (mucous plug) not relieved by bronchodilators. Symptoms of status asthmaticus are prolonged, severe, intractable wheezing, severe respiratory distress, asthma with respiratory failure, asthma attack with absence of breath sounds, lethargy, confusion, and failure to respond to the usual therapies.

Steroid Dependent Asthma: If there is no mention of side effects due to the steroid therapy, use a code from category 493. If, however, side effects are mentioned, both the asthma and the side effects of the steroid are coded. When the patient is being examined for adverse effects based on the long-term use of steroids, use code V58.65 *Long term (current) use of steroids* and a code from category 493 to identify the asthma.

The following fifth-digit subclassification is for use with category codes 493.0x-493.2x, 493.9x:

0 unspecified

1 with status asthmaticus

2 with acute exacerbation

493.0 ✓5th Extrinsic asthma — *caused by environmental factor (allergy)*
AHA: Nov-Dec, 1984, 17; July-Aug, 1985, 8; Q3, 1988, 5,9; Q1, 1991, 13; Q4, 2000, 42; Q4, 2001, 43

493.1 ✓5th Intrinsic asthma — *caused by body's response to infection or other factor*
AHA: Nov-Dec, 1984, 17; March-April, 1985, 7; July-Aug, 1985, 8; Q3, 1988, 9; Q3, 1988, 5,9; Q1, 1991, 13; Q4, 2000, 42; Q4, 2001, 43

493.2 ✓5th Chronic obstructive asthma — *persistent restriction of airflow and labored breathing*
AHA: Nov-Dec, 1984, 17; July-Aug, 1985, 8; Q3, 1988, 5,9; Q2, 1990, 20; Q1, 1991, 13; Q2, 1991, 21; Q4, 2000, 42; Q4, 2001, 43

493.81 Exercise induced bronchospasm — *physical activity causing spasms of the smooth muscle of the bronchi*

493.82 Cough variant asthma — *chronic cough (more than three weeks) is the only symptom; non-productive, nocturnal only cough is common; diagnosis only confirmed when cough resolves with asthma medication*

493.9 ✓5th Unspecified asthma — *unknown type*
AHA: Nov-Dec, 1984, 17; July-Aug, 1985, 8; Q3, 1988, 5,9; Q1, 1991, 13; Q4, 1997, 40; Q4, 2000, 42; Q4, 2001, 43

Documentation Issues

Documentation must always be clear and concise when identifying asthma with other conditions.

The physician must document the presence of "status asthmaticus" to promote coding accuracy. The admission of an asthma patient to the hospital is typically due to the patient's failure to respond to therapy, requiring more intensive therapy. Do not assume that since the patient was admitted, the diagnosis is status asthmaticus. Confirm the patient status with the physician before assigning the fifth digit 1.

Coding Clarification

Asthma with Associated Conditions: The following are common diagnostic statements and their associated code assignments:

- Asthma with COPD (493.2x)
- Asthma (493.0x-493.9x) and acute bronchitis (466.0)
- Chronic obstructive emphysema (492.8) associated with asthma (493.0x-493.9x)
- Either chronic obstructive bronchitis or asthma as comorbidity, such as chronic obstructive bronchitis (491.2x) superimposed on intrinsic asthma (493.10)
- Chronic pneumothorax (512.8) with intrinsic (493.10) or extrinsic (493.00) asthma
- Atelectasis (518.0) associated with asthma (493.0x-493.9x)
- Bronchiectasis (494) associated with asthma (493.0x-493.9x)

460–519

- Mediastinal or subcutaneous nontraumatic emphysema (518.1) with asthma (493.00 or 493.10)
- Wheezing (786.07) (commonly noted symptom of COPD with asthma)
- Pneumonia (486) with asthma (493.0x-493.9x)
- Reactive airway disease (493.90 *Asthma, type unspecified, status unspecified*)

Coding Scenario

A 49-year-old patient is seen in the clinic for adrenal-pituitary insufficiency secondary to steroids. The patient is a known steroid-dependent asthmatic.

> Code assignment: 255.4 *Corticoadrenal insufficiency,* 493.90 *Asthma, type unspecified, status unspecified,* and E932.0 *Drug causing adverse effects in therapeutic use, adrenal cortical steroids*

A 14-year-old male patient is seen in the emergency department with acute shortness of breath. The patient is a known asthmatic. The physician's diagnosis is asthma.

> Code assignment: 493.90 *Asthma, type unspecified, status unspecified*

A patient is admitted with acute respiratory insufficiency and asthma. The patient's history identifies that the patient has chronic obstructive asthma. The physician's final diagnosis on the discharge summary indicates chronic obstructive asthma with status asthmaticus and acute respiratory failure.

> Code assignment: 493.21 *Chronic obstructive asthma with status asthmaticus* and 518.81 *Acute respiratory failure*

A 20-year-old female patient, a collegiate track athlete, is admitted after collapsing during a track event with acute exacerbation of asthma. The patient's condition is brought under control with Albuterol and oxygen.

> Code assignment: 493.92 *Asthma, unspecified, with acute exacerbation*

494 Bronchiectasis

AHA: Q3, 1988, 5; Q4, 2000, 42

Bronchiectasis is the dilation of bronchi with mucous production and persistent cough. Mounier-Kuhn syndrome is a form of bronchiectasis. Code choice is determined by whether the patient also presents with acute bronchitis (acute exacerbation).

494.0 Bronchiectasis without acute exacerbation — *dilation of bronchi, mucous production, cough*
AHA: Q3, 1988, 5; Q4, 2000, 42

494.1 Bronchiectasis with acute exacerbation — *dilation of bronchi, mucous production, cough, with sudden worsening of condition*
AHA: Q3, 1988, 5; Q4, 2000, 42

Coding Clarification

Excluded from this rubric is bronchiectasis as a congenital disorder (748.61) and bronchiectasis in active tuberculosis (011.5).

495 Extrinsic allergic alveolitis

AHA: Q3, 1988, 5

Codes in this rubric report inflammation of the alveoli of the lung due to allergic reaction to the environment, including inhaled organic dust particles of fungal, thermophilic actinomycete, or other origin.

495.0 Farmers' lung — *antigen: Micropolyspora faeni or Thermoactinomyces vulgaris in moldy hay*
AHA: Q3, 1988, 5

495.1 Bagassosis — *antigen: Micropolyspora faeni or Thermoactinomyces vulgaris in sugarcane waste*
AHA: Q3, 1988, 5

495.2 Bird-fanciers' lung — *antigen: bird droppings from parakeets, pigeons and chickens*
AHA: Q3, 1988, 5

495.3 Suberosis — *antigen: moldy cork dust; "cork-handler's lung"*
AHA: Q3, 1988, 5

495.4 Malt workers' lung — *antigen: Aspergillus clavatus or Aspergillus fumigatus in moldy barley or malt*
AHA: Q3, 1988, 5

495.5 Mushroom workers' lung — *antigen: Micropolyspora faeni or Thermoactinomyces vulgaris in mushroom compost*
AHA: Q3, 1988, 5

495.6 Maple bark-strippers' lung — *antigen: Cryptostroma corticale in infected maple bark*
AHA: Q3, 1988, 5

495.7 "Ventilation" pneumonitis — *antigen: any of numerous organisms growing in ventilation systems*
AHA: Q3, 1988, 5

495.8 Other specified allergic alveolitis and pneumonitis — *wood asthma, coffee workers' lung, fish meal workers' lung, furrier's lung*
AHA: Q3, 1988, 5

495.9 Unspecified allergic alveolitis and pneumonitis — *unknown extrinsic alveolitis*
AHA: Q3, 1988, 5

460–519

 © 2004 Ingenix, Inc.

496 Chronic airway obstruction, not elsewhere classified OK

AHA: Q3, 1988, 5,56; Q2, 1991, 21; Q2, 1992, 16; Q2, 2000, 15; Q4, 2003, 109

Chronic airway obstruction is a nonspecific condition characterized by a chronic or recurrent reduction in expiratory airflow within the lung. Chronic obstructive pulmonary disease (COPD) and chronic obstructive lung disease (COLD) are the two most common descriptive diagnostic terms assigned to this code category.

Signs and symptoms of chronic airway obstruction, not elsewhere classified, include history of cigarette smoking and frequent respiratory infections, dyspnea on exertion with reduced exercise tolerance, sputum-productive cough, bronchi, decreased intensity of breath sounds, and prolonged expiration. Therapies include bronchodilators such as theophylline, corticosteroids such as prednisone, oxygen therapy and chest physiotherapy, and antibiotics for superimposed acute respiratory infections. Associated conditions include cor pulmonale (chronic pulmonary hypertension), sinus tachycardia, supraventricular arrhythmias, secondary polycythemia, acute bronchitis, pneumonia, left ventricular failure, pulmonary embolism, and acute respiratory insufficiency or failure.

Coding Clarification

Do not assign code 496 with any code from categories 491 through 493.

500–508 Pneumoconioses and Other Lung Diseases Due to External Agents

500 Coal workers' pneumoconiosis OK

Inhaling coal dust for prolonged periods can cause the disabling coal workers' pneumoconiosis, also known as black lung disease, which may produce: 1) asymptomatic anthracosis; 2) simple coal-workers pneumoconiosis (characterized by coal macules and nodules containing carbon-laden macrophages), with little or no pulmonary dysfunction; or 3) complicated coal-workers pneumoconiosis or progressive massive fibrosis (e.g., black scars in the lungs compromising pulmonary function). Symptoms include shortness of breath and a chronic cough. The diagnosis can be made with chest x-ray or a pulmonary function test. Most affected workers are older than age 50. Although some miners never develop the disease, others may develop the early signs after less than 10 years of mining experience. According to recent studies by the National Institute for Occupational Safety and Health (NIOSH), about one of every 20 miners studied has X-ray evidence of some pneumoconiosis. Pneumoconiosis is not reversible and federal laws require that mine dust levels be controlled to help prevent pneumoconiosis.

501 Asbestosis OK

Asbestosis is a serious lung inflammation caused by asbestos exposure (i.e., installed or removed insulation before 1975) that makes the lungs more susceptible to lung infections, such as the flu or pnuemococcus. In addition, asbestosis can lead to mesothelioma, a rare form of cancer in which malignant cells are found in the sac lining of the chest or abdomen. There is no cure for asbestosis, although symptoms can be treated. For example, the coughing can be treated with supplemental oxygen and treatments to remove secretions from the lung. According to the Occupational Safety and Health Administration: "OSHA is aware of no instance in which exposure to a toxic substance has more clearly demonstrated detrimental health effects on humans than has asbestos exposure. The diseases caused by asbestos exposure are life-threatening or disabling. Among these diseases are lung cancer, cancer of the mesothelial lining of the pleura and peritoneum, asbestosis, and gastrointestinal cancer."

502 Pneumoconiosis due to other silica or silicates OK

Silicosis is a pneumoconiosis that usually follows long-term inhalation of small particles of crystalline free silica in such industries as metal mining (lead, hard coal, copper, silver, gold), metal casting, pottery making, and sandstone and granite cutting. The etiology involves alveolar macrophages that engulf particles of free silica and enter the lymphatics and interstitial tissue. The macrophages cause the release of toxic enzymes, and fibrosis of the lung parenchyma occurs. When a macrophage dies, the silica particles are released and engulfed by other macrophages, and the process is repeated. Patients with simple nodular silicosis have no respiratory symptoms and usually no respiratory impairment. They may cough and raise sputum, but these symptoms are due to industrial bronchitis and occur as often in persons with normal x-rays. Conglomerate silicosis may lead to severe shortness of breath, cough, and sputum, with severity related to the size of the conglomerate in the lungs. Extensive masses can cause severe disability. Exposure of 20 to 30 years is necessary before the disease becomes apparent, although it can develop in less than 10 years when the exposure to dust is extremely high (i.e., in industries such as tunneling, abrasive soap making, and sandblasting). No effective treatment is known other than lung transplantation.

503 Pneumoconiosis due to other inorganic dust OK

Parenchymal lung diseases due to chronic inhalation of inorganic (mineral) dusts are called pneumoconioses. Several inert dusts, including iron oxide, barium, and tin, can produce conditions known as siderosis, baritosis, and stannosis, respectively. Berylliosis, also called beryllium disease, beryllium poisoning, or beryllium granulomatosis, is generalized granulomatous disease caused by inhalation of dust or fumes containing beryllium compounds and products. Acute berylliosis is a chemical pneumonitis, but other tissues (i.e., skin and conjunctivae) may be affected. Symptoms of chronic berylliosis include cough, chest pain, weight loss, and fatigue, although the patient may not develop any of these until 20 years after exposure has ceased. Diagnosis depends on a history of exposure and clinical manifestations. However, unless special immunologic techniques are used, distinguishing berylliosis from sarcoidosis (reported with ICD 9 CM code 135) is often impossible.

504 Pneumonopathy due to inhalation of other dust OK

505 Unspecified pneumoconiosis OK

506 Respiratory conditions due to chemical fumes and vapors

506.0 Bronchitis and pneumonitis due to fumes and vapors — (Use additional E code to identify cause) — *sudden, severe chemical bronchitis*

506.1 Acute pulmonary edema due to fumes and vapors — (Use additional E code to identify cause) — *sudden, severe edema*
AHA: Q3, 1988, 4

506.2 Upper respiratory inflammation due to fumes and vapors — (Use additional E code to identify cause) — *upper respiratory infection [URI] other than what is specified*

506.3 Other acute and subacute respiratory conditions due to fumes and vapors — (Use additional E code to identify cause) — *not specified elsewhere*

506.4 Chronic respiratory conditions due to fumes and vapors — (Use additional E code to identify cause) — *emphysema, obliterative bronchiolitis, pulmonary fibrosis*

506.9 Unspecified respiratory conditions due to fumes and vapors — (Use additional E code to identify cause)

507 Pneumonitis due to solids and liquids

AHA: Q3, 1991, 16

Pneumonitis due to solids and liquids is pneumonitis and pneumonia due to aspiration of foreign material into the tracheobronchial tree. Aspiration of inert material such as drinking water may cause asphyxia (category 934), but rarely results in pneumonia or pneumonitis. Aspiration of gastric contents or toxic materials such as petroleum distillates often causes pneumonia or pneumonitis due to an inflammatory response in the lungs and lung parenchyma.

"Cafe coronary syndrome" is an acute condition characterized by obstruction of the trachea or bronchi due to large particulate material such as meat and often results in a necrotizing pneumonitis. Signs and symptoms of pneumonitis due to inhalation of food or vomitus include a history of feeding disorder, convulsive disorder, marked debility or disturbance of consciousness, drug or alcohol intoxication, rales, dyspnea, cyanosis, hypotension, and tachycardia.

Diagnostic tests include chest x-ray to locate areas of multilobar infiltrates. ABGs suggest hypoxemia and gross exam may show blood-tinged sputum. Culture of sputum may reveal gram-positive and gram-negative organisms if infective nasopharyngeal organisms have been aspirated. Associated conditions include dehydration, concomitant bacterial pneumonia, bronchiectasis, pulmonary fibrosis, and acute respiratory failure.

Aspiration of gastric acid with a pH of less than 2.5, which can result in a life-threatening pneumonitis, may be referred to as "chemical pneumonitis."

507.0 Pneumonitis due to inhalation of food or vomitus — *aspiration pneumonia from food, saliva, vomit, not otherwise specified*
AHA: Q1, 1989, 10; Q3, 1991, 16

507.1 Pneumonitis due to inhalation of oils and essences — *exogenous lipoid pneumonia*
AHA: Q3, 1991, 16

507.8 Pneumonitis due to other solids and liquids — *detergent asthma*
AHA: Q3, 1991, 16

Coding Clarification

Although chemical pneumonitis usually is classified to rubric 506, when chemical pneumonitis is due to aspiration, assign 507.0.

Aspiration pneumonia or pneumonitis due to — or resulting from the presence of — a nasogastric tube, endotracheal tube, or tracheostomy is classified as a postoperative complication (997.3). The code for aspiration pneumonia may be used as a secondary code to further explain the nature of the respiratory complication. Note that in the case of aspiration pneumonia or pneumonitis following anesthesia, the proper cause and effect relationship needs to be determined. For example, if the aspiration pneumonia or pneumonitis is due to the induction of anesthesia (endotracheal intubation and aspiration, including Mendelson's syndrome), assign 997.3. If the aspiration pneumonia or pneumonitis is due to the anesthetic agent, follow ICD-9-CM coding rules regarding adverse reactions to drugs and chemicals.

 © 2004 Ingenix, Inc.

Subcategory 507.1 includes lipid (or "lipoid") pneumonia when due to an exogenous source. Lipid pneumonia is a chronic syndrome due to the repeated aspiration of oil-containing substances such as mineral oil, cod liver oil, and oily nose drops. This code excludes endogenous lipid pneumonia, which is caused by retention of lipids in the lung parenchyma released during the breakdown of tissue. Endogenous lipid pneumonia is reported with 516.8.

Subcategory 507.8 includes hydrocarbon pneumonitis and pneumonia due to inhalation or aspiration of solids and liquids. It excludes hydrocarbon pneumonitis and pneumonia due to fumes and vapors, which are classified in rubric 506.

508 Respiratory conditions due to other and unspecified external agents

508.0 Acute pulmonary manifestations due to radiation — (Use additional E code to identify cause) — *radiation pneumonitis*
AHA: Q2, 1988, 4

508.1 Chronic and other pulmonary manifestations due to radiation — (Use additional E code to identify cause) — *fibrosis of lung following radiation*

508.8 Respiratory conditions due to other specified external agents — (Use additional E code to identify cause) — *not elsewhere specified*

508.9 Respiratory conditions due to unspecified external agent — (Use additional E code to identify cause)

510–519 Other Diseases of Respiratory System

510 Empyema

Empyema is an infection in the pleural space. It is frequently accompanied by chest pain, shortness of breath, weakness, fever, and hemoptysis.

510.0 Empyema with fistula — (Use additional code to identify infectious organism: 041.00-041.9) — *including thoracic, pleural, mediastinal, hepatopleural, bronchopleural, bronchocutaneous*

510.9 Empyema without mention of fistula — (Use additional code to identify infectious organism: 041.00-041.9) — *with abscess, pyothorax, pyopneumothorax, empyema, fibrinopurulent pleurisy*
AHA: Q3, 1994, 6

Coding Clarification

A code for the infective agent in empyema can be found in Chapter 1 Infectious and Parasitic Diseases and should be reported secondarily. Empyema is classified according to whether a fistula is present.

511 Pleurisy

Pleurisy, also called pleuritic chest pain, is the inflammation of the pleura membrane that lines the chest cavity and contains the lung. Most cases are caused by infection, and many are associated with pneumonia in the underlying lung. Some cases are caused by viral infections or it may occur in other diseases such as tuberculosis, systemic lupus erythematosus, rheumatic fever, and kidney failure. Pleurisy may develop in conjunction with a blood clot on the lung; it may also be associated with the development of fluid in the pleural space between the chest wall and the lung. Sharp pain brought on by breathing and coughing is the most common symptom. If considerable fluid accumulates, the pain may subside, but the fluid may compress the lung and the patient may feel short of breath. In acute pleurisy, the pleura become reddened and covered by an exudate of lymph, fibrin, and cellular elements. The disease may advance to the second stage, in which adhesions, usually permanent, unite the inflamed surfaces. Diagnosis includes patient history about symptoms and previous illness and listening to the chest for sounds of irritated pleurae and pleural effusion. A chest x-ray may be required. A sample of fluid may be taken from the pleural space with a needle and syringe for microscopic examination in cases of suspected pleural effusion (fluid accumulation and bacterial infection). Since pleurisy and pleural effusion are symptoms of basic disorders, the treatment requires identifying and treating the underlying disease. The pain is controlled with analgesic drugs. For acute pleurisy accompanied by effusion, treatment includes drugs, including streptokinase and urokinase, cortisone and cefotetan, and fibrinolytic agents, and non-drug therapies such as shunts and chest drainage catheters, mini-invasive surgery, open thoracotomy, and decortication.

The definition of unspecified pleural effusion is abnormal accumulation of fluid in the pleural space, unspecified as to etiology. Included are transudative and exudative pleurisy and pleural effusions without further specification. Pleural effusion is a common manifestation of both systemic and intrathoracic diseases.

Signs and symptoms of unspecified pleural effusion include pleuritic chest pain, dyspnea, decreased tactile fremitus, pleural friction rub, dullness to percussion, egophony, and distant breath sounds. Therapies include thoracentesis (percutaneous) to remove excess fluid and relieve pain, tube thoracostomy for continuous drainage, and pleurodesis or pleurectomy for malignant pleural effusion.

511.0 Pleurisy without mention of effusion or current tuberculosis — *with adhesion, calcification, thickening of pleura*
AHA: Q3, 1994, 5

511.1 Pleurisy with effusion, with mention of bacterial cause other than tuberculosis — *pneumococcal, staphylococcal, streptococcal*

511.8 Pleurisy with other specified forms of effusion, except tuberculous — *encysted pleurisy, hemopneumothorax, hemothorax, hydropneumothorax, pleurorrhea, hydrothorax*
AHA: Q1, 1997, 10

511.9 Unspecified pleural effusion

Coding Clarification

Malignant pleural effusion (197.2) and pleurisy with tuberculosis (012.0) are excluded from this rubric.

512 Pneumothorax

Pneumothorax is air or other gas in the pleural space. This gas displaces lung capacity, and is commonly referred to as a "collapsed lung" because of the reduction in lung volume.

An iatrogenic pneumothorax occurs as the result of air introduced into the pleural space or lung puncture during a medical procedure. Most commonly, iatrogenic pneumothorax will occur during thoracentesis, catheter placement, arteriography, or intercostal nerve block.

Spontaneous pneumothorax is most common in adult males and has a high incidence of occurrence among patients with Marfan's syndrome. Nearly a third of patients with spontaneous pneumothorax have underlying chronic pulmonary disease.

Tension pneumothorax occurs when pressure in the pleural space is not sufficient to displace the mediastinum to the opposite side. Because this compromises venous return, tension pneumothorax is considered a medical emergency.

512.0 Spontaneous tension pneumothorax — *air leaking from the lung, and trapped in the lung lining*
AHA: Q3, 1994, 5

512.1 Iatrogenic pneumothroax — *air leaking from the lung, following surgery*
AHA: Q4, 1994, 40

512.8 Other spontaneous pneumothorax — *spontaneous or sucking pneumothorax, or pneumothorax not otherwise specified*
AHA: Q2, 1993, 3

513 Abscess of lung and mediastinum

513.0 Abscess of lung — *abscess, necrosis, or gangrene*
AHA: Q2, 1998, 7

513.1 Abscess of mediastinum — *pocket of pus in the tissue between the organs behind the sternum*

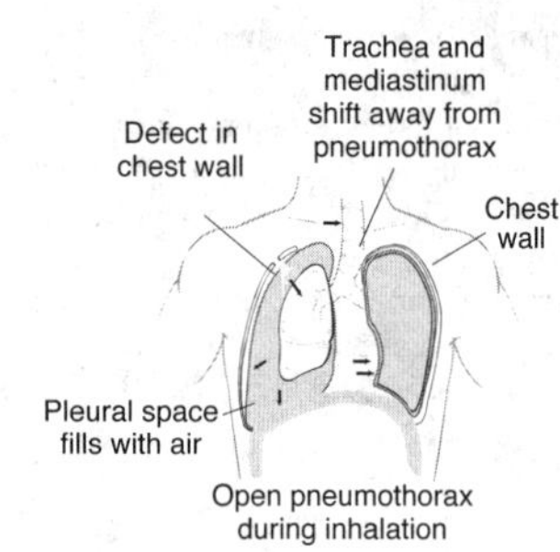

514 Pulmonary congestion and hypostasis OK

AHA: Q3, 1988, 5; Q2, 1998, 6

515 Postinflammatory pulmonary fibrosis OK

516 Other alveolar and parietoalveolar pneumonopathy

516.0 Pulmonary alveolar proteinosis — *chronic proteinaceous deposits in alveoli; Rosen-Castleman-Liebow syndrome*

516.1 Idiopathic pulmonary hemosiderosis — (Code first underlying disease, 275.0) — *essential brown induration of lung*

516.2 Pulmonary alveolar microlithiasis — *minute concretions in alveoli*

516.3 Idiopathic fibrosing alveolitis — *alveolar capillary block, diffuse pulmonary, Hamman-Rich syndrome*

516.8 Other specified alveolar and parietoalveolar pneumonopathies — *not otherwise classified, including endogenous lipoid pneumonia*
AHA: Q1, 1992, 12

516.9 Unspecified alveolar and parietoalveolar pneumonopathy

517 Lung involvement in conditions classified elsewhere

517.1 Rheumatic pneumonia — (Code first underlying disease, 390)

 © 2004 Ingenix, Inc.

517.2 Lung involvement in systemic sclerosis — (Code first underlying disease, 710.1)

517.3 Acute chest syndrome — (Code first sickle-cell disease in crisis: 282.42, 282.62, 282.64, 282.69)

517.8 Lung involvement in other diseases classified elsewhere — (Code first underlying disease: 135, 277.3, 710.0, 710.2, 710.4) — *not otherwise specified*
AHA: Q2, 2003, 7

Coding Clarification

Codes in this rubric should not be used as the principal or primary diagnosis. Code first the underlying disease.

518 Other diseases of lung

Pulmonary collapse is incomplete expansion of lobules (clusters of alveoli) or lung segments. Also called atelectasis, this condition may result in partial or complete lung collapse, which impairs gas exchange, resulting in hypoxia. Pulmonary collapse may be due to obstructions, such as mucous plugs, neoplasms and foreign bodies, or to external compression of the lungs from conditions such as pleural effusion, enlarged thoracic lymph nodes, and pneumothorax.

Signs and symptoms of pulmonary collapse include asymptomatic with slowly developing or minor atelectasis, decreased breath sounds, dull chest percussions with rapidly developing or massive atelectasis, sudden dyspnea, cyanosis, hypotension, tachycardia, elevated temperature, peripheral circulatory collapse or shock, diaphoresis, and substernal or intercostal retraction. Associated conditions include bronchiectasis, pulmonary fibrosis, infective pneumonitis, pleural effusion, enlarged thoracic lymph nodes, and pneumothorax.

518.0 Pulmonary collapse — *no air in a part of the lung; atelectasis, Brock's syndrome, middle lobe syndrome*
AHA: Q4, 1990, 25

518.1 Interstitial emphysema — *air trapped inappropriately in tissue outside bronchi, alveoli, or bronchioli; mediastinal emphysema or Hamman's syndrome*

518.2 Compensatory emphysema — *overdistension of lung tissue into a void created when adjacent tissue was excised or damaged*

518.3 Pulmonary eosinophilia — *transient infiltrations of lungs by eosinophilia; Löffler's syndrome, PIE syndrome, Weingarten's syndrome*

518.4 Unspecified acute edema of lung — *severe, sudden fluid retention within the lung, including postoperative*

518.5 Pulmonary insufficiency following trauma and surgery — *adult respiratory distress syndrome [ARDS], Woillez's disease*
AHA: Sept-Oct, 1987, 1; Q3, 1988, 3; Q3, 1988, 7

518.6 Allergic bronchopulmonary aspergillosis

Coding Clarification

Respiratory failure is failure of oxygenation and/or ventilation that is severe enough to impair or threaten the functioning of vital organs. With failure of oxygenation, the tissues of the lung are not functioning properly. An example of failure of oxygenation would be an acute exacerbation of bronchial asthma in a patient with emphysema. With failure of ventilation, airflow in and out of the lungs is impaired, for example, by compression of the trachea caused by metastatic carcinoma of the thoracic lymph nodes.

Signs and symptoms of respiratory failure include headache, cyanosis, dyspnea, impaired motor function, restlessness, confusion, anxiety, delirium, and occasionally symptoms of depressed consciousness, tachypnea, tachycardia, and tremor. Associated conditions include chronic obstructive lung disease such as chronic obstructive bronchitis, emphysema, cystic fibrosis, acute obstructive lung disease such as asthma, pneumonia, and acute bronchitis.

Diagnosis of respiratory failure based on ABG values is not absolute and may be adjusted according to the patient's baseline blood gas levels. Since some COPD patients have chronically abnormal values, the diagnosis of respiratory failure is made based on further decompensation from the patient's baseline.

518 Other diseases of lung

518.81 Acute respiratory failure — *not otherwise specified*
AHA: Sept-Oct, 1987, 1; Q3, 1988, 7; Q3, 1988, 10; Q2, 1990, 20; Q4, 1990, 25; Q2, 1991, 3; Q3, 1991, 14; Q4, 1998, 41; Q1, 2003, 15

518.82 Other pulmonary insufficiency, not elsewhere classified — *acute respiratory distress not elsewhere classified*
AHA: Q3, 1988, 7; Q2, 1991, 21; Q4, 2003, 105

518.83 Chronic respiratory failure — *persistent*
AHA: Q4, 2003, 103, 111

518.84 Acute and chronic respiratory failure — *sudden, severe*

518.89 Other diseases of lung, not elsewhere classified — *cyst, degeneration, scarring, pulmolithiasis, calcification, broncholithiasis, or occlusion*
AHA: Q4, 1988, 6; Q3, 1990, 18

Documentation Issues

When reviewing the documentation for supporting evidence of respiratory failure, the arterial blood gas pH is a helpful tool in making that determination in a patient with known chronic pulmonary disease. If the arterial blood gas pH is less than 7.35, it is a good indication of respiratory failure. Clarify with the physician before assigning a code for the respiratory failure. Additional documentation also must be provided to support the diagnosis.

If the documentation indicates that acute respiratory failure was the reason for the admission, then it is the principal/primary diagnosis for the hospital stay.

Coding Clarification

General: Four codes are used to separately classify respiratory failure:

- Respiratory failure following shock, trauma, and surgery — 518.5
- Acute and not otherwise specified respiratory failure — 518.81
- Chronic respiratory failure — 518.83
- Acute and chronic respiratory failure — 518.84

Adult Respiratory Distress Syndrome (ARDS): Noted as another term for respiratory failure due to shock, trauma, and surgery, this condition occurs in the presence of previously normal lungs. Other terms that identify adult respiratory distress syndrome are:

- Adult hyaline membrane disease
- DeNang lung syndrome
- White lung syndrome
- Postperfusion lung
- Capillary leak Syndrome
- Trauma wet lung
- Shock lung

To report ARDS, use code 518.5 *Pulmonary insufficiency following trauma and surgery.*

Drug Overdose with Respiratory Failure: If the patient is diagnosed with a drug overdose, the poisoning code is listed first, then the respiratory failure code. It is inappropriate to use the respiratory failure as the principal/primary diagnosis based on the requirement for ventilitory support. Keep in mind that poisoning codes take precedence over the code for the resulting condition.

Respiratory Failure Associated with Nonrespiratory Conditions: Sequencing is a common problem with coding respiratory failure with nonrespiratory conditions. Use the following guidelines when determining the principal/primary diagnosis:

- When the patient admission is for respiratory failure due to or associated with a chronic nonrespiratory condition, the respiratory failure is the principal/primary diagnosis.
- In cases where the patient is admitted for an acute exacerbation of a chronic condition with respiratory failure, the chronic condition code is listed first.
- When the patient is admitted with respiratory failure associated with or due to an acute nonrespiratory condition, code the acute condition first followed by the respiratory failure code.

Coding Scenario

A 63-year-old female is admitted to the facility in acute respiratory failure. The physician's final diagnostic statement identifies that the acute respiratory failure is due to mycoplasma pneumonia.

> Code assignment: 518.81 *Acute respiratory failure* and 483 *Mycoplasma pneumoniae*

A patient is admitted following an overdose of Valium. The patient is found to be in acute respiratory failure and is placed on ventilatory support.

> Code assignment: 969.4 *Poisoning by psychotropic agents, benzodiazepine-based tranquilizers,* 305.40 *Nondependent abuse of drugs, barbiturate and similarly acting sedative or hypnotic, unspecified,* 518.81 *Acute respiratory failure,* and E853.2 *Accidental poisoning by tranquilizers, benzodiazepine-based tranquilizers*

A patient is admitted to the facility via the emergency department with severe chest pain and shortness of breath. The final diagnosis is an acute nontransmural infarction, complicated by acute respiratory failure.

> Code assignment: 410.71 *Acute myocardial infarction, subendocardial infarction* and 518.81 *Acute respiratory failure*

519 Other diseases of respiratory system

This nonspecific code should be used only as a last resort when no other diagnosis can be made.

519.00 Unspecified tracheostomy complication

519.01 Infection of tracheostomy — (Use additional code to identify type of infection: 038.0-038.9, 682.1. Use additional code to identify organism: 041.00-041.9)

519.02 Mechanical complication of tracheostomy — *tracheal stenosis*

519.09 Other tracheostomy complications — *hemorrhage, fistula*

 © 2004 Ingenix, Inc.

519.1 Other diseases of trachea and bronchus, not elsewhere classified — *calcification, stenosis, ulcer*
AHA: Q3, 1988, 6; Q3, 2002, 18

519.2 Mediastinitis — *inflammation of the tissue between the organs behind the sternum*

519.3 Other diseases of mediastinum, not elsewhere classified — *fibrosis, hernia, retraction*

519.4 Disorders of diaphragm — *diaphragmitis, paralysis, relation*

519.8 Other diseases of respiratory system, not elsewhere classified — *cyst of pleura*
AHA: Q4, 1989, 12

519.9 Unspecified disease of respiratory system — *unknown, but including chronic respiratory disease not otherwise specified*

520–579
Diseases of the Digestive System

This chapter classifies diseases and disorders of all of the organs along the alimentary (digestive) tract — the long, muscular tube that begins at the mouth and ends at the anus. The major digestive organs include the pharynx, esophagus, stomach, and intestines. Accessory, or secondary, organs include the salivary and parotid glands, jaw, teeth, and the supporting structures of teeth, tongue, liver, gallbladder and biliary tract, pancreas, and peritoneum.

Structures that support the digestive process from outside this continuous tube are also included in this system: gallbladder, pancreas, and liver. These organs provide secretions that are critical to food absorption and use by the body.

The digestive system is a group of organs that breaks down and changes food chemically for absorption as simple, soluble substances by blood, lymph systems, and body tissues. The digestive system begins in the mouth, continues in the pharynx and esophagus, the stomach, the small and large intestines, the rectum, and the anus.

Digestion involves mechanical and chemical processes. Mechanical actions include chewing in the mouth, churning action in the stomach, and intestinal peristaltic action. These mechanical forces move the food through the digestive tract and mix it with secretions containing enzymes, which accomplish three chemical reactions: the conversion of carbohydrates to simple sugars, the breakdown of proteins into amino acids, and the conversion of fats into fatty acids and glycerol.

The stomach churns and mixes the food with hydrochloric acid and enzymes and gradually releases materials into the upper small intestine (the duodenum) through the pyloric sphincter.

The majority of the digestive process occurs in the small intestine where most foods are hydrolysed and absorbed. The products of digestion are actively or passively transported through the wall of the small intestine and assimilated into the body. The stomach and the large intestine (colon) can also absorb water, alcohol, certain salts and crystalloids, and some drugs. Water-soluble digestive products (minerals, amino acids, and carbohydrates) are transferred into the blood system and transported to the liver. Many fats, resynthesized in the intestinal wall, are picked up by the lymphatic system and enter the blood stream through the vena caval system, bypassing the liver.

Remaining undigested matter is passed into the large intestine (the colon) where water is extracted. This solid mass (the stool) is propelled into the rectum, where it is held until excreted through the anus.

Diseases and disorders that interfere with this function are classified here, along with diseases and disorders that affect the organs of the digestive tract, although they may have no direct affect on digestion. For example, dental caries have a direct effect on digestion because they interfere with mastication, the mechanical breakdown of food by chewing. Portal hypertension does not directly affect digestion, but is included because it represents a disease of a digestive system organ. Portal hypertension would have no discernible effect on the digestive process until the disease has progressed to the point that the liver can no longer perform its function as a digestive organ.

520–529 Diseases of Oral Cavity, Salivary Glands, and Jaws

This category includes diseases and disorders of the jaw, salivary and parotid glands, teeth, gingiva and periodontium, lips, oral mucosa, and tongue.

520 Disorders of tooth development and eruption

This rubric includes disorders of tooth development and eruption in all patients regardless of age. It is one of the few categories in ICD-9-CM that classifies congenital anomalies and hereditary disturbances outside of Chapter 14 Congenital Anomalies (740-759).

520.0 Anodontia — *absence of teeth*

520.1 Supernumerary teeth — *distomolar, fourth molar, mesiodens, paramolar*

520.2 Abnormalities of size and form of teeth — *fusion, concrescence, gemination, macrodontia, microdontia, dens evaginates, dens in dente, taurodontism, tuberculum paramolar*

520.3 Mottled teeth — *dental fluorosis, enamel opacities, mottling of enamel*

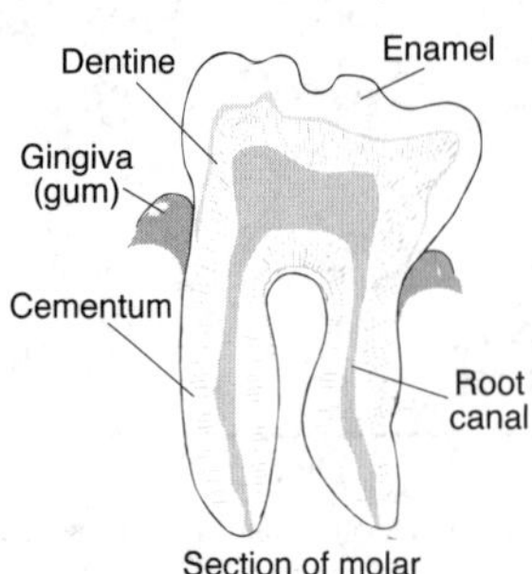

Section of molar

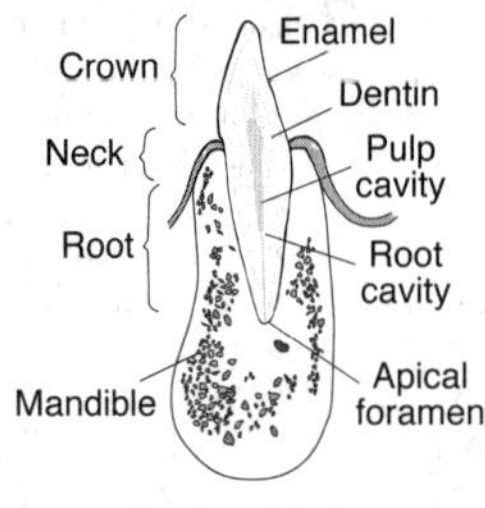

Section of incisor

Coding Clarification

Excessive use of fluoride can cause mottled bleaching of the enamel. The problem can be particularly evident in communities with drinking water containing greater than two parts per million, which can cause dental fluorosis. The signs are whitish flecks or spots, particularly on the front teeth, or dark spots or stripes in more severe cases. While tooth-whitening products can approve appearance in most cases, discoloration of enamel can also be a structural problem that requires proper diagnosis and treatment.

520.4 Disturbances of tooth formation — *aplasia and hypoplasia of cementum, dilaceration of tooth, enamel hypoplasia, Horner's or Turners tooth, hypocalcification*

520.5 Hereditary disturbances in tooth structure, not elsewhere classified — *amelogenesis, dentinogenesis, odontogenesis, dentinal dysplasia, shell teeth*

520.6 Disturbances in tooth eruption — *embedded, impacted, obstructed, premature eruption, premature shedding of deciduous tooth*

520.7 Teething syndrome

520.8 Other specified disorders of tooth development and eruption — *not otherwise specified, pre-eruptive color change*

520.9 Unspecified disorder of tooth development and eruption

Coding Clarification

Excluded from this rubric is exfoliation of teeth, classified to 525.0-525.19.

521 Diseases of hard tissues of teeth

This rubric includes the crown, dentin, enamel, and cementum of the tooth. This rubric includes caries of the cementum, dentin, enamel, as well as infantile melanodontia and white spot lesions of the teeth.v

Dental caries are a demineralization of a tooth's enamel caused by acids produced by bacteria, particularly *Streptococcus mutans*. Pit and fissure decay begins in the narrow grooves on the top of the crown and the cheek side of the back teeth and progresses rapidly. Smooth surface decay grows the slowest and begins as a white spot where bacteria are dissolving the calcium of the enamel. Root decay occurs in the cementum covering the root surface when gums have receded.

Attrition is the normal wearing away of the substance or structure of a tooth through regular use, while abrasion is wearing away of a tooth through an unnatural mechanical process. Erosion is a progressive eating away or destruction of the hard substance of a tooth by a chemical, not bacterial, process. Pathological resorption is a condition in which calcified tissue of the root is lost from the tooth through an absorption and removal process happening within the cementum and dentin, into the root canal, triggered by occlusive trauma and disease, such as neoplastic activity. Internal resorption is an unusual form of pathological resorption that begins in the center of the tooth, with inflamed and hyperplastic pulp tissue filling the resorbed central area and showing pink through the crown of the tooth.

Variations in intraoral mechanical forces, such as chewing or grinding of the teeth, determine the continued formation of bacteria on the teeth and the plaque that can lead to dental caries. Other causes are related to feeding behaviors, such as baby bottle tooth decay in infants, in addition to craniofacial problems, neurologic abnormalities, or impaired cognitive abilities that can interfere with proper dental care.

The bacteria that cause caries are microflora that are present not only in the oral cavity but also in the gastrointestinal tract and other parts of the body, increasing the risk of many disease states and changes in health status due to oral diseases. For example, poorly controlled diabetes (characterized by hyperglycemia and increased salivary glucose) is associated with an increased risk of several dental diseases and conditions.

Diagnosis of dental caries generally involves the use of a sharp explorer, a viewing mirror, and an artificial light source, as well as the drying of tooth surfaces to improve visibility. Radiographs or fiberoptic

 © 2004 Ingenix, Inc.

illumination may reveal smaller caries on the hidden surfaces between adjacent teeth. Four major types of primary prevention are fluoride therapy, fissure-sealant therapy, dietary counselling, and oral-hygiene measures.

521.00 Unspecified dental caries

521.01 Dental caries limited to enamel — *initial caries and white spot lesion*
AHA: Q4, 2001, 44

521.02 Dental caries extending into dentine

521.03 Dental caries extending into pulp

521.04 Arrested dental caries

521.05 Odontoclasia — *infantile melanodontia and melanodontoclasia*
AHA: Q4, 2001, 44

521.06 Dental caries pit and fissure

521.07 Dental caries of smooth surface

521.08 Dental caries of root surface

521.09 Other dental caries

521.10 Excessive attrition (approximal wear) (occlusal wear), unspecified

521.11 Excessive attrition (approximal wear) (occlusal wear), limited to enamel

521.12 Excessive attrition (approximal wear) (occlusal wear), extending into dentine

521.13 Excessive attrition (approximal wear) (occlusal wear), extending into pulp

521.14 Excessive attrition (approximal wear) (occlusal wear), localized

521.15 Excessive attrition (approximal wear) (occlusal wear), generalized

521.20 Diseases of hard tissues of teeth, abrasion, unspecified

521.21 Diseases of hard tissues of teeth, abrasion, limited to enamel

521.22 Diseases of hard tissues of teeth, abrasion, extending into dentine

521.23 Diseases of hard tissues of teeth, abrasion, extending into pulp

521.24 Diseases of hard tissues of teeth, abrasion,, localized

521.25 Diseases of hard tissues of teeth, abrasion,, generalized

521.30 Diseases of hard tissues of teeth, erosion, unspecified

521.31 Diseases of hard tissues of teeth, erosion, limited to enamel

521.32 Diseases of hard tissues of teeth, erosion, extending into dentine

521.33 Diseases of hard tissues of teeth, erosion, extending into pulp

521.34 Diseases of hard tissues of teeth, erosion, localized

521.35 Diseases of hard tissues of teeth, erosion, generalized

521.40 Diseases of hard tissues of teeth, pathological resorption, unspecified

521.41 Diseases of hard tissues of teeth, pathological resorption, internal

521.42 Diseases of hard tissues of teeth, pathological resorption, external

521.49 Diseases of hard tissues of teeth, other pathological resorption

521.5 Hypercementosis — *excessive deposits of cementum on the root of the tooth; cementation hyperplasia*

521.6 Ankylosis of teeth — *abnormal union of tooth to surrounding bone*

521.7 Intrinsic posteruptive color changes — *staining due to drugs, metal, pulpal bleeding, or not otherwise specified*

521.8 Other specified diseases of hard tissues of teeth — *not otherwise specified, irradiated enamel, sensitive dentin*

521.9 Unspecified disease of hard tissues of teeth

Coding Scenario

A 19-year old boy presents to his dentist for his semiannual oral exam after the recent removal of his orthodontic braces. The dentist discovers initial decay and white spots on the buccal smooth surface of his lower canines where the edge of the metal braces had been secured to the teeth for the last two years. He is advised to practice good brushing habits and informed that the initial decay will progress very slowly and not require filling for a while yet.

> Code assignment: 521.01 *Dental caries limited to enamel* and 521.07 *Dental caries of smooth surface*

522 Diseases of pulp and periapical tissues

The center of the tooth and its soft tissues are known as the pulp. It extends from the bottom of the crown to the bottom of the root and is made up of blood vessels that carry oxygen and nutrients back and forth from the heart. Nerves lining the pulp respond to heat, cold, and pressure.

An advanced bacterial infection of the pulp can, if untreated, spread to the root. If the root of the tooth dies, the toothache may stop, but the infection remains active and continues to spread and destroy tissue.

Signs and symptoms of acute apical periodontitis include swollen and red gum that may drain thick purulent material and often a throbbing pain that tends to radiate along the jaw. There is sensitivity of the teeth to hot or cold, possible fever and swollen glands of the neck, and a swollen area of the jaw in very serious cases. Biting or closing the mouth tightly also increases pain. The presence of an abscess, which is a collection of pus, requires immediate dental attention and antibiotics to control the infection, often prior to surgical intervention (e.g., root canal or, in extreme cases, an apicoectomy to drain the abscess prior to a root canal).

522.0 Pulpitis — *abscess, polyp; acute or chronic*

522.1 Necrosis of dental pulp — *death of pulp tissue; pulp gangrene*

522.2 Dental pulp degeneration — *denticles, pulp calcifications, pulp stones*

522.3 Abnormal hard tissue formation in dental pulp — *secondary or irregular dentin*

522.4 Acute apical periodontitis of pulpal origin — *severe inflammation of periodontal ligament, resulting from pulpal inflammation or necrosis*

522.5 Periapical abscess without sinus — *dental or dentoalveolar*

522.6 Chronic apical periodontitis — *persistent inflammation of periodontal ligament, from granuloma or not elsewhere specified*

522.7 Periapical abscess with sinus — *dental or alveolar process fistula*

522.8 Radicular cyst of dental pulp — *apical, periapical, radiculodental, periodontal cyst*

522.9 Other and unspecified diseases of pulp and periapical tissues — *not specified elsewhere or unknown*

Coding Clarification

Diseases of the pulp often begin with bacterial invasion of the pulp after attacking the dentin. Acute and chronic pulpitis (522.0) are conditions, often bacterial, accompanied by severe pain and acute inflammation causing pulp death and subsequent pulp extirpation or extraction. Necrosis of dental pulp (522.1) is a condition in which the pulp has been killed by acute or chronic inflammation; because the pulp is dead, pulp extirpation or tooth extraction is necessary. Periapical tissue surrounds the base of the tooth and a periapical abscess is an infection of the pulp and periapical tissue.

523 Gingival and periodontal diseases

Gingival and periodontal diseases include acute and chronic gingivitis, gingival recession, acute and chronic periodontitis, accretions on teeth, as well as other specified periodontal diseases such as gingival polyps and peripheral giant cell granuloma.

Gingivitis is the inflammation or swelling of the gum tissues. Gingivitis and periodontitis can be considered one disease complex caused by bacteria that incorporates into the dental plaque. Gingivitis often goes unnoticed in the early stages but once advanced, it spreads to the bony tissues, which lie under the gums and support the teeth. This is called periodontitis. In later stages of periodontitis, the teeth can become loose and severely infected with pus oozing from around the sockets. In very advanced periodontitis, the teeth can actually fall out or may have to be removed because of infection.

There are no symptoms in the early stages of gingivitis. Signs and symptoms of advanced gingivitis and periodontitis include blood on the tooth brush when brushing the teeth, swollen and red gums, tenderness when the gums are touched, pus around the teeth, bad taste in the mouth, and visible deposits of tartar or calculus on the teeth. A diagnosis of advanced gingivitis and periodontitis is by examination, gum probing, and dental x-rays. If untreated, gingivitis and periodontitis can lead to loss of teeth and infection of advanced periodontal disease can spread to other parts of the body, including the heart. Depending on the stage of the disease, treatment can range anywhere from simple cleaning, called prophylaxis, and home care to complex periodontal surgery. In advanced cases, some or all the teeth may have to be extracted.

523.0 Acute gingivitis — *severe inflammation of the gingiva*

523.1 Chronic gingivitis — *persistent inflammation of the gingiva*

523.20 Gingival recession, unspecified

523.21 Gingival recession, minimal

523.22 Gingival recession, moderate

523.23 Gingival recession, severe

523.24 Gingival recession, localized

523.25 Gingival recession, generalized

523.3 Acute periodontitis — *severe inflammation of the tissues that surround and support the teeth*

523.3 Acute periodontitis — *severe inflammation of the tissues that surround and support the teeth*

523.4 Chronic periodontitis — *persistent inflammation of the tissues that surround and support the teeth*

523.5 Periodontosis — *inflammation of the tissues that surround and support the teeth*

523.6 Accretions on teeth — *foreign material on surface of teeth, usually plaque or calculus*

523.8 Other specified periodontal diseases — *cysts, hemorrhage, occlusion, pocket, ulcer, pain, fibromatosis, lesions, giant cell granuloma*

523.9 Unspecified gingival and periodontal disease

Coding Clarification

Excluded from this category are acute necrotizing ulcerative gingivitis (101), herpetic gingivostomatitis

 © 2004 Ingenix, Inc.

(054.2), acute apical periodontitis (522.4), chronic apical periodontitis (522.6), periapical abscess (522.5, 522.7), and leukoplakia of gingiva (528.6).

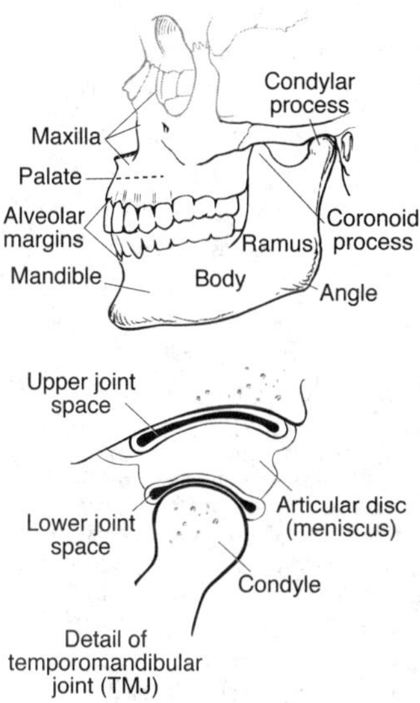

524 Dentofacial anomalies, including malocclusion

Malocclusion is an abnormal alignment of teeth and the way that the upper and lower teeth fit together (bite). It is often hereditary and may cause problems with biting and chewing but can usually be corrected with a brace on the teeth and proper orthodontic care.

Tuberosity of the jaw is seen as an elongated, raised, or protruding area on the angle of the jawbone. Sometimes the tuberosity can be raised or uneven after tooth extraction. Surgical correction of the tuberosity can be performed to correct a defect.

Dentofacial anomalies classified in this chapter may be acquired or due to congenital anomalies not classified to Chapter 14. Look in the ICD-9-CM index under both the condition and the main term "Anomaly, anomalous" to ensure proper code assignment.

Subcategory 524.0 classifies conditions affecting the size of the jaw, including hyperplasia, hypoplasia, macrogenia, and microgenia.

524.00 Unspecified major anomaly of jaw size

524.01 Maxillary hyperplasia — *overgrowth or overdevelopment of maxillary bone*

524.02 Mandibular hyperplasia — *overgrowth or overdevelopment of jaw bone*

524.03 Maxillary hypoplasia — *incomplete or underdevelopment of maxillary bone*

524.04 Mandibular hypoplasia — *incomplete or underdevelopment of jaw bone*

524.05 Macrogenia — *abnormal largeness of the chin*

524.06 Microgenia — *abnormal smallness of the chin*

524.07 Excessive tuberosity of jaw

524.09 Other specified major anomaly of jaw size — *not otherwise specified*

Subcategory 524.1 classifies inequality in the size or shape of one side of the maxilla and/or mandible compared with the other, or a difference in placement or arrangement of one of the jawbones about the craniofacial axis. These anomalies include prognathism, retrognathism, and maxillary asymmetry. Prognathism is anterior protrusion of the mandible or maxilla beyond the projection of the forehead. Retrognathism is the location of the maxilla or mandible behind the frontal plane of the forehead; it also is used as a general term meaning underdevelopment of the maxilla or mandible.

Subcategory 524.2 classifies dental arch anomalies. The dental arch is the curved structure of a line created by the buccal surfaces or the central grooves of all natural teeth and the residual ridge of missing teeth in the upper or lower jaw. Anomalies may occur as a malocclusion—an abnormal contact line between the biting and chewing tooth surfaces of the upper or lower teeth, an overbite or overlapping of upper teeth over the lower when biting down, or inadequate or excessive interarch distances—the vertical space defined between the upper and lower alveolar or residual arches, or ridges. Angle's class I is a malocclusion with correct mesiodistal relationship of the first permanent molars. Angle's class II, also called a distoclusion, is a posterior malocculsion in which the lower jaw and its first permanent molar is positioned further back than the upper. Angle's class III, also called a mesioclusion, is a protrusive malocculsion in which the lower jaw is more forward than the upper and its first permanent molar is positioned nearer to the center line of the arch than the upper. Returning the dental arch to proper positioning usually requires carefully planned orthodontic care, possibly concurrent with orthognathic surgery to reposition one or both jaws.

524.10 Unspecified anomaly of relationship of jaw to cranial base — *prognathism and retrognathism*

524.11 Maxillary asymmetry — *unequal development*

524.12 Other jaw asymmetry

524.19 Other specified anomaly of relationship of jaw to cranial base — *not otherwise specified*

524.20 Unspecified anomaly of dental arch relationship,

524.21 Anomaly of dental arch relationship, Angle's class I

524.22 Anomaly of dental arch relationship, Angle's class II

524.23 Anomaly of dental arch relationship, Angle's class III

524.24 Anomaly of dental arch relationship, open anterior occlusal relationship

524.25 Anomaly of dental arch relationship, open posterior occlusal relationship

524.26 Anomaly of dental arch relationship, excessive horizontal overlap

524.27 Anomaly of dental arch relationship, reverse articulation

524.28 Anomaly of dental arch relationship, anomalies of interarch distance

524.29 Other anomalies of dental arch relationship

Subcategory 524.3 classifies anomalies of tooth position. Crowding occurs when teeth come in too close to one another have no room for the normal spacing that should be present between the teeth. Crowding also causes overlapping and displacement of adjacent teeth in various directions. Excessive spacing is the opposite problem when a tooth is too far apart from its neighboring tooth, leaving an unfilled gap between them.

Horizontal displacement may be seen as crowns and roots out of the normal line, including "tipping" in their position. Vertical displacement may present as supra-eruption of a tooth in which it continues to grow out from the gingiva when the opposing tooth is missing in the other jaw, and may require placing the missing tooth and adjusting the height of the other. Infra-eruption of a tooth occurs when has not sufficiently erupted above the gum line. Tooth rotation is the malposition of a tooth that has turned about its own longitudinal axis. The interocclusal distance in teeth is determined from the biting/chewing contact surfaces of teeth in the maxilla (upper jaw) and the mandible (lower jaw) when the lower jaw is in the normal resting position. This natural space or clearance may be either greater than normal or insufficient. These problems may require orthodontic care to move the teeth into proper position and/or the strategic removal of certain teeth.

524.30 Anomaly of tooth position, unspecified

524.31 Crowding of teeth

524.32 Excessive spacing of teeth

524.33 Horizontal displacement of teeth

524.34 Vertical displacement of teeth

524.35 Rotation of teeth

524.36 Insufficient interocclusal distance of teeth (ridge)

524.37 Excessive interocclusal distance of teeth

524.39 Other anomalies of tooth position

524.4 Unspecified malocclusion

524.50 Dentofacial functional abnormality, unspecified

524.51 Abnormal jaw closure

524.52 Limited mandibular range of motion

524.53 Deviation in opening and closing of the mandible

524.54 Insufficient anterior guidance

524.55 Centric occlusion maximum intercuspation discrepancy

524.56 Dentofacial functional abnormality, non-working side interference

524.57 Lack of posterior occlusal support

524.59 Other dentofacial functional abnormalities

Subcategory 524.6 classifies temporomandibular joint disorders. The temporomandibular joints (TMJ) are located just in front of the ears and attach the mandible to the skull allowing the jaw to move. Symptoms of TMJ disorders include pain in the jaw, headache, stiffness in the jaw, earaches and popping or clicking sounds when opening the mouth. Symptoms may be often be alleviated with pain-relief medications and heat/cold, and other palliative measures. Oftentimes, such TMJ problems resolve themselves over time. In some instances, surgery is required to correct the problem.

524.60 Unspecified temporomandibular joint disorders — *TMJ syndrome; including Costen's syndrome*

524.61 Adhesions and ankylosis (bony or fibrous) of temporomandibular joint — *a union or stiffening of the TMJ due to bony or fibrous union across the joint*

524.62 Arthralgia of temporomandibular joint — *pain of TMJ, not inflammatory in nature*

524.63 Articular disc disorder (reducing or non-reducing) of temporomandibular joint

524.64 Temporomandibular joint sounds on opening and/or closing the jaw

524.69 Other specified temporomandibular joint disorders — *not otherwise specified, snapping jaw*

Subcategory 524.7 classifies anomalies of the dental alveoli and alveolar ridge, including hyperplasia and hypoplasia. Dental alveoli are the tooth sockets of the maxilla and mandible. The alveolar ridge is the bony process of the maxilla or mandible that contains the tooth sockets. Hyperplasia of the alveoli is an overgrowth or overdevelopment of bone, and hypoplasia of the alveoli is an underdevelopment or agenesis of bone.

A vertical displacement of the alveolus and teeth includes the extrusion or extended movement of the

 © 2004 Ingenix, Inc.

tooth and the root cavity, or socket in the jawbone where the tooth is held, beyond the normal occlusal plane when the opposing occlusal force is missing. The occlusal plane is the hypothetical surface on which upper and lower teeth meet when biting or chewing. The plane appears as a straight line to the lateral view, even though it is actually a compound curved surface, and the planar reference points are taken from specific points within the dental arches. A structural aberration that results in canting or tipping of the occlusal plane is a deviation that may require orthopedic and/or orthodontic care to achieve the true horizontal and vertical references for the occlusal plane that are the optimal end-point of treatment for the best mandibular maxillary relationship.

524.70 Unspecified alveolar anomaly

524.71 Alveolar maxillary hyperplasia — *overgrowth or underdevelopment of alveolar tissue of the maxillary bones*

524.72 Alveolar mandibular hyperplasia — *overgrowth or underdevelopment of alveolar tissue of the mandibular bones*

524.73 Alveolar maxillary hypoplasia — *incomplete or underdevelopment of alveolar tissue of the maxillary bones*

524.74 Alveolar mandibular hypoplasia — *incomplete or underdevelopment of alveolar tissue of the mandibular bones*

524.75 Vertical displacement of alveolus and teeth

524.76 Occlusal plane deviation

524.79 Other specified alveolar anomaly — *not otherwise specified*

524.81 Anterior soft tissue impingement

524.82 Posterior soft tissue impingement

524.89 Other specified dentofacial anomalies

524.9 Unspecified dentofacial anomalies

Coding Scenario

A 24-year-old female comes to her primary care physician to complain that her jaw continually pops when she makes a movement to open or close it in such a way that she actually feels the "pop". Sometimes she also experiences mobility problems with the jaw to get it open with increased loudness it the joint sounds, especially in the morning. She hasn't had pain in the jaw at this point, however. The physician listens for the joint sounds and gives the initial diagnosis of temporomandibular joint sounds.

> Code assignment: 524.64 *Temporomandibular joint sounds on opening and/or closing the jaw*

525 Other diseases and conditions of the teeth and supporting structures

Tooth loss can be caused by a variety of causes. Congenital conditions such as Papillon Lefevre syndrome, systemic conditions such as Langerhan's cell histiocytosis, loss of supporting structures, trauma, periodontal disease and dental caries may be responsible for loosing teeth.

A bacterium that spreads into the bony tissues which lie under the gums and support the teeth cause advanced gingivitis. This is called periodontitis.

Dental caries are a demineralization of a tooth's enamel caused by acids produced by bacteria. Advanced dental caries can cause decay and loss of a tooth.

The alveolar ridge is the line formed by the alveolar process, the root cavities or sockets of the jawbones. Edentulous ridges have lost the teeth that were once held in those sockets. Atrophy presents as a wasting and shrinking of the size of the alveolar ridge that previously held teeth. Severe atrophy may present as small, knife-like edges along the alveolar ridge and produce a sunken appearance to the mouth and lips, leaving a protruding chin, especially with anterior atrophy of the maxilla and mandible. Severe forms require oral maxillofacial surgery to reconstruct the maxilla and/or mandible. Bone grafts may be used for ridge augmentation, also possible orthopedic bone plates, a reconstruction of the vestibule of the mouth, and complete dentures.

525.0 Exfoliation of teeth due to systemic causes — *loss of teeth due to underlying condition*

525.10 Unspecified acquired absence of teeth — *edentulism and tooth extraction status, NOS*
AHA: Q4, 2001, 44

525.11 Loss of teeth due to trauma

525.12 Loss of teeth due to periodontal disease

525.13 Loss of teeth due to caries

525.19 Other loss of teeth

525.20 Unspecified atrophy of edentulous alveolar ridge

525.21 Minimal atrophy of the mandible

525.22 Moderate atrophy of the mandible

525.24 Minimal atrophy of the maxilla

525.25 Moderate atrophy of the maxilla

525.26 Severe atrophy of the maxilla

525.3 Retained dental root

525.53

525.8 Other specified disorders of the teeth and supporting structures — *not otherwise specified, cicatrix, cleft, hemorrhage, lesion, or enlargement of alveolar process or tissue; loose tooth; obliteration of vestibule*

525.9 Unspecified disorder of the teeth and supporting structures — *unknown cause of pain or other symptom*

526 Diseases of the jaws

Odontogenic cysts are developmental cysts arising from the enamel organ of teeth and include about 90 percent of all jaw cysts. While it is sometimes difficult to differentiate which type of odontogenic cyst is present, some have distinguishing features.

The radicular cyst is the most common of the odontogenic cysts; associated with a nonvital tooth, it is present at the apex of the root of a tooth or teeth. Other odontogenic cysts include residual cysts associated with the removal of teeth and primordial cysts associated with undeveloped teeth. Globulomaxillary cysts are located in the anterior region of the upper jaw and dentigerous cysts form in association with an unerupted permanent tooth, although they can occasionally surround a primary tooth, due to fluid accumulation.

Dentigerous cysts are found in children and adolescents. Adults can have dentigerous cysts associated with unerupted third molars. These cysts may expand, causing displacement or resorption of adjacent teeth. In a radiograph, dentigerous cysts appear as a dark area around the crown of the tooth.

Treatment for the dentigerous cyst includes removal and microscopic examination of the cyst wall since the cyst lining may have a neoplastic change, such as ameloblastoma, squamous cell carcinoma, or mucoepidermoid carcinoma. Marsupialization is a second method of treatment that involves removing the overlying soft tissue and bone, allowing discharge of matter.

526.0 Developmental odontogenic cysts — *dentigerous, eruption, follicular, lateral development, keratocyst, primordial cyst*

526.1 Fissural cysts of jaw — *globulomaxillary, incisor canal, median anterior maxillary, medial palatal, nasopalatine*

526.2 Other cysts of jaws — *aneurysmal, hemorrhagic, traumatic*

526.3 Central giant cell (reparative) granuloma

526.4 Inflammatory conditions of jaw — *abscess, osteitis, sequestrum of jawbone, periostitis*

526.5 Alveolitis of jaw — *inflammation of alveoli or tooth socket of jaw; dry socket; alveolar osteitis*

526.81 Exostosis of jaw — *bony projection that develops from cartilage of jaw*

526.89 Other specified disease of the jaws — *not otherwise specified, cherubism, fibrous dysplasia, latent bone cyst, fistula, perforation, unilateral condylar hyper- or hypoplasia of mandible*

526.9 Unspecified disease of the jaws — *unknown cause of pain or other symptom*

520–579

527 Diseases of the salivary glands

The salivary glands secrete a predominantly alkaline fluid that moistens the mouth, softens food, and aids in digestion. The three major salivary glands include the submaxillary glands around the mouth under the lower jaw, the sublingual glands beneath the tongue, and the parotid glands in front of each ear. Saliva is antimicrobal and works against a host of bacteria associated with oral and systemic diseases. Large salivary mucins are antiviral as are cystatins that are active against herpes viruses. Saliva also contains histatins, anti-fungal proteins that are potent inhibitors of candida, which is normally kept in check at extremely low levels in the mouth. The sublingual glands secrete the enzyme lysozyme, which destroys bacterial invasion with methods to include degrading bacterial membranes, inhibiting the growth and metabolism of certain bacteria, and disrupting bacterial enzyme systems. The saliva of the parotid gland contains the enzyme amylase that aids in the digestion of carbohydrates. In addition to these glands, there are hundreds of minor saliva glands in the lips, inner cheek area (buccal mucosa), and in other linings of the mouth and throat. Salivary calculi account for more than 50 percent of the major salivary gland diseases and are the most common cause of acute and chronic salivary gland infections.

527.0 Atrophy of salivary gland — *wasting away or death of tissue*

527.1 Hypertrophy of salivary gland — *overgrowth or over development of tissue; Mikulicz's syndrome*

527.2 Sialoadenitis — *inflammation*

527.3 Abscess of salivary gland — *pocket of pus*

527.4 Fistula of salivary gland — *abnormal sinus tract communicating between salivary gland and another site*

527.5 Sialolithiasis — *formation or presence of salivary calculus; stone, sialodocholithiasis*

527.6 Mucocele of salivary gland — *dilated salivary gland filled with accumulation of mucous*

527.7 Disturbance of salivary secretion — *hyposecretion, ptyalism, sialorrhea, xerostomia, Zagari's disease*

527.8 Other specified diseases of the salivary glands — *not otherwise specified, stenosis, stricture or obstruction of salivary duct; pneumoparotid; sialosis; obstruction of Stensen's or submaxillary duct; sialectasia*

527.9 Unspecified disease of the salivary glands — *unknown disorder*

Coding Clarification

Atrophy (527.0) in the diseases of the salivary glands is defined as a wasting away or death of tissue, while hypertrophy (527.1) is overgrowth or overdevelopment of tissue of the salivary glands.

© 2004 Ingenix, Inc.

Sialoadenitis (527.2) is the inflammation of a salivary gland and sialolithiasis (527.5) is the formation or presence of a salivary calculus.

528 Diseases of the oral soft tissues, excluding lesions specific for gingiva and tongue

Cancrum oris, or noma, is sudden, rapidly progressive tissue destruction. The mucous membranes (e.g., gums, lining of the cheeks) become inflamed and develop ulcers. The infection spreads from the mucous membranes to the skin. The tissues in the lips and cheeks die. Rapid, painless tissue breakdown continues and this gangrenous process can destroy the soft tissue and bone. Noma can also affect the mucous membranes of the genitals, spreading to the genital skin (this is sometimes called noma pudendi). Risk factors include Kwashiorkor and other forms of severe malnutrition, poor sanitation and poor cleanliness, disorders such as measles or leukemia, and living in an underdeveloped country.

Signs and symptoms include red and tender gums and inner cheeks, ulcers that develop a foul-smelling drainage, and eventual destruction of the bones around the mouth cause deformity and loss of teeth. A physical exam shows inflamed areas of the mucous membranes, mouth ulcers, and skin ulcers, and other signs of malnutrition. Noma can be fatal if left untreated or heal over time even without treatment. However, it can cause massive tissue destruction before healing. Treatment with penicillin and improving nutrition halts progression of the disease. Skin lesions eventually heal even without treatment, but severe scarring and deformity can develop.

Keratinized tissue is made up of keratin, the main protein constituent in the epidermis, hair, and nails. Soft keratin is found in epithelial tissue. Healthy attached keratinized mucosa that presents in an even thickness on residual ridge gingiva in the edentulous patient is ideal for denture stability, because dentures rely on the residual alveolar ridge and oral mucosa for support and retention. Sometimes the keratinized epithelium present on a residual ridge is not enough or is in excess. In these cases, the amount of tissue must either be augmented or decreased before restorative measures can be carried out.

528.0 Stomatitis — *inflammation of the mucous membrane of mouth*
AHA: Q2, 1999, 9

528.1 Cancrum oris — *gangrenous, ulcerative, inflammatory lesion of mouth*

528.2 Oral aphthae — *canker sore, aphthous stomatitis, periadenitis mucosa necrotica recurrens*

528.3 Cellulitis and abscess of oral soft tissues — *oral fistula, Ludwig's angina*

528.4 Cysts of oral soft tissues — *dermoid, epidermoid, Epstein's pearl, nasolabial, nasoalveolar, lymphoepithelial*

528.5 Diseases of lips — *abscess, cellulitis, fistula, hypertrophy; cheilitis, celiodynia, cheilosis*
AHA: Sept-Oct, 1986, 10

528.6 Leukoplakia of oral mucosa, including tongue — *white patch on oral mucosa which cannot be attributed to a specific disease; lip, tongue, mucosa, gingiva*

528.71 Minimal keratinized residual ridge mucosa

528.72 Excessive keratinized residual ridge mucosa

528.79 Other disturbances of oral epithelium, including tongue

528.8 Oral submucosal fibrosis, including of tongue

528.9 Other and unspecified diseases of the oral soft tissues — *cheek/lip biting; denture sore mouth; denture stomatitis, melanoplakia; buccal lesion; fistula in soft palate; redundant uvula; melanoplakia*

529 Diseases and other conditions of the tongue

Geographic tongue is described as a common and harmless condition in which one or more irregularly shaped patches appear on the tongue, in a design that may resemble a map of a country. The center area is redder than the rest of the tongue and the edges of the patch are whitish in color. The etiology is unknown, although a viral infection is assumed and it may be associated with a variety of inflammatory or allergic conditions as well. Geographic tongue often goes away without treatment, but can be treated with topical steroids such as topical Lidex gel.

529.0 Glossitis — *abscess or traumatic ulceration of tongue; Riga-Fede disease*

529.1 Geographic tongue — *benign migratory glossitis; glossitis areata exfoliativa*

529.2 Median rhomboid glossitis — *asymptomatic lesion of dorsum of tongue due to Candida albicans infection*

529.3 Hypertrophy of tongue papillae — *black hairy tongue; coated tongue, lingua villosa nigra, hypertrophy of foliate papillae*

529.4 Atrophy of tongue papillae — *bald tongue, glazed tongue, Hunter's or Moeller's glossitis, glossodynia exfoliativa, smooth atrophic tongue*

529.5 Plicated tongue — *fissured, furrowed, scrotal*

529.6 Glossodynia — *painful tongue; glossopyrosis*

529.8 Other specified conditions of the tongue — *not otherwise specified, cicatrix, hemorrhage, paralysis, glossoncus, glossoplegia, atrophy, crenated, enlargement, hypertrophy, hemiatrophy, glossocele, glossoptosis*

529.9 Unspecified condition of the tongue

530–537 Diseases of Esophagus, Stomach, and Duodenum

530 Diseases of esophagus

This category includes diseases and disorders of the esophagus, a muscular, tubular structure that serves as a conduit for the passage of food and water from the pharynx to the stomach. It functions by transporting food and fluids from the mouth to the stomach (and sometimes in the reverse direction) by a combination of gravity and peristaltic waves. The esophagus is equipped with two sphincters. The first is the pharyngeal-esophageal sphincter located at the level of the cricoid cartilage; the second is the gastroesophageal sphincter (also known as the lower esophageal sphincter) located at the level of the esophageal hiatus of the diaphragm.

Subcategory 530.0 classifies a neuromuscular disorder characterized by an absence of peristalsis, dilation of the body of the esophagus, and a conically narrowed cardioesophageal junction. The dominant symptom is dysphagia. Vigorous achalasia is a variant form characterized by recurring esophageal spasms.

Subcategory 530.1 classifies inflammation of the esophagus due to reflux, chemicals, and infection. Reflux esophagitis, sometimes referred to as peptic or regurgitant esophagitis, is the most common form of esophagitis and is caused by the reflux of acid and pepsin from the stomach into the esophagus. Normally, the gastroesophageal sphincter prevents the reflux of gastric juice into the esophagus, but a variety of conditions can compromise the sphincter's competency. Frequently, hiatal hernia is an underlying cause of sphincter incompetence. Other causes are pregnancy, certain drugs (anticholinergic agents, calcium channel blockers, beta-adrenergic agonists), scleroderma, obesity, placement of nasogastric tubes, and surgical vagotomy.

520–579

Chemical (corrosive) esophagitis is a chemical burn caused by ingestion and regurgitation of caustic liquids or solids. The caustic agent may result in sloughing of the mucous membrane, edema and inflammation of the submucosa, thrombosis of the esophageal vessels, secondary infection, perforation, and mediastinitis. Chemical esophagitis can cause severe damage and may constitute a medical emergency depending on the strength of the chemical and the length of time the chemical remains in the esophagus.

Esophagitis due to infection is relatively rare.

Signs and symptoms of esophagitis include heartburn after eating or while resting in recumbent position, chest pain sometimes masquerading as angina pectoris, regurgitation (water brash) and dysphagia due to inflammatory edema or stricture in the distal esophagus, and in patients with chemical esophagitis and a history of ingesting caustic liquids or solids, intense pain and chemical burns of the lips, buccal cavity, and tongue.

Esophagoscopy and biopsy may be performed to assess the severity of the esophagitis and rule out associated conditions such as strictures, ulcers, and carcinoma. Esophageal manometry may be performed to assess competency of the gastroesophageal sphincter. An acid perfusion test, also known as the Bernstein test, may be done to reproduce the pain associated with reflux and an acid reflux test may be performed to monitor the intraesophageal pH after instillation of hydrochloric acid into the stomach. Barium swallow and upper GI series are of limited diagnostic importance except in the most severe cases.

Therapies include alterations in diet and mealtimes, antacids, drugs to increase gastroesophageal sphincter tone such as bethanechol and metoclopramide, and avoidance of drugs known to decrease gastroesophageal sphincter pressure (anticholinergic agents, beta-adrenergic drugs). Surgical intervention includes antireflux surgery such as Nissen fundoplication, Belsey fundoplication, placement of an Angelchik ring (prosthesis) around the distal esophagus, and replacement of the esophagus with segments of stomach, jejunum, or colon in cases of severe damage.

An esophagostomy is an artificial opening from the esophagus to outside the body. Esophagostomies are performed on infants born with congenital esophageal atresia, as an interim treatment method to prepare the upper esophagus for a primary anastomosis procedure, by gradual elongation and lowered placement of the esophagostomy with traction on the distal end. Esophagostomies are also performed on patients with swallowing disorders, or dysphasia, when nonoral feedings are needed and the placement of other enteral feeding tubes is contraindicated. Patients with amyotrophic lateral sclerosis (Lou Gehrig's disease) or muscular dystrophy affecting their throat muscles and ability to eat may have an esophagostomy done to place a tube through the neck for feeding. A complication occurs when the stoma or skin surrounding it becomes infected, or when there is a malfunction occurring anywhere along the surgical opening from the esophagus to the skin surface.

530.0 Achalasia and cardiospasm — *failure of the esophagogastric sphincter to relax; aperistalsis of esophagus; megaesophagus*

 © 2004 Ingenix, Inc.

530.10 Unspecified esophagitis — (Use additional E code to identify cause, if induced by chemical or drug)

530.11 Reflux esophagitis — (Use additional E code to identify cause, if induced by chemical or drug) — *inflammation of the lower esophagus from regurgitation of acid gastric contents*
AHA: Q3, 1991, 20; Q1, 1992, 17; Q4, 1993, 27; Q4, 1995, 82

530.12 Acute esophagitis — (Use additional E code to identify cause, if induced by chemical or drug)

530.19 Other esophagitis — (Use additional E code to identify cause, if induced by chemical or drug) — *not otherwise specified, chemical burn, abscess, postoperative esophagitis*
AHA: Q3, 1991, 20; Q1, 1992, 17; Q4, 1993, 27; Q3, 2001, 10

Coding Clarification

Associated conditions include perforation and bleeding, ulcer formation, secondary infection, mediastinitis, tracheoesophageal fistulas, strictures, hiatal hernia, aspiration pneumonia, and carcinoma.

Assign code 530.10 for unspecified esophagitis, 530.11 for reflux esophagitis, and 530.19 for other specified types of esophagitis.

530.2 [5th] Ulcer of esophagus — (Use additional E code to identify cause, if induced by chemical or drug) — *fungal, peptic, due to ingestion of aspirin, chemicals, medicine*
AHA: Q4, 2003, 63

530.20 Ulcer of esophagus without bleeding — (Use additional E code to identify cause, if induced by chemical or drug)

530.21 Ulcer of esophagus with bleeding — (Use additional E code to identify cause, if induced by chemical or drug)

530.3 Stricture and stenosis of esophagus — *compression, obstruction*
AHA: Q1, 1988, 13; Q2, 1997, 3; Q2, 2001, 4

530.4 Perforation of esophagus — *rupture; Boerhaave's syndrome*

530.5 Dyskinesia of esophagus — *curling, corkscrew, spasm; Barsony-Polgar or Barsony-Teschendorf syndromes*
AHA: Nov-Dec, 1984, 19; Q1, 1988, 13

530.6 Diverticulum of esophagus, acquired — *herniated pouch or sac opening within the esophagus; epiphrenic, pharyngoesophageal, subdiaphragmatic, hypopharyngeal; esophagocele; traction, pulsion, pouch*
AHA: Jan-Feb, 1985, 3

530.7 Gastroesophageal laceration-hemorrhage syndrome — *Mallory-Weiss syndrome*

Coding Clarification

Subcategory 530.7 classifies mucosal laceration (or vertical tear) of the esophagus or cardioesophageal junction. More commonly known as Mallory-Weiss syndrome, this condition follows prolonged or forceful vomiting.

530.81 Esophageal reflux — *regurgitation of contents of stomach into the esophagus, without inflammation*
AHA: Q4, 1992, 27; Q1, 1995, 7; Q2, 2001, 4

530.82 Esophageal hemorrhage — *bleeding, except for varices*

530.83 Esophageal leukoplakia — *white patch in the esophagus which cannot be attributed to a specific disease*

530.84 Tracheoesophageal fistula — *acquired communication between trachea and esophagus*

530.85 Barrett's esophagus

530.86 Infection of esophagostomy

530.87 Mechanical complication of esophagostomy

Coding Clarification

Barrett's esophagus is a condition that develops in some people who have chronic gastroesophageal reflux disease (GERD) or inflammation of the esophagus (esophagitis). In Barrett's esophagus, the normal cells that line the esophagus, squamous cells, turn into a cell not typically found in humans, called columnar cells.

When normal squamous lining cells of the esophagus are replaced by columnar cells, the process is known as metaplasia. Barrett's esophagus is a kind of metaplasia. The metaplastic columnar lining comes in three types: two types are comparable to groups of cells found in regions of the stomach lining; the third type is comparable to groups of cells found in the small intestine. This intestinal type of metaplasia is important because it can potentially lead to the development of cancer.

530.89 Other specified disorder of the esophagus — *not otherwise specified, including cyst, deviation, erosion, fistula, pain, necrosis, relaxation, insufficiency*

530.9 Unspecified disorder of esophagus

531 Gastric ulcer

AHA: Q4, 1990, 27; Q1, 1991, 15

This rubric classifies a condition formed by discreet tissue destruction within the lumen of the stomach. The destruction is due to the action of hydrochloric (gastric) acid and pepsin on areas of gastric mucosa having a decreased resistance to ulceration.

Signs and symptoms of gastric ulcer include pain exacerbated by eating, weight loss, repeated vomiting

— which is a sign of possible gastric outlet obstruction — vomiting of frank red blood or "coffee ground" material, and black and tarry stools or heme positive stools if the ulcer is bleeding.

Lab work may show hypochromic blood loss anemia. Gastric analysis shows acid pH after administration of histamine or pentagastrin with usual finding of low to normal secretion of gastric acid. An upper GI series may be performed and an upper endoscopy with biopsy may be done to determine the ulcer's benign or malignant status.

Therapies include antacids, diet modification, H2 receptor antagonist drugs such as cimetidine and ranitidine, and other therapeutic agents (sucralfate, carbenoxolone, bismuth, certain prostaglandins, tricyclic antidepressants such as doxepin). In addition, gastric irradiation may be performed to reduce acid production temporarily in patients who cannot tolerate drugs or surgery. Other therapies include distal subtotal gastrectomy, subtotal gastrectomy with wedge resection of gastric ulcer, vagotomy with drainage, and vagotomy with antrectomy.

Associated conditions include acute and/or chronic blood loss anemia and gastric outlet obstruction.

The following fifth-digit subclassification is for use with categories 531-535:

0 without mention of obstruction

1 with obstruction

531.0 ✓5th Acute gastric ulcer with hemorrhage — (Use additional E code to identify drug, if drug induced) — *sudden, severe; prepyloric, pylorus, stomach; with bleeding*
AHA: Nov-Dec, 1984, 15; Q4, 1990, 27; Q1, 1991, 15

531.1 ✓5th Acute gastric ulcer with perforation — (Use additional E code to identify drug, if drug induced) — *sudden, severe; prepyloric, pylorus, stomach; with leaking stomach contents*
AHA: Q4, 1990, 27; Q1, 1991, 15

531.2 ✓5th Acute gastric ulcer with hemorrhage and perforation — (Use additional E code to identify drug, if drug induced) — *sudden, severe; prepyloric, pylorus, stomach; with bleeding and leaking stomach contents*
AHA: Q4, 1990, 27; Q1, 1991, 15

531.3 ✓5th Acute gastric ulcer without mention of hemorrhage or perforation — (Use additional E code to identify drug, if drug induced) — *sudden, severe; prepyloric, pylorus, stomach; without bleeding or leaking stomach contents*
AHA: Q4, 1990, 27; Q1, 1991, 15

531.4 ✓5th Chronic or unspecified gastric ulcer with hemorrhage — (Use additional E code to identify drug, if drug induced) — *persistent; prepyloric, pylorus, stomach; with bleeding*
AHA: Q4, 1990, 22; Q4, 1990, 27; Q1, 1991, 15

531.5 ✓5th Chronic or unspecified gastric ulcer with perforation — (Use additional E code to identify drug, if drug induced) — *persistent; prepyloric, pylorus, stomach; with leaking stomach contents*
AHA: Q4, 1990, 27; Q1, 1991, 15

531.6 ✓5th Chronic or unspecified gastric ulcer with hemorrhage and perforation — (Use additional E code to identify drug, if drug induced) — *persistent; prepyloric, pylorus, stomach; with bleeding and leaking stomach contents*
AHA: Q4, 1990, 27; Q1, 1991, 15

531.7 ✓5th Chronic gastric ulcer without mention of hemorrhage or perforation — (Use additional E code to identify drug, if drug induced) — *persistent; prepyloric, pylorus, stomach; without bleeding or leaking stomach contents*
AHA: Q4, 1990, 27; Q1, 1991, 15

531.9 ✓5th Gastric ulcer, unspecified as acute or chronic, without mention of hemorrhage or perforation — (Use additional E code to identify drug, if drug induced) — *unknown whether sudden or persistent; prepyloric, pylorus, stomach; unknown status of bleeding or leaking stomach contents*
AHA: Q4, 1990, 27; Q1, 1991, 15

Coding Clarification

A common factor in peptic ulcer is the presence of *Helicobacter pylori*, which is treated with bismuth salicylate and oral amoxicillin. The *H. pylori* should be reported secondarily with 041.86.

532 Duodenal ulcer

AHA: Q4, 1990, 27; Q1, 1991, 15

Duodenal ulcers are ulcers formed in the duodenum by discreet tissue destruction due to the actions of hydrochloric (gastric) acid and pepsin on areas of the mucosa having a decreased resistance to ulceration. Duodenal ulcers occur about five times more frequently than gastric ulcers. About 95 percent occur in the area of the duodenal bulb or cap.

Signs and symptoms of a duodenal ulcer include pain with cramps, burning, gnawing, heartburn, vomiting of highly acidic fluid with no retained food, deep epigastric tenderness, voluntary muscle guarding, unilateral rectus spasm over duodenal bulb, and melena and occult blood in stools in chronic ulcers.

 © 2004 Ingenix, Inc.

Pain diminishes by eating, but recurs two to three hours later.

Gastric analysis shows acid in all cases and a basal and maximal gastric hypersecretion of hydrochloric acid in some patients. Lab work may show hypochromic blood loss anemia. Radiographs demonstrate ulcer crater formation when the ulcer is not obscured by duodenal bulb formation. Esophagogastroduodenoscopy proves duodenal ulcer in cases not demonstrated radiographically.

Therapies include antacids, diet modification, H2 receptor antagonist drugs such as cimetidine and ranitidine, and other therapeutic agents (sucralfate, carbenoxolone, bismuth, certain prostaglandins, tricyclic antidepressants such as doxepin). Surgical interventions include subtotal gastrectomy, vagotomy, antrectomy, gastrojejunostomy, and total gastrectomy.

The following fifth-digit subclassification is for use with categories 531-535:

0 without mention of obstruction

1 with obstruction

532.0 5th Acute duodenal ulcer with hemorrhage — (Use additional E code to identify drug, if drug induced) — *sudden, severe; duodenum, postpyloric; with bleeding*
AHA: Q4, 1990, 22; Q4, 1990, 27; Q1, 1991, 15

532.1 5th Acute duodenal ulcer with perforation — (Use additional E code to identify drug, if drug induced) — *sudden, severe; duodenum, postpyloric; with leaking stomach contents*
AHA: Q4, 1990, 27; Q1, 1991, 15

532.2 5th Acute duodenal ulcer with hemorrhage and perforation — (Use additional E code to identify drug, if drug induced) — *sudden, severe; duodenum, postpyloric; with bleeding and leaking stomach contents*
AHA: Q4, 1990, 27; Q1, 1991, 15

532.3 5th Acute duodenal ulcer without mention of hemorrhage or perforation — (Use additional E code to identify drug, if drug induced) — *sudden, severe; duodenum, postpyloric; without bleeding or leaking stomach contents*
AHA: Q4, 1990, 27; Q1, 1991, 15

532.4 5th Chronic or unspecified duodenal ulcer with hemorrhage — (Use additional E code to identify drug, if drug induced) — *persistent; duodenum, postpyloric; with bleeding*
AHA: Q4, 1990, 27; Q1, 1991, 15

532.5 5th Chronic or unspecified duodenal ulcer with perforation — (Use additional E code to identify drug, if drug induced) — *persistent; duodenum, postpyloric; with leaking stomach contents*
AHA: Q4, 1990, 27; Q1, 1991, 15

532.6 5th Chronic or unspecified duodenal ulcer with hemorrhage and perforation — (Use additional E code to identify drug, if drug induced) — *persistent; duodenum, postpyloric; with bleeding and leaking stomach contents*
AHA: Q4, 1990, 27; Q1, 1991, 15

532.7 5th Chronic duodenal ulcer without mention of hemorrhage or perforation — (Use additional E code to identify drug, if drug induced) — *persistent; duodenum, postpyloric; without bleeding or leaking stomach contents*
AHA: Q4, 1990, 27; Q1, 1991, 15

532.9 5th Duodenal ulcer, unspecified as acute or chronic, without mention of hemorrhage or perforation — (Use additional E code to identify drug, if drug induced) — *unknown whether sudden or persistent; duodenum, postpyloric; unknown status of bleeding or leaking stomach contents*
AHA: Q4, 1990, 27; Q1, 1991, 15

533 Peptic ulcer, site unspecified

AHA: Q4, 1990, 27; Q1, 1991, 15

This rubric classifies acute or chronic benign ulcer occurring in a portion of the digestive tract accessible to gastric secretions. Peptic ulcers result from the corrosive action of acid gastric juice on vulnerable epithelium.

This rubric includes only peptic ulcers for which no site has been specified.

The following fifth-digit subclassification is for use with categories 531-535:

0 without mention of obstruction

1 with obstruction

533.0 5th Acute peptic ulcer, unspecified site, with hemorrhage — (Use additional E code to identify drug, if drug induced) — *sudden, severe; site unknown; with bleeding*
AHA: Q4, 1990, 27; Q1, 1991, 15

533.1 5th Acute peptic ulcer, unspecified site, with perforation — (Use additional E code to identify drug, if drug induced) — *sudden, severe; site unknown; with leaking stomach contents*
AHA: Q4, 1990, 27; Q1, 1991, 15

533.2 ✓5th Acute peptic ulcer, unspecified site, with hemorrhage and perforation — (Use additional E code to identify drug, if drug induced) — *sudden, severe; site unknown; with bleeding and leaking stomach contents*
AHA: Q4, 1990, 27; Q1, 1991, 15

533.3 ✓5th Acute peptic ulcer, unspecified site, without mention of hemorrhage and perforation — (Use additional E code to identify drug, if drug induced) — *sudden, severe; site unknown; without bleeding or leaking stomach contents*
AHA: Q4, 1990, 27; Q1, 1991, 15

533.4 ✓5th Chronic or unspecified peptic ulcer, unspecified site, with hemorrhage — (Use additional E code to identify drug, if drug induced) — *persistent; site unknown; with bleeding*
AHA: Q4, 1990, 27; Q1, 1991, 15

533.5 ✓5th Chronic or unspecified peptic ulcer, unspecified site, with perforation — (Use additional E code to identify drug, if drug induced) — *persistent; site unknown; with leaking stomach contents*
AHA: Q4, 1990, 27; Q1, 1991, 15

533.6 ✓5th Chronic or unspecified peptic ulcer, unspecified site, with hemorrhage and perforation — (Use additional E code to identify drug, if drug induced) — *persistent; site unknown; with bleeding and leaking stomach contents*
AHA: Q4, 1990, 27; Q1, 1991, 15

533.7 ✓5th Chronic peptic ulcer, unspecified site, without mention of hemorrhage or perforation — (Use additional E code to identify drug, if drug induced) — *persistent; site unknown; without bleeding or leaking stomach contents*
AHA: Q2, 1989, 16; Q4, 1990, 27; Q1, 1991, 15

533.9 ✓5th Peptic ulcer, unspecified site, unspecified as acute or chronic, without mention of hemorrhage or perforation — *unknown whether sudden or persistent; site unknown; unknown status of bleeding or leaking stomach contents*
AHA: Q4, 1990, 27; Q1, 1991, 15

Coding Clarification

Peptic ulcers may occur in the esophagus (subcategory 530.2), stomach (category 531), duodenum (category 532), jejunum and gastrojejunal area (category 534), and ileum (569.82).

534 *Gastrojejunal ulcer*

AHA: Q4, 1990, 27; Q1, 1991, 15

This rubric classifies ulcer formation at or proximal to the junction of a previous gastrojejunal anastomosis. The signs and symptoms, diagnostics, therapies, and associated conditions are virtually the same as for gastric or duodenal ulcers.

The following fifth-digit subclassification is for use with categories 531-535:

0 without mention of obstruction

1 with obstruction

534.0 ✓5th Acute gastrojejunal ulcer with hemorrhage — *sudden, severe; jejunal, gastrocolic, gastrointestinal, marginal, stomal, anastomotic; with bleeding*
AHA: Q4, 1990, 27; Q1, 1991, 15

534.1 ✓5th Acute gastrojejunal ulcer with perforation — *sudden, severe; jejunal, gastrocolic, gastrointestinal, marginal, stomal, anastomotic; with leaking stomach contents*
AHA: Q4, 1990, 27; Q1, 1991, 15

534.2 ✓5th Acute gastrojejunal ulcer with hemorrhage and perforation — *sudden, severe; jejunal, gastrocolic, gastrointestinal, marginal, stomal, anastomotic; with bleeding and leaking stomach contents*
AHA: Q4, 1990, 27; Q1, 1991, 15

534.3 ✓5th Acute gastrojejunal ulcer without mention of hemorrhage or perforation — *sudden, severe; jejunal, gastrocolic, gastrointestinal, marginal, stomal, anastomotic; without bleeding or leaking stomach contents*
AHA: Q4, 1990, 27; Q1, 1991, 15

534.4 ✓5th Chronic or unspecified gastrojejunal ulcer with hemorrhage — *persistent; jejunal, gastrocolic, gastrointestinal, marginal, stomal, anastomotic; with bleeding*
AHA: Q4, 1990, 27; Q1, 1991, 15

534.5 ✓5th Chronic or unspecified gastrojejunal ulcer with perforation — *persistent; jejunal, gastrocolic, gastrointestinal, marginal, stomal, anastomotic; with leaking stomach contents*
AHA: Q4, 1990, 27; Q1, 1991, 15

534.6 ✓5th Chronic or unspecified gastrojejunal ulcer with hemorrhage and perforation — *persistent; jejunal, gastrocolic, gastrointestinal, marginal, stomal, anastomotic; with bleeding and leaking stomach contents*
AHA: Q4, 1990, 27; Q1, 1991, 15

534.7 ✓5th Chronic gastrojejunal ulcer without mention of hemorrhage or perforation — *persistent; jejunal, gastrocolic, gastrointestinal, marginal, stomal, anastomotic; without bleeding or leaking stomach contents*
AHA: Q4, 1990, 27; Q1, 1991, 15

© 2004 Ingenix, Inc.

534.9 ✓5th Gastrojejunal ulcer, unspecified as acute or chronic, without mention of hemorrhage or perforation — *unknown whether sudden or persistent; jejunal, gastrocolic, gastrointestinal, marginal, stomal, anastomotic; unknown status of bleeding or leaking stomach contents*
AHA: Q4, 1990, 27; Q1, 1991, 15

535 Gastritis and duodenitis

AHA: Q4, 1991, 25; Q2, 1992, 9

Gastritis is an inflammation of the lining of the stomach and duodenitis is inflammation of the duodenum. Gastritis can take on several forms, including Watermelon gastritis, which is a hemorrhagic condition that has a watermelon like appearance. Ulcers of the duodenal bulb can often be hidden between the folds. Both diseases can progress to erosion, ulceration, and bleeding. Causes, which are the same for both disorders, include alcohol, prolonged irritation from the use of nonsteroidal anti-inflammatory drugs (NSAIDs), infection with the bacteria *Helicobacter pylori,* pernicious anemia, degeneration related to age, or chronic bile reflux. Symptoms include upper abdominal pain aggravated by eating, indigestion, nausea, vomiting, and dark stools. Complications include severe loss of blood and an increased risk of gastric or duodenal cancer. Diagnosis is by a gastroscopy, an esophagogastroduodenoscopy (EGD), a complete blood count for anemia, and a positive guaiac stool. Treatment for either gastritis or duodenitis depends on the cause, such as H2 blockers and antacids to reduce HCL production, unless the cause is from anti-inflammatory medications, antibiotic therapy for conditions caused by bacterial infection, and antacids to decrease gastric acid. Other treatments include vitamin B12 for pernicious anemia and laser therapy for severe forms (e.g., watermelon gastritis).

This rubric classifies self-limiting illnesses characterized by nausea, vomiting, anorexia, epigastric pain, and some systemic symptoms. Manifestations may be variable but anorexia is a consistent feature.

The following fifth-digit subclassification is for use with categories 531-535:

0 without mention of obstruction

1 with obstruction

535.0 ✓5th Acute gastritis — *severe inflammation of stomach*
AHA: Nov-Dec, 1986, 9; Q4, 1991, 25; Q2, 1992, 8; Q2, 1992, 9

535.1 ✓5th Atrophic gastritis — *inflammation of the stomach with atrophy of the mucous membrane and destruction of the peptic glands*
AHA: Q4, 1991, 25; Q2, 1992, 9; Q1, 1994, 18

535.2 ✓5th Gastric mucosal hypertrophy — *increase in size and number of cells in tissue of gastric mucosa; Menetrier's syndrome*
AHA: Q4, 1991, 25; Q2, 1992, 9

535.3 ✓5th Alcoholic gastritis

535.4 ✓5th Other specified gastritis — *including allergic, bile-induced, irritant, superficial, toxic*
AHA: Q4, 1990, 27; Q4, 1991, 25; Q2, 1992, 9

535.5 ✓5th Unspecified gastritis and gastroduodenitis — *unknown type*
AHA: Q4, 1991, 25; Q2, 1992, 9

535.6 ✓5th Duodenitis — *inflammation of the intestine between the pylorus and the jejunum*
AHA: Q4, 1991, 25; Q2, 1992, 9

536 Disorders of function of stomach

As food is eaten, it passes from the mouth through the esophagus and to the stomach. Acids in the stomach break down food, while the lower esophageal sphincter stops stomach acid from backing up into the esophagus. The contractile activity of the stomach helps to mix, grind, and evacuate small portions of chyme into the small bowel, while the rest of the chyme is mixed and ground. Anatomically, the stomach can be divided into three major regions: fundus (the most proximal), corpus, and antrum.

The term "functional" generally applies to disorders described by symptoms when no organic explanation is detected using common diagnostic procedures. Achlorhydria (536.0) is the absence of hydrochloric acid in the stomach. There are varying degrees of achlorhydria, although, the older the patient, the greater the deficiency up to a complete absence of hydrochloric acid. Symptoms frequently occur several hours after eating and include flatulence and often alternating constipation and diarrhea. Gastroparesis (536.3) is a disorder in which the stomach takes too long to empty its contents. Cause is unknown, although disruption of nerve stimulation to the intestine is a possible cause. Gastroparesis is often a complication of Type I diabetes; it occurs less often in people with Type II diabetes. Symptoms of gastroparesis are nausea, vomiting, an early feeling of fullness when eating, weight loss, abdominal bloating, and abdominal discomfort. In most cases, gastroparesis is usually a chronic condition, although treatment does help manage the condition. Risk factors include diabetes, systemic sclerosis, previous vagotomy, previous gastrectomy, visceral neuropathy, and use of anticholinergic medication.

536.0 Achlorhydria — *the absence of stomach acid, usually the result of atrophy of gastric mucosa; gastric anacidity*

536.1 Acute dilatation of stomach — *acute distention; Potain's syndrome*

536.2 Persistent vomiting — *habit, uncontrollable, Leyden's disease; not associated with pregnancy*

536.3 Gastroparesis — *a slight degree of paralysis within the muscular coat of the stomach*
AHA: Q4, 1994, 42; Q2, 2001, 4

536.40 Unspecified gastrostomy complication

536.41 Infection of gastrostomy — (Use additional code to specify type of infection: 038.0-038.9, 041.00-041.9. Use additional code to identify organism: 041.00-041.9)

536.42 Mechanical complication of gastrostomy

536.49 Other gastrostomy complications — *not otherwise specified*
AHA: Q4, 1998, 42

536.8 Dyspepsia and other specified disorders of function of stomach — *hypermotility, hourglass contraction, hyperacidity, indigestion, pain, hypertonicity, Reichmann's syndrome, spasms, hypochlorhydria, hyperchlorhydria, Rossbach's disease*
AHA: Nov-Dec, 1984, 9; Q2, 1989, 16; Q2, 1993, 6

536.9 Unspecified functional disorder of stomach — *unknown disorder or disturbance*

537 Other disorders of stomach and duodenum

537.0 Acquired hypertrophic pyloric stenosis — *construction, obstruction, stricture*
AHA: Jan-Feb, 1985, 14; Q2, 2001, 4

537.1 Gastric diverticulum — *herniated pouch or sac opening within the stomach or duodenum*
AHA: Jan-Feb, 1985, 4

537.2 Chronic duodenal ileus — *persistent obstruction between the pylorus and jejunum*

537.3 Other obstruction of duodenum — *cicatrix, stenosis, stricture, volvulus*

537.4 Fistula of stomach or duodenum — *gastrocolic, gastrojejunocolic*

537.5 Gastroptosis — *downward displacement of the stomach*

537.6 Hourglass stricture or stenosis of stomach — *cascade stomach*

537.81 Pylorospasm — *spasmodic contraction of the distal aperture of the stomach*
AHA: Q4, 1991, 25

537.82 Angiodysplasia of stomach and duodenum (without mention of hemorrhage) — *vascular abnormalities of stomach and duodenum, without bleeding*
AHA: Q4, 1990, 4; Q4, 1991, 25; Q3, 1996, 10

537.83 Angiodysplasia of stomach and duodenum with hemorrhage — *vascular abnormalities of stomach and duodenum, with bleeding*
AHA: Q4, 1991, 25

537.84 Dieulafoy lesion (hemorrhagic) of stomach and duodenum

537.89 Other specified disorder of stomach and duodenum — *not otherwise specified, prolapse, rupture, intestinal metaplasia of gastric mucosa, lesion, necrosis, gastrolith, hypertony, obstruction, volvulus, efferent loop syndrome, passive congestion, mechanical difficulty of gastroduodenal stoma*
AHA: Nov-Dec, 1984, 7; Q4, 1991, 25

537.9 Unspecified disorder of stomach and duodenum

540–543 Appendicitis

Appendicitis is inflammation of the vermiform appendix. It is usually initiated by obstruction of the appendiceal lumen by a fecalith, inflammation, neoplasm, or foreign body. The obstruction is followed by infection, edema, and frequently infarction of the appendiceal wall. Intraluminal tension develops rapidly and tends to cause mural necrosis and perforation.

Signs and symptoms of appendicitis include abdominal pain, usually beginning with epigastric or periumbilical pain associated with one or two episodes of vomiting. The abdominal pain may shift during the next 12 hours to the right lower quadrant (McBurney's point) where it persists as steady soreness aggravated by walking or coughing, anorexia, moderate malaise, slight to moderate fever, constipation (or occasionally diarrhea), rebound tenderness, and spasm.

Blood work may show moderate increase in white blood cells to 10,000/cu mm to 20,000/cu mm with an increase in neutrophils. Urinalysis may show a presence of microscopic hematuria and pyuria and barium enema may be used to visualize the entire appendix in uncertain cases.

Therapies include antibiotic therapy, nasogastric intubation, rehydration, and appendectomy with few exceptions.

Appendicitis is the most common nonobstetrical complication of pregnancy.

 © 2004 Ingenix, Inc.

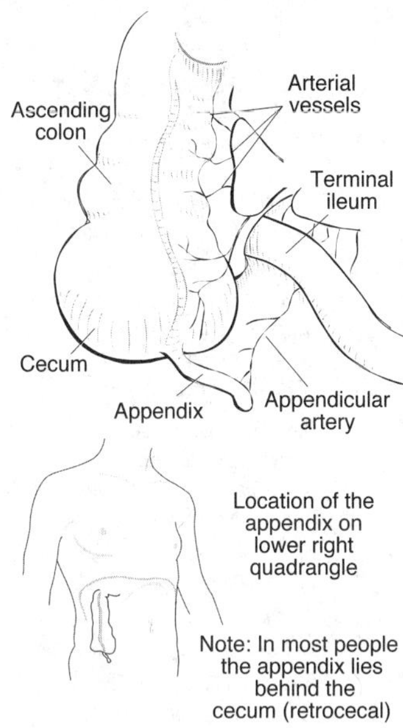

540 Acute appendicitis

AHA: Nov-Dec, 1984, 19

540.0 Acute appendicitis with generalized peritonitis — *fulminating, gangrenous, obstructive; with perforation, rupture*
AHA: Nov-Dec, 1984, 19

540.1 Acute appendicitis with peritoneal abscess — *generalized peritonitis; pocket of pus*
AHA: Nov-Dec, 1984, 19

540.9 Acute appendicitis without mention of peritonitis — *without rupture, perforation, peritonitis*
AHA: Nov-Dec, 1984, 19; Q4, 1997, 52; Q1, 2001, 15

543 Other diseases of appendix

543.0 Hyperplasia of appendix (lymphoid) — *increase in size and number of cells of appendix*

543.9 Other and unspecified diseases of appendix — *not otherwise specified, adhesion, cyst, mucocele, stercolith, fecalith, fistula, sloughing, strangulation, atrophy, intussusception, diverticulum, concretion*

550–553 Hernia of Abdominal Cavity

The definition of a hernia of the abdominal cavity is the protrusion of tissue, an organ, or part of an organ through an abnormal opening in the wall of the body cavity in which it is normally confined. The majority of hernias are abdominal resulting from herniation of abdominal contents through the internal or external inguinal rings, femoral rings, or defects in the abdominal wall resulting from trauma or improper healing after a surgical procedure.

550 Inguinal hernia

AHA: Nov-Dec, 1985, 12

An inguinal hernia is defined as a condition in which a loop of intestine enters the inguinal canal, a tubular passage through the lower layers of the abdominal wall. A hernia occurs when part of an organ protrudes through a weak point or tear in the thin muscular wall that holds the abdominal organs in place. A direct inguinal hernia creates a bulge in the groin area, and an indirect hernia descends into the scrotum. Inguinal hernias occur less often in women than men.

Hernias are caused by congenital (defects at birth) or age-related weaknesses in the abdominal walls. In males, they are often congenital and caused by an improper closure of the abdominal cavity. They can also be caused by an increase in pressure within the abdominal cavity due to heavy lifting, straining, violent coughing, obesity, or pregnancy.

Signs and symptoms include a protrusion in the groin area between the pubis and the top of the leg in the area known as the inguinal region of the abdomen or pain during urination or a bowel movement or when lifting a heavy object. The pain can be sharp and immediate. There may be a dull aching sensation, nausea, or constipation; these feelings typically get worse toward the end of the day or after standing for long periods of time and may disappear when lying down.q

A hernia that can be pushed back into the abdominal cavity (called a reducible hernia) is not considered an immediate health threat, though it does require surgery to repair the hernia. A hernia that cannot be pushed back in (called a nonreducible hernia) may lead to dangerous complications such as the obstruction of the flow of the intestinal contents or intestinal blood supply (strangulation), leading to tissue death, and requires immediate surgery.

The following fifth-digit subclassification is for use with category 550:

0 unilateral or unspecified (not specified as recurrent)

1 unilateral or unspecified, recurrent

2 bilateral (not specified as recurrent)3
bilateral, recurrent

550.0 ✓5th Inguinal hernia, with gangrene — *direct, double, indirect, oblique, sliding hernia; incarceration, irreducibility, strangulation*
AHA: Nov-Dec, 1985, 12

550.1 ✓5th Inguinal hernia, with obstruction, without mention of gangrene — *direct, double, indirect, oblique, sliding hernia; incarceration, irreducibility, strangulation*
AHA: Nov-Dec, 1985, 12

550.9 ✓5th Inguinal hernia, without mention of obstruction or gangrene — *direct, double, indirect, oblique, sliding hernia*
AHA: Nov-Dec, 1985, 12

551 Other hernia of abdominal cavity, with gangrene

551.00 Femoral hernia with gangrene, unilateral or unspecified (not specified as recurrent)

551.01 Femoral hernia with gangrene, recurrent unilateral or unspecified

551.02 Femoral hernia with gangrene, bilateral, (not specified as recurrent)

551.03 Femoral hernia with gangrene, recurrent bilateral

551.1 Umbilical hernia with gangrene — *abnormal protrusion of the intestine at the umbilicus*

551.20 Unspecified ventral hernia with gangrene — *abnormal protrusion of tissue through the abdominal wall, cause unknown*

551.21 Incisional ventral hernia, with gangrene — *abnormal protrusion of tissue through the abdominal wall, postoperative*

551.29 Other ventral hernia with gangrene — *abnormal protrusion of tissue through the abdominal wall, not otherwise specified*

551.8 Hernia of other specified sites, with gangrene — *Gruber's, Hesselbach's Rieux's; ischiorectal, lumbar, obturator, sciatic, retroperitoneal*

551.9 Hernia of unspecified site, with gangrene — *enterocele, epiplocele, interstitial, intestinal, intraabdominal, sacroepiplocele*

553.3 Diaphragmatic hernia without mention of obstruction or gangrene — *hiatal, paraesophageal, thoracic stomach*
AHA: Q1, 2000, 6; Q2, 2001, 6

552 Other hernia of abdominal cavity, with obstruction, but without mention of gangrene

552.00 Unilateral or unspecified femoral hernia with obstruction

552.01 Recurrent unilateral or unspecified femoral hernia with obstruction

552.02 Bilateral femoral hernia with obstruction

552.03 Recurrent bilateral femoral hernia with obstruction

552.1 Umbilical hernia with obstruction — *abnormal protrusion of the intestine of the umbilicus; incarcerated, irreducible, strangulated*

552.20 Unspecified ventral hernia with obstruction — *abnormal protrusion of tissue through the abdominal wall, cause unknown; incarcerated, irreducible, strangulated*

552.21 Incisional hernia with obstruction — *abnormal protrusion of tissue through the abdominal wall, postoperative; incarcerated, irreducible, strangulated*
AHA: Q3, 2003, 11

552.29 Other ventral hernia with obstruction — *abnormal protrusion of tissue through the abdominal wall, not otherwise specified; incarcerated, irreducible, strangulated*

552.3 Diaphragmatic hernia with obstruction — *hiatal, esophageal, paraesophageal, thoracic stomach; incarcerated, irreducible, strangulated*

552.8 Hernia of other specified site, with obstruction — *other sites including Gruber's, Hesselbach's Rieux's; Treitz's, ischiorectal, lumbar, obturator, retroperitoneal; incarcerated, irreducible, strangulated*

552.9 Hernia of unspecified site, with obstruction — *unknown site*

553 Other hernia of abdominal cavity without mention of obstruction or gangrene

Subcategory 553.3 reports a protrusion of part of the stomach through the esophageal hiatus of the diaphragm. The esophageal hiatus is the opening in the diaphragm between the central tendon and the hiatus aorticus where the esophagus and the two vagus nerves pass. Clinicians recognize two different types of esophageal hiatal hernias: paraesophageal and sliding (by far the more common type of hiatal hernia).

The paraesophageal hiatal hernia is characterized by all or part of the stomach herniating into the thorax immediately adjacent and to the left of a nondisplaced gastroesophageal junction. Reflux of the gastric contents does not occur because the gastroesophageal sphincter functions normal. Although this type of hiatal hernia is usually asymptomatic, complications can include hemorrhage, incarceration, obstruction, and strangulation.

With a sliding hiatal hernia, the upper stomach, along with the cardioesophageal junction, herniates upward into the posterior mediastinum. The stomach displacement may be stationary, or it may actually slide in and out of the thorax with movement, after a large meal, or with alterations of the pressure in the abdominal and thoracic cavities. Esophageal reflux and esophagitis are characteristic and due to

© 2004 Ingenix, Inc.

abnormalities in the esophageal sphincter. Sliding hiatal hernia may be complicated by development of ulcers or structure formation. Carcinoma is occasionally associated with sliding hiatal hernia.

Signs and symptoms of diaphragmatic hernia without mention of obstruction or gangrene include dysphagia, and retrosternal and epigastric burning in sliding hiatal hernia with reflux esophagitis.

Diagnostic tests include x-ray examination and fluoroscopy with or without contrast to demonstrate a protrusion of the stomach through the esophageal hiatus. Esophagoscopy and biopsy assess the severity of any esophagitis and rule out associated conditions such as strictures, polyps, ulcers, and carcinomas. Esophageal motility studies assess the competency of the esophageal sphincter and prolonged monitoring of the patient's pH in the lower esophagus establishes the presence of abnormal reflux.

Therapies include diet and antacids for esophagitis. There is no intervention for asymptomatic hiatal hernias. Surgery (for about 15 percent of patients with persistent and severe symptoms) includes Nissen fundoplication, Belsey fundoplication, and placement of a doughnut-shaped silicone prosthesis around the intraabdominal esophagus (Angelchik procedure) for uncomplicated hernias. The Collis procedure or Collis-Nissen operation, may be performed when the hernia is associated with acquired short esophagus. Other treatments include vagotomy, antrectomy, or a Roux-en-Y gastrojejunostomy when scar tissue around the gastroesophageal junction from previous surgery prevents a fundoplication.

Associated conditions include reflux esophagitis, esophageal stricture, polyps, ulcer formation with or without bleeding, carcinoma, and Saint's triad (hiatal hernia, gallbladder disease, and colon diverticulosis).

553.00 Unilateral or unspecified femoral hernia without mention of obstruction or gangrene, unilateral or unspecified

553.01 Femoral hernia without mention of obstruction or gangrene, recurrent unilateral or unspecified

553.02 Femoral hernia without mention of obstruction or gangrene, bilateral

553.03 Femoral hernia without mention of obstruction or gangrene, recurrent bilateral

553.1 Umbilical hernia without mention of obstruction or gangrene — *abnormal protrusion of the intestine at the umbilicus; paraumbilical*

553.20 Unspecified ventral hernia without mention of obstruction or gangrene — *abnormal protrusion of tissue through the abdominal wall; cause unknown*
AHA: Q3, 2003, 6

553.21 Incisional hernia without mention of obstruction or gangrene — *abnormal protrusion of tissue through the abdominal wall; postoperative*
AHA: Q3, 2003, 6

553.29 Other ventral hernia without mention of obstruction or gangrene — *not otherwise specified; including epigastric, spigelian*

553.3 Diaphragmatic hernia without mention of obstruction or gangrene — *hiatal, paraesophageal, thoracic stomach*
AHA: Q1, 2000, 6; Q2, 2001, 6

553.8 Hernia of other specified sites of abdominal cavity without mention of obstruction or gangrene — *appendix, obturator, pudendal, retroperitoneal, sciatic, lumbar, ischiatic, ischiorectal, duodenojejunal, mesenteric, mesocolon, omental*

553.9 Hernia of unspecified site of abdominal cavity without mention of obstruction or gangrene

555–558 Noninfectious Enteritis and Colitis

555 Regional enteritis

Regional enteritis is a form of inflammatory bowel disease characterized by a chronic granulomatous disease. Also known as Crohn's disease, regional enteritis most often affects the large intestines but may occur anywhere in the gastrointestinal tract (e.g., mouth, esophagus, stomach, duodenum, large intestine, appendix, and anus). The disease often results in multiple bowel resections.

Associated conditions include multiple strictures, bacterial overgrowth, and malabsorption.

555.0 Regional enteritis of small intestine — *Crohn's disease, granulomatous enteritis; duodenum, ileum, jejunum*

555.1 Regional enteritis of large intestine — *Crohn's disease, granulomatous enteritis; colon, large bowel, rectum*
AHA: Q3, 1999, 8

555.2 Regional enteritis of small intestine with large intestine — *Crohn's disease, granulomatous enteritis; regional ileocolitis*
AHA: Q1, 2003, 18

555.9 Regional enteritis of unspecified site

556 Ulcerative colitis

AHA: Q3, 1999, 8

Ulcerative colitis is a disease that causes inflammation and ulcers in the top layers of the lining of the large intestine. The inflammation usually occurs in the rectum and lower part of the colon, but it may affect the entire colon and makes the colon empty

520–579

frequently, causing diarrhea. Ulcers form in places where the inflammation has killed colon cells; the ulcers bleed and produce pus and mucous.

Ulcerative colitis rarely affects the small intestine except for the lower section, called the ileum. The disease can be difficult to diagnose because its symptoms are similar to other intestinal disorders such as irritable bowel syndrome and Crohn's disease, which usually occurs in the small intestine but may occur anywhere in the GI tract.

The most common symptoms of ulcerative colitis are abdominal pain and bloody diarrhea. Patients also may experience fatigue, weight loss, and rectal bleeding.

Blood tests may be performed to check for anemia, which could indicate bleeding in the colon or rectum. Blood tests may also reveal a high white blood cell count. A stool sample indicates whether there is bleeding or infection in the colon or rectum. A colonoscopy visualizes the inside of the colon and rectum. A barium enema x-ray of the colon allows a clear view of the colon, including any ulcers or other abnormalities. Treatment for ulcerative colitis depends on the seriousness of the disease. Most people are treated with medication, although in severe cases, a patient may need surgery to remove the diseased colon.

556.0 Ulcerative (chronic) enterocolitis — *persistent inflammation of the mucous membrane of small and large intestines*
AHA: Q3, 1999, 8

556.1 Ulcerative (chronic) ileocolitis — *persistent inflammation of the mucous membrane of ileum and colon*
AHA: Q3, 1999, 8

556.2 Ulcerative (chronic) proctitis — *persistent inflammation of the mucous membrane of the rectum*
AHA: Q3, 1999, 8

556.3 Ulcerative (chronic) proctosigmoiditis — *persistent inflammation of the mucous membrane of the sigmoid colon and rectum*
AHA: Q3, 1999, 8

556.4 Pseudopolyposis of colon

556.5 Left sided ulcerative (chronic) colitis

556.6 Universal ulcerative (chronic) colitis — *persistent inflammation of the mucous membrane of the entire colon*
AHA: Q3, 1999, 8

556.8 Other ulcerative colitis

556.9 Unspecified ulcerative colitis

557 Vascular insufficiency of intestine

Visceral ischemic syndromes are associated with atherosclerotic lesions obstructing the celiac trunk, superior mesenteric artery, and inferior mesenteric artery: embolism, mesenteric venous thrombosis, and aneurysms. Narrowing of the superior mesenteric artery often presents with intense abdominal pain that results in vomiting or loose bowel movements. Gradual occlusion of this artery causes severe pain around the navel within one hour of eating because of the increased demand for blood to the intestines for digestion. The abdomen becomes distended and the stool becomes bloody. The intestine turns gangrene because of the lack of blood being supplied to the area. Surgical intervention for embolectomy or bypass reconstruction of the obstructing lesions is usually necessary to avoid extensive intestinal necrosis or death. The major causes of small intestinal hemorrhage are infectious vascular infarctions, vascular anomalies, bleeding disorders, and tumors. Interference with blood flow to the colon is the cause of ischemic colitis (557.1), an inflammation disorder of the large intestine. Risks include a history of peripheral vascular disease, stroke, low blood pressure, congestive heart failure, diabetes, and abdominal radiation exposure. Other risk factors include previous aortic surgery with accidental damage to the artery supplying the colon.

557.0 Acute vascular insufficiency of intestine — *infarction, necrosis, hemorrhage, gangrene, thrombosis, embolism*
AHA: Q4, 2001, 53

557.1 Chronic vascular insufficiency of intestine — *abdominal angina, ischemic colitis or enteritis, stricture, artery syndrome, vascular insufficiency, Wilkie's syndrome*
AHA: Nov-Dec, 1984, 7; Nov-Dec, 1986, 11; Q4, 1990, 4; Q3, 1996, 9

557.9 Unspecified vascular insufficiency of intestine

558 Other noninfectious gastroenteritis and colitis

Other and unspecified noninfectious gastroenteritis and colitis include gastroenteritis and colitis that do not have an infectious or presumed infectious origin. The three most common forms are enteritis, gastroenteritis, and diarrhea, not otherwise specified.

Often, enteritis, gastroenteritis, and diarrhea, when specified as due to an underlying condition, should be classified to a different category. Infectious disease is the most frequent cause of gastritis and gastroenteritis and is classified to Chapter 1 Infectious and Parasitic Diseases (001-139).

Commonly caused by infection, diarrhea may also be caused by chronic bowel disease, malabsorption states, food poisoning, adverse reactions to medications, and dietary factors such as malnutrition and food allergy. Diarrhea also may be the result of cholestatic syndromes, pancreatic disease, metabolic disease, neurological disease, psychogenic disorders,

 © 2004 Ingenix, Inc.

heavy metal poisoning, laxative abuse, reflex from other viscera, and immunodeficiency disease.

558.1 Gastroenteritis and colitis due to radiation — *radiation enterocolitis*

558.2 Toxic gastroenteritis and colitis — (Use additional E code to identify cause)

558.3 Gastroenteritis and colitis, allergic — (Use additional code to identify type of food allergy: V15.01-V15.05)

558.9 Other and unspecified noninfectious gastroenteritis and colitis

560–569 Other Diseases of Intestines and Peritoneum

560 Intestinal obstruction without mention of hernia

This category includes functional obstruction of the intestines, usually the colon. Also known as adynamic ileus, this condition represents a neurogenic impairment of peristalsis that can lead to complete intestinal obstruction. The intraabdominal etiologies for paralytic ileus include gastrointestinal surgery (997.4), peritoneal irritations (such as intraabdominal hemorrhage, ruptured viscus, pancreatitis or peritonitis), or anoxic organic obstruction. Other etiologies include drugs with anticholinergic properties, renal colic, vertebral fractures, spinal cord injuries, uremia, severe infection, diabetic coma, and electrolyte imbalances.

Signs and symptoms of paralytic ileus include continuous mild to moderate abdominal pain, vomiting, constipation, and abdominal distention. There may be absent borborygmus, minimal to absent bowel sounds, and signs of dehydration. Lab work may show hemoconcentration and or electrolyte imbalances. Leukocytosis, anemia, or elevated serum amylase may be present depending on the initiating condition. X-ray of the abdomen shows distended gas-filled loops of bowel and may show air-fluid levels in the distended bowel.

Therapies include bed rest, restriction of oral intake, rehydration, and gastrointestinal suctioning. Surgical decompression via enterostomy or cecostomy may be performed in severe cases. Associated conditions include dehydration and other electrolyte imbalances.

When assigning 560.1, also classify any initiating diseases or disorders such as those outlined in the definition.

560.0 Intussusception — *prolapse of one section of bowel into an immediate adjacent section; invagination*
AHA: Q4, 1998, 82

560.1 Paralytic ileus — *adynamic, paralysis*
AHA: Jan-Feb, 1987, 13

560.2 Volvulus — *knotting, strangulation, torsion, twists*

560.30 Unspecified impaction of intestine

560.31 Gallstone ileus — *obstruction by gallstone*

560.39 Other impaction of intestine — *fecal reservoir syndrome, fecal impaction, enterolith, concretion*
AHA: Q4, 1998, 38

560.81 Intestinal or peritoneal adhesions with obstruction (postoperative) (postinfection) — *abnormal joining of separate tissue in the peritoneum or intestine*
AHA: Nov-Dec, 1987, 9; Q3, 1995, 6; Q4, 1995, 55

560.89 Other specified intestinal obstruction — *mural thickening causing obstruction, sympathicotonic obstruction, Ogilvie's syndrome*
AHA: Q1, 1988, 6; Q2, 1997, 3

560.9 Unspecified intestinal obstruction

562 Diverticula of intestine

AHA: Jan-Feb, 1985, 1; Q4, 1991, 25

Report any associated peritonitis with an additional code (567.0-567.9). Excluded from this rubric are congenital diverticulum of the colon (751.5), diverticulum of the appendix (543.9), and Meckel's diverticulum (751.0).

Use the codes in subclassification 562.1 to report formation of a pouch or sac in the colon due to pressure from within the colon. Diverticula and diverticulosis tend to occur in higher-pressure areas, such as the sigmoid colon, and dissect along the course of nutrient vessels. They consist of a mucosal coat and serosa and usually herniate through the muscularis of the colon.

Signs and symptoms of diverticula of the colon include left lower quadrant pain, either steady or severe lasting for days; cramping, intermittent and relieved by bowel movement; and constipation (or occasionally diarrhea). Guaiac testing shows occult blood in 20 percent of patients with diverticulosis. X-ray reveals diverticula and in some cases colonic spasm and interhaustral thickening or narrowing of the colonic lumen. Endoscopic exam with or without biopsy is performed when bleeding occurs to rule out other pathology. Therapies include increased bulk and fiber in diet, anticholinergic medications to control sigmoid colon spasm, and antibiotics for diverticulitis. Surgical resection of the involved portion of bowel may be performed when there are recurrent bouts of diverticulitis or to treat complications such as hemorrhage, perforation, and abscess formation.

True diverticula contain all layers of the bowel and are rare in the colon. False diverticula consist of mucosa and submucosa that have herniated through the muscularis. For coding purposes, the terms "true" and "false" have no significance and should be treated as nonessential modifiers.

Diverticula of the colon are considered pulsion type because they are pushed out by intraluminal pressure. In the ICD-9-CM index, the term "pulsion" is an essential modifier under the main term "Diverticula, diverticulosis, diverticulum," leading to code 530.6 for diverticula of the esophagus. Do not assign this code for a pulsion diverticula when it refers to other anatomic sites such as the colon.

562.00 Diverticulosis of small intestine (without mention of hemorrhage) — (Use additional code to identify any associated peritonitis: 567.0-567.9) — *sac-like herniations of the mucosal lining; duodenum, ileum, jejunum*
AHA: Jan-Feb, 1985, 1; Q4, 1991, 25

562.01 Diverticulitis of small intestine (without mention of hemorrhage) — (Use additional code to identify any associated peritonitis: 567.0-567.9) — *inflammation of sac-like herniations of mucosal lining; duodenum, ileum, jejunum*
AHA: Jan-Feb, 1985, 1; Q4, 1991, 25

562.02 Diverticulosis of small intestine with hemorrhage — (Use additional code to identify any associated peritonitis: 567.0-567.9) — *sac-like herniations of the mucosal lining; duodenum, ileum, jejunum; bleeding*
AHA: Jan-Feb, 1985, 1; Q4, 1991, 25

562.03 Divertulitis of small intestine with hemorrhage — (Use additional code to identify any associated peritonitis: 567.0-567.9) — *inflammation of sac-like herniations of mucosal lining; duodenum, ileum, jejunum; bleeding*
AHA: Jan-Feb, 1985, 1; Q4, 1991, 25

562.10 Diverticulosis of colon (without mention of hemorrhage) — (Use additional code to identify any associated peritonitis: 567.0-567.9) — *sac-like herniations of the mucosal lining*
AHA: Jan-Feb, 1985, 1; Jan-Feb, 1985, 5; Q4, 1990, 21; Q4, 1991, 25; Q3, 2002, 15

562.11 Diverticulitis of colon (without mention of hemorrhage) — (Use additional code to identify any associated peritonitis: 567.0-567.9) — *inflammation of sac-like herniations of mucosal lining*
AHA: Jan-Feb, 1985, 1; Jan-Feb, 1985, 5; Q4, 1991, 25; Q1, 1996, 14

562.12 Diverticulosis of colon with hemorrhage — (Use additional code to identify any associated peritonitis: 567.0-567.9) — *sac-like herniations of the mucosal lining; bleeding*
AHA: Jan-Feb, 1985, 1; Q4, 1991, 25

562.13 Diverticulitis of colon with hemorrhage — (Use additional code to identify any associated peritonitis: 567.0-567.9) — *inflammation of sac-like herniations of mucosal lining; bleeding*
AHA: Jan-Feb, 1985, 1; Q4, 1991, 25

564 Functional digestive disorders, not elsewhere classified

564.00 Unspecified constipation

564.01 Slow transit constipation

564.02 Outlet dysfunction constipation

564.09 Other constipation

564.1 Irritable bowel syndrome — *IBS, irritable bowel*
AHA: Q1, 1988, 6

564.2 Postgastric surgery syndromes — *dumping, jejunal, postgastrectomy, postvagotomy syndromes*
AHA: Q1, 1995, 11

564.3 Vomiting following gastrointestinal surgery

564.4 Other postoperative functional disorders — *diarrhea*

564.5 Functional diarrhea — *diarrhea with no detectable organic cause*

564.6 Anal spasm — *proctalgia fugax*

564.7 Megacolon, other than Hirschsprung's — *dilatation of colon; faulty bowel habit syndrome*

564.81 Neurogenic bowel

564.89 Other functional disorders of intestine — *atony of colon*
AHA: Q1, 1988, 6

564.9 Unspecified functional disorder of intestine

Coding Clarification

Excluded from this rubric are functional disorders of the stomach (536.0-536.9) and digestive disorders that have been specified as psychogenic (306.4).

565 Anal fissure and fistula

The last part of the rectum (anal canal) is a section about 1.5 inches long, which ends with the anus. An anal fissure is a tear in the lining of the anus frequently caused by constipation when a dry bowel movement results in a break in the tissue. However, fissures can also occur with severe bouts of diarrhea, inflammation, injury to the anal canal during childbirth, and laxative abuse. A fissure can be painful during and following bowel movements because of

520–579

© 2004 Ingenix, Inc.

the muscles that control the passage of stool and keep the anus tightly closed at other times. When those muscles expand, it stretches the fissure open. A fistula is a channel or tract that develops in the presence of inflammation and infection. The channel usually runs from the rectum to an opening in the skin around the anus. Since fistulas are infected channels, there is usually some drainage.

565.0 Anal fissure — *nontraumatic tear*

565.1 Anal fistula — *anorectal, rectum to skin*

Coding Clarification

Excluded from this rubric are traumatic fissures (863.89, 863.99), and fistulas of the rectum to internal organs. Refer to the ICD-9-CM index to classify fistulas of the rectum to internal organs.

567 Peritonitis

Use this rubric to report acute or chronic inflammation of the peritoneum. It may be in response to agents such as bacteria, viruses, bile, hydrochloric acid, and chemicals such as continuous ambulatory peritoneal dialysis (CAPD) fluid. Other causative agents include parasites, fungi, and foreign bodies such as barium sulfate, used in diagnostic roentgenographic studies. Ruptured viscus and surgical procedures are two common underlying factors in secondary peritonitis. Chronic peritonitis can lead to dense, widespread abdominal adhesions.

567.0 Peritonitis in infectious diseases classified elsewhere — (Code first underlying disease) — *secondary to underlying disease*

567.1 Pneumococcal peritonitis — *inflammation of peritoneal*

567.2 Other suppurative peritonitis — *abdominopelvic, mesenteric, omentum, peritoneum, retrocecal, retroperitoneal, subdiaphragmatic, subhepatic, subphrenic*
AHA: Q2, 1998, 19; Q3, 1999, 9; Q2, 2001, 11,12

567.8 Other specified peritonitis — *not otherwise specified, fat necrosis, peritonitis due to bile or urine*

567.9 Unspecified peritonitis

Coding Clarification

Excluded from this rubric are peritonitis defined as benign paroxysmal (277.3), female pelvic (614.5, 614.7), periodic familial (277.3), puerperal (670), or in cases of abortion (rubrics 634-638), appendicitis (540.0-540.1), or ectopic/molar pregnancy (639.0).

568 Other disorders of peritoneum

568.0 Peritoneal adhesions (postoperative) (postinfection) — *abdominal wall, diaphragm, intestine, male pelvis, mesenteric, omentum, stomach, adhesive bands*
AHA: Sept-Oct, 1985, 11; Q3, 1995, 7; Q4, 1995, 55; Q3, 2003, 7, 11

568.81 Hemoperitoneum (nontraumatic) — *blood in the peritoneal cavity*

568.82 Peritoneal effusion (chronic) — *persistent escape of fluid within the peritoneal cavity*

568.89 Other specified disorder of peritoneum — *not otherwise specified, including acquired deforming, hemorrhage, rupture, degeneration, cyst, granuloma, pneumatosis*

568.9 Unspecified disorder of peritoneum

569 Other disorders of intestine

569.0 Anal and rectal polyp — *not otherwise specified*

569.1 Rectal prolapse — *procidentia; anus, rectum*

569.2 Stenosis of rectum and anus — *stricture*

569.3 Hemorrhage of rectum and anus — *bleeding*

569.41 Ulcer of anus and rectum — *solitary, stercoral*

569.42 Anal or rectal pain — *proctalgia*
AHA: Q1, 1996, 13; Q1, 2003, 8

569.49 Other specified disorder of rectum and anus — *not otherwise specified, hypertrophy of anal papillae; granuloma, rupture, male proctocele/rectocele, relaxation, paralysis, cicatrix*

569.5 Abscess of intestine — *pocket of pus*

569.60 Unspecified complication of colostomy or enterostomy

569.61 Infection of colostomy or enterostomy — (Use additional code to identify organism: 041.00-041.9. Use additional code to specify type of infection: 038.0-038.9, 682.2)

569.62 Mechanical complication of colostomy and enterostomy — *malfunction*
AHA: Q4, 1995, 58; Q4, 1998, 44; Q1, 2003, 10

569.69 Other complication of colostomy or enterostomy — *not otherwise specified, fistula, hernia, stenosis, prolapse*
AHA: Q4, 1995, 58; Q3, 1998, 16

569.81 Fistula of intestine, excluding rectum and anus — *abnormal communication between intestine and other internal organ or site*
AHA: Q4, 1991, 25; Q3, 1999, 8

569.82 Ulceration of intestine

569.83 Perforation of intestine — *hole through the intestinal wall*
AHA: Q4, 1991, 25

569.84 Angiodysplasia of intestine (without mention of hemorrhage) — *degenerative dilation of vasculature of intestine, without bleeding*
AHA: Q4, 1990, 4; Q4, 1990, 21; Q4, 1991, 25; Q3, 1996, 10

569.85 Angiodysplasia of intestine with hemorrhage — *degenerative dilation of vasculature of intestine, with bleeding*
AHA: Q4, 1991, 25; Q3, 1996, 9

569.86 Dieulafoy lesion (hemorrhagic) of intestine

569.89 Other specified disorder of intestines — *not otherwise specified, enteroptosis, granuloma, prolapse, acquired deformity, sacculation, Lane's, Glenard's, or Payr's disease*
AHA: Q4, 1991, 25; Q3, 1996, 9

569.9 Unspecified disorder of intestine

Other Diseases of Digestive System

571 Chronic liver disease and cirrhosis

Use this rubric to report chronic liver disease and cirrhosis not due to infection. The liver is the largest gland in the body and serves many metabolic purposes including secretion of bile. Chronic alcohol use leads to three similar forms of liver disease: steatosis (fatty liver), hepatitis, and cirrhosis. The conditions have many overlapping features and each may occur without involvement of alcohol. Alcoholic cirrhosis accounts for about 60 percent of all cirrhosis cases and the risk appears to rise with the amount of alcohol consumed daily. The liver tends to shrink and become fibrotic.

Hepatitis is the inflammation of the liver, which is usually due to viral infection classified elsewhere or to toxic agents such as alcohol or drugs. Cirrhosis of the liver is a chronic, progressive disease characterized by damage to the hepatic parenchymal cells and nodular regeneration, fibrosis formation, and disturbance of the normal architecture. Two different types of cirrhosis have been described based on the amount of regenerative activity in the liver: chronic sclerosing cirrhosis in which the liver is small and hard and nodular cirrhosis in which the liver may be initially quite enlarged.

571.0 Alcoholic fatty liver

571.1 Acute alcoholic hepatitis — *severe inflammation of the liver due to alcoholic liver disease; Zieve's syndrome*
AHA: Q2, 2002, 4

571.2 Alcoholic cirrhosis of liver — *fibrosis and dysfunction of the liver due to alcoholic liver disease; Laennec's cirrhosis*
AHA: Nov-Dec, 1985, 14; Q1, 2002, 3; Q2, 2002, 4

571.3 Unspecified alcoholic liver damage

571.40 Unspecified chronic hepatitis

571.41 Chronic persistent hepatitis

571.49 Other chronic hepatitis — *not otherwise specified, Bearn-Kunkel-Slater syndrome, Wadenstrom's hepatitis*
AHA: Nov-Dec, 1985, 14; Q3, 1999, 19

571.5 Cirrhosis of liver without mention of alcohol — *fibrosis and dysfunction of the liver not due to alcohol consumption; cryptogenic, macronodular, micronodular; posthepatic, postnecrotic; Cruveilhier-Baumgarten cirrhosis*

571.6 Biliary cirrhosis — *fibrosis and dysfunction of the liver due to obstruction or infection of bile ducts; cholangitic, cholestatic*

571.8 Other chronic nonalcoholic liver disease — *not otherwise specified, fatty liver without alcohol, hardening liver, chronic yellow atrophy*
AHA: Q2, 1996, 12

571.9 Unspecified chronic liver disease without mention of alcohol — *unknown disease of liver*

572 Liver abscess and sequelae of chronic liver disease

Hepatic coma (572.2) is characterized by slow or rapid onset of bizarre behavior, disorientation, flapping tremors of extended arms, hyperactive reflexes, and later lethargy and coma. It seems to be caused by intoxication with ammonia, a product of protein digestion that the diseased liver fails to convert into urea. Hepatic encephalopathy is a complication of advanced liver disease probably caused by cerebral toxins, including ammonia, certain amines, and fatty acids. The symptoms are similar to those of a hepatic coma.

Hepatorenal syndrome (572.4) is combined liver and kidney failure that is usually caused by serious injury to the liver associated with hemorrhage, shock, and acute renal insufficiency. Hepatic necrosis is the destruction of functional liver tissue and can lead to the clinical syndrome hepatic failure, which may be induced by hepatotoxic drugs and may lead to progressive encephalopathy and death.

572.0 Abscess of liver — *pocket of pus*

572.1 Portal pyemia — *inflammation of portal vein or its branches; phlebitis, thrombophlebitis, pylephlebitis*

520–579

© 2004 Ingenix, Inc.

572.2 Hepatic coma — *portal-systemic encephalopathy*
AHA: Q3, 1995, 14; Q1, 2002, 3

572.3 Portal hypertension — *abnormally high blood pressure in the portal vein*

572.4 Hepatorenal syndrome — *kidney failure associated with liver disease; Heyd's syndrome*
AHA: Q3, 1993, 15

572.8 Other sequelae of chronic liver disease — *not elsewhere specified, adhesion, granuloma*

Coding Clarification

Excluded from this rubric is amebic liver abscess (006.3) and hepatorenal syndrome following delivery (674.8x).

573 Other disorders of liver

Code first underlying disease as appropriate.

573.0 Chronic passive congestion of liver — *persistent accumulation of escaped blood in liver tissue*

573.1 Hepatitis in viral diseases classified elsewhere — (Code first underlying disease: 074.8, 075, 078.5) — *secondary to underlying disease*

573.2 Hepatitis in other infectious diseases classified elsewhere — (Code first underlying disease, 084.9) — *secondary to underlying disease*

573.3 Unspecified hepatitis — (Use additional E code to identify cause)

573.4 Hepatic infarction — *area of dead liver tissue due to an interruption in circulation in that area*

573.8 Other specified disorders of liver — *hepatoptosis, hypertrophy, hemorrhage, obstruction, induration, lesion, prolapse, nontraumatic rupture*

573.9 Unspecified disorder of liver — *distention, palpable or torpid liver*

Coding Clarification

Excluded from this rubric are amyloid or lardaceous degeneration of liver (277.3), congenital cystic liver disease (751.62), glycogen infiltration of liver (271.0), hepatomegaly not otherwise specified (789.1), and portal vein obstruction (452).

574 Cholelithiasis

Use this rubric to report the presence or formation of concretions (calculi or "gallstones") in the gallbladder. The concretions contain cholesterol, calcium carbonate, or calcium bilirubinate either in pure forms or in various combinations. Many factors contribute to concretion formation, but they generally can be grouped into three categories: abnormal composition of bile, abnormal contractility of the gallbladder, and abnormal epithelial secretions. The disease is rare in children, and the rate of incidence is greater in people of native american ancestry and in women.

Choledocholithiasis is the presence or formation of concretions in any of the bile ducts. Common duct stones usually originate in the gallbladder, but may form spontaneously in the common duct following cholecystectomy. Features, in addition to those of cholecystitis, that suggest choledocholithiasis include Charcot's triad and cholangitis. Charcot's triad is a symptom complex consisting of frequently recurring attacks of severe, persistent, right upper quadrant pain lasting for hours; chills and fever associated with severe colic; and a history of jaundice chronologically associated with abdominal pain. Secondary pancreatitis, biliary cirrhosis, and hypoprothrombinemia may complicate choledocholithiasis.

Signs and symptoms of cholelithiasis include cramps or severe epigastric pain, nausea and vomiting, heartburn, eructation, flatulence, sensation of dullness in stomach, jaundice, distention of gallbladder, and pain on palpation of gallbladder. It is asymptomatic in many patients. X-rays of abdomen may show cholelithiasis, but most concretions are made up of cholesterol, which is radiolucent and cannot be visualized. Gallbladder ultrasound, HIDA scanning (a form of radionuclide excretion scan involving the intravenous injection of iminodiacetic acid), and oral cholecystography confirm the diagnosis. Lab work reveals cholesterol crystal formation in bile and granules of calcium bilirubinate in duodenal aspirate with acute cholecystitis. Lab work may reveal increased white blood cell count and serum bilirubin.

Therapies include administration of chenodeoxycholic acid for one to two years to dissolve concretions in asymptomatic patients; in asymptomatic diabetic patients, cholecystectomy is performed to avoid serious future complications. For acute cholecystitis, cholecystectomy (by open incision, laparoscopy, or endoscopically) is performed at the time of the acute cholecystitis, or electively four to six weeks after recovery in uncomplicated cases. A cholangiogram detects concretions blocking the common bile duct. If concretions are found, there is common bile duct exploration or insertion of T-tube with infusion of mono-octanoin to dissolve the stones.

Associated conditions include acute cholecystitis (including its major complications of empyema, perforations, pericholecystic abscess, bile peritonitis, and cholecystenteric fistulas), chronic cholecystitis, biliary adhesions, secondary pancreatitis, postcholecystectomy syndrome, Crohn's disease, liver damage, and obesity.

The following fifth-digit subclassification is for use with category 574:

0 without mention of obstruction

1 with obstruction

574.0 ✔5th Calculus of gallbladder with acute cholecystitis — *severe inflammation due to gallstone(s); cholelithiasis*
AHA: Q4, 1996, 32

574.1 ✔5th Calculus of gallbladder with other cholecystitis — *inflammation, persistent or unspecified, due to gallstone(s); cholelithiasis*
AHA: Q2, 1996, 13; Q4, 1996, 32,69; Q3, 1999, 9

574.2 ✔5th Calculus of gallbladder without mention of cholecystitis — *presence of gallstone(s) without inflammation*

574.3 ✔5th Calculus of bile duct with acute cholecystitis — *severe inflammation of gallbladder due to stone(s) in bile duct*

574.4 ✔5th Calculus of bile duct with other cholecystitis — *inflammation, persistent and unspecified, of gallbladder due to stone(s) in bile duct*

574.5 ✔5th Calculus of bile duct without mention of cholecystitis — *presence of bile duct stone(s) without inflammation of gallbladder*
AHA: Q3, 1994, 11

574.6 ✔5th Calculus of gallbladder and bile duct with acute cholecystitis — *presence of bile duct and gallbladder stones with severe inflammation*
AHA: Q4, 1996, 32

574.7 ✔5th Calculus of gallbladder and bile duct with other cholecystitis — *presence of bile duct and gallbladders stones, inflammation persistent and unspecified*
AHA: Q4, 1996, 32

574.8 ✔5th Calculus of gallbladder and bile duct with acute and chronic cholecystitis

574.9 ✔5th Calculus of gallbladder and bile duct without cholecystitis — *stones of gallbladder and bile duct without inflammation*
AHA: Q4, 1996, 32

575 *Other disorders of gallbladder*

Excluded from this rubric are cholelithiasis (rubric 574) and Hartmann's pouch of intestine (V44.3).

Acute cholecystitis is acute inflammation of the gallbladder without mention of cholelithiasis (calculi or "gallstones" of the gallbladder or bile ducts). This condition may be caused by obstruction of the cystic duct by another process (such as a malignant tumor), bile stasis ("sludge" formation, which is a precipitant of calcium bilirubinate calculi formation), or infection due to organisms such as *Escherichia coli, E. clostridia,* or *Salmonella typhi.*

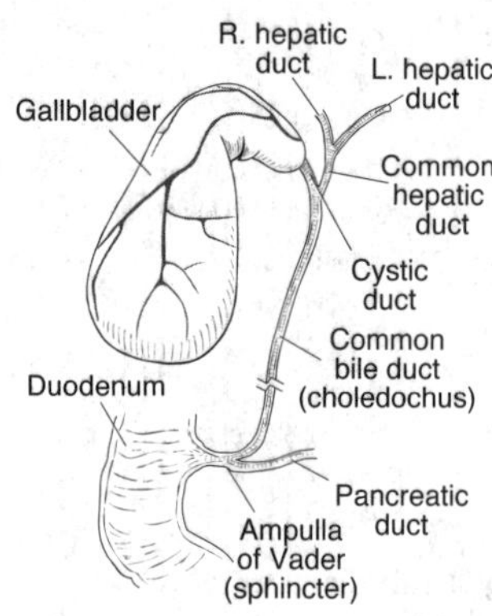

About 95 percent of acute cholecystitis is due to obstruction of the cystic duct by a gallstone impacted in Hartmann's pouch and classified to category 574.

Use subclassification 575.1 to report cholecystitis not otherwise specified and chronic cholecystitis without mention of cholelithiasis (calculi or "gallstones" of the gallbladder or bile ducts). Chronic cholecystitis rarely occurs in the absence of lithiasis but can occur in conditions such as cholesterolosis and adenomatous hyperplasia.

575.0 Acute cholecystitis — *severe inflammation gallbladder, no stones*
AHA: Q3, 1991, 17

575.10 Cholecystitis, unspecified — *inflammation of gallbladder of unknown type, no stones*
AHA: Q4, 1996, 32

575.11 Chronic cholecystitis — *persistent inflammation of gallbladder, no stones*
AHA: Q4, 1996, 32

575.12 Acute and chronic cholecystitis — *occlusion, stenosis, stricture, without stones*
AHA: Q4, 1996, 32; Q4, 1997, 52

575.2 Obstruction of gallbladder — *occlusion, stenosis, and stricture of cystic duct or gallbladder without mention of calculus*

575.3 Hydrops of gallbladder — *abnormal collection of fluid, gallbladder*
AHA: Q2, 1989, 13

575.4 Perforation of gallbladder — *hole in gallbladder wall*

575.5 Fistula of gallbladder — *abnormal communication between gallbladder and other tissue*

575.6 Cholesterolosis of gallbladder — *abnormal deposits of cholesterol in tissue of gallbladder*
AHA: Q4, 1990, 17

520–579

© 2004 Ingenix, Inc.

575.8 Other specified disorder of gallbladder — *adhesions, atrophy, cyst, hypertrophy, ulcer, calcification, infarct, sepsis, torsion, Hartmann's pouch, Rokitansky-Aschoff sinuses*
AHA: Q2, 1989, 13; Q4, 1990, 26

575.9 Unspecified disorder of gallbladder — *pain in gallbladder for unknown cause*

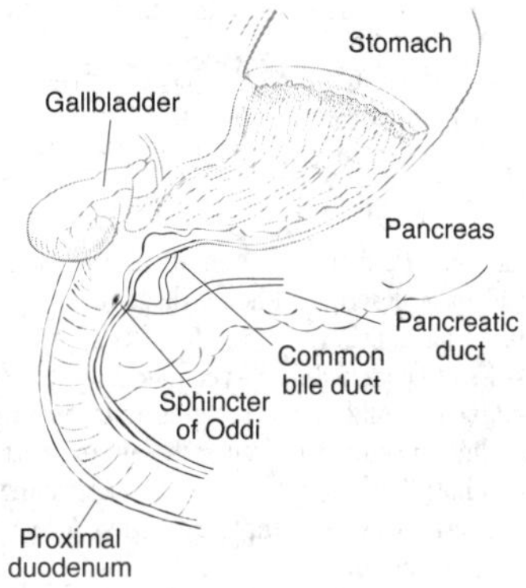

Location of the biliary tract

576 Other disorders of biliary tract

576.0 Postcholecystectomy syndrome — *jaundice or abnormal pain following cholecystectomy*
AHA: Q1, 1988, 10

576.1 Cholangitis — *inflammation of bile duct; recurrent, secondary, chronic, primary, acute, suppurative, sclerosing*
AHA: Q2, 1999, 13

576.2 Obstruction of bile duct — *occlusion, stenosis, stricture; Mirizzi's syndrome*
AHA: Q2, 1999, 13; Q1, 2001, 8; Q3, 2003, 17-18

576.3 Perforation of bile duct — *hole in the wall of bile duct*

576.4 Fistula of bile duct — *abnormal communication between bile duct and other tissue*

576.5 Spasm of sphincter of Oddi — *abnormal contraction in muscle of the threshold between bile duct and duodenum*

576.8 Other specified disorders of biliary tract — *adhesions, atrophy, cyst, hypertrophy, stasis, ulcer, cicatrix, obliteration, torsion of bile duct; abscess or inflammation of hepatic duct*
AHA: Q2, 1999, 14; Q3, 2003, 17

576.9 Unspecified disorder of biliary tract

Coding Clarification

Excluded from this rubric are disorders of the biliary tract involving the cystic duct or gallbladder (575.0-575.9).

577 Diseases of pancreas

Signs and symptoms of diseases of the pancreas include abdominal pain, weakness, dizziness, somnolence, grossly bloody or "coffee ground" vomitus, grossly bloody or black and tarry stools, and a history of bleeding diathesis. Other signs and symptoms include chronic conditions such as diverticulosis, fall in blood pressure of more than 10 mm Hg or rise in pulse rate of more than 20 beats per minute between supine and standing positions, altered level of consciousness, pallor, diaphoresis, and peripheral vasoconstriction.

577.0 Acute pancreatitis — *severe inflammation; necrotic, acute, hemorrhagic, subacute, suppurative, infective; including Fitz's syndrome*
AHA: Q2, 1989, 9; Q2, 1996, 13; Q2, 1998, 19; Q3, 1999, 9

577.1 Chronic pancreatitis — *persistent inflammation; infectious, interstitial, painless, recurrent, relapsing*
AHA: Q3, 1994, 11; Q2, 1996, 13; Q1, 2001, 8

577.2 Cyst and pseudocyst of pancreas

577.8 Other specified disease of pancreas — *atrophy, calculus, cirrhosis, fibrosis, necrosis, fistula, hyperfunction, insufficiency, sclerosis, nontraumatic rupture, duct obstruction; Hadfield-Clarke or Burke's syndrome*
AHA: Q1, 2001, 8

577.9 Unspecified disease of pancreas

Coding Clarification

Excluded from this rubric are mumps pancreatitis (072.3), islet cell tumor of pancreas (211.7), and pancreatic steatorrhea (579.4).

578 Gastrointestinal hemorrhage

AHA: Q4, 1990, 20; Q2, 1992, 9

Use this rubric to report bleeding of the stomach, ileum, jejunum, duodenum, and/or colon. The condition may be described as acute or chronic and involve a grossly bloody (visible) appearance or be detected by laboratory examination only (occult bleeding). GI bleeding is classified as either hematemesis (vomiting of blood), blood in stool which includes melena (partially digested blood showing as dark tarry stools) and hematochezia (passage of red blood in stools), and GI bleeding not specified as hematemesis or blood in stool.

Diagnostic tests may include a CBC to reveal normal hematocrit and hemoglobin for the first six hours of acute bleeding (the body can compensate for acute blood loss by vasoconstriction, delaying the intravascular fluids from entering the bloodstream). A peripheral blood smear in an acute hemorrhage longer than six hours often demonstrates normochromic and normocytic blood loss anemia. In chronic GI hemorrhage (acute exacerbation of chronic GI hemorrhage), a peripheral blood smear is characteristic of chronic blood loss showing microcytic, hypochromic anemia with marked increase in reticulocyte count. Abnormal BUN and creatinine levels suggest bleeding in the upper GI tract, and elevated liver enzymes indicate hypoperfusion of the liver following a bleeding episode. Nasogastric aspiration may be performed to confirm an upper GI bleed and an upper or lower endoscopy identifies the exact site and pathology of the bleeding. Upper GI series or barium enema locates the site when bleeding is inactive at the time of the test and a nuclear bleeding scan, such as technetium-labeled red cell scan and technetium sulfur-colloid scan, locates the site in the lower GI tract when bleeding is minimal. An angiography may be performed for both upper and lower GI bleeding and is often performed in anticipation of surgery.

Therapies include gastric lavage for upper GI bleeding confined to the stomach and medical management for lower GI bleeding unless the bleeding becomes life threatening. Therapeutic angiography using selective intra-arterial vasopressin or selective embolization of a bleeding vessel to control GI hemorrhage is also used. Use of an endoscopic laser or a heat probe induces coagulation, while surgery is directed at the etiology when bleeding is severe (e.g., gastrectomy and Billroth I reconstruction for GI bleeding due to perforated gastric ulcer or hemicolectomy for extensive diverticulosis of the colon).

Associated conditions include acute and/or chronic blood loss anemia, dehydration, gastritis, diverticulitis, neoplasms, arteriovenous malformations, chronic renal failure, diabetes mellitus, chronic obstructive lung disease, colitis, bleeding diathesis, chronic liver disease, Osler-Weber-Rendu syndrome, and valvular heart disease.

This category excludes bleeding of the anus and rectum for classification purposes. The terms "upper" and "lower" have no value as modifiers for classification of GI bleeding. GI bleeding must be assigned to code 578.9 *Hemorrhage of gastrointestinal tract, unspecified* when not further defined as hematemesis or blood in stool. Since upper GI bleeding may present not only as hematemesis but also as melena and even hematochezia in some cases, the codes are distinguished by the presentation of the GI bleeding, not the site.

Use subclassification 578.0 to report vomiting of frank red or partially digested blood. Hematemesis usually is indicative of bleeding of the upper gastrointestinal tract. Occult bleeding can be detected by analysis of vomitus or nasogastric tube aspiration. Gastric and gastroduodenal ulcers, gastritis, arteriovenous malformations, and neoplasms are the most common etiologies for hematemesis.

Certain conditions such as epistaxis may cause the patient to swallow and then vomit blood. Such vomiting of swallowed blood sometimes masquerades as hematemesis due to gastrointestinal hemorrhage.

Use subclassification 578.1 to report passage of frank red or partially digested blood in the stools which may be due to a condition in the upper or lower GI tract.

The general term "rectal bleeding" is used by clinicians to describe GI hemorrhage (classified here) or bleeding from sites within the rectum or anus classified to code 569.3. If the etiology of the rectal bleeding is a condition of the gastrointestinal tract excluding the anus and rectum, assign this code. Occult bleeding may be detected by performing a guaiac test on a stool sample. A positive guaiac test without further documentation of GI bleeding is classified to code 792.1 *Nonspecific abnormal findings in stool contents.*

578.0 Hematemesis — *vomiting blood*
AHA: Q4, 1990, 20; Q2, 1992, 9; Q2, 2002, 4

578.1 Blood in stool — *melena*
AHA: Q4, 1990, 20; Q2, 1992, 8; Q2, 1992, 9

578.9 Unspecified, hemorrhage of gastrointestinal tract — *not otherwise specified*
AHA: Nov-Dec, 1986, 9; Q4, 1990, 20; Q2, 1992, 9

Coding Clarification

Excluded from this rubric are gastrointestinal hemorrhage with angiodysplasia of stomach and duodenum (537.83), angiodysplasia of intestine (537.85), diverticulitis and diverticulosis (rubric 562), gastritis and duodenitis (535.0-535.6), and duodenal, gastric, gastrojejunal, or peptic ulcer (531.00-534.91).

579 Intestinal malabsorption

The mucosal layer of the intestine is crucial for the body to prevent bacteria, antigens, and undigested food from seeping through the gastrointestinal barrier and into the systemic circulation. Intestinal malabsorption (e.g., the inadequate absorption of nutrients from the small intestine) of the mucosal layer can result in weight loss and abnormal appearing stools. An increasingly permeable mucosal layer can result in a chronically overreactive immune system that can lead to inflammatory bowel disease (IBD) and its progression. Factors affecting permeability include lesions of the small intestine, amyloidosis, the lack of digestive enzymes (e.g., lactose intolerance), and surgical operations. Blockage

 © 2004 Ingenix, Inc.

of the intestinal lymphatic vessels, which are important in fat absorption, also may lead to malabsorption. A comprehensive digestive stool analysis can be performed in the diagnosis of malabsorption since the test evaluates a stool sample for digestion, absorption, intestinal function, and microbial flora. A small intestine biopsy is necessary for the diagnosis of many diseases of the intestinal mucosa such as celiac sprue, abetalipoproteinemia, and Whipple's disease. Certain diseases such as Crohn's have a patchy distribution and may yield a normal biopsy if normal mucosa is sampled.

Celiac disease (also called coeliac, nontropical sprue, celiac sprue, gluten intolerant enteropathy, or gluten sensitive enteropathy) is a condition in which there is a chronic reaction to certain proteins, commonly referred to as glutens, found in some cereal grains. This reaction destroys the villi in the small intestine, with resulting malabsorption of nutrients.

The disease affects both sexes and it can begin at any age, from infancy (as soon as cereal grains are introduced) to later life (even though the individual has consumed cereal grains all along). The onset of the disease seems to require genetic predisposition and some kind of trigger, such as overexposure to wheat, a pregnancy, an operation, or a viral infection.

579.0 Celiac disease — *crisis, rickets, gluten enteropathy, nontropical spur*

579.1 Tropical sprue — *diarrhea associated with enteric infection and nutritional deficiency*

579.2 Blind loop syndrome

579.3 Other and unspecified postsurgical nonabsorption

579.4 Pancreatic steatorrhea — *passage of large amounts of fat in the feces due to absence of pancreatic juice from intestine*

579.8 Other specified intestinal malabsorption

579.9 Unspecified intestinal malabsorption

580–629
Diseases of the Genitourinary System

This chapter classifies diseases and disorders of the kidney, ureter, bladder, urethra, prostate, male genital organs, female and male breast, and female genital organs.

Coding Clarification

Excluded from this chapter is hypertensive renal disease, found in rubric 403. Signs and symptoms of genitourinary system disorders that may describe the emerging nature of the patient's condition are found in rubric 788, which includes codes specific to incontinence of urine, painful or frequent urination, and kidney pain. Also, some genitourinary diseases are familial linked. Family history can be found in rubrics V16-V19.

580–589 Nephritis, Nephrotic Syndrome, and Nephrosis

The kidneys are behind the parietal peritoneum at the back of the abdominal cavity. They are located on either side of the vertebral column from the level of the 12th thoracic vertebra to the 3rd lumbar vertebra. The left kidney is often slightly larger than the right, and usually slightly higher in position, presumably because of the space taken by the liver. The kidneys are encased in heavy cushions of fat, which, with the renal fasciae connective tissue, anchors them in place. The average kidney is about 11.0 centimeters by 7.0 centimeters by 3.0 centimeters and roughly oval with a medial indentation (bean-shaped). The concave notch at this indentation is called the hilum, and is where structures enter and leave the kidney. Tough, white, fibrous connective tissue encapsulates each kidney.

The outer region of the kidney is the cortex. The medulla is the inner region, consisting of about a dozen distinct triangular wedges of tissue called the renal pyramids. The papilla (points) of the pyramids face inward and jut into cuplike structures, called calyces, where urine is collected for transport via the renal pelvis out of the kidney and into the ureter. The functional units of the kidney are the nephrons. Nephrons are microscopic units that process blood and form urine by filtration, reabsorption, and secretion. There are more than one million nephrons in each kidney, which make up the bulk of the organ's tissue.

580 Acute glomerulonephritis

Acute glomerulonephritis is acute inflammation in the glomeruli of the kidneys. Also known as acute hemorrhagic glomerulonephritis and acute nephritis, this condition frequently is a late complication of pharyngitis or skin infection.

Signs and symptoms of acute glomerulonephritis include a history of infection usually streptococcal, a history of concurrent systemic vasculitis or hypersensitivity reaction, malaise, headache, anorexia, low-grade fever, mild generalized edema, and retinal hemorrhages.

In acute glomerulonephritis, urinalysis reveals hematuria (may be microscopic or grossly bloody or coffee colored) and urine sediment containing protein, hyaline and granular casts in large numbers, and erythrocyte casts. Blood work reveals elevated BUN and creatinine, rapid sedimentation rate, and mild normochromic anemia. Therapies include antibiotics to eradicate the underlying infection (e.g., streptococcal pharyngitis), symptomatic treatment to prevent overhydration and hypertension, and dietary restriction of protein and sodium. Associated conditions include hypertension, hypertensive encephalopathy, congestive heart failure, infection (e.g., streptococcal pharyngitis, skin cellulitis), and retinal hemorrhage.

When acute glomerulonephritis does not heal within one to two years, or when it progresses to chronic renal failure or chronic renal insufficiency, it is designated as chronic glomerulonephritis.

Acute glomerulonephritis with lesion of proliferative glomerulonephritis is characterized by hypercellularity of the glomeruli. The condition is due to proliferation of endothelial and/or mesangial cells and infiltration of the tissues with neutrophils and monocytes.

Acute glomerulonephritis with lesion of rapidly progressive glomerulonephritis is acute glomerulonephritis with lesion characterized by rapid deterioration of kidney function, usually a few weeks to two months. Most patients who survive this condition, which is also known as acute crescentic glomerulonephritis, develop chronic renal failure within two years.

580.0 Acute glomerulonephritis with lesion of proliferative glomerulonephritis — *acute nephritis*

580.4 Acute glomerulonephritis with lesion of rapidly progressive glomerulonephritis — *acute nephritis with lesion of necrotizing glomerulitis*

580.81 Acute glomerulonephritis with other specified pathological lesion in kidney in disease classified elsewhere — (Code first underlying disease: 002.0, 070.0-070.9, 072.79, 421.0)

580.89 Other acute glomerulonephritis with other specified pathological lesion in kidney — *acute glomerulonephritis with lesion of exudative nephritis*

580.9 Acute glomerulonephritis with unspecified pathological lesion in kidney — *hemorrhagic glomerulonephritis specified as acute*

Coding Clarification

It is rare that a patient would be assigned codes from both categories 580 and 582 during the same episode of care. Acute exacerbation of chronic glomerulonephritis is classified to chronic glomerulonephritis (582) alone when the exacerbation refers to a progressive deterioration or worsening of symptoms of chronic glomerulonephritis. When the cause of the exacerbation is known, such as an intercurrent infection (e.g., streptococcal septicemia, 038.0), report the infection along with a code from category 582.

581 Nephrotic syndrome

Nephrotic syndrome is a condition characterized by proteinuria more than 3.5 g/100 ml, hypoalbuminemia less than 3 g/100 ml, hyperlipemia (cholesterol greater than 300 mg/100 ml), and massive edema. Usually due to some form of glomerulonephritis, nephrotic syndrome may result in chronic renal failure.

Nephrotic syndrome with lesion of proliferative glomerulonephritis is nephrotic syndrome with lesion characterized by hypercellularity of the glomeruli. The condition is due to proliferating endothelial and/or mesangial cells, and infiltration of the tissues with neutrophils and monocytes as a result of acute or membranoproliferative glomerulonephritis.

Nephrotic syndrome with lesion of membranous glomerulonephritis is nephrotic syndrome with lesion characterized by insidious onset of proteinuria. It is the result of protein deposits and diffuse thickening of the capillary basement membrane of the glomeruli.

Nephrotic syndrome with lesion of membranoproliferative glomerulonephritis is nephrotic syndrome with lesion characterized by infiltration of inflammatory cells, proliferating intrinsic glomerular cells, and altered structure and function of the basement membrane of the glomeruli.

581.0 Nephrotic syndrome with lesion of proliferative glomerulonephritis

581.1 Nephrotic syndrome with lesion of membranous glomerulonephritis — *epimembranous nephritis; idiopathic membranous glomerular disease*

581.2 Nephrotic syndrome with lesion of membranoproliferative glomerulonephritis — *nephrotic syndrome with lesion of lobular glomerulonephritis; nephrotic syndrome with lesion of mesangiocapillary glomerulonephritis*

581.3 Nephrotic syndrome with lesion of minimal change glomerulonephritis — *foot process disease; lipoid necrosis; minimal change nephrotic syndrome*

581.81 Nephrotic syndrome with other specified pathological lesion in kidney in diseases classified elsewhere — (Code first underlying disease: 084.9, 250.4, 277.3, 446.0, 710.0)

581.89 Other nephrotic syndrome with specified pathological lesion in kidney — *glomerulonephritis with edema and lesion of exudative nephritis*

581.9 Nephrotic syndrome with unspecified pathological lesion in kidney — *nephritis, nephrotic NOS; nephritis with edema NOS*

582 Chronic glomerulonephritis

Chronic glomerulonephritis is a slowly progressing disease (up to 30 years in some cases) characterized by chronic inflammation of the glomeruli, which results in sclerosis, scarring, and eventual chronic renal failure. Etiologies for chronic glomerulonephritis include primary renal disorders (classified to categories 580 and 581) and systemic diseases such as Goodpasture's syndrome, systemic lupus erythematosus, amyloidosis, and hemolytic-uremic syndrome.

Signs and symptoms of chronic glomerulonephritis include azotemia, nausea, vomiting, fatigue, malaise, pruritus, dyspnea, hematuria, and hypertension. An urinalysis reveals hematuria (may be microscopic or grossly bloody or coffee colored) and urine sediment containing protein, cylindruria (granular tube casts), and erythrocyte casts. Blood work reveals elevated BUN and creatinine, rapid sedimentation rate, and mild normochromic anemia. X-ray or renal ultrasound shows bilateral smaller kidneys and a renal biopsy identifies the underlying disease.

Therapies include antibiotics to treat any intercurrent infections, drugs such as diuretics to control hypertension, IV hydration, and fluid restriction or diuresis to correct fluid and electrolyte imbalances.

 © 2004 Ingenix, Inc.

There are dietary restrictions of sodium and protein and renal dialysis or renal transplant for patients with ESRD (end stage renal disease or chronic renal failure).

Associated conditions include congestive heart failure, and fluid, electrolyte, and acid-base imbalances. There may be hypertension, hypertensive encephalopathy, intercurrent infection, and underlying disease (e.g., systemic lupus erythematosus).

Chronic glomerulonephritis with lesion of proliferative glomerulonephritis is chronic glomerulonephritis with lesion characterized by hypercellularity of the glomeruli due to proliferation of endothelial and/or mesangial cells and infiltration of the tissues with neutrophils and monocytes as a result of repeated attacks of acute inflammation.

Chronic glomerulonephritis with lesion of membranous glomerulonephritis is chronic glomerulonephritis with lesion characterized by the insidious onset of proteinuria. It is the result of protein deposits and diffuse thickening of the capillary basement membrane of the glomeruli.

Chronic glomerulonephritis with lesion of membranoproliferative glomerulonephritis is chronic glomerulonephritis with lesion characterized by infiltration of inflammatory cells, proliferation of intrinsic glomerular cells, and altered structure and function of the basement membrane of the glomeruli.

Chronic glomerulonephritis with lesion of rapidly progressive glomerulonephritis is chronic glomerulonephritis with lesion characterized by rapid deterioration of kidney function, usually a few weeks to two months. Most patients with this condition, also known as chronic crescentic glomerulonephritis, develop chronic renal failure within one to two years.

582.0 Chronic glomerulonephritis with lesion of proliferative glomerulonephritis — *chronic (diffuse) proliferative glomerulonephritis*

582.1 Chronic glomerulonephritis with lesion of membranous glomerulonephritis — *focal glomerulonephritis; segmental hyalinosis*
AHA: Sept-Oct, 1984, 16

582.2 Chronic glomerulonephritis with lesion of membranoproliferative glomerulonephritis — *chronic endothelial glomerulonephritis; chronic mesangiocapillary glomerulonephritis*

582.4 Chronic glomerulonephritis with lesion of rapidly progressive glomerulonephritis — *chronic nephritis with lesion of necrotizing glomerulitis*

582.81 Chronic glomerulonephritis with other specified pathological lesion in kidney in diseases classified elsewhere

582.89 Other chronic glomerulonephritis with specified pathological lesion in kidney — *chronic glomerulonephritis with lesion of exudative nephritis*

582.9 Chronic glomerulonephritis with unspecified pathological lesion in kidney — *chronic hemorrhagic glomerulonephritis; small white kidney*
AHA: Q2, 2001, 12

Coding Clarification

Refer to the ICD-9-CM index under "Glomerulonephritis, due to or associated with" for a list of underlying (etiologic) conditions that can cause glomerulonephritis. The index refers you to codes in categories 580-583 in slanted brackets, indicating a manifestation code. Modify these suggested manifestation codes according to the amount of specificity in the physician's diagnostic statement. For example, for glomerulonephritis due to or associated with tuberculosis, the ICD-9-CM index lists codes 016.0x to classify the underlying disease of tuberculosis (add the appropriate fifth digit) and 583.81 for the manifestation of glomerulonephritis not specified as acute or chronic in diseases classified elsewhere. If the diagnostic statement specifies that the patient has chronic glomerulonephritis due to tuberculosis, the proper codes would be 016.0x and 582.81 for chronic glomerulonephritis in diseases classified elsewhere.

583 Nephritis and nephropathy, not specified as acute or chronic

Nephritis and nephropathy, not specific as acute or chronic, with lesion of proliferative glomerulonephritis are diseases with lesion characterized by hypercellularity of the glomeruli due to proliferating endothelial and/or mesangial cells, and infiltration of the tissues with neutrophils and monocytes as a result of acute inflammation.

Nephritis and nephropathy, not specified as acute or chronic, with lesion of membranous glomerulonephritis are diseases with lesion characterized by the insidious onset of proteinuria and unspecified nephritis or nephropathy. They are the result of protein deposits and diffuse thickening of the capillary basement membrane of the glomeruli.

Nephritis and nephropathy, not specified as acute or chronic, with lesion of membranoproliferative glomerulonephritis are diseases with lesion characterized by infiltration of inflammatory cells, proliferation of intrinsic glomerular cells, and alteration of the structure and function of the basement membrane of the glomeruli.

Nephritis and nephropathy, not specified as acute or chronic, with lesion of rapidly progressive glomerulonephritis are severe forms of glomerulonephritis with lesion characterized by rapid deterioration of kidney function, usually a few weeks to two months. Most patients with these diseases, also known as crescentic glomerulonephritis, develop chronic renal failure within one to two years.

583.0 Nephritis and nephropathy, not specified as acute or chronic, with lesion of proliferative glomerulonephritis — *proliferative nephritis NOS; proliferative nephropathy NOS*

583.1 Nephritis and nephropathy, not specified as acute or chronic, with lesion of membranous glomerulonephritis — *membranous glomerulonephritis NOS; membranous nephropathy NOS*

583.2 Nephritis and nephropathy, not specified as acute or chronic, with lesion of membranoproliferative glomerulonephritis — *membranoproliferative nephropathy NOS; nephritis NOS, with lesion of hypocomplementemic, lobular, or mesangiocapillary glomerulonephritis*

583.4 Nephritis and nephropathy, not specified as acute or chronic, with lesion of rapidly progressive glomerulonephritis — *necrotizing or rapidly progressive nephritis NOS; nephritis, unspecified, with lesion of necrotizing glomerulitis*

583.6 Nephritis and nephropathy, not specified as acute or chronic, with lesion of renal cortical necrosis — *nephritis NOS; renal cortical necrosis NOS*

583.7 Nephritis and nephropathy, not specified as acute or chronic, with lesion of renal medullary necrosis — *nephritis NOS with (renal) medullary [papillary] necrosis*

583.81 Nephritis and nephropathy, not specified as acute or chronic, with other specified pathological lesion in kidney, in diseases classified elsewhere

583.89 Other nephritis and nephropathy, not specified as acute or chronic, with specified pathological lesion in kidney — *glomerulitis with lesion of exudative nephritis; renal disease with lesion of interstitial nephritis*

583.9 Nephritis and nephropathy, not specified as acute or chronic, with unspecified pathological lesion in kidney — *glomerulitis NOS; nephritis NOS*

Coding Clarification

Refer to the ICD-9-CM index under "Glomerulonephritis, due to or associated with" for a list of underlying (etiologic) conditions that can cause glomerulonephritis. Note that the index will refer you to codes in categories 580-583 in slanted brackets, indicating a manifestation code. Modify these suggested manifestation codes according to the amount of specificity in the physician's diagnostic statement. For example, for glomerulonephritis due to or associated with tuberculosis, the ICD-9-CM index lists codes 016.0x to classify the underlying disease of tuberculosis (add the appropriate fifth digit) and 583.81 for the manifestation of glomerulonephritis not specified as acute or chronic in diseases classified elsewhere. If the diagnostic statement specifies that the patient has chronic glomerulonephritis due to tuberculosis, the proper codes would be 016.0x and 582.81 for chronic glomerulonephritis in diseases classified elsewhere.

Coding Scenario

The patient is admitted for hemodialysis. The patient is a Type I diabetic with progressive nephropathy. The physician also documents chronic renal failure in the medical history.

> Code assignment: 250.41 *Diabetes with renal manifestations*, 583.81 *Nephritis and nephropathy, not specified as acute or chronic, in diseases classified elsewhere*, and 585 *Chronic renal failure*

584 Acute renal failure

AHA: Q2, 1992, 5; Q4, 1992, 22; Q1, 1993, 18

Acute renal failure is sudden interruption of renal function following any one of a variety of conditions that insult the normal kidney. Although usually reversible with treatment, acute renal failure may progress to chronic renal insufficiency and chronic renal failure or death. Recovery from acute renal failure is marked by a conversion from an oliguric phase to a diuretic phase within a few days to six weeks.

The causes of acute renal failure are classified to prerenal, intrinsic (renal), or postrenal. Prerenal failure is due to diminished blood flow to the kidneys caused by conditions such as dehydration, shock, embolism, cardiac failure, hepatic failure, or sepsis. Intrinsic failure results from diseases and disorders of the kidneys. Acute tubular necrosis is the most common cause of renal failure, and results from conditions such as systemic lupus erythematosus, sickle cell disease, nephrotoxins, renal ischemia, acute pyelonephritis, and acute poststreptococcal glomerulonephritis. Postrenal failure is caused by bilateral obstruction of urinary outflow, as seen with ureteral calculi, blood clots, neoplasms, benign prostatic hypertrophy, and urethral strictures.

Signs and symptoms of acute renal failure include, in early stages, oliguria, sometimes anuria, azotemia, hypotension, electrolyte imbalances, fever and chills (indicating infection), anorexia, nausea, vomiting, diarrhea or constipation, uremic breath, headache, mental changes, pruritus, pallor, purpura, fluid overload, edema, and Kussmaul respirations. Blood work shows elevated BUN, serum creatinine, and potassium, decreased serum calcium, arterial pH, and bicarbonate. Urinalysis reveals urine specific gravity of approximately 1.010 (indicating isosthenuria) and sometimes protein and cellular debris. Radiology

580–629

 © 2004 Ingenix, Inc.

studies such as kidney ultrasound, intravenous pyelography, retrograde pyelography, and nephrotomography identify the pathology such as outflow obstruction or hydronephrosis. Therapies include dietary management and restriction of fluid intake with careful monitoring of electrolytes, and peritoneal dialysis or hemodialysis to control uremia.

584.5 Acute renal failure with lesion of tubular necrosis — *sudden onset of renal failure, compared to chronic, due to lower nephron necrosis; acute tubular necrosis*
AHA: Q2, 1992, 5; Q4, 1992, 22; Q1, 1993, 18

584.6 Acute renal failure with lesion of renal cortical necrosis — *severe decline in kidney function due to destruction of kidney filtering tissue, sudden onset*
AHA: Q2, 1992, 5; Q4, 1992, 22; Q1, 1993, 18

584.7 Acute renal failure with lesion of renal medullary (papillary) necrosis — *necrotizing renal papillitis*
AHA: Q2, 1992, 5; Q4, 1992, 22; Q1, 1993, 18

584.8 Acute renal failure with other specified pathological lesion in kidney — *acute renal failure with pathological lesion in kidney NEC*
AHA: Nov-Dec, 1985, 1; Q2, 1992, 5; Q4, 1992, 22; Q1, 1993, 18

584.9 Unspecified acute renal failure

Documentation Issues

Documentation in the record that may indicate the presence of renal failure could include:

- Markedly elevated values of serum creatinine or BUN, or diminished creatinine clearance.
- Clinical manifestations and laboratory findings of the degree of renal impairment primarily noted as the renal failure progresses. For example:
  - acidemia
  - anemia
  - hyperkalemia
  - hyperphosphatemia
  - hypocalcemia
  - renal osteodystrophy
  - uremic symptoms, (e.g., nausea, hemorrhagic conditions, vomiting, itching)

The above may be indicators of renal failure but confirmation and documentation from the physician must be obtained before assigning the code for renal failure.

If documentation identifies renal failure with hypertension, clarify with the physician as to whether the hypertension is malignant or accelerated. If the documentation identifies that the renal failure and hypertension are unrelated or the cause and effect relationship cannot be established, code each separately.

When the documentation identifies renal failure and diabetes but does not identify a cause and effect relationship, contact the physician for clarification. If the physician confirms that the renal failure is a manifestation of the diabetes, list the diabetes code first followed by the code identifying the specific type of renal failure.

When the physician documents azotemia, clarify whether or not the diagnosis of azotemia refers to the presence of acute renal failure or chronic renal failure. Unless acute or chronic renal failure is confirmed and documented by the physician, azotemia is reported with code 790.6 *Other abnormal blood chemistry.*

Coding Clarification

Excluded from this rubric are acute renal failure following labor and delivery (669.3x), posttraumatic (958.5), that complicating abortion (rubrics 634-638), or ectopic/molar pregnancy (639.3).

Diabetes Mellitus: Diabetes is one of a number of the ICD-9-CM classification categories that is used as a primary code to classify both the disease and its major manifestations. Additional codes should be used to provide more specificity in defining the manifestations. When a cause and effect relationship between the renal failure and the diabetes has been established, the diabetes code 250.4x is listed first with the appropriate renal failure code listed as an additional code. Accordingly, if the diagnosis does not indicate a cause and effect relationship between the diabetes and renal failure, the code for the renal failure may be listed first.

General Guidelines: Renal failure (category 584 *Acute renal failure,* 585 *Chronic renal failure,* and 586 *Renal failure, unspecified*) is the progression of renal insufficiency to the point at which renal function becomes further impaired and apparent clinical manifestations, such as anemia, develop. Renal insufficiency is more an abnormal laboratory assessment, while renal failure includes both the abnormal laboratory and the clinical findings.

Chronic renal failure is caused by a number of progressive diseases such as diabetes, primary hypertension, nephrosis, nephritis, obstructive uropathy, systemic lupus erythematosis (SLE), polycystic kidney disease, and other congenital disorders. In cases of chronic renal failure that becomes irreversible, the treatment may be either dialysis or transplantation.

© 2004 Ingenix, Inc.

It is possible for acute renal failure to be only temporary; the patient's renal function may be regained after interventions such as dialysis.

Hypertensive Heart and Renal Disease: Category 404 identifies hypertensive heart and renal disease and has a fifth-digit subclassification to identify renal failure. For example, in many cases renal failure is only seen in hypertensive heart and renal disease when the hypertension becomes malignant or accelerated. In these cases only one code is necessary: 404.02 *Hypertensive heart and renal disease, malignant, with renal failure.* Category 404 excludes acute renal failure; when this is noted, an additional code is required from category 584 *Acute renal failure.*

Hypertensive Renal Disease: Category 403 identifies hypertensive renal disease with renal failure with the fifth-digit assignment of "1." For example, in many cases renal failure is seen in hypertensive renal disease only when the hypertension becomes malignant or accelerated. In these cases only one code is necessary: 403.01 *Hypertensive renal disease, malignant, with renal failure.* Category 403 excludes acute renal failure; when this is noted, an additional code will be required from category 584 *Acute renal failure.*

Tumor Lysis Syndrome: This condition occurs as a result of massive doses of chemotherapy in the bloodstream. Two codes are required to report it accurately: 584.8 *Acute renal failure with other specified pathological lesion in kidney* and E933.1 *Adverse effect in therapeutic use, antineoplastic and immunosuppressive drugs,* or a code that would identify the specific drug used in therapy.

Secondary Hypertension: Category 405 *Secondary hypertension* does not include renal failure, so two codes are necessary to identify cases of renal failure with secondary hypertension.

Coding Scenario

A patient is admitted and treated for acute renal failure and essential hypertension.

> Code assignment: 584.9 *Acute renal failure, unspecified* and 401.9 *Essential hypertension, unspecified*

A patient is seen for acute renal failure that has an established hypertensive renal nephrosclerosis.

> Code assignment: 584.9 *Acute renal failure, unspecified* and 403.91 *Hypertensive renal disease, unspecified, with renal failure*

585 Chronic renal failure

AHA: Sept-Oct, 1984, 3; Nov-Dec, 1985, 15; Q4, 1989, 1; Q3, 1991, 8; Q1, 1993, 18; Q3, 1996, 9; Q2, 1998, 20; Q3, 1998, 6,7; Q4, 1998, 55; Q1, 2001, 3; Q2, 2001, 12,13; Q2, 2003, 7; Q4, 2003, 61, 111

Chronic renal failure is a multisystem disease due to a progressive loss of renal function. It usually develops gradually as a consequence of a wide spectrum of diseases such as primary and secondary glomerular disease, diabetes mellitus, and hereditary renal disease such as polycystic kidneys, hypertension, obstructive uropathy, chronic infection, and interstitial nephritis.

Signs and symptoms of chronic renal failure include weakness, fatigue, peripheral edema, headaches, pallor, thirst, anorexia, weight loss, nausea, vomiting, pruritus, polyuria (early stages), oliguria (late stages), nocturia, mental changes, and is asymptomatic until more than 75 percent of renal function is lost. Blood work shows elevated BUN, serum creatinine, and potassium; decreased serum calcium, arterial pH, and bicarbonate; and normochromic, normocytic anemia. An urinalysis reveals urine specific gravity of approximately 1.010 (indicating isosthenuria) and sometimes protein, glucose, WBCs, RBCs, waxy and granular casts. A chest x-ray may show cardiac enlargement, interstitial edema, lung edema, and frank pulmonary congestion. Other radiology, such as x-rays of the kidney-ureter-bladder, intravenous pyelography, renal arteriography, and renal scans such as selected radionuclide studies and ultrasound may aid in diagnosis and treatment. Kidney biopsy and histological examination identify underlying pathology.

Therapies include dietary management such as protein restriction, iron and/or folate supplements, and restriction of fluid intake with careful monitoring of urine volume and electrolytes. Other therapies include transfusion of blood or blood products to treat anemia, peritoneal dialysis or hemodialysis to control uremia in patients with ESRD, and renal transplant for patients with ESRD.

Associated conditions include normochromic, normocytic anemia, electrolyte imbalances, underlying disease (e.g., diabetes mellitus, hypertension), cardiovascular complications (congestive heart failure, dysrhythmias, uremic pericarditis, pericardial effusion), respiratory complications (Kussmaul respirations due to acidosis, uremic pleuritis, uremic pneumonitis, pleural effusion), renal osteodystrophy (bone disease), and gastrointestinal complications (gastritis, pancreatitis, duodenal ulcer, uremic colitis).

Documentation Issues

When the loss of renal function is incomplete, the term "chronic renal insufficiency" (593.9) is often used. When the loss of renal function is complete, the term "end-stage renal disease" or "chronic uremia" may be used. Because chronic renal failure causes major changes in all body systems, signs and symptoms may be widespread and varied.

Documentation in the record that may indicate the presence of renal failure could include:

 © 2004 Ingenix, Inc.

- Markedly elevated values of serum creatinine or BUN, or diminished creatinine clearance.
- Clinical manifestations and laboratory findings of the degree of renal impairment primarily noted as the renal failure progresses. For example:
  - acidemia
  - anemia
  - hyperkalemia
  - hyperphosphatemia
  - hypocalcemia
  - renal osteodystrophy
  - uremic symptoms, (e.g., nausea, hemorrhagic conditions, vomiting, itching)

The above may be indicators of renal failure but confirmation and documentation from the physician must be obtained before assigning the code for renal failure.

If documentation identifies renal failure with hypertension, clarify with the physician as to whether the hypertension is malignant or accelerated. If the documentation identifies that the renal failure and hypertension are unrelated or the cause and effect relationship cannot be established, code each separately.

When the documentation identifies renal failure and diabetes but does not identify a cause and effect relationship, contact the physician for clarification. If the physician confirms that the renal failure is a manifestation of the diabetes, list the diabetes code first followed by the code identifying the specific type of renal failure.

If the diagnostic statement identifies hypertension, chronic renal failure, and diabetes, verify the cause and effect relationship of the chronic renal failure with the physician. If the chronic renal failure is due to the diabetes, use codes 250.4x and code 585 as a secondary manifestation code; code also the specific type of hypertension. However, if the physician confirms that this is hypertensive renal disease (includes renal failure) due to diabetes, report with code 250.4x and a code from category 403, with a fifth digit of "1" to identify the renal failure.

Coding Clarification

Excluded from this code is chronic renal failure with any condition classifiable to 401 (403.0-403.9 with fifth-digit 1).

Dialysis Disequilibrium Syndrome: This condition is reported with code 276.9 *Electrolyte and fluid disorder not elsewhere classified.* Code also the underlying disease such as chronic renal failure (585), and also report the renal dialysis status (V45.1).

General Guidelines: Renal failure (category 584 *Acute renal failure,* category 585 *Chronic renal failure,* and 586 *Renal failure, unspecified*) is the progression of renal insufficiency to the point at which renal function becomes further impaired and apparent clinical manifestations, such as anemia, develop. Renal insufficiency is more an abnormal laboratory assessment, while renal failure includes both the abnormal laboratory and the clinical findings.

Chronic renal failure is caused by a number of progressive diseases such as diabetes, primary hypertension, nephrosis, nephritis, obstructive uropathy, systemic lupus erythematosis (SLE), polycystic kidney disease, and other congenital disorders. In cases of chronic renal failure that becomes irreversible, the treatment may be either dialysis or transplantation.

It is possible for acute renal failure to be only temporary; the patient's renal function may be regained after interventions such as dialysis.

Infection of Dialysis Catheter: If the patient develops an infection or an inflammatory reaction due to the dialysis catheter, report with code 996.68. Additional codes should also be reported to identify the bacterial agent (e.g., *Staphylococcus aureus,* 041.11) and the chronic renal failure (585).

Diabetes Mellitus: Diabetes is one of a number of the ICD-9-CM classification categories that is used as a primary code to classify both the disease and its major manifestations. Additional codes should be used to provide more specificity in defining the manifestations. When a cause and effect relationship between the renal failure and the diabetes has been established, the diabetes code 250.4x is listed first with the appropriate renal failure code listed as an additional code. Accordingly, if the diagnosis does not indicate a cause and effect relationship between the diabetes and renal failure, the code for the renal failure may be listed first.

Secondary Hypertension: Category 405 *Secondary hypertension* does not include renal failure, so two codes are necessary to identify cases of renal failure with secondary hypertension.

Coding Scenario

The patient is admitted for hemodialysis. The patient is an insulin-dependent, Type I diabetic with progressive nephropathy. The physician also documents chronic renal failure in the medical history.

> Code assignment: 250.41 *Diabetes with renal manifestations,* 583.81 *Nephritis and nephropathy, not specified as acute or chronic, in diseases classified elsewhere,* and 585 *Chronic renal failure*

A patient is diagnosed with chronic renal failure secondary to nephrosclerosis with uremia due to gout.

Code assignment: 274.10 *Gouty nephropathy, unspecified* and 585 *Chronic renal failure*

586 Unspecified renal failure OK

AHA: Q1, 1993, 18; Q3, 1998, 6

Documentation Issues

Documentation in the record that may indicate the presence of renal failure could include:

- Markedly elevated values of serum creatinine or BUN, or diminished creatinine clearance.
- Clinical manifestations and laboratory findings of the degree of renal impairment primarily noted as the renal failure progresses. For example:
  - acidemia
  - anemia
  - hyperkalemia
  - hyperphosphatemia
  - hypocalcemia
  - renal osteodystrophy
  - uremic symptoms, (e.g., nausea, hemorrhagic conditions, vomiting, itching)

The above may be indicators of renal failure but confirmation and documentation from the physician must be obtained before assigning the code for renal failure.

If documentation identifies renal failure with hypertension, clarify with the physician as to whether the hypertension is malignant or accelerated. If the documentation identifies that the renal failure and hypertension are unrelated, or the cause and effect relationship cannot be established, code each separately.

When the documentation identifies renal failure and diabetes but does not identify a cause and effect relationship, contact the physician for clarification. If the physician confirms that the renal failure is a manifestation of the diabetes, list the diabetes code first followed by the code identifying the specific type of renal failure.

Unless acute renal failure or chronic renal failure is confirmed and documented by the physician, azotemia is reported with code 790.6 *Other abnormal blood chemistry.*

Coding Clarification

Excluded from this rubric are renal failure following labor and delivery (669.3x), posttraumatic (958.5), that complicating abortion (rubrics 634-638) or ectopic/molar pregnancy (639.3x), extrarenal or prerenal uremia (788.9), or renal failure with any condition classifiable to 401 (403.0-403.9 with fifth-digit "1").

Diabetes Mellitus: Diabetes is one of a number of the ICD-9-CM classification categories that is used as a primary code to classify both the disease and its major manifestations. Additional codes should be used to provide more specificity in defining the manifestations. When a cause and effect relationship between the renal failure and the diabetes has been established, the diabetes code 250.4x is listed first with the appropriate renal failure code listed as an additional code. Accordingly, if the diagnosis does not indicate a cause and effect relationship between the diabetes and renal failure, the code for the renal failure may be listed first.

General Guidelines: Renal failure (category 584 *Acute renal failure,* 585 *Chronic renal failure,* and 586 *Renal failure, unspecified*) is the progression of renal insufficiency to the point at which renal function becomes further impaired and apparent clinical manifestations, such as anemia, develop. Renal insufficiency is more an abnormal laboratory assessment, while renal failure includes both the abnormal laboratory and the clinical findings.

Chronic renal failure is caused by a number of progressive diseases such as diabetes, primary hypertension, nephrosis, nephritis, obstructive uropathy, systemic lupus erythematosis (SLE), polycystic kidney disease, and other congenital disorders. In cases of chronic renal failure that becomes irreversible, the treatment may be either dialysis or transplantation.

Secondary Hypertension: Category 405 *Secondary hypertension* does not include renal failure, so two codes are necessary to identify cases of renal failure with secondary hypertension.

587 Unspecified renal sclerosis OK

Coding Clarification

Excluded from this rubric is arteriolar or arteriosclerotic nephrosclerosis (403.00-403.92).

588 Disorders resulting from impaired renal function

Secondary hyperparathyroidism results from releasing increased levels in response to deconditioning of the body to parathyroid hormone PTH due to another disease process, such as renal failure. PTH helps regulate the levels of calcium and phosphorus in the body, induces the release of calcium from bone, the amount of calcium taken from food, intestinal absorption of calcium, and the excretion of calcium in the urine. Renal osteodystrophy is caused by the kidney failing to maintain the appropriate level of

 © 2004 Ingenix, Inc.

calcium in the blood, which affect bone health. Nephrogenic diabetes is caused by the failure of the kidneys to absorb filtered fluids. Hypercalcemia, or increased levels of calcium in the blood, is a sign of hyperparathyroidism, when accompanied by a concurrent increase in the level of PTH hormone.

588.0 Renal osteodystrophy — *azotemic osteodystrophy; renal dwarfism; renal rickets*

588.1 Nephrogenic diabetes insipidus — *kidneys fail to resorb filtered fluids, leading to extreme thirst and frequent urination*

588.81 Secondary hyperparathyroidism (of renal origin)

588.89 Other specified disorders resulting from impaired renal function

588.9 Unspecified disorder resulting from impaired renal function — *disorder NOS due to impaired renal function*

Coding Clarification

Report 252.02 for hyperparathyroidism from non-renal causes.

589 Small kidney of unknown cause

589.0 Unilateral small kidney

589.1 Bilateral small kidneys

589.9 Unspecified small kidney — *of unknown cause*

Coding Clarification

These codes are considered nonspecific codes and should be used only when a more specific diagnosis of acquired or congenital small kidney cannot be determined.

590–599 Other Diseases of Urinary System

590 Infections of kidney

590.00 Chronic pyelonephritis without lesion of renal medullary necrosis — (Code, if applicable, any causal condition first. Use additional code to identify organism, such as E. coli, 041.4) — *chronic pyelitis, or pyonephrosis, without lesion of renal medullary necrosis use additional code to identify organism*

590.01 Chronic pyelonephritis with lesion of renal medullary necrosis — (Code, if applicable, any causal condition first. Use additional code to identify organism, such as E. coli, 041.4) — *chronic pyelitis or pyonephrosis with lesion of renal medullary necrosis use additional code to identify organism*

590.10 Acute pyelonephritis without lesion of renal medullary necrosis — (Use additional code to identify organism, such as E. coli, 041.4) — *acute pyelitis or acute pyonephrosis without lesion of renal medullary necrosis*

590.11 Acute pyelonephritis with lesion of renal medullary necrosis — (Use additional code to identify organism, such as E. coli, 041.4) — *acute pyelitis or acute pyonephrosis with lesion of renal medullary necrosis*

590.2 Renal and perinephric abscess — (Use additional code to identify organism, such as E. coli, 041.4) — *nephritic abscess; perirenal abscess*

590.3 Pyeloureteritis cystica — (Use additional code to identify organism, such as E. coli, 041.4) — *ureteritis cystica; infection of renal pelvis and ureter*

590.80 Unspecified pyelonephritis — (Use additional code to identify organism, such as E. coli, 041.4) — *pyelonephritis NOS*
AHA: Q4, 1997, 40; Q1, 1998, 10

590.81 Pyelitis or pyelonephritis in diseases classified elsewhere — (Code first underlying disease, 016.0. Use additional code to identify organism, such as E. coli, 041.4) — *in disease classified elsewhere*

590.9 Unspecified infection of kidney — (Use additional code to identify organism, such as E. coli, 041.4)

Coding Clarification

Use an additional code to identify infective agents, such as *Escherichia coli* (041.4).

591 Hydronephrosis OK

AHA: Q2, 1998, 9

Use this code to report dilation of the renal pelvis and calyces due to the obstruction of the flow of urine. Obstruction occurring at the ureteropelvic junction is sometimes referred to as primary hydronephrosis, and obstruction at any point distal to the ureteropelvic junction is sometimes referred to as secondary hydronephrosis.

Signs and symptoms of hydronephrosis include a history of any condition causing urinary obstruction, colicky pain in acute hydronephrosis, dull and aching flank pain in chronic hydronephrosis, and hematuria. Blood work may show azotemia (excess urea and other nitrogenous byproducts). Urinalysis may reveal red blood cells and pyuria if a concomitant urinary infection is present. Radiology, such as intravenous pyelography, cystoureterography, and kidney ultrasound, identify the site of the obstruction and confirm the diagnosis.

Therapies include cystoscopy to correct conditions such as benign prostatic hypertrophy and ureteral calculus (basket extraction of calculus or stent insertion), extracorporeal shock wave lithotripsy to break up calculi in the kidney or ureter, nephrostomy for severe obstructions, and surgery to correct conditions such as strictures, neoplasms, and congenital malformations.

Associated conditions include urinary tract infection, urinary calculus formation, benign prostatic hypertrophy or prostate cancer, urinary stricture formation, and congenital abnormalities.

Coding Clarification

Excluded from this code are congenital hydronephrosis (753.29) and hydroureter (593.5).

592 Calculus of kidney and ureter

Use this rubric to report stones of the kidney and ureter. Most stones are composed of calcium salts or magnesium/ammonium phosphate; most are idiopathic. Other stones may be composed of cystine or uric acid, and are a result of a defect in urinary acidification.

Nausea, infection, severe pain, and hematuria usually accompany kidney stones, if the stone is obstructing the flow of urine. If there is no obstruction, there may be no symptoms.

Ureteral calculi have migrated to the ureter from the kidney, and obstruction can compromise renal function. Symptoms are the same as for renal calculi.

592.0 Calculus of kidney — *renal calculus or stone; staghorn calculus*
AHA: Q1, 2000, 4

592.1 Calculus of ureter — *ureteric stone; ureterolithiasis*
AHA: Q1, 1991, 11; Q1, 1998, 10; Q2, 1998, 9

592.9 Unspecified urinary calculus — *renal or ureteral calculus NOS*
AHA: Q4, 1997, 40; Q1, 1998, 10

Coding Clarification

Excluded from this rubric is nephrocalcinosis (275.4).

593 Other disorders of kidney and ureter

The ureter is the tube leading from the kidney to the urinary bladder. It is approximately 28.0 centimeters long and is composed of three layers of tissue. The inner layer is a mucous lining. The smooth, muscular middle layer propels the urine from the kidney to the bladder by peristalsis. The outer layer is fibrous connective tissue. Each ureter leaves the kidney from the hilum, a concave notch on the middle surface, and enters the bladder through a narrow valvelike orifice that prevents backflow of urine to the kidney.

593.0 Nephroptosis — *floating kidney; mobile kidney*

593.1 Hypertrophy of kidney — *enlargement of kidney*

593.2 Acquired cyst of kidney — *peripelvic (lymphatic) cyst*
AHA: Q4, 1990, 3

593.3 Stricture or kinking of ureter — *stricture of pelviureteric junction*
AHA: Q2, 1998, 9

593.4 Other ureteric obstruction — *idiopathic retroperitoneal fibrosis; occlusion NOS of ureter*
AHA: Q2, 1997, 4

593.5 Hydroureter — *dilation of ureter due to obstructed urinary flow*

593.6 Postural proteinuria — *benign postural proteinuria; orthostatic proteinuria*

593.70 Vesicoureteral reflux, unspecified or without reflex nephropathy — *backflow of urine from bladder into ureter*
AHA: Q4, 1994, 42

593.71 Vesicoureteral reflux with reflux nephropathy, unilateral — *one-sided backflow of urine into ureter, causing renal scarring*
AHA: Q4, 1994, 42

593.72 Vesicoureteral reflux with reflux nephropathy, bilateral — *backflow of urine into ureters on both sides, causing renal scarring*
AHA: Q4, 1994, 42

593.73 Vesicoureteral reflux with reflux nephropathy, NOS — *backflow of urine into ureters, causing renal scarring*
AHA: Q4, 1994, 42

593.81 Vascular disorders of kidney — *renal artery embolism; renal artery hemorrhage; renal artery thrombosis; renal infarction*

593.82 Ureteral fistula — *intestinoureteral fistula*

593.89 Other specified disorder of kidney and ureter — *adhesions, kidney or ureter; periureteritis; ureteral polyp; ureterocele*

593.9 Unspecified disorder of kidney and ureter — *renal disease NOS; salt-losing nephritis or syndrome; Thorn's syndrome*
AHA: Q1, 1993, 17

Coding Clarification

Use this code series for kidney and ureter disorders that are not further specified as acute or chronic or are lacking a stated pathology or cause. Also classified to this code are syndromes of low salt, salt-losing, or salt depletion not further specified, as well as salt-losing or salt-wasting nephritis, nephropathy, or renopathy not further specified.

580–629

 © 2004 Ingenix, Inc.

594 Calculus of lower urinary tract

The lower urinary tract includes every part of the urinary system, except the kidneys. While the kidneys filter blood and produce urine, the remainder of the system stores and eliminates the waste liquid. The ureters carry urine from the kidneys to the bladder, the urinary bladder stores urine, and the urethra carries urine out of the body. Bladder stones are usually the result of another urologic problem such as urinary tract infection, bladder diverticulum, neurogenic bladder, or an enlarged prostate. Approximately 95 percent of all bladder stones occur in men. Bladder stones can cause irritation and damage inside the urinary tract, while chronic irritation with bladder calculi predisposes the bladder to cancer. Clinical signs include blood in the urine, frequent urination, increased thirst, abdominal distention or pain, and penile pain in males. Diagnosis is based on history; physical examination; x-rays, including x-rays taken with dye being placed into the bladder; urinalysis; and urine culture. Treatment includes drinking six to eight glasses of water each day to increase urinary output and help the stones pass. Stones that are not excreted spontaneously may be removed using a cystoscope or open surgery. Extracorporeal shock wave lithotripsy may be an alternative to surgery. Medications are rarely used to dissolve the stones.

594.0 Calculus in diverticulum of bladder — *stone in pouch of bladder wall*

594.1 Other calculus in bladder — *urinary bladder stone*

594.2 Calculus in urethra — *urinary stone in urethra*

594.8 Other lower urinary tract calculus — *suburethral urinary stone*
AHA: Jan-Feb, 1985, 16

594.9 Unspecified calculus of lower urinary tract

595 Cystitis

This rubric reports infections and inflammations of the bladder. An additional code should be reported to identify the infectious agent, as in *E. coli* 041.4. If the bladder inflammation or infection is due to a disease classified elsewhere, code first the underlying disease.

The urinary bladder is an expandable and collapsible bag located behind the symphysis pubis (pubic bone) and below the parietal peritoneum. This protective membrane covers only the top of the bladder. The bladder has a strong, specialized muscular layer called the detrusor muscle, a network of muscle bundles that run in all directions. The lining of the bladder is a mucous transitional epithelium that forms folds called rugae. These specialized tissue layers allow for the distension of the bladder as it fills with urine from the kidneys.

There are three openings in the floor of the bladder. The two ureters enter at the back of the bladder, guarded by the valvelike narrow regions that prevent backflow up to the kidneys. The opening into the urethra is in the front lower corner of the bladder. The bladder has two major functions: it stores urine before it leaves the body and, by means of the urethra, expels urine from the body.

Cystitis is a common complication of catheterization. When this occurs, report 996.64 *Infection and inflammatory reaction due to indwelling urinary catheter* and a cystitis code from this rubric.

595.0 Acute cystitis — (Use additional code to identify organism, such as E. coli, 041.4) — *acute infection of bladder*
AHA: Q2, 1999, 15

595.1 Chronic interstitial cystitis — (Use additional code to identify organism, such as E. coli, 041.4) — *Hunner's ulcer; panmural fibrosis of bladder; submucous cystitis*

595.2 Other chronic cystitis — (Use additional code to identify organism, such as E. coli, 041.4) — *chronic cystitis NOS; subacute cystitis*

595.3 Trigonitis — (Use additional code to identify organism, such as E. coli, 041.4) — *follicular cystitis; acute or chronic trigonitis; urethrotrigonitis*

595.4 Cystitis in diseases classified elsewhere — (Code first underlying disease: 006.8, 039.8, 120.0-120.9, 122.3, 122.6. Use additional code to identify organism, such as E. coli, 041.4)

595.81 Cystitis cystica — (Use additional code to identify organism, such as E. coli, 041.4) — *bladder inflammation due to multiple cysts*

595.82 Irradiation cystitis — (Use additional code to identify organism, such as E. coli, 041.4) — *bladder inflammation due to radiation*

595.89 Other specified types of cystitis — (Use additional code to identify organism, such as E. coli, 041.4) — *bladder abscess; emphysematous cystitis*

595.9 Unspecified cystitis — (Use additional code to identify organism, such as E. coli, 041.4)

Coding Clarification

Excluded from this rubric are prostatocystitis (601.3), cystitis in diphtheria (032.84), gonococcal cystitis (098.11, 098.31), monilial cystitis (112.2), trichomonal cystitis (131.09), and tuberculous cystitis (subclassification 016.1).

596 Other disorders of bladder

AHA: March-April, 1987, 10

Subclassification 596.0 reports a condition, also known as bladder outlet obstruction or vesicourethral obstruction, that occurs mostly in males and usually as a consequence of benign prostatic hypertrophy or prostatic cancer. It also may occur in either sex due to strictures (formed following radiation therapy, cystoscopy, catheterization injury, or infection), blood clots, bladder cancer, impacted calculi, extrinsic tumors, or disease compressing the bladder neck.

Bladder neck obstruction is associated with complications such as hydronephrosis, hydroureteronephrosis, or ureteronephrosis. The obstruction also may be due to bladder thickening and hypertrophy, trabeculation, or diverticula; hypertrophy and subsequent dilatation and atony of the renal pelvis; or renal parenchymal compression and ischemic atrophy.

Use subclassification 596.5 to report functional disorders of the bladder, the musculomembranous sac that serves as a reservoir for urine received from the kidneys through the ureters and as a contractile organ actively expelling its contents into the urethra. Functional disorders prevent the bladder from performing either or both of these functions. Included are hypertonicity, low bladder compliance, paralysis, neurogenic bladder, and detrusor sphincter dyssynergia.

Hypertonicity refers to excessive muscle tonus or tension. In the bladder, it usually refers to prolonged detrusor (bladder) muscle spasms and hypersensitivity or hyperreflexia of the detrusor muscle.

Low bladder compliance refers to the relative change in bladder volume when measured against bladder (detrusor muscle) pressure. Compliance can be measured by inflow cystometry. If the cystometry demonstrates a large bladder volume with little pressure change in the bladder, the patient has a bladder of high compliance; if the cystometry reveals a tense, firm bladder with high pressure, the bladder is of low compliance.

Paralysis of the bladder is a general term meaning loss of the ability of the detrusor muscles to contract. Such paralysis may have a variety of etiologies such as trauma, drugs, disease, or other structural or functional disorders in the bladder muscle or nerves.

Neurogenic bladder is due to a nervous system lesion. Terms used to describe neurogenic bladder are spastic bladder, reflex bladder, and flaccid bladder.

Detrusor sphincter dyssynergia, also known as bladder neck dyssynergia, is a condition in which urinary outflow is obstructed because the bladder neck fails to relax or tightens when the detrusor muscle contracts during micturition. The condition is rarely observed in females.

596.0 Bladder neck obstruction — (Use additional code to identify urinary incontinence: 625.6, 788.30-788.39) — *contracture of bladder neck or other vesicoureteral orifice*
AHA: Nov-Dec, 1986, 10; March-April, 1987, 10; Q2, 2001, 14; Q3, 2002, 28

596.1 Intestinovesical fistula — (Use additional code to identify urinary incontinence: 625.6, 788.30-788.39) — *enterovesical fistula; vesicorectal fistula*
AHA: March-April, 1987, 10

596.2 Vesical fistula, not elsewhere classified — (Use additional code to identify urinary incontinence: 625.6, 788.30-788.39) — *urethrovesical fistula; vesicocutaneous fistula*
AHA: March-April, 1987, 10

596.3 Diverticulum of bladder — (Use additional code to identify urinary incontinence: 625.6, 788.30-788.39) — *bladder diverticulitis*
AHA: March-April, 1987, 10

596.4 Atony of bladder — (Use additional code to identify urinary incontinence: 625.6, 788.30-788.39) — *hypotonicity of bladder; bladder inertia*
AHA: March-April, 1987, 10

596.51 Hypertonicity of bladder — (Use additional code to identify urinary incontinence: 625.6, 788.30-788.39) — *hyperactivity of bladder; overactivity of bladder*
AHA: March-April, 1987, 10

596.52 Low bladder compliance — (Use additional code to identify urinary incontinence: 625.6, 788.30-788.39) — *small or sensitive bladder that requires frequent emptying*
AHA: March-April, 1987, 10

596.53 Paralysis of bladder — (Use additional code to identify urinary incontinence: 625.6, 788.30-788.39) — *bladder unable to contract*
AHA: March-April, 1987, 10

596.54 Neurogenic bladder, NOS — (Use additional code to identify urinary incontinence: 625.6, 788.30-788.39) — *loss of bladder control most often due to spinal nerve damage from injury or neurological disease*
AHA: March-April, 1987, 10; Q1, 2001, 12

596.55 Detrusor sphincter dyssynergia — (Use additional code to identify urinary incontinence: 625.6, 788.30-788.39) — *loss of coordination between bladder emptying nerves and external urethral sphincter*
AHA: March-April, 1987, 10

© 2004 Ingenix, Inc.

596.59 Other functional disorder of bladder — (Use additional code to identify urinary incontinence: 625.6, 788.30-788.39) — *detrusor instability*
AHA: March-April, 1987, 10

596.6 Nontraumatic rupture of bladder — (Use additional code to identify urinary incontinence: 625.6, 788.30-788.39) — *spontaneous tear in bladder wall*
AHA: March-April, 1987, 10

596.7 Hemorrhage into bladder wall — (Use additional code to identify urinary incontinence: 625.6, 788.30-788.39) — *hyperemia of bladder*
AHA: March-April, 1987, 10

596.8 Other specified disorder of bladder — (Use additional code to identify urinary incontinence: 625.6, 788.30-788.39) — *calcified bladder; bladder hypertrophy*
AHA: Jan-Feb, 1985, 8; March-April, 1987, 10

596.9 Unspecified disorder of bladder — (Use additional code to identify urinary incontinence: 625.6, 788.30-788.39) — *bladder disease NOS*
AHA: Jan-Feb, 1985, 8; March-April, 1987, 10

Coding Clarification

Congenital bladder neck obstruction is excluded from this subclassification and should be reported with 753.6.

Use an additional code to report any urinary incontinence (625.6, 788.30-788.39).

Bladder Outlet Obstruction: In cases of benign prostatic hypertrophy with bladder outlet obstruction, the prostatic hypertrophy (600.00-600.01) is listed first and an additional code for the obstruction (596.0) is secondary, because the obstruction is typically a part of the condition due to the prostatic hypertrophy.

Urinary Retention: When urinary retention (788.20) is noted with benign prostatic hypertrophy (600.00-600.01), it is reported as a secondary code.

597 Urethritis, not sexually transmitted, and urethral syndrome

597.0 Urethral abscess — *periurethral abscess; bulbourethral gland abscess*

597.80 Unspecified urethritis — *urethritis NOS*

597.81 Urethral syndrome NOS

597.89 Other urethritis — *Cowperitis (males); urethral ulcer; para-urethritis; littritis (males); adenitis, Skene's glands (females)*

Coding Clarification

Excluded from this rubric is nonspecific urethritis, so stated, reported with 099.4.

598 Urethral stricture

A urethral stricture is a narrowing of the urethra. The urethra is a small tube lined with mucous membrane that leads from the bladder to the exterior of the body. In the male, it is approximately 20.0 centimeters long and passes through the prostate gland just below the bladder, where it joins the ejaculatory ducts. The tube extends forward and down to enter the base of the penis, and travels centrally through the length of the penis to end as a urinary meatus at the tip. In the female, the urethra lies directly behind the symphysis pubis and in front of the vagina, and is only about 3.0 centimeters long.

The function of the urethra in the female is to void urine from the bladder reservoir. In the male, the urethra is part of two different systems: in addition to voiding urine, the urethra also serves as the pathway for semen (fluid containing sperm) as it is ejaculated out of the body through the penis. Urine is prevented from mixing with semen during ejaculation by the reflex closure of the sphincter muscles guarding the opening into the bladder.

598.00 Urethral stricture due to unspecified infection — (Use additional code to identify urinary incontinence: 625.6, 788.30-788.39) — *urethral stricture due to infection NOS*

598.01 Urethral stricture due to infective diseases classified elsewhere — (Code first underlying disease: 095.8, 098.2, 120.0-120.9. Use additional code to identify urinary incontinence: 625.6, 788.30-788.39)

598.1 Traumatic urethral stricture — (Use additional code to identify urinary incontinence: 625.6, 788.30-788.39) — *postobstetric urethral stricture*

598.2 Postoperative urethral stricture — (Use additional code to identify urinary incontinence: 625.6, 788.30-788.39) — *postcatheterization stricture of urethra*
AHA: Q3, 1997, 6

598.8 Other specified causes of urethral stricture — (Use additional code to identify urinary incontinence: 625.6, 788.30-788.39) — *other specified cause of urethral stricture NEC*
AHA: Nov-Dec, 1984, 9

598.9 Unspecified urethral stricture — (Use additional code to identify urinary incontinence: 625.6, 788.30-788.39) — *pinhole meatus; ankylurethria*

Coding Clarification

Use an additional code to identify urinary incontinence (625.6; 788.30-788.39). Code first the underlying disease, as appropriate.

© 2004 Ingenix, Inc.

599 Other disorders of urethra and urinary tract

The definition of urinary tract infection, site not specified, is a wide variety of clinical conditions characterized by a significant number of microorganisms in an unspecified part of the urinary tract. Predisposing factors for urinary tract infection include, but are not limited to, calculi or other urinary tract obstruction, foreign bodies such as stents or catheters, congenital urinary anomalies, pregnancy, diabetes mellitus, neurogenic bladder, immunosuppression (such as following renal transplant), and vesicovaginal or intestinal fistulas. Many urinary tract infections recur due to bacterial persistence or reinfection from new organisms outside the urinary tract. Women are approximately 10 times more likely to develop a urinary tract infection than men.

Signs and symptoms of urinary tract infection, site not specified, include history of recurrent urinary tract infections, burning pain on urination, polyuria, suprapubic or abdominal pain, fever, and turbid, foul-smelling, dark urine. Urinalysis shows significant bacteriuria, often accompanied by proteinuria, hematuria, and pyuria, and urine culture reveals growth of more than 100,000 colonies of a single organism. Blood work may reveal neutrophilic leukocytosis and positive blood culture, especially if the infection involves the upper urinary tract. Radiology, such as intravenous urography or pyelography, voiding cystography, and renal ultrasound, may demonstrate complicating factors such as calculi, abscess formation, hydronephrosis, and congenital anomalies. Cystoscopy and ureteral catheterization to obtain differential urine specimens localize the infection site.

Therapies include antibiotics such as ampicillin, gentamicin, tetracycline, and tobramycin. Surgery can correct complications due to urinary tract infections (such as ureteral strictures) and conditions that predispose the patient to chronic or recurrent urinary tract infections (such as ureteral calculi or congenital abnormalities).

Associated conditions include urosepsis, diabetes mellitus, pregnancy (complicated), urinary tract obstruction (e.g., calculi, fibrosis), neurogenic bladder, congenital urinary tract anomalies, benign prostatic hypertrophy, prostatitis, infected diverticula, foreign bodies, vesicovaginal and intestinal fistulas, ureteral stump following nephrectomy, papillary necrosis, and urachal cyst.

Infections of the prostate, vagina, epididymis, and testis are classified elsewhere but may be swept into the nonspecific diagnosis of urinary tract infection by some clinicians.

Urinalysis and the urine culture are the most important indicators for urinary tract infection. Urine specimens, including the so-called "clean-catch" midstream specimen, are subject to contamination during collection from microorganisms surrounding the external urethra or by improper handling and storage. Thus, the presence of three or more species of microorganisms growing in large numbers suggests contamination, except in patients who have had an indwelling catheter for a long time. Also, patients who have received antibiotic therapy for any reason prior to testing may present false negative test results.

599.0 Urinary tract infection, site not specified — (Use additional code to identify organism, such as E. coli, 041.4) — *bacteriuria; pyuria*
AHA: Q1, 1992, 13; Q2, 1995, 7; Q2, 1996, 7; Q4, 1996, 33; Q1, 1998, 5; Q2, 1999, 15; Q4, 1999, 6; Q4, 2003, 79

Documentation Issues

When the documentation does not identify that the cause of the infection was due to the procedure (postoperative), clarification is required from the physician before a code is assigned identifying the infection as a procedural complication. If documentation cannot be obtained specifically stating the cause and effect relationship with the procedure, code 599.0 should be assigned.

When the documentation indicates urosepsis, the physician should be contacted to clarify whether the urosepsis is intended to mean generalized sepsis (septicemia) caused by leakage of urine or toxic urine by-products into the general vascular circulation, or that the urine is contaminated by bacteria, bacterial by-products, or perhaps other toxic material but without other findings (599.0). The alphabetic index refers the coder to urinary tract infection, but this may not be what the physician meant by this term. If the information is unobtainable, it is appropriate to use the index that defaults to code 599.0 for urosepsis.

Ask the physician if the site of the infection is known, and request an addendum to the medical record if the answer is affirmative.

Coding Clarification

This subcategory excludes urinary tract infection of newborn which is reported with code 771.82.

Secondary to Noncandidal Yeast: To properly report the urinary tract infection secondary to noncandidal yeast, use two codes: 599.0 *Urinary tract infection, site not specified* and 117.9 *Other and unspecified mycoses.*

Sepsis Secondary to Urinary Tract Infection: If a localized urinary infection has entered into the patient's blood stream and has developed into a generalized sepsis, use a code from category 038. Code 599.0 *Urinary tract infection, site not specified* is also reported as an additional code. If the code from category 038 identifies the causative organism, it is

© 2004 Ingenix, Inc.

not necessary to report a code from category 041 (e.g., pseudomonas septicemia 038.43).

Specified Organism: When the causative organism has been identified, it is reported as an additional code to the urinary tract infection (599.0). Using E. Coli as an example, a note is provided in the Tabular List, under category code 041 that states "This category is provided to be used as an additional code where it is desired to identify the bacterial agent in diseases classified elsewhere."

599.1 Urethral fistula — *urinary fistula NOS*
AHA: Q3, 1997, 6

599.2 Urethral diverticulum — *pouch in urethral wall*

599.3 Urethral caruncle — *urethral polyp*

599.4 Urethral false passage — *passage without opening at urethral meatus*

599.5 Prolapsed urethral mucosa — *urethrocele*

599.6 Unspecified urinary obstruction — (Use additional code to identify urinary incontinence: 625.6, 788.30-788.39) — *obstructive uropathy NOS*

599.7 Hematuria — *benign hematuria; essential hematuria*
AHA: Q3, 1995, 8; Q1, 2000, 5

Coding Clarification

Hematuria reports a condition in which blood appears in the urine. Also known as hemuresis, hematuria may present as gross, visible blood in the urine or as RBCs visible only under microscopy (microscopic hematuria). Hematuria may be due to a urethral infection; bladder neoplasms; or radiation injury, ureteral calculus, or kidney conditions such as polycystic disease, renal artery thrombosis, or trauma. Hematuria also can be caused by systemic disorders such as hemophilia, sickle cell crisis, thrombocytopenia, anaphylactoid purpura with renal involvement, and adverse effect of anticoagulant therapy.

Often the presentation of the hematuria gives clues as to the source of the bleeding. When blood appears only during the first fraction of voided urine (initial hematuria), the source is likely the anterior urethra or prostate gland. When blood appears during the terminal fraction of voided urine (terminal hematuria), the source is likely in the posterior urethra, vesicle neck, or trigone. Blood mixed in with the total urine volume (total hematuria) is from the kidneys, ureters, or bladder. Painful hematuria usually indicates infection, calculi, trauma, or foreign body in the lower urinary tract. Painless hematuria is often associated with a neoplasm or vascular disorder.

The definition of other specified disorders of urethra and urinary tract is disorders of the urethra and urinary tract not elsewhere classifiable, such as urethral hypermobility, intrinsic (urethral) sphincter deficiency, and urethral instability.

Urethral hypermobility refers to inferior and posterior motion of the urethra into the potential space of the vagina and is due to a loss of urethral supporting and backing structures of the pelvis and pelvic floor. Urethral hypermobility is associated with pathologies such as vaginal prolapse and cystoceles and is commonly seen in females with urinary stress incontinence.

Intrinsic (urethral) sphincter deficiency (ISD) is due to intrinsic sphincteric damage in which the urethra is usually well supported but there is a posterior rotation and opening of the bladder neck and posterior urethra during straining.

Urethral instability is a reflex relaxation of the urethral muscle with or without detrusor muscle contraction resulting in incontinence. This condition is commonly associated with females who have multiple sclerosis.

599.81 Urethral hypermobility — (Use additional code to identify urinary incontinence: 625.6, 788.30-788.39) — *hypermobility*

599.82 Intrinsic (urethral) sphincter deficiency (ISD) — (Use additional code to identify urinary incontinence: 625.6, 788.30-788.39) — *deficiency*
AHA: Q2, 1996, 15

599.83 Urethral instability — (Use additional code to identify urinary incontinence: 625.6, 788.30-788.39) — *instability*

599.84 Other specified disorders of urethra — (Use additional code to identify urinary incontinence: 625.6, 788.30-788.39) — *nontraumatic rupture of urethra; urethral cyst; malacoplakia of urethra*

599.89 Other specified disorders of urinary tract — (Use additional code to identify urinary incontinence: 625.6, 788.30-788.39) — *hymeno-urethral fusion; suburethral cyst*

599.9 Unspecified disorder of urethra and urinary tract

Coding Clarification

Excluded from this rubric is candidiasis of urinary tract (112.2). Use an additional code to identify the infective agent, as in *E. coli* (041.4).

Site Specificity: One of the most important aspects of coding urinary tract infections is site specificity in the medical record documentation. "UTI" is commonly used as a synonym for acute cystitis, acute pyelonephritis, and acute urethritis. Cystitis and urethritis are infections of the lower urinary tract, and pyelonephritis is an infection of the upper urinary tract. Cystitis is more often seen in females, whereas urethritis is more commonly seen in males.

If the site of the infection is known, do not use code 599.0. Code 599.0 is reserved for cases in which no attempt was made to document the site of the infection. Do not use 599.0 as an accompanying code to a specific urinary tract infection code. However, if two specific sites are named, it is correct to code them both (e.g., 595.0 *Acute cystitis* and 590.10 *Acute pyelonephritis without lesion of renal medullary necrosis*).

Remember that UTIs attributable to sexually transmitted diseases are coded to the infectious disease chapter.

Coding Scenario

A patient is seen in the clinic for painful urination and fever. A urine culture shows the bacterial agent *Pseudomonas*. The physician's diagnostic statement confirms a urinary tract infection due to *Pseudomonas*.

> Code assignment: 599.0 *Urinary tract infection, site not specified* and 041.7 *Pseudomonas*

A 79-year-old male is readmitted for a urinary tract infection due to a urinary retention catheter.

> Code assignment: 996.64 *Infection and inflammatory reaction due to internal prosthetic device, implant, and graft, indwelling urinary catheter* and 599.0 *Urinary tract infection, site not specified*

The patient's list of diagnoses reads acute pyelonephritis, acute cystitis, and urosepsis. After it is determined that urosepsis was not used as a synonym for septicemia.

> Code assignment: Code 590.10 *Acute pyelonephritis without lesion of renal medullary necrosis* and 595.0 *Acute cystitis*

600–608 Diseases of Male Genital Organs

The male reproductive system includes the two testes that produce spermatozoa (sperm) and male hormones. A system of ducts conveys sperm to the exterior of the body. This includes the epididymis and vas deferens, the seminal vesicles (glands which contribute secretions to semen), and the external genitalia, the scrotum, and penis. The prime function of the male genital system is sexual intercourse and propagation of the species.

600 Hyperplasia of prostate

AHA: Nov-Dec, 1986, 10; Q3, 1992, 7; Q3, 1994, 12; Q4, 2000, 43

This rubric classifies a condition believed to arise as fibrostromal proliferation in the periurethral glands. The etiology is unknown, but a relationship between aging and prostate enlargement is well documented. Most theories regarding the cause of benign prostatic hypertrophy focus on possible hormonal imbalances occurring in the male after age 50. The disease usually becomes symptomatic after age 60 and is due to median and/or lateral lobe (inner gland) enlargement. The outer prostate glands are pushed against the prostate capsule, resulting in a thick pseudocapsule referred to as the surgical capsule. As the enlargement continues and intracapsular pressure increases, urinary outflow is obstructed due to impingement of the urethra. Frequently, the typical signs and symptoms of benign prostatic hypertrophy are referred to as "prostatism."

Signs and symptoms of hyperplasia of the prostate include reduced urinary stream caliber and force, urinary hesitancy, feelings of incomplete voiding, nocturia, straining to initiate urination, severe urgency, suprapubic pain, bladder distention when in urinary retention, hematuria, increased urine residual, and prostate enlargement palpable with rectal exam. Urinalysis may reveal concomitant infection. Blood work may show elevated serum creatinine and BUN with prolonged obstruction. Excretory urograms reveal ureteral dilation, hydronephrosis or hydroureteronephrosis, or post voiding urinary retention. Pelvic ultrasound may be used to calculate exact amounts of residual urine. Cystoscopy shows enlargement of periurethral prostate glands and demonstrates secondary bladder wall changes such as trabeculation, vesicle calculi, acute and/or chronic inflammation due to infection, and bladder diverticula.

Therapies include sexual stimulation, prostatic massage, and catheterization for acute urine retention, which may result in a return to adequate voiding function. Other therapies include alpha-adrenergic drugs, such as terazosin and prazosin, to relax the external sphincter and prevent contractions of the prostatic capsule, prostatectomy (transurethral, retropubic, suprapubic, or peroneal) for patients with moderate to severe obstruction, and cryosurgery or transurethral balloon urethroplasty for patients who are poor surgical risks.

600.00 Hypertrophy (benign) of prostate without urinary obstruction — (Use additional code to identify urinary incontinence: 788.30-788.39) — *benign prostatic hypertrophy*
AHA: Q1, 2003, 6

600.01 Hypertrophy (benign) of prostate with urinary obstruction — (Use additional code to identify urinary incontinence: 788.30-788.39) — *benign prostatic hypertrophy*
AHA: Q1, 2003, 6; Q4, 2003, 64

600.10 Nodular prostate without urinary obstruction — (Use additional code to identify urinary incontinence: 788.30-788.39) — *small mass of tissue that swells, knots, or is a protuberance in the prostate*

© 2004 Ingenix, Inc.

600.11 Nodular prostate with urinary obstruction — (Use additional code to identify urinary incontinence: 788.30-788.39) — *small mass of tissue that swells, knots, or is a protuberance in the prostate, impeding the flow of urine*

600.20 Benign localized hyperplasia of prostate without urinary obstruction — (Use additional code to identify urinary incontinence: 788.30-788.39) — *associated with age, enlargement caused by proliferation of grandular and stromal elements; typically starting in the fifth decade of life*

600.21 Benign localized hyperplasia of prostate with urinary obstruction — (Use additional code to identify urinary incontinence: 788.30-788.39) — *associated with age, enlargement caused by proliferation of grandular and stromal elements; typically starting in the fifth decade of life, impeding the flow of urine*

600.90 Hyperplasia of prostate, unspecified, without urinary obstruction — (Use additional code to identify urinary incontinence: 788.30-788.39) — *associated with age, enlargement caused by proliferation of grandular and stromal elements; typically starting in the fifth decade of life*

600.91 Hyperplasia of prostate, unspecified, with urinary obstruction — (Use additional code to identify urinary incontinence: 788.30-788.39)

Coding Clarification

Use an additional code to identify urinary incontinence (788.30-788.39). Excluded from this rubric are benign neoplasm of the prostate (222.2) and malignant neoplasm of the prostate (185).

Bladder Outlet Obstruction: In cases of benign prostatic hypertrophy with bladder outlet obstruction, the prostatic hypertrophy with urinary obstruction (600.01) is listed.

Coding Scenario

A 69-year-old male is admitted to the facility with urinary retention and undergoes a transurethral resection of the prostate (TURP). The final diagnosis is benign prostatic hypertrophy.

> Code assignment: 600.01 *Hypertrophy (benign) of prostate, with urinary obstruction* and 788.20 *Retention of urine, unspecified*

601 Inflammatory diseases of prostate

601.0 Acute prostatitis — (Use additional code to identify organism: 041.0, 041.1) — *sudden onset of inflammation of prostate*

601.1 Chronic prostatitis — (Use additional code to identify organism: 041.0, 041.1) — *persistent inflammation of prostate*

601.2 Abscess of prostate — (Use additional code to identify organism: 041.0, 041.1) — *pus pocket in wall of prostate*

601.3 Prostatocystitis — (Use additional code to identify organism: 041.0, 041.1) — *inflammation of both prostate and bladder*

601.4 Prostatitis in diseases classified elsewhere — (Code first underlying disease: 016.5, 039.8, 095.8, 116.0. Use additional code to identify organism: 041.0, 041.1)

601.8 Other specified inflammatory disease of prostate — (Use additional code to identify organism: 041.0, 041.1) — *cavitary prostatitis; granulomatous prostatitis*

601.9 Unspecified prostatitis — (Use additional code to identify organism: 041.0, 041.1) — *prostatitis NOS*

Coding Clarification

Use an additional code to identify the infective agent, such as Staphylococcus (041.1) or Streptococcus (041.0). For prostatitis in diseases classified elsewhere, code first the underlying disease. Excluded from this rubric are gonococcal prostatitis (098.12, 098.32), monilial prostatitis (112.2), and trichomonal prostatitis (131.03).

602 Other disorders of prostate

602.0 Calculus of prostate — *prostatic stone*

602.1 Congestion or hemorrhage of prostate — *bleeding or collection of fluid in prostate*

602.2 Atrophy of prostate — *loss of prostatic tissue*

602.3 Dysplasia of prostate — *prostatic intraepithelial neoplasia I (PIN I) and prostatic intraepithelial neoplasia II (PIN II)*
AHA: Q4, 2001, 46

602.8 Other specified disorder of prostate — *prostatic fistula; prostatic infarction; periprostatic adhesions; prostatorrhea*

602.9 Unspecified disorder of prostate — *palpable prostate*

Coding Clarification

This subcategory excludes prostatic intraepithelial neoplasia III (PIN III), which is reported with code 233.4.

603 Hydrocele

Included in this rubric is a hydrocele of the spermatic cord, testis, or tunica vaginalis. The tunica vaginalis is the double-layer membrane that surrounds each testis; it consists of an outer parietal layer and an inner visceral serous layer. In the embryo, the tunica

© 2004 Ingenix, Inc.

vaginalis is an extension of the peritoneum, the membrane in the abdominal cavity. If, after it separates, the closure is not complete, fluid collects above the testes in a painless swelling called a hydrocele.

603.0 Encysted hydrocele

603.1 Infected hydrocele — (Use additional code to identify organism) — *infection in fluid-filled sac in testicular membrane*

603.8 Other specified type of hydrocele — *other specified hydrocele NEC*

603.9 Unspecified hydrocele — *hydrocele NOS*

Coding Clarification

Excluded from this rubric is a congenital hydrocele, reported with 778.6.

604 Orchitis and epididymitis

The testes are two small oval glands contained in the scrotum. The left testis is usually about 1.0 centimeter lower in the scrotal sac than the right. Both are suspended in the pouch by scrotal tissue and the spermatic cords; they are separated by a central partition. Dense, fibrous tissue, the tunica albuginea, encases each testis, enters the gland, and divides the glandular tissue into some 200 or 300 lobules. Each lobule contains coiled seminiferous tubules that produce sperm and which converge into about 20 small ducts that pass through the tunica albuginea and enter the epididymis.

The testes have two main functions: the production of sperm (spermatogenesis) and the secretion of hormones, mostly testosterone, which is responsible for the development of sexual characteristics in adolescent males and for the functioning of the male reproductive system.

Each epididymis lies along the top and back of the testis. It consists of a single, tightly coiled tube, enclosed in fibrous connective tissue casing. The epididymis tube is extremely small in diameter, but about 6.0 meters long. It forms a comma-shaped structure, with the blunt head at the top, a central body, and a tapered tail, which connects to the vas deferens.

The epididymis has three main functions, serving as one of the ducts through which the sperm pass, as a storage reservoir for maturing sperm, and as a contributor to seminal fluid.

604.0 Orchitis, epididymitis, and epididymo-orchitis, with abscess — (Use additional code to identify organism: 041.0, 041.1, 041.4) — *testicular abscess*

604.90 Unspecified orchitis and epididymitis — (Use additional code to identify organism: 041.0, 041.1, 041.4) — *orchitis and epididymitis NOS*

604.91 Orchitis and epididymitis in disease classified elsewhere — (Code first underlying disease: 032.89, 095.8, 125.0-125.9. Use additional code to identify organism: 041.0, 041.1, 041.4)

604.99 Other orchitis, epididymitis, and epididymo-orchitis, without mention of abscess — (Use additional code to identify organism: 041.0, 041.1, 041.4) — *orchitis, epididymitis and epididymo-orchitis, without mention of abscess NOS*

Coding Clarification

Use an additional code to identify the infective agent, such as *E. coli* (041.4), *Staphylococcus* (041.1), or *Streptococcus* (041.0). For orchitis and epididymitis in diseases classified elsewhere, code first the underlying disease. Excluded from this rubric are gonococcal orchitis (098.13, 098.33), mumps (072.0), tuberculous orchitis (016.5), and tuberculous epididymitis (016.4).

605 Redundant prepuce and phimosis OK

The prepuce is the double-layered sheath of skin covering the glans. Fused to the glans at birth by a shared membrane, the foreskin separates from the glans as the membrane dissolves. Phimosis refers to narrowness of the preputial sphincter that prevents the foreskin from being drawn back over the glans. A long foreskin, often due to redundant prepuce, may retain moisture, affecting the inner aspect of the prepuce and the glans. Balanitis, an inflammation of the glans, may develop in the devitalized tissues. Phimosis and persistent balanitis are the most common medical reasons for circumcision in the United States.

606 Male infertility

AHA: Q2, 1996, 9

A male is considered infertile when either of the two following conditions exists:

1. Inadequate sperm production: about 20 million sperm per milliliter of fluid is considered the lower limit of male fertility.
2. Abnormality in structure or motility of sperm that makes it unable to reach or penetrate the egg.

The most common male infertility factors include azoospermia (no sperm cells are produced) and oligospermia (few sperm cells are produced). Sometimes, sperm cells are malformed or they die before they can reach the egg. In some cases, a genetic disease such a cystic fibrosis or a chromosomal abnormality may be a factor.

Conditions that can cause male infertility include:

© 2004 Ingenix, Inc.

- Varicose veins in the spermatic cord since blood retained around the testes leads to an increase in temperature, which damages sperm
- Undescended testicles, which creates a higher temperature within the testes and, subsequently, impairs sperm production
- Radiation, chemotherapy, or removal of one or both testicles
- Hypothalamic or pituitary disorder
- Drug use, including alcohol, marijuana, female sex hormones, and the drugs used in chemotherapy

In addition, according to studies, the average sperm count is dropping worldwide, which may be due to both occupational and environmental exposure to chemicals that can disrupt hormone functions.

Tests for male infertility include sperm and semen analysis, physical exam for factors such as obstruction or congenital abnormality, a medical history as to the possibility of hormonal abnormality. The physical exam may indicate small, soft testicles, and hormone testing for FSH and testosterone may suggest that hormonal treatment may be beneficial. A biopsy can indicate if infection, injury, or other abnormality is interfering with the testis ability to produce sperm. Genetic testing may be performed to analyze whether azoospermia is associated with a chromosomal or DNA abnormality.

Between 30 and 50 percent of infertility in couples is attributable to the male.

606.0 Azoospermia — *Sertoli cell syndrome; Del Castillo's syndrome; infertility due to germinal cell aplasia*
AHA: Q2, 1996, 9

606.1 Oligospermia — *due to germinal cell desquamation; hypospermatogenesis*
AHA: Q2, 1996, 9

606.8 Infertility due to extratesticular causes — *due to drug therapy, infection, radiation*
AHA: Q2, 1996, 9

606.9 Unspecified male infertility

Coding Clarification

To report sperm count for fertility testing, see V26.21 *Fertility testing* or V26.22 *Aftercare following sterilization reversal.*

607 Disorders of penis

The penis is the organ of copulation and lies under the bladder, with the apex pointing downwards. It is composed of three cylindrical layers of tissue, which are enclosed in fibrous connective tissue, with an outer layer of skin. The smaller, lower cylinder is called the corpus spongiosum, through which the urethra passes to the external urinary meatus. The two upper and larger cylinders are the corpora cavernosa. At the end of the penis, the corpus spongiosum overlaps the ends of the corpora cavernosa, forming the bulging structure of the glans penis. Over this is a double fold of retractable skin called the prepuce, or foreskin. Surgical removal of foreskin is called circumcision.

The functions of the penis are copulation and to provide transport of semen through the urethra. Urine from the bladder is also excreted via the urethra.

Peyronie's disease is distinguished by plaque, or hard lump, that forms on the penis, due to causes unknown. The plaque develops on the upper or lower side of the penis in layers containing erectile tissue. It begins as a localized inflammation and can develop into a hardened scar.

Cases of Peyronie's disease range from mild to severe. Symptoms may develop slowly or appear overnight. Most of the time, the plaque that has hardened reduces flexibility, causing pain and forcing the penis to bend or arc during erection. The pain typically decreases over time, but the bend in the penis may remain a problem, making sexual intercourse complicated. In a small percentage of patients with the milder form of the disease, inflammation may resolve without pain or bending.

607.0 Leukoplakia of penis — *kraurosis*

607.1 Balanoposthitis — (Use additional code to identify organism) — *balanitis*

607.2 Other inflammatory disorders of penis — (Use additional code to identify organism) — *boil of corpus cavernosum*

607.3 Priapism — *painful erection*

607.81 Balanitis xerotica obliterans — *induratio penis plastica*

607.82 Vascular disorders of penis — *embolism of corpus cavernosum; hemorrhage of corpus cavernosum*

607.83 Edema of penis — *edema*

607.84 Impotence of organic origin — *impotence, organic*
AHA: Q3, 1991, 11

607.85 Peyronie's disease — *hardening of the corpora cavernosa of the penis, producing a fibrous chordee*
AHA: Q4, 2003, 64

607.89 Other specified disorder of penis — *atrophy of corpus cavernosum; cicatrix; phagedena*

607.9 Unspecified disorder of penis — *disorder NOS*

Coding Clarification

Excluded from this rubric is phimosis (605).

580–629

608 Other disorders of male genital organs

608.0 Seminal vesiculitis — (Use additional code to identify organism) — *abscess of seminal vesicle; vesiculitis (seminal)*

608.1 Spermatocele — *epididymal cyst filled with sperm-containing fluid*

608.2 Torsion of testis — *spermatic cord torsion; testicular torsion*

608.3 Atrophy of testis — *wasting of testicular tissue*

608.4 Other inflammatory disorder of male genital organs — (Use additional code to identify organism) — *scrotal boil; cellulitis of testicle*

608.81 Specified disorder of male genital organs in diseases classified elsewhere — (Code first underlying disease: 016.5, 125.0-125.9)

608.82 Hematospermia — *blood in ejaculate*
AHA: Q4, 2001, 46

608.83 Specified vascular disorder of male genital organs — *testicular hematoma; hematocele, NOS, male*
AHA: Q4, 2003, 110

608.84 Chylocele of tunica vaginalis — *chylocele*

608.85 Stricture of male genital organs — *stricture of vas deferens*

608.86 Edema of male genital organs — *fluid retention in male reproductive structure*

608.87 Retrograde ejaculation

608.89 Other specified disorder of male genital organs — *specified disorders NEC*

608.9 Unspecified disorder of male genital organs — *neuralgia; pain*

Coding Clarification
Use an additional code to identify the infective agent in infections and inflammatory disorders. In disorders of male genital organs in disease classified elsewhere, code first the underlying disease.

610–611 Disorders of Breast

The mammary glands are accessory organs of the female reproductive system, and are contained within the breast.

Each breast contains 15 to 20 lobes of glandular tissue consisting of smaller lobuli of alveoli (secreting cells) and ducts. The smaller ducts unite into a single milk-carrying duct for each lobe and these converge toward the nipple. The glandular tissue is contained within dense connective tissue that attaches to the pectoral muscle with suspensory ligaments, which extend from the skin to the pectoral muscle to provide support.

The nipple is located near the tip of each breast, surrounded by a circular area of pigmented and irregular surfaced skin called the areola.

The function of the mammary gland is lactation, which is the secretion of colostrum and subsequently milk for the nourishment of newborn infants. Successful lactation relies on pre- and postnatal production of hormones including progesterone, estrogen, prolactin, and oxytocin.

610 Benign mammary dysplasias

Benign mammary dysplasia, also known as chronic cystic mastitis or fibrocystic breast disease, is commonly found in normal breasts and believed to be a normal variant of tissue, and not a disease. Symptoms include a dense, irregular, and bumpy consistency in the breast tissue, especially in the outer upper quadrants and breast discomfort that is persistent or that occurs intermittently. Symptoms may range from mild to severe and typically peak just before each menstrual period and improve immediately after the menstrual period. Self-care may include restricting dietary fat and caffeine. Oral contraceptives may be prescribed because they often decrease the symptoms. Danazol, a synthetic androgen, may be used in severe cases.

610.0 Solitary cyst of breast — *cyst (solitary)*

610.1 Diffuse cystic mastopathy — *cysts scattered throughout*

610.2 Fibroadenosis of breast — *cystic fibroadenosis of breast; diffuse fibroadenosis*

610.3 Fibrosclerosis of breast — *fibrosclerosis*

610.4 Mammary duct ectasia — *periductal mastitis*

610.8 Other specified benign mammary dysplasias — *mazoplasia; sebaceous cyst*

610.9 Unspecified benign mammary dysplasia — *benign NOS*

611 Other disorders of breast

611.0 Inflammatory disease of breast — *acute or chronic abscess of areola; mammillary fistula; acute or subacute mastitis*

611.1 Hypertrophy of breast — *massive pubertal hypertrophy*

611.2 Fissure of nipple — *crack in nipple*

611.3 Fat necrosis of breast — *fat necrosis (segmental)*

611.4 Atrophy of breast — *wasting of breast tissue*

611.5 Galactocele

611.6 Galactorrhea not associated with childbirth — *flow of milk*

611.71 Mastodynia — *pain*

580–629

 © 2004 Ingenix, Inc.

611.72 Lump or mass in breast — *lump*
AHA: Q2, 2003, 4-5

611.79 Other sign and symptom in breast — *induration; inversion of nipple; thickening*

611.8 Other specified disorder of breast — *hematoma, (nontraumatic); infarction; pendulous*

611.9 Unspecified breast disorder — *disorder NOS*

614–616 Inflammatory Disease of Female Pelvic Organs

614 Inflammatory disease of ovary, fallopian tube, pelvic cellular tissue, and peritoneum

614.0 Acute salpingitis and oophoritis — (Use additional code to identify organism: 041.0, 041.1) — *any condition classifiable to 614.2, specified as acute or subacute*

614.1 Chronic salpingitis and oophoritis — (Use additional code to identify organism: 041.0, 041.1) — *hydrosalpinx; salpingitis follicularis*

614.2 Salpingitis and oophoritis not specified as acute, subacute, or chronic — (Use additional code to identify organism: 041.0, 041.1) — *pyosalpinx; tubo-ovarian inflammatory disease*
AHA: Q2, 1991, 5

614.3 Acute parametritis and pelvic cellulitis — (Use additional code to identify organism: 041.0, 041.1) — *acute inflammatory pelvic disease*

614.4 Chronic or unspecified parametritis and pelvic cellulitis — (Use additional code to identify organism: 041.0, 041.1) — *chronic inflammatory pelvic disease; abscess of broad ligament; pelvic cellulitis*

614.5 Acute or unspecified pelvic peritonitis, female — (Use additional code to identify organism: 041.0, 041.1) — *metroperitonitis*

614.6 Pelvic peritoneal adhesions, female (postoperative) (postinfection) — (Use additional code to identify any associated infertility, 628.2. Use additional code to identify organism: 041.0, 041.1) — *peritubal adhesions, tubo-ovarian adhesions*
AHA: Q3, 1994, 12; Q3, 1995, 7; Q1, 2003, 4; Q3, 2003, 6

614.7 Other chronic pelvic peritonitis, female — (Use additional code to identify organism: 041.0, 041.1)

614.8 Other specified inflammatory disease of female pelvic organs and tissues — (Use additional code to identify organism: 041.0, 041.1) — *specified inflammatory disease of female pelvic organs and tissues NEC*

614.9 Unspecified inflammatory disease of female pelvic organs and tissues — (Use additional code to identify organism: 041.0, 041.1)

615 Inflammatory diseases of uterus, except cervix

615.0 Acute inflammatory disease of uterus, except cervix — (Use additional code to identify organism: 041.0, 041.1) — *any condition classifiable to 615.9, specified as acute or subacute*

615.1 Chronic inflammatory disease of uterus, except cervix — (Use additional code to identify organism: 041.0, 041.1) — *any condition classifiable to 615.9, specified as chronic*

615.9 Unspecified inflammatory disease of uterus — (Use additional code to identify organism: 041.0, 041.1) — *endometritis; endomyometritis; perimetritis; pyometra*

616 Inflammatory disease of cervix, vagina, and vulva

616.0 Cervicitis and endocervicitis — (Use additional code to identify organism: 041.0, 041.1) — *cervicitis with or without mention of erosion or ectropion; Nabothian (gland) cyst of follicle*

616.10 Unspecified vaginitis and vulvovaginitis — (Use additional code to identify organism: 041.0, 041.1, 041.4) — *postirradiation vaginitis; vaginitis NOS*

616.11 Vaginitis and vulvovaginitis in diseases classified elsewhere — (Code first underlying disease, 127.4.)

616.2 Cyst of Bartholin's gland — (Use additional code to identify organism: 041.0, 041.1) — *fluid-filled sac within one of the paired glands*

616.3 Abscess of Bartholin's gland — (Use additional code to identify organism: 041.0, 041.1) — *pocket of pus within one of the paired glands*

616.4 Other abscess of vulva — (Use additional code to identify organism: 041.0, 041.1) — *vulvar carbuncle; vulvar boil*

616.50 Unspecified ulceration of vulva — (Use additional code to identify organism: 041.0, 041.1) — *ulcer NOS of vulva*

616.51 Ulceration of vulva in disease classified elsewhere — (Code first underlying disease: 016.7, 136.1.)

616.8 Other specified inflammatory disease of cervix, vagina, and vulva — (Use additional code to identify organism: 041.0, 041.1) — *caruncle of vagina or labium*

616.9 Unspecified inflammatory disease of cervix, vagina, and vulva — (Use additional code to identify organism: 041.0, 041.1) — *vaginal disorder NOS*

617–629 Other Disorders of Female Genital Tract

617 Endometriosis

Endometriosis is the presence of endometrial tissue (functioning endometrial glands and stoma) outside of its normal location (lining the uterine cavity). The etiology is unknown, though previous uterine surgery or heredity may be predisposing factors.

Signs and symptoms of endometriosis include acquired dysmenorrhea characterized by pain (that usually begins five to seven days before menstruation and lasts two to three days) in the lower abdomen, vagina, posterior pelvis, or back; bleeding from the vagina, rectum, or bladder depending on the site involved; dyspareunia; or cramps. A pelvic exam may locate sites of endometriosis, while laparoscopy confirms the diagnosis and stage of disease. Diagnostic radiology such as barium enema may rule out malignancy or inflammatory bowel disease.

Therapies include drugs such as progestins, danazol (a testosterone derivative), oral contraceptives, surgery ranging from local excision of endometrial tissue and preservation of the pelvic organs (for women who wish to bear children) to total abdominal hysterectomy with bilateral salpingo-oophorectomy (for older women and those with extensive disease).

Associated conditions include infertility, spontaneous abortion, and pelvic adhesions.

617.0 Endometriosis of uterus — *adenomyosis; cervical endometriosis*
AHA: Q3, 1992, 7

617.1 Endometriosis of ovary — *chocolate cyst of ovary; endometrial cystoma of ovary*

617.2 Endometriosis of fallopian tube — *aberrant uterine mucosal tissue inflaming tissues of fallopian tube*

617.3 Endometriosis of pelvic peritoneum — *aberrant uterine mucosal tissue inflaming tissues of peritoneum*

617.4 Endometriosis of rectovaginal septum and vagina — *aberrant uterine mucosal tissue inflaming tissues behind or in vagina*

617.5 Endometriosis of intestine — *endometriosis of appendix, colon or rectum*

617.6 Endometriosis in scar of skin — *aberrant uterine mucosal tissue inflaming scar tissues*

617.8 Endometriosis of other specified sites — *endometriosis of bladder, lung, umbilicus, vulva*

617.9 Endometriosis, site unspecified — *endometriosis NOS*

618 Genital prolapse

Genital prolapse is the protrusion or projection of pelvic organs into the vagina or outside the vaginal opening caused by weakening or damaged support structures. Types of prolapse include:

- Uterine prolapse: descent of the uterus and cervix down the vaginal canal due to weak or damaged pelvic support structures
- Cystocele: tissues supporting the wall between the bladder and the vagina weaken, allowing a portion of the bladder to descend and protrude into the vagina
- Urethrocele: urethra descends and presses into the vagina
- Rectocele: tissues supporting the wall between the vagina and the rectum weaken allowing the rectum to descend and protrude into the vagina
- Enterocele: portion of intestine herniates and protrudes into the vagina
- Vaginal vault prolapse: vagina descends, usually following a hysterectomy
- A perineocele in the female is a hernia in the perineum occurring between the rectum and the vagina. In the male, it is a hernia between the rectum and prostate.

Symptoms of prolapse vary according to the organs involved and the severity of the prolapse. Those commonly reported include aching discomfort in the pelvic region, urinary and bowel problems, and dull backache.

There are a number of contributing factors that can cause genital prolapse, including pregnancy and childbirth, menopause, raised pressure in the abdomen, and genetic predisposition.

Diagnosis involves a medical history and a physical examination, including a rectal exam if a rectocele or enterocele is suspected. The woman may be asked to cough or push down during the exam to raise the pressure in the abdomen and push any prolapse downwards, making it easier to see or feel.

There is a range of treatment options available for prolapse, both non-surgical and surgical. Non-surgical approaches include reducing pressure placed on the pelvis, pessaries (e.g., device that is inserted into the upper part of the vagina to provide support to the pelvic structures), and hormonal therapy. Surgical treatment includes vaginal repair, hysterectomy and vaginal repair, vaginal vault repair, and uterine preservation surgery (i.e., partial amputation of the cervix and the shortening of supporting ligaments).

© 2004 Ingenix, Inc.

618.00 Prolapse of vaginal walls without mention of uterine prolapse, unspecified

618.01 Cystocele without mention of uterine prolapse, midline

618.02 Cystocele without mention of uterine prolapse, lateral

618.03 Urethrocele without mention of uterine prolapse

618.04 Rectocele without mention of uterine prolapse

618.05 Perineocele without mention of uterine prolapse

618.09 Other prolapse of vaginal walls without mention of uterine prolapse

618.1 Uterine prolapse without mention of vaginal wall prolapse — (Use additional code to identify urinary incontinence: 625.6, 788.31, 788.33-788.39) — *descensus uteri; complete uterine prolapse*

618.2 Uterovaginal prolapse, incomplete — (Use additional code to identify urinary incontinence: 625.6, 788.31, 788.33-788.39) — *downward displacement of uterus into vagina*

618.3 Uterovaginal prolapse, complete — (Use additional code to identify urinary incontinence: 625.6, 788.31, 788.33-788.39) — *downward displacement and exposure of uterus within external genitalia*

618.4 Uterovaginal prolapse, unspecified — (Use additional code to identify urinary incontinence: 625.6, 788.31, 788.33-788.39) — *uterine prolapse NOS*

618.5 Prolapse of vaginal vault after hysterectomy — (Use additional code to identify urinary incontinence: 625.6, 788.31, 788.33-788.39) — *posthysterectomy vaginal vault prolapse*

618.6 Vaginal enterocele, congenital or acquired — (Use additional code to identify urinary incontinence: 625.6, 788.31, 788.33-788.39) — *pelvic enterocele, congenital or acquired*

618.7 Genital prolapse, old laceration of muscles of pelvic floor — (Use additional code to identify urinary incontinence: 625.6, 788.31, 788.33-788.39)

618.81 Incompetence or weakening of pubocervical tissue

618.82 Incompetence or weakening of rectovaginal tissue

618.83 Pelvic muscle wasting

618.89 Other specified genital prolapse

618.9 Unspecified genital prolapse — (Use additional code to identify urinary incontinence: 625.6, 788.31, 788.33-788.39) — *prolapsus*

Coding Scenario

A 37-year-old woman who gave birth one year ago is experiencing sensations of bladder fullness, or incomplete emptying after urination and urine leakage or incontinence upon changing position. Upon physical examination, the physician notes bulging in the anterior vaginal wall, some loss of normal vaginal rugae, but the lateral vaginal sulcus is intact and diagnoses her with a central defect cystocele with overflow incontinence.

> Code assignment: 618.01 *Cystocele, midline* and 788.38 *Overflow incontinence*

619 Fistula involving female genital tract

A fistula is an abnormal channel or duct connecting an organ to another organ, body cavity, or the surface. Types include:

- Blind (open on one end, but connects to two structures)
- Complete (external and internal openings)
- Incomplete (tube from the skin is closed on the inside and does not connect to any internal organ or structure)

Fistulas of the female genital tract include rectovaginal, vesicovaginal, vaginoperineal, cervicovesical, ureterovaginal, urethrovesico-vaginal, and enterovaginal.

619.0 Urinary-genital tract fistula, female — *cervicovesical, ureterovaginal, urethrovesicovaginal fistula*

619.1 Digestive-genital tract fistula, female — *intestinouterine, rectovulvar, uterorectal fistula*

619.2 Genital tract-skin fistula, female — *vaginoperineal fistula*

619.8 Other specified fistula involving female genital tract — *cervical, vaginal fistula*

619.9 Unspecified fistula involving female genital tract — *genital tract fistula NOS*

620 Noninflammatory disorders of ovary, fallopian tube, and broad ligament

620.0 Follicular cyst of ovary — *cyst of graafian follicle*

620.1 Corpus luteum cyst or hematoma — *lutein cyst*

620.2 Other and unspecified ovarian cyst — *corpus albicans cyst of ovary; retention cyst NOS of ovary*

620.3 Acquired atrophy of ovary and fallopian tube — *senile involution of ovary*

620.4 Prolapse or hernia of ovary and fallopian tube — *displacement of ovary and fallopian tube; salpingocele*

620.5 Torsion of ovary, ovarian pedicle, or fallopian tube — *torsion of accessory tube; torsion of hydatid of Morgagni*

620.6 Broad ligament laceration syndrome — *Masters-Allen syndrome*

620.7 Hematoma of broad ligament — *hematocele, broad ligament*

620.8 Other noninflammatory disorder of ovary, fallopian tube, and broad ligament — *cyst of broad ligament; infarction of ovary or fallopian tube; ovarian remnant syndrome; spastic fallopian tube*

620.9 Unspecified noninflammatory disorder of ovary, fallopian tube, and broad ligament — *broad ligament disorder NOS*

621 Disorders of uterus, not elsewhere classified

A uterine polyp is a growth from the endometrium. The polyp can contain endometrial, fibrous and muscular tissue. The polyp may cause pain and bleeding and may interfere with fertility. Surgical intervention may be required to treat a symptomatic polyp.

Uterine subinvolution is failure of the uterus to return to normal size after a physiological hypertrophy as in child birth or infection. Treatment may include curettage, methergine or antibiotics.

Endometrial hyperplasia is described as an abnormal overgrowth of the normal cells that line the uterus, called the endometrium. This overgrowth often causes heavy or prolonged menstrual flow (menorrhagia), bleeding after menopause, and bleeding between normal periods or at irregular intervals (metrorrhagia). Endometrial hyperplasia results from estrogen production in excess or prolonged amounts of estrogen, such as a reaction to hormone replacement therapy after menopause. The difference between simple and complex is determined by cytology studies where arborescent cell clusters are observed along with the types of branching and number of layers of stromal bundles inside the clusters.

621.0 Polyp of corpus uteri — *endometrial polyp*

621.1 Chronic subinvolution of uterus

621.2 Hypertrophy of uterus — *bulky uterus*

621.30 Endometrial hyperplasia, unspecified

621.31 Simple endometrial hyperplasia without atypia

621.32 Complex endometrial hyperplasia without atypia

621.33 Endometrial hyperplasia with atypia

621.4 Hematometra

621.5 Intrauterine synechiae — *adhesions of uterus; Asherman's syndrome*

621.6 Malposition of uterus — *anteversion of uterus; retroflexion of uterus*

621.7 Chronic inversion of uterus — *uterus is turned inside out*

621.8 Other specified disorders of uterus, not elsewhere classified — *boggy uterus; sclerotic endometrium*

621.9 Unspecified disorder of uterus — *uterine disorder NOS*

622 Noninflammatory disorders of cervix

Cervical dysplasia is described as abnormal cells in the cervix. These cells are precancerous and could lead to invasive carcinoma. Cervical dysplasia is usually asymptomatic and is usually diagnosed by annual Pap smears from the cervix. The difference between mild and moderate dysplasia of the cervix is based on cytology studies. CIN grade I is considered mild dysplasia and CIN grade II is considered moderate dysplasia.

622.0 Erosion and ectropion of cervix — *ulcer of cervix*

622.10 Dysplasia of cervix, unspecified

622.11 Mild dysplasia of cervix

622.12 Moderate dysplasia of cervix

622.2 Leukoplakia of cervix (uteri)

622.3 Old laceration of cervix — *adhesions of cervix*

622.4 Stricture and stenosis of cervix — *atresia (acquired) of cervix; cervical contracture*

622.5 Incompetence of cervix — *cervical incompetence*

622.6 Hypertrophic elongation of cervix — *overgrowth of cervix extends downward into vagina*

622.7 Mucous polyp of cervix — *polyp NOS of cervix*

622.8 Other specified noninflammatory disorder of cervix — *senile) atrophy of cervix; fibrosis of cervix*

622.9 Unspecified noninflammatory disorder of cervix — *noninflammatory NOS*

Coding Clarification

Report 233.1 for CIN grade III or severe cervical dysplasia.

Report 795.04 for Pap smear of the cervix with low grade squamous intraepithelial lesion (LGSIL).

Report 795.05 for Pap smear of the cervix with high grade squamous intraepithelial lesion (HGSIL).

© 2004 Ingenix, Inc.

623 Noninflammatory disorders of vagina

623.0 Dysplasia of vagina — *abnormal cells*

623.1 Leukoplakia of vagina — *thickened white patches*

623.2 Stricture or atresia of vagina — (Use additional E code to identify any external cause)

623.3 Tight hymenal ring — *rigid hymen, acquired or congenital; tight introitus*

623.4 Old vaginal laceration — *scarring*

623.5 Leukorrhea, not specified as infective — *thick, white discharge*

623.6 Vaginal hematoma — *blood pocket*

623.7 Polyp of vagina — *mucosal growth*

623.8 Other specified noninflammatory disorder of vagina

623.9 Unspecified noninflammatory disorder of vagina — *noninflammatory disease NOS*

624 Noninflammatory disorders of vulva and perineum

624.0 Dystrophy of vulva — *kraurosis; leukoplakia*

624.1 Atrophy of vulva — *wasting of external genitalia*

624.2 Hypertrophy of clitoris — *overgrowth of erectile body at anterior cleft of vulva*

624.3 Hypertrophy of labia — *vulvar hypertrophy NOS*

624.4 Old laceration or scarring of vulva

624.5 Hematoma of vulva — *pocket of blood in tussue*

624.6 Polyp of labia and vulva — *mucosal growth*

624.8 Other specified noninflammatory disorder of vulva and perineum — *cyst; edema; vitiligo*
AHA: Q1, 1995, 8; Q1, 2003, 13

624.9 Unspecified noninflammatory disorder of vulva and perineum — *unspecified*

625 Pain and other symptoms associated with female genital organs

625.0 Dyspareunia — *pain during sexual intercourse*

625.1 Vaginismus — *colpospasm; vulvismus*

625.2 Mittelschmerz — *ovulation pain*

625.3 Dysmenorrhea — *painful menstruation*
AHA: Q2, 1994, 12

625.4 Premenstrual tension syndromes — *premenstrual syndrome; menstrual migraine*
AHA: Q4, 2003, 116

625.5 Pelvic congestion syndrome — *congestion-fibrosis syndrome*

625.6 Female stress incontinence — *involuntary escape of urine during coughing, laughing or sneezing*

625.8 Other specified symptom associated with female genital organs — *palpable uterus; perineal swelling; vicarious (nasal) menstruation*
AHA: Nov-Dec, 1985, 16

625.9 Unspecified symptom associated with female genital organs — *pain in broad ligament, ovary, round ligament*

626 Disorders of menstruation and other abnormal bleeding from female genital tract

A woman's monthly cycle can be divided into three segments: menstruation, the follicular phase, and the luteal phase. During the middle, or follicular, segment, follicle stimulating hormone (FSH) prompts eggs in the ovary to mature and sprout a follicle, or layer of cells, which secrete estrogen. Estrogen levels then build until at their peak FSH is turned off and luteinizing hormone (LH) takes over. LH causes ovulation, the departure of the egg from the ovary. Progesterone, master hormone of the last, or luteal, stage continues development of the endometrium, the lining of the uterus. When conception does not occur, all hormone levels drop and menstruation begins. Uterine muscles contracting to squeeze out the lining may cause cramping; painful cramping is thought to be due to higher levels of prostaglandins. The egg bursting out of the ovary can cause pain on one side low in the abdomen 12 to 14 days after a period. Menstruation can begin at any time between the ages of 8 to 18; menopause generally occurs between the ages of 40 to 60.

626.0 Absence of menstruation — *amenorrhea (primary) (secondary)*

626.1 Scanty or infrequent menstruation — *hypomenorrhea; oligomenorrhea*

626.2 Excessive or frequent menstruation — *menometrorrhagia; menorrhagia; polymenorrhea*
AHA: Q2, 1994, 12

626.3 Puberty bleeding — *pubertal menorrhagia*

626.4 Irregular menstrual cycle — *irregular periods*

626.5 Ovulation bleeding — *regular intermenstrual bleeding*

626.6 Metrorrhagia — *irregular intermenstrual bleeding*

626.7 Postcoital bleeding — *vaginal bleeding after sexual intercourse*

626.8 Other disorder of menstruation and other abnormal bleeding from female genital tract — *delayed menstruation*

626.9 Unspecified disorder of menstruation and other abnormal bleeding from female genital tract — *paramenia*

627 Menopausal and postmenopausal disorders

Menopause refers to a process occurring in a female's reproductive life. Physically, this process has four stages:

1. Premenopause refers to the cusp of menopause. Periods may be irregular, but there are no classic menopausal symptoms such as hot flashes or vaginal dryness. Irregularity can run from shorter or longer periods with bouts of amenorrhea (no period).
2. Perimenopause refers to the onset of symptoms, such as erratic periods, hot flashes, and vaginal dryness, which are indicators of a drop in estrogen. This stage lasts about four years, covering the first two years prior to the last period to the next two years following the last menstrual period. Decreased levels of estrogen affects REM sleep, which precipitates the stress, depression, and anxiety associated with menopause.
3. Menopause refers to the final menstrual period, which is marked once the female has had no periods for one year. Vaginal bleeding after more than one year of a menstrual period is considered normal.
4. Postmenopause refers to the third of a woman's life, ranging from women who have been free of menstrual periods for at least one year to women celebrating a century birthday.

Use subclassification 627.1 to report bleeding from the female reproductive tract (vulva, vagina, cervix, or endometrium) occurring one year or more after menopause.

Signs and symptoms of postmenopausal bleeding include vaginal bleeding, excess cervical mucus, and atrophy of vaginal mucosa. Lab work such as analysis of cytologic smears from the cervix and endocervical canal, blood work to assess hormone levels, and dilation and curettage (D&C) may show pathological findings in the endometrium.

Therapies include estrogen creams to correct estrogen deficiency, D&C, and hysterectomy for endometrial carcinoma.

Associated conditions include hormonal imbalances, cancer, atrophic changes of the vagina or endometrium, and adverse effects of estrogen therapy.

627.0 Premenopausal menorrhagia — *climacteric menorrhagia; preclimacteric menorrhagia*

627.1 Postmenopausal bleeding — *bleeding after onset of menopause*

627.2 Symptomatic menopausal or female climacteric states — *climacteric syndrome*

627.3 Postmenopausal atrophic vaginitis — *senile (atrophic) vaginitis*

627.4 Symptomatic states associated with artificial menopause — *postartificial menopause syndromes*

627.8 Other specified menopausal and postmenopausal disorder — *atrophic menopausal cervix; postmenopausal endometrium (atrophic)*

627.9 Unspecified menopausal and postmenopausal disorder — *menopausal disorder NOS*

Coding Clarification

To report post-menopausal status without symptoms or disorder, see V49.81 *Postmenopausal status* (age-related) (natural). Excluded from this rubric is premature menopause NOS, classifiable to 256.31.

628 Female infertility

AHA: Q1, 1995, 7; Q2, 1996, 9

This rubric classifies the inability to conceive for at least a one year period after regular intercourse in the absence of contraceptive measures. There are three basic types of infertility: functional, anatomic, and psychogenic.

Functional infertility is due to impairment of the complex hormonal interactions involved in female reproduction. Anatomic infertility can be the result of congenital malformation, scarring or adhesions due to previous infection, atrophy due to hormone deficiency, or any other condition that mechanically impairs or prevents conception. An example of psychogenic infertility is the failure to ovulate due to the stress of marital discord (codes 628.0 and 306.59).

628.0 Female infertility associated with anovulation — (Use additional code for any associated Stein-Levanthal syndrome, 256.4) — *anovulatory cycle*
AHA: Q1, 1995, 7; Q2, 1996, 9

628.1 Female infertility of pituitary-hypothalamic origin — (Code first underlying disease: 253.0-253.4, 253.8)

628.2 Female infertility of tubal origin — (Use additional code for any associated peritubal adhesions, 614.6) — *tubal occlusion; tubal stenosis*
AHA: Q1, 1995, 7; Q2, 1996, 9

628.3 Female infertility of uterine origin — (Use additional code for any associated tuberculous endometriosis, 016.7) — *infertility associated with congenital anomaly of uterus; nonimplantation*
AHA: Q1, 1995, 7; Q2, 1996, 9

 © 2004 Ingenix, Inc.

628.4 Female infertility of cervical or vaginal origin — *infertility associated with anomaly of cervical mucus, or congenital structural anomaly*
AHA: Q1, 1995, 7; Q2, 1996, 9

628.8 Female infertility of other specified origin — *other specified cause*
AHA: Q1, 1995, 7; Q2, 1996, 9

628.9 Female infertility of unspecified origin — *unknown cause*
AHA: Q1, 1995, 7; Q2, 1996, 9

Coding Clarification

As appropriate, code first the underlying cause, as in adiposogenital dystrophy (253.8) or anterior pituitary disorder (253.0-253.4).

629 Other disorders of female genital organs

Although not practiced in this country, female circumcision or castration is practiced in other countries, from which the U.S. is receiving a number of immigrant populations. The World Health Organization has termed this as female genital mutilation, or FGM. Women who have undergone this type of mutilation present with a special set of serious problems and concerns not normally seen in relation to gynecological healthcare. Problems include difficult intercourse, childbirth, and pelvic infections. Those physicians who see a large immigrant population may have up to two thirds of their female patients present with some form of FGM.

Three levels of genital mutilation are practiced. The first type is known as clitoridectomy, with part or the entire clitoris removed. The second type involves the clitoris and the labia minora being amputated. These two types account for 85% of those who have had female castration performed. The third type is a severe form in which the clitoris is removed and most or all of the labia minora are also cut off. The labia majora are incised and made into a hood of skin to heal over the urethral and vaginal opening. After healing, another small opening is made for release of urine and menstrual blood. This third type is called infibulation. These patients require deinfibulation to permit intercourse, the deliver of a baby, or a pelvic exam. They also present with many more pelvic infections due to the interference of fluid drainage. Some women may also have had deinfibulation done to deliver a baby and then been reinfibulated. A greater risk of maternal and fetal death occurs for subsequent pregnancies.

629.0 Hematocele, female, not elsewhere classified

629.1 Hydrocele, canal of Nuck — *cyst of canal of Nuck (acquired)*

629.20 Female genital mutilation status, unspecified

629.21 Female genital mutilation, Type I status

629.22 Female genital mutilation, Type II status

629.23 Female genital mutilation, Type III status

629.8 Other specified disorder of female genital organs — *hydrocele of round ligament; ulcer of genital organ*

629.9 Unspecified disorder of female genital organs — *habitual aborter without current pregnancy*

Coding Scenario

A 25-year-old immigrant woman is seen by a physician with intense pelvic and vulvar pain. He suspects a severe pelvic inflammatory condition or infection and upon examination, notes that access to the introitus is severely compromised with external genitalia in a healed, but mutilated appearance. It is necessary for the artificially created covering to be surgically removed before any pelvic exam can be carried out. This is all performed at the same time under general anesthesia and a diagnosis of acute inflammatory pelvic disease is returned. The pathology report confirms the presence of group A streptococcus.

> Code assignment: 614.3 *Acute parametritis and pelvic cellulites*; 041.01 *Streptococcal infection, group A, in diseases classified elsewhere* ; 629.22 *Female genital mutilation status, Type III*

580–629

630–677 Complications of Pregnancy, Childbirth, and the Puerperium

This chapter classifies diseases and disorders that occur during pregnancy, childbirth, and the six weeks immediately following childbirth.

630–633 Ectopic and Molar Pregnancy

A molar pregnancy is abnormal products of conception and an ectopic pregnancy is the implantation of normal products of conception in an anatomic location other than the uterus. Use an additional code from rubric 639 to identify any complications.

630 Hydatidiform mole OK

Hydatidiform mole is an abnormal product of conception in which the epithelial covering of the chorionic villi proliferates with dissolution and cystic cavitation of the avascular stroma of the villi. The result is a mass of cells that resembles a bunch of grapes. This condition also is called cystic or vesicular mole.

Signs and symptoms of hydatidiform mole include bleeding, usually in the first trimester, larger than expected uterus for gestational age, nausea and vomiting, preeclampsia, and passage of vesicular tissue.

Lab work positive for hydatidiform mole reveals HCG greater than 100,000 mIU/ml. Amniography reveals a honeycomb appearance of the mole; an exam of a flat plate of the abdomen fails to show fetal skeleton after 15 weeks; and an ultrasound reveals abnormalities of the fetus and gestational sac. Therapies include suction curettage to evacuate the mole before completion of 20 weeks of gestation, primary hysterectomy in patients not desiring further pregnancies, and prophylactic chemotherapy in patients whose HCG titer rises or plateaus following pregnancy.

Coding Clarification

Associated conditions include malignancy in 20 percent of all patients with hydatidiform mole pregnancies. However, these malignancies are excluded from this rubric and are reported with 236.1.

631 Other abnormal product of conception OK

Included in this rubric are carneous mole, Breus' mole, and blighted ovum.

632 Missed abortion OK

AHA: Q1, 2001, 5

ICD-9-CM defines a missed abortion as the retention of a fetus for at least four weeks after fetal demise but before completion of 22 weeks of gestation. In the United States, this period of time varies according to state law and may be as few as 19 weeks.

Signs and symptoms of missed abortion include the disappearance of normal signs of pregnancy and failure of the uterus to grow.

Diagnostic tests include a pelvic exam that may reveal brownish vaginal discharge, no fresh bleeding, and a closed cervix, though no adnexal abnormalities. Lab work may reveal negative beta HCG and a significantly low plasma fibrinogen level in midtrimester missed abortion. An ultrasound will show there is no fetal cardiac activity. Therapies include dilation and curettage or dilation and evacuation if the pregnancy has not reached the second trimester. If the pregnancy is into the second trimester, laminaria, suppositories, or amniotic injections of prostaglandin are used to induce delivery of the products of conception.

A missed abortion may occur at any time during the pregnancy before completion of 22 weeks of gestation but usually occurs during the second trimester.

Coding Clarification

Retention of abnormal products of conception is excluded from this rubric and reported with 630 or 631. Also excluded from this rubric are failed induced abortion, classified to rubric 638, and fetal death (656.4).

633 Ectopic pregnancy

AHA: Q4, 2002, 61

Tubal pregnancy is the implantation of a fertilized ovum in the fallopian tube, more often on the right than the left. This condition is more common in women who have had previous tubal disease, such as endometriosis of the fallopian tube, tubal surgeries, or infertility due to tubal disease. A tubal pregnancy may occur in any patient, though approximately 40 percent of these pregnancies occur in women between the ages of 20 and 29.

Signs and symptoms of a tubal pregnancy include mild to severe abdominal pain and occasionally nausea and vomiting before rupture. Abnormal uterine bleeding after a rupture occurs in approximately 75 percent of cases. In a tubal pregnancy, the pelvic exam shows adnexal tenderness and possible severe pain on palpation or movement of the cervix and uterus. Pregnancy tests are positive in 82.5 percent of cases. Lab work shows elevated urine urobilinogen and an ultrasound may reveal an empty uterine cavity with products of conception outside the uterus. Laparoscopy may allow direct visualization of the ectopic pregnancy as will laparotomy (performed more often when profound hemorrhage is suspected).

Therapies include laparoscopy or laparotomy to remove the ectopic pregnancy. If the patient is concerned about fertility, fimbrioplasty and salpingostomy are performed to leave the fallopian tube in place. If fertility is not an issue, the tube is removed, the tubal disease corrected, and there is lysis of adhesions in the opposite adnexa. In cases with minimal or no bleeding and without rupture, there is milking of the pregnancy from the fimbriated end of the tube.

633.0 5th Abdominal pregnancy — (Use additional code from category 639 to identify any associated complications) — *intraperitoneal pregnancy*
AHA: Q4, 2002, 61

633.00 Abdominal pregnancy without intrauterine pregnancy — (Use additional code from category 639 to identify any associated complications)

633.01 Abdominal pregnancy with intrauterine pregnancy — (Use additional code from category 639 to identify any associated complications)

633.1 5th Tubal pregnancy — (Use additional code from category 639 to identify any associated complications) — *fallopian pregnancy; rupture of (fallopian) tube due to pregnancy*
AHA: Q2, 1990, 27; Q4, 2002, 61

633.10 Tubal pregnancy without intrauterine pregnancy — (Use additional code from category 639 to identify any associated complications)

633.11 Tubal pregnancy with intrauterine pregnancy — (Use additional code from category 639 to identify any associated complications)

633.2 5th Ovarian pregnancy — (Use additional code from category 639 to identify any associated complications) — *fertilized ovum implants on ovary*
AHA: Q4, 2002, 61

633.20 Ovarian pregnancy without intrauterine pregnancy — (Use additional code from category 639 to identify any associated complications)

633.21 Ovarian pregnancy with intrauterine pregnancy — (Use additional code from category 639 to identify any associated complications)

633.8 5th Other ectopic pregnancy — (Use additional code from category 639 to identify any associated complications) — *intraligamentous pregnancy; mesometric pregnancy*
AHA: Q4, 2002, 61

633.80 Other ectopic pregnancy without intrauterine pregnancy — (Use additional code from category 639 to identify any associated complications)

633.81 Other ectopic pregnancy with intrauterine pregnancy — (Use additional code from category 639 to identify any associated complications)

Coding Clarification

Subclassification 633.8 reports implantation of a fertilized ovum in other specified sites such as the cervix, the uterine musculature (mesometric), or uterine cornu (horn). Signs and symptoms of other ectopic pregnancy include mild to severe abdominal pain and occasionally nausea and vomiting before rupture. Frequently after rupture, there is abnormal uterine bleeding in approximately 75 percent of cases. Therapies, depending on the implantation site, include termination using such procedures as wedge resection of the uterus, fimbrioplasty, supracervical hysterectomy, unilateral salpingo-oophorectomy, and total abdominal hysterectomy.

633.9 5th Unspecified ectopic pregnancy — (Use additional code from category 639 to identify any associated complications) — *unknown*
AHA: Q4, 2002, 61

633.90 Unspecified ectopic pregnancy without intrauterine pregnancy — (Use additional code from category 639 to identify any associated complications)

633.91 Unspecified ectopic pregnancy with intrauterine pregnancy — (Use additional code from category 639 to identify any associated complications)

Coding Scenario

A 29-year-old female is admitted for tubal pregnancy. The patient undergoes a left salpingectomy for removal of the tubal pregnancy. A pathology report

© 2004 Ingenix, Inc.

confirms the diagnosis and identifies an embryonic cyst. The physician's final diagnostic statement is fallopian tube pregnancy and hydatid cyst of Morgagni.

> Code assignment: 633.10 *Tubal pregnancy without intrauterine pregnancy* and 752.11 *Embryonic cyst of fallopian tube*

634–639 Other Pregnancy with Abortive Outcome

Retained Products of Conception: When the patient is admitted following a spontaneous or legally induced abortion for retained products of conception, the patient is considered to have an incomplete abortion.

Septicemia and Septic Shock Associated With Abortion: Septicemia is defined as systemic disease caused by the presence of toxins or micro-organisms in the bloodstream. It is evidenced by infection with fever or hypothermia, tachypnea, tachycardia, and impaired organ system perfusion, such as altered mental status, oliguria, and relative hypotension. Metabolic acidosis may also be present secondary to impaired organ perfusion, as evidenced by either an increased lactate level, increased anion gap, or reduced blood pH. Because it is difficult to isolate the infectious organism in blood cultures, it may still be appropriate to code the septicemia in view of the clinical data. Report with a code from categories 634-638 with the appropriate fourth digit to identify the sepsis ("0") and/or septic shock ("5"). A fifth digit is also required to identify the stage of the abortion.

634 Spontaneous abortion

AHA: Q2, 1991, 16

The definition of spontaneous abortion is complete or incomplete expulsion of the products of conception before completion of 22 weeks of gestation. Spontaneous abortions may be complete with the expulsion of the entire products of conception, or incomplete with the retention of part of the products of conception, usually the placenta.

In an incomplete abortion, the amniotic sac and fetus may be expelled without the chorion and decidua, only the embryo may be expelled, or the amniotic sac may rupture with passage of the fetus alone. Incomplete abortion requires evacuation of the remaining tissue by curettage. Fever and abdominal pain may indicate infection.

Most spontaneous abortions are associated with abnormal products of conception such as abnormal karyotype. Overall, about 10 percent are thought to have chromosomal abnormalities.

In pregnancies of about 14 weeks or less, therapies include suction, sharp curettage, or both to remove remaining conceptus. If bleeding is brisk, a 5 percent dextrose solution is administered in lactated ringers with 10 units of oxytocin per 500 ml; antibiotics are used to control infection. In pregnancies greater than 14 weeks of gestation, oxytocin is administered intravenously or prostaglandin E2 is inserted by vaginal suppository to expedite the abortion.

The following fifth-digit suclassification is used to identify stage of abortion with categories 634-637:

0 unspecified
1 incomplete
2 complete

634.0 ✓5th Spontaneous abortion complicated by genital tract and pelvic infection — *miscarriage complicated by salpingitis*
AHA: Q2, 1991, 16

634.1 ✓5th Spontaneous abortion complicated by delayed or excessive hemorrhage — *miscarriage complicated by excessive bleeding*
AHA: Q2, 1991, 16

Severe hemorrhage must be present for codes from 634.1 to be assigned correctly.

634.2 ✓5th Spontaneous abortion complicated by damage to pelvic organs or tissues — *miscarriage complicated by uterine rupture*
AHA: Q2, 1991, 16

634.3 ✓5th Spontaneous abortion complicated by renal failure — *miscarriage complicated by renal failure*
AHA: Q2, 1991, 16

Spontaneous abortion complicated by renal failure is expulsion of the products of conception before completion of 22 weeks of gestation, complicated by renal failure in the mother.

634.4 ✓5th Spontaneous abortion complicated by metabolic disorder — *miscarriage complicated by diabetes mellitus*
AHA: Q2, 1991, 16

Spontaneous abortion complicated by metabolic disorder is expulsion of the products of conception before completion of 22 weeks of gestation, complicated by metabolic disorders such as diabetes mellitus.

634.5 ✓5th Spontaneous abortion complicated by shock — *miscarriage complicated by shock*
AHA: Q2, 1991, 16

Spontaneous abortion complicated by shock is expulsion of the products of conception before completion of 22 weeks of gestation, complicated by maternal shock, which is an acute peripheral circulatory failure due to an aberration of circulatory control or loss of circulating fluid. Signs and symptoms of spontaneous abortion complicated by shock include hypotension, coldness of skin, tachycardia, anxiety, or sudden disturbance of mental equilibrium.

634.6 5th Spontaneous abortion complicated by embolism — *miscarriage complicated by embolism*
AHA: Q2, 1991, 16

Spontaneous abortion complicated by embolism is expulsion of the products of conception before completion of 22 weeks of gestation, complicated by sudden blocking of an artery by a clot or foreign material in the mother.

The following fifth-digit suclassification is used to identify stage of abortion with categories 634-637:

0 unspecified

1 incomplete

2 complete

634.7 5th Spontaneous abortion with other specified complications — *miscarriage complicated by other specified complication*
AHA: Q2, 1991, 16

634.8 5th Spontaneous abortion with unspecified complication — *miscarriage with unspecified complication*
AHA: Q2, 1991, 16

634.9 5th Spontaneous abortion without mention of complication — *miscarriage without mention of complication*
AHA: Q2, 1991, 16

Coding Clarification

Threatened Abortion: The outcome of the encounter indicates the proper code assignment. If the products of conception are expelled, the appropriate code from category 634 is assigned. A code from categories 640-648 and 651-657 may be used to identify the condition causing the abortion. If the threatened abortion does not culminate in an abortion, the appropriate code from category 640 is assigned.

Coding Scenario

A patient is admitted for a D&C following spontaneous abortion of an 18-week gestational age fetus. The pathology report reveals products of conception were removed by curettage. The patient is discharged home.

Code assignment: 634.91 *Spontaneous abortion without mention of complication, incomplete*

635 Legally induced abortion

AHA: Q2, 1994, 14

A legally induced abortion is the intentional expulsion of the products of conception from the uterus by medical professionals working within the boundaries of the law.

The following fifth-digit suclassification is used to identify stage of abortion with categories 634-637:

0 unspecified

1 incomplete

2 complete

635.0 5th Legally induced abortion complicated by genital tract and pelvic infection — *therapeutic, complicated by salpingitis*
AHA: Q2, 1994, 14

635.1 5th Legally induced abortion complicated by delayed or excessive hemorrhage — *therapeutic, complicated by excessive bleeding*
AHA: Q2, 1994, 14

635.2 5th Legally induced abortion complicated by damage to pelvic organs or tissues — *therapeutic, complicated by uterine rupture*
AHA: Q2, 1994, 14

635.3 5th Legally induced abortion complicated by renal failure — *therapeutic, complicated by renal failure*
AHA: Q2, 1994, 14

635.4 5th Legally induced abortion complicated by metabolic disorder — *therapeutic, complicated by diabetes mellitus*
AHA: Q2, 1994, 14

635.5 5th Legally induced abortion complicated by shock — *therapeutic, complicated by shock*
AHA: Q2, 1994, 14

635.6 5th Legally induced abortion complicated by embolism — *therapeutic, complicated by embolism*
AHA: Q2, 1994, 14

635.7 5th Legally induced abortion with other specified complications — *therapeutic, with other specified complication*
AHA: Q2, 1994, 14

635.8 5th Legally induced abortion with unspecified complication — *therapeutic, with unknown complication*
AHA: Q2, 1994, 14

635.9 5th Legally induced abortion without mention of complication — *therapeutic abortion*
AHA: Q2, 1994, 14

Coding Scenario

Following a legally performed abortion, a patient is admitted for retained products of conception and septic shock. The causative organism is unknown.

Code assignment: 635.51 *Legally induced abortion complicated by shock, incomplete*

636 Illegally induced abortion

An illegally induced abortion is the intentional expulsion of the products of conception from the

 © 2004 Ingenix, Inc.

uterus by individuals working outside the boundaries of the law.

The following fifth-digit suclassification is used to identify stage of abortion with categories 634-637:

0 unspecified

1 incomplete

2 complete

636.0 5th Illegally induced abortion complicated by genital tract and pelvic infection — *criminal, complicated by salpingitis*

636.1 5th Illegally induced abortion complicated by delayed or exececessive hemorrhage — *criminal, complicated by excessive bleeding*

636.2 5th Illegally induced abortion complicated by damage to pelvic organs or tissue — *criminal, complicated by uterine rupture*

636.3 5th Illegally induced abortion complicated by renal failure — *criminal, complicated by renal failure*

636.4 5th Illegally induced abortion complicated by metabolic disorder — *criminal, complicated by diabetes mellitus*

636.5 5th Illegally induced abortion complicated by shock — *criminal, complicated by shock*

636.6 5th Illegally induced abortion complicated by embolism — *criminal, complicated by embolism*

636.7 5th Illegally induced abortion with other specified complications — *criminal, with other specified complication*

636.8 5th Illegally induced abortion with unspecified complication — *criminal, with unknown complication*

636.9 5th Illegally induced abortion without mention of complication — *criminal abortion*

637 Legally unspecified abortion

Use this rubric when documentation does not support a choice of a legally or an illegally induced abortion.

The following fifth-digit suclassification is used to identify stage of abortion with categories 634-637:

0 unspecified

1 incomplete

2 complete

637.0 5th Legally unspecified abortion complicated by genital tract and pelvic infection — *complicated by salpingitis*

637.1 5th Legally unspecified abortion complicated by delayed or excessive hemorrhage — *complicated by excessive bleeding*

637.2 5th Legally unspecified abortion complicated by damage to pelvic organs or tissues — *complicated by uterine rupture*

637.3 5th Legally unspecified abortion complicated by renal failure — *complicated by renal failure*

637.4 5th Legally unspecified abortion complicated by metabolic disorder — *complicated by diabetes mellitus*

637.5 5th Legally unspecified abortion complicated by shock — *complicated by shock*

637.6 5th Legally unspecified abortion complicated by embolism — *complicated by embolism*

637.7 5th Legally unspecified abortion with other specified complications — *with other specified complication*

637.8 5th Legally unspecified abortion with unspecified complication — *with unknown complication*

637.9 5th Legally unspecified abortion without mention of complication — *without mention of complication*

638 Failed attempted abortion

A failed attempted abortion is the attempted, although failed, intentional expulsion of the products of conception from the uterus.

638.0 Failed attempted abortion complicated by genital tract and pelvic infection — *failed therapeutic, complicated by salpingitis*

638.1 Failed attempted abortion complicated by delayed or excessive hemorrhage — *failed therapeutic, complicated by excessive bleeding*

638.2 Failed attempted abortion complicated by damage to pelvic organs or tissues — *failed therapeutic, complicated by ruptured fallopian tube*

638.3 Failed attempted abortion complicated by renal failure — *failed therapeutic, complicated by renal failure*

638.4 Failed attempted abortion complicated by metabolic disorder — *failed therapeutic, complicated by diabetes mellitus*

638.5 Failed attempted abortion complicated by shock — *failed therapeutic, complicated by shock*

638.6 Failed attempted abortion complicated by embolism — *failed therapeutic, complicated by embolism*

638.7 Failed attempted abortion with other specified complication — *failed therapeutic, with other specified complication*

638.8 Failed attempted abortion with unspecified complication — *failed therapeutic, with unspecified complication*

638.9 Failed attempted abortion without mention of complication — *failed therapeutic, without mention of complication*

639 Complications following abortion or ectopic and molar pregnancies

This rubric reports complications that follow an abortion or an ectopic or molar pregnancy. It is used when the complication (not the abortion or the ectopic or molar pregnancy) is the reason for the current episode of care. For example, a patient is readmitted one week after treatment for a tubal pregnancy, presenting with generalized sepsis. Codes 639.0x *General tract and pelvic infection* and 038.9 *Unspecified septicemia* would be used for the second admission. Code 633.1x *Tubal pregnancy* would not be used since it pertains only to the previous episode of care.

Genital tract and pelvic infection following an abortion, especially one performed illegally, is commonly caused by both aerobic and anaerobic organisms. The infection may be localized to the products of conception or it may result in endometritis, salpingo-oophoritis, peritonitis, or septicemia.

Signs and symptoms of genital tract and pelvic infection include pain, bleeding, fever, vaginal discharge, and recent illegal abortion. Lab work shows elevated white blood count and cultures identify organisms causing infection, generally gram-negative bacilli (most commonly *Escherichia coli* and *Bacteroides fragilis*) and gram-positive cocci (particularly *enterococci* and *beta-hemolytic streptococci*). The infective agent may be reported secondarily.

639.0 Genital tract and pelvic infection following abortion or ectopic and molar pregnancies — *endometritis, salpingitis, septicemia molar pregnancies*

639.1 Delayed or excessive hemorrhage following abortion or ectopic and molar pregnancies — *secondary*

639.2 Damage to pelvic organs and tissues following abortion or ectopic and molar pregnancies — *laceration or perforation of bladder, broad ligament, periurethral tissue or uterus molar pregnancies*

639.3 Renal failure following abortion or ectopic and molar pregnancies — *secondary*

639.4 Metabolic disorders following abortion or ectopic and molar pregnancies — *secondary*

639.5 Shock following abortion or ectopic and molar pregnancies — *secondary*

639.6 Embolism following abortion or ectopic and molar pregnancies — *secondary*

639.8 Other specified complication following abortion or ectopic and molar pregnancies — *secondary*

639.9 Unspecified complication following abortion or ectopic and molar pregnancies — *secondary*

Coding Clarification

This rubric also is used when the complication cannot be identified at the fourth-digit level in code categories 634-638. For example, a patient admitted for missed abortion also develops generalized sepsis during the same episode of care. Codes 632 *Missed abortion,* 639.0, and 038.9 would be used for this admission; the infection cannot be identified at the fourth-digit level for missed abortions.

Coding Scenario

A patient is diagnosed with sepsis and shock following an abortion performed two days prior.

> Code assignment: 639.0 *Genital and pelvic infection following abortion or ectopic and molar pregnancies* and 639.5 *Shock following abortion or ectopic and molar pregnancies*

640–648 Complications Mainly Related to Pregnancy

Codes in this section describe conditions that affect the management of pregnancy, labor or delivery, and the puerperium, even if the condition was present before pregnancy.

640 Hemorrhage in early pregnancy

AHA: Q2, 1990, 11

Early pregnancy is defined as before the completion of 22 weeks gestation.

Signs and symptoms of threatened abortion include bleeding and uterine cramping without cervical dilation.

Therapies include bed rest and observation. Use the fifth-digit 0 if the episode of care is unspecified or not applicable; fifth-digit 1 when the threatened abortion is treated successfully and the patient goes on to deliver at term; and fifth-digit 3 if the threatened abortion is treated successfully without delivery.

Subclassification 640.8 reports bleeding during pregnancy that does not pose a threat of aborting the fetus. Bleeding may occur at any time during the pregnancy, although it is most prevalent during the first trimester when the risk of aborting the fetus is greater than during either the second or third trimester. The patient's pelvic exam reveals no evidence of spontaneous abortion, either complete or incomplete; CBC may indicate anemia if heavy bleeding is present; and an ultrasound is negative for placental abnormalities. Associated conditions that would be reported instead of 640.8x include placenta previa (641.1x), premature separation of placenta (641.2x), and coagulation defects in mother (641.3x).

 © 2004 Ingenix, Inc.

Medical record documentation must indicate that the patient did not deliver during the current episode of care. If medical record documentation indicates that the physician was concerned about the likelihood of abortion, although there was no abortion, see 640.0x *Threatened abortion*. If medical record documentation such as ultrasound reports indicates an antepartum hemorrhagic condition affecting the placenta, see category 641 *Antepartum hemorrhage, abruptio placentae, and placenta previa* for alternative code selections.

The following fifth-digit subclassification is for use with category 640 to denote the current episode of care.

0 unspecified as to episode of care or not applicable

1 delivered, with or without mention of antepartum condition

3 antepartum condition or complication

640.0 5th Threatened abortion — *potential abortion marked by bloody uterine discharge*
AHA: Q2, 1990, 11

640.8 5th Other specified hemorrhage in early pregnancy — *menstruation during pregnancy*
AHA: Q2, 1990, 11

640.9 5th Unspecified hemorrhage in early pregnancy — *early pregnancy hemorrhage NOS*
AHA: Q2, 1990, 11

Coding Clarification

Only the fifth-digits 0, 1, and 3 apply to the 640 rubric.

Threatened Abortion: The outcome of the encounter indicates the proper code assignment. If the products of conception are expelled, the appropriate code from category 634 is assigned. A code from categories 640-648 and 651-657 may be used to identify the condition causing the abortion. If the threatened abortion does not culminate in an abortion, the appropriate code from category 640 is assigned.

641 Antepartum hemorrhage, abruptio placentae, and placenta previa

AHA: Q2, 1990, 11

Antepartum hemorrhage, abruptio placentae, and placenta previa present with bleeding before the onset of labor (antepartum hemorrhage), premature separation of a normal placenta (abruptio placentae), and implantation of the placenta over or near the internal cervical os (placenta previa).

The following fifth-digit subclassification is for use with category 641 to denote the current episode of care.

0 unspecified as to episode of care or not applicable

1 delivered, with or without mention of antepartum condition

3 antepartum condition or complication

641.0 5th Placenta previa without hemorrhage — *low implantation of placenta without hemorrhage*
AHA: Q2, 1990, 11

The definition of placenta previa without hemorrhage is implantation of the placenta over or near the internal os of the cervix. With total previa, the placenta completely covers the internal cervical os. Vaginal exam is contraindicated if placenta previa is suspected; ultrasound locates the exact position of the placenta. Therapies include bed rest if the patient is not near term; if the patient is at term, delivery of the fetus is usually by cesarean section.

If the fetus is not delivered during this episode of care, use the fifth digit 3 to indicate an antepartum condition.

641.1 5th Hemorrhage from placenta previa — *marginal placenta previa with hemorrhage; low lying placenta with hemorrhage*
AHA: Q2, 1990, 11

The definition of hemorrhage from placenta previa is implantation of the placenta over or near the internal os of the cervix with bleeding. With total previa, the placenta completely covers the internal cervical os. With partial previa, the placenta covers a portion of the internal cervical os.

Signs and symptoms of hemorrhage from placenta previa include sudden painless vaginal bleeding, beginning late in pregnancy, followed by painless massive bright red bleeding. Vaginal exam is contraindicated if placenta previa is suspected; ultrasound locates the exact position of the placenta. Therapies include bed rest if bleeding is minor and the patient is not near term, and if bleeding is substantial, blood transfusion and tocolytic agents are administered. If the fetus is not delivered during this episode of care, use the fifth digit 3 to indicate an antepartum condition.

Excluded from this subclassification is hemorrhage from vasa previa, reported with 663.5x.

641.2 5th Premature separation of placenta — *ablatio placentae; Couvelaire uterus; premature separation of normally implanted placenta; abruptio placentae*
AHA: Q2, 1990, 11

Premature separation of the placenta is separation of the placenta from the site of uterine implantation before delivery of the fetus. There are two forms of placental separation: concealed, in which the hemorrhage is confined to the uterine cavity; and external, in which blood drains through the cervix. The placenta may detach either entirely or partially. Etiologies are numerous and difficult to ascertain but include advanced maternal age, multiparity, uterine distention, vascular deficiency and/or deterioration, uterine anomalies, cigarette smoking, and alcohol abuse.

Signs and symptoms of premature separation of the placenta include abdominal or back pain and visible hemorrhage, depending on the degree of separation and blood loss, irritable abdomen, and tender and often hypertonic uterus.

To avoid precipitating greater hemorrhage, pelvic exam is contraindicated until diagnosis of abruptio placentae established. CBC may show reduced platelets and anemia, depending on the degree of hemorrhage; ultrasound determines the degree of separation and viability of the fetus. Therapies include fetal monitoring to determine if the fetus is in any distress, blood transfusion if severe hemorrhage is present, delivery of the fetus if either bleeding persists or separation is total.

641.3 ✓5th Antepartum hemorrhage associated with coagulation defects — *antepartum or intrapartum hemorrhage associated with afibrinogenemia, hyperfibrinolysis; hypofibrinogenemia*
AHA: Q2, 1990, 11

641.8 ✓5th Other antepartum hemorrhage — *antepartum or intrapartum hemorrhage associated with trauma or uterine leiomyoma*
AHA: Q2, 1990, 11

641.9 ✓5th Unspecified antepartum hemorrhage — *antepartum hemorrhage NOS; spots of pregnancy*
AHA: Q2, 1990, 11

642 Hypertension complicating pregnancy, childbirth, and the puerperium

AHA: Q2, 1990, 11

Hypertension complicating pregnancy, childbirth, and the puerperium may be benign, preexisting, chronic, or secondary to renal disease.

The following fifth-digit subclassification is for use with category 642 to denote the current episode of care.

0 unspecified as to episode of care or not applicable
1 delivered, with or without mention of antepartum condition
2 delivered, with mention of postpartum complication
3 antepartum condition or complication
4 postpartum condition or complication

642.0 ✓5th Benign essential hypertension complicating pregnancy, childbirth, and the puerperium — *elevated arterial blood pressure; essential or chronic hypertension specified as complicating, or as a reason for obstetric care during pregnancy, childbirth, or the puerperium*
AHA: Q2, 1990, 11

Benign essential hypertension complicating pregnancy, childbirth, and the puerperium is blood pressure of 140/90 or greater before the onset of pregnancy or in the first trimester of pregnancy. Signs and symptoms of benign essential hypertension complicating pregnancy, childbirth, and the puerperium include a history of chronic benign hypertension. Examination reveals hypertension without other signs of preeclampsia such as proteinuria or nondependent edema. EKG may reveal left ventricular hypertrophy and lab work often shows elevated serum creatinine. A chest x-ray may reveal cardiomegaly. Therapies include antihypertensive drugs of established long-term safety for mother and fetus such as methyldopa, clonidine, and labetalol.

642.1 ✓5th Hypertension secondary to renal disease, complicating pregnancy, childbirth, and the puerperium — *elevated arterial blood pressure due to kidney disease; hypertension secondary to renal disease*
AHA: Q2, 1990, 11

Hypertension secondary to renal disease, complicating pregnancy, childbirth, and the puerperium is preexisting renal disease that results in hypertension. Blood pressure is 140/90 or greater before the onset of pregnancy or in the first trimester of pregnancy. Signs and symptoms of hypertension secondary to renal disease, complicating pregnancy, childbirth, and the puerperium, include a history of chronic renal disease with resultant hypertension. Examination reveals hypertension, and edema. EKG may reveal left ventricular hypertrophy and lab work often shows elevated BUN and serum creatinine levels. A chest x-ray may reveal cardiomegaly. Fetal monitoring, fetal nonstress tests, and oxytocin challenge tests determine if pregnancy should be continued. Often, delivery, usually by cesarean section, is prescribed if blood pressure can no longer be controlled and the fetus has completed more than 22 weeks of gestation.

Therapies include antihypertensive drugs of established long-term safety for mother and fetus such as methyldopa, clonidine, and labetalol.

642.2 ✓5th Other pre-existing hypertension complicating pregnancy, childbirth, and the puerperium — *hypertensive heart and renal disease or malignant hypertension specified as complicating, or as a reason for obstetric care during pregnancy, childbirth, or the puerperium*
AHA: Q2, 1990, 11

© 2004 Ingenix, Inc.

642.3 5th Transient hypertension of pregnancy — *gestational hypertension; transient hypertension, so described, in pregnancy, childbirth, or the puerperium*
AHA: Q2, 1990, 11; Q3, 1990, 4

642.4 5th Mild or unspecified pre-eclampsia — *pre-eclampsia NOS or toxemia (pre-eclamptic) NOS*
AHA: Q2, 1990, 11

Mild or unspecified pre-eclampsia is the development of borderline hypertension, albuminuria, and unresponsive edema between the 20th week of pregnancy and the end of the first week postpartum. Signs and symptoms of mild or unspecified pre-eclampsia include weight gain of more than two pounds in one week and nondependent edema of the hands and feet. Examination shows hypertension of 140/90 or slightly higher or rise in systolic pressure of 20 mm Hg or diastolic of 15 mm Hg, and nondependent edema of the face or hands. Lab work reveals albuminuria of 1+ or greater and rising serum creatinine. Therapies include bed rest and delivery once the fetus has reached a suitable age of gestation to be viable and antihypertensive drugs of established long-term safety for mother and fetus such as methyldopa, clonidine, and labetalol.

Excluded from 642.4x are albuminuria in pregnancy without hypertension (646.2x) and edema in pregnancy without mention of hypertension (646.1x).

642.5 5th Severe pre-eclampsia — *HELLP syndrome; toxemia (pre-eclamptic), severe*
AHA: Nov-Dec, 1985, 3; Q2, 1990, 11

642.6 5th Eclampsia complicating pregnancy, childbirth or the puerperium — *toxemia with convulsions; eclamptic toxemia*
AHA: Q2, 1990, 11

642.7 5th Pre-eclampsia or eclampsia superimposed on pre-existing hypertension — *secondary*
AHA: Q2, 1990, 11

642.9 5th Unspecified hypertension complicating pregnancy, childbirth, or the puerperium — *childbirth, or the puerperium; hypertension NOS without mention of albuminuria or edema, complicating pregnancy, childbirth, or the puerperium*
AHA: Q2, 1990, 11

Documentation Issues

The physician must clearly indicate if the patient has eclampsia, pre-eclampsia, or hypertension during pregnancy for accurate code assignment to be made.

Pre-eclampsia or eclampsia may be accompanied by pulmonary edema. An additional code indicating the pulmonary edema is only assigned when the pulmonary edema is documented as cardiogenic.

Coding Clarification

Eclampsia: This is a condition occurring during pregnancy or the immediate post-partum period noted by convulsions, coma, and edema with associated pre-eclampsia. Report with code 642.6x *Eclampsia complicating pregnancy, childbirth or the puerperium.* A fifth digit must be assigned to indicate the episode of care.

Hypertension During Pregnancy: If the medical record states hypertension with mild proteinuria, report code 642.4x *Mild or unspecified pre-eclampsia.* If the hypertension is associated with severe proteinuria, this is indicated by code 642.5x *Severe pre-eclampsia.* When the medical record documentation states transient hypertension of pregnancy or gestational hypertension, code 642.3x. These codes require the assignment of a fifth digit to indicate the episode of care.

If the patient has pre-existing hypertension that is affecting or complicating the obstetrical care, code 642.0x is assigned. This coding guideline is supported by an includes note in the tabular chapter of the ICD-9-CM manual.

Hypertension secondary to renal disease that is complicating the obstetrical care during pregnancy, childbirth, or the postpartum period is assigned to code 642.1x. This code requires the assignment of a fifth digit to indicate the episode of care.

Pre-eclampsia: This is a condition affecting women during pregnancy with one or more of the following symptoms: hypertension, proteinuria, oliguria, cerebral or visual disturbances, and pulmonary edema.

Mild pre-eclampsia is defined as hypertension associated with mild edema and proteinuria late in pregnancy. Assign code 642.4x with the appropriate fifth digit to indicate the episode of care. Hypertension in the last trimester of pregnancy is also assigned code 642.4x.

Severe pre-eclampsia is specified as hypertension associated with either albuminuria or edema or both. Assign code 642.5x with the appropriate fifth digit indicating the episode of care. It may also be described as HELLP syndrome.

Coding Scenario

An inpatient delivers a liveborn female infant. Following the delivery, she has a blood pressure of 210/120, proteinuria, and edema. The patient suffers convulsions five hours post delivery.

> Code assignment: 642.62 *Eclampsia complicating pregnancy, childbirth or the puerperium, delivered, with mention of postpartum complication*

A patient who is 32 weeks pregnant is admitted due to severe hypertension, elevated liver function tests, and low platelet count. The diagnosis of HELLP is indicated.

Code assignment: 642.53 *Severe pre-eclampsia, antepartum condition or complication*

A patient at 35-week gestational age is seen in her physician's office with transient elevation of blood pressure during pregnancy.

Code assignment: 642.33 *Transient hypertension of pregnancy, antepartum condition or complication*

643 Excessive vomiting in pregnancy

AHA: Q2, 1990, 11

This category is used to describe vomiting that affects management of the pregnancy.

The following fifth-digit subclassification is for use with category 643 to denote the current episode of care.

0 unspecified as to episode of care or not applicable

1 delivered, with or without mention of antepartum condition

3 antepartum condition or complication

643.0 5th Mild hyperemesis gravidarum — *hyperemesis gravidarum, mild or unspecified, starting before the end of the 22nd week of gestation*
AHA: Q2, 1990, 11

643.1 5th Hyperemesis gravidarum with metabolic disturbance — *hyperemesis gravidarum starting before the end of the 22nd week of gestation, with metabolic disturbance, such as carbohydrate depletion, dehydration or electrolyte imbalance*
AHA: Q2, 1990, 11

643.2 5th Late vomiting of pregnancy — *excessive vomiting starting after 22 completed weeks of gestation*
AHA: Q2, 1990, 11

643.8 5th Other vomiting complicating pregnancy — (Use additional code to specify cause) — *vomiting due to organic disease or other cause, specified as complicating pregnancy, or as a reason for obstetric care during pregnancy*
AHA: Q2, 1990, 11

643.9 5th Unspecified vomiting of pregnancy — *vomiting as a reason for care during pregnancy, length of gestation unknown*
AHA: Q2, 1990, 11

Coding Clarification

Only fifth-digits 0, 1, and 3 apply to codes in the 643 rubric.

644 Early or threatened labor

AHA: Q2, 1990, 11

Threatened labor is regular, painful uterine contractions at least twice every 10 minutes for a 30-minute period of time with effacement or dilation of the cervix occurring after completion of 22 weeks of gestation but before completion of 37 weeks. There is neither rupture of membranes nor delivery of the fetus. The contractions cease and the cervix stops dilating.

The following fifth-digit subclassification is for use with category 644 to denote the current episode of care. Valid fifth-digits are in brackets [ ] after each code, unless noted at the rubric.

0 unspecified as to episode of care or not applicable

1 delivered, with or without mention of antepartum condition

3 antepartum condition or complication

644.0 5th Threatened premature labor — *premature labor after 22 weeks, but before 37 completed weeks of gestation*
AHA: Q2, 1990, 11

644.1 5th Other threatened labor — *false labor after 37 completed weeks of gestation; including Braxton Hicks contractions*
AHA: Q2, 1990, 11

644.2 5th Early onset of delivery — *onset (spontaneous) of delivery before 37 completed weeks of gestation*
AHA: Q2, 1990, 11; Q2, 1991, 16

Coding Clarification

Early onset of delivery is delivery of an infant after completion of 22 weeks of gestation but before completion of 37 weeks. Signs and symptoms of early onset of delivery include uterine contractions lasting at least 30 seconds and occurring at 10-minute intervals (at least) during a 30-minute period of time and continued dilation and effacement of the cervix over a period of time despite medications to stop.

Therapies include hydration and sedation once the patient is admitted in premature labor, tocolysis to try to prevent progression, and, when this fails, delivery of the infant.

Only the fifth-digits 0 or 1 are valid for 644.2. The fifth-digit 0, unspecified as to episode of care or not applicable, will rarely, if ever, be assigned as the subcategory implies delivery.

Abortion with Delivery of Liveborn Fetus: An attempt to terminate pregnancy may result in the delivery of a liveborn fetus. When this occurs, ICD-9-CM code 644.2x is assigned. Hospitals also assign the appropriate code from category V27 *Outcome of delivery* to indicate the live birth.

 © 2004 Ingenix, Inc.

Retained Products of Conception: When the patient is admitted following a spontaneous or legally induced abortion for retained products of conception, the patient is considered to have an incomplete abortion.

Threatened Abortion: The outcome of the encounter indicates the proper code assignment. If the products of conception are expelled, the appropriate code from category 634 is assigned. A code from categories 640-648 and 651-657 may be used to identify the condition causing the abortion. If the threatened abortion does not culminate in an abortion, the appropriate code from category 640 is assigned.

Coding Scenario

A patient is admitted for an induced abortion. Following prostaglandin suppositories and cervical dilation, a single liveborn male fetus is delivered.

> Code assignment: 644.21 *Early onset of delivery, with or without mention of antepartum condition.* Hospitals will also code V27.0 *Single liveborn*

645 Late pregnancy

AHA: Q2, 1990, 11; Q4, 1991, 26; Q4, 2000, 43

Post-term pregnancy is a normal pregnancy of more than 40 weeks, up to 42 weeks. A prolonged pregnancy is normal pregnancy that has advanced beyond 42 weeks of gestation. Postdatism may be treated by careful fetal monitoring with no intervention until there are indications the fetus is at risk. Postmaturity syndrome is a term that may be applied to both mothers and infants. In mothers, the syndrome is characterized by prolonged gestation, sometimes excessive fetal size, failing placental function, and impending fetal demise. When the term is used to describe infant pathology, it is classified to 766.2 *Post-term infant, not "heavy for dates."*

The following fifth-digit subclassification is for use with category 645 to denote the current episode of care.

0 unspecified as to episode of care or not applicable

1 delivered, with or without mention of antepartum condition

3 antepartum condition or complication

645.1 [5th] Post term pregnancy — *pregnancy over 40 completed weeks to 42 completed weeks gestation*
AHA: Q2, 1990, 11; Q4, 1991, 26; Q4, 2000, 43

645.2 [5th] Prolonged pregnancy — *pregnancy which has advanced beyond 42 completed weeks gestation*
AHA: Q2, 1990, 11; Q4, 1991, 26; Q4, 2000, 43

Coding Clarification

Only the fifth-digits 0, 1, and 3 apply to the 645 rubric.

646 Other complications of pregnancy, not elsewhere classified

AHA: Q2, 1990, 11; Q4, 1995, 59

The following fifth-digit subclassification is for use with category 646 to denote the current episode of care. Valid fifth-digits are in brackets [ ] after each code, unless noted at the rubric.

0 unspecified as to episode of care or not applicable

1 delivered, with or without mention of antepartum condition

2 delivered, with mention of postpartum complication

3 antepartum condition or complication

4 postpartum condition or complication

646.0 [5th] Papyraceous fetus — *skin of fetus resembles paper*
AHA: Q2, 1990, 11; Q4, 1995, 59

646.1 [5th] Edema or excessive weight gain in pregnancy, without mention of hypertension — *gestational edema; maternal obesity syndrome*
AHA: Q2, 1990, 11; Q4, 1995, 59

646.2 [5th] Unspecified renal disease in pregnancy, without mention of hypertension — *gestational proteinuria; albuminuria or nephropathy NOS in pregnancy or the puerperium*
AHA: Q2, 1990, 11; Q4, 1995, 59

646.3 [5th] Pregnancy complication, habitual aborter — *miscarried at least three times*
AHA: Q2, 1990, 11; Q4, 1995, 59

646.4 [5th] Peripheral neuritis in pregnancy

646.5 [5th] Asymptomatic bacteriuria in pregnancy

646.6 [5th] Infections of genitourinary tract in pregnancy — *secondary*
AHA: Q2, 1990, 11; Q4, 1995, 59

646.7 [5th] Liver disorders in pregnancy — *icterus gravis, or necrosis of liver, or acute yellow atrophy of liver (obstetric) (true)*
AHA: Q2, 1990, 11; Q4, 1995, 59

646.8 [5th] Other specified complications of pregnancy — *fatigue during pregnancy; herpes gestationis; pruritic gravidarum; ptyalism in pregnancy*
AHA: Jan-Feb, 1985, 15; Q2, 1990, 11; Q4, 1995, 59; Q3, 1998, 16

646.9 [5th] Unspecified complication of pregnancy — *pregnancy complication NOS*
AHA: Q2, 1990, 11; Q4, 1995, 59

Coding Clarification
Additional codes should be reported to further specify the complication. Do not report 646.3x *Pregnancy complication, habitual aborter* in the case of a current abortion (rubric 634) or if the patient is not currently pregnant (629.9). Report 646.9x *Unspecified complication of pregnancy* for herpes gestationis, insufficient weight gain in pregnancy, retinitis gravidarum, ptyalism pregnancy, pruritic gravidarum, or uterine size-date discrepancy.

647 Infectious and parasitic conditions in the mother classifiable elsewhere, but complicating pregnancy, childbirth, or the puerperium

AHA: Q2, 1990, 11

Subclassification 647.0 reports a pregnancy complicated by an infection of microorganism *Treponema pallidum,* which causes venereal disease that leads to many structural and cutaneous lesions and may be transmitted to the fetus in utero.

The following fifth-digit subclassification is for use with category 647 to denote the current episode of care. Valid fifth-digits are in brackets [ ] after each code, unless noted at the rubric.

0 unspecified as to episode of care or not applicable
1 delivered, with or without mention of antepartum condition
2 delivered, with mention of postpartum complication
3 antepartum condition or complication
4 postpartum condition or complication

647.0 5th Maternal syphilis complicating pregnancy, childbirth, or the puerperium — (Use additional code(s) to further specify complication) — *secondary*
AHA: Q2, 1990, 11

647.1 5th Maternal gonorrhea complicating pregnancy, childbirth, or the puerperium — (Use additional code(s) to further specify complication) — *secondary*
AHA: Q2, 1990, 11

647.2 5th Other maternal venereal diseases complicating pregnancy, childbirth, or the puerperium — (Use additional code(s) to further specify complication) — *secondary*
AHA: Q2, 1990, 11

647.3 5th Maternal tuberculosis complicating pregnancy, childbirth, or the puerperium — (Use additional code(s) to further specify complication) — *secondary*
AHA: Q2, 1990, 11

Subclassification 647.3 reports a pregnancy complicated by infection by mycobacterium and characterized by the formation of tubercles and caseous necrosis in the tissues.

647.4 5th Maternal malaria complicating pregnancy, childbirth, or the puerperium — (Use additional code(s) to further specify complication) — *secondary*
AHA: Q2, 1990, 11

Subclassification 647.4 reports a pregnancy complicated by a febrile disease caused by protozoa that are parasitic in the red blood cells. Symptoms, including fever, chills, and sweating, occur at intervals corresponding with a new generation of the parasites.

647.5 5th Maternal rubella complicating pregnancy, childbirth, or the puerperium — (Use additional code(s) to further specify complication) — *secondary*
AHA: Q2, 1990, 11

Subclassification 647.5 reports a pregnancy complicated by infection with a mild viral disease (German measles) known to cause birth defects.

647.6 5th Other maternal viral disease complicating pregnancy, childbirth, or the puerperium — (Use additional code(s) to further specify complication) — *secondary*
AHA: Jan-Feb, 1985, 15; Q2, 1990, 11

647.8 5th Other specified maternal infectious and parasitic disease complicating pregnancy, childbirth, or the puerperium — *secondary*
AHA: Q2, 1990, 11

647.9 5th Unspecified maternal infection or infestation complicating pregnancy, childbirth, or the puerperium — (Use additional code(s) to further specify complication) — *secondary*
AHA: Q2, 1990, 11

Coding Clarification
Use additional codes to further specify the complications.

648 Other current conditions in the mother classifiable elsewhere, but complicating pregnancy, childbirth, or the puerperium

AHA: Q2, 1990, 11

This rubric includes the listed conditions when complicating the pregnant state, aggravated by the pregnancy, or when it is the main reason for the obstetric care.

 © 2004 Ingenix, Inc.

The following fifth-digit subclassification is for use with category 648 to denote the current episode of care. Valid fifth-digits are in brackets [ ] after each code, unless noted at the rubric.

0 unspecified as to episode of care or not applicable

1 delivered, with or without mention of antepartum condition

2 delivered, with mention of postpartum complication

3 antepartum condition or complication

4 postpartum condition or complication

648.0 5th Maternal diabetes mellitus complicating pregnancy, childbirth, or the puerperium — (Use additional code(s) to identify the condition) — *secondary*
AHA: Q2, 1990, 11; Q3, 1991, 5,11

This subclassification reports pregnancy complicated by insulin- or non-insulin-dependent diabetes mellitus affecting the management and health of the mother and fetus during pregnancy. Signs and symptoms of diabetes mellitus include a history of diabetes, insulin- or non-insulin-dependent, with associated conditions such as ketoacidosis. Blood glucose may reveal hyper- or hypoglycemia during pregnancy. Urine culture and sensitivity may reveal asymptomatic urinary tract infection and markedly elevated glycosylated hemoglobin. Other lab work includes tests for electrolyte levels, BUN, and creatinine to evaluate any renal involvement. Ultrasound, fetal biophysical profiles, and other fetal tests may be performed to monitor fetal growth and detect any major congenital anomalies.

Patients with diabetes mellitus are more apt to develop pre-eclampsia or eclampsia. If medical record documentation indicates that either condition is present, assign an additional code.

This category excludes gestational diabetes (648.8x).

648.1 5th Thyroid dysfunction complicating pregnancy, childbirth, or the puerperium — (Use additional code(s) to identify the condition) — *secondary*
AHA: Q2, 1990, 11

648.2 5th Maternal anemia complicating pregnancy, childbirth, or the puerperium — (Use additional code(s) to identify the condition) — *secondary*
AHA: Q2, 1990, 11

Signs and symptoms of anemia include fatigue, palpitations, tachycardia, dyspnea, and pallor. In anemia, the CBC hemoglobin is 10g/100 ml. Red cells may be microcytic and hypochromic; reticulocytes and platelets may be normal or increased in number. For patients with iron deficiency anemia, lab work reveals serum iron below 30mcg/100 ml and elevated total iron binding capacity. For patients with folic acid anemia, lab work reveals low vitamin B12 levels. Therapies include iron therapy (oral, IV, or parenteral). Associated conditions include sickle cell anemia, sickle cell trait, and major and minor thalassemia. Anemia may be found in as many as 80 percent of pregnancies and is due mostly to dietary iron deficiency. Although rare, anemia also may be due to folic acid deficiency.

648.3 5th Maternal drug dependence complicating pregnancy, childbirth, or the puerperium — (Use additional code(s) to identify the condition) — *secondary*
AHA: Q4, 1988, 8; Q2, 1990, 11; Q2, 1998, 13

648.4 5th Maternal mental disorders complicating pregnancy, childbirth, or the puerperium — (Use additional code(s) to identify the condition) — *secondary*
AHA: Q2, 1990, 11; Q4, 1995, 63; Q2, 1998, 13

648.5 5th Maternal congenital cardiovascular disorders complicating pregnancy, childbirth, or the puerperium — (Use additional code(s) to identify the condition) — *secondary*
AHA: Q2, 1990, 11

648.6 5th Other maternal cardiovascular diseases complicating pregnancy, childbirth, or the puerperium — (Use additional code(s) to identify the condition) — *secondary*
AHA: Q2, 1990, 11; Q3, 1998, 11

648.7 5th Bone and joint disorders of maternal back, pelvis, and lower limbs, complicating pregnancy, childbirth, or the puerperium — *secondary*
AHA: Q2, 1990, 11

648.8 5th Abnormal maternal glucose tolerance, complicating pregnancy, childbirth, or the puerperium — (Use additional code(s) to identify the condition) — *secondary*
AHA: Q2, 1990, 11; Q3, 1991, 5

Subclassification 648.8 is reported when the patient has had abnormal glucose tolerance or gestational diabetes although a definitive diagnosis of diabetes mellitus has not been made.

648.9 5th Other current maternal conditions complicating pregnancy, childbirth, or the puerperium — (Use additional code(s) to identify the condition) — *secondary*
AHA: Nov-Dec, 1987, 10; Q2, 1990, 11

Coding Clarification

Use an additional code to describe the condition. Excluded from this rubric are conditions both known or suspected of having affected the fetus, which are reported with codes from rubric 655 *Known or suspected fetal abnormality affecting management of mother.*

This subclassification reports conditions affecting the management of the pregnancy and delivery in the absence of combination codes. This code and the appropriate code from another chapter of ICD-9-CM indicate the treatment of the condition that is affecting management of the pregnancy.

650–659 Normal Delivery, and Other Indications for Care in Pregnancy, Labor, and Delivery

650 Normal delivery OK

AHA: Q4, 1995, 28,59; Q3, 2000, 5; Q3, 2001, 12; Q2, 2002, 10

The definition of delivery in a completely normal case is spontaneous vaginal delivery of a single live infant after completion of 38 to 42 weeks of gestation, with cephalic presentation, without instrumentation, and with no antepartum or postpartum conditions or complications.

Documentation Issues

Examine the medical record documentation to determine if there were any conditions, early in the pregnancy, that affected management of the patient.

Coding Clarification

This category is appropriate to use if an episiotomy was performed, membranes were ruptured artificially, or the placenta was extracted manually. If forceps or vacuum extraction were used to assist delivery, see category 669 *Other complications of labor and delivery, not elsewhere classified.* Rubric 650 is for use as a single diagnosis code and is not to be used with any other code in the range 630-676. Use an additional code to indicate the outcome of delivery (V27).

Threatened Abortion: The outcome of the encounter indicates the proper code assignment. If the products of conception are expelled, the appropriate code from category 634 is assigned. A code from categories 640-648 and 651-657 may be used to identify the condition causing the abortion. If the threatened abortion does not culminate in an abortion, the appropriate code from category 640 is assigned.

651 Multiple gestation

The following fifth-digit subclassification is for use with category 651 to denote the current episode of care.

0 unspecified as to episode of care or not applicable

1 delivered, with or without mention of antepartum condition

3 antepartum condition or complication

651.0 5th Twin pregnancy — *two fetuses*

651.1 5th Triplet pregnancy — *three fetuses*

651.2 5th Quadruplet pregnancy — *four fetuses*

651.3 5th Twin pregnancy with fetal loss and retention of one fetus — *vanishing twin syndrome (651.33)*

651.4 5th Triplet pregnancy with fetal loss and retention of one or more

651.5 5th Quadruplet pregnancy with fetal loss and retention of one or more

651.6 5th Other multiple pregnancy with fetal loss and retention of one or more fetus(es)

651.8 5th Other specified multiple gestation

651.9 5th Unspecified multiple gestation — *superfecundation; superfetation*

Coding Clarification

Use an additional code from rubric V27 to indicate the outcome of delivery in multiple births, identifying livebirths and stillborn births in cases of multiple births. If one or more fetus is malpositioned, also report a code from subclassification 652.6. Only the fifth-digits 0, 1, and 3 apply to the 651 rubric.

652 Malposition and malpresentation of fetus

The following fifth-digit subclassification is for use with category 652 to denote the current episode of care.

0 unspecified as to episode of care or not applicable

1 delivered, with or without mention of antepartum condition

3 antepartum condition or complication

652.0 5th Unstable lie of fetus — (Code first any associated obstructed labor, 660.0) — *changing fetal position*

652.1 5th Breech or other malpresentation successfully converted to cephalic presentation — (Code first any associated obstructed labor, 660.0) — *cephalic version NOS*

652.2 5th Breech presentation without mention of version — (Code first any associated obstructed labor, 660.0) — *breech delivery (assisted) (spontaneous) NOS*

Breech presentation without mention of version is presentation of buttocks first without successful version. There are three forms of breech presentation: frank, in which the legs of the fetus extend over the abdomen and thorax so that the feet lie beside the face; complete, in which the fetal position is maintained so that the legs are flexed and crossed; and incomplete, in which one or both lower legs and feet are prolapsed into the vagina. Foot or knee presentations are subdivisions of incomplete breech presentation and are coded to 652.8x.

In breech presentation, the abdominal exam (four maneuvers of Leopold) identifies the fetal back on one side and the small parts on the opposite side. Lower fetal pole is less distinct, especially if

 © 2004 Ingenix, Inc.

engagement has occurred. Fetal heart tones are heard near the midline, slightly above and to one side of the umbilicus. If the cervix is slightly dilated and the membranes are ruptured, vaginal exam may allow palpation and identification of the presenting part; ultrasound reveals breech presentation. Delivery may be by cesarean section, breech extraction, manual assist, or spontaneous, depending on various obstetrical factors, including age and weight of the fetus and type of breech.

652.3 5th Transverse or oblique presentation of fetus — (Code first any associated obstructed labor, 660.0) — *oblique lie; transverse lie*

652.4 5th Fetal face or brow presentation of fetus — (Code first any associated obstructed labor, 660.0) — *mentum presentation*

652.5 5th High fetal head at term — (Code first any associated obstructed labor, 660.0) — *failure of head to enter pelvic brim*

652.6 5th Multiple gestation with malpresentation of one fetus or more — (Code first any associated obstructed labor, 660.0)

652.7 5th Prolapsed arm of fetus — (Code first any associated obstructed labor, 660.0) — *arm protrudes through birth canal*

652.8 5th Other specified malposition or malpresentation of fetus — (Code first any associated obstructed labor, 660.0) — *compound presentation; nuchal hitch (arm)*

652.9 5th Unspecified malposition or malpresentation of fetus — (Code first any associated obstructed labor, 660.0) — *malpresentation NOS*

Coding Clarification

Any obstructed labor (660.0x) would be sequenced first, followed by a code from this rubric to identify malposition of the fetus. Only the fifth-digits 0, 1, and 3 apply to the 652 rubric.

653 Disproportion in pregnancy, labor, and delivery

Disproportion in this rubric refers to maternal and fetal structural abnormalities or disproportions that interfere with normal delivery. Cephalopelvic disproportion is a disparity between the size of the maternal pelvis and the fetal head that precludes vaginal delivery. In fetopelvic disproportion, the presenting part of the baby is too large to fit through the mother's pelvis; labor progresses to a certain degree and then labor stops. The cervix stops dilating and delivery is by forceps, vacuum extractor, or cesarean section. When an attempt at forceps delivery proves too difficult, the obstetrician should perform a cesarean section. The fetus may be seriously injured or the infant may die if fetopelvic disproportion is encountered after the body has been delivered and the head is trapped. Prolonged labor due to cephalopelvic disproportion (CPD) is a leading cause of maternal death in the developing world. An unusually large fetus increases the likelihood of cephalopelvic disproportion requiring hospitalization for Cesarean delivery or shoulder dystocia during vaginal birth. Fetal anomalies such as hydrocephaly, encephalocele, and soft tissue tumors may obstruct labor and require fetal imaging based on vaginal or abdominal exam or when the fetus presents. Caesarean section is a way to reduce mortality resulting from obstructed labor. In addition, efforts to widen the birth canal are used to save the life of both mother and fetus, especially in third world countries where a Caesarean may increase the incidence of infection and maternal death. Perineotomy is a procedure to widen the lower portion of the birth canal, and symphysiotomy is a surgical widening at the upper level of the birth canal.

The following fifth-digit subclassification is for use with category 653 to denote the current episode of care.

0 unspecified as to episode of care or not applicable

1 delivered, with or without mention of antepartum condition

3 antepartum condition or complication

653.0 5th Major abnormality of bony pelvis, not further specified, in pregnancy — (Code first any associated obstructed labor, 660.1) — *pelvic deformity NOS*

653.1 5th Generally contracted pelvis in pregnancy — (Code first any associated obstructed labor, 660.1) — *contracted pelvis NOS*

653.2 5th Inlet contraction of pelvis in pregnancy — (Code first any associated obstructed labor, 660.1) — *inlet contraction (pelvis)*

653.3 5th Outlet contraction of pelvis in pregnancy — (Code first any associated obstructed labor, 660.1) — *outlet contraction (pelvis)*

653.4 5th Fetopelvic disproportion — (Code first any associated obstructed labor, 660.1) — *cephalopelvic disproportion NOS; disproportion of mixed maternal and fetal origin, with normally formed fetus*

Fetopelvic disproportion is a condition in which the presenting part of a normally formed fetus is too large to pass through the pelvic canal. Upon palpation of the abdomen, a large presenting part of the fetus in proportion to the mother's pelvic canal is revealed. Ultrasound determines fetal size, with therapy that includes cesarean delivery.

653.5 5th Unusually large fetus causing disproportion — (Code first any associated obstructed labor, 660.1) — *disproportion of fetal origin with normally formed fetus*

Use this subclassification to report an unusually large fetus too large to pass through the pelvic canal. Upon palpation of the abdomen, a disproportionately large fetus is revealed. Ultrasound determines fetal size. Therapies include cesarean delivery.

653.6 ✓5th Hydrocephalic fetus causing disproportion — (Code first any associated obstructed labor, 660.1) — *large head of fetus disproportionate to maternal pelvis*

653.7 ✓5th Other fetal abnormality causing disproportion — (Code first any associated obstructed labor, 660.1) — *conjoined twins; fetal ascites; fetal myelomeningocele; fetal sacral teratoma*

653.8 ✓5th Fetal disproportion of other origin — (Code first any associated obstructed labor, 660.1)

653.9 ✓5th Unspecified fetal disproportion — (Code first any associated obstructed labor, 660.1) — *disproportion NOS*

Coding Clarification

If labor is obstructed, sequence the obstruction (660.1x) first, followed by a code from this rubric to report the disproportion. Only the fifth-digits 0, 1, and 3 apply to the 653 rubric.

654 Abnormality of organs and soft tissues of pelvis complicating pregnancy, childbirth, or the puerperium

The following fifth-digit subclassification is for use with category 654 to denote the current episode of care. Valid fifth-digts are in brackets [ ] at the end of each code, unless noted at the rubric.

0 unspecified as to episode of care or not applicable

1 delivered, with or without mention of antepartum condition

2 delivered, with mention of postpartum complication

3 antepartum condition or complication

4 postpartum condition or complication

654.0 ✓5th Congenital abnormalities of pregnant uterus complicating pregnancy, childbirth, or the puerperium — (Code first any associated obstructed labor, 660.2) — *double uterus; uterus bicornis*

654.1 ✓5th Tumors of body of pregnant uterus — (Code first any associated obstructed labor, 660.2) — *fibroids*

654.2 ✓5th Previous cesarean section complicating pregnancy, childbirth, or the puerperium — (Code first any associated obstructed labor, 660.2) — *scar from previous cesarean delivery*
AHA: Q1, 1992, 8

Use codes in 654.2 to report pregnancy, childbirth, or the puerperium complicated by a uterine scar caused by a previous cesarean section. Therapies include vaginal or repeat cesarean delivery.

654.3 ✓5th Retroverted and incarcerated gravid uterus — (Code first any associated obstructed labor, 660.2) — *uterus is tilted so that it cannot rise above the sacral promontory*

654.4 ✓5th Other abnormalities in shape or position of gravid uterus and of neighboring structures — (Code first any associated obstructed labor, 660.2) — *cystocele; pendulous abdomen; rectocele*

654.5 ✓5th Cervical incompetence complicating pregnancy, childbirth, or the puerperium — (Code first any associated obstructed labor, 660.2) — *presence of Shirodkar suture with or without cervical incompetence*

Use codes in subclassification 654.5 to report dilation of the cervix, usually leading to second-trimester abortion. The etiology may be congenital or due to acquired causes such as previous surgical dilation, conization, breech extraction, or other trauma of delivery. Signs and symptoms of cervical incompetence include a history of previous late spontaneous abortions. A cervical exam allows passage of No. 8 Hegar dilator past the internal cervical os. Hysterosalpingostomy demonstrates a widened cervical os. Therapies include McDonald, Shirodkar, or other cerclage procedure (placement of encircling suture about the cervical os using heavy nonabsorbable suture or mercilene tape) to prevent protrusion and consequent rupture of the amniotic sac, followed by removal of the suture at 38 weeks or when labor begins.

654.6 ✓5th Other congenital or acquired abnormality of cervix complicating pregnancy, childbirth, or the puerperium — (Code first any associated obstructed labor, 660.2) — *cicatricial cervix; cervical polyp; stenosis or stricture of cervix*

654.7 ✓5th Congenital or acquired abnormality of vagina complicating pregnancy, childbirth, or the puerperium — (Code first any associated obstructed labor, 660.2) — *septate vagina; vaginal stenosis or stricture*

654.8 ✓5th Congenital or acquired abnormality of vulva complicating pregnancy, childbirth, or the puerperium — (Code first any associated obstructed labor, 660.2) — *fibrosis of perineum; persistent hymen; rigid perineum*
AHA: Q1, 2003, 14

654.9 ✓5th Other and unspecified abnormality of organs and soft tissues of pelvis complicating pregnancy, childbirth, and the puerperium — *uterine scar NEC; dystocia syndrome*

If labor is obstructed, sequence the obstruction (660.2x) first, followed by a code from this rubric to report the abnormality of organs and soft tissues of the pelvis.

 © 2004 Ingenix, Inc.

655 Known or suspected fetal abnormality affecting management of mother

AHA: Q3, 1990, 4

The following fifth-digit subclassification is for use with category 655 to denote the current episode of care.

0 unspecified as to episode of care or not applicable

1 delivered, with or without mention of antepartum condition

3 antepartum condition or complication

655.0 5th Central nervous system malformation in fetus affecting management of mother — *fetal or suspected fetal; anencephaly, hydrocephalus or spina bifida (with myelomeningocele)*

655.1 5th Chromosomal abnormality in fetus affecting management of mother — *known to have damaged or mutated chromosome resulting in abnormality*

655.2 5th Hereditary disease in family possibly affecting fetus, affecting management of mother

655.3 5th Suspected damage to fetus from viral disease in mother, affecting management of mother — *maternal rubella*

655.4 5th Suspected damage to fetus from other disease in mother, affecting management of mother — *maternal alcohol addiction or maternal listerosis or maternal toxoplasmosis*

655.5 5th Suspected damage to fetus from drugs, affecting management of mother — *drug damage*

655.6 5th Suspected damage to fetus from radiation, affecting management of mother — *radiation damage*

655.7 5th Decreased fetal movements — *reduction in fetal movements*
AHA: Q4, 1997, 41

655.8 5th Other known or suspected fetal abnormality, not elsewhere classified, affecting management of mother — *suspected damage to fetus from environmental toxins or intrauterine contraceptive device*

655.9 5th Unspecified fetal abnormality affecting management of mother

Coding Clarification

Report codes in this rubric when the listed conditions in the fetus are reasons for observation or obstetrical care of the mother or for termination of the pregnancy. Only the fifth-digits 0, 1, and 3 apply to the 655 rubric.

656 Other fetal and placental problems affecting management of mother

The following fifth-digit subclassification is for use with category 656 to denote the current episode of care.

0 unspecified as to episode of care or not applicable

1 delivered, with or without mention of antepartum condition

3 antepartum condition or complication

656.0 5th Fetal-maternal hemorrhage affecting management of mother — *leakage (microscopic) of fetal blood into maternal circulation*

656.1 5th Rhesus isoimmunization affecting management of mother — *anti-D [Rh] antibodies; Rh incompatibility*

656.2 5th Isoimmunization from other and unspecified blood-group incompatibility affecting management of mother — *ABO isoimmunization*

656.3 5th Fetal distress affecting management of mother — *metabolic acidemia*
AHA: Nov-Dec, 1986, 4

The definition of fetal distress is metabolic abnormalities, notably hypoxia, and acidosis, which affect the functions of vital organs of the fetus. Fetal distress can occur at any time during pregnancy, or during or because of the stress of uterine contractions and medications. In fetal distress, the fetal heart monitor reveals acceleration or deceleration of fetal heart rate, flattened heart rate baseline, and extreme and variable deceleration of uterine tachysystole and tetanic contractions. Fetal scalp blood sampling (blood pH) reveals fetal distress. Therapies include administration of oxygen to the mother.

Excluded from this subclassification are abnormal fetal acid-base balance (656.8x), abnormality in fetal heart rate or rhythm (659.7x), or meconium in liquor (656.8x).

656.4 5th Intrauterine death affecting management of mother — *fetal death NOS; fetal death after completion of 22 weeks' gestation; missed delivery*

656.5 5th Poor fetal growth affecting management of mother — *"light for dates"; "placental insufficiency"; "small for dates"*

656.6 5th Excessive fetal growth affecting management of mother — *"large for dates"*

656.7 5th Other placental conditions affecting management of mother — *abnormal placenta; placental infarct*

656.8 5th Other specified fetal and placental problems affecting management of mother — *abnormal acid-base balance; intrauterine abscess; lithopedion*

656.9 ✓5th Unspecified fetal and placental problem affecting management of mother

Coding Clarification

Report codes in this rubric when the listed conditions in the fetus are a reason for observation or obstetrical care of the mother or for termination of the pregnancy. Only the fifth-digits 0, 1, and 3 apply to the 656 rubric.

657 Polyhydramnios

Polyhydramnios is excess amniotic fluid surrounding the fetus and can occur when the fetus fails to swallow and absorb amniotic fluid in excess of normal amounts due to, among other causes, gastrointestinal obstruction and neurological problems. Decreases or excessive amounts of amniotic fluid may be associated with abnormalities in the fetus. This condition is discovered at or before delivery and is evaluated during the infant's hospital stay. Documenting polyhydramnios may include:

- History of the pregnancy
- History of past pregnancies and the health of children delivered
- Other family history

If there is a concern regarding polyhydramnios, the amount of amniotic fluid can be estimated using ultrasound. The amount of fluid that is normal changes with gestational age; however, polyhydramnios is typically defined as a total fluid volume of greater than 24.0 centimeters.

The following fifth-digit subclassification is for use with category 657 to denote the current episode of care.

0 unspecified as to episode of care or not applicable

1 delivered, with or without mention of antepartum condition

3 antepartum condition or complication

657.0 ✓5th Polyhydramnios — *excessive amniotic fluid*
AHA: Q4, 1991, 26

Coding Clarification

This code requires a fifth-digit. Assign a 0 for fourth-digit placement with this code, and then assign the appropriate fifth-digit. Only the fifth-digits 0, 1, and 3 apply to the 657 rubric.

658 Other problems associated with amniotic cavity and membranes

The following fifth-digit subclassification is for use with category 658 to denote the current episode of care.

0 unspecified as to episode of care or not applicable

1 delivered, with or without mention of antepartum condition

3 antepartum condition or complication

658.0 ✓5th Oligohydramnios — *presence of abnormally low amount of amniotic fluid*

658.1 ✓5th Premature rupture of membranes in pregnancy — *rupture of amniotic sac less than 24 hours prior to onset of labor*

658.2 ✓5th Delayed delivery after spontaneous or unspecified rupture of membranes — *prolonged rupture of membranes NOS; rupture of amniotic sac 24 hours or more prior to the onset of labor*

658.3 ✓5th Delayed delivery after artificial rupture of membranes

658.4 ✓5th Infection of amniotic cavity — *amnionitis; membranitis; chorioamnionitis*

658.8 ✓5th Other problems associated with amniotic cavity and membranes — *amnion nodosum; amniotic cyst; infarct of amnion; cyst of chorion*

Coding Clarification

Amniotic fluid embolism (673.1x) is excluded from this rubric. Only the fifth-digits 0, 1, and 3 apply to the 658 rubric.

659 Other indications for care or intervention related to labor and delivery, not elsewhere classified

An "elderly" pregnant woman is one who is 35 years of age or older. A primigravida is pregnancy with a first child, while a multigravida is pregnancy with a second or greater pregnancy.

The following fifth-digit subclassification is for use with category 659 to denote the current episode of care.

0 unspecified as to episode of care or not applicable

1 delivered, with or without mention of antepartum condition

3 antepartum condition or complication

659.0 ✓5th Failed mechanical induction of labor — *failure of induction of labor by surgical or other instrumental methods*

659.1 ✓5th Failed medical or unspecified induction of labor — *failed induction NOS; failure of induction of labor by medical methods, such as oxytocic drugs*

659.2 ✓5th Maternal pyrexia during labor, unspecified — *fever while the patient is in labor*

659.3 ✓5th Generalized infection during labor — *septicemia during labor*

659.4 ✓5th Grand multiparity, with current pregnancy — *birth to six or more children previously*

© 2004 Ingenix, Inc.

659.5 5th Elderly primigravida — *beyond the age norm for a first pregnancy*
AHA: Q3, 2001, 12

659.6 5th Elderly multigravida — *age at delivery at least 35, and has experienced at least one pregnancy previously*
AHA: Q3, 2001, 12

659.7 5th Abnormality in fetal heart rate or rhythm — *depressed fetal heart tones, including brachycardia, tachycardia*
AHA: Q4, 1998, 48

659.8 5th Other specified indications for care or intervention related to labor and delivery — *age less than 16 years at expected date of delivery*
AHA: Q3, 2001, 12

659.9 5th Unspecified indication for care or intervention related to labor and delivery

Coding Clarification

Supervision only of the pregnancy of an elderly primigravida is reported with V23.81; supervision of an elderly multigravida with V23.82. Only the fifth-digits 0, 1, and 3 apply to the 659 rubric.

660–669 Complications Occurring Mainly in the Course of Labor and Delivery

660 Obstructed labor

AHA: Q3, 1995, 10

Labor is described in stages. The latent phase lasts from several hours to as long as three days with uterine contractions and passage of the mucus plug. During the first stage, the contractions come at intervals and may be accompanied by mild pain. The cervix dilates until its opening is large enough to allow the passage of the infant and by the end of the first stage, the amniotic sac breaks. The first stage can last many hours in obstructed labor, where the baby is unusually large or badly angled. Obstructed labor may be due to anatomical abnormalities, prematurity, and unusual orientation of the child in the uterus, such as breech presentation (e.g., head last in the birth canal) and transverse presentation (e.g., sideways position in the birth canal). Obstructed labor is a leading cause of maternal and fetal death.

The following fifth-digit subclassification is for use with category 660 to denote the current episode of care.

0 unspecified as to episode of care or not applicable

1 delivered, with or without mention of antepartum condition

3 antepartum condition or complication

660.0 5th Obstruction caused by malposition of fetus at onset of labor — (Use additional code from 652.0-652.9 to identify condition) — *secondary*
AHA: Q3, 1995, 10

660.1 5th Obstruction by bony pelvis during labor and delivery — (Use additional code from 653.0-653.9 to identify condition) — *secondary*
AHA: Q3, 1995, 10

660.2 5th Obstruction by abnormal pelvic soft tissues during labor and delivery — (Use additional code from 654.0-654.9 to identify condition) — *secondary*
AHA: Q3, 1995, 10

660.3 5th Deep transverse arrest and persistent occipitoposterior position during labor and delivery

660.4 5th Shoulder (girdle) dystocia during labor and delivery — *impacted shoulders*
AHA: Q3, 1995, 10

660.5 5th Locked twins — *one twin is in breech position, the other high in head position, rendering vaginal delivery impossible*
AHA: Q3, 1995, 10

660.6 5th Unspecified failed trial of labor — *failed trial of labor*
AHA: Q3, 1995, 10

660.7 5th Unspecified failed forceps or vacuum extractor — *application of ventouse or forceps*
AHA: Q3, 1995, 10

660.8 5th Other causes of obstructed labor — *other specified causes of obstructed labor NEC*
AHA: Q3, 1995, 10

660.9 5th Unspecified obstructed labor — *dystocia NOS or fetal dystocia NOS or maternal dystocia NOS*
AHA: Q3, 1995, 10

Coding Clarification

Additional codes may be required to report the cause of the obstruction and should be sequenced secondarily to the code from this rubric. Only the fifth-digits 0, 1, and 3 apply to the 660 rubric.

661 Abnormality of forces of labor

Labor is diagnosed when there is regular uterine activity in association with cervical dilatation or effacement. Labor can be obstructed due to weak uterine muscle contractions and other problems during the stages of labor. Uterine inertia, or poor contraction strength, is a common reason for prolonged latent phase. Uterine inertia can be primary (e.g., when few contractions are initiated or do not start) or secondary (e.g., the slowing down of labor). Slow progress at the end of the first stage may be due to cephalopelvic disproportion, malposition, or poor

© 2004 Ingenix, Inc.

contraction strength. An oxytocin infusion helps overcome malposition or poor contraction strength. In the third stage, the uterus may be prevented from contracting effectively by fragments of placenta that remain in the uterus after delivery or by benign growths of uterine muscle within the uterine wall; however, in most cases, the uterine muscle simply fails to contract adequately.

The following fifth-digit subclassification is for use with category 661 to denote the current episode of care.

0 unspecified as to episode of care or not applicable

1 delivered, with or without mention of antepartum condition

3 antepartum condition or complication

661.0 5th Primary uterine inertia — *weakness of uterus during first stage of labor; including failure of cervical dilation; hypotonic uterine dysfunction, primary*

661.1 5th Secondary uterine inertia — *weakness of uterus in second stage of labor; including arrested active phase of labor; hypotonic uterine dysfunction, secondary*

661.2 5th Other and unspecified uterine inertia — *desultory labor; irregular labor; slow slope active phase of labor*

661.3 5th Precipitate labor — *rapid labor and delivery*

Precipitate labor is cervical dilation of 5.0 centimeters or more per hour for primigravidas and 10.0 centimeters or more per hour for multigravidas. Usually, precipitate labor is the result of extraordinary forceful uterine contractions or low birth canal resistance.

661.4 5th Hypertonic, incoordinate, or prolonged uterine contractions — *cervical spasm; dyscoordinate labor; hourglass contraction of uterus; retraction ring (Band's) (pathological); uterine spasm*

661.9 5th Unspecified abnormality of labor

Coding Clarification

Only the fifth-digits 0, 1, and 3 apply to the 661 rubric.

662 Long labor

Labor is described in stages. During the first stage, the cervix dilates until its opening is large enough to allow the passage of the infant. The first stage can last many hours in obstructed labor, where the baby is unusually large or badly angled. The second stage begins with the complete dilation and effacement of the cervix and ends at the birth. During the third stage of labor, which occurs within the first hour of birth, placental material is expelled through the birth canal. Labor averages about 13 hours for first deliveries and about eight hours for subsequent deliveries. Dystocia, or difficult labor, includes labor that fails to progress, prolonged labor, or difficult childbirth. Dysfunctional labors due to cephalopelvic disproportion (CPD) occur when the baby is too large to pass safely through the mother's pelvis.

The following fifth-digit subclassification is for use with category 662 to denote the current episode of care.

0 unspecified as to episode of care or not applicable

1 delivered, with or without mention of antepartum condition

3 antepartum condition or complication

662.0 5th Prolonged first stage of labor

662.1 5th Unspecified prolonged labor — *unknown stage*

662.2 5th Prolonged second stage of labor

662.3 5th Delayed delivery of second twin, triplet, etc.

Coding Clarification

Only the fifth-digits 0, 1, and 3 apply to the 662 rubric.

663 Umbilical cord complications during labor and delivery

This rubric covers umbilical complications at birth, which include:

- Occult prolapse — occurs with intact membranes when the cord is expelled before the presenting part or is trapped in front of a shoulder.
- Overt prolapse — occurs with ruptured membranes when the cord is in front of the presenting part. It most commonly occurs spontaneously with breech presentation but also occurs with vertex presentation, particularly when membranes are ruptured and the presenting part is not engaged. Treatment is immediate delivery and the practitioner must hold the presenting part up off the prolapsed cord to prevent further, prolonged compression. The cord is kept in the vagina to prevent drying.
- Vasa previa — the umbilical cord is the presenting part, a dangerous condition since the umbilical vessels can become pinched off or rupture as they are compressed between the fetus and the walls of the birth canal.

The following fifth-digit subclassification is for use with category 663 to denote the current episode of care.

0 unspecified as to episode of care or not applicable

1 delivered, with or without mention of antepartum condition

3 antepartum condition or complication

663.0 5th Prolapse of cord, complicating labor and delivery — *presentation of cord; an emergent situation*

 © 2004 Ingenix, Inc.

663.1 ✓5th Cord around neck, with compression, complicating labor and delivery — *cord tightly around neck*

663.2 ✓5th Other and unspecified cord entanglement, with compression, complicating labor and delivery — *entanglement of cords of twins in mono-amniotic sac; knot in cord (with compression)*

663.3 ✓5th Other and unspecified cord entanglement, without mention of compression, complicating labor and delivery

663.4 ✓5th Short cord complicating labor and delivery — *lacks appropriate amount of slack, increasing risk of placental abruption*

663.5 ✓5th Vasa previa complicating labor and delivery — *umbilical cord is presenting part*

663.6 ✓5th Vascular lesions of cord complicating labor and delivery — *bruising; hematoma; thrombosis of vessels*

663.8 ✓5th Other umbilical cord complications during labor and delivery — *velamentous insertion of umbilical cord; ruptured umbilical cord*

663.9 ✓5th Unspecified umbilical cord complication during labor and delivery

Coding Clarification

Only the fifth-digits 0, 1, and 3 apply to the 663 rubric.

664 Trauma to perineum and vulva during delivery

AHA: Nov-Dec, 1984, 10; Q1, 1992, 11

This category includes a laceration, rupture, or a tear of the perineum and vulva during delivery due to damage from instruments such as forceps or from an extension of an episiotomy.

The following fifth-digit subclassification is for use with category 664 to denote the current episode of care.

0 unspecified as to episode of care or not applicable

1 delivered, with or without mention of antepartum condition

3 antepartum condition or complication

664.0 ✓5th First-degree perineal laceration during delivery — *perineal laceration, rupture or tear involving fourchette, hymen, labia, skin, vagina or vulva*
AHA: Nov-Dec, 1984, 10; Q1, 1992, 11

664.1 ✓5th Second-degree perineal laceration during delivery — *perineal laceration, rupture or tear (following episiotomy) involving pelvic floor, perineal muscles, or vaginal muscles*
AHA: Nov-Dec, 1984, 10; Q1, 1992, 11

664.2 ✓5th Third-degree perineal laceration during delivery — *perineal laceration, rupture or tear (following episiotomy) involving anal sphincter, rectovaginal septum or sphincter, NOS*
AHA: Nov-Dec, 1984, 10; Q1, 1992, 11

664.3 ✓5th Fourth-degree perineal laceration during delivery — *se*[illegible]*ry*
AHA: Nov-D[illegible], 10; Q1, 1992, 11

664.4 ✓5th Unspecified perineal laceration during delivery — *central laceration*
AHA: Nov-Dec, 1984, 10; Q1, 1992, 8; Q1, 1992, 11

664.5 ✓5th Vulvar and perineal hematoma during delivery

664.8 ✓5th Other specified trauma to perineum and vulva during delivery

664.9 ✓5th Unspecified trauma to perineum and vulva during delivery

Coding Clarification

Only the fifth-digits 0, 1, and 3 apply to the 664 rubric.

665 Other obstetrical trauma

The following fifth-digit subclassification is for use with category 665 to denote the current episode of care. Valid fifth-digts are in brackets [ ] at the end of each code, unless noted at the rubric.

0 unspecified as to episode of care or not applicable

1 delivered, with or without mention of antepartum condition

2 delivered, with mention of postpartum complication

3 antepartum condition or complication

4 postpartum condition or complication

665.0 ✓5th Rupture of uterus before onset of labor

665.1 ✓5th Rupture of uterus during and after labor — *rupture of uterus NOS*

665.2 ✓5th Obstetrical inversion of uterus — *failure of placenta to separate from uterus, facilitating the turning of the uterus inside out*

665.3 ✓5th Obstetrical laceration of cervix

665.4 ✓5th High vaginal laceration during and after labor — *laceration of vaginal wall or sulcus without mention of perineal laceration*

665.5 ✓5th Other obstetrical injury to pelvic organs — *injury to bladder or urethra*
AHA: March-April, 1987, 10

665.6 ✓5th Obstetrical damage to pelvic joints and ligaments — *avulsion of inner symphyseal cartilage; damage to coccyx; separation of symphysis pubis*
AHA: Nov-Dec, 1984, 12

665.7 ✓5th Obstetrical pelvic hematoma — *hematoma of vagina*

665.8 ✓5th Other specified obstetrical trauma

665.9 ✓5th Unspecified obstetrical trauma — *obstetrical trauma NOS*

666 Postpartum hemorrhage

AHA: Q1, 1988, 14

Postpartum hemorrhage is vaginal bleeding in excess of 500 ml during the third stage of labor, in the immediate postpartum period, or after the first 24 hours following delivery. Therapies include manual exploration of the uterine cavity for retained placenta and curettage of the uterine cavity.

Postpartum hemorrhage due to etiologies other than a retained placenta or membranes is classified elsewhere. Other etiologies for postpartum hemorrhage include lacerations of the cervix, vagina, or perineum, rupture of the uterus, a hypotonic myometrium due to general anesthesia, and overdistension of the uterus due to an abnormally large fetus or multiple gestation.

The following fifth-digit subclassification is for use with category 666 to denote the current episode of care.

0 unspecified as to episode of care or not applicable

2 delivered, with mention of postpartum complication

4 postpartum condition or complication

666.0 ✓5th Third-stage postpartum hemorrhage — *hemorrhage associated with retained, trapped, or adherent placenta; retained placenta NOS*
AHA: Q1, 1988, 14

666.1 ✓5th Other immediate postpartum hemorrhage — *atony of uterus; hemorrhage within the first 24 hours following delivery of placenta; postpartum hemorrhage (atonic) NOS*
AHA: Q1, 1988, 14

666.2 ✓5th Delayed and secondary postpartum hemorrhage — *hemorrhage after the first 24 hours following delivery; hemorrhage associated with retained portions of placenta or membranes; postpartum hemorrhage specified as delayed or secondary; retained products of conception NOS*
AHA: Q1, 1988, 14

666.3 ✓5th Postpartum coagulation defects — *postpartum afibrinogenemia or fibrinolysis*
AHA: Q1, 1988, 14

Coding Clarification

Postpartum hemorrhage may be associated with a retained, trapped, or adherent placenta (666.0x). It also may occur within the first 24 hours following delivery of the fetus but not be associated with a retained portion of the placenta and/or membranes (code 666.1x). Delayed or secondary postpartum hemorrhage refers to hemorrhage occurring after the first 24 hours after delivery of the fetus and usually is associated with a retained portion of the placenta and/or membranes (666.2x). Code 666.3x includes postpartum coagulation defects, as seen in hypofibrinogenemia or thrombocytonia. Only the fifth-digits 0, 2, and 4 apply to the 666 rubric.

667 Retained placenta or membranes, without hemorrhage

AHA: Q1, 1988, 14

The placenta is normally delivered within 30 minutes of the birth. If the placenta does not deliver spontaneously, the practitioner will administer an analgesic and reach into the uterus to retrieve the placenta. If the placenta delivers spontaneously, the practitioner will check the placenta for completeness. If the placenta is not complete, the practitioner will examine the uterus and try to remove the residual pieces. In some cases, the uterus will be suctioned or scraped to remove residual tissues. If retained placenta is left untreated, there is a high risk of maternal death. However, manual removal of the placenta is an invasive procedure with its own serious complications of hemorrhage, infection, or genital tract trauma. Noninvasive techniques include injecting saline solution and oxytocin into the umbilical vein. This code reports the diagnosis without hemorrhage.

The following fifth-digit subclassification is for use with category 667 to denote the current episode of care.

0 unspecified as to episode of care or not applicable

2 delivered, with mention of postpartum complication

4 postpartum condition or complication

667.0 ✓5th Retained placenta without hemorrhage — *placenta accreta, retained placenta NOS, or retained placenta, total, no hemorrhage*
AHA: Q1, 1988, 14

667.1 ✓5th Retained portions of placenta or membranes, without hemorrhage — *retained products of conception, following delivery, without hemorrhage*
AHA: Q1, 1988, 14

Coding Clarification

Only the fifth-digits 0, 2, and 4 apply to the 667 rubric.

© 2004 Ingenix, Inc.

668 Complications of the administration of anesthetic or other sedation in labor and delivery

This rubric includes complications arising from the administration of a general or local anesthetic, analgesic, or other sedation in labor or delivery.

The following fifth-digit subclassification is for use with category 668 to denote the current episode of care.

0 unspecified as to episode of care or not applicable

1 delivered, with or without mention of antepartum condition

2 delivered, with mention of postpartum complication

3 antepartum condition or complication

4 postpartum condition or complication

668.0 5th Pulmonary complications of the administration of anesthesia or other sedation in labor and delivery — (Use additional code(s) to further specify complication) — *pressure collapse of lung or inhalation or aspiration of stomach contents or secretions following anesthesia or other sedation; Use additional code to further specify complication*

668.1 5th Cardiac complications of the administration of anesthesia or other sedation in labor and delivery — (Use additional code(s) to further specify complication)

668.2 5th Central nervous system complications of the administration of anesthesia or other sedation in labor and delivery — *cerebral anoxia following anesthesia or other sedation; Use additional code to further specify complication*

668.8 5th Other complications of the administration of anesthesia or other sedation in labor and delivery — (Use additional code(s) to further specify complication) — *other specified complications of anesthesia or other sedation use additional code to further specify complication*
AHA: Q2, 1999, 9

668.9 5th Unspecified complication of the administration of anesthesia or other sedation in labor and delivery — (Use additional code(s) to further specify complication) — *anesthesia complication NOS, obstetric use additional code to further specify complication*

Coding Clarification

Additional codes may be required to further identify the specific complications. This rubric excludes a reaction to a spinal or lumbar puncture or a spinal headache (349.0).

669 Other complications of labor and delivery, not elsewhere classified

The following fifth-digit subclassification is for use with category 669 to denote the current episode of care. Valid fifth-digts are in brackets [ ] at the end of each code, unless noted at the rubric.

0 unspecified as to episode of care or not applicable

1 delivered, with or without mention of antepartum condition

2 delivered, with mention of postpartum complication

3 antepartum condition or complication

4 postpartum condition or complication

669.0 5th Maternal distress — *metabolic disturbance*

669.1 5th Shock during or following labor and delivery — *obstetric shock*

669.2 5th Maternal hypotension syndrome — *low arterial blood pressure in the mother*

669.3 5th Acute renal failure following labor and delivery

669.4 5th Other complications of obstetrical surgery and procedures — *cardiac arrest or failure following cesarean or other obstetrical surgery or procedure, including delivery NOS*

669.5 5th Forceps or vacuum extractor delivery without mention of indication — *delivery by ventouse*

669.6 5th Breech extraction, without mention of indication

669.7 5th Cesarean delivery, without mention of indication

669.8 5th Other complications of labor and delivery

669.9 5th Unspecified complication of labor and delivery — *sudden death during childbirth*

670–677 Complications of the Puerperium

Categories 671 and 673-676 include the listed conditions even if they occur during pregnancy or childbirth.

670 Major puerperal infection

Puerperal infection refers to bacterial infection following childbirth. The bacteria are normally found in the mother's genital tract, but may be introduced from the woman's intestine and skin or from the practitioner. The genital tract, particularly the uterus, is the most commonly infected site and in a major episode, the infection can spread to other parts of the body. The primary symptom is a fever between birth and 10 days postpartum. Endometritis is the most prominent of these infections and can occur if the uterus has retained a piece of the placenta.

The following fifth-digit subclassifications are for use with category 670 to denote the current episode of care.

0 unspecified as to episode of care or not applicable

2 delivered, with mention of postpartum complication

4 postpartum condition or complication

670.0 5th Major puerperal infection — *infection and inflammation in the days following childbirth; puerperal endometritis, fever, pelvic cellulitis or sepsis*
AHA: Q2, 1991, 7; Q4, 1991, 26

Coding Clarification
Select the appropriate fifth-digit subclassification for this code and use a 0 as the fourth-digit.

This rubric excludes infection following abortion (639.0), minor genital tract infection following delivery (646.6x), puerperal pyrexia (672), and urinary tract infection following delivery (646.6x). Only the fifth-digits 0, 2, and 4 apply to the 670 rubric.

671 Venous complications in pregnancy and the puerperium

The following fifth-digit subclassifications are for use with category 671 to denote the current episode of care.

0 unspecified as to episode of care or not applicable

1 delivered, with or without mention of antepartum condition

2 delivered, with mention of postpartum complication

3 antepartum condition or complication

4 postpartum condition or complication

671.0 5th Varicose veins of legs in pregnancy and the puerperium — *distended tortuous veins of the lower extremities associated with pregnancy*

671.1 5th Varicose veins of vulva and perineum in pregnancy and the puerperium — *distended tortuous veins on the external female genitalia and perineum associated with pregnancy*

671.2 5th Superficial thrombophlebitis in pregnancy and the puerperium — *inflammation and blood clot of superficial vein following childbirth; thrombophlebitis (superficial)*

671.3 5th Deep phlebothrombosis, antepartum — *inflammation and blood clot of deep vein in pregnant patient; deep-vein thrombosis, antepartum*

671.4 5th Deep phlebothrombosis, postpartum — *inflammation and blood clot of deep vein in pregnant patient; deep-vein thrombosis, postpartum*

671.5 5th Other phlebitis and thrombosis in pregnancy and the puerperium — *cerebral venous thrombosis; thrombosis of intracranial venous sinus*

671.8 5th Other venous complications in pregnancy and the puerperium — *hemorrhoids*

671.9 5th Unspecified venous complication in pregnancy and the puerperium — *phlebitis NOS; thrombosis NOS*

672 Pyrexia of unknown origin during the puerperium

Select the appropriate fifth-digit subclassification for this code, and use a 0 as the fourth-digit.

The following fifth-digit subclassifications are for use with category 672 to denote the current episode of care.

0 unspecified as to episode of care or not applicable

2 delivered, with mention of postpartum complication

4 postpartum condition or complication

672.0 5th Pyrexia of unknown origin during the puerperium — *postpartum fever NOS; puerperal fever NOS; puerperal pyrexia NOS*
AHA: Q4, 1991, 26

673 Obstetrical pulmonary embolism

This rubric reports pulmonary emboli in pregnancy, childbirth, or the puerperium, or specified as puerperal.

The following fifth-digit subclassifications are for use with category 673 to denote the current episode of care.

0 unspecified as to episode of care or not applicable

1 delivered, with or without mention of antepartum condition

2 delivered, with mention of postpartum complication

3 antepartum condition or complication

4 postpartum condition or complication

673.0 5th Obstetrical air embolism — *bubble of air blocking artery in the lung, associated with pregnancy*

673.1 5th Amniotic fluid embolism — *bubble of amniotic fluid blocking artery in mother's lung*

673.2 5th Obstetrical blood-clot embolism — *puerperal pulmonary embolism NOS*

673.3 5th Obstetrical pyemic and septic embolism — *blockage of the artery in the lung, associated with infection in pregnancy*

673.8 5th Other obstetrical pulmonary embolism — *fat embolism*

Coding Clarification
Excluded are emboli following abortion (639.6).

 © 2004 Ingenix, Inc.

674 Other and unspecified complications of the puerperium, not elsewhere classified

The following fifth-digit subclassifications are for use with category 674 to denote the current episode of care. Valid fifth-digts are in brackets [ ] at the end of each code, unless noted at the rubric.

0 unspecified as to episode of care or not applicable
1 delivered, with or without mention of antepartum condition
2 delivered, with mention of postpartum complication
3 antepartum condition or complication
4 postpartum condition or complication

674.0 5th Cerebrovascular disorders in the puerperium — *secondary*

674.1 5th Disruption of cesarean wound — *dehiscence or disruption of uterine wound*

674.2 5th Disruption of obstetrical perineal wound — *breakdown of perineum; secondary perineal tear; disruption of episiotomy wound*

674.3 5th Other complications of obstetrical surgical wounds — *hematoma, hemorrhage or infection of cesarean or perineal wound*
AHA: Q2, 1991, 7

674.4 5th Placental polyp

674.5 5th Peripartum cardiomyopathy

674.8 5th Other complications of the puerperium — *hepatorenal syndrome, following delivery; subinvolution of the uterus; puerperal cardiac thrombosis*
AHA: Q3, 1998, 16

674.9 5th Unspecified complications of the puerperium — *sudden death of unknown cause during the puerperium*

675 Infection of the breast and nipple associated with childbirth

Included in this rubric are the listed conditions as they occur during childbirth, pregnancy, or in the puerperium.

The following fifth-digit subclassifications are for use with category 675 to denote the current episode of care.

0 unspecified as to episode of care or not applicable
1 delivered, with or without mention of antepartum condition
2 delivered, with mention of postpartum complication
3 antepartum condition or complication
4 postpartum condition or complication

675.0 5th Infection of nipple associated with childbirth — *abscess of the nipple*

675.1 5th Abscess of breast associated with childbirth — *mammary abscess; purulent abscess*

675.2 5th Nonpurulent mastitis associated with childbirth — *lymphangitis of breast; interstitial mastitis*

675.8 5th Other specified infection of the breast and nipple associated with childbirth

675.9 5th Unspecified infection of the breast and nipple associated with childbirth

676 Other disorders of the breast associated with childbirth and disorders of lactation

Included in this rubric are the listed conditions as they occur during childbirth, pregnancy, or in the puerperium.

The following fifth-digit subclassifications are for use with category 676 to denote the current episode of care.

0 unspecified as to episode of care or not applicable
1 delivered, with or without mention of antepartum condition
2 delivered, with mention of postpartum complication
3 antepartum condition or complication
4 postpartum condition or complication

676.0 5th Retracted nipple associated with childbirth — *drawing back of the projected surface of the mammary gland*

676.1 5th Cracked nipple associated with childbirth — *fissure of nipple*

676.2 5th Engorgement of breasts associated with childbirth — *abnormally high accumulation of milk in the breast ducts*

676.3 5th Other and unspecified disorder of breast associated with childbirth — *absence of milk secretion by the breast*

676.4 5th Failure of lactation — *agalactia*

676.5 5th Suppressed lactation

676.6 5th Galactorrhea — *Chiari-Frommel syndrome*

676.8 5th Other disorders of lactation — *galactocele*

676.9 5th Unspecified disorder of lactation

677 Late effect of complication of pregnancy, childbirth, and the puerperium OK

AHA: Q4, 1994, 42; Q1, 1997, 9

Documentation Issues

Documentation must clearly indicate that the condition is a result of a complication that initially developed during the pregnancy, delivery, or the postpartum period to substantiate a late effect code selection.

Coding Clarification

Code first any sequelae. This category is to be used to indicate conditions in 632-648.9x and 651-676.9x as the cause of the late effect classifiable elsewhere. The "late effects" include conditions specified as such, or as sequelae, which may occur at any time after the puerperium.

Etiology: A late effect of pregnancy, childbirth, and the puerperium is a condition identified as being caused by or the sequel of a complication initially arising during this period (e.g., conditions classified to categories 632-648.9x and 651-676.9x). It does not include those conditions treated during the pregnancy, delivery, and postpartum period.

To report the late effect of complication of pregnancy, childbirth, and the puerperium, use code 677. This code does not require a fourth or fifth digit. Code also any sequelae of the complication.

Coding Scenario

A patient who is six months post-delivery of an infant is seen for rectal dilation. She has scarring secondary to a third degree laceration resulting from delivery.

> Code assignment: 677 *Late effect of complication of pregnancy, childbirth, and the puerperium* and 569.2 *Stenosis of rectum and anus*

680–709
Diseases of the Skin and Subcutaneous Tissue

This chapter classifies diseases and disorders of the epidermis, dermis, subcutaneous tissue, nails, sebaceous glands, sweat glands, and hair and hair follicles.

680–686 Infections of Skin and Subcutaneous Tissue

This range of codes classifies infections of the skin and subcutaneous tissue into diseases and disorders such as boils, carbuncles, furuncles, cellulitis, abscess, lymphadenitis, local infections, and pilonidal cysts. When assigning a code from categories 680-686, also assign a code (as a secondary code) to identify the infective organism, such as staphylococcus (code 041.1).

680 Carbuncle and furuncle

Carbuncles and furuncles are infections caused by either aerobic or anaerobic bacterial organisms. A carbuncle is a collection of pus contained in a cavity or sac. A furuncle is a painful nodule formed by circumscribed inflammation of the skin and subcutaneous tissue that encloses a central core.

Signs and symptoms of carbuncles and furuncles include pain, fluctuating or fixed mass, fever, chills, and malaise with furuncle in active stage. A gram stain and culture (if open wound or pus is present) may be performed to identify the infective organism. Therapies include antimicrobials (penicillin).

680.0 Carbuncle and furuncle of face — *single boil or cluster of boils on sites including ear, nose, temple*

680.1 Carbuncle and furuncle of neck — *single boil or cluster of boils, neck*

680.2 Carbuncle and furuncle of trunk — *back, breast, chest, flank, groin, perineum, umbilicus, abdominal wall*

680.3 Carbuncle and furuncle of upper arm and forearm — *arm, axilla, shoulder*

680.4 Carbuncle and furuncle of hand — *finger, thumb, wrist*

680.5 Carbuncle and furuncle of buttock — *anus, gluteal region*

680.6 Carbuncle and furuncle of leg, except foot — *ankle, knee, thigh, hip*

680.7 Carbuncle and furuncle of foot — *heel, toe*

680.8 Carbuncle and furuncle of other specified sites — *head except face; scalp*

680.9 Carbuncle and furuncle of unspecified site — *unknown site*

Coding Clarification

Use an additional code to identify the infective organism, typically streptococcus or staphylococcus. Use the appropriate fourth digit to indicate the anatomic location of the furuncle or carbuncle. Excluded from this rubric are carbuncles of the eye, lacrimal apparatus, and orbit, classified to rubrics in the nervous system chapter of ICD-9-CM, and those of the genital system, classified to the chapter on diseases of the genitourinary system.

Excluded from this range are certain infections of the skin classified to Chapter 1 Parasitic and Infectious Diseases of ICD-9-CM, including erysipelas (035), erysipeloid of Rosenbach (027.1), herpes (rubrics 053 and 054), molluscum contagiosum (078.0), and viral warts (078.1).

681 Cellulitis and abscess of finger and toe

AHA: Jan-Feb, 1987, 12; Q2, 1991, 5

Cellulitis and abscess of the finger and toe are infections often caused by group A streptococci or *Staphylococcus aureus* but may be caused by other organisms. Cellulitis is an infection of the dermis and subcutaneous tissues. An abscess is a collection of pus resulting from an acute or chronic localized infection associated with tissue destruction.

Signs and symptoms of cellulitis and abscess of the finger and toe include erythema, warmth, edema, and pain.

Lab work reveals elevated sedimentation rate and mild leukocytosis with left shift. A gram stain and culture of the lesion identify the infective organism. Therapies include antimicrobials (penicillin or cephalosporin). Associated conditions include surgical wounds, cutaneous ulcers of the skin, and diabetes mellitus.

681.00 Unspecified cellulitis and abscess of finger — (Use additional code to identify organism) — *sudden, severe inflammation of finger not otherwise specified*
AHA: Jan-Feb, 1987, 12; Q2, 1991, 5

681.01 Felon — (Use additional code to identify organism) — *cellulitis in fleshy tip of finger; Whitlow*
AHA: Jan-Feb, 1987, 12; Q2, 1991, 5

681.02 Onychia and paronychia of finger — (Use additional code to identify organism) — *in or around fingernail; panaritium, perionychia*
AHA: Jan-Feb, 1987, 12; Q2, 1991, 5

681.10 Unspecified cellulitis and abscess of toe — (Use additional code to identify organism) — *sudden, severe inflammation of toe not otherwise specified*
AHA: Jan-Feb, 1987, 12; Q2, 1991, 5

681.11 Onychia and paronychia of toe — (Use additional code to identify organism) — *in or around toenail; panaritium, perionychia*
AHA: Jan-Feb, 1987, 12; Q2, 1991, 5

681.9 Cellulitis and abscess of unspecified digit — (Use additional code to identify organism)

Documentation Issues

If the documentation has an unclear diagnostic statement as to the site or type of injury, it will be necessary to obtain clarification from the physician to make an accurate code selection.

When the documentation identifies cellulitis following the repair of a laceration, clarification should be made with the physician whether the cellulitis is a postoperative infection or solely a complicated wound infection. Do not assume that the wound is the problem and the origin of the infection rather than the surgical procedure.

Coding Clarification

Use an additional code to identify the infective organism, typically streptococcus or staphylococcus. When cellulitis occurs with a chronic skin ulcer (category 707), code both conditions.

Cellulitis Associated with Pregnancy or Delivery: There are times when a patient will develop pelvic cellulitis after delivery or following an abortion. In these instances, only codes indicating the puerperal infection (codes from chapter 22) are indicated. The cellulitis is not coded separately.

Cellulitis Secondary to Superficial Injury: When cellulitis is the result of a superficial injury, burn, or frostbite, two codes are required: one for the cellulitis and one describing the injury.

Gangrenous Cellulitis: If the documentation indicates that gangrenous cellulitis is present, code 785.4 is assigned with the injury or ulcer code and not a code from categories 681-682.

Open Wound with Cellulitus: When cellulitis is associated with an open wound, the code for a complicated open wound is assigned followed by the code for cellulitis when the patient is being seen primarily for treatment of the open wound. However, if the patient is being seen primarily for treatment of the cellulitis and the open wound is minor and does not require specific treatment, the appropriate code for cellulitis is indicated followed by an additional code identifying the complicated open wound.

Postoperative Cellulitis: Cellulitis resulting from a postoperative wound infection requires two codes: 998.59 *Other postoperative infection* and the appropriate code from categories 681 and 682 identifying the cellulitis.

Skin Ulcers and Cellulitus: A frequent complication of chronic skin ulcers is cellulitis. Since the codes identifying chronic skin ulcers (707.0-707.9) do not include any mention of cellulitis, two codes are necessary. Code both the chronic skin ulcer and the cellulitis.

Coding Scenario

A patient is being treated for a gangrenous abscess of the big toe of the right foot.

> Code assignment: 785.4 *Gangrene* and 681.10 *Unspecified cellulitis and abscess of toe*

682 Other cellulitis and abscess

AHA: Sept-Oct, 1985, 10; Jan-Feb, 1987, 12; Q2, 1991, 5

Cellulitis and abscess are infections caused by streptococci, staphylococci, or other organisms. Cellulitis is an infection of the dermis and subcutaneous tissues, more severe in patients with lower resistance to infection (e.g., diabetics). An abscess is a collection of pus resulting from an acute or chronic localized infection associated with tissue destruction.

Signs and symptoms of other cellulitis and abscess include edema, warmth, redness, pain, and interference with function. A gram stain and culture of the lesion identify the infective organism. Blood work usually reveals negative cultures, while serological testing, specifically measurement of anti-DNAse B, confirms streptococcal etiology. Therapies include antimicrobials (penicillin).

682.0 Cellulitis and abscess of face — (Use additional code to identify organism) — *cheek, chin, forehead, nose, temple, submandibular region*
AHA: Sept-Oct, 1985, 10; Jan-Feb, 1987, 12; Q2, 1991, 5

682.1 Cellulitis and abscess of neck — (Use additional code to identify organism) — *sudden severe suppurative inflammation and edema in muscle or subcutaneous tissue*
AHA: Sept-Oct, 1985, 10; Jan-Feb, 1987, 12; Q2, 1991, 5

 © 2004 Ingenix, Inc.

682.2 Cellulitis and abscess of trunk — (Use additional code to identify organism)

682.3 Cellulitis and abscess of upper arm and forearm — (Use additional code to identify organism) — *axilla, shoulder*
AHA: Sept-Oct, 1985, 10; Jan-Feb, 1987, 12; Q2, 1991, 5; Q2, 2003, 7

682.4 Cellulitis and abscess of hand, except fingers and thumb — (Use additional code to identify organism) — *wrist*
AHA: Sept-Oct, 1985, 10; Jan-Feb, 1987, 12; Q2, 1991, 5

682.5 Cellulitis and abscess of buttock — (Use additional code to identify organism) — *gluteal region*
AHA: Sept-Oct, 1985, 10; Jan-Feb, 1987, 12; Q2, 1991, 5

682.6 Cellulitis and abscess of leg, except foot — (Use additional code to identify organism) — *ankle, knee, thigh, hip*
AHA: Sept-Oct, 1985, 10; Jan-Feb, 1987, 12; Q2, 1991, 5; Q4, 2003, 108

682.7 Cellulitis and abscess of foot, except toes — (Use additional code to identify organism) — *heel*
AHA: Sept-Oct, 1985, 10; Jan-Feb, 1987, 12; Q2, 1991, 5

682.8 Cellulitis and abscess of other specified site — (Use additional code to identify organism) — *scalp, pterygopalatine fossa, head, except face*
AHA: Sept-Oct, 1985, 10; Jan-Feb, 1987, 12; Q2, 1991, 5

682.9 Cellulitis and abscess of unspecified site — (Use additional code to identify organism) — *unknown site*
AHA: Sept-Oct, 1985, 10; Jan-Feb, 1987, 12; Q2, 1991, 5

Documentation Issues

If the documentation has an unclear diagnostic statement as to the site or type of injury, it will be necessary to obtain clarification from the physician to make an accurate code selection.

When the documentation identifies cellulitis following the repair of a laceration, clarification should be made with the physician whether the cellulitis is a postoperative infection or solely a complicated wound infection. Do not assume that the wound is the problem and the origin of the infection rather than the surgical procedure.

Coding Clarification

Use an additional code to identify the infective organism, typically streptococcus. Abscess and lymphangitis are included in this code category. Sequencing should follow the guidelines for selection of the principal diagnosis. When cellulitis or abscess occurs with chronic skin ulcer (category 707), code both conditions.

Cellulitis Associated with Pregnancy or Delivery: There are times when a patient will develop pelvic cellulitis after delivery or following an abortion. In these instances, only codes indicating the puerperal infection (codes from chapter 22) are indicated. The cellulitis is not coded separately.

Cellulitis Secondary to Superficial Injury: When cellulitis is the result of a superficial injury, burn, or frostbite, two codes are required: one for the cellulitis and one describing the injury.

Gangrenous Cellulitis: If the documentation indicates that gangrenous cellulitis is present, code 785.4 is assigned with the injury or ulcer code and not a code from categories 681-682.

Open Wound with Cellulitus: When cellulitis is associated with an open wound, the code for a complicated open wound is assigned followed by the code for cellulitis when the patient is being seen primarily for treatment of the open wound. However, if the patient is being seen primarily for treatment of the cellulitis and the open wound is minor and does not require specific treatment, the appropriate code for cellulitis is indicated followed by an additional code identifying the complicated open wound.

Postoperative Cellulitis: Cellulitis resulting from a postoperative wound infection requires two codes: 998.59 *Other postoperative infection* and the appropriate code from categories 681 and 682 identifying the cellulitis.

Septic Leukocytoclastic Vasculitis: Two codes are required to report this condition: 446.29 *Other specified hypersensitivity angiitis* and a code from category 682 *Other cellulitis and abscess.*

Skin Ulcers and Cellulitus: A frequent complication of chronic skin ulcers is cellulitis. Since the codes identifying chronic skin ulcers (707.0-707.9) do not include any mention of cellulitis, two codes are necessary. Code both the chronic skin ulcer and the cellulitis.

Coding Scenario

An 8-year-old male is seen in the physician's office with cellulitis of the left forearm. The patient's mother states that there was an insect bite in the area and believes the skin infection resulted from scratching the bite.

> Code assignment: 682.3 *Other cellulitis and abscess of upper arm and forearm* and 913.5 *Superficial injury of elbow, forearm, and wrist, insect bite, nonvenomous, infected*

A patient has an open wound of the left upper leg with the development of cellulitis.

680–709

Code assignment: 682.6 *Other cellulitis and abscess of leg, except foot* and 890.1 *Open wound of hip and thigh, complicated*

A patient had a coronary bypass graft 10 days ago and is admitted today with cellulitis of the incision site.

Code assignment: 998.5 *Postoperative infection* and 682.2 *Cellulitis and abscess of trunk*

683 Acute lymphadenitis OK

Acute lymphadenitis is sudden, severe inflammation of the lymph nodes. The infection may be due to streptococci, staphylococci, or other organisms. Therapies include antimicrobials (penicillin).

680–709

Coding Clarification

Use an additional code to identify the infective organism, typically streptococcus. Abscess and acute lymphangitis are included in this code category. Chronic or subacute, mesenteric, and unspecified lymphadenitis are excluded. Sequencing should follow the guidelines for selection of the principal diagnosis. When cellulitis or abscess associated with acute lymphadenitis occurs with a chronic skin ulcer (category 707), code both conditions.

684 Impetigo OK

Impetigo is a superficial skin infection. There are two types of impetigo: bullous and vesicular. With bullous impetigo, fragile bullae form rapidly, break early, and heal centrally, leaving crusted erosions. Vesicular impetigo originates as small vesicles or pustules that break, exposing a red, moist base, and secrete a honey-yellow to white-brown crust. Usually caused by streptococci, staphylococci, or both, impetigo occurs most frequently after a minor skin injury such as a cut, scrape, or insect bite but infrequently may also develop on healthy skin.

Signs and symptoms of impetigo include skin lesions, itching, and mild pain. Blood work reveals elevated sedimentation rate. A gram stain and culture of the lesion identify the infective organism, and antistreptolysin-O (ASO) titers detect streptococcal infection. Therapies include triple antibiotic ointment (bacitracin, Polysporin, and neomycin applied three times daily).

Coding Clarification

Excluded from this rubric is impetigo herpetiformis, reported with 694.3.

685 Pilonidal cyst

A pilonidal cyst is a hair-containing cyst or sinus located at the sacrococcygeal area, which often has a sinus that opens at a postanal dimple.

Signs and symptoms of pilonidal cyst include edema, warmth, redness, pain, and interference with function. A gram stain and culture of the lesion identify the infective organism. Blood work usually identifies negative culture. Therapies include incision and drainage or circumferential excision. Use the appropriate fourth digit to indicate the presence or absence of an abscess.

685.0 Pilonidal cyst with abscess — *cyst and abscess in sacrococcygeal tissue, including sinus or fistula*

685.1 Pilonidal cyst without mention of abscess — *cyst in sacrococcygeal tissue, including sinus or fistula*

686 Other local infection of skin and subcutaneous tissue

This rubric classifies other local infections of the skin and subcutaneous tissue including pyoderma, pyogenic granuloma, granuloma, or dermatitis due to a pus-forming organism such as those classified to rubric 041. Therapies include antibiotics and incision and drainage of larger lesions.

686.00 Unspecified pyoderma — *dermatitis unknown*

686.01 Pyoderma gangrenosum — *persistent, debilitating dermatitis with boggy blue-red ulcers*
AHA: Q4, 1997, 42

686.09 Other pyoderma — *not elsewhere classified*

686.1 Pyogenic granuloma of skin and subcutaneous tissue — *septic, suppurative, telangiectaticum*

686.8 Other specified local infections of skin and subcutaneous tissue — *dermatitis vegetans; Andrew's pustular bacteride; Brandt's syndrome; Danbold-Closs syndrome; Spiegler-Fendt sarcoid*

686.9 Unspecified local infection of skin and subcutaneous tissue — *skin infection or fistula, unknown*

690–698 Other Inflammatory Conditions of Skin and Subcutaneous Tissue

Excluded from this range of codes is panniculitis, classified to 739.30-739.39.

690 Erythematosquamous dermatosis

Erythematosquamous dermatosis is an inflammatory, scaly condition of the skin predominantly affecting the scalp and face.

Signs and symptoms of erythematosquamous dermatosis include dandruff, itching, dry skin, and crusted scalp lesion ("cradle cap") in infants. Therapies include hydrocortisone cream for facial lesions and dandruff shampoo for scalp and other hairy areas.

 © 2004 Ingenix, Inc.

690.10 Unspecified seborrheic dermatitis — *not otherwise specified*
AHA: Q4, 1995, 58

690.11 Seborrhea capitis — *exclusive to scalp; cradle cap*
AHA: Q4, 1995, 58

690.12 Seborrheic infantile dermatitis — *itchy and scaly inflammation of skin in infants*
AHA: Q4, 1995, 58

690.18 Other seborrheic dermatitis — *not otherwise specified, including Unna's disease*
AHA: Q4, 1995, 58

690.8 Other erythematosquamous dermatosis — *parakeratosis*

Coding Clarification

Excluded from this rubric are eczematous dermatitis of the eyelid (373.31), parakeratosis variegata (696.2), psoriasis (rubric 696), and seborrheic keratosis (702).

691 Atopic dermatitis and related conditions

691.0 Diaper or napkin rash — *psoriasiform napkin eruption; ammonia dermatitis*

691.8 Other atopic dermatitis and related conditions — *atopic dermatitis; Besnier's prurigo; atopic neurodermatitis; prurigo-asthma syndrome; intrinsic eczema*

692 Contact dermatitis and other eczema

This rubric classifies rash as a result of a substance that comes in contact with the skin. Initially, the rash is limited to the site of contact but may spread.

Signs and symptoms of contact dermatitis and other eczema include transient redness to severe swelling, itching, and vesiculation. Therapies include identification and elimination of the offending agent, topical corticosteroid gel in less acute situations, emollient, and other protective ointment for dry dermatitis.

692.0 Contact dermatitis and other eczema due to detergents — *allergic reaction*

692.1 Contact dermatitis and other eczema due to oils and greases — *allergic reaction*

692.2 Contact dermatitis and other eczema due to solvents — *chlorocompound, cyclohexane, ester, glycol, hydrocarbon, ketone groups*

692.3 Contact dermatitis and other eczema due to drugs and medicines in contact with skin — (Use additional E code to identify drug) — *arnica, fungicides, iodine, keratolytics, mercurials, neomycin, pediculocides, phenols, scabicides; dermatitis medicamentosa*

692.4 Contact dermatitis and other eczema due to other chemical products — *acids, adhesive plaster, alkalis, caustics, dichromate, insecticide, nylon, plastic, rubber*
AHA: Q2, 1989, 16

692.5 Contact dermatitis and other eczema due to food in contact with skin — *cereals, fish, flour, fruit, meat, milk*

692.6 Contact dermatitis and other eczema due to plants (except food) — *lacquer tree; poison ivy, oak, sumac; primrose; ragweed*

Subcategory 692.7 reports photodamage to the skin. Photodamage is a serious medical condition that has been identified with an increased risk of premalignant skin lesions, such as actinic keratosis, and skin malignancies such as basal cell carcinoma and melanoma.

692.70 Unspecified dermatitis due to sun

692.71 Contact dermatitis and other eczema due to sunburn — *first degree and sunburn NOS*
AHA: Q4, 2001, 47

Interestingly, no differentiation is made between first, second, and third degree sunburn in ICD-9-CM.

Do not use a sunburn code to report a burn received in a tanning booth. Instead, report that burn with 692.82.

692.72 Acute dermatitis due to solar radiation — (Use additional E code to identify drug, if drug-induced) — *Berlogue dermatitis, photoallergic response, phototoxic response, polymorphus light eruption*

Use subclassification 692.72 to report acute contact photosensitive reaction due to solar radiation. Contact photosensitive reaction is categorized as photoallergic or phototoxic. Sunburn is excluded from this code, see 692.71 and 692.76-692.77.

Photoallergic contact dermatitis is an allergic dermatitis caused by a photosensitizing substance plus sunlight in a sensitized person. The clinical presentation is similar to allergic contact dermatitis except that sunlight must be present to induce the reaction. If the photosensitizer acts internally, it is photodrug dermatitis; if it acts externally, it is a photocontact dermatitis. Some examples of oral photodrug dermatitis photosensitizers are diuretics such as Diuril, hypoglycemics such as Orinase, and phenothiazine such as Thorazine. Examples of topical photocontact dermatitis photosensitizers are antimicrobials such as bithionol and antihistamines such as Benadryl. Report an E code secondarily to identify the drug if the dermatitis is drug-induced.

Phototoxic contact dermatitis is a nonimmunologic reaction that occurs two to six hours after the skin has been exposed to a photosensitizing agent and solar radiation. The clinical presentation is similar to sunburn. Some examples of phototoxic dermatitis are phototoxic tar dermatitis (dermatitis associated with coal tar, creosote, or pitch), phytophotodermatitis, dermatitis bullosa striata pratensis (grass or meadow dermatitis), and berloque (perfume) dermatitis.

692.73 Actinic reticuloid and actinic granuloma — *skin growths the result of persistent inflammation of the skin as a reaction to solar rays*

Use subclassification 692.73 to report a severe and chronic form of photosensitivity (actinic reticuloid) and skin lesion (actinic granuloma). Usually affecting males between the ages of 45 and 70, actinic reticuloid requires complete avoidance of sunlight and other forms of ultraviolet radiation since it is resistant to treatment with sunscreens and steroids.

Actinic granuloma begins as papules and nodules. These lesions grow very slowly and eventually become annular. Persistent for years, actinic granuloma is believed to be due to defective repair of connective tissue damaged by sun and heat.

692.74 Other chronic dermatitis due to solar radiation — *solar elastosis, chronic solar skin damage*

Use subclassification 692.74 to report other specified and unspecified forms of chronic dermatitis due to solar radiation. Included are conditions such as actinic cheilitis, actinic solar elastosis, Favre-Racouchot syndrome, "sailor's skin," and "farmer's skin."

692.75 Disseminated superficial actinic porokeratosis (DSAP)

692.76 Sunburn of second degree

692.77 Sunburn of third degree

692.79 Other dermatitis due to solar radiation — *hydroa aestivale; photodermatitis, photosensitiveness*

692.81 Dermatitis due to cosmetics

692.82 Dermatitis due to other radiation — *infrared lights, ultraviolet lights, tanning beds, x-rays*
AHA: Q3, 2000, 5; Q4, 2001, 47

Coding Clarification

Use subclassification 692.82 to report dermatitis due to forms of radiation other than solar radiation, such as x-rays, radiation from tanning beds, infrared rays, ionizing radiation, ultraviolet light (excluding sunlight), and gamma rays.

692.83 Dermatitis due to metals — *jewelry*

Use subclassification 692.83 to report dermatitis due to exposure to or contact with metals or metallic salts. Nickel, the chromates, and mercury are the most common causes of metal dermatitis in the United States. Other metals associated with dermatitis are rhodium, platinum, cobalt, tungsten, cadmium, beryllium, vanadium, and zinc. Metals and metal salts can occur in soap and detergents, cosmetics, hair dyes, and tattoos.

692.84 Contact dermatitis and other eczema due to animal (cat) (dog) dander

Contact dermatitis is an allergic reaction of the skin characterized by a rash or hives. This is usually an immune reaction to a protein found in animal dander. This may be a result of direct contact with an animal or contact with fabric containing the animal dander.

692.89 Contact dermatitis and other eczema due to other specified agent — *not elsewhere specified, including dermatitis due to weather, dyes, preservatives, blister beetle dermatitis, enema rash, caterpillar dermatitis*

692.9 Contact dermatitis and other eczema, due to unspecified cause

Coding Clarification

Use the appropriate fourth digit to indicate the causative agent. An E code from the table of drugs and chemicals should be reported secondarily to report an adverse effect from a drug or chemical.

Excluded from this rubric are allergy NOS (995.3), contact dermatitis of the eyelids (373.32), dermatitis due to a substance taken internally (rubric 693), eczema of the external ear (380.22), perioral dermatitis (695.3), urticarial reactions (708.0-708.9, 995.1), and seborrheic keratosis (702.11-702.19).

693 Dermatitis due to substances taken internally

Use this rubric to report dermatitis due to the ingestion of drugs, chemicals, foodstuffs, or other substances. The condition usually manifests with an abrupt onset of diffuse, symmetric erythematous eruptions. The cause may be an allergic reaction, adverse effect, drug interaction, idiosyncratic reaction, or some other cause.

693.0 Dermatitis due to drugs and medicines taken internally — (Use additional E code to identify drug) — *dermatitis medicamentosa not otherwise specified*

The definition of dermatitis due to drugs and medicines taken internally is systemic erythematous inflammation of the skin, also known as dermatitis medicamentosa or drug eruption. The condition may mimic inflammatory skin conditions such as eczema, toxic erythema, and erythroderma. Onset may be sudden (e.g., urticaria or angioedema after penicillin) or delayed.

Signs and symptoms of dermatitis due to drugs and medicines taken internally include mild rash to toxic epidermal microlysis, malaise, fever, arthralgia, and headache. Therapies include cessation of the offending drug; lubricant for dry, itching,

 © 2004 Ingenix, Inc.

maculopapular eruption; and corticosteroid for the existing rash.

ICD-9-CM coding rules regarding poisonings and adverse effects must be followed using the table of drugs and chemicals.

693.1 Dermatitis due to food taken internally — *infested food*

693.8 Dermatitis due to other specified substances taken internally — *not specified elsewhere*

693.9 Dermatitis due to unspecified substance taken internally

Coding Clarification

Excluded from this rubric are adverse effect NOS of drugs and medicines (995.2), allergy NOS (995.3), contact dermatitis (rubric 692), and urticarial reactions (708.0-708.9, 995.1).

694 Bullous dermatoses

Use this rubric to report cutaneous lesions of bullous dermatoses. The primary lesion in many diseases, bullae are large blisters that form at some level of the skin.

694.0 Dermatitis herpetiformis — *dermatosis herpetiformis; Duhring's disease, Brocq-Duhring disease; hydroa herpetiformis*

694.1 Subcorneal pustular dermatosis — *Sneddon-Wilkinson disease*

694.2 Juvenile dermatitis herpetiformis — *juvenile pemphigoid*

694.3 Impetigo herpetiformis — *rare dermatosis of third trimester with multiply symptoms*

694.4 Pemphigus — *erythematosus, foliaceus, vegetans, vulgaris; Senear-Usher syndrome*

694.5 Pemphigoid — *bullous, herpes circinatus bullosus, senile dermatitis herpetiformis*

The definition of pemphigoid is chronic, benign eruption, including benign pemphigus and bullous pemphigoid. Pemphigoid is seen chiefly in the elderly and in individuals with autoimmune disease. Signs and symptoms of pemphigoid include tense bullae on normal or reddened skin. Immunofluorescence studies confirm the diagnosis. Therapies include prednisone.

694.60 Benign mucous membrane pemphigoid without mention of ocular involvement — *cicatricial pemphigoid, mucosynechial atrophic bullous dermatitis*

694.61 Benign mucous membrane pemphigoid with ocular involvement — *cicatricial pemphigoid, mucosynechial atrophic bullous dermatitis*

694.8 Other specified bullous dermatosis — *not specified elsewhere*

694.9 Unspecified bullous dermatosis

695 Erythematous conditions

Erythema has many causes, including an immunologic reaction triggered by circulating immune complexes, drugs (penicillin, barbiturates, sulfonamides), and infection (herpes simplex, Mycoplasma pneumoniae). Etiology is unknown in many of the erythematous conditions. Treatments include painkillers and ice packs to ease the pain of nodules and medical attention directed toward the underlying disease.

Papules, plaques, and bulls eye (target) lesions are diagnostic of erythema multiforme (695.1). On mucous membranes, it begins as blisters and progresses to ulcers. A more advanced form, Stevens-Johnson syndrome, can be fatal.

Recurring mouth and genital ulcers, and inflammation of the uvea are characteristic of Behcet's syndrome (695.2), which can also affect the retina, brain, joints, skin, and bowels.

Rosacea (695.3) is a hereditary, chronic disorder characterized by groups of arterioles, capillaries, and venules that become dilated, resulting in small papules and pustules, especially around the nose, forehead, cheekbones, and chin. Patients with progressive rosacea may be seen by an ophthalmologist to detect early subclinical complications.

Red plaques with an expanding inflammatory border and hypopigmented atrophic scarring is characteristic of discoid lupus erythematosus (695.4), which is not usually associated with systemic manifestations. Lesions are commonly in areas exposed to sunlight such as the face, ears, neck, and scalp.

695.0 Toxic erythema — *erythema venenatum*

Use subcategory 695.0 to report erythematous eruptions of a wide anatomic area caused by bacterial or other toxins or administration of medications in toxic dosages.

695.1 Erythema multiforme — *toxic epidermal necrolysis, erythema iris; herpes iris; syndromes: Lyell's; Stevens-Johnson, Baader', Flessinger-Rendu, Klauder's*

695.2 Erythema nodosum — *painful inflammation of tissue of lower extremities usually caused by a hypersensitivity reaction, and sometimes seen as a manifestation of disease, as in sarcoidosis*

695.3 Rosacea — *erythematosa acne; rhinophyma; perioral dermatitis; rosacea acne*

695.4 Lupus erythematosus — *discoid lupus erythematosus, not disseminated*

Coding Clarification

Use subcategory 695.4 to report lupus erythematosus, a chronic disease that causes inflammation of the connective tissue of the skin only. Occurring worldwide, this disease affects nine times as many women as men, usually those of childbearing age, and can lead to scarring and permanent disfigurement.

Signs and symptoms of lupus erythematosus include erythematous, round scaling papules usually on malar prominences, the bridge of the nose, scalp, and external auditory canals. Thickened areas of skin may later scar.

Lab work reveals leukopenia, positive LE cells test in only 10 percent of patients. A skin biopsy shows immunoglobulins or complement components. Therapies include reduced exposure to sunlight, topical corticosteroid for lesions, and antimalarials (Plaquenil).

This subcategory includes discoid lupus erythematosus but excludes lupus vulgaris NOS (017.0) and systemic lupus erythematosus (710.0).

695.81 Ritter's disease — *generalized staph syndrome causing exfoliation and raw skin in infants*

695.89 Other specified erythematous condition — *erythema intertrigo; pityriasis rubra; dermatitis epidemica; syndromes: Savill's; Sweet's, Wilson-Brocq, Bury's, Leiner's*
AHA: Sept-Oct, 1986, 10

695.9 Unspecified erythematous condition

696 Psoriasis and similar disorders

Use this category to report a common skin disease characterized by patches of inflamed, red skin, covered by silvery scales and sometimes accompanied by painful swelling and stiffness of the joints (arthritis). With psoriasis, new cells are produced 10 times faster than normal, but the rate at which old cells are shed is unchanged. Consequently, the stratum corneum becomes thickened with flaky, immature skin cells. Occurring predominantly over the elbows, knees, scalp, and trunk, psoriasis tends to run in families, affects men and women equally, and usually appears between the ages of 10 and 30.

Therapies include moderate exposure to sunlight or phototherapy and the use of an emollient for mild cases, ointment containing coal tar or anthralin for moderate cases, and topical corticosteroids and oral methotrexate for severe cases.

696.0 Psoriatic arthropathy — *psoriasis associated with joint disease*

696.1 Other psoriasis and similar disorders — *acrodermatitis continua, dermatitis repens, Willan-Plumbe syndrome*

696.2 Parapsoriasis — *parakeratosis variegata; parapsoriasis lichenoides chronica; pityriasis lichenoides et varioliformis; Brocq's parapsoriasis; Mucah-Haberman syndrome; Wise's disease*

696.3 Pityriasis rosea — *pityriasis circinata (et maculata)*

696.4 Pityriasis rubra pilaris — *Devergie's disease, lichen ruber acuminatus*

696.5 Other and unspecified pityriasis — *not otherwise specified*

696.8 Other psoriasis and similar disorders — *not otherwise specified*

697 Lichen

This rubric describes papular skin diseases characterized by small lesions set close together. A biopsy is performed to make the diagnosis of the particular form of the disease and treatments include topical corticosteroids to reduce itching and induce regression of the lesions. Hyperpigmented areas may persist after the lesions have resolved. An example from this rubric is lichen sclerosus, which is a skin disorder that affects the vulva. The cause is unknown and, similar to other diseases in this rubric, the condition resembles the appearance of lichens (mixture of fungi and algae) found in nature.

697.0 Lichen planus — *planopilaris, ruber planus*

Use subcategory 697.0 to report an inflammatory cutaneous and mucous membrane condition characterized by pruritic, violaceous, and flattop papules with fine white streaks and symmetric distribution. Signs and symptoms of lichen planus include chronic papules, acute lesions of the skin and mucous membranes, and severe itching. Histopathology of the skin lesion confirms the diagnosis. Therapies include topical, intralesional, and systemic steroids, antihistamines, psoralens plus long-wave ultraviolet light, and oral griseofulvin.

697.1 Lichen nitidus — *Pinkus' disease*

697.8 Other lichen, not elsewhere classified — *ruber moniliforme, striata*

697.9 Unspecified lichen

Coding Clarification

Excluded from this rubric are obtusus corneus (698.3), congenital pilaris (757.39), ruber acuminatus (696.4), sclerosus of atrophicus (701.9), scrofulosus (017.0), simplex chronicus (698.3), congenital spinulosus (757.39), and urticatus (698.2).

698 Pruritus and related conditions

Use this rubric to report conditions characterized by an intense itching and/or burning sensation of the skin. Most cases of generalized pruritus are due to dry skin but may be due to a variety of dermatologic or systemic conditions. Therapies include elimination of soaps or detergents, cessation of all but necessary medications, the application of moisturizers while the skin is wet, tranquilizers in severe cases, and topical or systemic corticosteroids as well as antihistamines and antiserotonin drugs.

 © 2004 Ingenix, Inc.

Pruritus (itching) may be related to a wide variety of conditions classifiable elsewhere, such as scabies, atopic dermatitis, sunburn, uremia, and contact dermatitis. In most cases, the pruritus is an integral part of the disease and is not reported separately. Excluded from this rubric is pruritus that is psychogenic in nature (306.3).

698.0 Pruritus ani — *intense anal itch*

698.1 Pruritus of genital organs — *intense genital itch*

698.2 Prurigo — *lichen urticatus; Hebra's prurigo; urticaria papulosa; mitis prurigo; prurigo simplex*

698.3 Lichenification and lichen simplex chronicus — *neurodermatitis; prurigo nodularis; Brocq's lichen simplex chronicus; Hyde's or Vidal's disease*

698.4 Dermatitis factitia (artefacta) — (Use additional code to identify any associated mental disorder) — *dermatitis ficta, neurotic excoriation*

698.8 Other specified pruritic conditions — *not classified elsewhere, including hiemalis, senilis, winter itch*

698.9 Unspecified pruritic disorder

700–709 Other Diseases of Skin and Subcutaneous Tissue

Excluded from this range of codes are conditions confined to the eyelids (373.0-374.9) and congenital conditions of the hair, skin, and nails (759.0-759.9).

700 Corns and callosities OK

Calluses and corns are knobs of hyperkeratotic tissue caused by pressure or friction, most commonly seen in the bony prominences of the feet or hands. Benign conditions, they can cause pain that requires treatment by a podiatrist or physician.

701 Other hypertrophic and atrophic conditions of skin

701.0 Circumscribed scleroderma — *Addison's keloid, morphea, localized dermatosclerosis, von Zambusch's disease, lichen sclerosus et atrophicus*

701.1 Acquired keratoderma — *elastosis perforans serpiginosa; acquired ichthyosis, acquired keratoderma palmaris et plantaris; keratosis blennorrhagica*
AHA: Q4, 1994, 48

701.2 Acquired acanthosis nigricans — *keratosis nigricans*

701.3 Striae atrophicae — *atrophic skin spots; striae disease; senile degenerative atrophy; atrophy blanche of Milian*

701.4 Keloid scar — *hypertrophic scar, cheloid*

Keloid scars are tumors consisting of actively growing hypertrophic cutaneous scar tissue. They occur as a result of trauma or irritation such as burns, incisions, vaccinations, insect bites, and other stimuli. Ulcerated keloids are prone to carcinomatous transformation, but the majority behave as benign neoplasms. Dark-skinned races are particularly susceptible to keloid formation. Hypertrophic scars are similar to keloids except they lack the characteristic tumor formation of keloids and do not grow beyond the margins of the original injury.

Signs and symptoms of keloid scar include a history of surgery or skin trauma, overreactive visible scar formation, itching, and burning. A skin biopsy may be performed to determine the histopathology. Therapies include surgical or laser excision, z-plasty when the scar crosses a flexion surface, cryotherapy (freezing with liquid nitrogen), radiation therapy, and injection of corticosteroid such as Kenalog-10.

In many cases, keloids and hypertrophic scars are residuals of previous trauma or surgery. If the etiology of the keloid or hypertrophic scar is known and described as a late effect, assign a secondary code describing the late effect. For example, if the diagnosis were residual keloid due to a previously treated burn of the hand, codes 701.4 and 906.6 would be assigned.

701.5 Other abnormal granulation tissue — *excessive granulation*

701.8 Other specified hypertrophic and atrophic condition of skin — *atrophia cutis senilis, cutis laxa senilis, acantholysis, pachydermatitis, Pick-Herxheimer or Gougerot-Carteaud syndrome, elastosis senilis, folliculitis ulerythematosa reticulata, confluent and reticulate papillomatosis*

701.9 Unspecified hypertrophic and atrophic condition of skin — *skin tag, atrophoderma, pendulous abdomen, redundant skin, or unknown*

Coding Clarification

Excluded form this rubric are dermatomyositis (710.0), hereditary edema of the legs (757.0), and scleroderma (generalized) (710.3).

702 Other dermatoses

702.0 Actinic keratosis — *sharply outlined warty growth usually caused by sun damage to skin*
AHA: Q1, 1992, 18

Use subcategory 702.0 to report precancerous warty lesions due to the cumulative effect of overexposure to sunlight. These lesions also are known as solar or senile keratosis, keratoderma, keratoma, acanthosis verrucosa, verruca senilis, and plana senilis. Therapies include cryotherapy (freezing with liquid nitrogen) and 5-Fluorouracil.

680–709

Use subcategory 702.1 to report superficial noninvasive tumors (usually multiple) originating in the epidermis. Characterized by numerous yellow or brown sharply marginated, oval, raised lesions, these tumors also are known as seborrheic warts or verrucae. They occur commonly in middle-aged or older patients. Therapies include shaving the lesions.

702.11 Inflamed seborrheic keratosis — *warty growth of basaloid sells not otherwise specified*
AHA: Q4, 1994, 48

702.19 Other seborrheic keratosis

702.8 Other specified dermatoses — *acanthotic nevus, cutaneous horn, sebaceous nevus, or not otherwise specified*

Coding Clarification

Excluded from this rubric is carcinoma in situ (232.0-232.9).

703 Diseases of nail

Nails are hard, keratinized cells of epidermis that consist of a nail body, a free edge, and a nail root. Vascular tissue gives the visible nail body its pink color, except at the whitish lunula where the vascular tissue does not show through. The nail groove is between the nail fold and the nail bed, which is the epidermis beneath the nail. The cuticle, or eponychium, is a narrow band of epidermis that adheres to the nail wall. The thickened stratum corneum below the free edges is referred to as the hyponychium. The nail matrix, at the proximal end of the nail bed, promotes nail growth, which occurs when superficial cells of the matrix transform into nail cells. In the process, the harder layer is pushed forward over the stratum germinativum. The average growth rate for fingernails is about 1.0 millimeter per week; growth is slower for the toenails. Onychomycosis (703.8) is an infection of the nail or nail bed caused by pathogenic fungi.

An ingrowing nail is a painful condition, usually of the big toe, in which one or both edges of the nail press into the adjacent skin, leading to infection and inflammation. Common causes include poor personal hygiene, tight-fitting shoes, and incorrect nail cutting. Therapies include soaking, antibiotics to control infection, and removal of the nail edge. Excluded from this subclassification is nail infection, reported with 681.9.

703.0 Ingrowing nail — *unguis incarnatus; with infection*

703.8 Other specified disease of nail — *dystrophia unguium, hypertrophy, leukonychia, onychauxis, onycholysis, acquired polyunguia; subungual hemorrhage; horn of nail; Beau's lines; acquired anonychia; koilonychia, acquired pachyonychia, or not otherwise specified*

703.9 Unspecified disease of nail

Coding Clarification

Excluded from this rubric are congenital anomalies of the nail (757.5) and onychia and paronychia (681.02, 681.11).

704 Diseases of hair and hair follicles

The primary function of hair is protection (i.e., eyebrows and eyelashes protect the eyes from foreign objects). Hair follicles (downgrowths into the dermis) develop during the third and fourth months of fetal life and by the sixth month the follicles produce lanugo, which is shed from the trunk prior to birth. Several months after birth, a coarser hair, vellus, develops and the remaining lanugo is shed from the eyebrows, eyelids, and scalp and replaced by terminal hairs. Terminal hairs also develop in the axillary and pubic regions and on the face at puberty.

The hair shaft, which projects above the surface of the skin, is made up of the inner medulla, which consists of cells containing eleidin and air spaces; the cortex, which contains pigment granules in dark hair but mostly are in white hair; and the cuticle, the outermost layer of the shaft. The root is the portion below the surface that penetrates into the dermis and, like the shaft, consists of a medulla, cortex, and cuticle. The color of hair is due primarily to melanin.

704.00 Unspecified alopecia — *loss of hair, type unknown*

704.01 Alopecia areata — *patchy loss of hair; usually temporary*

704.02 Telogen effluvium — *temporary excessive hair loss due to stressor like childbirth, surgery, weight loss*

704.09 Other alopecia — *folliculitis decalvans; oligotrichia, Quinquaud's disease, tinea decalvans, pseudopelade*

704.1 Hirsutism — *excessive hair growth; acquired lanuginosa, polytrichia*

704.2 Abnormalities of the hair — *atrophic hair, clastothrix, fragilitas crinium, trichorrhexis nodosa*

704.3 Variations in hair color — *canities, premature gray, heterochromia, acquired poliosis circumscripta*

704.8 Other specified disease of hair and hair follicles — *ingrown hair, folliculitis, perifolliculitis, sycosis, Bockhart's impetigo, mentagra*

704.9 Unspecified disease of hair and hair follicles

Coding Clarification

Excluded from this rubric are congenital anomalies (757.4).

 © 2004 Ingenix, Inc.

705 Disorders of sweat glands

A sweat, or sudoriferous, gland is a type of exocrine gland that eliminates perspiration to cool the skin. The sweat glands are a simple cuboidal or columnar epithelium with pale-staining cells. The base of the sweat glands has a row of myoepithelial cells wrapped around the outside of the gland. Eccrine sweat glands are found in skin throughout the body, particularly on the forehead, scalp, axillae, palms, and soles and produce watery and neutral or slightly acidic sweat. Apocrine sweat glands are in the axilla, areola, and circumanal region and begin to function in puberty and produce viscid milky secretions in response to external stimuli. Apocrine glands accumulate secretory products at the outer margin of the cell and that portion pinches off to form the secretion; the remaining part of the cell repairs itself and repeats the process.

705.0 Anhidrosis — *diminished sweating; hypohidrosis, oligohidrosis*

705.1 Prickly heat — *heat rash, sudamina, miliaria rubra, sweat retention syndrome*

705.21 Primary focal hyperhidrosis

705.22 Secondary focal hyperhidrosis

705.81 Dyshidrosis — *usually affecting hands and feet; cheiropompholyx, pompholyx*

705.82 Fox-Fordyce disease — *rare eruption of follicular papules of axillae, nipples, pubic region*

705.83 Hidradenitis — *inflammation of sweat gland; Pollitzer's disease, hidradenitis suppurativa*

Hyperhidrosis is the clinical disorder of excessive sweating, beyond what the body requires to maintain thermal control. This condition may be generalized, often called secondary hyperhidrosis, occurring with another associated condition such as metabolic or endrocine disorder, malignancies, drugs, substance abuse, toxins, infections, cardiovascular disorders, or respiratory failure.

Primary hyperhidrosis occurs in the absence of any underlying or causative condition, and is almost always focal, confined to one or more specific areas of the body, like the axilla, the soles of the feet, the palms, or the face. Secondary hyperhidrosis may also occur as focal, however, when it is caused by a local condition or treatment, such as radiation therapy to a specific tumor location, or spinal disease or injury. Hyperhidrosis is first treated by a trial of topical medication applications with surgery as a final step.

Use subclassification 705.83 to report inflammation of the apocrine sweat glands occurring in the axillae, anogenital regions, nipples, and under the female breast. The condition may produce chronic abscesses or sinus tract formation. In most cases, hidradenitis is caused by the obstruction of the apocrine sweat pores due to the application of underarm deodorants, irritant depilatories, or other topical ointments or creams. Signs and symptoms of hidradenitis include large painful abscesses resulting from double comedones and extensive deep dermal inflammation, weight loss, fever, malaise, local pain, and tenderness. A gram stain and culture of the lesion identify the infective organism. Therapies include antimicrobials (penicillin), surgical excision, and plastic repair of the affected area in chronic conditions.

Sequence an additional code secondarily to identify the infective organism, typically streptococcus or staphylococcus.

705.89 Other specified disorder of sweat glands — *not otherwise specified, including bromhidrosis, chromhidrosis, abscess, cyst, granulosis rubra nasi, urhidrosis, osmidrosis, hematidrosis*

705.9 Unspecified disorder of sweat glands

Coding Clarification

Report 780.8 for generalized hyperhidrosis.

Coding Scenario

A 17-year-old male comes to his primary care physician complaining of sweating under the arms and on his palms. He says his shirts seem to be continually wet, and his hands may drip with sweat, but this occurs only during waking hours and seems to stop when he is asleep. It is now interfering with daily activities as he cannot maintain a proper grip on the ball during sports and his embarrassing underarms are causing him social anxieties. The physician diagnoses him with focal primary hyperhidrosis and informs him of treatment choices such as topical and systemic agents, iontophoresis, and botox injections to be considered before surgical sweat gland resection

Code assignment: 705.21 *Primary focal hyperhidrosis*

706 Diseases of sebaceous glands

A sebaceous gland is one of several types of glands located in the skin and occurs most commonly in association with hair follicles (i.e., on the face and scalp and in the genital area). These glands produce sebum, a thick, slightly oily secretion that conditions the skin, which empties into the hair follicle.

Acne (706.0, 706.1) is an inflammatory skin condition characterized by superficial skin eruptions that occur when sebaceous glands within the hair follicles become plugged, because secretion occurs faster than the oil and skin cells can exit the follicle. If the plug ruptures the wall of the follicle, the oil, dead skin cells, and bacteria found on the surface of the skin can enter to form the infected pustules (e.g., pimples). The condition usually begins at puberty and affects 75 percent of all teenagers to some extent, probably due to hormonal changes that stimulate the sebaceous glands. Sebaceous hyperplasia (706.8) describes sebaceous glands enlarged by a central hair follicle that can appear on the forehead or cheeks as small yellow bumps up to 3.0 millimeters in diameter.

706.0 Acne varioliformis — *frontalis, necrotica*

706.1 Other acne — *conglobata, cystic, pustular, vulgaris, comedo, blackhead*

706.2 Sebaceous cyst — *atheroma, keratin cyst, infected steatoma, wen*

Coding Clarification

A sebaceous cyst is a slowly developing, benign cystic tumor of the skin containing follicular, keratinous, and sebaceous material. Frequently found on the scalp, ears, face, back, or scrotum, sebaceous cysts may grow very large and become infected by bacteria. An exam reveals a firm, globular, movable, and nontender tumor. Therapies include incision and expression of contents for small lesions (milium); for larger lesions, surgical excision of the cyst walls.

706.3 Seborrhea — *excessive production of sebum*

Coding Clarification

Excluded from this subclassification are dermatitis (690.10) and keratosis (702.11-702.19).

706.8 Other specified disease of sebaceous glands — *asteatosis cutis, xerosis cutis*

706.9 Unspecified disease of sebaceous glands

707 Chronic ulcer of skin

Use this rubric to report a chronic defect of the skin, deeper than erosion or excoriation, extending at least into the dermal layer. Chronic ulcers usually are due to chronic inflammation, ischemia, or both.

707.00 Decubitus ulcer, unspecified site

707.01 Decubitus ulcer, elbow

707.02 Decubitus ulcer, upper back

707.03 Decubitus ulcer, lower back

707.04 Decubitus ulcer, hip

707.05 Decubitus ulcer, buttock

707.06 Decubitus ulcer, ankle

707.07 Decubitus ulcer, heel

707.09 Decubitus ulcer, other site

Documentation Issues

Documentation may identify synonymous terms for decubitus ulcers such as bed sores, plaster ulcer, pressure sore, or ulcer.

There are six stages to a decubitus ulcer that may be documented but have no effect on code selection. Code selection is based on the location of the decubitus ulcer.

Coding Clarification

Use subclassification 707.0x to report a condition, also known as a bedsore or pressure sore, that affects superficial tissues and may also deepen to affect muscle and bone. Usually occurring over a bony prominence at the sacrum, hip, heel, shoulder, or elbow, decubitus ulcers develop in patients who are bedridden, unconscious, or immobile, for example, stroke or spinal cord injury victims. Intrinsic loss of pain and pressure sensations, disuse atrophy, malnutrition, anemia, and infection play roles in the formation of decubitus ulcers. Herpes simplex virus is suspected in immunocompromised patients. In early stages, the condition is reversible, but left untended, a decubitus ulcer can become extensively infected, necrotic, and, ultimately, irreversible.

Signs and symptoms of decubitus ulcer include: in the first stage, deep pink, red, or mottled skin that is warm, firm, or stretched tightly across the area; in the second stage, blistering, cracking, or abrasion of the skin; in the third stage, a crater-like sore with involvement of underlying structures, and exposure of fat; in the fourth stage, necrosis extended through skin and fat to the muscle; in the fifth stage, advanced fat and muscle necrosis; and in the sixth stage, bone destruction and osteomyelitis.

Therapies include a high protein, well-balanced diet, application of absorbable gelatin sponges (Gelfoam), a change in the patient's position every two hours, and the use of egg-crate mattresses and protective padding (sheepskin). Other therapies include stimulation of the affected area by gentle massage to facilitate circulation (thus healing), debridement (excisional, chemical, and whirlpool), or deeper surgery with closure or skin grafting for advanced stages.

Recurrent Decubitus Ulcer with Failed Graft: A recurrent decubitus ulcer that has had multiple failed grafts is reported with a code from 707.0 subcategory and 996.52 *Mechanical complication of device, implant or graft.*

Residual Pressure Sore with Recurrent Ischial Sinus: This condition is classified as a decubitus ulcer. The formation of the ischial sinus in the decubitus ulcer is an integral component of the disease progression and no additional code is assigned.

Coding Scenario

A patient has had multiple grafting procedures for treatment of an extensive decubitus ulcer of the buttock. The patient is being readmitted for complications of the skin graft.

> Code assignment: 707.05 *Decubitus ulcer, buttock* and 996.52 *Mechanical complication of device, implant, or graft*

An elderly patient is transferred from an extended care facility for treatment of a decubitus ulcer of the

© 2004 Ingenix, Inc.

heel. The physician also identifies the patient as a Type I diabetic with related progressive peripheral vascular disease.

Code assignment: 707.07 *Decubitus ulcer, heel,* 250.71 *Diabetes with peripheral circulatory disorders, Type I [insulin dependent type], not stated as uncontrolled,* and 443.81 *Peripheral angiopathy in diseases classified elsewhere*

707.10 Ulcer of lower limb, unspecified — *unknown site, not calf*
AHA: Q4, 1999, 15; Q4, 2000, 44; Q4, 2002, 43

707.11 Ulcer of thigh — *between hip and knee*
AHA: Q4, 1999, 15; Q4, 2000, 44

707.12 Ulcer of calf

707.13 Ulcer of ankle

707.14 Ulcer of heel and midfoot — *plantar surface of midfoot*
AHA: Q4, 1999, 15; Q4, 2000, 44

707.15 Ulcer of other part of foot — *toes*
AHA: Q4, 1999, 15; Q4, 2000, 44

707.19 Ulcer of other part of lower limb — *not otherwise specified*
AHA: Q4, 1999, 15; Q4, 2000, 44

707.8 Chronic ulcer of other specified site — *groin, hand, neck, perineum, sacrum, scalp, submental*

707.9 Chronic ulcer of unspecified site — *unknown skin site*

Coding Clarification

Code, if applicable, any causal condition first, as in atherosclerosis with ulceration (440.23), chronic venous hypertension with ulcer (459.31), chronic venous hypertension with ulcer and inflammation (459.33), postphlebitic syndrome with ulcer (459.11), postphlebitic syndrome with ulcer and inflammation (459.13), and diabetes (250.80-250.83). Codes are chosen according to ulcer site. In some cases, multiple codes may be required.

708 Urticaria

Use this rubric to report eruption of itching edema of the skin (hives). Often due to hypersensitivity to a drug, food, or insect stings or bites, urticaria also may be due to such stimuli as physical exercise, heat, cold, sunlight, anxiety, and tension. Most episodes are acute and self-limiting over a period of one to two weeks.

Signs and symptoms of urticaria include pruritus, wheals that may remain small or may enlarge, rings of erythema, and edema. Therapies include cessation of nonessential medication or other causative factors, oral antihistamine (Benadryl, Atarax, and Periactin), and prednisone in more severe cases (associated with angioedema).

708.0 Allergic urticaria — *allergic hives*

708.1 Idiopathic urticaria — *hives of unknown cause*

708.2 Urticaria due to cold and heat — *hives due to heat or cold*

708.3 Dermatographic urticaria — *hives raised as a result of scratching*

708.4 Vibratory urticaria — *hives as a response to vibration*

708.5 Cholinergic urticaria

708.8 Other specified urticaria — *nettle rash, recurrent periodic rash, chronic hives*

708.9 Unspecified urticaria — *hives of unknown cause*

Coding Clarification

Excluded from this rubric are angioneurotic edema (995.1), Quincke's edema (995.1), hereditary angioedema (277.6), giant urticaria (995.1), papulosa urticaria (698.2), and urticaria pigmentosa (757.33).

709 Other disorders of skin and subcutaneous tissue

709.00 Dyschromia, unspecified — *variation of skin pigmentation of unknown cause*

709.01 Vitiligo

709.09 Other dyschromia — *Civatte's poikiloderma, classic piebaldism, café au lait spots, xanthosis, Sutton's or Schamberg's disease, liver spots*

709.1 Vascular disorder of skin — *angioma serpiginosum, purpura annularis telangiectodes, Gougerot-Blum syndrome, Majocchi's disease*

709.2 Scar condition and fibrosis of skin — *adherent scar, cicatrix, disfigurement*
AHA: Nov-Dec, 1984, 19

709.3 Degenerative skin disorder — *calcinosis circumscripta or cutis, colloid milium, Miescher-Leder syndrome, Wagner's disease, skin deposits*

709.4 Foreign body granuloma of skin and subcutaneous tissue

709.8 Other specified disorder of skin — *epithelial hyperplasia, menstrual dermatosis, vesicular eruption, dermatosis papulosa nigra, macules, papules, sclerosing lipogranuloma*
AHA: Nov-Dec, 1987, 6

709.9 Unspecified disorder of skin and subcutaneous tissue

710–739

Diseases of the Musculoskeletal System and Connective Tissue

This chapter classifies diseases and disorders of the bones, muscles, cartilage, fascia, ligaments, synovia, tendons, and bursa.

Connective tissue disorders classified to Chapter 13 are those primarily affecting the musculoskeletal system. Injuries and certain congenital disorders of the musculoskeletal system are classified elsewhere.

Many codes for the manifestation of musculoskeletal diseases due to specified infections and other diseases and disorders classified elsewhere are included in this chapter. Also included are many codes describing the residuals of previous diseases, disorders, and injuries classified as late effects. These codes often can be identified by the term "acquired" in the description.

710–719 Arthropathies and Related Disorders

Excluded from this section are disorders of the spine (720.0-724.9).

710 Diffuse diseases of connective tissue

This rubric reports a group of diseases in which the primary lesion appears to be damage to collagen, a protein that is the major component of connective tissue. Collagen (rheumatoid) diseases, attributed largely to disorders of the immune complex mechanism, include myositis, sclerosis, dermal atrophy, arthritis, vasculitis, nephritis, carditis, subcutaneous nodules, polyserositis, and lupus erythematosus. Many of these conditions, such as polyarteritis nodosa (a connective tissue disease that is a form of vasculitis), are classified to other chapters.

Category 710 includes diffuse diseases of connective tissues; most are collagen diseases whose effects are not mainly confined to a single body system. For proper code assignment, follow the ICD-9-CM index carefully and read the includes and excludes notes pertaining to this category. Also excluded are those diffuse diseases affecting mainly the cardiovascular system, as in polyarteritis and other allied conditions (446.0-446.7).

710.0 Systemic lupus erythematosus — (Use additional code to identify manifestation: 424.91, 581.81, 582.81, 583.81) — *disseminated, Libman-Sacks disease, L.E. cell phenomenon*
AHA: Q2, 1997, 8; Q2, 2003, 7-8

Use subclassification 710.0 to report an inflammatory autoimmune disorder that may affect multiple organ systems. The disease is usually chronic, and the clinical course is mild to fulminating. Clinical exacerbations and remissions of manifestations involving the skin, serosal surfaces, central nervous system, kidneys, and blood cells are characteristic. Arthralgia, symmetrical arthritis, and inflammatory muscle involvement are common musculoskeletal features of acute systemic lupus erythematosus. The disease is most prevalent in women, particularly black women, of childbearing age.

No single etiology for the disease has been discovered, but initiation and expression of the disease has been associated with hormonal influences, genetic factors, loss of tolerance to autoantigens, and certain viruses and drugs. The hands and wrist are two sites commonly affected by lupus arthritis.

Signs and symptoms of systemic lupus erythematosus include fever, anorexia, malaise, weight loss, and skin lesions identical to chronic discoid lupus erythematosus, redness and edema affecting the nose and cheeks revealing a classic butterfly rash, photosensitivity and other ocular manifestations, and joint symptoms with or without acute synovitis. Lab work may show mild normochromic, normocytic anemia, or occasionally autoimmune hemolytic anemia. Lab work also may reveal leukopenia, lymphopenia, and thrombocytopenia. Therapies include limited, symptomatic intervention, such as topical sunscreens for photosensitivity, in mild, benign forms of the disease, in addition to nonsteroidal antiinflammatory medications to control fever, joint complaints, and serositis, as well as antimalarial drugs (chloroquine, hydroxychloroquine) and topical corticosteroids for skin manifestations. Systemic corticosteroids are prescribed for more severe manifestations involving the heart and kidneys. Immunosuppressive agents (such as cyclophosphamide, chlorambucil, and azathioprine) may be prescribed in cases resistant to corticosteroids.

© 2004 Ingenix, Inc.

Associated conditions include endocarditis, renal failure due to proliferative glomerulonephritis, nephritis or nephritis syndrome, Raynaud's phenomenon, anemia, pleurisy and pleural effusion, bronchopneumonia, restrictive lung diseases, vasculitis (with resulting ileus and peritonitis), and Hashimoto's thyroiditis.

Excluded from this code is lupus erythematosus (discoid) not otherwise specified (695.4).

710.1 Systemic sclerosis — (Use additional code to identify manifestation: 359.6, 517.2) — *acrosclerosis, CRST or Weissenbach-Thibierge syndrome, scleroderma, progressive systemic sclerosis*
AHA: Q1, 1988, 6

Use 710.1 to report widespread small vessel obliteration and fibrotic thickening of the skin and multiple organs, including the alimentary tract, kidneys, lungs, muscles, joints, nerves, and heart. When localized to the face and extremities (with Raynaud's phenomena), it is called acrosclerosis. A distinct form of systemic sclerosis is CREST syndrome, which stands for subcutaneous Calcinosis, Raynaud's phenomenon, Esophageal motility dysfunction, Sclerodactyly, and Telangiectasia.

Associated conditions include Raynaud's phenomena, subcutaneous calcinosis (nodular deposition of calcium salts in the subcutaneous tissues or muscles), ulcers and infection of the finger tips, telangiectasia, malabsorption syndrome, and carpal tunnel syndrome.

Excluded from this code is circumscribed scleroderma (701.0).

710.2 Sicca syndrome — *keratoconjunctivitis sicca, including Sjögren's disease*

Use 710.2 to report Sjögren's syndrome resulting from lymphocytic infiltration of lacrimal and salivary glands. An idiopathic, autoimmune disorder, Sjögren's syndrome is characterized by xerostomia (dry mouth), keratoconjunctivitis sicca (dry eyes), and parotid gland enlargement. Primary Sjögren's syndrome presents a wide variety of clinical manifestations due to a wider involvement of the exocrine glands. The organs involved may include the skin, lung, GI tract, kidney, muscles, nerves, spleen, and thyroid. Secondary Sjögren's syndrome is limited to symptoms of the lacrimal and salivary glands.

Lab work may reveal a higher frequency of human lymphocytic antigen HLA-DR3 in primary Sjögren's syndrome and of HLA-DR4 in secondary Sjögren's syndrome.

Associated conditions include rheumatoid arthritis and other collagen diseases.

710.3 Dermatomyositis — *poikilodermatomyositis, polymyositis with skin involvement, Petges-Cléjat or Unverricht-Wagner syndromes*

Use 710.3 to report nonsuppurative inflammation of the skin, subcutaneous tissues, and muscles with necrosis of muscle fibers. The disease complex is differentiated from polymyositis by the presence of a characteristic rash of edema and erythema and a heliotrope discoloration particularly around the eyes.

Physical exam reveals prominent proximal muscle weakness. Lab work shows elevated muscle enzymes. Electromyograph (EMG) reveals myopathic patterns and muscle biopsy reveals inflammatory infiltrates.

Associated conditions include malignancy of visceral organs in adults.

710.4 Polymyositis — *chronic, progressive, inflammatory symmetrical weakness of limb girdles, with pain*

Use 710.4 to report a condition identical to dermatomyositis without the characteristic skin lesions.

710.5 Eosinophilia myalgia syndrome — (Use additional E code to identify drug, if drug-induced) — *toxic oil syndrome*
AHA: Q4, 1992, 21

Use 710.5 to report a multisystem inflammatory and fibrosing illness associated with ingestion of L-tryptophan, an oral nutritional substance of amino acids. It includes toxic oil syndrome and eosinophilic fasciitis.

Signs and symptoms of eosinophilia myalgia syndrome include a history of over-the-counter use of nutritional supplements containing L-tryptophan, muscle and joint pain, weakness, swelling of the arms and legs, fever, and rash. Blood work shows increased circulating eosinophils.

Associated conditions include pneumonia, cardiac arrhythmia, pulmonary hypertension (cor pulmonale), and polyneuropathy.

710.8 Other specified diffuse disease of connective tissue — *not elsewhere classified*
AHA: March-April, 1987, 12

Subcategory 710.8 includes carpal tunnel osteolysis syndrome.

710.9 Unspecified diffuse connective tissue disease — *unknown collagen disease*

Coding Clarification

Category 710 includes diffuse diseases of connective tissues; most are collagen diseases whose effects are not mainly confined to a single body system. For proper code assignment, follow the ICD-9-CM index read the includes and excludes notes pertaining to

 © 2004 Ingenix, Inc.

this category. Also excluded are those diffuse diseases affecting mainly the cardiovascular system, as in polyarteritis and other allied conditions (446.0-446.7).

711 Arthropathy associated with infections

AHA: Q1, 1992, 17

This rubric includes infections of the articular joints of bones, and must be differentiated from infections of the bones classifiable to category 730.

Direct microbial contamination may cause a primary infection of the articular joints. The routes of infection include open fractures, surgical procedures, diagnostic needle aspirations, and therapeutic drug injections.

The following fifth-digit subclassification is for use with categories 711-712, 715-716, 718-719, and 730. Valid fifth-digits are in brackets [ ] at the end of each code.

- 0 site unspecified
- 1 shoulder region (acromioclavicular joint, clavicle, glenohumeral joint, scapula, sternoclavicular joint)
- 2 upper arm (elbow joint, humerus)
- 3 forearm (radius, ulna, wrist joint)
- 4 hand (carpus, metacarpus, phalanges)
- 5 pelvic regions and thigh (buttock, femur, hip joint)
- 6 lower leg (fibula, knee joint, patella, tibia)
- 7 ankle and foot (ankle joint, metatarsus, phalanges, tarsus, other joints in foot)
- 8 other specified sites (head, neck, ribs, skull, trunk, vertebral column)
- 9 multiple sites

711.0 5th Pyogenic arthritis — (Use additional code to identify infectious organism: 041.0-041.8) — *due to infectious organism, including staph, strep, H. influenzae, E. coli, pneumococcus*
AHA: Q1, 1991, 15; Q1, 1992, 16; Q1, 1992, 17

Use codes in subcategory 711.0 to report an acute, destructive bacterial process in a joint following infection, usually occurring as acute monoarticular (single joint) arthritis. The knee and large joints are most often involved.

Signs and symptoms of pyogenic arthritis include fever, joint pain, decreased range of motion, and swelling and redness over the affected joint. Gross examination of aspirated synovial (joint) fluid confirms the presence of pus (pyarthrosis); a gram stain and culture may detect microorganisms and crystals; an examination with polarizing microscope reveals crystals. Therapies include removal of inflammatory material by aspiration or incision and drainage, antibiotic therapy that may be prolonged, and resting the joint in a stable position.

Associated conditions include systemic or localized infections, intravenous drug abuse, recent trauma or surgery, pyogenic arthropathy, septicemia, and osteomyelitis.

Not all pyogenic joint infections are classifiable to subcategory 711.0. Before assigning code 711.0, carefully review the entries in the ICD-9-CM index under the terms "Arthritis, arthritic," "due to or associated with," and the includes note under subcategory 711.4 for any bacterial organism not specifically referenced under category 041. List a code from category 041 as a secondary code to identify the specific organism responsible for the arthritis or arthropathy.

711.1 5th Arthropathy associated with Reiter's disease and nonspecific urethritis — (Code first underlying disease: 099.3, 099.4) — *arthritis, arthropathy, polyarthritis, polyarthropathy code first underlying disease as: 099.4, 099.3*
AHA: Q1, 1992, 17

Use codes in subcategory 711.1 to report seronegative reactive arthritis. Occurring predominantly in the lower extremities, it is triggered by urethritis, cervicitis, or dysenteric infections. The syndrome consists of a triad of nonspecific (nongonococcal or simple) urethritis, conjunctivitis (or sometimes uveitis), and arthritis, and sometimes appears with mucocutaneous lesions. There is a close correlation between this disease and the presence of the histocompatibility antigen HLA-B27.

These manifestation codes include arthropathy with Reiter's disease and nonspecific urethritis. ICD-9-CM classifies etiology first, then manifestation, to remain compatible with the dual classification concept used in the international version of ICD-9.

711.2 5th Arthropathy in Behcet's syndrome — (Code first underlying disease, 136.1) — *arthritis, arthropathy, polyarthritis, polyarthropathy code first underlying disease 136.1*
AHA: Q1, 1992, 17

Use codes in subcategory 711.2 to report a multisystem disorder of unknown etiology named after the Turkish dermatologist who first described it. Recurrent oral and genital ulcers, uveitis, seronegative arthritis, and central nervous system abnormalities characterize the syndrome. The arthritic component involves large and small joints with a nonspecific, self-limiting synovitis and, in more than two-thirds of the patients, commonly affects the knees and ankles. The arthritic changes resemble those of rheumatoid arthritis but are milder and lead only to shallow erosions of the articular cartilage in the more severe cases. Therapies include immunomodulating drugs and corticosteroids.

Associated conditions include cranial nerve palsies, encephalitis, mental disturbances, spinal cord lesions, convulsions, and, although rarely, death.

These manifestation codes include arthropathy associated with Behcet's syndrome (136.1). ICD-9-CM classifies etiology first, then manifestation, to remain compatible with the dual classification concept used in the international version of ICD-9.

711.3 5th Postdysenteric arthropathy — (Code first underlying disease: 002.0-002.9, 008.0-009.3) — *secondary to gastrointestinal infection*
AHA: Q1, 1992, 17

Use codes in subcategory 711.3 to report rare enteropathic arthropathies due to a wide range of specific dysentery-causing organisms, Shigella, and typhoid fever.

These manifestation codes include postdysenteric arthropathy, and are distinguished from subcategory 713.1 by an infectious or parasitic etiology for the enteropathic arthritis. ICD-9-CM classifies etiology first, then manifestation, to remain compatible with the dual classification concept used in the international version of ICD-9.

Excluded from this subclassification is salmonella arthritis (003.23).

711.4 5th Arthropathy associated with other bacterial diseases — (Code first underlying disease, such as: diseases classifiable to 010-040 (except 036.82), 090-099 (except 098.50)) — *secondary*
AHA: Q1, 1992, 17

Use codes in subcategory 711.4 to report arthropathy due to a wide variety of bacteria, excluding the pyogenic organisms identified under subcategory 711.0 and bacterial arthropathies classified elsewhere.

These manifestation codes include arthropathy associated with other bacterial diseases. ICD-9-CM classifies etiology first, then manifestation, to remain compatible with the dual classification concept used in the international version of ICD-9.

Excluded from this rubric are gonococcal arthritis (098.50) and meningococcal arthritis (036.82).

711.5 5th Arthropathy associated with other viral diseases — (Code first underlying disease, such as: diseases classifiable to 045-049, 050-079 (except 056.71), 480, 487) — *secondary*
AHA: Q1, 1992, 17

Use codes in subcategory 711.5 to report arthropathy associated with a wide variety of other viral diseases including rubella, mumps, infectious mononucleosis, lymphogranuloma venereum, variola, and many others.

These manifestation codes include arthropathy associated with other viral diseases. Arthropathy associated with viral hepatitis should also be classified here. ICD-9-CM classifies etiology first, then manifestation, to remain compatible with the dual classification concept used in the international version of ICD-9.

Excluded from this subclassification is arthropathy due to rubella (056.7).

711.6 5th Arthropathy associated with mycoses — (Code first underlying disease: 110.0-118) — *secondary*
AHA: Q1, 1992, 17

Use codes in subcategory 711.6 to report arthropathy due to mycoses. Mycoses are diseases caused by fungi. A variety of fungal organisms may lodge in the synovium and create suppurative or granulomatous lesions. The synovium usually is the primary site of joint involvement, but secondary infection can spread from the marrow cavity to the subchondral bone and then into the articular tissues.

These manifestation codes includes arthropathy associated with mycoses. ICD-9-CM classifies etiology first, then manifestation, to remain compatible with the dual classification concept used in the international version of ICD-9.

711.7 5th Arthropathy associated with helminthiasis — (Code first underlying disease: 125.0-125.9) — *secondary*
AHA: Q1, 1992, 17

Use codes in subcategory 711.7 to report arthropathy due to parasitic infection of helminths (worms), hydatid cysts, or helminth larvae.

These manifestation codes include arthropathies associated with helminthiases. ICD-9-CM classifies etiology first, then manifestation, to remain compatible with the dual classification concept used in the international version of ICD-9.

711.8 5th Arthropathy associated with other infectious and parasitic diseases — (Code first underlying disease, such as: diseases classifiable to 080-088, 100-104, 130-136) — *secondary*
AHA: Q3, 1990, 14; Q4, 1991, 15; Q1, 1992, 17

The manifestation codes in subcategory 711.8 include arthropathy associated with other infectious and parasitic diseases. ICD-9-CM classifies etiology first, then manifestation, to remain compatible with the dual classification concept used in the international version of ICD-9.

Excluded from this subclassification is arthropathy associated with sarcoidosis (713.7).

© 2004 Ingenix, Inc.

711.9 [5th] Unspecified infective arthritis — *infective agent unknown*
AHA: Q1, 1992, 17

Coding Clarification

Direct microbial infections resulting from surgical, diagnostic, and therapeutic procedures are classified to categories 996-999.

Excluded from this rubric is rheumatic fever (390).

Most of the arthropathies classified here are due to indirect (secondary) infections, and require a second code to identify the infectious organism or the underlying disease.

Arthritis as a Late Effect: As mentioned earlier, arthritis can be a late effect or a residual of a disease process or injury.

In most circumstances, the residual condition or nature of the late effect is coded first, followed by the late effect code for the cause of the residual condition, except when instructed otherwise by the alphabetic index of the ICD-9-CM manual.

Arthritis Associated with Other Diseases: Arthritis can be a manifestation or symptom of other diseases or conditions. For example:

Arthritis due to Lyme Disease: A common manifestation of Lyme disease is joint pain (arthralgia) and arthritis. These symptoms occur early in the disease process and each should be separately coded.

In instances when the patient has both Lyme disease and the clinical manifestation of arthritis, code 088.81 is assigned as well as the code indicating arthritis associated with other parasitic diseases (711.8x).

Multiple Coding: There are times when arthritis will require multiple codes. In these instances, the alphabetic index of the ICD-9-CM manual will identify a code for both the etiology and the manifestation following the subentry term, with the second code italicized and in slanted brackets. Both codes should be assigned and in the sequence that the patient presents.

Type of Arthritis: The term arthritis is used by medical personnel to describe more than 100 various forms of rheumatic disease. Arthritis can affect multiple body systems and/or sites including joints, muscles, connective tissues, skin, and internal organs. The most widespread forms of arthritis are osteoarthritis and rheumatoid arthritis. This disease can also be the sequelae of other disease processes or caused by infectious organisms.

Osteoarthritis: The most common form of arthritis is osteoarthritis (OA). Physicians often call this form of arthritis by various terms including degenerative joint disease (DJD), osteoarthrosis, degenerative arthritis, and hypertrophic arthritis.

Osteoarthritis noted as generalized is a chronic noninflammatory arthritis that affects multiple sites, commonly of older patients, marked by degeneration of articular cartilage and enlargement of bone, and pain and stiffness occurring with any type of activity but subsiding when the patient rests. This form should be reported with subcategory code 715.0x. Only three of the 10 fifth digits available for osteoarthritis may be used with this subcategory: 0, 4, and 9.

There are two categories of localized osteoarthritis: primary and secondary.

- Primary osteoarthritis is also known as idiopathic or polyarticular degenerative arthritis. Primarily this form affects joints of the spine, knee, hip, and small joints of the hands and feet.
- Secondary osteoarthritis, also known as monarticular arthritis, is due to an illness or injury and affects the joint of one area. Possible causes include, but are not limited to, infectious, metabolic, endocrine, or neuropathic diseases; diseases that alter the normal function and structure of the cartilage (e.g., Paget's disease, gout, chondrocalcinosis, etc.); and acute or chronic injuries or trauma.

Rheumatoid Arthritis: Rheumatoid arthritis is a disease of the autoimmune system that can affect the entire body. This disease can occur during childhood (called juvenile rheumatoid arthritis) or adulthood. Single or multiple sites may be affected.

Pyogenic Arthritis: This form of arthritis is due to an acute inflammation of the synovial membranes with purulent effusion into the joint caused by a bacterial infection. It may also be referred to in the medical record documentation as suppurative arthritis or suppurative synovitis. It may progress and become chronic resulting in sinus formation, osteomyelitis, and joint deformity.

When reporting pyogenic arthritis, use subcategory code 711.0 with the appropriate fifth digit to identify the specific site. An additional code indicating the infectious organism is assigned if it is known.

Pyogenic arthritis can also affect other tissues and organs. When this occurs, the code for the condition responsible for the encounter is assigned as well as a code for the pyogenic arthritis (711.0x).

Gout: This is an acute recurrent arthritis in which excessive uric acid in the blood is deposited in the peripheral joints. It may be chronic, which can cause progressive debilitation. However, all hyperuricemia is not gout, and all hyperuricemia does not progress to gout.

Coding Scenario

A patient with recently diagnosed Lyme disease is seen in the office for follow-up. She is now complaining of joint pain and swelling of the knees. The physician states that arthritis due to the Lyme disease is now present.

> Code assignment: 088.81 *Lyme disease* and 711.86 *Arthropathy associated with other infectious and parasitic diseases, lower leg (fibula, knee joint, patella, tibia)*

A patient who was treated five years ago for Lyme disease is now seen in the office for residual arthritic pain. After examination, the physician's diagnostic statement indicates that the patient has arthritis secondary to Lyme disease. The medical record identifies that the patient is cured of Lyme disease, but still has the residual arthritis of multiple sites from the disease.

> Code assignment: 139.8 *Late effect of other and unspecified infectious and parasitic diseases* and 711.89 *Arthropathy associated with other infectious and parasitic diseases, multiple sites*

712 Crystal arthropathies

Use this rubric to report chondrocalcinosis, arthritis, and synovitis, as well as pseudogout and calcium pyrophosphate dehydrate deposition (CPDD) disease. The presence, and not the chemical composition, of crystals (apatite and hydroxyapatite, calcium pyrophosphate, calcium and dicalcium phosphate, calcium oxalate, and lipid crystals) acts as irritants. The mechanisms of initial precipitation are unknown, but predisposing conditions such as degradation of the cartilage matrix may be involved. Once the crystals have accumulated, they are taken up by phagocytic cells, initiating the inflammatory sequence. This in turn causes additional damage to the affected tissues.

The term chondrocalcinosis refers to calcification of articular cartilage. Articular chondrocalcinosis also is known as pseudogout since the disease is characterized by calcified deposits in the cartilage, but is free of the urate crystals found in gout. Aspiration and examination of synovial fluid allows precise diagnosis. Therapies include aspiration of the acutely inflamed joint; drugs such as corticosteroid injections; nonsteroidal, anti-inflammatory drugs; and intravenous colchicine.

The following fifth-digit subclassification is for use with categories 711-712, 715-716, 718-719, and 730. Valid fifth-digits are in brackets [ ] at the end of each code.

- 0 site unspecified
- 1 shoulder region (acromioclavicular joint, clavicle, glenohumeral joint, scapula, sternoclavicular joint)
- 2 upper arm (elbow joint, humerus)
- 3 forearm (radius, ulna, wrist joint)
- 4 hand (carpus, metacarpus, phalanges)
- 5 pelvic regions and thigh (buttock, femur, hip joint)
- 6 lower leg (fibula, knee joint, patella, tibia)
- 7 ankle and foot (ankle joint, metatarsus, phalanges, tarsus, other joints in foot)
- 8 other specified sites (head, neck, ribs, skull, trunk, vertebral column)
- 9 multiple sites

712.1 5th Chondrocalcinosis due to dicalcium phosphate crystals — (Code first underlying disease, 275.4) — *crystal-induced arthritis*

The manifestation codes in subcategory 712.1 include chondrocalcinosis due to dicalcium phosphate crystals. ICD-9-CM classifies etiology first, then manifestation, to remain compatible with the dual classification concept used in the international version of ICD-9.

712.2 5th Chondrocalcinosis due to pyrophosphate crystals — (Code first underlying disease, 275.4) — *crystal-induced arthritis*

Use codes in subcategory 712.2 to report chondrocalcinosis due to pyrophosphate crystals, which is a calcium pyrophosphate dehydrate deposition (CPPD) disease and type II crystal deposition disease.

The manifestation codes include chondrocalcinosis due to pyrophosphate crystals. ICD-9-CM classifies etiology first, then manifestation, to remain compatible with the dual classification concept used in the international version of ICD-9.

712.3 5th Chondrocalcinosis, cause unspecified — (Code first underlying disease, 275.4)

Codes in subcategory 712.3 include chondrocalcinosis due to unspecified cause. ICD-9-CM classifies etiology first, then manifestation, to remain compatible with the dual classification concept used in the international version of ICD-9.

712.8 5th Other specified crystal arthropathies

Use codes in subcategory 712.8 to report other specified crystal arthropathies due to lipid crystals, apatite and hydroxyapatite, calcium oxalate, calcium phosphate, and other identifiable crystals not elsewhere classifiable.

712.9 5th Unspecified crystal arthropathy — *crystal-induced arthritis, type unknown*

 © 2004 Ingenix, Inc.

Coding Clarification

This category includes crystal (mineral) deposition arthropathies with the exception of gouty arthropathy, which is classified to code 274.0. Crystal deposition disease type I refers to gouty arthropathy due to uric acid crystals and should be classified to subcategory 274.0; type II crystal deposition disease includes the disorders classified to subcategory 712.2.

713 Arthropathy associated with other disorders classified elsewhere

This rubric includes manifestation codes used to classify arthropathy associated with other disorders classified elsewhere. ICD-9-CM classifies etiology first, then manifestation, to remain compatible with the dual classification concept used in the international version of ICD-9.

713.0 Arthropathy associated with other endocrine and metabolic disorders — (Code first underlying disease: 243-244.9, 252.0, 253.0, 270.2, 272.0-272.9, 275.0, 279.00-279.09) — *secondary*

713.1 Arthropathy associated with gastrointestinal conditions other than infections — (Code first underlying disease: 555.0-555.9, 556.0-556.9) — *secondary*

713.2 Arthropathy associated with hematological disorders — (Code first underlying disease: 202.3, 203.0, 204.0-208.9, 282.4-282.7, 286.0-286.2) — *secondary*

713.3 Arthropathy associated with dermatological disorders — (Code first underlying disease: 695.1, 695.2) — *secondary*

713.4 Arthropathy associated with respiratory disorders — (Code first underlying disease, such as: diseases classifiable to 490-519) — *secondary*

713.5 Arthropathy associated with neurological disorders — (Code first underlying disease: 094.0, 250.6, 336.0) — *secondary*

713.6 Arthropathy associated with hypersensitivity reaction — (Code first underlying disease: 287.0, 999.5) — *secondary*

713.7 Other general diseases with articular involvement — (Code first underlying disease: 135, 277.3) — *secondary*
AHA: Q2, 1997, 12

713.8 Arthropathy associated with other conditions classifiable elsewhere — (Code first underlying disease) — *secondary*

Coding Clarification

Whenever the physician's diagnostic statement specifies etiology for the patient's arthropathy, a code from category 713 should be used as a secondary code. For example, the diagnosis "arthropathy due to hemochromatosis" is assigned codes 275.0 and 713.0, and the diagnosis "arthropathic multiple myeloma of the hip" is assigned codes 203.0x and 713.2. In the first case, the cause and effect relationship is stated; in the second, the relationship is implied. The term "associated with" in the code title indicates that both parts of the title may be in the physician's diagnostic statement. The word "as" in the notation *"code first underlying disease as"* under each subcategory indicates an incomplete list of etiologies.

Coding Scenario

A patient develops arthritis of multiple joints as a result of her ulcerative colitis.

> Code assignment: 556.9 *Ulcerative colitis, unspecified* and 713.1 *Arthropathy associated with gastrointestinal conditions other than infectious*

714 Rheumatoid arthritis and other inflammatory polyarthropathies

AHA: Q2, 1995, 3

714.0 Rheumatoid arthritis — (Use additional code to identify manifestation: 357.1, 359.6) — *chronic rheumatic polyarthritis*
AHA: Q1, 1990, 5; Q2, 1995, 3

Rheumatoid arthritis is a chronic, systemic inflammatory disease of unknown etiology, characterized by a variable but prolonged course with exacerbations and remissions of joint pains and swelling. In early stages, the disease attacks the joints of the hands and feet. As the disease progresses, more joints become involved. Also known as primary progressive arthritis and proliferative arthritis, the disease often leads to progressive deformities, which may develop rapidly and cause permanent disability.

Clinical manifestations of rheumatoid arthritis are highly variable, particularly in the mode of onset, distribution, degree of severity, and rate of progression. Joint disease is the major manifestation; systemic involvement (spleen, liver, eyes, etc.) is rare.

Signs and symptoms of rheumatoid arthritis include articular inflammation, malaise, weight loss, paresthesia, Raynaud's phenomenon, periarticular pain and stiffness, symmetrical joint swelling and stiffness, warmth, and tenderness (most severe in the morning, somewhat subsiding during the day).

Lab work includes a complete blood count (CBC) to reveal anemia, elevated white blood cell count (WBC), and elevated erythrocyte sedimentation rate (ESR). Various serological tests may be used to detect rheumatoid factor, but false positive and false negative results are not unusual; typically, tests show elevated gamma globulins IgM and IgC during both acute and chronic phases. X-rays of affected joints early in the disease reveal evidence of periarticular soft tissue swelling and joint effusion. As the disease progresses, x-rays show regional osteoporosis, osteolysis of subchondral bone, narrowing of cartilage spaces, and, in the late stages, subluxation, dislocation, and ankylosis.

Therapies include medical treatment directed toward pain relief and reduction of inflammation with a wide variety of drugs including gold salts, corticosteroids, and nonsteroidal antiinflammatory drugs for preservation of function and prevention of deformities. Physical and occupational therapy and splinting of joints are other therapies, as well as surgery such as arthrodesis, synovectomy, tendon grafts and transplantations, arthroplasty, capsulectomy, and capsulotomy.

Associated conditions include nonspecific pericarditis and pleuritis, pulmonary fibrosis, secondary amyloidosis, leukopenia, arteritis, and adverse effect of medications used to treat rheumatoid arthritis.

714.1 Felty's syndrome — *rheumatoid arthritis with splenoadenomegaly and leukopenia*
AHA: Q2, 1995, 3

The definition of Felty's syndrome is the association of rheumatoid arthritis with splenomegaly and leukopenia. Mild anemia and thrombocytopenia may accompany the variable severe neutropenia, and skin and pulmonary infections are frequent complications.

714.2 Other rheumatoid arthritis with visceral or systemic involvement — *rheumatoid carditis*
AHA: Q2, 1995, 3

Other rheumatoid arthritis with visceral or systemic involvement occurs in the connective tissue components of the cardiovascular, reticuloendothelial, digestive, and respiratory system.

714.3 5th Juvenile chronic polyarthritis

Juvenile chronic polyarthritis is a rheumatoid-like disorder occurring in children (onset prior to age 17), involving one or more joints. Juvenile rheumatoid arthritis has a much more favorable prognosis than adult-onset disease.

The disease process for juvenile rheumatoid arthritis and polyarthritis is different genetically and immunologically from rheumatoid arthritis in adults, but the condition is still classified to subcategory 714.3 with the appropriate fifth digit, depending on the clinical presentation.

714.30 Polyarticular juvenile rheumatoid arthritis, chronic or unspecified — *number of joints affected unspecified, Still's disease*
AHA: Q2, 1995, 3

Polyarticular juvenile rheumatoid arthritis, chronic or unspecified, is systemic juvenile arthritis or polyarthritis, also known as Still's disease, that interferes with growth and development.

714.31 Polyarticular juvenile rheumatoid arthritis, acute — *affecting many joints*
AHA: Q2, 1995, 3

Polyarticular juvenile rheumatoid arthritis, acute, is systemic juvenile arthritis or polyarthritis, also known as Still's disease, described as acute. Typically, the acute phase includes high fever, erythematous rash, anemia, generalized lymphadenopathy, and, in some cases, hepatosplenomegaly, iridocyclitis, and pericarditis.

714.32 Pauciarticular juvenile rheumatoid arthritis — *affecting only a few joints*
AHA: Q2, 1995, 3

Pauciarticular juvenile rheumatoid arthritis is a disease, also known as oligoarticular juvenile arthritis, affecting a small number of joints, usually two to five. It is associated with chronic iridocyclitis in 25 to 30 percent of patients and can lead to blindness.

714.33 Monoarticular juvenile rheumatoid arthritis — *affecting one joint*
AHA: Q2, 1995, 3

Monoarticular juvenile rheumatoid arthritis is juvenile arthritis limited to one joint.

Pauciarticular juvenile arthritis may be used to describe monoarticular juvenile arthritis. In such cases, verify the diagnosis with the physician to ensure proper code assignment.

714.4 Chronic postrheumatic arthropathy — *chronic rheumatoid nodular fibrositis, Jaccoud's syndrome*
AHA: Q2, 1995, 3

The definition of chronic postrheumatic arthropathy is a form of arthropathy of the hands and feet caused by repeated attacks of rheumatic arthritis. Also called Jaccoud's syndrome, this disease is characterized by flexion deformities, particularly of the metacarpophalangeal joints, and is associated with pronounced ulnar deviation of the fingers. Chronic rheumatoid nodular fibrositis is a variation of this disease characterized by the presence of subcutaneous nodules in the region of the previously involved joints.

714.81 Rheumatoid lung — *Caplan's syndrome, diffuse interstitial rheumatoid lung disease, fibrosing alveolitis*
AHA: Q2, 1995, 3

Rheumatoid lung is diseases of the lung associated with rheumatoid arthritis, including Hamman-Rich syndrome (when associated with rheumatoid arthritis) and Caplan's syndrome, a syndrome of rheumatoid pneumoconiosis seen in patients with concomitant coal worker's pneumoconiosis.

 © 2004 Ingenix, Inc.

714.89 Other specified inflammatory polyarthropathies — *not otherwise specified*
AHA: Q2, 1995, 3

714.9 Unspecified inflammatory polyarthropathy

Documentation Issues

The physician should clearly indicate the type of arthritis and the sites affected by the condition for appropriate code selection to be made.

When pyogenic arthritis is documented and the infectious organism has not been identified, contact the physician for clarification as an additional code should be used to identify the infectious organism.

If conditions that are integral to the disease process of the arthritis are mentioned in the final diagnostic statement, they should not be assigned as additional codes (e.g., pain, joint swelling).

Coding Scenario

A 10-year-old patient in seen in the rheumatology clinic complaining of joint pain and swelling with early morning fatigue. After a comprehensive evaluation, it is determined that she is in the early stages of juvenile rheumatoid arthritis.

> Code assignment: 714.30 *Polyarticular juvenile rheumatoid arthritis, chronic or unspecified*

715 Osteoarthrosis and allied disorders

Osteoarthrosis and allied disorders are degenerative, rather than inflammatory, diseases of one or more joints. Also known as osteoarthritis and degenerative joint disease, osteoarthrosis is most conspicuous in the large joints and initiated by local deterioration of the articular cartilage. It progressively destroys the cartilage, remodels the subchondral bone, and causes a secondary inflammation of the synovial membrane.

Signs and symptoms of osteoarthrosis and allied disorders include pain in the affected joints, muscle spasm, crepitation, and atrophy of surrounding muscles without evidence of inflammation.

Lab work is usually of little value, although examination of synovial fluid may demonstrate increased mucin content. X-rays of affected joints readily show narrowing of articular space, subchondral sclerosis and cysts, osteophyte formation, and joint remodeling.

Therapies include pain and weight management, reduction of secondary inflammation of the synovial membrane, and physical and occupational therapy to help the patient maintain joint function and prevent or correct joint deformities. Surgery such as osteotomy near the joint improves biomechanics and soft tissue operations such as release of muscle contractions and neurectomy may help relieve intractable pain. For osteoarthritis of the hip, therapy includes hip preserving surgery (excision of osteophytes, curettage and bone grafting of acetabular cysts, proximal femoral osteotomy and muscle release) or hip reconstruction (cup arthroplasty, total hip replacement, femoral head replacement, and arthrodesis).

Assignment of the fourth digit to codes in this category is based on whether the disease is generalized or localized and whether it is primary or secondary.

The following fifth-digit subclassification is for use with categories 711-712, 715-716, 718-719, and 730. Valid fifth-digits are in brackets [ ] at the end of each code.

0 site unspecified
1 shoulder region (acromioclavicular joint, clavicle, glenohumeral joint, scapula, sternoclavicular joint)
2 upper arm (elbow joint, humerus)
3 forearm (radius, ulna, wrist joint)
4 hand (carpus, metacarpus, phalanges)
5 pelvic regions and thigh (buttock, femur, hip joint)
6 lower leg (fibula, knee joint, patella, tibia)
7 ankle and foot (ankle joint, metatarsus, phalanges, tarsus, other joints in foot)
8 other specified sites (head, neck, ribs, skull, trunk, vertebral column)
9 multiple sites

715.0 5th Osteoarthrosis, generalized — *degenerative joint disease, multiple joints; primary generalized hypertrophic osteoarthrosis*

Generalized disease is osteoarthrosis involving many joints without any known preexisting abnormality. Localized osteoarthrosis is disease confined to a limited number of sites, generally one or two of the larger weight-bearing joints, such as the hip or knee.

715.1 5th Osteoarthrosis, localized, primary — *idiopathic localized osteoarthropathy*

Primary osteoarthrosis is idiopathic or due to some constitutional or genetic factor.

715.2 5th Osteoarthrosis, localized, secondary — *coxae malum senilis*

Secondary osteoarthrosis is due to some identifiable initiating factor. These factors include obesity, trauma, congenital malformations, superimposition of fibrosis and scarring from previous inflammatory disease or infection, foreign bodies, malalignment of joints, metabolic or circulatory bone diseases, and iatrogenic factors such as osteoarthrosis caused by continuous pressure on the joint surfaces during orthopedic treatment of congenital deformities. Secondary osteoarthroses should be paired with a second code describing the causative injury, disorder, or disease.

© 2004 Ingenix, Inc.

715.3 5th Osteoarthrosis, localized, not specified whether primary or secondary — *Otto's pelvis*

715.8 5th Osteoarthrosis involving or with mention of more than one site, but not specified as generalized

715.9 5th Osteoarthrosis, unspecified whether generalized or localized

Documentation Issues

The physician should clearly indicate the type of arthritis and the sites affected by the condition for appropriate code selection to be made.

When pyogenic arthritis is documented and the infectious organism has not been identified, contact the physician for clarification as an additional code should be used to identify the infectious organism.

If conditions that are integral to the disease process of the arthritis are mentioned in the final diagnostic statement, they should not be assigned as additional codes (e.g., pain, joint swelling).

Coding Clarification

Type of Arthritis: The term arthritis is used by medical personnel to describe more than 100 various forms of rheumatic disease. Arthritis can affect multiple body systems and/or sites including joints, muscles, connective tissues, skin, and internal organs. The most widespread forms of arthritis are osteoarthritis and rheumatoid arthritis. This disease can also be the sequelae of other disease processes or caused by infectious organisms.

Osteoarthritis: The most common form of arthritis is osteoarthritis (OA). Physicians often call this form of arthritis by various terms including degenerative joint disease (DJD), osteoarthrosis, degenerative arthritis, and hypertrophic arthritis.

Osteoarthritis noted as generalized is a chronic noninflammatory arthritis that affects multiple sites, commonly of older patients, marked by degeneration of articular cartilage and enlargement of bone, and pain and stiffness occurring with any type of activity but subsiding when the patient rests. This form should be reported with subcategory code 715.0x. Only three of the 10 fifth digits available for osteoarthritis may be used with this subcategory: 0, 4, and 9.

Coding Scenario

A patient is seen in the office for a follow-up examination of her osteoarthritis in the right knee.

> Code assignment: 715.96 *Osteoarthritis, unspecified whether generalized or localized, lower leg (fibula, knee joint, patella, tibia)*

716 *Other and unspecified arthropathies*

AHA: Q2, 1995, 3

The following fifth-digit subclassification is for use with categories 711-712, 715-716, 718-719, and 730. Valid fifth-digits are in brackets [ ] at the end of each code.

0 site unspecified

1 shoulder region (acromioclavicular joint, clavicle, glenohumeral joint, scapula, sternoclavicular joint)

2 upper arm (elbow joint, humerus)

3 forearm (radius, ulna, wrist joint)

4 hand (carpus, metacarpus, phalanges)

5 pelvic regions and thigh (buttock, femur, hip joint)

6 lower leg (fibula, knee joint, patella, tibia)

7 ankle and foot (ankle joint, metatarsus, phalanges, tarsus, other joints in foot)

8 other specified sites (head, neck, ribs, skull, trunk, vertebral column)

9 multiple sites

716.0 5th Kaschin-Beck disease — *endemic polyarthritis*
AHA: Q2, 1995, 3

716.1 5th Traumatic arthropathy — *following injury*
AHA: Q2, 1995, 3

716.2 5th Allergic arthritis — *immunological reaction following exposure to antigen*
AHA: Q2, 1995, 3

Allergic arthritis is associated with a hypersensitive state acquired through exposure to an allergen.

Loosening of orthopedic implants (including prostheses and other devices) due to an allergic or inflammatory reaction to chromium, cobalt, or nickel in the implant is classified as a postoperative complication. In such cases, use code 996.66 or 996.67 to classify the postoperative complication, followed by 716.2x to further describe the nature of the complication.

Excluded from this subclassification is arthritis associated with Henoch-Schonlein purpura or serum sickness (713.6).

716.3 5th Climacteric arthritis — *menopausal*
AHA: Q2, 1995, 3

716.4 5th Transient arthropathy

716.5 5th Unspecified polyarthropathy or polyarthritis

716.6 5th Unspecified monoarthritis — *unknown type*
AHA: Q2, 1995, 3

716.8 5th Other specified arthropathy — *not otherwise specified, including due to old epiphyseal slip, villous arthritis*
AHA: Q2, 1995, 3

 © 2004 Ingenix, Inc.

716.9 ✓5th Unspecified arthropathy

Coding Scenario

A patient with a previous fracture of the left wrist is diagnosed with osteoarthritis due to the fracture.

> Code assignment: 716.13 *Traumatic arthropathy, forearm (radius, ulna, wrist joint)* and 905.2 *Late effect of fracture of upper extremities*

717 Internal derangement of knee

This rubric includes degenerative disorders of the articular cartilage or meniscus of the knee, as well as the late effects of acute trauma to the knee classifiable to category 836.

717.0 Old bucket handle tear of medial meniscus — *old bucket handle tear of unspecified cartilage*

717.1 Derangement of anterior horn of medial meniscus

717.2 Derangement of posterior horn of medial meniscus

717.3 Other and unspecified derangement of medial meniscus — *degeneration of internal semilunar cartilage*

Code 717.3 includes tears of the medial cartilage, or the meniscus, of the knee that may be described as radial, peripheral, horizontal cleavage type, flap, and complex tears.

717.40 Unspecified derangement of lateral meniscus

717.41 Bucket handle tear of lateral meniscus

717.42 Derangement of anterior horn of lateral meniscus

717.43 Derangement of posterior horn of lateral meniscus

717.49 Other derangement of lateral meniscus — *not otherwise specified*

Code 717.49 includes tears of the lateral meniscus of the knee that may be described as radial, peripheral, horizontal cleavage type, flap, and complex tears.

717.5 Derangement of meniscus, not elsewhere classified — *congenital discoid meniscus, cyst of semilunar cartilage*

Code 717.5 includes other forms of meniscal derangements, such as cysts of any meniscus and congenital discoid lateral or medial meniscus.

717.6 Loose body in knee — *joint mice, rice bodies*

Loose body in knee is joint mice, rice bodies, and debris described as cartilaginous (cartilage only, radiolucent on x-rays), osseous (bony), osteocartilaginous, and fibrous. Osteochondritis dissecans is commonly the cause; other causes include synovial chondromatosis, osteophytes, fractured articular surfaces, and damaged menisci.

717.7 Chondromalacia of patella — *degeneration or softening of articular cartilage of patella*
AHA: Nov-Dec, 1984, 9; March-April, 1985, 14

717.81 Old disruption of lateral collateral ligament

717.82 Old disruption of medial collateral ligament

717.83 Old disruption of anterior cruciate ligament

717.84 Old disruption of posterior cruciate ligament

717.85 Old disruption of other ligament of knee — *capsular ligament*

717.89 Other internal derangement of knee — *not otherwise specified, calcification, derangement of ligament, slipped patella, intraligamentous cyst, Haglund-Lawen-Frund syndrome, Budinger-Ludloff-Lawen disease*

Code 717.89 includes old disruptions of the arcuate complex, medial capsule, lateral capsule, and popliteus.

717.9 Unspecified internal derangement of knee

Coding Clarification

This rubric excludes acute derangement of the knee and current injury (836.0-836.6), ankylosis (718.5x), contracture (718.4x), deformity (736.4-736.6), and recurrent dislocation (718.3x).

718 Other derangement of joint

The following fifth-digit subclassification is for use with categories 711-712, 715-716, 718-719, and 730. Valid fifth-digits are in brackets [ ] at the end of each code.

0 site unspecified
1 shoulder region (acromioclavicular joint, clavicle, glenohumeral joint, scapula, sternoclavicular joint)
2 upper arm (elbow joint, humerus)
3 forearm (radius, ulna, wrist joint)
4 hand (carpus, metacarpus, phalanges)
5 pelvic regions and thigh (buttock, femur, hip joint)
6 lower leg (fibula, knee joint, patella, tibia)
7 ankle and foot (ankle joint, metatarsus, phalanges, tarsus, other joints in foot)
8 other specified sites (head, neck, ribs, skull, trunk, vertebral column)
9 multiple sites

718.0 ✓5th Articular cartilage disorder — *meniscus old rupture, old tear*

718.1 ✓5th Loose body in joint — *joint mice*

Loose body in joint is joint mice, rice bodies, and debris described as cartilaginous, osseous (bony), osteocartilaginous, or fibrous in joints other than the knee.

718.2 5th Pathological dislocation — *spontaneous; not recurrent and not from injury*

Pathological dislocation is dislocation of an articular joint due to a disease process (e.g., poliomyelitis), rather than trauma.

Code 718.2 should be accompanied by a second ICD-9-CM code identifying the specific pathology (etiology of the pathological dislocation).

718.3 5th Recurrent dislocation of joint — *occurring again and again*
AHA: Nov-Dec, 1987, 7

Recurrent dislocation of a joint is chronic, subsequent, additional, and repeated dislocations or subluxations of a joint due to trauma.

718.4 5th Contracture of joint — *strong resistance to stretch*
AHA: Q4, 1998, 40

Contracture of a joint is a disorder characterized by restriction of joint motion due to contraction of the muscles that articulate the joint. The condition may be due to tonic spasm, fibrosis, loss of musculature equilibrium, or disuse atrophy.

718.5 5th Ankylosis of joint — *immobility*

718.6 5th Unspecified intrapelvic protrusion of acetabulum — *protrusio acetabuli, cause unknown*

718.7 5th Developmental dislocation of joint

Excluded from this subclassification are congenital dislocation of joint (754.0-755.8) and traumatic dislocation of joint (830-839).

718.8 5th Other joint derangement, not elsewhere classified — *flail joint, instability of joint*

The codes in this subclassification may be used as an additional code to classify instability of a joint secondary to removal of a prosthesis. Use code 909.3 when the instability is described as a late effect of the prosthesis removal.

718.9 5th Unspecified derangement of joint — *unknown cause*

719 Other and unspecified disorders of joint

The following fifth-digit subclassification is for use with codes 719.0-719.6 and 719.8-719.9. Valid fifth-digits are in brackets [ ] at the end of each code.

0 site unspecified

1 shoulder region (acromioclavicular joint, clavicle, glenohumeral joint, scapula, sternoclavicular joint)

2 upper arm (elbow joint, humerus)

3 forearm (radius, ulna, wrist joint)

4 hand (carpus, metacarpus, phalanges)

5 pelvic regions and thigh (buttock, femur, hip joint)

6 lower leg (fibula, knee joint, patella, tibia)

7 ankle and foot (ankle joint, metatarsus, phalanges, tarsus, other joints in foot)

8 other specified sites (head, neck, ribs, skull, trunk, vertebral column)

9 multiple sites

719.0 5th Effusion of joint — *hydrarthrosis, swelling of joint*

Effusion of joint is the escape of fluid from blood vessels or lymphatics into joint spaces. Hemorrhagic effusion is from blood. Hydrarthrosis is the accumulation of watery fluid in a joint. Effusion indicates synovial irritation due to disease or trauma (excluding current injury).

Therapies include aspiration of a tense effusion.

719.1 5th Hemarthrosis — *blood in the joint*

Hemarthrosis is the presence of gross blood in the joint spaces, excluding that due to current injury or hemophilia.

719.2 5th Villonodular synovitis

Villonodular synovitis is a form of inflammation involving the synovial membranes of joints. There are two types of villonodular synovitis: pigmented and nonpigmented.

Therapies include steroidal and nonsteroidal medication to reduce inflammation and synovectomy when nonoperative therapy fails.

Villonodular synovitis may be a form of benign neoplasm of the connective tissue of the synovium, or be representative of granulomatous disease. The term "villonodular synovitis" is sometimes used to describe conditions such as xanthofibroma, giant cell tumor of tendon sheath, and benign synovioma, which are classified elsewhere.

719.3 5th Palindromic rheumatism — *Hench-Rosenberg syndrome, intermittent hydrarthrosis*

 © 2004 Ingenix, Inc.

Palindromic rheumatism is sudden and recurring attacks of moderate to severe joint pain and swelling. The etiology is unknown but the condition has been associated with irritants and allergic reactions.

719.4 5th Pain in joint — *arthralgia*

719.5 5th Stiffness of joint, not elsewhere classified

719.6 5th Other symptoms referable to joint — *joint crepitus, snapping hip*
AHA: Q1, 1994, 15

719.7 Difficulty in walking

719.8 5th Other specified disorders of joint — *not otherwise specified, including calcification, fistula*

719.9 5th Unspecified disorder of joint

720–724 Dorsopathies

720 Ankylosing spondylitis and other inflammatory spondylopathies

Ankylosing spondylitis is a form of chronic inflammation of the spine and the sacroiliac joints. Chronic inflammation in these areas causes pain and stiffness in and around the spine and can lead to a complete fusion of the vertebrae, a process called ankylosis. Ankylosis causes total loss of mobility of the spine and it is a systemic rheumatic disease, causing inflammation in joints away from the spine, as well as inflammation in organs such as the eyes, heart, lungs, and kidneys. The disease is more common in males. In women, joints away from the spine are more frequently affected. Although ankylosing spondylitis can occur at any age, onset usually falls in the second and third decades; the cause is believed to be genetic. Common symptoms include back pain and stiffness over a period of weeks or months and lasting longer than three months, and early morning stiffness improved by warm shower or light exercise. Diagnosis depends on the history of symptoms, physical examination, and x-ray findings. X-rays are taken of the sacroiliac joints to note changes in tissues caused by inflammation, although tissue changes do not always appear on x-rays in the early stages of the disease. There is no cure and treatment consists of medicines to alleviate the pain and stiffness (i.e., non-steroidal anti-inflammatory drugs), daily exercises that incorporate stretching and strengthening, and good posture habits.

Ankylosing spondylitis shares many features with other arthritic conditions, such as psoriatic arthritis, reactive arthritis, arthritis associated with Crohn's disease, and ulcerative colitis. The conditions are collectively referred to as spondyloarthropathies.

720.0 Ankylosing spondylitis — *arthritis primarily of the sacroiliac joints and to varying degree, the rest of the spine and peripheral joints, with no new bone formation; Marie-Strumpell spondylitis*

Ankylosing spondylitis is a chronic, progressive inflammatory disease of unknown etiology involving primarily the small apophyseal and costovertebral joints of the spine and sacroiliac. This disease also is known as Marie-Strumpell or Bekhterev disease.

720.1 Spinal enthesopathy — *Romanus lesion; disorder of peripheral ligamentous or muscular attachments of spine*

720.2 Sacroiliitis, not elsewhere classified — *pain and inflammation within the joint or the junction of sacrum and hip*

720.81 Inflammatory spondylopathies in diseases classified elsewhere — (Code first underlying disease, 015.0) — *secondary to underlying disease*

720.89 Other inflammatory spondylopathies — *not otherwise specified*

720.9 Unspecified inflammatory spondylopathy — *unknown type*

721 Spondylosis and allied disorders

AHA: Q2, 1989, 14

Spondylosis and allied disorders are degenerative, rather than inflammatory conditions. Myelopathy is a qualifying term describing diseases and disturbances of the spinal cord. Paresthesia, loss of sensation, and loss of sphincter control are among the most common forms of myelopathy.

721.0 Cervical spondylosis without myelopathy — *cervical or cervicodorsal; in the neck*
AHA: Q2, 1989, 14

721.1 Cervical spondylosis with myelopathy — *spondylogenic compression of cervical spinal cord; vertebral artery compression or anterior spinal artery compression syndromes*
AHA: Q2, 1989, 14

721.2 Thoracic spondylosis without myelopathy — *upper back, T1-T12*
AHA: Q2, 1989, 14

721.3 Lumbosacral spondylosis without myelopathy — *lower back, L1-L5*
AHA: Q2, 1989, 14; Q4, 2002, 107

721.41 Spondylosis with myelopathy, thoracic region — *upper back, T1-T12*
AHA: Q2, 1989, 14

721.42 Spondylosis with myelopathy, lumbar region — *lower back, L1-L5*
AHA: Q2, 1989, 14

721.5 Kissing spine — *Baastrup's, Michotte's syndromes*
AHA: Q2, 1989, 14

721.6 Ankylosing vertebral hyperostosis — *hypertrophy or exostosis causing immobility*
AHA: Q2, 1989, 14

721.7 Traumatic spondylopathy — *Kummell's disease*
AHA: Q2, 1989, 14

721.8 Other allied disorders of spine — *not otherwise specified, arthritis of coccyx*
AHA: Q2, 1989, 14

721.90 Spondylosis of unspecified site without mention of myelopathy — *unknown cause, but without compression of spinal cord*
AHA: Q2, 1989, 14

721.91 Spondylosis of unspecified site with myelopathy — *unknown cause, but with compression of spinal cord*
AHA: Q2, 1989, 14

Coding Clarification

Assignment of a fourth digit to codes in this category is based on the presence or absence of myelopathy. For coding purposes, myelopathy includes any symptomatic impingement, compression, disruption, or disturbance of the spinal cord or blood supply of the spinal cord due to spondylosis.

Neurogenic Bladder: Many conditions may result in neurogenic bladder including cauda equina syndrome, injury to the spine and spinal cord, spondylitis, neoplasms, fractures, and congenital defects. When the neurogenic bladder is not due to a spinal condition, it is classified to one of the bladder dysfunction categories.

Spondylosis: This is a compression of any or all of the nerve roots of the cauda equina and causes a variety of sensory and motor deficits. Spondylosis with myelopathy indicates deficits due to nerve compression and would include neurogenic bladder. However, it is appropriate to code lumbar or sacral spondylosis with neurogenic bladder by reporting both codes 721.42 and 344.61.

Pain or neuritis is a symptom of spondylosis and therefore does not need to be coded in addition to a code from categories 721-722.

722 Intervertebral disc disorders

AHA: Q1, 1988, 10

An intervertebral disk is the flexible plate that connects any two adjacent vertebrae in the spine; they cushion the spinal cord from the impact produced by the body's movements. Each disk is composed of a gelatinous material in the center, called the nucleus pulposus, surrounded by rings of a fibrous tissue. With age, these disks can degenerate and dry out, and the fibers holding them in place can tear. Eventually, the disk torn from the tissue can rupture the fibrocartilagenous material, which releases the nucleus pulpsus. Pressure may force the nucleus pulposus outward, placing pressure on the spinal cord and causing pain. Disk herniation most commonly affects the lumbar region between the fifth lumbar vertebra and the first sacral vertebra. However, disk herniation also occurs in the cervical spine. Muscle weakness or bladder and bowel function interference because of the pressure on a nerve root often requires a diskectomy.

722.0 Displacement of cervical intervertebral disc without myelopathy — *neuritis or radiculitis due to displacement or rupture of cervical intervertebral disc; neck, C1-C7; without compression of spinal cord*
AHA: Q1, 1988, 10

722.10 Displacement of lumbar intervertebral disc without myelopathy — *lumbago, neuritis, radiculitis, or sciatica due to displacement of intervertebral disc; lower back, L1-L5; without compression of spinal cord*
AHA: Q1, 1988, 10; Q4, 2002, 107; Q1, 2003, 7; Q3, 2003, 12

722.11 Displacement of thoracic intervertebral disc without myelopathy — *lumbago, neuritis, radiculitis, or sciatica due to displacement of intervertebral disc; upper back, T1-T12; without compression of spinal cord*
AHA: Q1, 1988, 10

722.2 Displacement of intervertebral disc, site unspecified, without myelopathy — *lumbago, neuritis, radiculitis, or sciatica due to displacement of intervertebral disc; unknown site in spine; without compression of spinal cord*
AHA: Q1, 1988, 10

722.3 [5th] Schmorl's nodes

Schmorl's nodes describe the prolapse of the nucleus pulposus into an adjoining vertebra, as seen on x-rays of the spine.

722.30 Schmorl's nodes, unspecified region — *nodule caused by prolapse of disk pulp into adjacent vertebra, unknown site in spine*
AHA: Q1, 1988, 10

722.31 Schmorl's nodes, thoracic region — *nodule caused by prolapse of disk pulp into adjacent vertebra, upper back, T1-T12*
AHA: Q1, 1988, 10

722.32 Schmorl's nodes, lumbar region — *nodule caused by prolapse of disk pulp into adjacent vertebra, lower back, L1-L5*
AHA: Q1, 1988, 10

722.39 Schmorl's nodes, other spinal region — *nodule caused by prolapse of disk pulp into adjacent vertebra, cervical, C1-C7, or not otherwise specified*
AHA: Q1, 1988, 10

722.4 Degeneration of cervical intervertebral disc — *cervicothoracic intervertebral disc*
AHA: Q1, 1988, 10

© 2004 Ingenix, Inc.

722.51 Degeneration of thoracic or thoracolumbar intervertebral disc

722.52 Degeneration of lumbar or lumbosacral intervertebral disc

722.6 Degeneration of intervertebral disc, site unspecified — *unknown site*
AHA: Q1, 1988, 10

722.70 Intervertebral disc disorder with myelopathy, unspecified region — *with compression on spine, unknown site in spine*
AHA: Q1, 1988, 10

722.71 Intervertebral cervical disc disorder with myelopathy, cervical region — *with compression on spine, in neck, C1-C7*
AHA: Q1, 1988, 10

722.72 Intervertebral thoracic disc disorder with myelopathy, thoracic region — *with compression on spine, upper back, T1-T12*
AHA: Q1, 1988, 10

722.73 Intervertebral lumbar disc disorder with myelopathy, lumbar region — *with compression on spine, lower back, L1-L5*
AHA: Q1, 1988, 10

722.8 5th Postlaminectomy syndrome

Postlaminectomy syndrome is a complex of symptoms following laminectomy surgery. It includes conditions and syndromes described as postfusion, postmicrosurgery, and postchemonucleolysis.

722.80 Postlaminectomy syndrome, unspecified region — *unknown site on spine*
AHA: Jan-Feb, 1987, 7; Q1, 1988, 10

722.81 Postlaminectomy syndrome, cervical region — *neck, C1-C7*
AHA: Jan-Feb, 1987, 7; Q1, 1988, 10

722.82 Postlaminectomy syndrome, thoracic region — *upper back, T1-T12*
AHA: Jan-Feb, 1987, 7; Q1, 1988, 10

722.83 Postlaminectomy syndrome, lumbar region — *lower back, L1-L5*
AHA: Jan-Feb, 1987, 7; Q1, 1988, 10; Q2, 1997, 15

722.90 Other and unspecified disc disorder of unspecified region — *calcification, discitis, unknown site on spine*
AHA: Nov-Dec, 1984, 19; Q1, 1988, 10

722.91 Other and unspecified disc disorder of cervical region — *calcification, discitis, neck, C1-C7*
AHA: Q1, 1988, 10

722.92 Other and unspecified disc disorder of thoracic region — *calcification, discitis, upper back, T1-T12*
AHA: Q1, 1988, 10

722.93 Other and unspecified disc disorder of lumbar region — *calcification, discitis, lower back, L1-L5*
AHA: Q1, 1988, 10

Coding Clarification

Herniated Disc: When sciatica is the result of a slipped or degenerative intervertebral disc, the sciatica is a symptom of the disc disease and does not need to be coded separately. For lateral disc herniation, assign an appropriate code from the 722.0-722.2 subcategories.

Intervertebral Disc Space Infection: An intervertebral disc space infection is a condition also known as discitis and is classified to category 722.

Neurogenic Bladder: Many conditions may result in neurogenic bladder including cauda equina syndrome, injury to the spine and spinal cord, spondylitis, neoplasms, fractures, and congenital defects. When the neurogenic bladder is not due to a spinal condition, it is classified to one of the bladder dysfunction categories.

Posterior midline disk prolapse: A compression of the nerve roots at the level of L2-3 may result in acute cauda equina syndrome. In these instances, code 722.73 should be reported as well as code 344.61 to indicate both the prolapsed disc and the cauda equina syndrome with neurogenic bladder.

Postoperative Back Pain: A patient who has post-laminectomy lumbar back pain with no herniated disc or other condition causing this pain should be classified to code 722.83 *Postlaminectomy syndrome, lumbar region.* However, if after diagnostic testing it is determined that there is a condition present, such as a herniated disc that is causing that pain, then code the causative condition.

Spinal Stenosis: There are two forms of spinal stenosis: degeneration of the intervertebral disc (arthritic) and congenital. Degenerative spinal stenosis is classified to category 722. Congenital spinal stenosis is classified to categories 723-724.

Spondylosis: Pain or neuritis is a symptom of spondylosis and therefore does not need to be coded in addition to a code from categories 721-722.

Coding Scenario

A patient is seen with herniation of the L3-L4. The medical record indicates that no myelopathy is present.

> Code assignment: 722.10 *Displacement of lumbar intervertebral disc without myelopathy*

A 69-year-old female is seen with acute mid-back pain. It is determined by x-ray that she has degenerative disc disease of the thoracic spine.

Code assignment: 722.51 *Degeneration of thoracic or thoracolumbar intervertebral disc*

A 54-year-old male is seen by his neurologist 10 weeks post laminectomy. He is complaining of back pain radiating down the right leg. An MRI reveals no further herniation. The physician indicates in the medical record that the patient has postlaminectomy syndrome.

Code assignment: 722.83 *Postlaminectomy syndrome, lumbar region*

723 Other disorders of cervical region

AHA: Q2, 1989, 14; Q3, 1994, 14

723.0 Spinal stenosis in cervical region — *stricture in neck region, C1-C7*
AHA: Q2, 1989, 14; Q3, 1994, 14; Q4, 2003, 101

723.1 Cervicalgia — *pain in neck region,*
AHA: Q2, 1989, 14; Q3, 1994, 14

723.2 Cervicocranial syndrome — *Barre-Lieou, craniovertebral, or posterior cervical sympathetic syndromes*
AHA: Q2, 1989, 14; Q3, 1994, 14

723.3 Cervicobrachial syndrome (diffuse)

723.4 Brachial neuritis or radiculitis nos — *radicular syndrome of upper limbs*
AHA: Q2, 1989, 14; Q3, 1994, 14

723.5 Torticollis, unspecified — *contracture of neck*
AHA: Q2, 1989, 14; Q3, 1994, 14; Q1, 1995, 7; Q2, 2001, 21

723.6 Panniculitis specified as affecting neck — *cutaneous nodules caused by subcutaneous inflammatory reaction*
AHA: Q2, 1989, 14; Q3, 1994, 14

723.7 Ossification of posterior longitudinal ligament in cervical region

723.8 Other syndromes affecting cervical region — *not otherwise specified, including, video display tube syndrome, occipital neuralgia, Klippel's disease*
AHA: Q2, 1989, 14; Q3, 1994, 14; Q1, 2000, 7

Code 723.8 includes cervical instability syndromes, including C1-2 rotary instability syndrome.

723.9 Unspecified musculoskeletal disorders and symptoms referable to neck

Documentation Issues

To ensure correct code assignment of a herniated disc, the physician should include in the documentation the presence or absence of myelopathy.

Spinal stenosis that is not documented as being degenerative or congenital is classified to categories 723-724; however, it is advisable to ask for clarification from the physician before assigning a nonspecific code. The physician should document the type of spinal stenosis, such as degenerative or congenital, in the medical record.

Coding Clarification

Spinal Stenosis: There are two forms of spinal stenosis: degeneration of the intervertebral disc (arthritic) and congenital. Degenerative spinal stenosis is classified to category 722. Congenital spinal stenosis is classified to categories 723-724.

Misnomer: Occipital neuralgia is actually a neuropathy. The condition is characterized by pain in the occiput and suboccipital region, involving nerve entrapment or impingement. It may be a consequence of injury, arthritis, trauma, compression of the occipital nerves, or tumors of the second and third cervical dorsal roots. Treatment depends on symptoms if the cause of the neuralgia is unknown. If the cause is known, treatment is directed to it. Some treatments include anticonvulsants for atypical facial pain, tricyclic antidepressants for pain similar to tic douleroux, local nerve blocks, injections of local anesthetics, and steroids.

Coding Scenario

A 24-year-old female presents with throbbing pain in the back of the head, toward the base of the skull. Her history is negative for any head trauma. After workup, the diagnosis is documented to be occipital neuralgia.

Code assignment: Code 723.8 *Other syndromes affecting cervical region*

A 48-year-old male is seen in the emergency department with numbness over the base of the skull. His history is negative for any head trauma and is currently being treated for arthritis. The diagnosis is documented as occipital neuralgia. There is no documentation found in the medical record that would warrant reporting the arthritis as the underlying condition.

Code assignment: 723.8 *Other syndromes affecting cervical region*

724 Other and unspecified disorders of back

AHA: Q2, 1989, 14

724.00 Spinal stenosis, unspecified region other than cervical — *stricture, unknown site in spine*
AHA: Q2, 1989, 14

724.01 Spinal stenosis of thoracic region — *stricture, upper back, T1-T12*
AHA: Q2, 1989, 14

 © 2004 Ingenix, Inc.

724.02 Spinal stenosis of lumbar region — *stricture, lower back, L1-L5*
AHA: Q2, 1989, 14; Q4, 1999, 13

724.09 Spinal stenosis, other region other than cervical — *stricture, other site, cervical site excluded*
AHA: Q2, 1989, 14

724.1 Pain in thoracic spine — *upper back, T1-T12*
AHA: Q2, 1989, 14

724.2 Lumbago — *lower back, L1-L5*
AHA: Nov-Dec, 1985, 12; Q2, 1989, 14

724.3 Sciatica — *neuralgia of sciatic nerve*
AHA: Q2, 1989, 12; Q2, 1989, 14

724.4 Thoracic or lumbosacral neuritis or radiculitis, unspecified — *vertebral bodies impingement syndrome, radicular syndrome of lower limbs*
AHA: Q2, 1989, 14; Q2, 1999, 3

724.5 Unspecified backache — *specifics unknown*
AHA: Q2, 1989, 14

724.5 Unspecified backache — *specifics unknown*
AHA: Q2, 1989, 14

724.6 Disorders of sacrum — *ankylosis, instability, or Thiele syndrome*
AHA: Q2, 1989, 14

724.70 Unspecified disorder of coccyx

724.71 Hypermobility of coccyx

724.79 Other disorder of coccyx — *pain, coccygodynia*
AHA: Q2, 1989, 14

724.8 Other symptoms referable to back — *ossification of posterior longitudinal ligament, sacral panniculitis, muscle spasm, stiffness in back*
AHA: Q2, 1989, 14

724.9 Other unspecified back disorder

Documentation Issues

To ensure correct code assignment of a herniated disc, the physician should include in the documentation the presence or absence of myelopathy.

Spinal stenosis that is not documented as being degenerative or congenital is classified to categories 723-724; however, it is advisable to ask for clarification from the physician before assigning a nonspecific code. The physician should document the type of spinal stenosis, such as degenerative or congenital, in the medical record.

Coding Clarification

Spinal Stenosis: There are two forms of spinal stenosis: degeneration of the intervertebral disc (arthritic) and congenital. Degenerative spinal stenosis is classified to category 722. Congenital spinal stenosis is classified to categories 723-724.

725–729 Rheumatism, Excluding the Back

725 Polymyalgia rheumatica OK

Polymyalgia rheumatica is a self-limiting disease of the elderly which often develops abruptly with joint and muscle pain and stiffness of the pelvis and shoulder girdle in association with fever, malaise, fatigue, weight loss, and anemia. The disease bears a close relationship with giant cell arteritis, and the two conditions often occur concomitantly.

726 Peripheral enthesopathies and allied syndromes

Peripheral enthesopathies and allied syndromes are disorders of peripheral ligamentous or muscular attachments. The term "enthesopathy" is an obscure medical term meaning disease of the ligamentous or muscular attachments of a joint.

726.0 Adhesive capsulitis of shoulder

Adhesive capsulitis of the shoulder is frozen shoulder syndrome, characterized by development of diffuse capsulitis of the glenohumeral joint with subsequent adherence of the inflamed capsule to the humeral head. Contracture due to the shrunken, adherent capsule prevents motion in the glenohumeral joint; that is, the joint is "frozen" in one position. The capsulitis may be caused by a variety of intrinsic and extrinsic disorders such as bicipital tendinitis, calcific supraspinatus tendinitis, basal pleurisy, and subphrenic inflammation.

Therapies include arthroscopic lavage, distension, and instillation of cortisone.

726.1 5th Rotator cuff syndrome of shoulder and allied disorders

Rotator cuff syndrome of the shoulder and allied disorders are disorders of the ligamentous or muscular attachments of the shoulder joint and allied syndromes of the rotator cuff. The rotator cuff is a musculotendinous structure that blends with the joint capsule and is attached to the humerus. The supraspinatus is the major muscle that contributes to the formation of the rotator cuff.

726.10 Unspecified disorders of bursae and tendons in shoulder region — *rotator cuff or supraspinatus syndromes*
AHA: Q2, 2001, 11

726.11 Calcifying tendinitis of shoulder — *hardening and inflammation of tendons due to calcium deposits*

726.12 Bicipital tenosynovitis — *inflammation of the tendon and tendon sheath surrounding the long head of the biceps*

710–739

726.19 Other specified disorders of rotator cuff syndrome of shoulder and allied disorders — *not otherwise specified, including painful arc syndrome*

726.2 Other affections of shoulder region, not elsewhere classified — *periarthritis, scapulohumeral fibrositis, Duplay's or shoulder impingement syndromes*

726.30 Unspecified enthesopathy of elbow — *disorder of the attachment of muscle or tendon to bone, site unknown*

726.31 Medial epicondylitis of elbow — *disorder of the attachment of muscle or tendon to bone*

726.32 Lateral epicondylitis of elbow — *disorder of the attachment of muscle or tendon to bone, tennis/golfer's elbow*

726.33 Olecranon bursitis — *inflammation of bursa; elbow*

Olecranon bursitis is inflammation of the olecranon bursa. There are two olecranon bursae: one lies deep to the triceps tendon and the other between the skin and olecranon process. The latter is more commonly inflamed.

726.39 Other enthesopathy of elbow region — *not otherwise specified*

726.4 Enthesopathy of wrist and carpus — *disorder of the attachment of muscle or tendon to bone, bursitis, periarthritis*

726.5 Enthesopathy of hip region — *disorder of the attachment of muscle or tendon to bone, bursitis, periarthritis; gluteal, trochanteric, or psoas tendinitis, iliac crest spur*

Enthesopathy of the hip region is a complex of conditions such as iliotibial band syndrome of the hip, trochanteric bursitis, subgluteal bursitis, iliopectineal bursitis, trochanteric tendinitis (with calcification), psoas and tibiopsoas tendinitis, iliac crest spur, and snapping hip syndrome.

726.60 Unspecified enthesopathy of knee — *disorder of the attachment of muscle or tendon to bone, bursitis, periarthritis, site unknown*

726.61 Pes anserinus tendinitis or bursitis — *inflammation of the combined insertion of tendinous expansions of satirise, gracilis, and semitendinosus muscles*

726.62 Tibial collateral ligament bursitis — *Pellegrini-Stieda syndrome*

726.63 Fibular collateral ligament bursitis — *inflammation of bursa*

726.64 Patellar tendinitis — *inflammation of patellar tendon*

726.65 Prepatellar bursitis — *inflammation of bursa*

726.69 Other enthesopathy of knee — *infrapatellar, subpatellar*

Code 726.69 includes iliotibial band syndrome of the knee, infrapatellar bursitis, subpatellar bursitis, medial gastrocnemius bursitis, and semimembranosus bursitis.

726.70 Unspecified enthesopathy of ankle and tarsus — *disorder of the attachment of muscle or tendon to bone, site unknown*

726.71 Achilles bursitis or tendinitis — *Albert's disease*

726.72 Tibialis tendinitis — *anterior or posterior*

726.73 Calcaneal spur

726.79 Other enthesopathy of ankle and tarsus — *not otherwise specified, peroneal tendinitis*

Subclassification 726.79 includes peroneal tendinitis, "pump bump" and tendinitis of the flexor hallucis longus, flexor digitorum longus, extensor hallucis longus, and extensor digitorum longus.

726.8 Other peripheral enthesopathies — *not otherwise specified*

726.90 Enthesopathy of unspecified site — *unknown site*

726.91 Exostosis of unspecified site — *bone spur NOS*
AHA: Q2, 2001, 15

727 Other disorders of synovium, tendon, and bursa

727.0 ✓5th Synovitis and tenosynovitis

Synovitis is inflammation of a synovial membrane, especially the synovium that lines articular joints. In a normal synovial joint, the smooth and reciprocally shaped cartilaginous opposing surfaces permit a fluid, frictionless, and painless articulation. Irregularities, disease, and damage to the articular surfaces lead to progressive degenerative changes resulting in pain and limitation of movement. The joint capsule is particularly sensitive to stretching and increased fluid pressure.

Tenosynovitis is the inflammation of a tendon and its synovial sheath. It is also known as tendosynovitis, tendovaginitis, tenontothecitis, tenontolemmitis, and vaginal or tendinous synovitis. At the site of friction, the tendon is enveloped by a sheath consisting of a visceral and parietal layer of synovial membrane and is lubricated by a synovial-like fluid containing hyaluronate. The synovial sheath is in turn covered by a dense, fibrous tissue sheath. Irregularities, disease, and damage to the tendon's attachment to the articular joints may lead to progressive degenerative changes with resultant limitation of movement and pain. The synovial membranes of tendon sheaths and bursae are capable of the same inflammatory reactions to abnormal conditions as the synovial membranes of joints.

727.00 Unspecified synovitis and tenosynovitis — *synovitis NOS, tenosynovitis NOS*

© 2004 Ingenix, Inc.

727.01 Synovitis and tenosynovitis in diseases classified elsewhere — (Code first underlying disease: 015.0-015.9) — *secondary to an underlying disease*

727.02 Giant cell tumor of tendon sheath

727.03 Trigger finger (acquired)

727.04 Radial styloid tenosynovitis — *de Quervain's disease*

727.05 Other tenosynovitis of hand and wrist — *not otherwise specified*

727.06 Tenosynovitis of foot and ankle

727.09 Other synovitis and tenosynovitis — *buttock, elbow, hip, knee*

727.1 Bunion — *enlargement of the first metatarsal head caused by inflammation of bursa, frequently resulting in lateral displacement of the great toe*

A bunion is a localized friction-type bursitis located at either the medial or dorsal aspect of the first metatarsophalangeal joint. Bunions of the medial aspect are usually associated with hallux valgus.

727.2 Specific bursitides often of occupational origin — *chronic crepitant synovitis of wrist, miner's elbow or knee*

Specific bursitides often of occupational origin is friction-type bursitis of various sites excluding bunions. Examples of these bursitides are "housemaid's knee," "student's elbow," and "weaver's bottom."

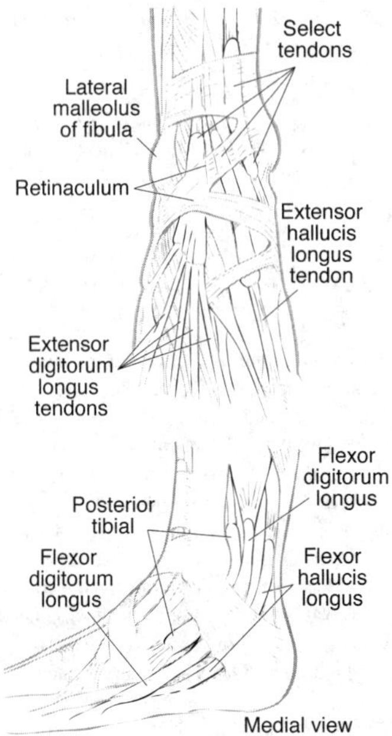

Medial view

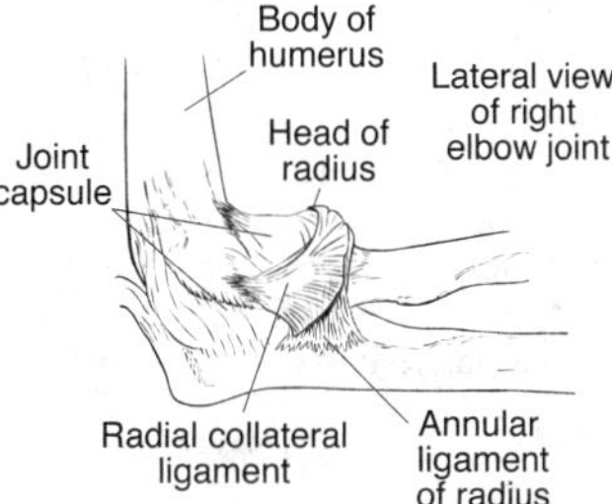

Synovial membranes are contained within the joint capsule

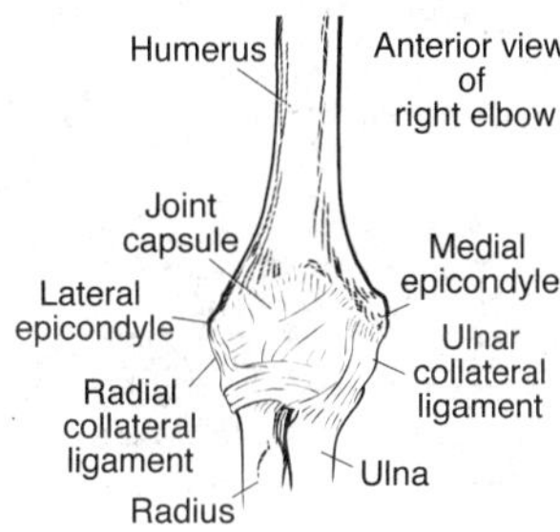

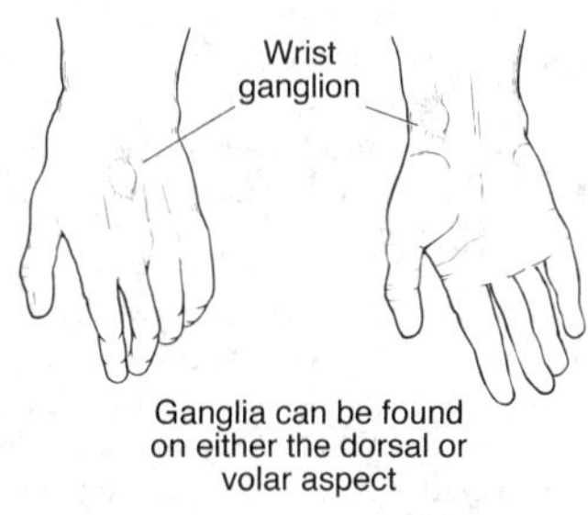

Ganglia can be found on either the dorsal or volar aspect

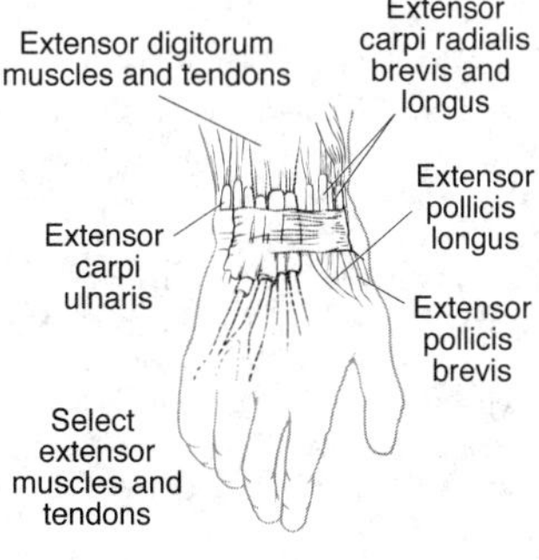

710–739

727.3 Other bursitis disorders — *not otherwise specified*

727.4 ✓5th Ganglion and cyst of synovium, tendon, and bursa

Ganglion and cyst of synovium, tendon, and bursa are thin-walled cystic lesions of unknown etiology containing thick, clear, mucinous fluid, possibly due to mucoid degeneration. Arising in relation to periarticular tissues, joint capsules, and tendon sheaths, ganglia are limited to the hands and feet and are most common in the dorsum of the wrist.

727.40 Unspecified synovial cyst — *round, cystic swelling of unspecified synovial site*
AHA: Q2, 1997, 6

727.41 Ganglion of joint — *round, cystic swelling*

727.42 Ganglion of tendon sheath — *round, cystic swelling*

727.43 Unspecified ganglion — *round, cystic swelling of unspecified site*

727.49 Other ganglion and cyst of synovium, tendon, and bursa — *round cystic swelling of bursa*

727.50 Unspecified rupture of synovium — *nontraumatic, unknown site*

727.51 Synovial cyst of popliteal space — *Baker's cyst of knee*

Synovial cyst of the popliteal space is Baker's cysts, sometimes called popliteal cysts. In children, Baker's cysts are common but usually are asymptomatic and regress spontaneously. In adults, Baker's cysts, in conjunction with synovial effusion due to rheumatoid arthritis or degenerative joint disease, may produce significant impairment. When a Baker's cyst interferes with normal knee function, surgical exploration and excision of the cyst is indicated.

Baker's cysts are classified under subcategory 727.5 for rupture of synovium because the cysts usually communicate with the knee joint through a long and tortuous duct, allowing the cyst to become distended by any synovial effusion and possibly extend down as far as the mid calf.

727.59 Other rupture of synovium — *other*

Rupture of tendon, nontraumatic, is a rupture due to pathology rather than trauma or injury. A normal tendon seldom ruptures even with strenuous activity, but if it has become damaged by disease (e.g., secondary to tenosynovitis) or degenerated due to the fraying caused by friction (e.g., due to bony erosion), it may rupture even with normal activity. Degeneration occurs in rheumatic arthritis, lupus erythematosus, hyperparathyroidism, and systemic steroid use, or when steroids are injected directly into a tendon.

Therapies include reconstructive surgery to repair or replace the abnormal part of the ruptured tendon.

727.60 Nontraumatic rupture of unspecified tendon — *unknown tendon*

727.61 Complete rupture of rotator cuff

727.62 Nontraumatic rupture of tendons of biceps (long head)

727.63 Nontraumatic rupture of extensor tendons of hand and wrist

Subclassification 727.63 includes the extensor pollicis longus, extensor pollicis brevis, extensor digitorum communis, extensor indicis, and the abductor pollicis longus tendons.

727.64 Nontraumatic rupture of flexor tendons of hand and wrist

Subclassification 727.64 includes the flexor digitorum superficialis, flexor digitorum profundus, and the flexor pollicis longus tendons.

727.65 Nontraumatic rupture of quadriceps tendon

727.66 Nontraumatic rupture of patellar tendon

727.67 Nontraumatic rupture of Achilles tendon

727.68 Nontraumatic rupture of other tendons of foot and ankle — *not otherwise specified*

727.69 Nontraumatic rupture of other tendon — *not otherwise specified*

727.81 Contracture of tendon (sheath) — *acquired short Achilles tendon*

727.82 Calcium deposits in tendon and bursa — *calcification or calcific tendonitis, not otherwise specified*

727.83 Plica syndrome — *plica knee*
AHA: Q4, 2000, 44

727.89 Other disorders of synovium, tendon, and bursa — *abscess, hemorrhage, union of bursa or tendon, pseudobursa*
AHA: Q2, 1989, 15

727.9 Unspecified disorder of synovium, tendon, and bursa — *specifics unknown, including sloughing tendon, slipped tendon, degeneration of synovial membrane, tenophyte*

728 Disorders of muscle, ligament, and fascia

Muscle is an organ composed of one of three types of muscle tissue (skeletal, cardiac, or smooth) that is specialized for contraction to produce voluntary or involuntary movements. Ligament is dense, regularly arranged connective tissue that attaches bone to bone. The fascia is thin connective tissue covering, or separating, the muscles and internal organs of the body. It varies in thickness, density, elasticity, and composition. Fascia, muscles, and ligaments are normally exposed to stress throughout life. Damage occurs when the muscle or connective tissue is exposed to higher-than-usual stress levels, such as sudden excessive stress, or the result of repetitive stress. Whether damaged by repetitive overuse or by acute injury, treatment includes a brief period of

© 2004 Ingenix, Inc.

relative rest, with length depending on the extent of injury, followed by gradual movement and activity.

728.0 Infective myositis — *purulent, suppurative*

Infective myositis is inflammation of the voluntary muscles due to infection. It is usually secondary to osteomyelitis or a penetrating wound, but hematogenous infection can occur in debilitated patients or patients with suppressed immunity.

Signs and symptoms of infective myositis include marked swelling and pain, usually confined to shoulder girdle and arms, but may affect any part of the body.

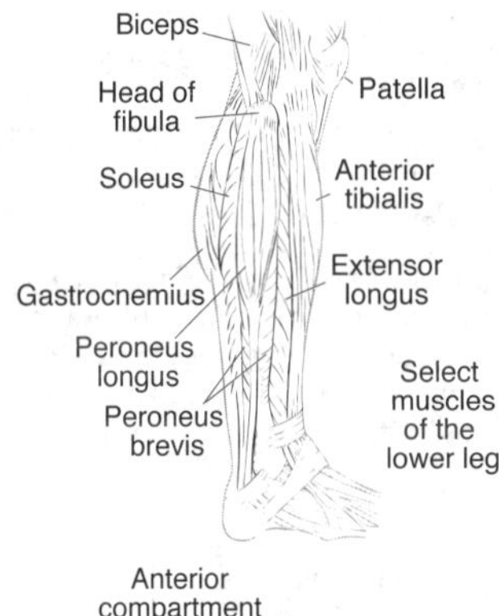

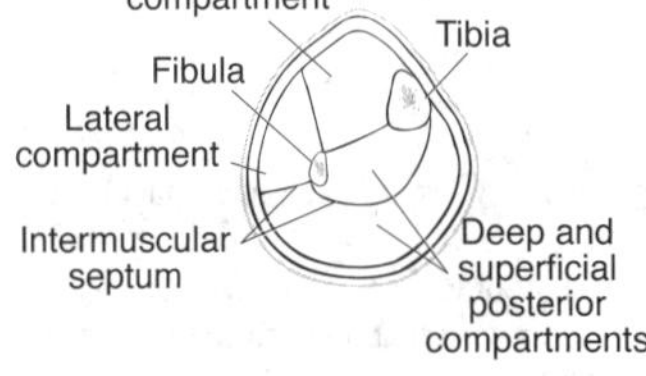

Cross section depicting compartments of lower leg

728.10 Unspecified calcification and ossification — *massive calcification*

728.11 Progressive myositis ossificans — *Munchmeyer's syndrome*

728.12 Traumatic myositis ossificans — *myositis ossificans (circumscripta)*

728.13 Postoperative heterotopic calcification — *occurring at the site of surgery*

728.19 Other muscular calcification and ossification — *not otherwise specified, including polymyositis ossificans*

728.2 Muscular wasting and disuse atrophy, not elsewhere classified — *hemiatrophy of leg, myofibrosis*

728.3 Other specific muscle disorders — *arthrogryposis, immobility syndrome*

728.4 Laxity of ligament — *looseness or relaxation*

728.5 Hypermobility syndrome

728.6 Contracture of palmar fascia — *Dupuytren's contracture*

728.71 Plantar fascial fibromatosis — *plantar fascia syndrome, contracture, traumatic fasciitis*

728.79 Other fibromatoses of muscle, ligament, and fascia — *not otherwise specified, Garrod's or knuckle pads, nodular fasciitis, subcutaneous or proliferative pseudosarcomatous fibromatosis*

728.81 Interstitial myositis

728.82 Foreign body granuloma of muscle — *talc granuloma of muscle*

728.83 Rupture of muscle, nontraumatic

728.84 Diastasis of muscle — *diastasis recti*

728.85 Spasm of muscle

728.86 Necrotizing fasciitis — (Use additional code to identify infectious organism, 041.00-041.89, 785.4, if applicable)

728.87 Muscle weakness — *weariness and fatigue of muscles*
AHA: Q4, 2003, 66

728.88 Rhabdomyolysis — *muscle breakdown or dissolution of muscle, related to myoglobin in the urine; may be due to extreme and prolonged physical exertion*
AHA: Q4, 2003, 66

728.89 Other disorder of muscle, ligament, and fascia — (Use additional E code to identify drug, if drug-induced) — *not otherwise specified, thecal abscess; cicatrix of muscle; calcification, contraction or cyst of ligament; contraction, eosinophilic, hernia of fascia*
AHA: Q2, 2001, 14,15; Q3, 2002, 28

728.9 Unspecified disorder of muscle, ligament, and fascia

Report 618.83 for pelvic muscle wasting and disuse atrophy.

729 Other disorders of soft tissues

729.0 Rheumatism, unspecified and fibrositis — *specifics unknown*

729.1 Unspecified myalgia and myositis — *unspecified generalized musculoskeletal pain, stiffness and easy fatigability*

729.2 Unspecified neuralgia, neuritis, and radiculitis — *pain along an inflamed nerve, with inflammation of the root of the associated spinal nerve, site unspecified*

Coding Clarification

Panniculitis, unspecified, is inflammation of subcutaneous fat. The term often is used solely to refer to an inflammation of the panniculus adiposa of the abdominal wall. Miscellaneous forms of panniculitis include those resulting from trauma,

© 2004 Ingenix, Inc.

insulin injections, pancreatitis, allergic reactions, insect toxins, angiitis, idiopathic cold agglutinins, and sclerosing lipogranulomas.

Many variations of panniculitis, such as erythema nodosum (tuberculous and nontuberculous) and erythema pernio, are classified elsewhere. When coding panniculitis, obtain as much specific information as possible and follow the ICD-9-CM index carefully.

729.30 Panniculitis, unspecified site — *Weber-Christian disease*

729.31 Hypertrophy of fat pad, knee — *infrapatellar fat pad*

729.39 Panniculitis of other sites — *not otherwise specified*

729.4 Unspecified fasciitis — *inflammation of the fibrous tissue that acts to compartmentalize muscle*
AHA: Q2, 1994, 13

729.5 Pain in soft tissues of limb — *not otherwise specified*

729.6 Residual foreign body in soft tissue

729.81 Swelling of limb

729.82 Cramp of limb

729.89 Other musculoskeletal symptoms referable to limbs

729.9 Other and unspecified disorders of soft tissue — *not otherwise specified, polyalgia, nontraumatic compartment or Profichet's syndrome*

730–739 Osteopathies, Chondropathies, and Acquired Musculoskeletal Deformities

730 Osteomyelitis, periostitis, and other infections involving bone

AHA: Q4, 1997, 43

Osteomyelitis, periostitis, and other infections involving bone is a broad spectrum of bone infections. Osteomyelitis is an inflammation of bone and bone marrow. The condition is commonly due to a pathogen such as bacteria, virus, protozoa, or fungus. Periostitis is an inflammation of the periosteum, the thick fibrous membrane covering all of the surfaces of bones except at the articular cartilage. The combination of osteomyelitis and periostitis is periosteomyelitis.

The pathogenesis of osteomyelitis, periostitis, and periosteomyelitis follows three general routes of infection. Hematogenous osteomyelitis (acute) is a form of osteomyelitis common to children where blood-borne organisms settle in the metaphyseal vascular bed of the rapidly developing long bones. Osteomyelitis may develop as an extension of a contiguous infection, particularly infections involving ischemic, diabetic, or neurotrophic ulcers. The third route of infection is by direct inoculation of pathogens through an open wound created by injury or a surgical procedure.

Signs and symptoms of osteomyelitis, periostitis, and other infections involving bone include pain and unwillingness to move the affected area and, occasionally, malaise, fever, chills, and anorexia. Sometimes the site of infection closest to the surface may be detected by palpation.

Lab work includes aspiration with a large bore needle for gram stain and a culture to confirm the diagnosis and reveal the pathogenic agent. Blood cultures may be positive in patients with acute hematogenous osteomyelitis. Bone scans such as scintigraphy are useful, although other factors may cause false positive results and false negative results are possible with acute hematogenous osteomyelitis.

Therapies include long-term antibiotic therapy and surgery to incise and drain the involved area and remove necrotic debris in severe acute cases. Other surgery includes sequestrectomy, excision of multiple sinus tracts, craterization, saucerization, partial excision of bone, and bone grafting for chronic osteomyelitis.

Associated conditions include skin ulcers of various types, septicemia, diabetes, tuberculosis, poliomyelitis, neuropathy, septic arthritis, and trauma (such as compound fractures).

Osteomyelitis may result from direct inoculation from a traumatic or surgical wound. In these cases, follow the Department of Health and Human Services (DHHS) definitions regarding principal and other diagnoses code sequencing and ICD-9-CM coding rules regarding late effects and complications of surgical and medical care where applicable.

The following fifth-digit subclassification is for use with categories 711-712, 715-716, 718-719, and 730. Valid fifth-digits are in brackets [ ] at the end of each code.

0 site unspecified

1 shoulder region (acromioclavicular joint, clavicle, glenohumeral joint, scapula, sternoclavicular joint)

2 upper arm (elbow joint, humerus)

3 forearm (radius, ulna, wrist joint)

4 hand (carpus, metacarpus, phalanges)

5 pelvic regions and thigh (buttock, femur, hip joint)

6 lower leg (fibula, knee joint, patella, tibia)

7 ankle and foot (ankle joint, metatarsus, phalanges, tarsus, other joints in foot)

8 other specified sites (head, neck, ribs, skull, trunk, vertebral column)

9 multiple sites

© 2004 Ingenix, Inc.

730.0 ✓5th Acute osteomyelitis — (Use additional code to identify organism, 041.1) — *abscess of any bone except accessory sinus, jaw, or mastoid*
AHA: Q4, 1997, 43

Acute osteomyelitis is diseases including periostitis and periosteomyelitis in acute and subacute forms. Clinically, patients fall into two groups: those who respond to intravenous antibiotics and those who require surgical intervention.

730.1 ✓5th Chronic osteomyelitis — (Use additional code to identify organism, 041.1) — *Brodie's abscess, Busquet's disease, sequestrum, sclerosing osteomyelitis of Garre*
AHA: Q4, 1997, 43

Chronic osteomyelitis is persistent, recurring infection of bone and/or draining sinuses, often regarded as controllable but incurable.

730.2 ✓5th Unspecified osteomyelitis — (Use additional code to identify organism, 041.1) — *osteitis or osteomyelitis of unknown origin, with or without periostitis*
AHA: Q4, 1997, 43

730.3 ✓5th Periostitis without mention of osteomyelitis — (Use additional code to identify organism, 041.1) — *abscess without mention of osteomyelitis*
AHA: Q4, 1997, 43

730.7 ✓5th Osteopathy resulting from poliomyelitis — (Code first underlying disease: 045.0-045.9. Use additional code to identify organism) — *secondary to polio*
AHA: Q4, 1997, 43

730.8 ✓5th Other infections involving bone in diseases classified elsewhere — (Code first underlying disease: 002.0, 015.0-015.9. Use additional code to identify organism) — *secondary to underlying disease*
AHA: Q3, 1991, 10; Q2, 1997, 16; Q4, 1997, 43

730.9 ✓5th Unspecified infection of bone — (Use additional code to identify organism, 041.1)

731 Osteitis deformans and osteopathies associated with other disorders classified elsewhere

Osteitis deformans and osteopathies associated with other disorders classified elsewhere include the disseminated bone disorder known as Paget's disease. Characterized by slow and progressive enlargement and deformity of multiple bones, Paget's disease is associated with unexplained acceleration of both deposition and resorption of bone. During the early (osteolytic) phase of the disease, resorption exceeds deposition, and the bone, although enlarged, becomes sponge-like, weakened, and deformed. The second (osteosclerotic) phase is marked by deposition exceeding resorption resulting in the bones becoming thick and dense. The disease sometimes is associated with an invariably fatal form of malignant osteogenic sarcoma as a result of hyperactive osteoblast activity. Etiology is unknown, but there is some evidence that it may be triggered by a "slow virus" that affects primarily the osteoclasts.

731.0 Osteitis deformans without mention of bone tumor — *Paget's disease of bone*

731.1 Osteitis deformans in diseases classified elsewhere — (Code first underlying disease: 170.0-170.9) — *secondary to underlying disease*

731.2 Hypertrophic pulmonary osteoarthropathy — *Bamberger-Marie disease, Minkowski's, Pierre Marie-Bamberger, or thoracogenous rheumatic syndromes*

731.8 Other bone involvement in diseases classified elsewhere — (Code first underlying disease, 250.8. Use additional code to specify bone condition: 730.00-730.09) — *secondary to underlying disease*
AHA: Q2, 1997, 16; Q4, 1997, 43

732 Osteochondropathies

Osteochondropathies are self-limiting disorders of unknown etiology that mostly affect children (juvenile osteochondrosis) 3 to 10 years of age. Four phases in the pathogenesis of the disease have been identified: necrosis, revascularization with bone deposition and resorption, bone healing, and bone deformity. The fourth phase often is associated with degenerative arthropathy and is subject to ICD-9-CM coding rules regarding late effects, where applicable.

732.0 Juvenile osteochondrosis of spine — *marginal or vertebral epiphysis of Scheuermann or spine; vertebral epiphysitis*

732.1 Juvenile osteochondrosis of hip and pelvis — *acetabulum, head of femur, iliac crest, symphysis pubis; coxa plana, ischiopubic synchondrosis of van Neck, Wadenstrom's disease, pseudocoxalgia*

732.2 Nontraumatic slipped upper femoral epiphysis — *slipped upper femoral epiphysis, not otherwise specified*

732.3 Juvenile osteochondrosis of upper extremity — *capitulum of humerus if Panner, carpal lunate of Kienbock, head of humerus of Haas, heads of metacarpals of Mauclaire, lower ulna of Burns, radial head of Brailsford*

732.4 Juvenile osteochondrosis of lower extremity, excluding foot — *primary patellar center of Köhler, proximal tibia of Blount, secondary patellar center of Sinding-Larsen, tibial tubercle of Osgood-Schlatter; tibia vara, Blount-Barber or Erlacher-Blount syndromes*

732.5 Juvenile osteochondrosis of foot — *astragalus of Diaz, calcaneum of Sever, second metatarsal of Freiberg, fifth metatarsal of Iselin, os tibiale externum of Haglund, tarsal navicular of Köhler, calcaneal apophysitis, epiphysitis os calcis, Mouchet's disease*

732.6 Other juvenile osteochondrosis — *apophysitis, epiphysitis, osteochondritis, osteochondrosis of site not otherwise specified*

732.7 Osteochondritis dissecans

Osteochondritis dissecans is a form of osteochondropathy in which the convex surfaces of certain pressure epiphyses are susceptible to avascular necrosis. When a small tangential segment of subchondral bone becomes separated or "dissected" from the remaining portion of the epiphysis by reactive fibrous and granulation tissue, it is designated an osteochondritis or osteochondrosis dissecans.

732.8 Other specified forms of osteochondropathy — *adult osteochondrosis of spine*

732.9 Unspecified osteochondropathy — *apophysitis, epiphysitis, osteochondritis, osteochondrosis, not specified as adult or juvenile, of site not otherwise specified*

Coding Clarification

Many osteochondroses are identified by their eponyms (e.g., Kienbock's disease of the carpal lunate) and can be found under the main terms "Disease," "Osteochondrosis," and "Syndrome" in the ICD-9-CM index.

733 Other disorders of bone and cartilage

Osteoporosis is generalized bone disease characterized by decreased osteoblastic formation of matrix combined with increased osteoclastic resorption of bone, resulting in a marked decrease in bone mass. Osteoporosis often presents with osteopenia, which is a decrease in bone mineralization. Osteoporosis is classified into two major groups: primary and secondary. Primary osteoporosis implies that the condition is a fundamental disease entity and may be further broken down into involutional disease (e.g., juvenile). Secondary osteoporosis attributes the condition to an underlying clinical disease, medical condition, or medication.

Signs and symptoms of osteoporosis include chronic and intermittent back pain (due to vertebral microfractures), skeletal remodeling such as dorsal kyphosis, or loss of height.

Lab work usually shows normal results although metabolic studies may reveal a negative calcium balance. Radiographs and bone scans determine the extent and severity of osteoporosis and osteopenia and may reveal fresh or old evidence of pathological fractures. Quantitative computed tomography (CT) and single and dual energy x-ray absorptiometry (DEXA) measure bone density, and bone biopsy occasionally is done for histological studies.

Therapies include medical management such as dietary manipulation, calcitonin, diphosphonate's, vitamin D, calcium and sodium fluoride, and estrogen therapy following menopause.

Associated conditions include pathological fractures; in the case of secondary osteoporosis, a wide range of underlying factors such as anemia, hormone-related disorders, hepatic disease, starvation and anorexia, small intestine disease, mastocytosis, hemochromatosis, acromegaly, and conditions resulting from gastrectomy and treatment with anticonvulsants may be involved.

733.00 Unspecified osteoporosis — *wedging of vertebra not otherwise specified*
AHA: Q2, 1998, 12; Q3, 2001, 19

733.01 Senile osteoporosis — *bone mass reduction, usually without abnormality of mineral or organic content, in postmenopausal women*

733.02 Idiopathic osteoporosis — *bone mass reduction, usually without abnormality of mineral or organic content, not the result of disease or trauma*

733.03 Disuse osteoporosis

733.09 Other osteoporosis — (Use additional E code to identify drug) — *not otherwise specified, including drug-induced osteoporosis, Preiser's disease*
AHA: Q4, 2003, 108

A pathological fracture occurs at a site weakened by preexisting disease. These fractures are often differentiated from traumatic fractures by clinically assessing the magnitude of the trauma or stress causing the fracture. A relatively minor trauma or stress can cause a pathological fracture in bones diseased by osteoporosis and other metabolic bone disease, disseminated bone disorders, inflammatory bone diseases, Paget's disease, neoplasms, or any other condition that can compromise bone strength and integrity.

733.10 Pathologic fracture, unspecified site — *spontaneous fracture, site unknown*
AHA: Nov-Dec, 1985, 16; Nov-Dec, 1986, 10; Q4, 1993, 25

 © 2004 Ingenix, Inc.

733.11 Pathologic fracture of humerus — *spontaneous fracture*
AHA: Nov-Dec, 1985, 16; Nov-Dec, 1986, 10; Q4, 1993, 25

733.12 Pathologic fracture of distal radius and ulna — *spontaneous fracture*
AHA: Nov-Dec, 1985, 16; Nov-Dec, 1986, 10; Q4, 1993, 25

733.13 Pathologic fracture of vertebrae — *spontaneous fracture*
AHA: Nov-Dec, 1985, 16; Nov-Dec, 1986, 10; Q4, 1993, 25; Q3, 1999, 5

733.14 Pathologic fracture of neck of femur — *spontaneous fracture*
AHA: Nov-Dec, 1985, 16; Nov-Dec, 1986, 10; Q4, 1993, 25; Q1, 1996, 16; Q1, 2001, 1

733.15 Pathologic fracture of other specified part of femur — *spontaneous fracture*
AHA: Nov-Dec, 1985, 16; Nov-Dec, 1986, 10; Q4, 1993, 25; Q2, 1998, 12

733.16 Pathologic fracture of tibia or fibula — *spontaneous fracture*
AHA: Nov-Dec, 1985, 16; Nov-Dec, 1986, 10; Q4, 1993, 25

733.19 Pathologic fracture of other specified site — *spontaneous fracture, site not otherwise specified*
AHA: Nov-Dec, 1985, 16; Nov-Dec, 1986, 10; Q4, 1993, 25

Excluded from this subclassification is stress fracture (733.93-733.95).

When a fracture is due to a minor injury, the physician must determine if the injury was sufficient to cause the fracture or if the fracture is pathologic. Documentation must support the code selection of a pathological fracture (733.1x).

733.20 Unspecified cyst of bone (localized) — *unknown site*

733.21 Solitary bone cyst — *unicameral bone cyst*

733.22 Aneurysmal bone cyst

733.29 Other cyst of bone — *not otherwise specified, fibrous dysplasia*

733.3 Hyperostosis of skull — *formation of new, abnormal bone on the inner aspect of cranial bones; leontiasis ossium, Buchem's, Morel-Moore, and Morgagni-Stewart-Morel syndromes*

Aseptic necrosis of bone is infarction of bone tissue due to noninfectious etiologies such as fractures (avascular necrosis due to fracture), ischemic disorders, and immunosuppressive agents such as corticosteroids following renal transplants. It leads to degenerative joint disease or nonunion of fracture.

Osteonecrosis can be used to describe a wide variety of disorders, both infectious and noninfectious, resulting in bone infarction.

Some conditions falling under the general category of osteonecrosis are due to infectious etiologies and should be classified elsewhere. For example, osteonecrosis associated with acute staphylococcal osteomyelitis is classified to subcategories 730.0x and 041.1. Osteonecrosis unspecified as to infectious or noninfectious etiology is classified to subcategory 730.1x.

733.40 Aseptic necrosis of bone, site unspecified — *death of bone tissue not due to infection, unknown site*

733.41 Aseptic necrosis of head of humerus — *death of bone tissue not due to infection*

733.42 Aseptic necrosis of head and neck of femur — *death of bone tissue not due to infection*

733.43 Aseptic necrosis of medial femoral condyle — *death of bone tissue not due to infection*

733.44 Aseptic necrosis of talus — *death of bone tissue not due to infection*

733.49 Aseptic necrosis of other bone site — *death of bone tissue not due to infection, site not otherwise specified*

733.5 Osteitis condensans — *piriform sclerosis of ilium*

733.6 Tietze's disease — *painful swell and inflammation of unknown origin of rib cartilage; costochondral junction syndrome, costochondritis*

733.7 Algoneurodystrophy — *disuse atrophy of bone, Sudeck's atrophy*

733.81 Malunion of fracture — *broken bone heals in misalignment*
AHA: Q2, 1994, 5

733.82 Nonunion of fracture — *broken bone fails to heal*
AHA: Nov-Dec, 1984, 18; Q2, 1994, 5

733.90 Disorder of bone and cartilage, unspecified — *specifics unknown*

733.91 Arrest of bone development or growth — *Harris lines, epiphyseal arrest*

733.92 Chondromalacia — *localized, except patella, systemic, tibial plateau*

733.93 Stress fracture of tibia or fibula — *stress reaction of tibia or fibular*
AHA: Q4, 2001, 48

733.94 Stress fracture of the metatarsals — *stress reaction of metatarsals*
AHA: Q4, 2001, 48

733.95 Stress fracture of other bone — *stress reaction of other bone*
AHA: Q4, 2001, 48

733.99 Other disorders of bone and cartilage — *not otherwise specified, diaphysitis, hypertrophy of bone, relapsing polychondritis, Bruck's disease, slipped rib, xiphoiditis, ossification of cartilage*
AHA: Jan-Feb, 1987, 14

Coding Clarification

Nature of Pathological Fractures: A pathological fracture is a spontaneous fracture that occurs without external injury or by a minor or slight injury to a weakened bone. Bone density may become weakened by a number of conditions including but not limited to bone cysts, bone tumors, hyperparathyroidism, nutritional maladies, congenital anomalies, osteoporosis, Paget's disease, or osteomyelitis.

Because a fracture must either be traumatic (due to an injury) or pathological (due to weakened bone), a code from categories 800-829 must never accompany a code from category 733.

Report 380.03 for chondritis of pinna.

Coding Scenario

A 92-year-old female patient is seen complaining of pain of her left leg and back. She denies any traumatic injury. Upon x-ray examination, the physician determines that the patient has a pathological compression fracture of the L-3 vertebral body.

> Code assignment: 733.13 *Pathologic fracture of vertebrae*

734 Flat foot OK

Flat feet have a low arch and leave a nearly complete imprint; there is only a slight inward curve where the arch should be. The stretching or tearing of the posterior tibial tendon, which supports the arch and helps lift the heel off the ground, can lead to an adult acquired flatfoot deformity. Causes include trauma, overuse, and medical conditions such as obesity, diabetes, previous surgery, and steroid injections. The condition progresses from pain, swelling, and weakness to the tendon to a rigid flattening of the foot and ankle pain. Treatment depends on the stage of progression at the time of examination. Early stages can be treated non-surgically by rest and anti-inflammatory drugs. Orthotics and minor tendon surgery can help in advanced states, while later stages may require reconstructive surgery to stabilize the foot and ankle.

735 Acquired deformities of toe

735.0 Hallux valgus (acquired) — *deformity in which the great toe angles toward other toes of that foot*

735.1 Hallux varus (acquired) — *deformity in which the great toe angles away from other toes of that foot*

735.2 Hallux rigidus — *limited motion of great toe due to painful flexion; also called hallux rigidus*

735.3 Hallux malleus — *hammer toe of big toe*

735.4 Other hammer toe (acquired) — *hammer toe, other than big toe*

735.5 Claw toe (acquired) — *contracture of toe*

735.8 Other acquired deformity of toe — *hypertrophic, overriding, overlapping, or pigeon toe*

735.9 Unspecified acquired deformity of toe

736 Other acquired deformities of limbs

736.00 Unspecified deformity of forearm, excluding fingers

736.01 Cubitus valgus (acquired) — *deformity in which the forearm angles away from the body*

736.02 Cubitus varus (acquired) — *deformity in which the forearm angles toward the body*

736.03 Valgus deformity of wrist (acquired) — *deformity in which the wrist angles away from the body*

736.04 Varus deformity of wrist (acquired) — *deformity in which the wrist angles toward the body*

736.05 Wrist drop (acquired) — *paralysis or injury of extensor muscles of hand and fingers causing flexion of wrist*

Wrist drop is a condition in which the wrist remains flexed downward and is unable to be extended. It is often caused by injury to the radial nerve of the forearm or paralysis of the muscles in the hand and wrist.

736.06 Claw hand (acquired) — *contracture of hand*

A claw hand is characterized by curved or bent fingers, making the hand appear claw-like. Claw hand can be something that a child is born with (congenital) or can develop as a consequence of disorders (acquired).

736.07 Club hand, acquired

736.09 Other acquired deformities of forearm, excluding fingers — *not otherwise specified, intrinsic swan neck hand*

736.1 Mallet finger — *constant flexion of distal joint*

736.20 Unspecified deformity of finger

736.21 Boutonniere deformity — *fixed flexion of proximal interphalangeal joint and hyperextension of distal interphalangeal joint*

736.22 Swan-neck deformity

© 2004 Ingenix, Inc.

736.29 Other acquired deformity of finger — *not otherwise specified, shallow acetabulum, acquired short ip, wandering acetabulum*
AHA: Q2, 1989, 13

736.30 Unspecified acquired deformity of hip

736.31 Coxa valga (acquired) — *angle formed by the head and neck of the femur and axis of the shaft is increased*

736.32 Coxa vara (acquired) — *angle formed by the head and neck of the femur and axis of the shaft is decreased*

736.39 Other acquired deformities of hip — *not otherwise specified*
AHA: Q2, 1991, 18

736.41 Genu valgum (acquired) — *"knock-knee;" knees close together, ankles far apart*

736.42 Genu varum (acquired) — *"bowleg," knees far apart, ankles close together*

736.5 Genu recurvatum (acquired) — *"back-knee," hyperextension of knee*

736.6 Other acquired deformities of knee — *not otherwise specified*

736.70 Unspecified deformity of ankle and foot, acquired

736.71 Acquired equinovarus deformity — *clubfoot*

736.72 Equinus deformity of foot, acquired — *tip-toe walking deformity*

736.73 Cavus deformity of foot, acquired — *abnormally high arch*

736.74 Claw foot, acquired — *contracture deformity*

736.75 Cavovarus deformity of foot, acquired

736.76 Other acquired calcaneus deformity — *not otherwise specified*

736.79 Other acquired deformity of ankle and foot — *not otherwise specified, pronation of ankle or foot, varus talipes, valgus talipes*

736.81 Unequal leg length (acquired)

736.89 Other acquired deformity of other parts of limb — *not otherwise specified, including angulation or torsion of tibia; bowing of femur, fibula, tibia, winged scapula*

736.9 Acquired deformity of limb, site unspecified

737 Curvature of spine

Curvature of the spine is a deformity of the spine when it is not in straight alignment or with proper convexity. Kyphosis is an abnormal increase in the thoracic convexity as viewed from the side. Lordosis is the anterior convexity of the cervical and lumbar spine as viewed from the side.

737.0 Adolescent postural kyphosis — *acquired abnormal convex curve of spine*

737.10 Kyphosis (acquired) (postural)

737.11 Kyphosis due to radiation

737.12 Kyphosis, postlaminectomy

737.19 Other kyphosis (acquired) — *not otherwise specified*

737.20 Lordosis (acquired) (postural) — *not due to disease or injury*

737.21 Lordosis, postlaminectomy

737.22 Other postsurgical lordosis

737.29 Other lordosis (acquired)

Scoliosis is lateral curvature of the spine and kyphoscoliosis is a lateral curvature of the spine with extensive flexion. Scoliosis may be described as structural or nonstructural depending on whether the condition is reversible. Etiologies for nonstructural scoliosis include poor posture, pain, muscle spasms, and uneven limb lengths.

Specific etiologies for osteopathic scoliosis include fractures and dislocations of the spine, rickets, osteomalacia, and thoracogenic conditions such as unilateral pulmonary disease, or deformities caused by unilateral surgical procedures. Neuropathic scoliosis etiologies include acquired conditions such as poliomyelitis, paraplegia, syringomyelia, and Friedreich's ataxia.

737.30 Scoliosis (and kyphoscoliosis), idiopathic — *not due to disease or injury*
AHA: Q3, 2003, 19

737.31 Resolving infantile idiopathic scoliosis

737.32 Progressive infantile idiopathic scoliosis

737.33 Scoliosis due to radiation

737.34 Thoracogenic scoliosis

737.39 Other kyphoscoliosis and scoliosis — *not otherwise specified*
AHA: Q2, 2002, 16

737.40 Unspecified curvature of spine associated with other condition — (Code first associated condition: 015.0, 138, 237.7, 252.0, 277.5, 356.1, 731.0, 733.00-733.09) — *unknown type, secondary to underlying disease*

737.41 Kyphosis associated with other condition — (Code first associated condition: 015.0, 138, 237.7, 252.0, 277.5, 356.1, 731.0, 733.00-733.09) — *abnormal convex curve of the spine as seen in profile, secondary to underlying disease*

737.42 Lordosis associated with other condition — (Code first associated condition: 015.0, 138, 237.7, 252.0, 277.5, 356.1, 731.0, 733.00-733.09) — *abnormal concave curve of the spine as seen in profile*

710-739

737.43 Scoliosis associated with other condition — (Code first associated condition: 015.0, 138, 237.7, 252.0, 277.5, 356.1, 731.0, 733.00-733.09) — *abnormal lateral curve of the spine*

737.8 Other curvatures of spine associated with other conditions — *not otherwise specified*

737.9 Unspecified curvature of spine associated with other condition

ICD-9-CM coding rules for late effects are applicable for osteopathic and neuropathic etiologies when scoliosis represents the residual of the etiology. Etiologies for myopathic scoliosis are all congenital scolioses classified in ICD-9-CM Chapter 14 Congenital Anomalies (740-759).

738 Other acquired musculoskeletal deformity

Other acquired musculoskeletal deformity is a noncongenital deformity due to a variety of conditions such as degenerative disease; a late effect of fracture, dislocation, or other soft tissue injury or infection; or pathological weakness of a musculoligamentous structure.

Deformities due to acute injury or illness are classified only to the acute injury or illness to which they pertain; an "acquired deformity" of the nasal septum due to acute fracture of the septum requires one code only (802.0).

738.0 Acquired deformity of nose — *overdevelopment of nasal bones*

Other acquired deformity of the head includes deformities of the zygoma and zygomatic arch. The zygoma is the long slender process of the temporal and malar bones on each side of the skull. The bridge formed by the articulation of the temporal and malar processes is the zygomatic arch to which the masseter muscle, which moves the lower jaw (mandible), is attached.

738.10 Unspecified acquired deformity of head

738.11 Zygomatic hyperplasia — *overgrowth*

738.12 Zygomatic hypoplasia — *undergrowth*

738.19 Other specified acquired deformity of head — *not otherwise specified*
AHA: Q2, 2003, 13

738.2 Acquired deformity of neck

738.3 Acquired deformity of chest and rib — *thorax, chest, rib, xiphoid process, pectus carinatum, pectus excavatum*

738.4 Acquired spondylolisthesis

Acquired spondylolisthesis is forward slipping of one vertebral body (with the remainder of the spinal column above it) in relation to the vertebral segment immediately below, not due to congenital deformity or fracture. Acquired spondylolisthesis may be secondary to degenerative disk disease, a late effect of fracture, or due to spondylolysis (not qualified as congenital) or pathological weakness of bone.

The subterm "traumatic" listed in the ICD-9-CM index under the main term "Spondylolisthesis" refers to spondylolisthesis due to birth or intrauterine trauma, rather than as a late effect of trauma occurring any time after birth. Traumatic spondylolisthesis is considered a congenital anomaly and is classified to code 756.12. Spondylolisthesis due to acute trauma is classified as a current injury and coded as an acute fracture of the vertebra. Spondylolisthesis as a late effect of trauma, such as a prior fracture of the vertebra, is classified as acquired using the appropriate ICD-9-CM code for late effect (e.g., 905.1).

738.5 Other acquired deformity of back or spine

738.6 Acquired deformity of pelvis — *pelvic obliquity*

738.7 Cauliflower ear

738.8 Acquired musculoskeletal deformity of other specified site — *not otherwise specified, clavicle*
AHA: Q2, 2001, 15

738.9 Acquired musculoskeletal deformity of unspecified site

739 Nonallopathic lesions, not elsewhere classified

739.0 Nonallopathic lesion of head region, not elsewhere classified — *occipitocervical*

739.1 Nonallopathic lesion of cervical region, not elsewhere classified — *cervicothoracic*

739.2 Nonallopathic lesion of thoracic region, not elsewhere classified — *thoracolumbar*

739.3 Nonallopathic lesion of lumbar region, not elsewhere classified — *lumbosacral*

739.4 Nonallopathic lesion of sacral region, not elsewhere classified — *sacrococcygeal, sacroiliac*

739.5 Nonallopathic lesion of pelvic region, not elsewhere classified — *hip, pubic*

739.6 Nonallopathic lesion of lower extremities, not elsewhere classified — *thigh, knee, calf, foot*

739.7 Nonallopathic lesion of upper extremities, not elsewhere classified — *forearm, wrist, hand, upper arm*

739.8 Nonallopathic lesion of rib cage, not elsewhere classified

739.9 Nonallopathic lesion of abdomen and other sites, not elsewhere classified

© 2004 Ingenix, Inc.

740–759
Congenital Anomalies

Congenital anomalies may be the result of genetic factors (chromosomes), teratogens (agents causing physical defects in the embryo), or both. The anomalies may be apparent at birth or hidden and identified sometime after birth. Whatever the cause, congenital anomalies can be attributed to nearly 50 percent of deaths to full-term newborn infants.

Codes in Chapter 14 are classified according to a principal or defining defect rather than to the cause (chromosome abnormalities are the exception). Regardless of the origin, dysmorphology — clinical structural abnormality — is generally the primary indication of a congenital anomaly and, in many cases, a syndrome may be classified according to a single anatomic anomaly rather than a complex of symptoms. For example, Apert's syndrome is classified to 755.55 *Acrocephalosyndactyly.* Rubric 755 classifies reduction deformities of the lower limb, and abnormal bony fusion in the feet is a single anatomic anomaly of the multi-complex syndrome that can include fusion in the hands and facial anomalies.

Coding Clarification

ICD-9-CM does not differentiate between abnormalities that are intrinsic — related to the fetus — or extrinsic — as a result of intrauterine problems, although a note in ICD-9-CM prior to rubric 754 *Certain congenital musculoskeletal deformities* identifies codes as specific to extrinsic factors. However, ICD-9-CM does make a distinction in the classification of an anomaly as compared to a deformity. An anomaly is a malformation caused by abnormal fetal development, as in transposition of great vessels or spina bifida. A deformity is an alteration in structure caused by an extrinsic force, as in intrauterine compression. The force may cause a disruption in a normal fetal structure, including congenital amputations from amniotic bands.

In some cases, two codes are necessary to describe the condition. For example, the condition thalidomide phocomelia (thalidomide influence on the developing fetus during the perinatal period) requires two codes: 755.23 *Longitudinal deficiency, combined, involving humerus, radius, and ulna (complete or incomplete)* and 760.79 *Noxious influences affecting fetus via placenta or milk.*

There is no clear distinction between what is classified to Chapter 14 and a congenital anomaly classified to another chapter in ICD-9-CM. For example, oligohydramnios, a condition caused by a complication of pregnancy, is classified to Chapter 15 Certain Conditions Originating in the Perinatal Period (760-779). Retinoblastoma, a tumor arising in the fetal retina and diagnosed after birth, is reported with 190.5 *Malignant neoplasm of the retina* from Chapter 2 Neoplasms. The congenital absence of clotting factors is reported with codes in the rubric 286 *Coagulation defects.*

740 Anencephalus and similar anomalies

Anencephalus is a usually fatal brain defect of the newborn caused by a closure of the neural groove early in the first trimester of pregnancy. It can present in several forms:

- The cranial vault may be absent
- The cerebral hemispheres are missing or exist as masses attached to the base of the skull
- The brain is abnormally shaped

Anencephalus is identified in the patient record as acrania, partial or total absence of the skull; amyelencephalus, the absence of the brain and spinal cord; hemianencephaly, absence of half the brain; and hemicephaly, absence of one of the brain hemispheres.

740.0 Anencephalus — *anencephalus; acrania; amyelencephalus; hemicephaly; hemiencephaly*

740.1 Craniorachischisis — *craniorachischisis; Antley- Bixler syndrome*

740.2 Iniencephaly — *Iniencephaly; protrusion of brain into cord space*

Coding Clarification

Medical management in rubric 740 is attuned to a fatal outcome, whereas the conditions falling into rubric 741 are not necessarily terminal.

Condition	Antomy Displaced	Nature of Defect	Structural Defect Location
Craniorhachischisis	C + B	Fissure	Skull and Vertebral column
Encephalocystocele	B	Hernia of brain, filled with CSF	Skull
Holoprosencephaly	B	Forebrain defect	Brain
Hydroencephalocele	B	Brain protrudes in a sac	Skull
Hydromeningocele	M	Meninges protrude, filled with CSF	Vertebral column
Iniencephaly	B	brain protrudes into cord space	Skull
Meningoencephalocele	B + M	Brain and meninges protrude	Skull
Micrencephaly	B	abnormally small brain	Brain
Microgyria	B	abnormally small convolutions of brain	Brain
Myelomeningocele	C +M	Meninges and cord protrude	Vertebral column
Hydrocephalus	B	CSF volume too great	Brain (CSF circulation)
Syringomyelocele	C	Hernia cavity communicates with cord	Cord
Myelocystocele	C	Cord substance protrudes	Cord
Myelocele	C	Cord protrudes	Vertebral column
B= Brain		C= Skull	M= Meninges

741 *Spina bifida*

AHA: Q3, 1994, 7

Citing the location of the lesion is mandatory when coding spina bifida; the unspecified fifth digit should be avoided. The presence or absence of hydrocephalus is a second axis in the rubric, while spina bifida occulta is excluded from this rubric and is reported with 756.17.

Spina bifida, a defect in the vertebral column, presents in conjunction with several anomalies or it may occur as a solitary anomaly. Prognosis depends both on the number and severity of anomalies and on the size and location of the vertebral defect. Paralysis at the level below the defect is always present when the cord or spinal nerve roots are involved. Defects at the lumbosacral level can cause bladder and rectal problems. The child will often have orthopedic problems such as kyphosis or clubfoot. Death is usually ascribed to shunt complications, including infection and renal failure.

The circulation of the cerebrospinal fluid (CSF) is impeded, causing additional fluid pressure on the brain, in hydrocephalus, a condition that may be categorized as either communicating or non-communicating. In communicating hydrocephalus, there is no obstruction.

Type II is the most serious of the four types of malformations found in Arnold-Chiari or Chiari disease and the only type assigned to this subcategory. In this variation, the inferior poles of the cerebellum and the medulla protrude through the foramen magnum into the spinal canal. It is typically associated with other anomalies such as polymicrogyria, meningomyelocele, and hydrocephalus.

Subclassification 741.9 includes:

- Spinal hydromeningocele: fluid-filled sac composed of meninges protruding through the vertebral column defect
- Hydromyelocele: sac filled with CSF protruding through the wall of the spinal cord
- Meningocele: sac of meninges protruding through the skull or vertebral column
- Meningomyelocele: sac of meninges and cord protruding through the spinal column
- Myelocele: protrusion of the cord through the vertebral column
- Myelocystocele: protrusion of cord substance through the spinal canal
- Rachischisis: complete fissure in the vertebral column
- Syringomyelocele: saclike protrusion of the cord that remains in communication with the central canal of the cord

The following fifth-digit subclassification is for use with category 741:

0 unspecified region

1 cervical region

2 dorsal (thoracic) region

3 lumbar region

740–759

© 2004 Ingenix, Inc.

741.0 ✓5th Spina bifida with hydrocephalus

741.9 ✓5th Spina bifida without mention of hydrocephalus

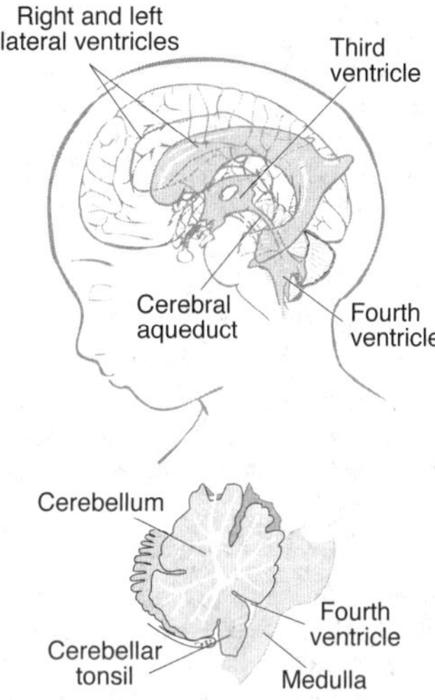

Detail of section through brain stem showing part of cerebellum herniating into the brain stem (Chiari malformation)

742 Other congenital anomalies of nervous system

742.0 Encephalocele

An encephalocele is a neural herniation of brain parenchyma and meninges that protrudes through a cranial defect. Encephalocele is also known as cranium bifidum with encephalocele, hydrencephalocele, and hydrencephalomeningocele. Lesions occur in the occipital region or anywhere in the cranial vault.

742.1 Microcephalus

In microcephalus, the head circumference is more than two standard deviations below the mean for age, sex, race, and gestation. Anomalous development, such as a chromosomal disorder or maternal phenylketonuria, during the first seven months of gestation causes primary microcephaly. Secondary microcephaly results from an insult, such as infection, trauma, anoxia, or metabolic disorders, during the last two months of gestation or during the perinatal period.

742.2 Congenital reduction deformities of brain

742.3 Congenital hydrocephalus

Ventricular enlargement, abundant cerebral spinal fluid, and, in most cases, increasing pressure are present in congenital hydrocephalus. In addition, the foramen of Magendie and the foramen of Luschka may be undeveloped, resulting in the obstruction of fluid through the aqueduct of Sylvius, which carries the cerebrospinal fluid between the midbrain and the fourth ventricle. An obstruction of the fourth ventricle outlet, as seen in Dandy-Walker syndrome (741.0 with spina bifida) describes noncommunicating hydrocephalus. Other conditions that may present include arachnoiditis and lesions such as neoplasms, cysts, and hematomas. In addition, the obstruction may be secondary to exudate, hemorrhage, or parasites.

Communicating hydrocephalus may be due to adhesions of the basilar cisterns or surface subarachnoid space following infection or hemorrhage, post developmental adhesions, vitamin A deficiency, developmental failure or erythrocyte obstruction of the arachnoid villi, or Arnold Chiari malformation (741.0).

Cerebral cysts, macroencephaly, (synonym for megalencephaly) an abnormally large head, large convolutions of the cerebrum, ulegyria, — abnormal convolutions of the cerebrum due to scarring — and porencephaly — a cerebral cyst with an opening into a ventricle — are abnormalities that may progress to hydrocephalus. These conditions are reported with 742.4.

742.4 Other specified congenital anomalies of brain

742.51 Diastematomyelia

Diastematomyelia reports a longitudinal fissure in the spinal cord that results in gait disturbance, muscular atrophy, and lack of sphincter control.

742.53 Hydromyelia

Hydromyelia reports a dilated spinal canal. It is a synonym for hydrorhachis.

Amyelia is the absence of a spinal cord, whereas atelomyelia is an incompletely developed cord. Myelodysplasia and myelatelia are synonymous terms describing a defective spinal cord.

742.59 Other specified congenital anomaly of spinal cord

742.8 Other specified congenital anomalies of nervous system

Marcus-Gunn syndrome, also known as jaw-winking syndrome, is characterized by the onset of rapid eyelid movement, producing a winking effect, when the jaw moves. The cause is unknown.

Riley-Day syndrome, or familial dysautonomia, is primarily found in families of European-Jewish extraction. Poor sucking ability, sweating while eating, hypotonia, and insensitivity to pain characterize the condition.

742.9 Unspecified congenital anomaly of brain, spinal cord, and nervous system

Coding Clarification

Acquired hydrocephalus (331.3-331.4) is excluded from this rubric, as is hydrocephalus due to congenital toxoplasmosis (771.2).

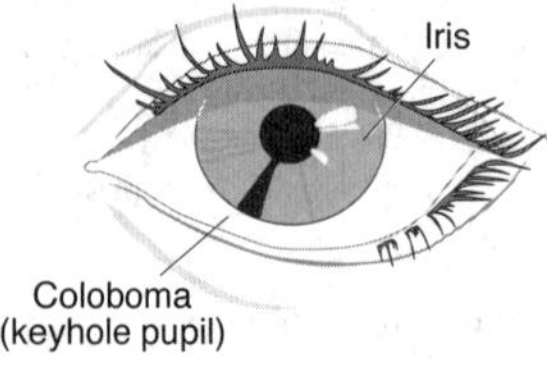

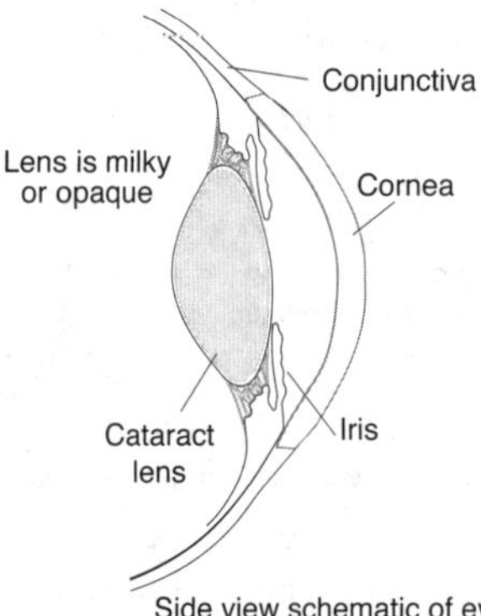

Side view schematic of eye

743 Congenital anomalies of eye

Any structure or organ of the body is subject to a failure or deviation in development. Congenital anomalies of the eye are classified according to the specific site affected and the type of defect. They include:

- Anophthalmos: absence of an eye
- Cryptophthalmos: uninterrupted extension of an eyelid across the eyeball
- Microphthalmos: abnormally small eye

743.00	Unspecified clinical anophthalmos
743.03	Cystic eyeball, congenital
743.06	Cryptophthalmos
743.10	Unspecified microphthalmos
743.11	Simple microphthalmos
743.12	Microphthalmos associated with other anomalies of eye and adnexa

Physicians assess microphthalmos according to levels of debility. Pure microphthalmos, a condition of a small eye with a tendency to angle-closing glaucoma, is reported with 743.12 if the condition causes vision complications. Simple microphthalmos (743.11) is a small eye, which is essentially normal in functionality.

Buphthalmos is congenital glaucoma. In affected infants, a defect in the iridocorneal angle, an outlet in the anterior chamber of the eye, impedes aqueous circulation.

Glaucoma is an elevated pressure in the aqueous humor. Undetected, glaucoma can lead to nerve damage and blindness. Surgery, directed toward restoring the natural circulation of the aqueous, can prevent loss of sight. A genetic abnormality or an inflammation of the eye prior to birth can cause congenital glaucoma.

743.20	Unspecified buphthalmos
743.21	Simple buphthalmos
743.22	Buphthalmos associated with other ocular anomaly

Excluded from these subclassifications are glaucoma of childhood (365.14) and traumatic glaucoma due to birth injury (767.8).

Cataracts are milky or opaque areas on the lens of the eye that translate into milky or opaque disturbances in the field of vision. Infection during development, genetic error, or metabolites residing within the lens may be the cause. Other anomalies of the lens include aphakia, or congenital absence of the lens, and anomalies of shape including spherophakia (sphere shaped) or microphakia (small lens). An ectopic lens is a displaced lens.

A coloboma describes a part absent from an ophthalmological structure, due usually to a chromosomal defect, which presents as a fissure of the iris, the ciliary body, or the choroid (thus the common name "keyhole pupil"). It is typically associated with CHARGE syndrome (C=coloboma; H=heart; A=atresia of choanae, R=retarded growth and development, G=genital hypoplasia, E=ear anomalies). Coloboma may increase the risk of iridial tearing and often includes iris and choroid flaws.

743.30	Unspecified congenital cataract
743.31	Congenital capsular and subcapsular cataract
743.32	Congenital cortical and zonular cataract
743.33	Congenital nuclear cataract
743.34	Congenital total and subtotal cataract
743.35	Congenital aphakia
743.36	Congenital anomalies of lens shape
743.37	Congenital ectopic lens
743.39	Other congenital cataract and lens anomalies

Excluded from these subclassifications are cataracts that are associated with syndromes congenital in nature although not present at birth, as in craniofacial dystosis (756.0). These cataracts are reported with 366.44.

© 2004 Ingenix, Inc.

743.41 Congenital anomaly of corneal size and shape

743.42 Congenital corneal opacity, interfering with vision

743.43 Other congenital corneal opacity

743.44 Specified congenital anomaly of anterior chamber, chamber angle, and related structures

743.45 Aniridia

Aniridia, the incomplete formation of the iris, results in vision loss. Typically, aniridia is bilateral and gives the appearance of black irises though it is the pupil — and not the iris — which is dark. An autosomal-dominant or autosomal-recessive gene can be a cause and, if so determined, the child may have other health or developmental problems.

743.46 Other specified congenital anomaly of iris and ciliary body

Anisocoria, or unequal pupils, is a common condition. In corectopia, the pupil is asymmetrically placed in the iris. Children with iris colobomata should be checked for fissure of the optic nerve and of the fundus.

743.47 Specified congenital anomaly of sclera

743.48 Multiple and combined congenital anomalies of anterior segment of eye

743.49 Other congenital anomaly of anterior segment of eye

743.51 Vitreous anomaly, congenital

743.52 Fundus coloboma

743.53 Congenital chorioretinal degeneration

743.54 Congenital folds and cysts of posterior segment of eye

743.55 Congenital macular change

743.56 Other congenital retinal changes

743.57 Specified congenital anomalies of optic disc

743.58 Congenital vascular anomalies of posterior segment of eye

743.59 Other congenital anomalies of posterior segment of eye

743.61 Congenital ptosis of eyelid

A severe case of ptosis is treated immediately after birth since it can disrupt visual development. In less severe cases, treatment is delayed until the child reaches 3 to 5 years of age.

743.62 Congenital deformity of eyelid

Ablepharon, the congenital absence of an eyelid, seldom appears as a solitary variant, which is typical of agenesis anomalies.

An accessory eyelid is an additional eyelid.

Entropion is inversion of the lower eyelid, whereas ectropion is the eversion of the lower eyelid. Both conditions require surgical correction since rubbing caused by the displacement often scars the cornea.

743.63 Other specified congenital anomaly of eyelid

743.64 Specified congenital anomaly of lacrimal gland

743.65 Specified congenital anomaly of lacrimal passages

The lacrimal glands produce the tears that moisten the eyes to keep them healthy. Tears are produced at each blink and pumped down and across the eye. Any excess tears drain through the tear duct and into the nose, which explains why noses run when crying. Excess tears can also create problems. Surgery may be required to open ducts obstructed by pus in an infection resulting from stagnant tears.

743.66 Specified congenital anomaly of orbit

743.69 Other congenital anomalies of eyelids, lacrimal system, and orbit

743.8 Other specified congenital anomalies of eye

743.9 Unspecified congenital anomaly of eye

744 Congenital anomalies of ear, face, and neck

Codes in this rubric are classified according to site and the impairment associated with the anomaly. The most significant codes in this rubric are those reporting hearing impairments, classified to subcategory 744.0. Congenital deafness, without mention of cause, is excluded from this rubric and is reported with codes from the series 389.0-389.9.

744.00 Unspecified congenital anomaly of ear causing impairment of hearing

744.01 Congenital absence of external ear causing impairment of hearing

744.02 Other congenital anomaly of external ear causing impairment of hearing

744.03 Congenital anomaly of middle ear, except ossicles, causing impairment of hearing

744.04 Congenital anomalies of ear ossicles

744.05 Congenital anomalies of inner ear

744.09 Other congenital anomalies of ear causing impairment of hearing

744.1 Congenital anomalies of accessory auricle

744.21 Congenital absence of ear lobe

744.22 Macrotia

744.23 Microtia

Microtia, external auditory canal atresia, and ossicular fusion often occur together. Auricle atresia is associated with craniofacial syndromes such as Treacher-Collins and Nager syndromes, but may occur in solitary.

744.24 Specified congenital anomaly of Eustachian tube

744.29 Other congenital anomaly of ear

Large and protruding ears, called Bat ear, can be surgically modified. Polyotia is the presence of an accessory auricle. Pointed ear, Stahl's ear, and Spoke ear describe ears pointed at the top. Darwin's tubercle, a prominence on the upper posterior of the superior ridge of the auricle; is a vestigial remnant of a folded ear.

744.3 Unspecified congenital anomaly of ear

Branchial cleft relates to embryonic development of the external auricle, the external auditory meatus, and the tympanic membrane. A sinus is a blind ending tract. A fistula is an open-ended tract.

744.41 Congenital branchial cleft sinus or fistula

744.42 Congenital branchial cleft cyst

744.43 Congenital cervical auricle

744.46 Congenital preauricular sinus or fistula

744.47 Congenital preauricular cyst

744.49 Other congenital branchial cleft cyst or fistula; preauricular sinus

744.5 Congenital webbing of neck

Pterygium colli is a webbed effect produced by an anomalous band of fascia extending from the mastoid process to the clavicle.

744.81 Macrocheilia

744.82 Microcheilia

Microcheilia is an abnormally small lip.

744.83 Macrostomia

744.84 Microstomia

Microstomia is an abnormally small mouth.

744.89 Other specified congenital anomaly of face and neck

744.9 Unspecified congenital anomaly of face and neck

745–747 Congenital Anomalies of the Cardiovascular System

One percent of all births has a cardiac anomaly. The evaluation of an infant or child with a cardiac anomaly must determine the anomalous pattern of vascularity, cardiac enlargement, whether cyanosis is present, or a combination of the possible irregularities. An anomalous vascular pattern indicates abnormal circulation. An anomalous vascularity is characterized as a transposition or transposition complex anomaly. The term transposition refers to the normal anterior-to-posterior relationships of the vessels. An enlarged heart requires an evaluation of the chambers to determine the extent of the anomaly. Cyanosis is the most common variant, followed by volume load disorders.

745 Bulbus cordis anomalies and anomalies of cardiac septal closure

Bulbus cordis relates to embryological development of the fetal heart. Persistent truncus arteriosus is the failure of the aorticopulmonary trunk to divide at the correct developmental stage. There are four classifications and an infant born with the condition presents as cyanotic and tachypneic, and may be struggling with congestive heart failure due to the effects of the abnormally increased pulmonary artery blood flow. The infant may require the Rastelli procedure, which involves separating the pulmonary artery from the primitive truncus to create a right ventricle-to-pulmonary artery conduit.

745.0 Bulbus cordis anomalies and anomalies of cardiac septal closure, common truncus

745.10 Complete transposition of great vessels

745.11 Transposition of great vessels, double outlet right ventricle

Double outlet right ventricle is a cyanotic congenital heart disease, affecting more males than females, and presents within the first 24 hours after birth. The infant is often cyanotic and tachypneic, and congestive heart failure is probable. Survival depends on the existence of a ventricular septal defect, an atrial septal defect, or a patent ductus arteriosus, which allow communication between the pulmonary and systemic circulations. Many of the operative procedures work with the anomalous anatomy to achieve operational pulmonary and systemic circulations. For example, the Jantene operation creates a corrective arterial switch.

In Taussig-Bing syndrome, the aorta is in the right ventricle, the pulmonary artery is located in both ventricles, and a ventricular septal defect is present. The child is often cyanotic due to the oxygen insufficiency resulting from the anomalies.

745.12 Corrected transposition of great vessels

Report 745.12 to identify a newborn with a transposition syndrome subsequently corrected since this transposition often involves sequelae.

745.19 Other transposition of great vessels

745.2 Tetralogy of Fallot

The tetralogy of Fallot represents 8 percent of all congenital heart diseases. The anomaly, which presents by 6 months, is a cyanotic and transposition syndrome. A right aortic arch, abnormal origin of coronary arteries, a left superior vena cava, and an enlarged bronchial artery are characteristic. Palliative repairs are performed in the early years, with definitive repair reserved until 5 to 7 years of age, using the Blalock-Taussig, Pohl's, or Waterston-Cooley operations. This code excludes Fallot's triad, which is reported with 746.09.

© 2004 Ingenix, Inc.

745.3 Bulbus cordis anomalies and anomalies of cardiac septal closure, common ventricle

A common ventricle anomaly occurs when a single ventricle arises from the absence of a ventricular septum. Typically, there is transposition of the great vessels, cardiomegaly, cyanosis, congestive heart failure, and mixed pulmonary and system circulation.

745.4 Ventricular septal defect

Ventricular septal defects (VSD) may appear as solitary anomalies or present as part of a syndrome, such as Holt-Roan syndrome, trisomy 13, 18, and 21, and tetralogy of Fallot. A VSD may involve both the membranous and muscular portions of the ventricles. Approximately 80 percent involve the membranous septum. Within two to three months of birth, the infant presents with congestive heart failure. Treatment includes patching the VSD, pulmonary artery banding, and medical therapy. Common atrioventricular canal type anomalies (745.69) and single ventricle anomalies (745.3) are excluded from this code.

Eisenmenger's syndrome is a progressive cyanotic condition characterized by a VSD, pulmonary hypertension, and combined pulmonary and systemic circulations. A small, asymptomatic VSD is a primary characteristic of Roger's disease, also reported with 745.4.

745.5 Ostium secundum type atrial septal defect

Ostium secundum accounts for 90 percent of all atrial septal defects (ASD). Treatment depends on the age of the patient at evaluation and usually involves applying a patch to the ASD. An ASD left untreated can cause right heart failure, atrial fibrillation later in life, and the increased risk of blood clots leading to a stroke.

Lutembacher's syndrome, reported with 745.5, is an ASD in conjunction with mitral rheumatic stenosis. A patent foramen ovale, also reported with 745.5, is treated when other heart defects are present. The foramen ovale normally closes shortly after birth.

There are three classifications of cushion defects: complete, partial, and intermediate. A complete defect presents with congestive heart failure and all types demonstrate ostium primum. A partial defect is the most common. About 40 percent of cushion anomalies are associated with trisomy-21 (Down's syndrome), which is separately reported with 758.0.

745.60 Unspecified type congenital endocardial cushion defect

745.61 Ostium primum defect

745.69 Other congenital endocardial cushion defect

745.7 Cor biloculare

Cor biloculare describes a heart lacking both an atrial and a ventricular septum. A two-chambered heart severely compromises the newborn and few born with the condition live to the first year.

745.8 Other bulbus cordis anomalies and anomalies of cardiac septal closure

745.9 Unspecified congenital defect of septal closure

746 Other congenital anomalies of heart

Endocardial fibroelastosis is excluded from this rubric and is reported with 425.3.

746.00 Unspecified congenital pulmonary valve anomaly

746.01 Congenital atresia of pulmonary valve

Absence of the pulmonary valve is associated with hypoplastic right heart structures. An infant becomes critically ill when the foramen ovale and PDA close and result in impaired pulmonary circulation. A shunt may be placed between the aorta and the pulmonary artery or a pulmonary artery may be implanted to correct the problem.

746.02 Congenital stenosis of pulmonary valve

A ventricle may become enlarged to compensate for the slow down of blood circulation due to a narrowed valve. Severe stenosis, reported with 746.02, requires surgical repair and lifelong antibiotic prophylaxis.

746.09 Other congenital anomalies of pulmonary valve

Other pulmonary insufficiencies are managed medically. The trilogy or triad of Fallot involves pulmonary stenosis, ASD, and right ventricular hypertrophy.

746.1 Congenital tricuspid atresia and stenosis

746.2 Ebstein's anomaly

In Ebstein's anomaly, the tricuspid valve is displaced downward, which can lead to fatigue palpitations and dyspnea. A portion of the RV is atrialized (i.e., thinned and dysplastic). Dilated tricuspid annulus and a dilated RA are present. Of the four classifications, "D" is the most severe, manifesting with nearly total atrialization of the RV and other cardiac anomalies such as ASD and Wolff-Parkinson-White syndrome.

746.3 Congenital stenosis of aortic valve

746.4 Congenital insufficiency of aortic valve

Thickened and stiffened valves may cause the stenosis or it may be due to the valve having only one or two cusps. If severe, the stenosis produces fatigue, dizziness, and fainting.

746.5 Congenital mitral stenosis

Fusion of the commissures of the valve causes mitral stenosis. The valves are not calcific and the treatment is a commissurotomy.

746.6 Congenital mitral insufficiency

Mitral insufficiency is regurgitation or back flow into the RA leading to decreased systemic flow. The condition overworks the heart in its efforts to pump blood to the body's periphery.

746.7 Hypoplastic left heart syndrome

Hypoplastic left heart syndrome accounts for 10 percent of all heart defects. The LV is tiny and symptoms include stenosis or atresia of the aortic and mitral valves and coarctation of the aorta. The condition can be critical and treatments include heart transplant and palliative reconstruction. If a transplant is necessary, large amounts of donor aorta must be used in the reconstruction of the aorta. If reconstruction is the selected treatment, it is performed in stages (i.e., the Norwood procedure is performed immediately, followed by the Glenn procedure three to six months later, and the Fontan reconstructive procedure at 18 to 24 months of age).

746.81 Congenital subaortic stenosis

In subaortic stenosis, the LV works hard to push the blood past the coarctation of the aorta, a condition that leads to cardiomegaly and congestive heart failure. A mild condition requires no surgery unless, over time, the stenosis worsens and leads to severe tachycardia, tachypnea, and eventually into congestive heart failure. Other milder complications include fatigue, chest pain, and fainting.

746.82 Cor triatriatum

In cor triatriatum, a small extra chamber above the LA receives the blood from the pulmonary vein. This extra chamber hampers the force of the blood entering the LA and, as a result, congestive heart failure may result.

746.83 Congenital infundibular pulmonic stenosis

Infundibular pulmonic stenosis is a narrowing of the outflow tract of the right ventricle below the pulmonary valve within the infundibulum. The condition is due to a fibrous diaphragm or to a long, narrow fibromuscular channel.

746.84 Congenital obstructive anomalies of heart, not elsewhere classified

Uhl's disease is a RV spongiform dysplasia, characteristically with paper-thin ventricle walls.

746.85 Congenital coronary artery anomaly

Anomalous Left Coronary Artery Originating from Pulmonary Artery (ALCAPA) is a serious condition and, if left untreated, only about 20 percent of children survive beyond adolescence. A single coronary artery is inadequate for perfusion and infarctions leave the heart dependent on collateral circulation to perfuse the left ventricle. Surgery establishes a two-coronary artery system through re-vascularization.

746.86 Congenital heart block

Congenital heart block appears as both a sole congenital variant and as part of a syndrome of congenital anomalies. An isolated variant may be associated with autoimmune diseases in the mother. In these situations, the infants are born with neonatal lupus syndrome, which disappears after 6 months of age. The heart block does not disappear. Whatever the origin of the disorder, diminished cardiac output progresses to congestive heart failure. The infant is surgically treated with pacemaker implantation.

746.87 Congenital malposition of heart and cardiac apex

There are four types of dextrocardia:

1. Dextroposition: extrinsic factor causes the heart to shift to the right, leading to hypoplastic right lung, a partial anomaly of the pulmonary venous connection to the inferior vena cava, and right-sided pulmonary collaterals.
2. Dextroversion: abnormal rotation of the cardiac loops in embryological development leads to atrioventricular or ventriculoatrial discordance, or a single ventricle, which may be part of Cantrell syndrome: omphalocele or other midline defect, lower sternal defect, anterior inferior diaphragmatic defect, parietal pericardial defect, and left ventricular diverticulum.
3. Ventriculoatrial situs inversus: associated with tetralogy of Fallot, and Kartagener's syndrome. Excluded from 746.87 is dextrocardia with complete transposition of viscera, which is reported with 759.3.
4. Levocardia: includes four variants: 1) situs solitus with normal heart, 2) levoposition (heart shifts left in the mediastinum due to dysgenesis of the left lung), 3) levoversion of situs inversus, atrioventricular and ventriculoatrial discordance, 4) situs ambiguous.

Dextrocardia and levocardia are both reported with 746.87 in ICD-9-CM.

Ectopic cordis is a serious anomaly in which the sternum is split and the heart protrudes (most common form) or the heart is displaced to the abdomen or neck. A newborn with the condition generally dies within a few days of birth in nearly 100 percent of cases. Ectopic cordis is reported with 746.87.

746.89 Other specified congenital anomaly of heart

In diverticulum of the left ventricle, the diverticulum protrudes into the epigastrium. It may or may not be an isolated anomaly.

Brugada syndrome is a combination of right bundle branch block, ST elevation, and arrhythmic right ventricular dysplasia (ARVD), which results in abnormal left ventricular electrophysiology and

 © 2004 Ingenix, Inc.

sudden death. The condition runs in families and is treated by implantation of an automatic cardioverter-defibrillator.

746.9 Unspecified congenital anomaly of heart

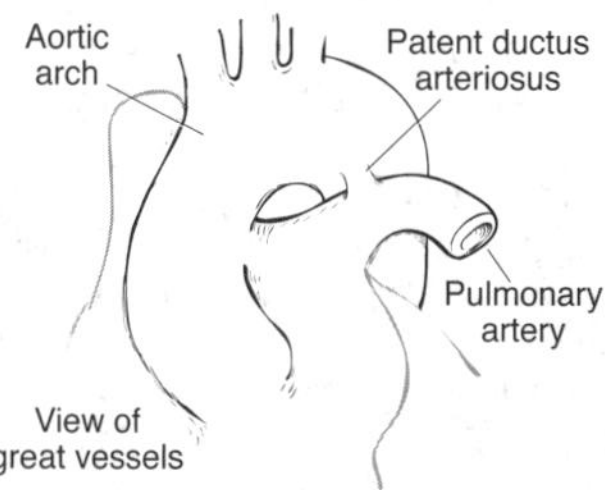

The ductus arteriosus is the natural shunt that bypasses lung circulation in the prenatal phase

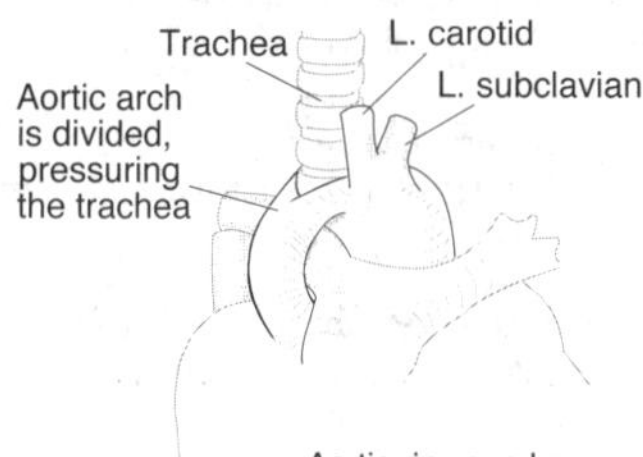

Aortic ring syndrome

747 Other congenital anomalies of circulatory system

747.0 Patent ductus arteriosus

Other terms for patent ductus arteriosus (PDA) are persistent ductus arteriosus or patent ductus Botallo. The incidence is greater in females and it is one of the most common cardiovascular anomalies. The ductus arteriosus is patent during fetal life for breathing through the umbilical cord and, in most infants, closes within a few weeks of birth. A patent ductus arteriosus allows the lungs to be bypassed until birth, shunting right ventricular blood to the aorta. The condition presents two ways: if the infant is premature, the patency typically closes once the infant reaches the appropriate developmental stage. If the infant is term, with persistent patency, the infant will experience elevated left heart pressures and increased pulmonary circulation, putting undue strain on the left heart and pulmonary vasculature, leading to pulmonary vascular disease and congestive heart failure. There is an increased risk of bacterial endocarditis. PDAs are surgically corrected, no matter their size, due to probable complications.

747.10 Coarctation of aorta (preductal) (postductal)

Coarctation refers to a pinching of the aortic arch, forcing the left heart to pump past the obstruction, which leads to enlargement, increased blood pressure in arteries behind the obstruction, decreased pressure in arteries post obstruction, and congestive heart failure. In post obstruction, the aorta may enlarge to increase the risk of dilation, aneurysm, rupture, and stroke. Patients with coarctation are at lifelong risk for bacterial endocarditis and for myocardial infarction. The obstruction is resected as soon as possible after birth and the same procedure may need to be repeated in adulthood. The congestive failure subsides after corrective surgery, although there may be persistent pulmonary hypertension.

747.11 Congenital interruption of aortic arch

747.20 Unspecified congenital anomaly of aorta

747.21 Congenital anomaly of aortic arch

An anomalous arch in double aortic arch encircles the trachea or the esophagus, leading to tracheal compression and subsequent proclivity to repeated respiratory infections. The anomalous arch may be patent and always causes difficulty because of its position.

747.22 Congenital atresia and stenosis of aorta

Aortic stenosis is a progressive condition that rarely produces symptoms in the young. Progressive elevated resistance to the pumping action of the left ventricle leads to increased LV pressure and hypertrophy. Hypertrophy weakens the heart and is prodromal to heart failure. The thicker and stiffer the ventricle walls, the weaker the pumping action. The two most common forms of aortic stenosis are valvular obstruction resulting from a defect in the valve, and subaortic obstruction, found in the Left Ventricular Outlet Tract. The condition may be an isolated phenomenon or appear in conjunction with VSD, PDA, and coarctation of the aorta.

747.29 Other congenital anomaly of aorta

Aneurysms of the sinus of Valsalva may not be apparent until adulthood. If rupture occurs, the patient is subject to congestive heart failure and sudden death. Typically, the rupture occurs in either the right or left coronary sinus leading to an acute right-to-left shunt.

747.3 Congenital anomalies of pulmonary artery

Agenesis of the pulmonary artery is rare, occurring on the left more than on the right, and is usually a benign variation. When symptomatic, it results in frequent respiratory tract infections with bronchiectasis.

747.40 Congenital anomaly of great veins unspecified

747.41 Total congenital anomalous pulmonary venous connection

Total anomalous pulmonary venous return (TAPVR) allows oxygenated blood to drain into the right atrium (normally the recipient of deoxygenated blood). ASD often accompanies the condition. It is

740–759

treated by severing the pulmonary return to the RA and creating a return to the LA.

747.42 Partial congenital anomalous pulmonary venous connection

Partial anomalous pulmonary venous return (PAPVR) is rarely clinically significant unless associated with sinus venosus ASD, which elevates it to significant importance.

747.49 Other congenital anomalies of great veins

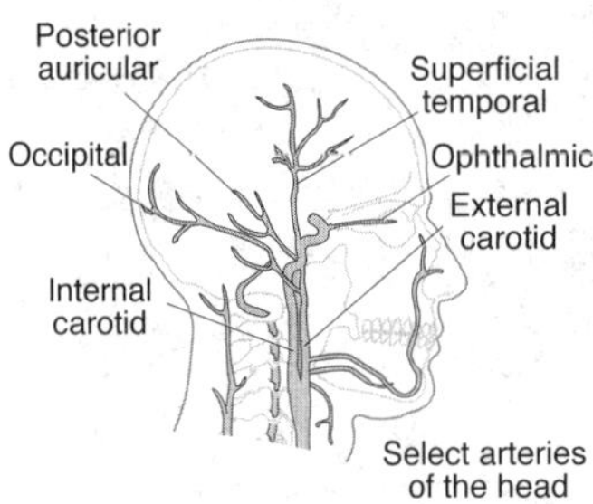

Select arteries of the head

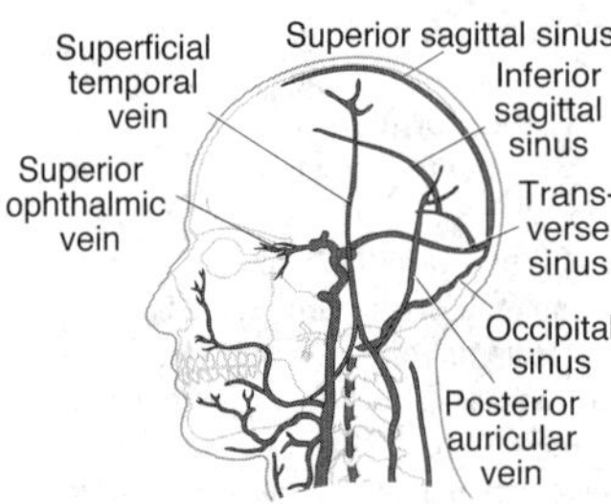

Select veins of the head

In Scimitar syndrome, one lobe of the left lung is hypoplastic leading to a right shift by the heart. PAPVR is usually present, the thoracic aorta or the celiac axis supplies blood to the aorta, and there are diaphragmatic and thoracic defects.

Persistent left superior vena cava (LSVC), the most common thoracic venous anomaly, is a remnant of a structure normally disappearing during embryological development and, if a solitary variant, is seldom symptomatic or significant.

747.5 Congenital absence or hypoplasia of umbilical artery

747.60 Congenital anomaly of the peripheral vascular system, unspecified site

747.61 Congenital gastrointestinal vessel anomaly

747.62 Congenital renal vessel anomaly

747.63 Congenital upper limb vessel anomaly

747.64 Congenital lower limb vessel anomaly

747.69 Congenital anomaly of other specified site of peripheral vascular system

747.81 Congenital anomaly of cerebrovascular system

747.82 Congenital spinal vessel anomaly

747.83 Persistent fetal circulation

747.89 Other specified congenital anomaly of circulatory system

747.9 Unspecified congenital anomaly of circulatory system

Documentation Issues

Documentation must be clear and concise for accurate code selection. The physician must identify the specific vessel involved in the arteriovenous malformation for the most appropriate code to be assigned.

Coding Clarification

Cardiac Outflow Tract Obstruction: This congenital anomaly should be reported with code 747.3 *Congenital anomalies of pulmonary artery.* Included in this code are other anomalies such as atresia, agenesis, stenosis, coarctation, and hypoplasia of the pulmonary artery as well as pulmonary arteriovenous aneurysms.

Spinal Arteriovenous Malformation: Spinal A-V malformations are anomalous communications between a vein and an artery that are congenital in nature. Congenital A-V malformations are caused by persistent embryonic vessels that fail to differentiate into veins and arteries. Spinal dural A-V malformations are the most common type in adults. These lesions develop progressive sensory motor symptoms ranging from painful paraparesis to acute quadriplegia. Report with code 747.82 *Congenital spinal vessel anomaly.*

Coding Scenario

A patient is admitted for a resection of a spinal dural arteriovenous malformation.

> Code assignment: 747.82 *Congenital spinal vessel anomaly*

A patient is diagnosed with right outflow tract obstruction.

> Code assignment: 747.3 *Congenital anomalies of pulmonary artery*

748 Congenital anomalies of respiratory system

748.0 Congenital choanal atresia

748.1 Other congenital anomaly of nose

748.2 Congenital web of larynx

748.3 Other congenital anomaly of larynx, trachea, and bronchus

748.4 Congenital cystic lung

 © 2004 Ingenix, Inc.

748.5	Congenital agenesis, hypoplasia, and dysplasia of lung
748.60	Unspecified congenital anomaly of lung
748.61	Congenital bronchiectasis
748.69	Other congenital anomaly of lung
748.8	Other specified congenital anomaly of respiratory system
748.9	Unspecified congenital anomaly of respiratory system

Coding Clarification

Excluded from this rubric is congenital defect of the diaphragm, which is reported with 756.6.

749 Cleft palate and cleft lip

Cleft palate is the fourth most common birth defect and the most common facial birth defect, affecting approximately one out of every 700 infants. While it is associated with multiple defect syndromes, it is typically associated with a cleft lip, occurring in the first few weeks of fetal development, and is multifactorial in cause. A cleft palate is repaired at 6 to 12 months of age and may require follow up surgery at a later age. If the cleft involves the gum line, an alveolar bone graft is used in the restorative surgery.

749.00	Unspecified cleft palate
749.01	Unilateral cleft palate, complete
749.02	Unilateral cleft palate, incomplete
749.03	Bilateral cleft palate, complete
749.04	Bilateral cleft palate, incomplete
749.10	Unspecified cleft lip
749.11	Unilateral cleft lip, complete
749.12	Unilateral cleft lip, incomplete
749.13	Bilateral cleft lip, complete
749.14	Bilateral cleft lip, incomplete
749.20	Unspecified cleft palate with cleft lip
749.21	Unilateral cleft palate with cleft lip, complete
749.22	Unilateral cleft palate with cleft lip, incomplete
749.23	Bilateral cleft palate with cleft lip, complete
749.24	Bilateral cleft palate with cleft lip, incomplete
749.25	Other combinations of cleft palate with cleft lip

750 Other congenital anomalies of upper alimentary tract

750.0	Tongue tie
750.10	Congenital anomaly of tongue, unspecified
750.11	Aglossia

Aglossia is absence of the tongue. It is seen in Hanhart syndrome, a condition marked by absent tongue and serious anomalies of the limbs.

750.12	Congenital adhesions of tongue
750.13	Congenital fissure of tongue

Bifid tongue occurs when the tongue buds fail to develop normally. It is seen most often in South America.

750.15	Macroglossia

Macroglossia is an abnormally large tongue.

750.16	Microglossia

Microglossia is an abnormally small tongue.

750.19	Other congenital anomaly of tongue
750.21	Congenital absence of salivary gland
750.22	Congenital accessory salivary gland
750.23	Congenital atresia, salivary duct
750.24	Congenital fistula of salivary gland
750.25	Congenital fistula of lip
750.26	Other specified congenital anomalies of mouth
750.27	Congenital diverticulum of pharynx

A pharyngeal pouch is an abnormal pocket in the wall of the pharynx, causing difficulty in swallowing.

750.29	Other specified congenital anomaly of pharynx
753.3	Other specified congenital anomalies of kidney

A tracheoesophageal fistula, which is an abnormal opening between the trachea and the esophagus, must be repaired immediately after birth. In esophageal atresia, the esophagus ends in a blind pouch. Even though the esophagus ends in a blind pouch, it is essential that newborns are able to suck and swallow. Surgical intervention temporarily diverts the esophagus to an opening in the neck, while the infant's nutrition is maintained by IV feedings.

Esophageal stenosis is an abnormally narrowed lumen of the esophagus associated with vomiting and dysphagia.

750.4	Other specified congenital anomaly of esophagus
750.5	Congenital hypertrophic pyloric stenosis

Hypertrophic pyloric stenosis is the most common cause of surgery in the young infant, excluding hernia surgery. In this condition, the outlet to the intestines becomes blocked, leading to projectile vomiting, electrolyte imbalances, and dehydration. The condition is often diagnosed between 2 and 4 weeks of age. Pyloromyotomy may be delayed until an electrolyte disturbance or dehydration is corrected.

750.6 Congenital hiatus hernia

A hiatal hernia is an upward displacement of the stomach through the esophageal hiatus into the mediastinal cavity, leading to esophageal reflux disease. It is always corrected.

750.7 Other specified congenital anomalies of stomach

Cardiospasm is the failure of the cardiac sphincter to relax, leading to aperistalsis. In hourglass stomach, fibrous bands pinch in the stomach, giving it an hourglass appearance. When the stomach is transposed, it lies on the right side of the abdomen. Megalogastria is an abnormally large stomach and microgastria is an abnormally small stomach.

750.8 Other specified congenital anomalies of upper alimentary tract

750.9 Unspecified congenital anomaly of upper alimentary tract

Coding Clarification

This rubric excludes congenital dentofacial anomalies classified to 524.0-524.9.

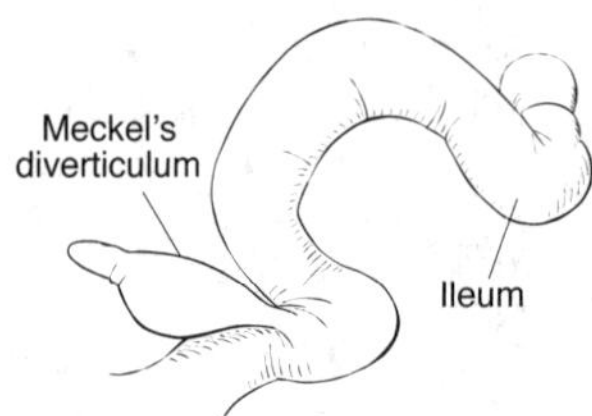

The diverticulum pouch is often found about 50 cm from the ileocecal junction

751 *Other congenital anomalies of digestive system*

751.0 Meckel's diverticulum

Meckel's diverticulum is a sacculation of the distal ileum caused by failure of the vitelline duct to atrophy. It is the most frequently occurring digestive malformation and usually presents with massive dark red rectal bleeding which is often painless to the child. Strangulation or intussusception can occur.

751.1 Congenital atresia and stenosis of small intestine

Atresia of the small intestine usually affects the ileum and is associated with trisomy-21 (Down syndrome) if it appears in the duodenum. It is diagnosed in utero through ultrasound or shortly after birth and treated with resection and primary anastomosis.

751.2 Congenital atresia and stenosis of large intestine, rectum, and anal canal

Imperforate anus is diagnosed on birth. The infant is given a diverting colostomy and corrective surgery is performed later.

751.3 Hirschsprung's disease and other congenital functional disorders of colon

Hirschsprung's disease is a massive distention of the colon with associated inability to defecate due to lack of innervation of the affected portion of the colon. It has familial associations and is more commonly seen in males. The condition is often diagnosed about 48 hours after birth, as the infant is unable to pass meconium, and treatment is immediate to prevent the onset of enterocolitis.

751.4 Congenital anomalies of intestinal fixation

Volvulus is a potential symptom of malrotation of the intestine, leading to strangulation and intestinal infarction through choking off the mesenteric artery.

751.5 Other congenital anomalies of intestine

Dolichocolon is an abnormally long colon.

A persistent cloaca is the third level of a developmental anomaly involving the persistence of a urogenital sinus. In this condition, there is a single orifice behind the clitoris and agenesis of the anus and vagina. Treatment is delayed until the child is at least 1 year of age. A colostomy is performed after birth as a temporary measure and the infant is catheterized intermittently until corrective surgery is performed.

751.60 Unspecified congenital anomaly of gallbladder, bile ducts, and liver

751.61 Congenital biliary atresia

Biliary atresia is the lack of patency of the extrahepatic ducts thought to be an obliterative process rather than a developmental anomaly. It is a serious condition, which may lead to cirrhosis of the liver. Approximately 10 percent of the cases are associated with multiple malformations, the most common being polysplenia (multiple right-sided spleens, a midline liver, a pre-duodenal portal vein, and cardiac malformations).

751.62 Congenital cystic disease of liver

Congenital polycystic disease of the liver involves the formation of numerous cysts that block the drainage of bile.

751.69 Other congenital anomaly of gallbladder, bile ducts, and liver

When the liver or gallbladder is characterized as floating, the organ is displaced and moveable.

751.7 Congenital anomalies of pancreas

If the pancreas either does not develop (agenesis) or is extremely underdeveloped (hypoplasia), intrauterine growth is retarded due to lack of the

740–759

 © 2004 Ingenix, Inc.

insulin, which would normally be secreted by the pancreas.

751.8 Other specified congenital anomalies of digestive system

751.9 Unspecified congenital anomaly of digestive system

752 Congenital anomalies of genital organs

752.0 Congenital anomalies of ovaries

Ovarian agenesis is associated with low set ears, a high palate, mental retardation, and edema of the extremities. The genitalia may be ambiguous. Without the estrogen produced by the ovaries, breast development and menarche do not occur.

A streak ovary contains streaks of fibrous stroma where germ cells should reside. Germ cells are absent.

752.10 Unspecified congenital anomaly of fallopian tubes and broad ligaments

752.11 Embryonic cyst of fallopian tubes and broad ligaments

Gartner's duct stretches from the parovarium to the vagina. The epoophoron is a rudimentary structure composed of Gartner's duct and up to 15 transverse ducts.

752.19 Other congenital anomaly of fallopian tubes and broad ligaments

752.2 Congenital doubling of uterus

A didelphic uterus is associated with a septate vagina. It has two cervices and two small uteri. An expectant mother with a didelphic uterus may have a difficult time bringing a child to term.

752.3 Other congenital anomaly of uterus

A bicornuate uterus has two uterine cavities correctable by surgery.

A unicornuate uterus has only one lateral half and usually only one fallopian tube. This condition is associated with a high rate of miscarriage.

752.40 Unspecified congenital anomaly of cervix, vagina, and external female genitalia

752.41 Embryonic cyst of cervix, vagina, and external female genitalia

752.42 Imperforate hymen

752.49 Other congenital anomaly of cervix, vagina, and external female genitalia

Synechia vulvae are fused labia minora. There is a tiny opening that permits the flow of urine from the urethra.

752.51 Undescended testis

In true cryptorchism, the testis is concealed within the abdominal cavity. In incomplete cryptorchism, the testis has partially descended within the inguinal canal and arrested. Both conditions are associated with low birth weight, with incidence increasing as birth weights decrease. Cryptorchism must be corrected through orchiopexy by age 2 or sterility will result.

752.52 Retractile testis

A retractile testis can be manipulated into the scrotum without strain.

752.61 Hypospadias

In hypospadias, the urethral meatus lies on the ventral portion of the penile shaft. Corrective surgery should be performed by 8 to 12 months of age.

752.62 Epispadias

Epispadias is rare, with the urethral meatus on the dorsal portion of the penile shaft. The penis curves upward.

752.63 Congenital chordee

Chordee is the downward bowing of the penis and is associated with hypospadias, although it may occur as a solitary variant.

752.64 Micropenis

Micropenis, a form of ambiguous genitalia, is caused by a lack of endocrine output during fetal life, specifically lack of testosterone. Typically the penis, though small, is normal in function. Testosterone shots administered in infancy allow the penis to obtain normal size.

752.65 Hidden penis

752.69 Other penile anomalies

Penile agenesis is so rare that it occurs in one out of 30 million births. The scrotum is usually normal, though the testicles are undescended.

Penile duplication presents as a bifid penis with two corpora cavernosa and two hemialgias and may range from the glans only to duplication of the entire urogenital tract.

In torsion of the penis, the rotation is typically to the left.

752.7 Indeterminate sex and pseudohermaphroditism

Indeterminate sex, pseudohermaphroditism, and intersex are interchangeable terms. This category excludes all forms of this condition but gonadal dysgenesis. As in other forms of the condition, in hermaphroditism due to gonadal dysgenesis, the external genitalia do not match the genetic makeup of the individual. The fetus begins as a female and, if the chromosome pattern is XY, develops as a boy. For reasons unrelated to the other causes of the condition, gonadal development is subpart, leading to the birth of an infant of ambiguous sex.

752.81 Scrotal transposition

752.89 Other specified anomalies of genital organs

752.9 Unspecified congenital anomaly of genital organs

Documentation Issues

If the documentation identifies congenital chordee with hypospadias, both should be coded separately. Congenital chordee (752.63) is commonly noted as an associated condition with hypospadias (752.61).

Coding Clarification

Excluded from this rubric are syndromes associated with anomalies in the number and form of chromosomes (758.0-758.9) and testicular feminization syndrome (257.8).

Epispadias: This condition is a partial or complete dorsal fusion anomaly of the urethra. It may appear in both male and female patients, but is typically seen in males. As a male defect it is marked by the urethral opening on the dorsal surface of the penis; in females it appears as a slit in the upper wall of the urethra. Classically this condition is seen in patients with exstrophy of the bladder. Report with code 752.62 *Epispadias*.

Hydatid Cyst of Morgagni: In female patients, this condition would be reported with code 752.11 *Embryonic cyst of fallopian tubes and broad ligaments*. If identified in a male patient, report with code 752.89 *Other specified anomalies of genital organs*.

Hypospadias: A male developmental defect characterized by an a abnormal opening of the urethra on the ventral surface of the penis or on the perineum; it is also a rare defect in the vagina of females. Report with code 752.61 *Hypospadias*.

Micropenis or Microphallus: This condition is due to the developmental failure of the penis caused by either failure of testosterone to stimulate the tissues or failure of the tissues to respond to testosterone stimulation. Report with code 752.64 *Micropenis*.

Coding Scenario

A 16-month-old boy is admitted for surgical repair of hypospadias and congenital chordee.

> Code assignment: 752.63 *Congenital chordee* and 752.61 *Hypospadias*

A 29-year-old female is admitted for tubal pregnancy. The patient undergoes a left salpingectomy for removal of the tubal pregnancy. A pathology report confirms the diagnosis and identifies an embryonic cyst. The physician's final diagnostic statement is fallopian tube pregnancy and hydatid cyst of Morgagni.

> Code assignment: 633.10 *Tubal pregnancy* and 752.11 *Embryonic cyst of fallopian tubes and broad ligaments*

753 Congenital anomalies of urinary system

753.0 Congenital renal agenesis and dysgenesis

Renal agenesis can be either bilateral or unilateral. When bilateral, the condition is terminal due to its affect on other organs. In bilateral agenesis of the kidneys, the fetus lives in an environment of oligohydramnios, which prevents normal development of the lungs. (The lungs are dependent on a moist environment for normal development.)

753.10 Unspecified congenital cystic kidney disease

753.11 Congenital single renal cyst

There is evidence that a single congenital renal cyst is a marker for polycystic kidney disease.

753.12 Congenital polycystic kidney, unspecified type

753.13 Congenital polycystic kidney, autosomal dominant

Polycystic kidney disease, autosomal-dominant, is a progressive disease of adult onset characterized by bilateral cysts. The kidneys are enlarged and their function is impaired.

753.14 Congenital polycystic kidney, autosomal recessive

Polycystic kidney disease, autosomal-recessive, has early childhood onset. There are multiple cysts in the kidneys and liver, leading to failure of both organs.

753.15 Congenital renal dysplasia

753.16 Congenital medullary cystic kidney

Medullary cystic kidney is a disease of the renal tubules leading to proteinuria and renal failure.

753.17 Congenital medullary sponge kidney

A medullary sponge kidney demonstrates dilation of the tubules. It may be symptomatic if calcinosis develops in the tubules, leading to renal insufficiency.

753.19 Other specified congenital cystic kidney disease

753.20 Unspecified obstructive defect of renal pelvis and ureter

753.21 Congenital obstruction of ureteropelvic junction

Congenital obstruction of the ureteropelvic junction is the most common urinary tract anomaly. Its appearance is associated with other anomalies of the urinary tract such as horseshoe kidney, ectopic kidney, multicystic, and dysplastic kidney. The condition may be diagnosed antenatally and is corrected within the first few months of life. A pyeloplasty promotes normal growth and development of urinary tract structures.

753.22 Congenital obstruction of ureterovesical junction

740–759

© 2004 Ingenix, Inc.

Obstruction of the ureterovesical junction often occurs with ureteropelvic obstruction.

753.23 Congenital ureterocele

753.29 Other obstructive defect of renal pelvis and ureter

753.3 Other specified congenital anomalies of kidney

Horseshoe and discoid kidneys are the products of fusion anomalies. A discoid kidney is fused medially at both poles, while a horseshoe kidney is fused at the lower poles. Horseshoe kidney may be associated with Wilms' tumor and anomalies of a number of body systems. An ectopic kidney is on the opposite side of its ureter.

753.4 Other specified congenital anomalies of ureter

Duplication occurs most frequently among ureteral anomalies.

753.5 Exstrophy of urinary bladder

Exstrophy of the bladder is the absence of part of the lower abdominal wall and part of the anterior bladder wall, allowing the posterior bladder wall to protrude. The bladder must be closed immediately after birth, a first stage of complex reconstructive surgeries.

753.6 Congenital atresia and stenosis of urethra and bladder neck

Urethral atresia is successfully treated antenatally by placement of a vesicoamniotic shunt.

753.7 Congenital anomalies of urachus

A urachal cyst presents as an extraperitoneal mass near the umbilicus. It may become infected or rupture, possibly causing peritonitis if it drains into the peritoneum rather than through the umbilicus.

753.8 Other specified congenital anomaly of bladder and urethra

Congenital diverticulum of the bladder, also known as Hutch diverticulum, occurs where the ureter enters the bladder and may cause obstruction and deviation. The diverticulum threatens the competence of the ureterovesical valve, leading to vesicoureteral reflux.

Female hypospadias presents the urinary meatus fairly near its normal position; however, it is associated with other anomalies of the urinary-genital tract.

753.9 Unspecified congenital anomaly of urinary system

754 Certain congenital musculoskeletal deformities

Defects in this rubric are limited by ICD-9-CM notes to those defects caused by extrinsic factors (e.g., intrauterine problems including malposition and pressure).

754.0 Congenital musculoskeletal deformities of skull, face, and jaw

Dolichocephaly is a skull that is long in relation to the anterior/posterior axis. Plagiocephaly is a lopsided and twisted skull. Potter's facies is a facial appearance characterized by deep folds under the eyes. The folds are caused by oligohydramnios related to agenesis of the kidneys.

754.1 Congenital musculoskeletal deformity of sternocleidomastoid muscle

Sternocleidomastoid torticollis is apparent after birth. Because there are other non-muscular causes of congenital torticollis, the pediatrician must ascertain the cause. If it is muscular, the child should be checked for hip dysplasia, as it is frequently associated with muscular torticollis. Treatment involves daily stretching for the first year of life. If torticollis persists, surgery is necessary to correct the asymmetrical tilt to the face.

754.2 Congenital musculoskeletal deformity of spine

Congenital scoliosis, an anterior/posterior plane vertebral malformation, may appear in three variants. It can be an isolated deformity or be associated with other multi-system deformities. Approximately 20 percent of the cases include genitourinary malformations, while another 20 percent show coexistent cord defects.

Lordosis is an exaggerated inward curve in the low back.

Dislocation and subluxation of the hip occur in conjunction with ligamentous laxity of the hip joint capsules. Females are affected nine times out of 10 and there is a 30 to 50 percent incidence among breech births. Osteoarthritis, gait abnormalities, pains, and unequal leg length may result if left untreated.

754.30 Congenital dislocation of hip, unilateral

754.31 Congenital dislocation of hip, bilateral

754.32 Congenital subluxation of hip, unilateral

754.33 Congenital subluxation of hip, bilateral

754.35 Congenital dislocation of one hip with subluxation of other hip

Bowing of the long bones can occur alone or as part of a series of anomalies, of which osteogenesis imperfecta is the most known.

754.40 Congenital genu recurvatum

754.41 Congenital dislocation of knee (with genu recurvatum)

754.42 Congenital bowing of femur

754.43 Congenital bowing of tibia and fibula

754.44 Congenital bowing of unspecified long bones of leg

754.50 Congenital talipes varus

740–759

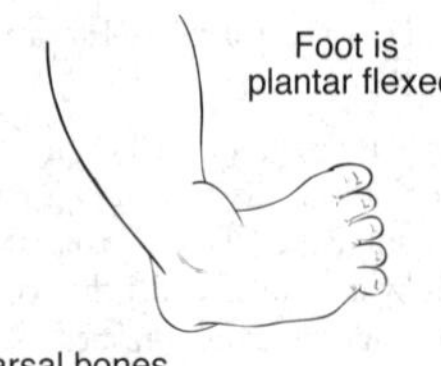

The congenital deformity known as clubfoot is usually bilateral. The bones and soft tissues may be normal in shape but are locked in a tortured position.

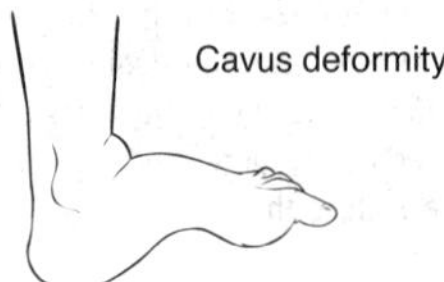

In talipes varus, the foot rotates outward, promoting walking on the outside of the sole.

754.51 Congenital talipes equinovarus

Also known as clubfoot, talipes equinovarus is a condition in which the sole points straight back. As is the case with the other foot deformities, talipes equinovarus arises from improper alignment of the baby in utero.

754.52 Congenital metatarsus primus varus

Metatarsus primus varus is a deformity of the cuneiform bone.

754.53 Congenital metatarsus varus

Metatarsus varus is a toeing-in deformity.

754.59 Other congenital varus deformity of feet

Talipes calcaneovarus has the foot pointing out and down.

754.60 Congenital talipes valgus

Talipes valgus is a deformity in which the foot toes in, promoting walking on the inside of the soles.

754.61 Congenital pes planus

Congenital flat foot is a more severe problem than acquired flat foot.

754.62 Talipes calcaneovalgus

Talipes calcaneovalgus, in which the foot toes out, is the most common foot deformity.

754.69 Other congenital valgus deformity of feet

Talipes equinovalgus is a form of clubfoot in which the heel points outward.

754.70 Unspecified talipes

754.71 Talipes cavus

In talipes cavus, there is muscle imbalance and weakness due to many causes. The forefoot is adducted and the heel is valgus.

754.79 Other congenital deformity of feet

Pectus excavatum produces a deep indentation in the chest at the level of the breastbone. It may be a solitary phenomenon, but has a strong association with Marfan's syndrome and cardiac anomalies. More males than females are affected by the condition. Pectus carinatum, which causes the chest to curve outward like a pigeon's breast, is associated with other anomalies and is primarily a cosmetic problem.

754.81 Pectus excavatum

754.82 Pectus carinatum

754.89 Other specified nonteratogenic anomalies

755 Other congenital anomalies of limbs

Intrinsic and extrinsic factors may cause the anomalies reported by this rubric. Intrinsic factors include errors of fetal development. Extrinsic factors are the result of intrauterine problems including malposition and pressure and comprise only 2 percent of all congenital anomalies.

Polydactyly may be genetic, solitary, or part of numerous syndromes. The supernumerary digits may be rudimentary or normally formed.

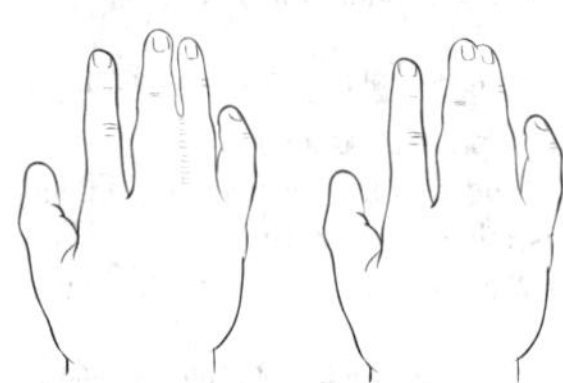

Syndactyly of digits (webbing)
Image at right depicts a case involving fusion of bone and nail

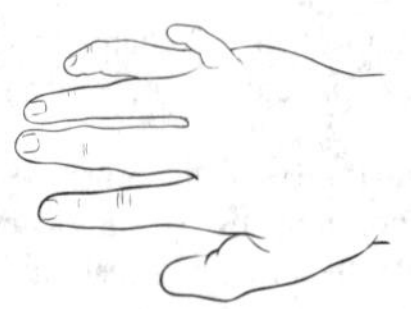

Supernumerary digit

755.00 Polydactyly, unspecified digits

755.01 Polydactyly of fingers

755.02 Polydactyly of toes

Syndactyly is genetically linked and may appear in conjunction with other syndromes. When the webbing is confined to the skin, surgery is generally performed at 6 months of age to enhance normal digit

740–759

© 2004 Ingenix, Inc.

development. The corrective operation involves splitting the webbing and applying skin grafts. When all five bones are fused, the situation is more complex and surgery rarely is able to provide optimal function.

755.10 Syndactyly of multiple and unspecified sites

755.11 Syndactyly of fingers without fusion of bone

755.12 Syndactyly of fingers with fusion of bone

755.13 Syndactyly of toes without fusion of bone

755.14 Syndactyly of toes with fusion of bone

755.20 Congenital unspecified reduction deformity of upper limb

Ectromelia is hypoplasia of the long bones in the upper limb. In hemimelia, a part of the bone of the upper limb is missing.

755.21 Congenital transverse deficiency of upper limb

Amelia is the congenital absence of the upper limb.

Congenital amputation of any limb may be due to constriction by fibrous amniotic bands or to teratogenic factors.

755.22 Congenital longitudinal deficiency of upper limb, not elsewhere classified

In complete phocomelia, the hands are attached to the trunk. In incomplete phocomelia, there may be a rudimentary long bone.

755.23 Congenital longitudinal deficiency, combined, involving humerus, radius, and ulna (complete or incomplete)

755.24 Congenital longitudinal deficiency, humeral, complete or partial (with or without distal deficiencies, incomplete)

Proximal phocomelia means the absence of a humerus.

755.25 Congenital longitudinal deficiency, radioulnar, complete or partial (with or without distal deficiencies, incomplete)

755.26 Congenital longitudinal deficiency, radial, complete or partial (with or without distal deficiencies, incomplete)

755.27 Congenital longitudinal deficiency, ulnar, complete or partial (with or without distal deficiencies, incomplete)

755.28 Congenital longitudinal deficiency, carpals or metacarpals, complete or partial (with or without incomplete phalangeal deficiency)

755.29 Congenital longitudinal deficiency, phalanges, complete or partial

755.30 Congenital unspecified reduction deformity of lower limb

Ectromelia is hypoplasia of the long bones in the lower limb. In hemimelia, a part of the bone of the lower limb is missing.

755.31 Congenital transverse deficiency of lower limb

Amelia is the congenital absence of one or more lower limbs.

755.32 Congenital longitudinal deficiency of lower limb, not elsewhere classified

755.33 Congenital longitudinal deficiency, combined, involving femur, tibia, and fibula (complete or incomplete)

Complete phocomelia of the lower limb means the direct attachment of the feet to the trunk.

755.34 Congenital longitudinal deficiency, femoral, complete or partial (with or without distal deficiencies, incomplete)

Proximal phocomelia of the lower limb means the absence of a femur.

755.35 Congenital longitudinal deficiency, tibiofibular, complete or partial (with or without distal deficiencies, incomplete)

755.36 Congenital longitudinal deficiency, tibia, complete or partial (with or without distal deficiencies, incomplete)

755.37 Congenital longitudinal deficiency, fibular, complete or partial (with or without distal deficiencies, incomplete)

755.38 Congenital longitudinal deficiency, tarsals or metatarsals, complete or partial (with or without incomplete phalangeal deficiency)

755.39 Congenital longitudinal deficiency, phalanges, complete or partial

755.4 Congenital reduction deformities, unspecified limb

755.50 Unspecified congenital anomaly of upper limb

755.51 Congenital deformity of clavicle

755.52 Congenital elevation of scapula

Sprengel's deformity connotes a hypoplastic and elevated scapula. Often, the hypoplastic trapezius, deltoid, or rhomboid is absent. The result may be torticollis, scoliosis, or limb length discrepancy.

755.53 Radioulnar synostosis

The forearm is permanently pronated in radioulnar synostosis. Most cases do not require surgery.

755.54 Madelung's deformity

Madelung's deformity is a dysplasia of the radius involving an exaggerated radial inclination, a short forearm, dorsal dislocation of the ulnar head, and a "V" shaped proximal carpal row. The condition may arise from an abnormal fibrous band tethering the sigmoid notch of the radius proximally to the ulna.

755.55 Acrocephalosyndactyly

Apert's syndrome involves premature fusing of the cranial sutures, asymmetrical facies, webbed hands, and progressive calcification and fusion of the bones of the hands, feet, and cervical spine.

755.56 Accessory carpal bones

755.57 Macrodactylia (fingers)

755.58 Congenital cleft hand

Lobster-claw hand, a rare disorder, affects the phalanges of the middle finger. The corresponding metacarpal may be absent and the hand is separated into medial and lateral sections by a deep cleft.

755.59 Other congenital anomaly of upper limb, including shoulder girdle

Cleidocranial dysostosis, or Scheutthauer-Marie-Sainton syndrome, is a genetic disease most often characterized by the absence or hypoplastic development of the collarbone.

In cubitus valgus, the forearm deviates away from the midline on extension. In cubitus varus, the forearm deviates inward when extended.

The angle between the long axes of the neck and shaft of the femur is 120-125 degrees in the normal individual. In coxa valga, this angle is increased to approximately 140 degrees, creating extreme adduction with the possibility of a superior dislocation in the immature hip. In coxa vara, this angle is abnormally decreased, creating an extreme abduction. Coxa vara is much more common than coxa valga.

755.60 Unspecified congenital anomaly of lower limb

755.61 Congenital coxa valga

755.62 Congenital coxa vara

755.63 Other congenital deformity of hip (joint)

755.64 Congenital deformity of knee (joint)

Genu valgum (knock-knee) is a normal part of development that may require surgical intervention if it persists beyond 10 or 12 years of age and if there are more than three inches between the ankles.

755.65 Macrodactylia of toes

755.66 Other congenital anomaly of toes

The correction of hallux valgus is postponed until skeletal maturity.

755.67 Congenital anomalies of foot, not elsewhere classified

"Coalition" and "bar" refer to an abnormal union of bones that are normally separated.

755.69 Other congenital anomaly of lower limb, including pelvic girdle

755.8 Other specified congenital anomalies of unspecified limb

Larsen's syndrome is a genetic, multi-system disorder that presents with multiple dislocations and other bony irregularities, as well as cylindrical fingers and unusual facies. Other symptoms include mental retardation, short stature, and cardiac abnormalities.

755.9 Unspecified congenital anomaly of unspecified limb

756 Other congenital musculoskeletal anomalies

756.0 Congenital anomalies of skull and face bones

Acrocephaly is a pointed vault of the skull.

Craniosynostosis is an abnormal fusing of the cranial sutures. In the newborn, the cranial sutures are open, serving two desired outcomes: normal delivery with a malleable head and the ability of the skull to grow to accommodate the growing brain. The sagittal suture is the most frequently occurring site of synostosis and is the least likely to be associated with genetics. Any bilateral craniosynostosis is a flag for a possible genetic relationship.

Corrective surgery is performed primarily for cosmetic reasons, although in some cases, the facial bones are affected or the brain does not have enough room and the surgery is justified for both cosmetic and medical reasons.

Oxycephaly describes a cone-shaped head.

Platybasia is an upward thrust of the odontoid bone through the foramen magnum, causing pressure on the midbrain.

Trigonocephaly is a triangular-shaped head.

Crouzon's disease combines craniosynostosis, exophthalmos, hypoplastic midface, flat sphenoids, and a large mandible. Genetic and spontaneous causes are split 50 percent. Asymmetrical exophthalmos and the large jaw are correctable.

Hypertelorism is an abnormal distance between the eyes.

First arch syndrome refers to the developmental stage of the first arch, and involves numerous craniofacial anomalies.

Oculo-auricle-vertebral (OAV) syndrome is synonymous with Goldenhar's syndrome and is non-hereditary.

Greig's syndrome is a hereditary disease involving multiple deformities of the hands and feet, macrocephaly, hypertelorism, mild mental retardation, and a broad, flat nose.

Hallman Streiff syndrome is an oculo-mandibula-facial syndrome inclusive of short stature and congenital cataracts.

Treacher-Collins, synonymous with Franceschetti's syndrome, is genetically driven and involves an eye slant, lip coloboma, micrognathia, microtia, hypoplastic zygomatic arches, and macrostomia.

756.10 Congenital anomaly of spine, unspecified

756.11 Congenital spondylolysis, lumbosacral region

Spondylolysis is a defect in the vertebra, usually L5, filled with fibrous tissue containing nerve endings that are painful due to compression.

756.12 Congenital spondylolisthesis

Spondylolisthesis is the slipping forward of one vertebra over another, often L5, and is usually associated with a spinal defect such as spina bifida occulta. Females are more often affected.

756.13 Congenital absence of vertebra

756.14 Hemivertebra

A hemivertebra, a condition that can promote scoliosis, is treated with fusion and bone graft to render it equal in height.

756.15 Congenital fusion of spine (vertebra)

Bertolotti's syndrome involves sacralization of the L4-L5 vertebrae. An L5 transverse process forms a pseudoarthrosis with the ala of S1, increasing the tilt of the vertebra and enhancing the possibility of scoliosis.

756.16 Klippel-Feil syndrome

A short neck caused by the fusion of existing cervical vertebrae and the absence of at least one cervical vertebra characterize Klippel-Feil syndrome, also known as brevicollis. It has a high rate of associated malformations or syndromes and affects females.

756.17 Spina bifida occulta

Spina bifida occulta is fairly benign in adults if not causing apparent problems during childhood. The disorder is vertebral, as in spina bifida aperta; however, skin covers the defect in the occulta form. In severe forms, which accounts for about 2 percent of the occulta cases, the condition is called spinal dysraphism to distinguish it from its benign presentation.

756.19 Other congenital anomaly of spine

756.2 Cervical rib

A cervical rib is a supernumerary rib in the cervical region, which can lead to thoracic outlet syndrome.

756.3 Other congenital anomaly of ribs and sternum

756.4 Chondrodystrophy

Chondrodystrophy, a defect of the cartilage growth mechanism, is the primary cause of short limb dwarfism, a condition characterized by decreased length of the long bones, although the diameter is not affected. The condition is hereditary.

Dyschondroplasia typically affects unilateral joints and involves knobby fingers and genu valgus.

Jeune's syndrome is an asphyxiating thoracic dystrophy.

Maffucci's syndrome, another term for Kast's syndrome, is a non-hereditary dyschondroplasia and involves soft tissue hemangiomata, cyst-like bone lesions, and multiple phleboliths. The hemangiomata can enhance dysplastia.

756.50 Unspecified congenital osteodystrophy

756.51 Osteogenesis imperfecta

Osteogenesis imperfecta is a hereditary collagen disorder that produces very brittle bones. Type 1 is the most common and mildest form, with the affected person's stature being normal or near normal. Multiple fractures may occur prior to puberty, decreasing later in life. Type II is the most severe, causing death at or soon after birth. Types III and IV are treated with intramedullary rods inserted into the long bones.

756.52 Osteopetrosis

Osteopetrosis produces an overgrowth of bone that spills into the marrow and obliterates the marrow of the bones below the head and the foramina. The loss of marrow leads to anemia and heptad-splenomegaly. Osteopetrosis can lead to sight and hearing impairments because the nerves cannot emerge through their foramina in the skull.

756.53 Osteopoikilosis

Osteopoikilosis, a rare genetic disorder, manifests in multiple areas of increased bone density, although the disorder is often asymptomatic. It is associated with other disorders such as dwarfism or scleroderma.

756.54 Polyostotic fibrous dysplasia of bone

756.55 Chondroectodermal dysplasia

Chondroectodermal dysplasia is characterized by abnormal development of hair, skin, teeth, and cartilage. Polydactyly and heart anomalies are also present.

756.56 Multiple epiphyseal dysplasia

756.59 Other congenital osteodystrophy

McCune-Albright syndrome, which usually affects females, involves bone disease with enhanced potential for fractures, leg deformities, endocrine disease, and skin changes. There is wide variability in the degree of severity.

756.6 Congenital anomaly of diaphragm

756.70 Unspecified congenital anomaly of abdominal wall

756.71 Prune belly syndrome

Prune belly syndrome, also known as Eagle-Barrett disease, manifests in the absence of the lower rectus

740–759

abdominus and the medial portions of the oblique muscles. There are urinary tract anomalies. About 95 percent of infants affected are males and 50 percent of all affected newborns are stillborn or die within two years of birth.

756.79 Other congenital anomalies of abdominal wall

An omphalocele is a defect in the abdominal wall involving the umbilicus. Large omphaloceles contain parts of the intestines that are reduced over time. The condition may be associated with a syndrome or may appear as a solitary variant.

756.81 Congenital absence of muscle and tendon

756.82 Accessory muscle

756.83 Ehlers-Danlos syndrome

Ehlers-Danlos syndrome, a genetic collagen disorder, causes hyperelasticity of the skin, hypermobility of the joints, and fragility of blood vessels. Wound healing is impaired.

756.89 Other specified congenital anomaly of muscle, tendon, fascia, and connective tissue

Use this code for amyotrophia congenita, congenital shortening of tendon, Ayala's disease, Bakwin-Krida syndrome, elongated ligamentum patellae, Fong's syndrome, HOOD syndrome, Krabbe's syndrome, Oestreicher-Turner syndrome, popliteal web syndrome, Pyle-Cohn disease, Schwartz- (Jambul) syndrome, Touraine's syndrome, congenital trigger finger, Turner-Kieser syndrome, and Waardenburg's syndrome.

756.9 Other and unspecified congenital anomaly of musculoskeletal system

Documentation Issues

Because it is not unusual for multiple anomalies to be present, the physician should clearly indicate in the medical record documentation those anomalies that are related vs. those that do not appear to be due to a disease process.

Coding Clarification

Craniosynostosis: This is the premature closure of one or more of the cranial sutures. This premature closure is usually incomplete and affects one suture. It can result in abnormalities of the cranial contour. This condition is classified to code 756.0.

Nager Syndrome: This is a congenital disorder that is also known as preaxial acrofacial dysostosis. In addition to anomalies of the face, patients with this condition may also have cleft palate, hypoplastic or aplastic thumb, hip dislocation, reduced stature, and mild mental retardation.

Code 756.0 is assigned to indicate the congenital anomalies of the skull and face. If any other features of the disease are present that do not appear to be indicated by using this code, those anomalies should be coded separately.

757 Congenital anomalies of the integument

757.0 Hereditary edema of legs

Congenital lymphedema is a disorder of the lymph drainage system affecting the legs. Infection is a constant threat. Garments that avoid compression and the use of gradient pumps are the common treatments.

757.1 Ichthyosis congenita

Ichthyosis congenita refers to scaly skin as a result of an excessive production of skin cells.

Sjögren-Larsson syndrome manifests with dry, scaly skin, as well as mental retardation, speech abnormalities, and spasticity. Retinal degeneration is characteristic in about 50 percent of all cases.

757.2 Dermatoglyphic anomalies

757.31 Congenital ectodermal dysplasia

Congenital ectodermal dysplasia, or hidrotic ED, is an inherited disorder primarily affecting the French. The nails are thick and there is thick skin on the palms and soles, and dark skin on the elbows and knees.

757.32 Congenital vascular hamartomas

Port wine stain, or nevus flammeus, is a hemangioma that is red and flat at birth, which thickens over time.

757.33 Congenital pigmentary anomaly of skin

Urticaria pigmentosa is a self-limiting rash that tends to disappear after puberty.

757.39 Other specified congenital anomaly of skin

Congenital pachydermatocele, or cutis pendula, causes the skin to hang in wrinkled folds.

757.4 Specified congenital anomalies of hair

Congenital alopecia is the failure of hair to grow or develop.

757.5 Specified congenital anomalies of nails

Anonychia is the absence of one or more fingernails.

757.6 Specified congenital anomalies of breast

757.8 Other specified congenital anomalies of the integument

757.9 Unspecified congenital anomaly of the integument

758 Chromosomal anomalies

Chromosomes are divided into two types: autosomes and sex-linked. Of the 23 pairs, only one pair, the 23rd, is related to sex and is distributed as XX in girls and XY in boys. The other 22 pairs are called

© 2004 Ingenix, Inc.

autosomes. The conditions in the 758 category involve anomalies in either the sex chromosome or autosome arrangements.

758.0 Down's syndrome

Down's syndrome is the result of an extra chromosome (trisomy) on the 21st pair of chromosomes. Characteristics include hypertrophy, hearing loss due to the angle of the ear canals, developmental delay, delay in language acquisition, and heart defects.

758.1 Patau's syndrome

Patau's syndrome is also a trisomic condition involving the 13th pair of autosomes. The brain's failure to divide into lobes is a primary characteristic that can affect the senses of sight, smell, and hearing. Lip and palate (typically cleft) anomalies may be present.

758.2 Edwards' syndrome

Edwards' syndrome, a trisomic autosome 18, involves delays in growth, the respiratory system, craniofacial malformations, skeletal defects, and webbing. Mental retardation is another characteristic.

758.31 Cri-du-chat syndrome

Cri-du-chat syndrome, also called cat cry syndrome, results from a deletion of the short arm of the fifth chromosome and may vary from a tiny deletion of one band to the entire small arm. Incidence makes it one of the most common autosomal deletions with variability between 1 in 20,000-50,000 births. Children with cri-du-chat present with an abnormally small head (microcephaly), with accompanying small jaw and chin (micrognathia), low set ears, wide set eyes (hypertelorism), and profound or severe mental retardation and psychomotor problems. The identifying characteristic diagnosed in infants is the unusual, high-pitched, cat cry.

758.32 Velo-cardio-facial syndrome

Velo-cardio-facial syndrome (VCFS) refers to the palate, the heart, and the face, where the most common, identifying signs and symptoms of this syndrome are manifested, although not in every child with VCFS. These characteristic problems include: cleft palate, heart defects, and an elongated face with almond-shaped eyes, a wide nose, and small ears. VCFS is caused by deletion of genes on a specific part of the 22nd chromosome. There is still great variation in the presentation of this disease—up to 30 different problems have been related to it, including feeding problems, weak immune systems, weak musculature, hypothyroidism, short stature, and scoliosis. It affects about 130,000 individuals in the U.S., occurring in approximately 5-8% of all those born with a cleft palate, around 1 in 700 live births.

758.39 Autosomal deletion syndromes, other autosomal deletions

Microdeletions, such as Miller-Dieker and Smith-Magenis syndromes are included under 758.33 other microdeletions. Miller-Dieker syndrome is seen when there is a deletion from the short arm of chromosome 17, sometimes in combination with duplication of the long arm. Also known as agyria (lack of sulci and gyri) and lissencephaly (smooth surface of the brain), it causes death in infancy or early childhood with an array or problems from the multiple developmental defects and abnormalities of the brain that it produces: retarded mental, speech, and motor development, neurological complications, and multiple abnormalities affecting the kidneys, heart, gastrointestinal tract, and other organs.

Smith-Magenis syndrome is also due to a deletion in a certain area of chromosome 17 that results in craniofacial changes, speech delay, hoarse voice, hearing loss in many, and behavioral problems, such as self-destructive head banging, wrist biting, and tearing at nails.

758.4 Balanced autosomal translocation in normal individual

758.5 Other conditions due to autosomal anomalies

758.6 Gonadal dysgenesis

Turner's syndrome, also known as XO syndrome, affects females. It is sex chromosome linked, occurring once every 2,500 births. Characteristics include short stature, ovarian dysgenesis, and associated heart, kidney, and thyroid disorders. Growth hormone and estrogen are used to treat the symptoms.

758.7 Klinefelter's syndrome

Klinefelter's syndrome affects only males, and involves an additional X chromosome, creating a pattern of XXY instead of XY. The condition is divided in mosaic and non-mosaic patients (mosaic implies that not all cells are affected). Characteristics include delayed language development. Injections of testosterone can counter the physical anomalies of the syndrome. Associated disorders are asthma, hypostatic leg ulcers, thrombophlebitis, and osteoporosis. Male breast cancer presents a risk 20 times that of the non-Klinefelter male and there is also an increased incidence of mediastinal germ cell cancer.

A variant of Klinefelter syndrome produces two sets of abnormal sex chromosomes, for an XX YY arrangement. Another variant is XXXXY.

758.81 Other conditions due to sex chromosome anomalies

758.89 Other conditions due to chromosome anomalies

MELAS syndrome is a mitochondrial myopathy that can lead to stroke-like episodes and encephalomyopathy. Patients are increasingly fatigued in this progressive disease.

758.9 Conditions due to anomaly of unspecified chromosome

759 Other and unspecified congenital anomalies

759.0 Congenital anomalies of spleen

Asplenia is a serious condition associated with congenital heart anomalies.

759.1 Congenital anomalies of adrenal gland

Use code 759.1 to report adrenal hypoplasia, or an absent, accessory, or aberrant adrenal gland. Excluded from this code are congenital disorders of steroid metabolism (255.2) and adrenogenital disorders (255.2).

759.2 Congenital anomalies of other endocrine glands

A thyroglossal duct cyst is a fluid-filled connective duct extending from the tongue base to the thyroid. The thyroglossal duct generally disappears during fetal development. This code reports thyroglossal duct cyst, absent parathyroid gland, accessory thyroid gland, or persistent thyroglossal or thyrolingual duct. Excluded from this code are congenital goiter (246.1) and congenital hypothyroidism (243).

759.3 Situs inversus

Situs inversus, or Kartagener's syndrome, is a condition in which the abdominal and/or thoracic organs are in reverse position.

759.4 Conjoined twins

Conjoined twins are born from a single ovum and a shared single placenta. They are always identical. The incidence is one in every 50,000 to 80,000 births, with the highest incidence in Africa and India. The twins can be joined at various sites, the most common being the thoracopagus arrangement of sharing a heart, joined at the chest, followed by omphalopagus, an anterior union at the midtrunk. Most conjoined twins miscarry or are stillborn.

759.5 Tuberous sclerosis

Tuberous sclerosis promotes benign tumors in the vital organs as well as in the eyes and skin, and affects both sexes. This condition can cause epileptic seizures and developmental delays and may be referred to as Bourneville's disease, Epiloia, Bourneville-Pringle syndrome, or Pringle's disease.

759.6 Other congenital hamartoses, not elsewhere classified

Von Hippel-Lindau syndrome involves abnormal growth of the blood vessels leading to hemangiomata and hemangioblastomata. They tend to grow in the retina, brain, cord, and adrenals. Predisposing the affected individuals to kidney cancer, it appears in the fourth decade.

Also use this code to report Jahnke's syndrome, Peutz-Jeghers syndrome, Sturge-Weber (-Dimitri) syndrome, Kalischer's syndrome, Krabbe's cutaneocerebral angioma syndrome, Lawford's syndrome, Milles' syndrome, Shimmer's syndrome, Sturge-Kalischer-Weber syndrome, and Weber-Dimitri syndrome.

759.7 Multiple congenital anomalies, so described

759.81 Prader-Willi syndrome

Prader-Willi syndrome is characterized by several conditions, including hypotonia, hypogonadism, hyperphagia, cognitive impairments, behavioral difficulties, and morbid obesity. The hypothalamus dysfunction leads to the disordered appetite (hyperphagia), which in turn causes the morbid obesity. The disorder is considered to be a deletion error in the genes.

759.82 Marfan's syndrome

Marfan syndrome is a connective tissue disorder, affecting the long limbs, fingers, and toes. Arm span often exceeds height. The face is narrow and sharply featured and the chest may be excavatum or carinatum. The lens may be displaced, causing myopia. Other symptoms include loose joints, weakened aorta and cardiac valves, decreased lung elasticity, and scoliosis.

759.83 Fragile X syndrome

Fragile X syndrome occurs in males and females and involves mental retardation that is often more profound in males.

759.89 Other specified multiple congenital anomalies, so described

This code can be reported to describe congenital malformation syndromes affecting multiple systems, not elsewhere classified, including Alport's syndrome, bird-headed dwarf (Seckel's syndrome), Brachmann-de Lange syndrome, Brachymorphism with ectopic lentis (Marchesani -(Weil) syndrome, Craniocarpotarsal dystrophy (Freeman-Sheldon syndrome), whistling-face syndrome, microencephaly, and dwarfism (Cockayne's syndrome). Other conditions reported with this code include Noonan's syndrome, Orodigitofacial dystosis (Bardet-Biedl) syndrome, Papillon-Lege and Psaume syndrome, Rubinstein-Taybi's syndrome, Smith-Lemli Opitz syndrome, Synophthalmus, and a congenital thoracogastroschisis, umbilical fistula, or cyst.

Laurence-Moon-Biedl syndrome, reported with this code, involves obesity, mental retardation, polydactyly or syndactyly, renal disease, retinitis pigmentosa, genital hypoplasia, and, in males, hypogonadism.

759.9 Unspecified congenital anomaly

740–759

© 2004 Ingenix, Inc.

760–779

Certain Conditions Originating in the Perinatal Period

This chapter classifies conditions that begin during the perinatal period even if death or morbidity occur later. The perinatal period is defined as the period of time occurring before, during, and up to 28 days following birth. These codes are used to classify causes of morbidity and mortality in the fetus or newborn and should never be used on the mother's coding profile. Additional codes can be used to further specify the newborn's condition.

760–763 Maternal Causes of Perinatal Morbidity and Mortality

Use these codes to report fetal or newborn conditions caused by systemic, metabolic, or infectious diseases of the mother. Maternal diseases that can affect the health or life of the fetus or newborn include hypertension, renal disease, urinary or respiratory tract infections, and circulatory diseases (pulmonary embolism, thrombophlebitis). Categories 760-763 also include fetal or newborn conditions caused by maternal nutritional disorders; maternal injury, surgery, or death; maternal ingestion of drugs, chemicals, or alcohol; and maternal complications of labor, delivery, or both.

These codes are reserved for use on the newborn coding profile as a secondary diagnosis to follow a code from rubrics V30-V39 for liveborn infants. They also may be used as a principal diagnosis for a newborn that has been transferred or readmitted for a condition classifiable to codes 760-763. Assign a code from these categories only when there is evidence documented in the chart that the maternal condition has in fact affected the fetus or newborn.

760 Fetus or newborn affected by maternal conditions which may be unrelated to present pregnancy

AHA: Nov-Dec, 1984, 11; Q2, 1989, 14; Q3, 1990, 5; Q2, 1992, 12; Q1, 1994, 8

760.0 Fetus or newborn affected by maternal hypertensive disorders — *fetus or newborn affected by maternal hypertension*
AHA: Nov-Dec, 1984, 11; Q2, 1989, 14; Q3, 1990, 5; Q2, 1992, 12; Q1, 1994, 8

Use code 760.0 to report a fetal or newborn condition caused by maternal hypertension. The hypertension may be benign or malignant, preexisting, transient or gestational, chronic, or secondary (such as that due to renal artery stenosis). The incidence of maternal hypertension varies from 0.5 to 4 percent depending on the race and age of the mother, and averages 2.5 percent. The fetus or infant of a mother with hypertension has a 25 to 30 percent risk of prematurity and a 10 to 15 percent chance of being small for gestation age (SGA).

Therapies include resuscitation at birth for anoxia. Associated conditions include prematurity, alveolar conditions, respiratory distress syndrome, inadequate or erratic brain perfusion, acute tubular necrosis, necrotizing enterocolitis, hypotension, blood pressure peaks, hypovolemia, SGA, hypermagnesemia, thrombocytopenia, and neutropenia.

Use code 760.0 for the fetus or newborn when the maternal conditions have been classified to rubric 642.

760.1 Fetus or newborn affected by maternal renal and urinary tract diseases — *fetus or newborn affected by renal and urinary tract diseases*
AHA: Nov-Dec, 1984, 11; Q2, 1989, 14; Q3, 1990, 5; Q2, 1992, 12; Q1, 1994, 8

Use code 760.1 for the fetus or newborn when the maternal conditions have been classified to rubrics 580-599.

760.2 Fetus or newborn affected by maternal infections — *fetus or newborn affected by maternal infectious disease, but fetus not manifesting that disease*
AHA: Nov-Dec, 1984, 11; Q2, 1989, 14; Q3, 1990, 5; Q2, 1992, 12; Q1, 1994, 8

Use code 760.2 for the fetus or newborn when the maternal infectious disease has been classified to 001-136 and 487, but the fetus or newborn is not manifesting the disease. Excluded from this subcategory are congenital infectious diseases (771.0-771.8) and maternal genital tract and other localized infection (780.8).

760.3 Fetus or newborn affected by other chronic maternal circulatory and respiratory diseases — *fetus or newborn affected by chronic maternal circulatory and respiratory diseases*
AHA: Nov-Dec, 1984, 11; Q2, 1989, 14; Q3, 1990, 5; Q2, 1992, 12; Q1, 1994, 8

Use code 760.3 for the fetus or newborn when the maternal conditions are classifiable to 390-459, 490-519, or 745-748.

760.4 Fetus or newborn affected by maternal nutritional disorders — *fetus or newborn affected by nutritional disorders*
AHA: Nov-Dec, 1984, 11; Q2, 1989, 14; Q3, 1990, 5; Q2, 1992, 12; Q1, 1994, 8

Use code 760.4 for the fetus or newborn when the maternal disorders are classifiable to 260-269. Excluded from this code is fetal malnutrition (764.10-764.29).

760.5 Fetus or newborn affected by maternal injury — *fetus or newborn affected by maternal injury*
AHA: Nov-Dec, 1984, 11; Q2, 1989, 14; Q3, 1990, 5; Q2, 1992, 12; Q1, 1994, 8

Use code 760.5 for the fetus or newborn when the maternal disorders are classifiable to 800-995.

760.6 Fetus or newborn affected by surgical operation on mother

Excluded from code 760.6 are cesarean section for present delivery (763.4); damage to placenta from amniocentesis, cesarean section, or surgical induction (762.1); or previous surgery to uterus or pelvic organs (763.89).

760.70 Noxious influences affecting fetus or newborn via placenta or breast milk, unspecified noxious substance — *fetus or newborn affected by drug NEC*
AHA: Nov-Dec, 1984, 11; Q2, 1989, 14; Q3, 1990, 5; Q3, 1991, 21; Q2, 1992, 12; Q1, 1994, 8

Use code 760.70 when the fetal or newborn condition is caused by maternal ingestion of drugs or chemicals. This includes drugs taken for therapeutic purposes during pregnancy (but excludes drugs taken during labor and delivery, classified to code 763.5), drugs taken before pregnancy is known, and exposure to chemicals through the maternal work place while the fetus is in utero. Most drugs ingested during pregnancy, including their metabolites, cross the placenta and reach the fetus. Therefore, many substances have the potential for affecting the fetus. The specific effects on the fetus or newborn depend on the type of noxious substance.

Associated conditions include limb defects, skeletal and facial anomalies, mental retardation, chromosomal abnormalities, cardiac defects, and central nervous system defects.

760.71 Noxious influences affecting fetus or newborn via placenta or breast milk, alcohol — *fetal alcohol syndrome*
AHA: Nov-Dec, 1984, 11; Q2, 1989, 14; Q3, 1990, 5; Q3, 1991, 21; Q2, 1992, 12; Q1, 1994, 8

Use code 760.71 to report a fetal or newborn condition caused by maternal ingestion of alcohol during pregnancy. This code includes fetal alcohol syndrome (FAS), a condition diagnosed in patients born to chronic alcoholics who drank heavily during pregnancy. Lesser alcohol abuse results in a decreased severity of the manifestations of FAS. It is not known how much alcohol can be consumed safely.

Signs and symptoms of alcohol abuse include jitteriness, diaphoresis, and convulsions; with acute intoxication, stupor or coma, confusion, lethargy, and poor reflex responses; with fetal alcohol syndrome, pre- and postnatal growth retardation, short palpebral fissures, midfacial hypoplasia, low unparallel ears, flattened nasal bridge, and abnormal palmar creases. Toxicology tests of blood or urine reveal the presence of alcohol. Associated conditions include cardiac defects, joint contractures, and mental retardation.

This code is used to report the effects of alcohol on the fetus or newborn, including alcohol withdrawal syndrome. Note that some newborns may suffer from both fetal alcohol syndrome and alcohol withdrawal syndrome, or fetal alcohol syndrome and acute alcohol intoxication.

760.72 Noxious influences affecting fetus or newborn via placenta or breast milk, narcotics

Use code 760.72 to report fetal or newborn conditions caused by maternal ingestion of narcotics during pregnancy. Narcotics include opium, heroin, morphine, codeine, papaverine, and their many synthetics such as Demerol and methadone.

Signs and symptoms of narcotics abuse include drowsiness and "nodding," small or pinpoint pupils, urinary retention, shallow irregular respirations or apnea, and, in severe cases, hypotension, hypothermia, and pulmonary edema. Toxicology tests of blood or urine reveal the presence of narcotics. Therapies include drugs such as naloxone (Narcan).

This subclassification is used to report the effects of narcotics on the fetus or newborn. It excludes drug withdrawal syndrome, which is classified to code 779.5. Note that some newborns may suffer from both drug withdrawal syndrome and other physiopathological effects of narcotics in the perinatal period such as acute intoxication; both conditions should be coded.

760.73 Noxious influences affecting fetus or newborn via placenta or breast milk, hallucinogenic agents

Use code 760.73 to report the fetal or newborn condition caused by maternal ingestion of hallucinogenic agents during pregnancy. Hallucinogenic agents include lysergide (LSD), mescaline, psilocybin, sodium thiopental (STP),

 © 2004 Ingenix, Inc.

marijuana, phencyclidine (PCP), tetrahydrocannabinol (THC), and hashish.

Signs and symptoms of using hallucinogenic agents include dilated pupils, restlessness, hyperreflexia, easy distractibility, and tachycardia. Toxicology tests of blood or urine reveal the presence of hallucinogenics. Therapies include drugs such as diazepam and ammonium chloride.

This subclassification is used to report the effects of hallucinogens on the fetus or newborn. It excludes drug withdrawal syndrome, which is classified to code 779.5. Medical literature indicates that, of all hallucinogens, only chronic marijuana abuse has been associated with drug withdrawal symptoms.

760.74 Noxious influences affecting fetus or newborn via placenta or breast milk, anti-infectives — *fetus affected by antibiotics via placenta or breast milk*
AHA: Nov-Dec, 1984, 11; Q2, 1989, 14; Q3, 1990, 5; Q3, 1991, 21; Q2, 1992, 12; Q1, 1994, 8

Use code 760.74 to report a fetal or newborn condition caused by maternal ingestion of anti-infectives, such as antibiotics, during pregnancy. Antibiotics that have been associated with birth defects include sulfonamides, metronidazole, and tetracycline as well as antibiotics that inhibit deoxyribonucleic acid (DNA) or ribonucleic acid (RNA) synthesis such as actinomycin D, mitomycin C, adenine arabinoside, and idoxuridine.

Associated conditions include nerve damage, inhibition of bone growth, discoloration of teeth due to demineralization of enamel, and connective tissue defects.

760.75 Noxious influences affecting fetus or newborn via placenta or breast milk, cocaine

The physician should document the specific effects of the mother's cocaine use on the newborn, that is, if the newborn exhibited manifestations or mortality, tested positive for cocaine, or is experiencing drug withdrawal syndrome.

Cocaine Addiction in Newborns: Two scenarios may present in newborns who are born to cocaine-addicted mothers. The newborn may exhibit no manifestations of the drug but test positive for cocaine. In this instance, code 760.75 *Cocaine affecting fetus or newborn via placenta or breast milk* is reported. However, the infant may experience drug withdrawal. In these instances, code 779.5 *Drug withdrawal syndrome in newborn* is reported.

Newborn Delivered by Cocaine Abuser/Dependent: When a newborn is affected by the mother's use of cocaine, specified as a cause of mortality or morbidity, or when the infant has a positive drug screen, assign code 760.75.

If the infant does not exhibit an associated complication or test positive for cocaine in a drug screen, code 760.75 is not assigned.

Signs and symptoms of cocaine use include hyperactivity, hyperthermia, tachycardia, dilated pupils, and, in severe cases, convulsions, coma, and circulatory collapse. Toxicology tests of blood or urine reveal the presence of cocaine.

Therapies include drugs such as diazepam or chlorpromazine.

Associated conditions include infant drug withdrawal, renal system anomalies, central nervous system anomalies, and sudden infant death syndrome (SIDS).

760.76 Noxious influences affecting fetus or newborn via placenta or breast milk, diethylstilbestrol [DES]

760.79 Noxious influences affecting fetus or newborn via placenta or breast milk, other — *fetus or newborn affected by immune sera, medicinal agents NEC, or toxic substance NEC*
AHA: Nov-Dec, 1984, 11; Q2, 1989, 14; Q3, 1990, 5; Q3, 1991, 21; Q2, 1992, 12; Q1, 1994, 8

These codes may be used regardless of the patient's age. For example, it is not uncommon for the daughters of women who ingested diethylstilbestrol (DES) during pregnancy to develop ovarian cancer from exposure to the drug through the placenta while in utero.

In addition, these codes may be used when the fetus or newborn shows signs and symptoms of acute intoxication of the noxious influence.

Excluded from these subclassifications are anesthetic and analgesic drugs administered during labor and delivery (763.5) and drug withdrawal syndrome in newborn (779.5).

760.8 Other specified maternal conditions affecting fetus or newborn — *genital tract and other localized infection affecting fetus or newborn, but fetus or newborn manifesting that disease*
AHA: Nov-Dec, 1984, 11; Q2, 1989, 14; Q3, 1990, 5; Q2, 1992, 12; Q1, 1994, 8

760.9 Unspecified maternal condition affecting fetus or newborn

Coding Clarification

Excluded from this rubric is maternal endocrine and metabolic disorders affecting fetus or newborn (775.0-775.9).

Coding Scenario

A newborn male is delivered in the hospital to a mother who has a past history of cocaine abuse. The newborn has no manifestations from the drug abuse; however, the infant tests positive for cocaine.

Code assignment: V30.00 *Single liveborn, born in hospital, delivered without mention of cesarean delivery* and 760.75 *Cocaine affecting fetus or newborn via placenta or breast milk*

761 Fetus or newborn affected by maternal complications of pregnancy

AHA: Q2, 1989, 14; Q3, 1990, 5

761.0 Fetus or newborn affected by incompetent cervix of mother

761.1 Fetus or newborn affected by premature rupture of membranes of mother

761.2 Fetus or newborn affected by oligohydramnios

Coding Clarification

Associated conditions include Potter's syndrome, fetal urinary tract obstruction, intrauterine growth retardation, amniotic band syndrome, fetal compression, and fetal demise.

Use code 761.2 *Fetus or newborn affected by oligohydramnios* to report a fetus or newborn affected by the presence of less than 300 ml of amniotic fluid at term.

761.3 Fetus or newborn affected by polyhydramnios — *hydramnios (acute) (chronic)*
AHA: Q2, 1989, 14; Q3, 1990, 5

Coding Clarification

Polyhydramnios is often associated with maternal diabetes; however, the cause is unknown in approximately a third of all cases.

Associated conditions include esophageal atresia, anencephaly, spinal bifida, and isoimmunization.

Use code 761.3 to report a fetus or newborn affected by the presence of an excessive amount of amniotic fluid during pregnancy.

761.4 Fetus or newborn affected by ectopic pregnancy of mother — *abdominal, intraperitoneal, and tubal*
AHA: Q2, 1989, 14; Q3, 1990, 5

Coding Clarification

This condition frequently occurs when the mother has some type of infertility. The most frequent site of ectopic pregnancy is within the fallopian tube. It is rare for the fetus to complete the weeks of gestation necessary to be viable.

Use code 761.4 to report a fetus or newborn affected by implantation of the fertilized ovum in an area other than the uterus, for example, the cervix, uterine tube, ovary, or abdominal or pelvic cavity.

761.5 Fetus or newborn affected by multiple pregnancy of mother — *triplet, twin births*
AHA: Q2, 1989, 14; Q3, 1990, 5

761.6 Fetus or newborn affected by maternal death

761.7 Fetus or newborn affected by malpresentation before labor — *breech presentation, external version, oblique lie, transverse lie, unstable lie*
AHA: Q2, 1989, 14; Q3, 1990, 5

761.8 Fetus or newborn affected by other specified maternal complications of pregnancy — *spontaneous abortion, fetus*
AHA: Q2, 1989, 14; Q3, 1990, 5

761.9 Fetus or newborn affected by unspecified maternal complication of pregnancy

762 Fetus or newborn affected by complications of placenta, cord, and membranes

AHA: Q2, 1989, 14; Q3, 1990, 5; Q1, 1994, 8

762.0 Fetus or newborn affected by placenta previa

Use code 762.0 to report a fetus or newborn affected by the implantation of the placenta over or near the internal os of the cervix. There are two forms of placental previa: total, in which the placenta completely covers the internal cervical os; and partial, in which the placenta covers a portion of the internal cervical os. Placenta previa often results in a fetus being delivered prior to term.

Associated conditions include prematurity, alveolar conditions, respiratory distress syndrome, inadequate or erratic brain perfusion, hypotension, blood pressure peaks, infections including meningitis and sepsis, and SGA.

762.1 Fetus or newborn affected by other forms of placental separation and hemorrhage — *abruptio placentae; antepartum hemorrhage; damage to placenta from amniocentesis; cesarean section or surgical induction; blood loss; premature separation of placenta; rupture of marginal sinus*
AHA: Q2, 1989, 14; Q3, 1990, 5; Q1, 1994, 8

762.2 Fetus or newborn affected by other forms of other and unspecified morphological and functional abnormalities of placenta — *dysfunction, infarction, insufficiency; yellow vernix syndrome*
AHA: Q2, 1989, 14; Q3, 1990, 5; Q1, 1994, 8

© 2004 Ingenix, Inc.

762.3 Fetus or newborn affected by placental transfusion syndromes — (Use additional code to indicate resultant condition in fetus or newborn: 772.0, 776.4) — *placental and cord abnormality resulting in twin-to-twin or other transplacental transfusion*
AHA: Q2, 1989, 14; Q3, 1990, 5; Q1, 1994, 8

762.4 Fetus or newborn affected by prolapsed cord — *cord presentation*
AHA: Q2, 1989, 14; Q3, 1990, 5; Q1, 1994, 8

762.5 Fetus or newborn affected by other compression of umbilical cord — *cord around neck; entanglement; knot, torsion*
AHA: Q2, 1989, 14; Q3, 1990, 5; Q1, 1994, 8; Q2, 2003, 9

762.6 Fetus or newborn affected by other and unspecified conditions of umbilical cord — *short cord, thrombosis, varices, velamentous insertion, vasa previa*
AHA: Q2, 1989, 14; Q3, 1990, 5; Q1, 1994, 8

762.7 Fetus or newborn affected by chorioamnionitis — *amnionitis, membranitis, placentitis*
AHA: Q2, 1989, 14; Q3, 1990, 5; Q1, 1994, 8

762.8 Fetus or newborn affected by other specified abnormalities of chorion and amnion — *not elsewhere classified*
AHA: Q2, 1989, 14; Q3, 1990, 5; Q1, 1994, 8

762.9 Fetus or newborn affected by unspecified abnormality of chorion and amnion

763 Fetus or newborn affected by other complications of labor and delivery

AHA: Q2, 1989, 14; Q3, 1990, 5; Q1, 1994, 8

763.0 Fetus or newborn affected by breech delivery and extraction

763.1 Fetus or newborn affected by other malpresentation, malposition, and disproportion during labor and delivery — *abnormality of bony pelvis, contracted pelvis, persistent occipitoposterior position, shoulder presentation, transverse lie*
AHA: Q2, 1989, 14; Q3, 1990, 5; Q1, 1994, 8

763.2 Fetus or newborn affected by forceps delivery — *fetus or newborn affected by forceps extraction*
AHA: Q2, 1989, 14; Q3, 1990, 5; Q1, 1994, 8

763.3 Fetus or newborn affected by delivery by vacuum extractor

763.4 Fetus or newborn affected by cesarean delivery

763.5 Fetus or newborn affected by maternal anesthesia and analgesia — *reactions and intoxications from maternal opiates and tranquilizers during labor and delivery*
AHA: Q2, 1989, 14; Q3, 1990, 5; Q1, 1994, 8

763.6 Fetus or newborn affected by precipitate delivery — *rapid second stage*
AHA: Q2, 1989, 14; Q3, 1990, 5; Q1, 1994, 8

763.7 Fetus or newborn affected by abnormal uterine contractions — *fetus or newborn affected by contraction ring, hypertonic labor, hypotonic uterine dysfunction, uterine inertia or dysfunction*
AHA: Q2, 1989, 14; Q3, 1990, 5; Q1, 1994, 8

763.81 Abnormality in fetal heart rate or rhythm before the onset of labor

763.82 Abnormality in fetal heart rate or rhythm during labor

763.83 Abnormality in fetal heart rate or rhythm, unspecified as to time of onset

763.89 Other specified complications of labor and delivery affecting fetus or newborn — *fetus or newborn affected by abnormality of maternal soft tissues, destructive operation on live fetus to facilitate delivery, induction of labor (medical), previous surgery to uterus or pelvic organs*
AHA: Q2, 1989, 14; Q3, 1990, 5; Q1, 1994, 8; Q4, 1998, 46

763.9 Unspecified complication of labor and delivery affecting fetus or newborn

764–779 Other Conditions Originating in the Perinatal Period

764 Slow fetal growth and fetal malnutrition

AHA: Q2, 1989, 15; Q2, 1991, 19; Q1, 1994, 8; Q4, 2002, 63

This category reports conditions in which the fetus is considerably below the normal weight of offspring of the same gestational age. Malnutrition in a fetus may be due to defective assimilation or utilization of foods or to a maternal diet that is unbalanced or insufficient. Other factors that may cause an infant to be light for dates are genetic disorders, drugs, small maternal stature, placenta previa, multiple pregnancies, hypertension, anemia, and renal disease.

This condition may be described with such terms as "small for gestational age," "low birth weight," or "intrauterine growth retardation" (IUGR).

Associated conditions include genetic disorders such as Down's syndrome, Edwards' syndrome, autosomal trisomy, and Turner syndrome.

The following fifth-digit subclassification is for use with categories 764-765 to denote birthweight:

0 unspecified
1 less than 500 grams (less than 1.1 lbs)
2 500-749 grams (1.11 to 1.67 lbs)
3 750-999 grams (1.68 to 2.23 lbs)
4 1000-1249 grams (2.24 to 2.78 lbs)
5 1250-1499 grams (2.79 to 3.34 lbs)
6 1500-1749 grams (3.35 to 3.9 lbs)
7 1750-1999 grams (3.91 to 4.5 lbs)
8 2000-2499 grams (4.51 to 5.59 lbs)
9 2500 grams or more (5.6 lbs and over)

764.0 5th "Light-for-dates" without mention of fetal malnutrition — *infants underweight for gestational age; "small for dates"*
AHA: Q2, 1989, 15; Q2, 1991, 19; Q1, 1994, 8; Q4, 2002, 63

764.1 5th "Light-for-dates" with signs of fetal malnutrition — *infants "light-for-dates;" infant showing signs of fetal malnutrition, such as dry peeling skin and loss of subcutaneous tissue; intrauterine malnutrition*
AHA: Q2, 1989, 15; Q2, 1991, 19; Q1, 1994, 8; Q4, 2002, 63

764.2 5th Fetal malnutrition without mention of "light-for-dates" — *infants, not underweight for gestational age, showing signs of fetal malnutrition, such as dry peeling skin and loss of subcutaneous tissue; intrauterine malnutrition*
AHA: Q2, 1989, 15; Q2, 1991, 19; Q1, 1994, 8; Q4, 2002, 63

764.9 5th Unspecified fetal growth retardation — *intrauterine growth retardation; undeveloped fetus or newborn*
AHA: Q2, 1989, 15; Q2, 1991, 19; Q1, 1994, 8; Q4, 2002, 63

765 Disorders relating to short gestation and unspecified low birthweight

AHA: Q2, 1989, 15; Q2, 1991, 19; Q1, 1994, 8; Q1, 1997, 6

Use this category to report short gestation and low birthweight disorders in a viable infant.

Associated conditions include alveolar conditions, respiratory distress syndrome, inadequate or erratic brain perfusion, hypotension, blood pressure peaks, infections including meningitis and sepsis, and SGA.

The following fifth-digit subclassification is for use with categories 764-765 to denote birthweight:

0 unspecified
1 less than 500 grams (less than 1.1 lbs)
2 500-749 grams (1.11 to 1.67 lbs)
3 750-999 grams (1.68 to 2.23 lbs)
4 1000-1249 grams (2.24 to 2.78 lbs)
5 1250-1499 grams (2.79 to 3.34 lbs)
6 1500-1749 grams (3.35 to 3.9 lbs)
7 1750-1999 grams (3.91 to 4.5 lbs)
8 2000-2499 grams (4.51 to 5.59 lbs)
9 2500 grams or more (5.6 lbs and over)

765.0 5th Extreme fetal immaturity — (Use additional code for weeks of gestation: 765.20-765.29) — *usually implies a birthweight of less than 1000 grams*
AHA: Q2, 1989, 15; Q2, 1991, 19; Q1, 1994, 8; Q1, 1997, 6; Q4, 2002, 63

765.1 5th Other preterm infants — (Use additional code for weeks of gestation: 765.20-765.29) — *usually implies a birthweight of 1000 to 2499 grams*
AHA: Q2, 1989, 15; Q2, 1991, 19; Q1, 1994, 8; Q1, 1997, 6; Q4, 2002, 63

765.20 Unspecified weeks of gestation
765.21 Less than 24 completed weeks of gestation
765.22 24 completed weeks of gestation
765.23 25-26 completed weeks of gestation
765.24 27-28 completed weeks of gestation
765.25 29-30 completed weeks of gestation
765.26 31-32 completed weeks of gestation
765.27 33-34 completed weeks of gestation
765.28 35-36 completed weeks of gestation
765.29 37 or more completed weeks of gestation

766 Disorders relating to long gestation and high birthweight

Category 766 reports disorders in a viable infant born after 42 weeks of gestation and/or described as "heavy," "large-for-dates," or greater than 4,500 grams birthweight.

766.0 Exceptionally large baby relating to long gestation — *implies a birthweight of 4500 grams or more*

Use code 766.0 to report an infant weighing over the 90th percentile for gestational age. Approximately 1 to 3 percent of neonates in the United States are considered large for gestational age. A baby may be exceptionally large when the mother has a large frame, is obese, or has diabetes. Associated conditions include hypoxia during labor and birth trauma.

© 2004 Ingenix, Inc.

766.1 Other "heavy-for-dates" infants not related to gestation period — *fetus or infant "heavy-" or "large-for-dates," regardless of period of gestation*

766.21 Post-term infant — *over 40 completed weeks to 42 completed weeks*

766.22 Prolonged gestation of infant — *beyond 42 completed weeks of gestation, postmaturity*

767 Birth trauma

The definition of birth trauma is injury to the fetus or newborn during delivery. Such injury may be due to breech presentation or forceps delivery.

767.0 Subdural and cerebral hemorrhage, birth trauma — (Use additional code to identify cause) — *due to birth trauma or to intrapartum anoxia or hypoxia; including subdural hematoma (localized), tentorial tear; secondary code to identify cause*

Subdural and cerebral hemorrhage is hemorrhage in or around the brain.

Signs and symptoms of subdural and cerebral hemorrhage include seizures, abnormally large head, diminished tone and/or resistance of skeletal muscles, retinal hemorrhage, positive transillumination of skull, or poor Moro's response (reaction to sudden loud noises).

Lab work reveals red blood cells in cerebral spinal fluid. A computed tomography (CT) scan of the head confirms the diagnosis.

Therapies include fluid removal by daily subdural taps.

Associated conditions include hypoxia while in utero, anoxia while in utero, and prematurity.

Excluded from this subcategory is intraventricular hemorrhage (772.10-772.14).

767.11 Birth trauma, Epicranial subaponeurotic hemorrhage (massive)

Epicranial subaponeurotic hemorrhage is the rupture of the emissary veins, connections between the dural sinuses and scalp veins. Blood accumulates in the space between the epicranial aponeurosis of the scalp and the periosteum, typically caused by vacuum extraction during delivery. The aponeurosis is a structure that connects the frontal and occipital bellies of the occipitalfrontalis muscle and epicranial.

767.19 Birth trauma, Other injuries to scalp

Injuries to the scalp include caput succedaneum, subgaleal hemorrhage, and cephalhematoma. Caput succedaneum, edema of the presenting portion of the scalp, usually is a mild trauma resulting from the pressure of the fetal scalp against the uterine cervix during labor and delivery. Subgaleal hemorrhage is a greater trauma manifested by a boggy feeling over the entire scalp, and cephalhematoma is hemorrhage of the periosteum of the skull.

767.2 Fracture of clavicle, birth trauma

767.3 Other injuries to skeleton, birth trauma — *fracture of long bones, skull*

767.4 Injury to spine and spinal cord, birth trauma — *dislocation, fracture, laceration, rupture*

767.5 Facial nerve injury, birth trauma — *facial palsy, Bell's paralysis of newborn*

767.6 Injury to brachial plexus, birth trauma — *brachial, Erb (-Duchenne), and Klumpke (-Déjérine) paralysis or palsy*

Use code 767.6 to report injury of the brachial plexus nerve during delivery. Damage of this nerve can affect the muscles of the arm and shoulder.

767.7 Other cranial and peripheral nerve injuries, birth trauma — *phrenic nerve paralysis*

767.8 Other specified birth trauma — *eye damage; hematoma or liver (subcapsular), testes, vulva; rupture of liver, spleen; scalpel wound; traumatic glaucoma; hematoma of sternocleidomastoid; ruptured stomach due to injury at birth; ruptured viscera; torticollis due to birth injury*

767.9 Unspecified birth trauma — *birth injury NOS*

768 Intrauterine hypoxia and birth asphyxia

AHA: Q4, 1992, 20

Use codes in category 768 to report reduction of oxygen resulting in impending or actual cessation of life. The condition may be brought on by events such as acute blood loss, aspiration of meconium, or a tight nuchal cord.

Signs and symptoms of intrauterine hypoxia and birth asphyxia include low Apgar score, pale or cyanotic color, poor or absent respirations, and poor reflexes and muscle tone. Fetal monitor shows irregular heart rhythm. Blood gases show hypercapnia and hypoxia. Therapies include endotracheal intubation and ventilation, and IV fluids with glucose.

Associated conditions include hypoglycemia, respiratory or metabolic acidosis, coma and seizures due to anoxic brain damage, fluid retention and hyponatremia due to acute tubular necrosis, sepsis, and bowel disorders, such as necrotizing enterocolitis.

768.0 Fetal death from asphyxia or anoxia before onset of labor or at unspecified time — (Use only when associated with newborn morbidity classifiable elsewhere) — *secondary*
AHA: Q4, 1992, 20

768.1 Fetal death from asphyxia or anoxia during labor — (Use only when associated with newborn morbidity classifiable elsewhere) — *secondary*
AHA: Q4, 1992, 20

768.2 Fetal distress before onset of labor, in liveborn infant — (Use only when associated with newborn morbidity classifiable elsewhere) — *secondary; fetal metabolic acidemia first noted during labor, in liveborn infant*
AHA: Q4, 1992, 20

Use code 768.2 to report hypoxia and acidosis affecting the functions of vital organs, such as the heart and lungs, of a fetus to the point of temporary injury, permanent injury, or death.

768.3 Fetal distress first noted during labor, in liveborn infant — (Use only when associated with newborn morbidity classifiable elsewhere)

768.4 Fetal distress, unspecified as to time of onset, in liveborn infant — (Use only when associated with newborn morbidity classifiable elsewhere) — *secondary, fetal metabolic acidemia unknown as to time of onset, in liveborn infant*
AHA: Nov-Dec, 1986, 10; Q4, 1992, 20

768.5 Severe birth asphyxia — (Use only when associated with newborn morbidity classifiable elsewhere) — *secondary; birth asphyxia with neurologic involvement*
AHA: Nov-Dec, 1986, 3; Q4, 1992, 20

768.6 Mild or moderate birth asphyxia — (Use only when associated with newborn morbidity classifiable elsewhere) — *secondary;*
AHA: Nov-Dec, 1986, 3; Q4, 1992, 20

768.9 Unspecified birth asphyxia in liveborn infant — (Use only when associated with newborn morbidity classifiable elsewhere) — *anoxia NOS, asphyxia NOS, hypoxia NOS*
AHA: Q4, 1992, 20

769 Respiratory distress syndrome in newborn OK

AHA: Nov-Dec, 1986, 6; Q1, 1989, 10

Use code 769 to report insufficient lung maturity of the fetus or newborn resulting in severe hypoxemia and multiple organ failure or death if left untreated. Also known as hyaline membrane disease and respiratory distress syndrome of the premature infant, this condition occurs primarily in premature infants (before completion of 37 weeks of gestation) or infants whose mothers are diabetic. It also may develop in infants whose mothers have toxemia or hypertension.

Signs and symptoms of respiratory distress syndrome include rapid labored respirations, substernal retractions, nasal alae flaring and "grunting" retractions, and low Apgar scores. Chest x-ray shows diffuse pulmonary atelectasis with overdistended alveolar ducts; blood gases show hypoxia. Therapies include IV fluids and electrolytes, oxygen therapy via nasal prongs, facemask, nasopharyngeal tube and endotracheal tube, and ventilation (CPAP, IPPV, and PEEP).

Associated conditions include respiratory or metabolic acidosis, hypoxemia, multiple organ failure, and atelectasis.

This category includes Type I respiratory distress syndrome or distress of the newborn. Type II respiratory distress syndrome or distress of the newborn is reported with 770.6, as is transient tachypnea of newborn.

770 Other respiratory conditions of fetus and newborn

770.0 Congenital pneumonia — *infective pneumonia acquired prenatally*

770.1 Meconium aspiration syndrome — *aspiration of contents of birth canal NOS; meconium aspiration below vocal cords; fetal aspiration and meconium pneumonitis*

770.2 Interstitial emphysema and related conditions of newborn — *pneumomediastinum, pneumopericardia, and pneumothorax originating in the perinatal period*

770.3 Pulmonary hemorrhage of fetus or newborn — *hemorrhage of alveolar, intraalveolar, and massive pulmonary originating in the perinatal period*

770.4 Primary atelectasis of newborn — *pulmonary immaturity NOS*

770.5 Other and unspecified atelectasis of newborn — *atelectasis NOS, partial, and secondary originating in the perinatal period; pulmonary collapse*

770.6 Transitory tachypnea of newborn — *idiopathic tachypnea, wet lung syndrome*
AHA: Nov-Dec, 1986, 6; Q1, 1989, 10; Q3, 1993, 7; Q1, 1994, 12; Q4, 1995, 4

770.7 Chronic respiratory disease arising in the perinatal period — *bronchopulmonary dysplasia, interstitial pulmonary fibrosis of prematurity, Wilson-Mikity syndrome, bubbly lung syndrome*
AHA: Nov-Dec, 1986, 11; Q2, 1991, 19

770.81 Primary apnea of newborn — *apneic spells NOS, essential and sleep apnea of newborn*
AHA: Q2, 1996, 10; Q2, 1998, 10; Q4, 2002, 65

 © 2004 Ingenix, Inc.

770.82 Other apnea of newborn — *obstructive apnea of newborn*
AHA: Q2, 1996, 10; Q2, 1998, 10; Q4, 2002, 65

770.83 Cyanotic attacks of newborn

770.84 Respiratory failure of newborn — *excluding respiratory distress syndrome (769)*
AHA: Q2, 1996, 10; Q2, 1998, 10; Q4, 2002, 65

770.89 Other respiratory problems of newborn after birth

770.9 Unspecified respiratory condition of fetus and newborn

771 Infections specific to the perinatal period

AHA: Nov-Dec, 1985, 4

771.0 Congenital rubella — *congenital rubella pneumonitis*
AHA: Nov-Dec, 1985, 4

Use code 771.0 to report a fetal infection of the virus rubella while in utero. Maternal rubella infection that occurs within a month before conception and through the second trimester is associated with newborn disease.

Signs and symptoms of congenital rubella include hepatosplenomegaly, "blueberry muffin" skin, and purpuric lesions. Lab work, such as immunofluorescence or enzyme immunoassays, reveals elevated antirubella IgM or IgG titers. Therapies include management of complications.

Associated conditions include hemolytic and hypoplastic anemia, pneumonia, meningoencephalitis, glaucoma and cataracts, thrombocytopenia, cardiac deformities such as patent ductus arteriosus, and other birth defects such as microcephaly and mental retardation.

771.1 Congenital cytomegalovirus infection — *congenital cytomegalic inclusion disease*
AHA: Nov-Dec, 1985, 4

Code 771.1 reports fetal infection with cytomegalovirus (CMV), a member of the herpes virus family, while in utero.

This subcategory includes only congenital CMV infections; that is, those acquired up until the moment of birth, including passage through the birth canal. Noncongenital CMV infections of the newborn — for example, those acquired through breast milk, in the nursery or home, or through postnatal blood transfusion — are classified elsewhere.

771.2 Other congenital infection specific to the perinatal period — *herpes simplex, listeriosis, malaria, toxoplasmosis, tuberculosis*
AHA: Nov-Dec, 1985, 4

771.3 Tetanus neonatorum — *tetanus omphalitis*
AHA: Nov-Dec, 1985, 4

771.4 Omphalitis of the newborn — *infection of naval cord and umbilical stump*
AHA: Nov-Dec, 1985, 4

771.5 Neonatal infective mastitis

771.6 Neonatal conjunctivitis and dacryocystitis — *ophthalmia neonatorum NOS*
AHA: Nov-Dec, 1985, 4

771.7 Neonatal Candida infection — *neonatal moniliasis, thrush in newborn*
AHA: Nov-Dec, 1985, 4

771.81 Septicemia (sepsis) of newborn — (Use additional code to identify organism)

771.82 Urinary tract infection of newborn — (Use additional code to identify organism)

771.83 Bacteremia of newborn — (Use additional code to identify organism)

771.89 Other infections specific to the perinatal period — (Use additional code to identify organism) — *intra-amniotic infection of fetus NOS, infection of newborn NOS*
AHA: Nov-Dec, 1985, 4; Q4, 2002, 66

Coding Clarification

Excluded from this rubric are congenital pneumonia (770.1), congenital syphilis (090.0-090.9), maternal infectious disease as a cause of mortality or morbidity in fetus or newborn, but fetus or newborn not manifesting the disease (760.2), ophthalmia neonatorum due to gonococcus (098.40), and other infections not specifically classified to this category.

772 Fetal and neonatal hemorrhage

Blood loss in this rubric is classified according to the site of hemorrhage. Typically, in fetal and neonatal hemorrhage, the infant will be hypotensive and pale. Hypovolemic shock should be corrected immediately.

772.0 Fetal blood loss — *fetal blood loss from cut end of co-twin's cord, placenta, ruptured cord, and vasa previa; exsanguination; hemorrhage into co-twin, mother's circulation*

772.10 Intraventricular hemorrhage, unspecified grade

772.11 Intraventricular hemorrhage, Grade I — *includes bleeding into germinal matrix*
AHA: Q4, 1988, 8; Q3, 1992, 8; Q4, 2001, 49

772.12 Intraventricular hemorrhage, Grade II — *includes bleeding into ventricle*
AHA: Q4, 1988, 8; Q3, 1992, 8; Q4, 2001, 49

772.13 Intraventricular hemorrhage, Grade III — *includes bleeding with enlargement of ventricle*
AHA: Q4, 1988, 8; Q3, 1992, 8; Q4, 2001, 49; Q4, 2001, 51

772.14 Intraventricular hemorrhage, Grade IV — *includes bleeding into cerebral cortex*
AHA: Q4, 1988, 8; Q3, 1992, 8; Q4, 2001, 49

772.2 Fetal and neonatal subarachnoid hemorrhage of newborn — *from any perinatal cause*

772.3 Umbilical hemorrhage after birth — *slipped umbilical ligature*

772.4 Fetal and neonatal gastrointestinal hemorrhage

772.5 Fetal and neonatal adrenal hemorrhage

772.6 Fetal and neonatal cutaneous hemorrhage — *bruising, ecchymoses, petechiae, superficial hematoma in fetus or newborn*

772.8 Other specified hemorrhage of fetus or newborn — *hemopericardium, hemothorax of newborn*

772.9 Unspecified hemorrhage of newborn

Coding Clarification

Excluded from this rubric are hematological disorders of the fetus and newborn (776.0-776.9).

773 Hemolytic disease of fetus or newborn, due to isoimmunization

In isoimmunization, the mother develops antibodies against an antigen derived from a genetically dissimilar fetus.

773.0 Hemolytic disease due to Rh isoimmunization of fetus or newborn — *premature destruction of red blood cells due to incompatibility of Rh fetal-maternal blood grouping and positive Coombs test; including anemia, erythroblastosis, hemolytic disease, jaundice due to Rh antibodies, isoimmunization, and maternal/fetal incompatibility; Rh hemolytic disease, Rh isoimmunization*

Code 773.0 reports incompatibility that occurs when an Rh-negative mother carries an Rh-positive fetus. Antibodies cross the placenta into the fetus and lead to hemolysis of the fetal blood.

Signs and symptoms of hemolytic disease due to Rh isoimmunization include scalp edema, cardiomegaly, hepatomegaly, splenomegaly, pale skin, and severe generalized edema.

Associated conditions include erythroblastosis fetalis, hydrops fetalis, ascites, polyhydramnios, pleural effusion, heart failure, anemia, and asphyxia during delivery due to an enlarged liver.

773.1 Hemolytic disease due to abo isoimmunization of fetus or newborn — *ABO hemolytic disease, ABO isoimmunization; anemia, erythroblastosis, hemolytic disease, jaundice due to ABO antibodies, isoimmunization, maternal/fetal incompatibility*
AHA: Q3, 1992, 8

Use code 773.1 to report incompatibility that occurs when a mother with blood type O carries a fetus with blood type A or B. Antibodies cross the placenta into the fetus and cause hemolysis of the fetal blood.

Signs and symptoms of hemolytic disease due to ABO isoimmunization include scalp edema, cardiomegaly, hepatomegaly, splenomegaly, pale skin, and severe generalized edema.

Associated conditions include erythroblastosis fetalis, hydrops fetalis, ascites, polyhydramnios, pleural effusion, heart failure, anemia, and asphyxia during delivery due to an enlarged liver.

773.2 Hemolytic disease due to other and unspecified isoimmunization of fetus or newborn — *erythroblastosis NOS, hemolytic disease NOS, jaundice or anemia due to unknown blood-group incompatibility*
AHA: Q1, 1994, 13

773.3 Hydrops fetalis due to isoimmunization — (Use additional code to identify type of isoimmunization: 773.0-773.2) — *secondary to identify type of isoimmunization*

Use code 773.3 to report gross edema of the entire body of the fetus with associated anemia due to mother-fetus blood incompatibility. The condition has a high mortality rate, especially in premature infants. Blood work reveals mother-fetus Rh and ABO incompatibility. Therapies include exchange blood transfusions, resuscitation and mechanical ventilation at birth, and thoracentesis.

Associated conditions include erythroblastosis fetalis, respiratory failure, pleural effusion, alloimmune hemolytic anemia, high output cardiac failure, and hypoproteinemia.

773.4 Kernicterus due to isoimmunization of fetus or newborn — (Use additional code to identify type of isoimmunization: 773.0-773.2) — *secondary to identify type of isoimmunization*

Kernicterus is a significantly large accumulation of bilirubin in the brain that may result in brain damage because of an incompatibility of fetal and maternal blood.

Signs and symptoms of kernicterus due to isoimmunization include jaundice, high fever, seizures, blunted Moro reflex, opisthotonic posturing, incomplete flexion of extremities, vomiting, and high-

 © 2004 Ingenix, Inc.

pitched cry. Therapies include phototherapy and exchange blood transfusions.

Associated conditions include mental retardation and hemolytic disease.

773.5 Late anemia due to isoimmunization of fetus or newborn

Documentation Issues

Abnormal Bilirubin: When a laboratory result indicates an elevation of the bilirubin, but the medical record lacks evidence that the infant was treated, these abnormal findings should not be coded. The physician can be queried to determine if jaundice was present.

Coding Clarification

Due to Blood-group Incompatibility: When the documentation specifies that the infant has jaundice due to blood-group incompatibility, code 773.1 *Hemolytic disease due to ABO isoimmunization* should be reported. Do not use codes 774.2 or 774.6 as additional codes because code 773.1 already includes jaundice.

Preterm Jaundice: This condition is a form of jaundice identified in an infant born before the completion of 36 weeks gestation. When the medical record documentation indicates this condition, code 774.2 *Neonatal jaundice associated with preterm delivery* should be reported.

774 Other perinatal jaundice

Jaundice is also known as hyperbilirubinemia, which refers to the excess of bilirubin. The excess bilirubin may be caused by an overproduction of bilirubin, an impaired ability to secrete bilirubin, or a mixture of both causes.

774.0 Perinatal jaundice from hereditary hemolytic anemias — (Code first underlying disease: 282.0-282.9) — *secondary to underlying disease*

774.1 Perinatal jaundice from other excessive hemolysis — (Use additional code to identify cause) — *secondary to identify cause; including jaundice from bruising, drugs or toxins transmitted from mother, infection, polycythemia, swallowed maternal blood*

774.2 Neonatal jaundice associated with preterm delivery — *hyperbilirubinemia of prematurity; jaundice due to delayed conjugation associated with preterm delivery*
AHA: Q3, 1991, 21

774.30 Neonatal jaundice due to delayed conjugation, cause unspecified — *Lucey-Driscoll syndrome*

774.31 Neonatal jaundice due to delayed conjugation in diseases classified elsewhere — (Code first underlying disease: 243, 277.4) — *secondary to underlying disease*

774.39 Other neonatal jaundice due to delayed conjugation from other causes — *jaundice due to delayed conjugation from causes such as breast milk inhibitors and delayed development of conjugating system*

774.4 Perinatal jaundice due to hepatocellular damage — *fetal or neonatal hepatitis, giant cell hepatitis, inspissated bile syndrome*

774.5 Perinatal jaundice from other causes — (Code first underlying cause: 271.1, 277.00-277.09, 751.61) — *Code first underlying cause, as: 271.1, 277.00-277.09, 751.61*

774.6 Unspecified fetal and neonatal jaundice — *icterus neonatorum, neonatal hyperbilirubinemia (transient), physiologic jaundice NOS*
AHA: Q2, 1989, 15; Q1, 1994, 13

774.7 Kernicterus of fetus or newborn not due to isoimmunization — *bilirubin encephalopathy, kernicterus of newborn NOS*

Documentation Issues

When a laboratory result indicates an elevation of the bilirubin, but the medical record lacks evidence that the infant was treated, these abnormal findings should not be coded. The physician can be queried to determine if jaundice was present.

Coding Clarification

Use code 774.7 to report a significantly large accumulation of bilirubin in the brain that may result in brain damage not due to a fetal/maternal blood incompatibility (ABO incompatibility). The condition may be caused by a large influx of red blood cells through the umbilicus at the time of delivery.

Signs and symptoms of kernicterus not due to isoimmunization include jaundice, high fever, seizures, blunted Moro reflex, opisthotonic posturing, incomplete flexion of the extremities, vomiting, and high-pitched cry. Therapies include phototherapy and exchange blood transfusions.

Associated conditions include mental retardation.

Due to Blood-group Incompatibility: When the documentation specifies that the infant has jaundice due to blood-group incompatibility, code 773.1 *Hemolytic disease due to ABO isoimmunization* should be reported. Do not use codes 774.2 or 774.6 as additional codes; code 773.1 already includes jaundice.

Preterm Jaundice: This condition is a form of jaundice identified in an infant born before the completion of 36 weeks gestation. When the medical record documentation indicates this condition, code

774.2 *Neonatal jaundice associated with preterm delivery* should be reported.

Coding Scenario

A 35-week-gestational age male is delivered via cesarean delivery. The physician indicates that the infant has preterm jaundice.

> Code assignment: V30.01 *Single liveborn, born in hospital, delivered by cesarean delivery* and 774.2 *Neonatal jaundice associated with preterm delivery*

775 Endocrine and metabolic disturbances specific to the fetus and newborn

This rubric includes transitory endocrine and metabolic disturbances caused by the infant's response to maternal endocrine and metabolic factors, the infant's removal from them, or the infant's adjustment to extrauterine existence.

775.0 Syndrome of "infant of diabetic mother" — *maternal diabetes mellitus affecting fetus or newborn (with hypoglycemia)*
AHA: Q3, 1991, 5

This code reports a syndrome with manifestations including macrosomia, birth asphyxia, hypoglycemia, cardiorespiratory disorders, and congenital malformations.

Signs and symptoms of syndrome of "infant of a diabetic mother" include large size, obesity, listlessness, limpness, poor feeding, and red florid complexion due to excessive amount of blood.

775.1 Neonatal diabetes mellitus — *diabetes mellitus syndrome in newborn*
AHA: Q3, 1991, 6

775.2 Neonatal myasthenia gravis

775.3 Neonatal thyrotoxicosis — *hyperthyroidism (transient)*

775.4 Hypocalcemia and hypomagnesemia of newborn — *cow's mile hypocalcemia, hypocalcemic tetany, hypoparathyroidism, phosphate-loading hypocalcemia*

775.5 Other transitory neonatal electrolyte disturbances — *dehydration*

775.6 Neonatal hypoglycemia

775.7 Late metabolic acidosis of newborn

775.8 Other transitory neonatal endocrine and metabolic disturbances — *amino acid metabolic disorders described as transitory; including tyrosinemia*

775.9 Unspecified endocrine and metabolic disturbances specific to the fetus and newborn

776 Hematological disorders of fetus and newborn

776.0 Hemorrhagic disease of newborn — *diathesis, vitamin K deficiency, Minot's disease*

776.1 Transient neonatal thrombocytopenia — *due to exchange transfusion, idiopathic maternal thrombocytopenia, isoimmunization*

776.2 Disseminated intravascular coagulation in newborn

776.3 Other transient neonatal disorders of coagulation — *transient coagulation defect, newborn*

776.4 Polycythemia neonatorum — *plethora; polycythemia due to donor twin transfusion, maternal-fetal transfusion*

776.5 Congenital anemia — *anemia following fetal blood loss*

776.6 Anemia of neonatal prematurity

Use code 776.6 to report anemia in a viable infant born before completing 37 weeks of gestation in which the number of erythrocytes per cu mm and the quantity of hemoglobin are reduced. The hemoglobin nadir for premature infants is 6.5-9.0 g/100 ml as opposed to 9.5-11.0 g/100 ml for term infants. The extent of the anemia is directly related to the birth weight.

Signs and symptoms of anemia of prematurity include tachycardia, tachypnea, poor feeding, apnea, and dyspnea. Lab work shows abnormally low hemoglobin. Therapies include packed red blood cells, particularly when blood removed for testing exceeds 10 percent of estimated volume, and iron supplement.

Associated conditions include alveolar conditions, respiratory distress syndrome, inadequate or erratic brain perfusion, hypotension, blood pressure peaks, and infections including meningitis and sepsis.

776.7 Transient neonatal neutropenia — *isoimmune and maternal transfer neutropenia*

776.8 Other specified transient hematological disorders of fetus or newborn — *other specified*

776.9 Unspecified hematological disorder specific to fetus or newborn

777 Perinatal disorders of digestive system

777.1 Fetal and newborn meconium obstruction — *congenital fecaliths, meconium ileus NOS, meconium plug syndrome, delayed passage of meconium*

Meconium obstruction is obstruction of the digestive tract due to the fetal tar-like meconium.

© 2004 Ingenix, Inc.

Signs and symptoms of meconium obstruction include no stools for the first 24 to 48 hours of life, abdominal distention, symptoms of distal intestinal obstruction and incomplete obstruction, and vomiting. Radiology tests, such as a contrast enema, locate the obstruction. Therapies include contrast enema (therapeutic) and saline enemas.

This subcategory includes meconium plug syndrome but excludes meconium ileus (277.01).

777.2 Neonatal intestinal obstruction due to inspissated milk

777.3 Neonatal hematemesis and melena due to swallowed maternal blood — *swallowed blood syndrome in newborn*

777.4 Transitory ileus of newborn

777.5 Necrotizing enterocolitis in fetus or newborn — *pseudomembranous enterocolitis in newborn*

777.6 Perinatal intestinal perforation — *meconium peritonitis*

777.8 Other specified perinatal disorder of digestive system — *other specified*

777.9 Unspecified perinatal disorder of digestive system

Excluded from this rubric is intestinal obstruction classifiable to 560.0-560.9.

778 Conditions involving the integument and temperature regulation of fetus and newborn

778.0 Hydrops fetalis not due to isoimmunization — *idiopathic hydrops*

Use this code to report gross edema of the entire body of the fetus with associated anemia. Nonimmune fetal hydrops can be caused by a wide variety of diseases and disorders involving many different body systems. The infant mortality rate is very high, particularly with premature infants. Therapies include vigorous resuscitation including mechanical ventilation at birth, thoracentesis for pleural effusion, and diuresis. Associated conditions include erythroblastosis fetalis, anemia, hypoproteinemia, respiratory failure, and pleural effusion.

Most diagnostic studies, such as fetal ultrasounds and maternal blood examination, are performed in utero and are not reported in the newborn's chart.

Excluded from this subclassification is hydrops fetalis due to isoimmunization (773.3).

778.1 Sclerema neonatorum — *subcutaneous fat necrosis, Underwood's disease*

778.2 Cold injury syndrome of newborn

778.3 Other hypothermia of newborn

778.4 Other disturbance of temperature regulation of newborn — *dehydration fever, environmentally-induced pyrexia, hyperthermia, transitory fever*

778.5 Other and unspecified edema of newborn — *edema neonatorum*

778.6 Congenital hydrocele — *congenital hydrocele of tunica vaginalis*

Use code 778.6 to report a collection of fluid in the tunica vaginalis of the testicle or along the spermatic cord, or a serous dilation of a cervical duct of an infant. Almost all neonatal hydroceles are communicating and close spontaneously.

Therapies include surgery to repair persistent hydrocele (lasting more than one year) by inguinal incision and ligation of sac.

778.7 Breast engorgement in newborn — *noninfective mastitis*

778.8 Other specified condition involving the integument of fetus and newborn — *urticaria neonatorum*

778.9 Unspecified condition involving the integument and temperature regulation of fetus and newborn

779 Other and ill-defined conditions originating in the perinatal period

779.0 Convulsions in newborn — *fits and seizures in newborn*
AHA: Nov-Dec, 1994, 11

779.1 Other and unspecified cerebral irritability in newborn — *other and unknown*

779.2 Cerebral depression, coma, and other abnormal cerebral signs in fetus or newborn — *CNS dysfunction in newborn NOS*

779.3 Feeding problems in newborn — *regurgitation, slow feeding, and vomiting in newborn*
AHA: Q2, 1989, 15

779.4 Drug reactions and intoxications specific to newborn — *Gray syndrome from chloramphenicol administration in newborn*

Use code 779.4 to report toxic conditions and adverse drug reactions in neonates, especially premature infants, caused by the body's immature detoxification and excretion mechanisms. Gray syndrome, or gray baby syndrome, is a condition caused by an infant's inability to efficiently conjugate and eliminate the antibiotic chloramphenicol.

779.5 Drug withdrawal syndrome in newborn — *drug withdrawal syndrome in infant of dependent mother*
AHA: Q3, 1994, 6

Code 799.5 reports a syndrome in newborns adversely affected by mothers who are addicted to, or frequent abusers of, drugs. Narcotics, cocaine, and coca plant derivatives are the most frequently abused drugs capable of causing withdrawal symptoms in the newborn, but barbiturates, other tranquilizers, amphetamines, other stimulants, and other addictive substances can cause the syndrome.

Signs and symptoms of drug withdrawal syndrome in the newborn include irritability, tremulousness, tachypnea, vomiting or diarrhea, fever, and convulsions. Toxicology tests of blood or urine identify the drug. Therapies include close monitoring for seizure activity or arrhythmias, detoxification tailored for the drug of dependence, drugs such as phenytoin sodium (Dilantin) or phenobarbital for seizures, and exchange transfusions in emergencies.

Associated conditions include fetal alcohol syndrome, dehydration, hypocalcemia, and seizures.

779.6 Termination of pregnancy (fetus) — *fetal death due to induced abortion and termination of pregnancy*

779.7 Periventricular leukomalacia

779.81 Neonatal bradycardia

779.82 Neonatal tachycardia

779.83 Delayed separation of umbilical cord

779.89 Other specified conditions originating in the perinatal period — *atheromatosis of colon, toxemia, uremia, Harlequin color change syndrome, hypertonicity of infancy, papyraceous fetus, strophulus*
AHA: Q1, 1994, 15; Q4, 2002, 67

779.9 Unspecified condition originating in the perinatal period — *congenital debility NOS, stillbirth NEC*

Coding Clarification

Cocaine Addiction in Newborns: Two scenarios may present in newborns who are born to cocaine-addicted mothers. The newborn may exhibit no manifestations of the drug but test positive for cocaine. In this instance, code 760.75 *Cocaine affecting fetus or newborn via placenta or breast milk* is reported. However, the infant may experience drug withdrawal. In these instances, code 779.5 *Drug withdrawal syndrome in newborn* is reported.

Coding Scenario

A mother addicted to cocaine comes to the hospital and delivers a newborn that is in drug withdrawal.

> Code assignment: V30.00 *Single liveborn, born in hospital, delivered without mention of cesarean delivery* and 779.5 *Drug withdrawal syndrome in newborn*

© 2004 Ingenix, Inc.

780–799
Symptoms, Signs, and Ill-Defined Conditions

This chapter includes symptoms, signs, and abnormal results of laboratory or other investigative procedures, as well as ill-defined conditions for which there are no other, more specific diagnoses classifiable elsewhere.

In general, codes from this chapter are used to report symptoms, signs, and ill-defined conditions that point with equal suspicion to two or more diagnoses or represent important problems in medical care that may affect management of the patient. In addition, this chapter provides codes to classify abnormal findings that are reported without a corresponding definitive diagnosis. Codes for such findings can be located in the alphabetic index under such terms as "Abnormal, abnormality, abnormalities," "Decrease, decreased," "Elevation," and "Findings, abnormal, without diagnosis."

Codes from this chapter also are used to report symptoms and signs that existed on initial encounter but proved to be transient and without a specified cause. Also included are provisional diagnoses for patients who fail to return for further investigation, cases referred elsewhere for further investigation before being diagnosed, and cases in which a more definitive diagnosis was not available for other reasons.

Do not assign a code from categories 780-799 when the symptoms, signs, and abnormal findings pertain to a definitive diagnosis. For example, a patient with acute appendicitis would not need additional codes for abdominal pain (rubric 789) and abdominal rigidity (789.4). These signs and symptoms are integral to acute appendicitis and add no value to the patient's coding profile when assigned as secondary codes.

However, you may use a code from this chapter to report symptoms, signs, and abnormal findings that pertain to a particular clinical diagnosis if they represent important problems in medical care. Such problems may be useful to record because they may affect length of stay or level of nursing care and/or monitoring. Such problems also may require additional diagnostic or clinical evaluation or may affect treatment plans. In these cases, list the definitive condition as the principal diagnosis and the symptoms secondarily.

List as a secondary diagnosis any symptoms, signs, and abnormal findings that are not integral to the principal diagnosis but provide important clinical information. For example, a patient with benign prostatic hypertrophy (rubric 600) admitted in acute urinary retention might have acute urinary retention listed as a secondary diagnosis (788.2). Acute urinary retention is not integral to the disease process for benign prostatic hypertrophy, but is an indication for catheterization or surgery. Acute urinary retention can be viewed as an "important medical problem" when the medical record documentation shows the need for clinical evaluation or diagnostic procedures to rule out pathology other than benign prostatic hypertrophy as the etiology. Therapeutic treatment (e.g., catheterization prior to surgery) includes increased nursing care and/or monitoring such as catheter care or extended length of hospital stay.

List as the principal diagnosis any symptoms, signs, and abnormal findings that, after study, cannot be attributed to a definitive diagnosis classifiable to another ICD-9-CM chapter. Also, list as the principal diagnosis any symptom, sign, or abnormal finding that points to contrasting or comparative diagnoses (e.g., it points with equal suspicion to two or more diagnoses). List the contrasting or comparative diagnoses as secondary.

780–789 Symptoms

The definition of a symptom is a subjective observation reported to the physician by the patient but not confirmed by the physician. These observations depart from the structure, function, or sensation that the patient normally experiences.

780 General symptoms

AHA: March-April, 1985, 3; Q2, 1990, 3; Q2, 1990, 5; Q2, 1990, 15; Q1, 1991, 12

These subclassifications report impaired consciousness due to dysfunction of the cerebral hemispheres, the upper brainstem, or both. These codes include coma, transient alteration of awareness, persistent vegetative state, and other alterations such as drowsiness, semicoma, somnolence, stupor, or suppressed or impaired awareness or unconsciousness.

Coma is a state of profound stupor or unconsciousness from which the patient cannot be aroused by external stimuli. The etiology may be trauma, intracranial neoplasm, infection and toxic reaction to infection, poisoning and adverse effects of drugs and chemicals, hypertensive and atherosclerotic cerebrovascular disease, or thrombosis.

Transient alteration of awareness refers to symptoms of staring or transient loss of awareness. This condition has been associated with migraines, epileptic seizures, transient ischemic attacks, or psychological disorders, but in many cases the etiology is unknown.

Lab work may identify the cause based on blood work (hematocrit, respiratory gases, WBC, BUN), urinalysis (sugar, acetone, albumin, sedatives), and levels of glucose, sodium, potassium, bicarbonate, chloride, alcohol, and bromide. A gastric lavage reveals suspected poisoning. A lumbar puncture (if infection is suspected as the etiology) and culture identify the presence of white blood cells and the infective organism.

Therapies depend on etiology and may include, if the cause is unknown, temperature, pulse, respirations and blood pressure checked at frequent intervals, and glucose infusion.

Associated conditions include epidural/subdural hematoma, cerebral infarct or hemorrhage, brain tumor or abscess, brain stem infarction, tumor, hemorrhage, trauma, concussion, cerebral lacerations or contusion, cardiac arrhythmia, shock, epilepsy, infection, subarachnoid hemorrhage, catatonia, hypoglycemia, and diabetic acidosis.

780.01 Coma — *persistent unconsciousness*
AHA: March-April, 1985, 3; Q2, 1990, 3; Q2, 1990, 5; Q2, 1990, 15; Q1, 1991, 12; Q4, 1992, 20; Q3, 1996, 16

780.02 Transient alteration of awareness — *alternating states of consciousness and unconsciousness*
AHA: March-April, 1985, 3; Q2, 1990, 3; Q2, 1990, 5; Q2, 1990, 15; Q1, 1991, 12; Q4, 1992, 20

780.03 Persistent vegetative state — *awake without consciousness*
AHA: March-April, 1985, 3; Q2, 1990, 3; Q2, 1990, 5; Q2, 1990, 15; Q1, 1991, 12; Q4, 1992, 20

780.09 Other alteration of consciousness — *not specified elsewhere, including drowsiness, semicoma, somnolence, stupor*
AHA: March-April, 1985, 3; Q2, 1990, 3; Q2, 1990, 5; Q2, 1990, 15; Q1, 1991, 12; Q4, 1992, 20

780.1 Hallucinations — *auditory, visual, gustatory, olfactory, tactile*
AHA: March-April, 1985, 3; Q2, 1990, 3; Q2, 1990, 5; Q2, 1990, 15; Q1, 1991, 12

Use code 780.1 to report sensory perception of an object or event without corresponding external stimuli. Hallucinations generally take one of five forms, as follows:

- Auditory (perception of nonexistent voices or sounds)
- Visual (perception of nonexistent people, places, or other visual stimuli such as flashes of light)
- Olfactory (perception of nonexistent odors)
- Tactile (perception of nonexistent contact stimuli such as crawling insects on skin)
- Gustatory (perception of unpleasant tastes)

Hallucinations may be due to drugs or toxic substances or due to chronic conditions such as schizophrenia, depression, bipolar affective disorders, and organic brain syndromes.

780.2 Syncope and collapse — *blackout, fainting, Gower's syndrome*
AHA: March-April, 1985, 3; Nov-Dec, 1985, 12; Q2, 1990, 3; Q2, 1990, 5; Q2, 1990, 15; Q1, 1991, 12; Q3, 1995, 14; Q3, 2000, 12; Q1, 2002, 6

Signs and symptoms of syncope and collapse include motionlessness, paleness, diaphoresis, weak pulse, and shallow breathing. Physical exam reveals hypotension and postural changes in heart rate and blood pressure. Lab work may show elevated fasting blood sugar (confirming hyperglycemia) and elevated cardiac serum isoenzyme (identifying acute myocardial infarction). Hematocrit may detect anemia. An electrocardiogram (EKG) may suggest arrhythmia, conduction abnormality, ventricular hypertrophy, or myocardial infarction. A computed tomography (CT) scan of the head and brain confirms focal neurological deficit or intracranial process. Therapies depend on the etiology.

Associated conditions include seizure disorder, arrhythmias, hypovolemia, myocardial infarction, drug toxicity, and transient ischemic attack.

If the cause of the syncope is not documented, verify with the physician as to whether the cause has been established. If so, be sure the medical record is updated to support code selection. For example, if syncope is due to bradycardia, then bradycardia should be documented for accurate reporting.

Definition: Syncope is a transient loss of consciousness due to inadequate blood flow to the brain. The patient experiences generalized weakness, an inability to continue standing, and loss of consciousness. It can last anywhere from a few seconds to as long as 30 minutes. Any form of syncope is reported with code 780.2 if no specific disease process can be identified as causing the condition.

© 2004 Ingenix, Inc.

Neurocardiogenic Syncope: This type of syncope is also known as vasodepressor or vasovagal syncope. It is a condition that results from a drop in blood pressure due to failure of peripheral resistance with concomitant reduced venous return. It may also be due to slowing of the heart, emotional stress, pain, acute loss of blood, or assuming an upright position after having been supine for a prolonged period. It is not uncommon for patients who have just donated blood to experience this form of syncope.

Reaction or Hypersensitivity to Medications: When this occurs, code first the syncope (780.2) followed by an E-code to identify the type of medication.

Convulsions are a series of jerking movements of the face, trunk, or extremities, with involuntary contracture of voluntary muscles. Etiology is an acute focal or generalized disturbance in cerebral function. A small focus of diseased tissue in the cerebrum discharges abnormally in response to certain endogenous or exogenous stimuli. Spread of the discharge to other portions of the cerebrum results in convulsive activity and loss of consciousness. Codes in this subclassification are selected based on whether the convulsions are febrile in origin.

Associated conditions include hyperpyrexia (acute infection, heat stroke), central nervous system infections (meningitis, encephalitis, brain abscess), cerebral trauma (skull fracture, birth injury), cerebral edema (hypertensive encephalopathy, eclampsia), metabolic disturbances (hypoglycemia, hypoparathyroidism), and cerebral hypoxia (Adams-Stokes syndrome, anesthesia).

Codes in subcategory 780.3 classify convulsive disorders and seizures that are ill-defined, as well as sudden, acute symptomatic manifestations of other conditions. Excluded from this subclassification is neonatal convulsion (779.0). Classify convulsive or seizure disorders described as irreversible, intractable, recurrent, repetitive, chronic, or requiring maintenance with phenobarbital or Dilantin for control to rubric 345 *Epilepsy.*

780.31 Febrile convulsions — *pyrexial seizure*
AHA: March-April, 1985, 3; Nov-Dec, 1987, 12; Q2, 1990, 3; Q2, 1990, 5; Q2, 1990, 15; Q1, 1991, 12; Q4, 1992, 23; Q1, 1993, 24; Q3, 1994, 9; Q1, 1997, 12; Q2, 1997, 8; Q4, 1997, 45

780.39 Other convulsions — *not originating with fever*
AHA: March-April, 1985, 3; Nov-Dec, 1987, 12; Q2, 1990, 3; Q2, 1990, 5; Q2, 1990, 15; Q1, 1991, 12; Q4, 1992, 23; Q1, 1993, 24; Q3, 1994, 9; Q1, 1997, 12; Q2, 1997, 8; Q4, 1998, 39; Q2, 1999, 17; Q1, 2003, 7

Only if the diagnosis specifically indicates epilepsy should it be coded as such. Assign code 780.3x unless the documentation states epilepsy.

In cases where repeated admissions for seizures have occurred during the first three years after birth, verify with the physician if the patient's diagnosis of "convulsions" or "seizures" should be classified as infantile spasms, code 345.6x. If the physician does not verify that the condition is infantile spasms, and no underlying pathology is found, use code 780.39 for convulsions of unknown etiology.

When the documentation indicates the diagnosis of posttraumatic seizure disorder only, clarify with the physician if the seizure disorder is to be coded seizure (780.39) or as epilepsy (345.9x).

Benign Shuddering Attacks: This movement disorder noted in young children is not coded as an epileptic or convulsive condition. It is a nonepileptic disorder that may occur as frequently as several times a day, but typically decreases in frequency as the child ages. Use code 333.93 to classify this condition.

Drug Withdrawal: Patients may experience convulsions as a result of inappropriate use of drugs and medications.

Code 780.39 should be used to identify the physical disturbance of convulsions due to drug withdrawal. Code 292.0 would also be used to identify the drug withdrawl. Assign an additional code for the associated drug dependence (304).

If a patient experiences convulsions as a result of discontinuing a medication, use code V58.69 *Long-term (current) drug use,* in addition to the code for the convulsions. If the convulsions are a result of the patient not taking a medication as prescribed, code V15.81 *Noncompliance with medical treatment* should be identified as an additional diagnosis.

Febrile Convulsions: This is the most common seizure disorder of children; 40 percent of first time seizures are febrile. Treatment includes temperature control with acetaminophen and control of the seizures with diazepam or Ativan suppositories. This condition is identified with code 780.31 *Febrile convulsions.*

Neurocysticercosis: This condition is caused by an infestation of the larval form of the parasite Taenia solium. Brain involvement of the parasite can result in epilepsy, increased intracranial pressure, and other neurologic conditions. Two codes should be indicated: 123.1 to identify the parasitic infection and code 780.3x indicating the convulsions.

Newborn Convulsions: Convulsions of a newborn are serious and can be caused by such conditions as hypoglycemia, hypocalcemia, sepsis, or central nervous system damage. If no etiology has been determined during the newborn stay, report with code 779.0 *Convulsions in newborn.*

Code 780.3x is assigned only when repeated admissions have occurred following birth and the etiology of the convulsions is unknown.

780.4 Dizziness and giddiness — *light-headedness, vertigo not otherwise specified*
AHA: March-April, 1985, 3; Q2, 1990, 3; Q2, 1990, 5; Q2, 1990, 15; Q1, 1991, 12; Q2, 1991, 17; Q2, 1997, 9; Q3, 2000, 12; Q2, 2003, 11

Use code 780.4 to report the illusion of movement or a feeling of unsteadiness or light-headedness.

Associated conditions include brain stem ischemia, head trauma, multiple sclerosis, posterior fossa tumor, acoustic neuroma, labyrinthitis, Meniére's disease, vestibular neuritis, herpes zoster, and toxic levels of drugs.

Excluded from this subcategory are sleep disturbances that are not organic in nature (307.40-307.49).

780.50 Unspecified sleep disturbance

780.51 Insomnia with sleep apnea — *cessation of breathing causes sleeplessness*
AHA: March-April, 1985, 3; Q2, 1990, 3; Q2, 1990, 5; Q2, 1990, 15; Q1, 1991, 12

There are three types of sleep apnea: obstructive, central, and mixed; of the three, obstructive sleep apnea (OSA) is the most common. Despite the difference in the root cause of each type, people with untreated sleep apnea stop breathing repeatedly during their sleep, sometimes hundreds of times during the night and often for a minute or longer, according to the American Sleep Apnea Association.

Obstructive sleep apnea is caused by a blockage of the airway, usually when the soft tissue in the rear of the throat collapses and closes during sleep. In central sleep apnea, the airway is not blocked but the brain fails to signal the muscles to breathe. Mixed sleep apnea is a combination of the two. The condition arouses sleep apnea victims from sleep in order for them to resume breathing, resulting in fragmented sleep.

Sleep apnea affects more than 12 million Americans, according to the National Institutes of Health. Males are more prone to sleep apnea than females. Risk of sleep apnea increases for those overweight and older than 40 years of age, although sleep apnea can strike anyone at any age.

Untreated, sleep apnea can cause high blood pressure and other cardiovascular disease, memory problems, weight gain, impotency, and headaches. Several treatment options exist, and research into additional options continues.

780.52 Other insomnia — *sleeplessness not associated with apnea*
AHA: March-April, 1985, 3; Q2, 1990, 3; Q2, 1990, 5; Q2, 1990, 15; Q1, 1991, 12

780.53 Hypersomnia with sleep apnea — *cessation of breathing causes sleepiness*
AHA: March-April, 1985, 3; Nov-Dec, 1985, 4; Q2, 1990, 3; Q2, 1990, 5; Q2, 1990, 15; Q1, 1991, 12; Q1, 1993, 28

780.54 Other hypersomnia — *sleepiness not associated with apnea*
AHA: March-April, 1985, 3; Q2, 1990, 3; Q2, 1990, 5; Q2, 1990, 15; Q1, 1991, 12

780.55 Disruptions of 24-hour sleep-wake cycle — *inversion of sleep rhythm, irregular sleep-wake cycle*
AHA: March-April, 1985, 3; Q2, 1990, 3; Q2, 1990, 5; Q2, 1990, 15; Q1, 1991, 12

780.56 Dysfunctions associated with sleep stages or arousal from sleep

780.57 Other and unspecified sleep apnea — *unknown or not elsewhere classified*
AHA: March-April, 1985, 3; Q2, 1990, 3; Q2, 1990, 5; Q2, 1990, 15; Q1, 1991, 12; Q1, 1993, 28; Q1, 1997, 5; Q1, 2001, 6

Other and unspecified sleep apnea involves the abnormal cessation of breathing during sleep not classified elsewhere. Sleep apnea is due to either a failure of the ventilatory drive as seen in diseases of the central nervous system or an obstruction of the upper airway as seen in massive obesity or tonsillar hypertrophy. Central sleep apnea is a form of apnea due to a hereditary failure of the ventilatory drive in males.

780.58 Sleep related movement disorder

Sleep related movement disorder, also known as nocturnal myoclonus, is characterized by involuntary movement during sleep. This can range from slight movement of small continuous movements of the ankle or toes to wild flailing of the legs and arms. The patient may initially present with poor sleep or daytime sleepiness. The disorder is characterized by repetitive, involuntary movement during the night. The cause of this disorder is not known. Sleep studies are required for definitive diagnosis. Currently there is no cure, but medication may alleviate the symptoms.

780.59 Other sleep disturbances

780.6 Fever — *pyrexia, PUO, FUO, chills with fever*
AHA: March-April, 1985, 3; Q2, 1990, 3; Q2, 1990, 5; Q2, 1990, 15; Q1, 1991, 12; Q2, 1991, 8; Q4, 1999, 26; Q3, 2000, 13

Fever is an abnormal elevation of body temperature (at least 38.3 C or 101 F) for a minimum of three weeks without the etiology being determined despite exhaustive investigation. Fever that is ill-defined or unspecified also is classified here.

Therapies depend on the etiology, but include cooling blankets, cold compresses, antibiotics, and antipyretics (aspirin, acetaminophen). Associated conditions include infections, connective tissue

© 2004 Ingenix, Inc.

disorders, and occult neoplasm (leukemia, lymphoma).

Excluded from this subcategory is fatigue during combat (308.0-308.9), heat (992.6), and pregnancy (646.8x); and fatigue or malaise related to neurasthenia (300.5) and senile asthenia (797).

780.71 Chronic fatigue syndrome — *severe, prolonged fatigue impairing daily function, without proven physical or psychological cause*
AHA: March-April, 1985, 3; March-April, 1987, 8; Q4, 1988, 12; Q2, 1990, 3; Q2, 1990, 5; Q2, 1990, 15; Q1, 1991, 12; Q4, 1998, 48

Chronic fatigue syndrome (CFS) also is known as myalgic encephalomyelitis, postviral fatigue syndrome, and chronic fatigue and immune dysfunction syndrome. It is marked by unrelenting exhaustion, muscle pain, cognitive disorders that patients call "brain fog," and a profound weakness that does not go away with a few good nights of sleep. There is no known cause. CFS may begin after a bout with a cold, bronchitis, hepatitis, or an intestinal bug. For some, it follows a bout of infectious mononucleosis or during a period of high stress. Unlike flu symptoms, CFS symptoms, such as a chronic headache, muscle and joint aches, and fatigue, either hang on or come and go frequently for more than six months. Some patients are bedridden; others can work or attend school at least part time, since any exertion typically worsens symptoms.

CFS is diagnosed two to four times more often in females than males and it is estimated that as many as 500,000 people in the United States have a CFS-like condition. There is no effective treatment for CFS. However, nonsteroidal anti-inflammatory drugs, such as ibuprofen, reduce body aches or fever, and nonsedative antihistamines relieve any prominent allergic symptoms, such as a runny nose.

780.79 Other malaise and fatigue — *asthenia, postviral syndrome, Stiller's asthenia, neurasthenia, albionarc*
AHA: March-April, 1985, 3; March-April, 1987, 8; Q4, 1988, 12; Q2, 1990, 3; Q2, 1990, 5; Q2, 1990, 15; Q1, 1991, 12; Q4, 1999, 26; Q1, 2000, 6

780.8 Generalized hyperhidrosis — *night sweats, diaphoresis, excessive sweating*
AHA: March-April, 1985, 3; Q2, 1990, 3; Q2, 1990, 5; Q2, 1990, 15; Q1, 1991, 12

780.91 Fussy infant (baby)

780.92 Excessive crying of infant (baby)

780.93 Memory loss

780.94 Early satiety

780.99 Other general symptoms — *chill(s) NOS, generalized pain, hypothermia not associated with environmental temperature*
AHA: March-April, 1985, 3; Nov-Dec, 1985, 12; Q2, 1990, 3; Q2, 1990, 5; Q2, 1990, 15; Q1, 1991, 12; Q3, 1993, 11; Q4, 1999, 10; Q4, 2002, 67; Q4, 2003, 103

Report 705.21 for primary focal hyperhidrosis. Report 705.22 for secondary focal hyperhidrosis. Report 333.99 for restless leg syndrome.

Coding Scenario

A 72-year-old female is seen with complaints of transient dizziness. She must sit down immediately when experiencing this symptom. She states that she may have lost consciousness for a few seconds but is unsure. The physician documents syncope and will order further diagnostic testing if the patient experiences recurrence of the symptoms.

Code assignment: 780.2 *Syncope and collapse*

A patient is seen in the physician's office complaining of persistent fainting spells upon rising in the morning. She notes no other symptoms. The physician documents neurocardiogenic syncope and recommends further testing.

Code assignment: 780.2 *Syncope and collapse*

A 5-year-old male is seen in the emergency department. His mother states that he suffered a seizure. Upon examination the child is found to have acute nonsuppurative otitis media and a temperature of 104.2.

Code assignment: 780.31 *Febrile convulsions* and 381.00 *Acute nonsuppurative otitis media, unspecified*

A 2-year-old female is admitted via the emergency department for recurrent seizures. The physician's final diagnostic statement states recurrent seizure disorder.

Code assignment: 780.39 *Other convulsions*

A 45-year-old male presents for the result of his recent polysomnography. Initially, the patient presented with symptoms of feeling tired during the day. The patient's wife stated that the patient had continuous leg movement during the night. Urine and blood tests were normal. Sleep study confirms the patient's leg movement several times during the night awakening the patient. Diagnosis: Sleep related movement disorder.

Code assignment: 780.58 *Sleep related movement disorder*

781 Symptoms involving nervous and musculoskeletal systems

AHA: March-April, 1985, 3; Q2, 1990, 3; Q2, 1990, 5; Q2, 1990, 15; Q1, 1991, 12

781.0 Abnormal involuntary movements — *spasms, tremors, head movements, fasiculations; not otherwise specified*
AHA: March-April, 1985, 3; Q2, 1990, 3; Q2, 1990, 5; Q2, 1990, 15; Q1, 1991, 12

781.1 Disturbances of sensation of smell and taste — *anosmia, parageusia, parosmia*
AHA: March-April, 1985, 3; Q2, 1990, 3; Q2, 1990, 5; Q2, 1990, 15; Q1, 1991, 12

781.2 Abnormality of gait — *ataxic, paralytic, spastic, staggering*
AHA: March-April, 1985, 3; Q2, 1990, 3; Q2, 1990, 5; Q2, 1990, 15; Q1, 1991, 12

781.3 Lack of coordination — *muscular incoordination, ataxia not otherwise specified*
AHA: March-April, 1985, 3; Q2, 1990, 3; Q2, 1990, 5; Q2, 1990, 15; Q1, 1991, 12; Q3, 1997, 12

781.4 Transient paralysis of limb — *transient monoplegia*
AHA: March-April, 1985, 3; Q2, 1990, 3; Q2, 1990, 5; Q2, 1990, 15; Q1, 1991, 12

781.5 Clubbing of fingers — *enlargement of soft tissues of distal fingers*
AHA: March-April, 1985, 3; Q2, 1990, 3; Q2, 1990, 5; Q2, 1990, 15; Q1, 1991, 12

781.6 Meningismus — *irritation of lining of brain or spinal cord; Dupre's syndrome, meningism*
AHA: March-April, 1985, 3; Jan-Feb, 1987, 7; Q2, 1990, 3; Q2, 1990, 5; Q2, 1990, 15; Q1, 1991, 12; Q3, 2000, 13

781.7 Tetany — *extremity muscle spasms; carpopedal spasm, magnesium deficiency syndrome*
AHA: March-April, 1985, 3; Q2, 1990, 3; Q2, 1990, 5; Q2, 1990, 15; Q1, 1991, 12

Tetany is a type of cramp that causes the muscles of the hands and feet to cramp rhythmically, as well as spasms of the larynx with difficulty in breathing, nausea, vomiting, convulsions, and considerable pain. The disorder stems from a mineral imbalance, such as a lack of calcium, potassium, or magnesium, or an acid or alkaline condition of the body.

Associated conditions include poorly controlled hypoparathyroidism, hypophosphatemia, osteomalacia, renal disorders, or malabsorption syndromes. Treatment is directed at restoring metabolic balance, as by intravenous administration of calcium in cases of hypocalcemia (calcium deficiency).

781.8 Neurological neglect syndrome — *asomatognosia, hemi-akinesia, hemi-spatial neglect, sensory neglect, visuospatial neglect*
AHA: March-April, 1985, 3; Q2, 1990, 3; Q2, 1990, 5; Q2, 1990, 15; Q1, 1991, 12; Q4, 1994, 37

781.91 Loss of height — *not due to osteoporosis*
AHA: March-April, 1985, 3; Q2, 1990, 3; Q2, 1990, 5; Q2, 1990, 15; Q1, 1991, 12; Q4, 2000, 45

781.92 Abnormal posture

781.93 Ocular torticollis

781.94 Facial weakness — *facial droop*
AHA: Q4, 2003, 72

781.99 Other symptoms involving nervous and musculoskeletal systems — *acragnosis, acroagnosis, acute catatonia, floppy infant syndrome, growing pains; not otherwise specified*
AHA: March-April, 1985, 3; Q2, 1990, 3; Q2, 1990, 5; Q2, 1990, 15; Q1, 1991, 12; Q4, 2000, 45

Excluded from this rubric are depression not otherwise specified (311); pain in the limb (729.5); and disorders relating to the back (724.0-724.9), hearing (388.0-389.9), joint (718.0-719.9), limb (729.0-729.9), neck (723.0-723.9), or vision (368.0-369.9).

782 Symptoms involving skin and other integumentary tissue

AHA: March-April, 1985, 3; Q2, 1990, 3; Q2, 1990, 5; Q2, 1990, 15; Q1, 1991, 12

782.0 Disturbance of skin sensation — *anesthesia, burning, prickling, numbness, tingling, hyperesthsia, hypoesthesia, paresthesia, Berger's paresthesia, pseudohemianesthesia*
AHA: March-April, 1985, 3; Q2, 1990, 3; Q2, 1990, 5; Q2, 1990, 15; Q1, 1991, 12

782.1 Rash and other nonspecific skin eruption — *exanthem*
AHA: March-April, 1985, 3; Q2, 1990, 3; Q2, 1990, 5; Q2, 1990, 15; Q1, 1991, 12

782.2 Localized superficial swelling, mass, or lump — *subcutaneous nodules*
AHA: March-April, 1985, 3; Q2, 1990, 3; Q2, 1990, 5; Q2, 1990, 15; Q1, 1991, 12

782.3 Edema — *fluid in soft tissue; localized, anasarca, dropsy, Secretan's syndrome*
AHA: March-April, 1985, 3; Q2, 1990, 3; Q2, 1990, 5; Q2, 1990, 15; Q1, 1991, 12; Q2, 2000, 18

Edema is the accumulation of excessive amounts of fluid (water and sodium) in the intercellular tissue spaces of the body. Edema results when the balance of the lymphatic system, which normally transports excess interstitial fluid back to the intravascular space, is compromised. Pitting edema is a type of edema that retains for a time the indentation produced by pressure that forces fluid into the underlying tissues. Nonpitting edema is a type of edema that leaves no indentation when pressure is applied because fluid has coagulated in the tissues.

 © 2004 Ingenix, Inc.

Edema may occur at any site of the body, indicating different causes.

Excluded from this code are ascites (789.5), edema of newborn (778.5), edema of pregnancy (642.0x-642.9x, 646.1x), fluid retention (276.6), hydrops fetalis (773.3, 778.0), hydrothorax (511.8), and nutritional edema (260, 262).

782.4 Jaundice, unspecified, not of newborn — *bilirubin causing yellow cast to skin; cholemia, icterus*
AHA: March-April, 1985, 3; Q2, 1990, 3; Q2, 1990, 5; Q2, 1990, 15; Q1, 1991, 12

Use this code to report yellow discoloration of the skin and/or mucous membranes due to excessive levels of bilirubin in the blood. Pruritus, dark urine, and clay-colored stools commonly accompany jaundice. Etiologies for jaundice include congestive heart failure, carcinoma of the papilla of Vater or pancreas, cholecystitis and cholelithiasis, Kaye or Byler cholestasis, Laennec's or primary cirrhosis of the liver, liver abscess, hepatitis, acute or chronic pancreatitis, Dubin-Johnson syndrome, hemolytic anemia, glucose-6-phosphate dehydrogenase (G6PD) deficiency, and drug-induced hepatic insult. Lab work may include urine and fecal urobilinogen, serum bilirubin, liver enzyme tests, serum cholesterol, prothrombin, and complete blood count (CBC). Liver biopsy may rule out hepatic etiology.

Therapies depend on the etiology, such as cholecystectomy for jaundice due to cholecystitis; dietary management, including increased carbohydrates, decreased proteins, and fewer high-fat foods; frequent skin cleansing; and topical antipruritic medications for pruritus.

Jaundice in newborn (774.0-774.7) and jaundice due to isoimmunization (773.0-773.2, 773.4) are excluded from this code.

782.5 Cyanosis — *deficient oxygen in blood, causing blue cast to skin*
AHA: March-April, 1985, 3; Q2, 1990, 3; Q2, 1990, 5; Q2, 1990, 15; Q1, 1991, 12

Cyanosis in newborn (770.83) is excluded from this code.

782.61 Pallor — *pale skin*
AHA: March-April, 1985, 3; Q2, 1990, 3; Q2, 1990, 5; Q2, 1990, 15; Q1, 1991, 12

782.62 Flushing — *ruddy skin, excessive blushing*
AHA: March-April, 1985, 3; Q2, 1990, 3; Q2, 1990, 5; Q2, 1990, 15; Q1, 1991, 12

782.7 Spontaneous ecchymoses — *hemorrhagic spots with the appearance of freckles; petechiae*
AHA: March-April, 1985, 3; Q2, 1990, 3; Q2, 1990, 5; Q2, 1990, 15; Q1, 1991, 12

Ecchymoses is defined as a purplish, flat bruise that occurs when blood leaks out into the top layers of skin; the bruise is not raised but may be irregular in shape. Spontaneous ecchymoses is often a symptom of a coagulation disorder. Sometimes diagnostic tests are necessary to determine the diagnosis, such as serologic tests, biopsies, culture plus antimicrobial sensitivity, dermatrophy, and test media-ring worm.

782.8 Changes in skin texture — *induration, thickening, scabs, scales*
AHA: March-April, 1985, 3; Q2, 1990, 3; Q2, 1990, 5; Q2, 1990, 15; Q1, 1991, 12

782.9 Other symptoms involving skin and integumentary tissues — *not otherwise specified*
AHA: March-April, 1985, 3; Q2, 1990, 3; Q2, 1990, 5; Q2, 1990, 15; Q1, 1991, 12

Symptoms relating to possible breast disorders (611.71-611.79) are excluded from this rubric.

783 Symptoms concerning nutrition, metabolism, and development

AHA: March-April, 1985, 3; Q2, 1990, 3; Q2, 1990, 5; Q2, 1990, 15; Q1, 1991, 12

783.0 Anorexia — *loss of appetite*
AHA: March-April, 1985, 3; Q2, 1990, 3; Q2, 1990, 5; Q2, 1990, 15; Q1, 1991, 12

This code reports loss of appetite. This is a common symptom of gastrointestinal (GI) and endocrine disorders as well as psychological disturbances. Investigation of organ-specific pathology (function studies of thyroid, liver, kidney, upper GI, gallbladder), barium enema, and blood work allow assessment of nutritional status.

Associated conditions include hypopituitarism, hypothyroidism, ketoacidosis, appendicitis, cirrhosis, Crohn's disease, gastritis, hepatitis, chronic renal failure, pernicious anemia, alcoholism, anorexia nervosa, and cancer.

This subcategory does not include anorexia nervosa. Anorexia nervosa is a psychophysiological condition classified to 307.1. Also excluded is loss of appetite with a nonorganic origin (307.59).

Polyphagia refers to eating to the point of being focused only on eating (or excessive eating) before feeling full. This can be a symptom of various disorders. It can be intermittent or persistent and depending on the cause, it may or may not result in weight gain. Common causes include anxiety, premenstrual syndrome, bulimia, diabetes mellitus, gestational diabetes, Graves' disease, hyperthyroidism, hypoglycemia, and drugs such as corticosteroids, cyproheptadine, and tricyclic antidepressants.

783.1 Abnormal weight gain

783.21 Loss of weight

783.3 Feeding difficulties and mismanagement — *typically in elderly, infants*
AHA: March-April, 1985, 3; Q2, 1990, 3; Q2, 1990, 5; Q2, 1990, 15; Q1, 1991, 12; Q3, 1997, 12

783.40 Lack of normal physiological development, unspecified — *inadequate development, lack of development in childhood*
AHA: March-April, 1985, 3; Q2, 1990, 3; Q2, 1990, 5; Q2, 1990, 15; Q1, 1991, 12; Q3, 1997, 4; Q4, 2000, 45

783.41 Failure to thrive — *failure to gain weight in childhood*
AHA: March-April, 1985, 3; Q2, 1990, 3; Q2, 1990, 5; Q2, 1990, 15; Q1, 1991, 12; Q3, 1997, 4; Q4, 2000, 45; Q1, 2003, 12

783.42 Delayed milestones — *late walker, late talker*
AHA: March-April, 1985, 3; Q2, 1990, 3; Q2, 1990, 5; Q2, 1990, 15; Q1, 1991, 12; Q3, 1997, 4; Q4, 2000, 45

783.43 Short stature — *growth failure, physical retardation in childhood*
AHA: March-April, 1985, 3; Q2, 1990, 3; Q2, 1990, 5; Q2, 1990, 15; Q1, 1991, 12; Q3, 1997, 4; Q4, 2000, 45

783.5 Polydipsia

783.6 Polyphagia

Excluded from this subcategory are disorders of eating of nonorganic origin (307.50-307.59).

783.7 Adult failure to thrive

783.9 Other symptoms concerning nutrition, metabolism, and development

784 Symptoms involving head and neck

AHA: March-April, 1985, 3; Q2, 1990, 3; Q2, 1990, 5; Q2, 1990, 15; Q1, 1991, 12

784.0 Headache

Use code 784.0 to report pain in the cranial vaults, orbits, or nape of neck. About 90 percent of all headaches are benign. The basic etiologies of the headache are muscle contraction (tension headache), vascular (migraine or cluster headache), or a combination.

Excluded from this subcategory are atypical face pain (350.2), migraine (346.0x-346.9x), and tension headache (307.81).

784.1 Throat pain

784.2 Swelling, mass, or lump in head and neck

784.3 Aphasia

Aphasia is impaired expression or comprehension of written or spoken language due to disease or injury of one or more of the brain's language centers: Broca's area, Wernicke's area, or arcuate fasciculus. Broca's area controls the muscle for speech (expressive aphasia). Wernicke's area controls the auditory and visual comprehension for speech (receptive aphasia). The arcuate fasciculus aids in control of the content of speech and enables repetition.

Associated conditions include Alzheimer's disease, brain tumor, cerebrovascular accident, encephalitis, head trauma, and heroin overdose.

784.40 Unspecified voice disturbance

784.41 Aphonia — *loss of voice*
AHA: March-April, 1985, 3; Q2, 1990, 3; Q2, 1990, 5; Q2, 1990, 15; Q1, 1991, 12

784.49 Other voice disturbance — *change, hoarseness, hypernasality, dysphonia, plicae dysphonia ventricularis, rhinolalia, trachyphonia; not otherwise specified*
AHA: March-April, 1985, 3; Q2, 1990, 3; Q2, 1990, 5; Q2, 1990, 15; Q1, 1991, 12

784.5 Other speech disturbance — *dysarthria, dysphasia, slurred speech*
AHA: March-April, 1985, 3; Q2, 1990, 3; Q2, 1990, 5; Q2, 1990, 15; Q1, 1991, 12

784.60 Symbolic dysfunction, unspecified — *unknown variety*
AHA: March-April, 1985, 3; Q2, 1990, 3; Q2, 1990, 5; Q2, 1990, 15; Q1, 1991, 12

784.61 Alexia and dyslexia — *organic inability or difficulty in reading*
AHA: March-April, 1985, 3; Q2, 1990, 3; Q2, 1990, 5; Q2, 1990, 15; Q1, 1991, 12

784.69 Other symbolic dysfunction — *acalculia, agnosia, Bianchi's or Gerstmann's syndrome, palilalia, agraphia, apraxia*
AHA: March-April, 1985, 3; Q2, 1990, 3; Q2, 1990, 5; Q2, 1990, 15; Q1, 1991, 12

784.7 Epistaxis — *nosebleed*
AHA: March-April, 1985, 3; Q2, 1990, 3; Q2, 1990, 5; Q2, 1990, 15; Q1, 1991, 12

Use code 784.7 to report nosebleed. Typically occurring unilaterally, epistaxis may be spontaneous or induced from the front or back of the nose. The majority of nosebleeds occur within the anterior-inferior nasal septum (Kiesselbach's plexus), but they also can occur at the point where the inferior turbinates meet the nasopharynx. In nonsevere cases, a complete blood count may reveal acute blood loss anemia, prothrombin, and activated partial thromboplastin time measurements. Therapies include application of external pressure, insertion of cotton treated with vasoconstrictor and local anesthetic, and humidified oxygen. In severe cases, therapies may include IV hydration, pinching in of the nares to control bleeding in the absence of nasal fracture, and anterior or posterior nasal packing if other measures prove ineffective in controlling bleeding.

Associated conditions include maxillofacial injury, nasal fracture, nasal tumors, orbital floor fracture,

© 2004 Ingenix, Inc.

acute sinusitis, hypertension, cirrhosis, hepatitis, renal failure, skull fracture, aplastic and acute blood loss anemia, coagulation disorders, hereditary hemorrhagic telangiectasia (Rendu-Osler-Weber disease), leukemia, polycythemia vera, systemic lupus erythematosus, infectious mononucleosis, influenza, and anticoagulant use (adverse effect).

784.8 Hemorrhage from throat — *bleeding*
AHA: March-April, 1985, 3; Q2, 1990, 3; Q2, 1990, 5; Q2, 1990, 15; Q1, 1991, 12

784.9 Other symptoms involving head and neck — *choking sensation, sternutation, mouth breathing, sneezing, or halitosis; not otherwise specified*
AHA: March-April, 1985, 3; Q2, 1990, 3; Q2, 1990, 5; Q2, 1990, 15; Q1, 1991, 12

Excluded from this rubric are encephalopathy not otherwise specified (348.3) and specific symptoms involving neck classifiable to rubric 723.

785 Symptoms involving cardiovascular system

AHA: March-April, 1985, 3; Q2, 1990, 3; Q2, 1990, 5; Q2, 1990, 15; Q1, 1991, 12

785.0 Unspecified tachycardia — *rapid heart beat*
AHA: March-April, 1985, 3; Q2, 1990, 3; Q2, 1990, 5; Q2, 1990, 15; Q1, 1991, 12; Q2, 2003, 11

This code reports a heart rate greater than 100 beats per minute caused by the heart making an effort to deliver more oxygen to the body tissues by increasing the rate at which blood passes through the vessels. Usually, the patient will complain of palpitations or racing of the heart. Tachycardia may be the result of excitement, exercise, pain, or fever as well as caffeine and tobacco. However, it may be an early sign of a life-threatening disorder such as cardiogenic or septic shock.`

Associated conditions include neurogenic shock, adult respiratory distress syndrome, chronic obstructive pulmonary disease, pneumothorax, pulmonary embolism, cardiac dysrhythmia, cardiogenic shock, congestive heart failure, hypertensive crisis, myocardial infarction, thyrotoxicosis, anemia, diabetic ketoacidosis, hyponatremia, anaphylactic shock, and septic shock.

Excluded from this subcategory is paroxysmal tachycardia (427.0-427.2) and neonatal tachycardia (779.82).

785.1 Palpitations — *awareness of heart beat*
AHA: March-April, 1985, 3; Q2, 1990, 3; Q2, 1990, 5; Q2, 1990, 15; Q1, 1991, 12

785.2 Undiagnosed cardiac murmurs — *mitral or systolic click syndrome, heart murmur not otherwise specified*
AHA: March-April, 1985, 3; Q2, 1990, 3; Q2, 1990, 5; Q2, 1990, 15; Q1, 1991, 12; Q4, 1992, 16

785.3 Other abnormal heart sounds — *cardiac dullness, friction fremitus, precardial friction*
AHA: March-April, 1985, 3; Q2, 1990, 3; Q2, 1990, 5; Q2, 1990, 15; Q1, 1991, 12

785.4 Gangrene — (Code first any associated underlying condition:250.7, 443.0) — *phagedena, spreading cutaneous gangrene, gangrenous cellulitis*
AHA: March-April, 1985, 3; March-April, 1986, 12; Q2, 1990, 3; Q2, 1990, 5; Q2, 1990, 15; Q3, 1990, 15; Q1, 1991, 12; Q3, 1991, 12

Gangrene is the death of tissue due to loss of vascular supply. Gangrene may be wet (bacterial infection with cellulitis) or dry (affected area is dry and shriveled).

Associated conditions include diabetes with microangiopathy, ischemia due to atherosclerosis or embolism, and Raynaud's phenomenon. Code first any associated underlying disease.

This subcategory excludes gas gangrene due to tissue invasion by *Clostridium perfringens* or other clostridia (classified to code 040.0) and gangrene to a variety of specific sites. Refer to the ICD-9-CM index under "Gangrene, gangrenous" for specific code assignments since some specific types of gangrene are classified to other chapters.

Use codes in this subclassification to report a condition in which the blood flow to peripheral tissues and perfusion are inadequate to sustain life due to insufficient cardiac output or maladapted distribution of peripheral blood flow. The principal deficiency is a reduction in perfusion of vital tissues resulting in inadequate oxygen delivery. This facilitates aerobic metabolism, which results in anaerobic respiration. The result is increased production and accumulation of lactic acid (metabolic acidosis) with compensatory hyperventilation and respiratory alkalosis. Eventually, the homeostatic mechanisms that serve to maintain acid-base balance fail, leading to cell death and subsequent organ failure.

Cardiogenic shock is shock resulting from decreased cardiac output in heart disease. Associated conditions include disturbance of heart rate or rhythm, acute myocardial infarction, valvular heart disease, cardiomyopathy, hypoxemia secondary to pulmonary or neurologic disease, tension pneumothorax, pericardial tamponade, massive pulmonary embolism, prosthetic valve malfunction, and mixed acid-base balance disorder.

Shock due to anesthetic (995.4), anaphylactic shock (995.0), electric shock (994.8), shock following abortion (639.5), shock from lightning (994.0), shock following an obstetrical procedure (669.1), postoperative shock (998.0), or traumatic shock (958.4) are excluded from this classification.

785.50 Unspecified shock — *unknown cause*
AHA: March-April, 1985, 3; Q2, 1990, 3; Q2, 1990, 5; Q2, 1990, 15; Q1, 1991, 12; Q2, 1996, 10

785.51 Cardiogenic shock — *failure of peripheral circulation due to heart insufficiency*
AHA: March-April, 1985, 3; Q2, 1990, 3; Q2, 1990, 5; Q2, 1990, 15; Q1, 1991, 12

785.52 Septic shock — (Code first systemic inflammatory response syndrome due to infectious process with organ dysfunction, 995.92) — *infection in the blood stream or other tissues that is usually circulated throughout the body; the infectious agent(s) in the vascular system causes large amounts of blood sit in the capillaries and veins, with cytokines, prostaglandins, and/or other intermediaries possibly involved in the process*
AHA: Q4, 2003, 73, 79

785.59 Other shock without mention of trauma — *hypervolemic, septic shock; not otherwise specified*
AHA: March-April, 1985, 3; Q2, 1990, 3; Q2, 1990, 5; Q2, 1990, 15; Q1, 1991, 12; Q2, 2000, 3

785.6 Enlargement of lymph nodes — *lymphadenopathy, swollen glands*
AHA: March-April, 1985, 3; Q2, 1990, 3; Q2, 1990, 5; Q2, 1990, 15; Q1, 1991, 12

785.9 Other symptoms involving cardiovascular system — *strong pulse, weak pulse, bruit; not otherwise specified*
AHA: March-April, 1985, 3; Q2, 1990, 3; Q2, 1990, 5; Q2, 1990, 15; Q1, 1991, 12

Excluded from this rubric is heart failure, not otherwise specified (428.9).

786 Symptoms involving respiratory system and other chest symptoms

AHA: March-April, 1985, 3; Q2, 1990, 3; Q2, 1990, 5; Q2, 1990, 15; Q1, 1991, 12

786.00 Unspecified respiratory abnormality

786.01 Hyperventilation — *rapid breathing*
AHA: March-April, 1985, 3; Q2, 1990, 3; Q2, 1990, 5; Q2, 1990, 15; Q1, 1991, 12

786.02 Orthopnea — *difficult respiration except when patient is upright*
AHA: March-April, 1985, 3; Q2, 1990, 3; Q2, 1990, 5; Q2, 1990, 15; Q1, 1991, 12

786.03 Apnea — *momentary cessation in breathing*
AHA: March-April, 1985, 3; Q2, 1990, 3; Q2, 1990, 5; Q2, 1990, 15; Q1, 1991, 12; Q4, 1998, 50

This subclassification excludes sleep apnea (780.51, 780.53, and 780.57) and apnea of newborn (770.81, 770.82).

786.04 Cheyne-Stokes respiration

Cheyne-Stokes respiration is defined as an abnormal breathing pattern that is first shallow and infrequent and then increases gradually to abnormally deep and rapid, before fading away completely for about five to 30 seconds, before the next cycle of shallow breathing begins. Cheyne-Stokes respiration is often accompanied by changes in the level of consciousness; it most commonly occurs in seriously ill patients with brain or heart disorders. It may occur during sleep.

Therapies include treating the associated heart or brain disorder and prescribing the drug aminophylline.

786.05 Shortness of breath

786.06 Tachypnea — *quick, shallow breathing*
AHA: March-April, 1985, 3; Q2, 1990, 3; Q2, 1990, 5; Q2, 1990, 15; Q1, 1991, 12; Q4, 1998, 50

786.07 Wheezing — *whistling noises during breathing*
AHA: March-April, 1985, 3; Q2, 1990, 3; Q2, 1990, 5; Q2, 1990, 15; Q1, 1991, 12; Q4, 1998, 50

786.09 Other dyspnea and respiratory abnormalities — *snoring, yawning, paroxysmal dyspnea, respiratory distress; not otherwise specified*
AHA: March-April, 1985, 3; Q1, 1990, 9; Q2, 1990, 3; Q2, 1990, 5; Q2, 1990, 15; Q1, 1991, 12; Q1, 1997, 7; Q2, 1998, 10

This subclassification excludes respiratory distress of newborn (770.89) and respiratory failure of newborn (770.84).

786.1 Stridor — *harsh sound associated with respiration in patients with airway obstruction*
AHA: March-April, 1985, 3; Q2, 1990, 3; Q2, 1990, 5; Q2, 1990, 15; Q1, 1991, 12

786.2 Cough

786.3 Hemoptysis — *cough with hemorrhage*
AHA: March-April, 1985, 3; Q2, 1990, 3; Q2, 1990, 5; Q2, 1990, 15; Q4, 1990, 26; Q1, 1991, 12

Hemoptysis is coughing up or spitting out of blood or bloody sputum from the lungs or tracheobronchial tree. Expectoration of 200 ml of blood in a single episode suggests severe bleeding. Expectoration of 400 ml in three hours, or more than 600 ml in 16 hours, is life threatening. Bleeding into the respiratory tract by bronchial or pulmonary vessels causes

 © 2004 Ingenix, Inc.

hemoptysis, which reflects changes in the vascular walls and blood-clotting mechanisms. Lab work, including complete count, sputum culture and smear, and coagulation studies, may reveal anemia or infection. Chest x-ray, pulmonary arteriography, or lung scan may rule out disease such as carcinoma, tuberculosis, and pneumonia. Bronchoscopy (with biopsy), in severe hemoptysis, locates bleeding site. Therapies include placement of the patient in Trendelenburg position to promote drainage of blood from the lungs and cough suppressants to prevent blood from spreading throughout the lungs.

Associated conditions include chronic bronchitis, bronchogenic carcinoma, bronchiectasis, laryngeal cancer, bronchial adenoma, lung abscess, pneumonia (Klebsiella, pneumococcal), pulmonary arteriovenous fistula, pulmonary contusion, pulmonary edema, pulmonary embolism with infarction, pulmonary hypertension (primary), pulmonary tuberculosis and silicosis, tracheal trauma, ruptured aortic aneurysm, Wegener's granulomatosis, systemic lupus erythematosus, and coagulation disorder.

786.4 Abnormal sputum — *in color, amount, odor, quantity*
AHA: March-April, 1985, 3; Q2, 1990, 3; Q2, 1990, 5; Q2, 1990, 15; Q1, 1991, 12

786.50 Unspecified chest pain — *unknown cause*
AHA: March-April, 1985, 3; Q2, 1990, 3; Q2, 1990, 5; Q2, 1990, 15; Q1, 1991, 12; Q4, 1999, 25; Q1, 2002, 4; Q1, 2003, 6

Use code 786.50 to report localized discomfort occurring in the chest. Among possible etiologies are acute myocardial infarction, angina, chest trauma, and peptic ulcer disease. Studies vary depending on the suspected etiology (e.g., electrocardiogram (EKG) for acute myocardial infarction, chest x-ray for chest trauma). Therapies include analgesics for pain control.

786.51 Precordial pain — *chest pain near heart*
AHA: March-April, 1985, 3; Q2, 1990, 3; Q2, 1990, 5; Q2, 1990, 15; Q1, 1991, 12

786.52 Painful respiration — *pleurodynia, Prinzmetal-Massumi syndrome, pleuritic pain*
AHA: Nov-Dec, 1984, 17; March-April, 1985, 3; Q2, 1990, 3; Q2, 1990, 5; Q2, 1990, 15; Q1, 1991, 12

Use this code to report a form of chest pain due to painful inhalation, expiration, or both. It may be due to pain in the chest wall (rib cage and sternum), pleura, or accessory muscles of respiration.

786.59 Other chest pain — *not otherwise specified, including discomfort, pressure, tightness in chest*
AHA: March-April, 1985, 3; Q2, 1990, 3; Q2, 1990, 5; Q2, 1990, 15; Q1, 1991, 12; Q1, 2002, 6

786.6 Swelling, mass, or lump in chest

786.7 Abnormal chest sounds — *rales, tympany, friction sounds, abnormal percussion*
AHA: March-April, 1985, 3; Q2, 1990, 3; Q2, 1990, 5; Q2, 1990, 15; Q1, 1991, 12

786.8 Hiccough — *singultus, spastic diaphragm*
AHA: March-April, 1985, 3; Q2, 1990, 3; Q2, 1990, 5; Q2, 1990, 15; Q1, 1991, 12

A hiccough, or hiccups, is defined as repetitive, involuntary, spasmodic contractions of the diaphragm. Hiccups are a symptom, not a disease. Hiccups involve the diaphragm (large, thin muscle that separates the chest from the abdomen) and phrenic nerve (nerve that connects the diaphragm to the brain). Almost everybody gets hiccups, even a fetus in a mother's womb.

Hiccups are caused by an irritation of nerves from the brain that control breathing muscles, especially the diaphragm. Causes are numerous for prolonged or recurrent hiccup episodes and include diseases of the pleura, pneumonia, uremia, alcoholism, use of certain prescription or non-prescription drugs, pregnancy, and disorders of the stomach, esophagus, bowel, or pancreas. There is no known prevention for hiccups, though prolonged episodes may require surgery to cut the phrenic nerve.

786.9 Other symptoms involving respiratory system and chest — *breath-holding spell*
AHA: March-April, 1985, 3; Q2, 1990, 3; Q2, 1990, 5; Q2, 1990, 15; Q1, 1991, 12

787 Symptoms involving digestive system

AHA: March-April, 1985, 3; Q2, 1990, 3; Q2, 1990, 5; Q2, 1990, 15; Q1, 1991, 12

Often, nausea and vomiting are symptoms of metabolic or microbial toxins or reactions to drugs, radiation, or motion (i.e., seasickness). Therapies depend on the etiology and include antiemetics (Inapsine, Reglan, Compazine, and Norzine).

Excluded from this subclassification are hematemesis not otherwise specified (578.0), excessive vomiting in pregnancy (643.0x-643.9x), regurgitation of food in newborn (779.3), habitual vomiting (536.2), psychogenic vomiting not otherwise specified (307.54), and constipation (564.00-564.09).

787.01 Nausea with vomiting

787.02 Nausea alone

787.03 Vomiting alone

787.1 Heartburn — *pyrosis, waterbrash*
AHA: March-April, 1985, 3; Q2, 1990, 3; Q2, 1990, 5; Q2, 1990, 15; Q1, 1991, 12; Q2, 2001, 6

787.2 Dysphagia — *difficulty in swallowing, cricopharyngeal syndrome*
AHA: March-April, 1985, 3; Q2, 1990, 3; Q2, 1990, 5; Q2, 1990, 15; Q1, 1991, 12; Q2, 2001, 4; Q4, 2003, 103, 109

Dysphagia is difficulty in swallowing. Pre-esophageal dysphagia is difficulty in emptying material from the oral pharynx into the esophagus. Esophageal dysphagia is difficulty in passing food down the esophagus. The most common symptom of esophageal disorders, dysphagia is classified as phase 1, 2, or 3. Phase 1, transfer phase, typically results from a neuromuscular disorder. Phase 2, transport phase, usually indicates spasm or carcinoma. Phase 3, entrance phase, results from lower esophageal narrowing by diverticula, esophagitis, and other disorders. Endoscopy with biopsy visualizes any gross pathology and provides specimens. Esophageal manometry measures esophageal pressure of upper and lower sphincters and detects abnormal contractions and peristalsis. Esophageal acidity test (usually performed with manometry) or acid perfusion test (Bernstein test) detects gastric acid reflux.

Associated conditions include amyotrophic lateral sclerosis, myasthenia gravis, Parkinson's disease, oral cavity tumor, carcinoma (laryngeal, esophageal, gastric), pharyngitis (chronic), airway obstruction, progressive systemic sclerosis, achalasia, and dysphagia lusoria. Associated esophageal conditions include esophageal compression (external), esophageal diverticulum, esophageal leiomyoma, esophageal obstruction by foreign body, esophagitis (corrosive, monilial, reflux), and lower esophageal ring. Other associated conditions include mediastinitis, Plummer-Vinson syndrome, systemic lupus erythematosus, hypocalcemia, syphilis, botulism, lead poisoning, and tetanus.

787.3 Flatulence, eructation, and gas pain — *bloating, tympanites, abdominal distension*
AHA: March-April, 1985, 3; Q2, 1990, 3; Q2, 1990, 5; Q2, 1990, 15; Q1, 1991, 12

787.4 Visible peristalsis — *hyperperistalsis*
AHA: March-April, 1985, 3; Q2, 1990, 3; Q2, 1990, 5; Q2, 1990, 15; Q1, 1991, 12

787.5 Abnormal bowel sounds — *absent or hyperactive*
AHA: March-April, 1985, 3; Q2, 1990, 3; Q2, 1990, 5; Q2, 1990, 15; Q1, 1991, 12

787.6 Incontinence of feces — *encopresis, incontinence of sphincter ani*
AHA: March-April, 1985, 3; Q2, 1990, 3; Q2, 1990, 5; Q2, 1990, 15; Q1, 1991, 12; Q1, 1997, 9

787.7 Abnormal feces — *bulky stools*
AHA: March-April, 1985, 3; Q2, 1990, 3; Q2, 1990, 5; Q2, 1990, 15; Q1, 1991, 12

787.91 Diarrhea — *loose, copious stools*
AHA: March-April, 1985, 3; Q2, 1990, 3; Q2, 1990, 5; Q2, 1990, 15; Q1, 1991, 12; Q4, 1995, 54

787.99 Other symptoms involving digestive system — *tenesmus, swelling, neuralgia, change in bowel habits*
AHA: March-April, 1985, 3; Q2, 1990, 3; Q2, 1990, 5; Q2, 1990, 15; Q1, 1991, 12

788 Symptoms involving urinary system

AHA: March-April, 1985, 3; Q2, 1990, 3; Q2, 1990, 5; Q2, 1990, 15; Q1, 1991, 12

Signs and symptoms of retention of urine include distended abdomen, pain, and urgency. Therapies include catheterization and surgery, such as transurethral resection of the prostate in males. Associated conditions include benign prostatic hypertrophy, neurogenic bladder, carcinoma of the prostate, urethral stricture, and urinary tract infection.

Inability to void is a common sequela to pelvic and perineal surgery or surgery performed under spinal anesthesia. The condition is not necessarily a postoperative complication. Documentation should support the condition as a medical management problem and not solely reflect prophylactic measures such as bladder catheterization.

788.0 Renal colic — *kidney or ureter*
AHA: March-April, 1985, 3; Q2, 1990, 3; Q2, 1990, 5; Q2, 1990, 15; Q1, 1991, 12

788.1 Dysuria — *painful urination, strangury*
AHA: March-April, 1985, 3; Q2, 1990, 3; Q2, 1990, 5; Q2, 1990, 15; Q1, 1991, 12

788.20 Unspecified retention of urine — *unknown type*
AHA: March-April, 1985, 3; Q2, 1990, 3; Q2, 1990, 5; Q2, 1990, 15; Q1, 1991, 12; Q3, 1996, 10; Q1, 2003, 6; Q3, 2003, 12-13

788.21 Incomplete bladder emptying

788.29 Other specified retention of urine — *not otherwise specified*
AHA: March-April, 1985, 3; Q2, 1990, 3; Q2, 1990, 5; Q2, 1990, 15; Q1, 1991, 12

Signs and symptoms of incontinence of urine include stress, urge, overflow or total incontinence; intermittent leakage resulting from sudden physical strain; dribble resulting from urinary retention; inability to suppress the sudden urge to urinate; and continuous leakage. Cystoscopy with biopsy visualizes any gross pathology and provides specimens. Cystometry tests bladder compliance, capacity, and residual volume. Therapies include bladder retraining and surgery such as creation of urinary diversion.

Associated conditions include cerebrovascular accident, diabetic neuropathy, Guillain-Barré

 © 2004 Ingenix, Inc.

syndrome, multiple sclerosis, spinal cord injury, benign prostatic hypertrophy, bladder calculi, bladder cancer, prostatic cancer, chronic prostatitis, and urethral stricture.

Code, if applicable, any causal condition first, such as congenital ureterocele (753.23).

Excluded from this subclassification is urinary incontinence of nonorganic origin (307.6). Female stress incontinence is reported with 625.6.

788.3 ✓5th Urinary incontinence — (Code, if applicable, any causal condition first: 618.0-618.9, 753.23)
AHA: March-April, 1985, 3; Q2, 1990, 3; Q2, 1990, 5; Q2, 1990, 15; Q1, 1991, 12; Q4, 1992, 22

788.30 Unspecified urinary incontinence — *unknown type of enuresis, bladder neck syndrome*

788.31 Urge incontinence — *inability to control flow upon urge*

788.32 Stress incontinence, male — *inability to control flow upon pressure*

788.33 Mixed incontinence urge and stress (male)(female) — *urge and stress*

788.34 Incontinence without sensory awareness — *no sensory warning*

788.35 Post-void dribbling — *inability to control flow after urination*

788.36 Nocturnal enuresis — *bed-wetting*

788.37 Continuous leakage — *constant flow*

788.38 Overflow incontinence

788.39 Other urinary incontinence — *not otherwise specified*

788.41 Urinary frequency — *frequent micturition*

788.42 Polyuria — *copious micturition*

788.43 Nocturia — *frequent nighttime micturition*

788.5 Oliguria and anuria — *deficient secretion or suppression of urine*

788.61 Splitting of urinary stream — *intermittent urinary stream*

788.62 Slowing of urinary stream — *weak stream*

788.63 Urgency of urination

788.69 Other abnormality of urination — *not otherwise specified*

788.7 Urethral discharge — *penile discharge, urethrorrhea*

788.8 Extravasation of urine — *escape of urine into adjacent tissues*

788.9 Other symptoms involving urinary system — *not otherwise specified, including extrarenal uremia, tenesmus*

Excluded from this rubric are hematuria (599.7), nonspecific findings on examination of the urine (791.0-791.9), small kidney of unknown cause (589.0-589.9), and uremia not otherwise specified (586).

789 Other symptoms involving abdomen and pelvis

AHA: March-April, 1985, 3; Q2, 1990, 3; Q2, 1990, 5; Q2, 1990, 15; Q1, 1991, 12

The following fifth-digit subclassification is to be used for codes 789.0, 789.3, 789.4, and 789.6:

0 unspecified site
1 right upper quadrant
2 left upper quadrant
3 right lower quadrant
4 left lower quadrant
5 periumbilic
6 epigastric
7 generalized
9 other specified site or multiple sites

789.0 ✓5th Abdominal pain — *cramps, colic*
AHA: March-April, 1985, 3; Q2, 1990, 3; Q2, 1990, 5; Q2, 1990, 15; Q1, 1991, 12; Q1, 1995, 3

Use this subclassification to report localized pain or discomfort affecting the abdominal area. It may be due to drug use, the effect of toxins, or disorders of the gastrointestinal, reproductive, genitourinary, musculoskeletal, or vascular system. Blood work shows hematocrit, WBC, and differential and platelet counts. Urinalysis may identify urinary tract infection or kidney disease. Other lab work may reveal elevated liver enzymes (in hepatic disease), elevated serum bilirubin (in hepatobiliary disease), elevated serum amylase (in pancreatitis), or bacteria and parasites in stool culture (in acute diarrhea). Abdominal x-ray (supine and upright or decubitus and flat) may reveal intestinal disease or obstruction, while an ultrasound may identify aneurysms. Intravenous pyelogram (IVP) may identify renal disease or ureteral obstruction, while a sigmoidoscopy reveals condition of sigmoid colon and rectum. Associated conditions include peritonitis, perforated peptic ulcer, gallbladder disease, appendicitis, colitis, pancreatitis, lymphadenitis, pelvic inflammatory disease, intestinal obstruction, ruptured liver or spleen, ovarian cyst, ectopic pregnancy, endometriosis, pneumonia, myocardial ischemia, leukemia, nephritis, uremia, herpes zoster, and ureteral obstruction.

789.1 Hepatomegaly — *enlarged liver*
AHA: March-April, 1985, 3; Q2, 1990, 3; Q2, 1990, 5; Q2, 1990, 15; Q1, 1991, 12

789.2 Splenomegaly — *enlarged spleen*
AHA: March-April, 1985, 3; Q2, 1990, 3; Q2, 1990, 5; Q2, 1990, 15; Q1, 1991, 12

789.3 5th Abdominal or pelvic swelling, mass, or lump — *diffuse or generalized swelling or mass*
AHA: March-April, 1985, 3; Q2, 1990, 3; Q2, 1990, 5; Q2, 1990, 15; Q1, 1991, 12

789.4 5th Abdominal rigidity — *inflexibility, turgidity*
AHA: March-April, 1985, 3; Q2, 1990, 3; Q2, 1990, 5; Q2, 1990, 15; Q1, 1991, 12

789.5 Ascites — *fluid in peritoneal cavity*
AHA: March-April, 1985, 3; Q4, 1989, 11; Q2, 1990, 3; Q2, 1990, 5; Q2, 1990, 15; Q1, 1991, 12

Ascites is accumulation of serous fluid in the peritoneal cavity. Signs and symptoms of ascites include abdominal discomfort, distention, dyspnea, and a flat or an inverted umbilicus. Abdominal percussion transmits fluid wave and reveals shifting dullness. Paracentesis to remove fluid (typically 50 ml to 100 ml) may reveal the following:

- High WBC (more than 300 cells/ml to 500 cells/ml suggests infection)
- Sanguineous fluid (indicative of neoplasm or tuberculosis)
- Milky or chylous fluid (common with lymphoma)
- Concentrations of protein (less than 3 g/100 ml suggests liver disease or systemic disorder)

Therapies include bed rest, sodium restriction (20 mEq/day to 40 mEq/day), spironolactone such as Aldactone (100 mg/day to 300 mg/day, orally), monitoring of body weight and urinary sodium, and peritoneal-jugular shunting.

Associated conditions include chronic or subacute liver disease (most commonly cirrhosis from alcoholism), chronic active hepatitis, severe alcoholic hepatitis without cirrhosis, hepatic vein obstruction, systemic disease (heart failure, nephrotic syndrome), carcinomatosis, and tubercular peritonitis.

If the physician documents malignant ascites, assign code 197.6 instead.

789.6 5th Abdominal tenderness — *rebound tenderness*
AHA: March-April, 1985, 3; Q2, 1990, 3; Q2, 1990, 5; Q2, 1990, 15; Q1, 1991, 12

789.9 Other symptoms involving abdomen and pelvis — *umbilical bleeding or discharge; not otherwise specified*
AHA: March-April, 1985, 3; Q2, 1990, 3; Q2, 1990, 5; Q2, 1990, 15; Q1, 1991, 12

790–796 Nonspecific Abnormal Findings

790 Nonspecific findings on examination of blood

AHA: Q2, 1990, 16

790.01 Precipitous drop in hematocrit — *drop in red blood cell count*
AHA: Q2, 1990, 16; Q4, 2000, 46

790.09 Other abnormality of red blood cells — *morphology, volume, anisocytosis, poikilocytosis; not otherwise specified*
AHA: Q2, 1990, 16; Q4, 2000, 46

790.1 Elevated sedimentation rate — *sed rate*
AHA: Q2, 1990, 16

790.21 Impaired fasting glucose — *elevated fasting glucose*

790.22 Impaired glucose tolerance test (oral) — *a metabolic test that measures carbohydrate tolerance; which includes the measurement of active insulin, a test on the liver based on the ability and power to absorb and store large quantities of glucose; elevated glucose tolerance test*

790.29 Nonspecific findings, Other abnormal glucose — *abnormal non-fasting glucose, pre-diabetes*

790.3 Excessive blood level of alcohol — *indicative of alcohol consumption*
AHA: Sept-Oct, 1986, 3; Q2, 1990, 16

790.4 Nonspecific elevation of levels of transaminase or lactic acid dehydrogenase (LDH) — *a marker for hemolysis, pulmonary embolism, liver malignancy*
AHA: Q2, 1990, 16

790.5 Other nonspecific abnormal serum enzyme levels — *acid phosphatase, alkaline phosphate, amylase, lipase*
AHA: Q2, 1990, 16

790.6 Other abnormal blood chemistry — *cobalt, copper, iron, lithium, magnesium, mineral, zinc*
AHA: Q4, 1988, 1; Q2, 1990, 16

Use code 790.6 to report an abnormal finding on blood chemistry tests for which there is no corresponding diagnosis, such as copper, iron, lithium, and magnesium.

790.7 Bacteremia — (Use additional code to identify organism) — *bacteria in the blood*
AHA: Q3, 1988, 12; Q2, 1990, 16; Q4, 1993, 29; Q2, 2003, 7

Use code 790.7 to report the presence of live bacteria circulating in the bloodstream. Bacteremia frequently results from surgical procedures (e.g., incision and drainage of an abscess or dental extractions). It also

 © 2004 Ingenix, Inc.

may result from colonization of indwelling urinary catheters or other invasive apparatus. Therapies include antibiotics.

Associated conditions include abscessed teeth, urinary tract infection, and infected medical device.

The term "bacteremia" is sometimes used ambiguously by clinicians to mean septicemia, which is bacteremia with clinical signs and symptoms of systemic infection and classified to rubric 038. To ensure proper classification, verify with the physician any reports of bacteremia with signs and symptoms of systemic infection such as fever, chills, prostration, nausea and vomiting, diarrhea, metastatic abscesses, and skin eruptions.

Bacteremia of newborn (771.83) is excluded from this code.

790.8 Unspecified viremia — *virus in the blood*
AHA: Q4, 1988, 10; Q2, 1990, 16

790.91 Abnormal arterial blood gases

790.92 Abnormal coagulation profile — *bleeding time, coagulation time, PTT, PT*
AHA: Q2, 1990, 16; Q4, 1993, 29

790.93 Elevated prostate specific antigen (PSA)

790.94 Euthyroid sick syndrome

790.95 Other nonspecific findings on examination of blood, elevated C-reactive protein (CRP)

The presence of inflammation in an arterial wall has been found to contribute to plaque rupture and artery obstruction, thereby also contributing to heart attacks and strokes, even when the patient has none of the other classic risk factors involved in atherosclerosis. Elevated C-reactive protein (CRP) found in blood as this is a marker for inflammation occurring anywhere in the body. This level can vary from day to day and tends to increase with aging, low levels of physical activity, diabetes, depression, and even sleep disorders.

C-reactive protein is recognized as a risk factor in cardiovascular disease and is becoming more and more a risk assessment factor of heart disease and stroke along with cholesterol screening. This means that patients screened for this may come from several different patient groupings, including those with hypothyroidism and/or progressive thyroid failure, premature atherosclerosis, those undergoing peritoneal dialysis, middle aged men and women with and without other risk factors, and those with periodontal disease. Patients presenting with periodontal disease, especially, are at risk for cardiovascular problems. The inflammation from periodontal disease allows oral bacteria to enter the bloodstream, and causes the liver to produce proteins, such as CRP, that inflame arteries and promote blood clot formation.

790.99 Other nonspecific findings on examination of blood — *not otherwise specified, including proteinemia*
AHA: Q2, 1990, 16; Q4, 1993, 29; Q2, 2003, 14

Excluded from this rubric are abnormalities of platelets (287.0-287.9), thrombocytes (287.0-287.9), or white blood cells (288.0-288.9).

791 Nonspecific findings on examination of urine

AHA: Q2, 1990, 16

791.0 Proteinuria — *protein in urine; albuminuria, Bence-Jones proteinuria*
AHA: Q2, 1990, 16; Q3, 1991, 8

Proteinuria is defined as urinary protein excretion of greater than 150 mg per day. The types of proteinuria can be classified as glomerular, tubular, or overflow. Glomerular disease is the most common cause, resulting in urinary loss of albumin and immunoglobulins. Tubular proteinuria occurs when tubulointerstitial disease prevents the proximal tubule from reabsorbing low-molecular-weight proteins. Tubular diseases include hypertensive nephrosclerosis and tubulointerstitial nephropathy caused by nonsteroidal anti-inflammatory drugs. In overflow proteinuria, low-molecular-weight proteins inhibit the reabsorption of filtered proteins.

Lab tests include a quantitative measurement of protein excretion, which can be done with a 24-hour urine specimen or the urine protein-to-creatinine ratio (UPr/Cr). Dipstick analysis is used in most outpatient settings to semiquantitatively measure the urine protein concentration. The sulfosalicylic acid (SSA) turbidity test qualitatively screens for proteinuria.

Therapy depends on urine to protein concentration. Proteinuria of more than two g per 24 hours (moderate to heavy) requires aggressive work-up. If the creatinine clearance is normal and if there is a clear diagnosis such as diabetes or uncompensated congestive heart failure, the underlying medical condition can be treated with close follow-up of proteinuria and renal function (creatinine clearance). Benign causes include fever, intense activity or exercise, dehydration, emotional stress, and acute illness. More serious causes include glomerulonephritis and multiple myeloma. Common secondary causes are diabetic nephropathy, amyloidosis, and systemic lupus erythematosus.

This subcategory excludes postural proteinuria (593.6) and proteinuria arising during pregnancy or the puerperium (642.0x-642.9x, 646.2x).

791.1 Chyluria — *excess lymphatic fluid in urine*
AHA: Q2, 1990, 16

791.2 Hemoglobinuria — *blood in urine seen in a lab exam*
AHA: Q2, 1990, 16

791.3 Myoglobinuria — *myoglobin in the urine*
AHA: Q2, 1990, 16

791.4 Biliuria — *bile pigments in the urine*
AHA: Q2, 1990, 16

791.5 Glycosuria — *sugar in the urine*
AHA: Q2, 1990, 16

791.6 Acetonuria — *acetone in the urine; ketonuria*
AHA: Q2, 1990, 16

791.7 Other cells and casts in urine — *not otherwise specified*
AHA: Q2, 1990, 16

791.9 Other nonspecific finding on examination of urine — *crystalluria, melanuria, cocciurea, uricosuria, elevated 18-ketosteriods, catecholamines, indolacetic acid, or VMA*
AHA: Q2, 1990, 16

Excluded from this rubric are hematuria (599.7), specific findings indicating abnormality of amino-acid transport and metabolism (270.0-270.9), and specific findings indicating abnormality of carbohydrate transport and metabolism (271.0-271.9).

792 Nonspecific abnormal findings in other body substances

AHA: Q2, 1990, 16

792.0 Nonspecific abnormal finding in cerebrospinal fluid

792.1 Nonspecific abnormal finding in stool contents — *mucus, pus, fat, abnormal color, occult stool*
AHA: Q2, 1990, 16; Q2, 1992, 9

792.2 Nonspecific abnormal finding in semen — *abnormal spermatozoa*
AHA: Q2, 1990, 16

792.3 Nonspecific abnormal finding in amniotic fluid — *fluid surround fetus*
AHA: Nov-Dec, 1986, 4; Q2, 1990, 16

792.4 Nonspecific abnormal finding in saliva

792.5 Cloudy (hemodialysis) (peritoneal) dialysis affluent

792.9 Other nonspecific abnormal finding in body substances — *peritoneal, pleural, synovial, vaginal or other fluid, not elsewhere specified*
AHA: Q2, 1990, 16

A nonspecific abnormal finding in chromosomal analysis (795.2) is excluded from the rubric.

793 Nonspecific abnormal findings on radiological and other examination of body structure

AHA: Q2, 1990, 16

This rubric includes nonspecific abnormal findings in thermography, ultrasound (echogram), and x-ray.

793.0 Nonspecific abnormal findings on radiological and other examination of skull and head — *upon x-ray, ultrasound, thermography*
AHA: Q2, 1990, 16

793.1 Nonspecific abnormal findings on radiological and other examination of lung field — *coin lesion or shadow upon x-ray, ultrasound, thermography*
AHA: Q2, 1990, 16

793.2 Nonspecific abnormal findings on radiological and other examination of other intrathoracic organs — *heart shadow, mediastinal shift upon x-ray, ultrasound, thermography*
AHA: Q2, 1990, 16

793.3 Nonspecific abnormal findings on radiological and other examination of biliary tract — *nonvisualization of gallbladder upon x-ray, ultrasound, thermography*
AHA: Q2, 1990, 16

793.4 Nonspecific abnormal findings on radiological and other examination of gastrointestinal tract — *upon x-ray, ultrasound, thermography*
AHA: Q2, 1990, 16

793.5 Nonspecific abnormal findings on radiological and other examination of genitourinary organs — *filling defect of bladder, kidney or ureter upon x-ray, ultrasound, thermography*
AHA: Q2, 1990, 16; Q4, 2000, 46

793.6 Nonspecific abnormal findings on radiological and other examination of abdominal area, including retroperitoneum — *upon x-ray, ultrasound, thermography*
AHA: Q2, 1990, 16

793.7 Nonspecific abnormal findings on radiological and other examination of musculoskeletal system — *upon x-ray, ultrasound, thermography*
AHA: Q2, 1990, 16

793.80 Unspecified abnormal mammogram

793.81 Mammographic microcalcification

793.89 Other abnormal findings on radiological examination of breast

© 2004 Ingenix, Inc.

793.9 Nonspecific abnormal findings on radiological and other examination of other site of body — *placenta, skin, subcutaneous tissue upon x-ray, ultrasound, thermography*
AHA: Q2, 1990, 16

Abnormal results of function studies and radioisotope scans (794.0-794.9) are excluded from the rubric.

794 Nonspecific abnormal results of function studies

AHA: Q2, 1990, 16

This rubric includes nonspecific abnormal findings in radioisotope scans, uptake studies, and scintiphotography.

794.00 Unspecified abnormal function study of brain and central nervous system

794.01 Nonspecific abnormal echoencephalogram

794.02 Nonspecific abnormal electroencephalogram (EEG)

794.09 Other nonspecific abnormal result of function study of brain and central nervous system — *brain scan; not otherwise specified*
AHA: Q2, 1990, 16

794.10 Nonspecific abnormal response to unspecified nerve stimulation

794.11 Nonspecific abnormal retinal function studies — *ERG*
AHA: Q2, 1990, 16

794.12 Nonspecific abnormal electro-oculogram (EOG)

794.13 Nonspecific abnormal visually evoked potential — *VEP*
AHA: Q2, 1990, 16

794.14 Nonspecific abnormal oculomotor studies

794.15 Nonspecific abnormal auditory function studies

794.16 Nonspecific abnormal vestibular function studies

794.17 Nonspecific abnormal electromyogram (EMG)

794.19 Other nonspecific abnormal result of function study of peripheral nervous system and special senses

794.2 Nonspecific abnormal results of pulmonary system function study — *lung scan, ventilatory capacity, vital capacity*
AHA: Q2, 1990, 16

794.30 Nonspecific abnormal unspecified cardiovascular function study

794.31 Nonspecific abnormal electrocardiogram (ecg) (ekg) — *Q-T interval prolongations, Romano-Ward syndrome*
AHA: Q2, 1990, 16

794.39 Other nonspecific abnormal cardiovascular system function study — *ballistocardiogram, phonocardiogram, vectorcardiogram*
AHA: Q2, 1990, 16

794.4 Nonspecific abnormal results of kidney function study — *renal function test*
AHA: Q2, 1990, 16

794.5 Nonspecific abnormal results of thyroid function study — *thyroid scan, thyroid uptake*
AHA: Q2, 1990, 16

794.6 Nonspecific abnormal results of other endocrine function study — *pituitary, thymus, adrenal, hypothalamus*
AHA: Q2, 1990, 16

794.7 Nonspecific abnormal results of basal metabolism function study — *BMR*
AHA: Q2, 1990, 16

794.8 Nonspecific abnormal results of liver function study — *liver scan*
AHA: Q2, 1990, 16

794.9 Nonspecific abnormal results of other specified function study — *bladder, pancreas, placenta, spleen*
AHA: Q2, 1990, 16

795 Other and nonspecific abnormal cytological, histological, immunological and DNA test findings

AHA: Q2, 1990, 16

795.0 [5th] Abnormal Papanicolaou smear of cervix and cervical HPV — *Pap smear*
AHA: Q2, 1990, 16; Q4, 2002, 69

795.00 Abnormal glandular Papanicolaou smear of cervix

795.01 Papanicolaou smear of cervix with atypical squamous cells of undetermined significance (ASC-US)

795.02 Papanicolaou smear of cervix with atypical squamous cells cannot exclude high grade squamous intraepithelial lesion (ASC-H)

795.03 Papanicolaou smear of cervix with low grade squamous intraepithelial lesion (LGSIL)

795.04 Papanicolaou smear of cervix with high grade squamous intraepithelial lesion (HGSIL)

795.05 Cervical high risk human papillomavirus (HPV) DNA test positive

795.08 Nonspecific abnormal papanicolaou smear of cervix, unsatisfactory smear

795.09 Other abnormal Papanicolaou smear of cervix and cervical HPV

Women who have abnormal results of a Pap smear test returned have some kind of atypical cellular changes occurring in the cervix uteri. These changes include abnormal glandular cell changes, and high and low grade squamous intraepithelial lesions. Positive results for a DNA test to detect the presence of the human papilloma virus can be very effective in helping doctors determine which patients who have had an abnormal smear result have cancer or precancer and need immediate attention. High risk types of this virus are the cause of most cervical cancers and can now be detected with certain DNA tests. Those patients who test positive are carefully followed for cervical cancer.

The histological and immunological cell changes reported with the Bethesda system are determined by cytology studies of the cell samples taken in smear tests. Dysplasias are more definitive results returned from biopsy samples of the cervical tissue taken during colposcopy exams and not Pap smears. Colposcopy with biopsy is the next step in diagnosing abnormal smear results in high-risk patients. Pap smears are screening tests and the actual changes occurring in the cells could be more or less severe. A Pap smear that results in a low grade squamous intraepithelial lesion usually indicates there is mild dysplasia, CIN I and koilo cytotic atypia. A Pap smear result of high grade squamous intraepithelial lesion usually indicates there is a moderate dysplasia. Dysplasias can progress to cancerous conditions that may require treatments such as removal or destruction of cervical tissue, cervicectomy, or even hysterectomy.

Excluded from this subcategory (795.0) are carcinoma of cervix (233.1), cervical intraepithelial neoplasia I (622.11), cervical intraepithelial neoplasia II (622.12), cervical intraepithelial neoplasia III (233.1), dysplasia (histologically confirmed) of cervix NOS (622.10), mild dysplasia (histologically confirmed) (622.12), severe dysplasia (histologically confirmed) (233.1).

795.1 Nonspecific abnormal Papanicolaou smear of other site — *Pap smear other than cervical*
AHA: Q2, 1990, 16

795.2 Nonspecific abnormal findings on chromosomal analysis — *abnormal karyotype*
AHA: Q2, 1990, 16

795.3 ✓5th Nonspecific positive culture findings — *nose, sputum, throat, wound*
AHA: Q2, 1990, 16

795.31 Nonspecific positive findings for anthrax

795.39 Other nonspecific positive culture findings

795.4 Other nonspecific abnormal histological findings

795.5 Nonspecific reaction to tuberculin skin test without active tuberculosis — *Mantoux test, PPD positive, positive TB skin test*
AHA: Q2, 1990, 16

795.6 False positive serological test for syphilis — *Wassermann reaction*
AHA: Q2, 1990, 16

795.71 Nonspecific serologic evidence of human immunodeficiency virus (HIV) — (This code is only to be used when a test finding is reported as nonspecific. Asymptomatic positive findings are coded to V08. If any HIV infection symptom or condition is present, see code 042. Negative findings are not coded.) — *nonspecific findings only*
AHA: July-Aug, 1987, 24; Q2, 1990, 16; Q2, 1992, 11; Q1, 1993, 21, 22; Q2, 1993, 6

When the medical record documentation indicates "possible," "probable," or "questionable" AIDS, not confirmed, without manifestations, the record should be returned to the physician for further clarification. Physicians also need to be aware that unacceptable terminology and abbreviations in the medical record should not be used. These terms only cause confusion in code selection.

Positive Newborn Testing: If a newborn has a positive ELISA or Western Blot test for HIV, the correct code to use is 795.71 *Nonspecific serologic evidence of human immunodeficiency virus [HIV]*. These tests may reflect the antibodies of the mother and not the baby. If the mother is positive for HIV, the antibody may cross the placenta to the newborn. The antibodies may be carried up to 18 months producing a false-positive result. These false-positive results during the newborn's first 18 months are due to the mother's antibodies carried by the newborn. The baby may later lose those antibodies, indicating that he/she was actually never infected.

795.79 Other and unspecified nonspecific immunological findings — *raised antibody titer, raised immunoglobulin level*
AHA: Q2, 1990, 16; Q2, 1993, 6

Excluded from this rubric are nonspecific abnormalities of red blood cells (790.01-790.09).

The nonspecific abnormal smear results are reported with codes in this chapter under subcategory 795.0, while the dysplasias are reported under subcategory 622.1. Severe or high grade squamous intraepithelial cervical dysplasia is excluded and is reported in the neoplasm chapter with code 233.1.

Coding Scenario

A 39-year-old female presents to her OB/GYN physician for a colposcopy and biopsy. Her recent Pap smear returned with a diagnosis of atypical high grade squamous intraepithelial lesion (HGSIL) identified. He performs a colposcopy and biopsy. Her visit is recorded as high grade squamous intraepithelial lesion (HGSIL).

© 2004 Ingenix, Inc.

Coding Assignment: 795.04 *Papanicolaou smear of cervix with high grade squamous intraepithelial lesion (HGSIL)*

796 Other nonspecific abnormal findings

AHA: Q2, 1990, 16

796.0 Nonspecific abnormal toxicological findings — *heavy metals or drugs in blood, urine or other tissue*
AHA: Q2, 1990, 16; Q1, 1997, 16

796.1 Abnormal reflex

796.2 Elevated blood pressure reading without diagnosis of hypertension — *no formal diagnosis of hypertension; incidental finding*
AHA: July-Aug, 1984, 12; Q2, 1990, 16; Q3, 1990, 4; Q2, 2003, 11

796.3 Nonspecific low blood pressure reading

796.4 Other abnormal clinical finding

796.5 Abnormal finding on antenatal screening

796.6 Nonspecific abnormal findings on neonatal screening

This code represents a status determination or laboratory findings result and not an actual presenting diagnosis. It denotes simply that some condition for which the infant was screened during normal newborn testing, came back with positive results that the infant may possibly have an abnormal condition for which the infant will need to be tested more extensively so a specific determination or an actual diagnosis can be made.

796.9 Other nonspecific abnormal finding — *not elsewhere specified*
AHA: Q2, 1990, 16

Refer to the ICD-9-CM Index before assigning a code from this rubric to ensure a more specific code cannot be found.

When the documentation identifies a postoperative hypertension, the physician needs to document whether it was caused by inadequate control of pain or patient agitation, and if the hypertension was merely an elevation in blood pressure without mention of hypertension (796.2) or a benign hypertension (401.1).

Elevated Blood Pressure: Also known as transient hypertension, this condition is an elevated blood pressure reading without a diagnosis of hypertension and may be characteristic of older age groups or due to emotional stress. For these cases, report code 796.2 *Elevated blood pressure reading without diagnosis of hypertension.*

Coding Scenario

A patient is seen for blood pressure checks three times a week due to transient elevated blood pressure readings.

Code assignment: 796.2 *Elevated blood pressure reading without diagnosis of hypertension*

797–799 Ill–Defined and Unknown Causes of Morbidity and Mortality

797 Senility without mention of psychosis OK

Senility is triggered by mental decline and its cause is related to the neurons of the nervous system. With age, some shrinkage of the brain occurs due to the loss of neurons throughout life. The shrinkage is often insignificant, but in roughly 10 percent of the elderly, the brain atrophy is severe and senility results. The five major symptoms of senility are forgetfulness, irritability, poor judgment, disorientation, and general intellectual decline. The first signs are lapses in recent memory and an inability to grasp new information. As the illness progresses, abstract thinking is impaired, judgment becomes poor, and verbal communication becomes difficult. In time, the person is unable to perform ordinary activities and becomes completely dependent on others for physical needs. Diagnosis includes personal history, physical exam, and neurological testing. In many patients, the condition is one that mimics senility and is due to causes such as toxic drug reactions or high blood pressure. There is no cure for senility and the standard management is to delay the progression of symptoms.

Senile psychoses (290.0-290.9) are excluded from this category.

798 Sudden death, cause unknown

798.0 Sudden infant death syndrome — *crib death, SIDS*

Sudden infant death syndrome (SIDS) is defined as the sudden death of an infant younger than 1 year of age that remains unexplained after a thorough case investigation, including performance of a complete autopsy, examination of the death scene, and review of the clinical history.

According to the National SIDS Resource Center, most researchers now believe that babies who die of SIDS are born with one or more conditions that make them especially vulnerable to stresses that occur in the normal life of an infant, including both internal and external influences. Maternal risk factors include cigarette smoking during pregnancy, maternal age under 20 years, poor prenatal care, low weight gain, anemia, use of illegal drugs, and a history of sexually transmitted disease or urinary tract infection.

Most deaths from SIDS occur by the end of the sixth month, with the greatest number occurring between two and four months of age. A SIDS death occurs quickly and is often associated with sleep, with no signs of suffering. More deaths are reported in the fall and winter (in both the Northern and Southern Hemispheres) and there is a 60 to 40 percent male-to-female ratio. A death is diagnosed as SIDS only after all other alternatives have been eliminated: SIDS is a diagnosis of exclusion and includes investigations of the autopsy, death scene, and a review of the victim and family case history.

798.1 Instantaneous death

798.2 Death occurring in less than 24 hours from onset of symptoms, not otherwise explained — *without sign of disease or trauma*

798.9 Unattended death — *found dead*

799 Other ill-defined and unknown causes of morbidity and mortality

799.0 Asphyxia — *lack of oxygen*

Use this code to report a lack of oxygen in respiration resulting in threatened or actual cessation of breath.

Therapies depend on the etiology (e.g., removal of foreign body obstructing the trachea or electrical defibrillation for cardiopulmonary arrest) and may include closed cardiac massage if a heart beat and carotid pulse are absent, and the placement of the

patient in Trendelenburg position to promote drainage of water from the lungs (fresh water victim). Other therapies include mechanical ventilation, intensive respiratory therapy, IV administration of sodium bicarbonate, inhalation or injection of beta-agonists (epinephrine, Isuprel, Alupent, Brethine) to reduce bronchospasm, and administration of corticosteroids and antibiotics.

799.1 Respiratory arrest — *cardiorespiratory failure*

Use code 799.1 to report a cessation of breathing, identified as primary, secondary, or complete. Primary respiratory arrest may be due to airway obstruction, decreased respiratory drive, or respiratory muscle weakness. Secondary respiratory arrest may be a result of cardiac arrest. Therapies include cardiopulmonary resuscitation, intubation, and ventilation.

This code excludes respiratory distress of newborn (770.89) and respiratory failure of newborn (770.84).

799.2 Nervousness

799.3 Unspecified debility — *specifics unknown*

799.4 Cachexia — *wasting disease; general ill health and poor nutrition*
AHA: Q3, 1990, 17

The protein-wasting syndrome called cachexia most commonly occurs with lung, pancreatic, stomach, bowel, and prostate cancers, and rarely with breast cancer. It also affects people with AIDS, uncontrolled rheumatoid arthritis, severe infections, chronic lung and bowel disease, and heart failure. The cause is usually related to liver metastasis with resulting pain and loss of appetite. Sometimes the cause is mechanical, such as when a tumor grows into the stomach or blocks the intestine.

Undiagnosed and untreated cachexia is life threatening. It can decrease the effectiveness of cancer treatments such as chemotherapy and radiation therapy, and magnify their side effects.

799.81 Decreased libido — *drop off in sexual desire*
AHA: Q4, 2003, 75

799.89 Other ill-defined conditions

799.9 Other unknown and unspecified cause of morbidity or mortality — *unknown cause of morbidity or mortality*
AHA: Q1, 1990, 20; Q1, 1998, 4

© 2004 Ingenix, Inc.

800–999
Injury and Poisoning

800–829 Fractures

A fracture is a break in a bone resulting from two possible causes: the direct or indirect application of undue force against the bone and pathological changes resulting in spontaneous fractures. This chapter includes only those fractures that have arisen as a result of an injury. It excludes malunions and nonunions of fractured bones.

The clinician always determines whether a fracture is open or closed; this is one of the first determinations that should be made.

Closed fractures are contained beneath the skin, while open or compound fractures connote an associated open wound.

Terms that typically describe closed fractures include:

- Comminuted — a splintering of the fractured bone
- Depressed — a portion of the skull broken and driven inward from a forceful blow
- Fissured — a fracture that does not split the bone
- Greenstick — occurs in children; the bone is somewhat bent and partially broken
- Impacted — one fractured bone end wedged into another
- Linear — straight line
- Simple — intact ligaments and skin
- Slipped epiphysis — separation of the growing end of the bone (epiphysis) from the shaft of the bone that occurs in children and young adults who still have active epiphyses
- Spiral — resembles a helix

Open fractures have a distinctive vocabulary. They are always compound, with a wound leading to the fracture or the broken bone ends protruding through the skin. There is a very high risk of infection with open fractures since the tissues are exposed to contaminants. Also, there may be missiles or foreign bodies embedded in the tissues that must be removed during surgery. Puncture wounds may be present.

Both open and closed fractures may earn the descriptive term of "complicated." A complicated fracture is one in which a bone fragment has injured an internal organ. For example, the ribs may injure the lungs, liver, and spleen, depending on the nature and direction of the force causing the fracture.

800 Fracture of vault of skull

AHA: Sept-Oct, 1985, 3; Q2, 1989, 15; Q2, 1990, 7; Q3, 1990, 5; Q3, 1990, 13; Q4, 1990, 26; Q4, 1996, 36

The vault of the skull is composed of three bones: the frontal bone and two parietal bones. Fractures of the vault may be accompanied by cerebral contusion or laceration; subarachnoid, subdural, or extradural hemorrhage; or an unspecified cause of hemorrhage.

Cerebral contusions and lacerations constitute severe injury. One of the great problems associated with head trauma is that the brain sustains a double blow — the initial blow that causes the brain to travel to the opposite side of the skull, smiting the interior skull with significant force. This second blow is called contrecoup. Such force applied to the brain causes swelling and increased intracranial pressure that is very dangerous. Serious head trauma has a high mortality rate, nearly 50 percent. In addition to edema, a second complication is hemorrhage resulting from laceration of blood vessels. If the fracture is open, the brain is exposed to bacteria, compounding the danger.

Major trauma to the forebrain with no injury to the brainstem may result in survival of the patient in a chronic vegetative state for several years.

Patients who have survived severe head trauma often deal with posttraumatic epilepsy for many years.

The following fifth-digit subclassification is for use with the appropriate codes in categories 800, 801, 803, and 804:

0 unspecified state of consciousness
1 with no loss of consciousness
2 with brief [less than one hour] loss of consciousness
3 with moderate [1-24 hours] loss of consciousness
4 with prolonged [more than 24 hours] loss of consciousness and return to pre-existing conscious level
5 with prolonged [more than 24 hours] loss of consciousness, without return to pre-existing conscious level
6 with loss of consciousness of unspecified duration
9 with concussion, unspecified

800.0 5th Closed fracture of vault of skull without mention of intracranial injury

800.1 5th Closed fracture of vault of skull with cerebral laceration and contusion

800.2 5th Closed fracture of vault of skull with subarachnoid, subdural, and extradural hemorrhage

800.3 5th Closed fracture of vault of skull with other and unspecified intracranial hemorrhage

800.4 5th Closed fracture of vault of skull with intercranial injury of other and unspecified nature

800.5 5th Open fracture of vault of skull without mention of intracranial injury

800.6 5th Open fracture of vault of skull with cerebral laceration and contusion

800.7 5th Open fracture of vault of skull with subarachnoid, subdural, and extradural hemorrhage

800.8 5th Open fracture of vault of skull with other and unspecified intracranial hemorrhage

800.9 5th Open fracture of vault of skull with intracranial injury of other and unspecified nature

801 Fracture of base of skull

AHA: Sept-Oct, 1985, 3; Q2, 1989, 15; Q2, 1990, 7; Q3, 1990, 5; Q3, 1990, 13; Q4, 1990, 26; Q4, 1996, 36

Included in the description for the base of the skull are the following bones:

- Occiput — bone at the base of the skull; contains the foramen magnum, the opening in the bone that allows the spinal cord to join the brain.
- Orbital roof — the orbit has a roof and a floor. The roof is considered part of the skull base, an exception is the frontal bone that forms part of the roof of the orbit as part of the skull vault.
- Sphenoid bone — large bone containing the sphenoid sinus, forming part of the back of the orbit.
- Temporal bones (2) — adjoin the parietal, sphenoid, and occipital bones.
- Cranial fossae — anterior, middle, and posterior — The three fossae form the floor of the cranial cavity (on the superior aspect of the base of the skull) and provide a surface to support the various lobes of the brain. The frontal lobes rest on the anterior fossa, the temporal lobes on the middle fossa, and the pons and medulla oblongata are contained within the posterior fossa, with the cerebellum expanding over the medulla oblongata.

The following fifth-digit subclassification is for use with the appropriate codes in categories 800, 801, 803, and 804:

0 unspecified state of consciousness
1 with no loss of consciousness
2 with brief [less than one hour] loss of consciousness
3 with moderate [1-24 hours] loss of consciousness
4 with prolonged [more than 24 hours] loss of consciousness and return to pre-existing conscious level
5 with prolonged [more than 24 hours] loss of consciousness, without return to pre-existing conscious level
6 with loss of consciousness of unspecified duration
9 with concussion, unspecified

801.0 5th Closed fracture of base of skull without mention of intracranial injury

801.1 5th Closed fracture of base of skull with cerebral laceration and contusion

801.2 5th Closed fracture of base of skull with subarachnoid, subdural, and extradural hemorrhage

801.3 5th Closed fracture of base of skull with other and unspecified intracranial hemorrhage

801.4 5th Closed fracture of base of skull with intracranial injury of other and unspecified nature

801.5 5th Open fracture of base of skull without mention of intracranial injury

801.6 5th Open fracture of base of skull with cerebral laceration and contusion

801.7 5th Open fracture of base of skull with subarachnoid, subdural, and extradural hemorrhage

801.8 5th Open fracture of base of skull with other and unspecified intracranial hemorrhage

801.9 5th Open fracture of base of skull with intracranial injury of other and unspecified nature

© 2004 Ingenix, Inc.

802 Fracture of face bones

AHA: Sept-Oct, 1985, 3; Q2, 1989, 15; Q2, 1990, 7; Q3, 1990, 5; Q3, 1990, 13; Q4, 1990, 26; Q4, 1996, 36

The facial bones comprise the following bones:

- Nasal bone — adjoins the frontal bone to form the superior aspect of the nose
- Mandible — lower jawbone
- Maxilla — upper jawbone
- Zygomatic bones — two bones of the cheek
- Lacrimal bones — two bones of the tear ducts
- Vomer — inferior and interior support for nasal conchae
- Orbital plate — two bones in the area of the eye
- Palate — the roof of the mouth

The orbit is one of the most complex bony structures in the skull. The frontal, mandible, lacrimal, orbital plate, zygomatic, and sphenoid bones fit together to form support and protection for the eyeball.

The following fifth-digit subclassification is for use with the appropriate codes in categories 800, 801, 803, and 804:

0 unspecified state of consciousness
1 twith no loss of consciousness
2 with brief [less than one hour] loss of consciousness
3 with moderate [1-24 hours] loss of consciousness
4 with prolonged [more than 24 hours] loss of consciousness and return to pre-existing conscious level
5 with prolonged [more than 24 hours] loss of consciousness, without return to pre-existing conscious level
6 with loss of consciousness of unspecified duration
9 with concussion, unspecified

802.0 Nasal bones, closed fracture
802.1 Nasal bones, open fracture
802.2 5th Mandible, closed fracture
802.3 5th Mandible, open fracture
802.4 Malar and maxillary bones, closed fracture
802.5 Malar and maxillary bones, open fracture
802.6 Orbital floor (blow-out), closed fracture
802.7 Orbital floor (blow-out), open fracture
802.8 Other facial bones, closed fracture
802.9 Other facial bones, open fracture

803 Other and unqualified skull fractures

AHA: Sept-Oct, 1985, 3; Q2, 1989, 15; Q2, 1990, 7; Q3, 1990, 5; Q3, 1990, 13; Q4, 1990, 26; Q4, 1996, 36

Use these codes when the record lacks specific information regarding the trauma to the head.

The following fifth-digit subclassification is for use with the appropriate codes in categories 800, 801, 803, and 804:

0 unspecified state of consciousness
1 twith no loss of consciousness
2 with brief [less than one hour] loss of consciousness
3 with moderate [1-24 hours] loss of consciousness
4 with prolonged [more than 24 hours] loss of consciousness and return to pre-existing conscious level
5 with prolonged [more than 24 hours] loss of consciousness, without return to pre-existing conscious level
6 with loss of consciousness of unspecified duration
9 with concussion, unspecified

803.0 5th Other closed skull fracture without mention of intracranial injury
803.1 5th Other closed skull fracture with cerebral laceration and contusion
803.2 5th Other closed skull fracture with subarachnoid, subdural, and extradural hemorrhage
803.3 5th Closed skull fracture with other and unspecified intracranial hemorrhage
803.4 5th Other closed skull fracture with intracranial injury of other and unspecified nature
803.5 5th Other open skull fracture without mention of intracranial injury
803.6 5th Other open skull fracture with cerebral laceration and contusion
803.7 5th Other open skull fracture with subarachnoid, subdural, and extradural hemorrhage
803.8 5th Other open skull fracture with other and unspecified intracranial hemorrhage
803.9 5th Other open skull fracture with intracranial injury of other and unspecified nature

804 Multiple fractures involving skull or face with other bones

AHA: Sept-Oct, 1985, 3; Q2, 1989, 15; Q2, 1990, 7; Q3, 1990, 5; Q3, 1990, 13; Q4, 1990, 26; Q4, 1996, 36

This category is used when bones of the skull or face are fractured, together with bones in other parts of the body. If there is more specific information about the nature of the various fractures, code more specifically.

800–999

The following fifth-digit subclassification is for use with the appropriate codes in categories 800, 801, 803, and 804:

0 unspecified state of consciousness

1 twith no loss of consciousness

2 with brief [less than one hour] loss of consciousness

3 with moderate [1-24 hours] loss of consciousness

4 with prolonged [more than 24 hours] loss of consciousness and return to pre-existing conscious level

5 with prolonged [more than 24 hours] loss of consciousness, without return to pre-existing conscious level

6 with loss of consciousness of unspecified duration

9 with concussion, unspecified

804.0 5th Closed fractures involving skull or face with other bones, without mention of intracranial injury

804.1 5th Closed fractures involving skull or face with other bones, with cerebral laceration and contusion

804.2 5th Closed fractures involving skull or face with other bones with subarachnoid, subdural, and extradural hemorrhage

804.3 5th Closed fractures involving skull or face with other bones, with other and unspecified intracranial hemorrhage

804.4 5th Closed fractures involving skull or face with other bones, with intracranial injury of other and unspecified nature

804.5 5th Open fractures involving skull or face with other bones, without mention of intracranial injury

804.6 5th Open fractures involving skull or face with other bones, with cerebral laceration and contusion

804.7 5th Open fractures involving skull or face with other bones with subarachnoid, subdural, and extradural hemorrhage

804.8 5th Open fractures involving skull or face with other bones, with other and unspecified intracranial hemorrhage

804.9 5th Open fractures involving skull or face with other bones, with intracranial injury of other and unspecified nature

805–809 Fracture of Neck and Trunk

805 Fracture of vertebral column without mention of spinal cord injury

AHA: Sept-Oct, 1985, 3; Q2, 1989, 15; Q2, 1990, 7; Q3, 1990, 5; Q3, 1990, 13; Q4, 1990, 26

The vertebral column forms a protective shield around the spinal column, much as the cranium protects the brain. It allows movement through articulation of the cervical, thoracic, and lumbar vertebrae (sacral vertebrae are fused). Each vertebra has a body and a neural arch, which encase the spinal cord. Each vertebra has several prominent aspects called processes for the attachment of muscles, tendons, and other soft tissues.

The two transverse processes of the cervical vertebrae have a small foramen, the foramen transversarium, through which the vertebral artery and vein and a plexus of sympathetic nerves travel. The first cervical vertebra is called the atlas and supports the globe of the head; it has no vertebral body; instead, the part of the vertebra that would have been the body is fused with the second cervical vertebra to form an osseous pivot around which the head turns. The second cervical vertebra is called the axis.

The thoracic (dorsal) vertebrae accept the heads of the ribs. The lumbar vertebrae are the largest of the moveable vertebrae, or true vertebrae.

Below the thoracic vertebrae are the five lumbar vertebrae, which are larger than the thoracic and cervical vertebrae and support a great amount of weight.

The sacrum consists of five large vertebrae that are fused in the adult. The female sacrum is shorter and wider than the male sacrum.

The composition of the coccyx varies from three to five fused segments, though the typical configuration is four.

The spinal cord, protected by the vertebral column, shares the three meningeal layers, the dura, arachnoid, and pia maters with the brain. It is described anatomically in relation to the vertebrae at each level, but the cord is not identical to the column. In addition to nerve tracts to the brain, enclosed within the column, the spinal nerves exit the column to innervate specific muscle groups bilaterally, according to their level on the vertebral column. The part of the cord that extends below the lumbar level resembled a horse's tail to early anatomists, hence its name — cauda equina.

Similar to the brain, the cord has both gray and white matter. Hemorrhage into the gray matter is known as hematomyelia; its symptoms, which are often permanent, include muscle wasting, diminished tendon reflexes, and muscle weakness. Spinal concussion, the same contrecoup action described in the brain, can result in loss of cord function after a very severe blow or jarring.

 © 2004 Ingenix, Inc.

The following fifth-digit subclassification is for use with codes 805.0-805.1:

0 cervical vertebra, unspecified level
1 first cervical vertebra
2 second cervical vertebra
3 third cervical vertebra
4 fourth cervical vertebra
5 fifth cervical vertebra
6 sixth cervical vertebra
7 seventh cervical vertebra
8 multiple cervical vertebra

805.0 5th Closed fracture of cervical vertebra without mention of spinal cord injury

805.1 5th Open fracture of cervical vertebra without mention of spinal cord injury

805.2 Closed fracture of dorsal (thoracic) vertebra without mention of spinal cord injury

805.3 Open fracture of dorsal (thoracic) vertebra without mention of spinal cord injury

805.4 Closed fracture of lumbar vertebra without mention of spinal cord injury

805.5 Open fracture of lumbar vertebra without mention of spinal cord injury

805.6 Closed fracture of sacrum and coccyx without mention of spinal cord injury

805.7 Open fracture of sacrum and coccyx without mention of spinal cord injury

805.8 Closed fracture of unspecified part of vertebral column without mention of spinal cord injury

805.9 Open fracture of unspecified part of vertebral column without mention of spinal cord injury

806 Fracture of vertebral column with spinal cord injury

AHA: Sept-Oct, 1985, 3; Q2, 1989, 15; Q2, 1990, 7; Q3, 1990, 5; Q3, 1990, 13; Q4, 1990, 26

A transverse cord injury will cause immediate total paralysis and sensory loss below the level of the injury. It is sometimes referred to as a complete injury. An incomplete lesion will result in partial motor and sensory loss. Depending on the site of injury, outcomes vary, ranging from respiratory paralysis (injury above C5 level); quadriplegia, which is paralysis of four limbs (C4-C5); and paralysis of the legs and partial paralysis of the arms, with abduction and flexion of the arms as movement potentials (C5-C6). C6-C7 allows shoulder movement and elbow flexion, though the lower limbs are paralyzed. Complete loss of bowel and bladder control is associated with injury to the third, fourth, and fifth sacral nerve roots or to the juncture at L1. Posterior cord syndrome is an incomplete injury resulting in motor paralysis and loss of posterior spinal column sensory function.

Paralysis to both legs and the lower portion of the body is termed paraplegia.

The documentation in the medical record should be clear for coding these injuries as either complete or incomplete. Resort to "unspecified" only if the physician fails to make the distinction.

806.00 Closed fracture of C1-C4 level with unspecified spinal cord injury

806.01 Closed fracture of C1-C4 level with complete lesion of cord

806.02 Closed fracture of C1-C4 level with anterior cord syndrome

806.03 Closed fracture of C1-C4 level with central cord syndrome

806.04 Closed fracture of C1-C4 level with other specified spinal cord injury

806.05 Closed fracture of C5-C7 level with unspecified spinal cord injury

806.06 Closed fracture of C5-C7 level with complete lesion of cord

806.07 Closed fracture of C5-C7 level with anterior cord syndrome

806.08 Closed fracture of C5-C7 level with central cord syndrome

806.09 Closed fracture of C5-C7 level with other specified spinal cord injury

806.10 Open fracture of C1-C4 level with unspecified spinal cord injury

806.11 Open fracture of C1-C4 level with complete lesion of cord

806.12 Open fracture of C1-C4 level with anterior cord syndrome

806.13 Open fracture of C1-C4 level with central cord syndrome

806.14 Open fracture of C1-C4 level with other specified spinal cord injury

806.15 Open fracture of C5-C7 level with unspecified spinal cord injury

806.16 Open fracture of C5-C7 level with complete lesion of cord

806.17 Open fracture of C5-C7 level with anterior cord syndrome

806.18 Open fracture of C5-C7 level with central cord syndrome

806.19 Open fracture of C5-C7 level with other specified spinal cord injury

806.20 Closed fracture of T1-T6 level with unspecified spinal cord injury

806.21 Closed fracture of T1-T6 level with complete lesion of cord

806.22 Closed fracture of T1-T6 level with anterior cord syndrome

806.23 Closed fracture of T1-T6 level with central cord syndrome

806.24 Closed fracture of T1-T6 level with other specified spinal cord injury

806.25 Closed fracture of T7-T12 level with unspecified spinal cord injury

806.26 Closed fracture of T7-T12 level with complete lesion of cord

806.27 Closed fracture of T7-T12 level with anterior cord syndrome

806.28 Closed fracture of T7-T12 level with central cord syndrome

806.29 Closed fracture of T7-T12 level with other specified spinal cord injury

806.30 Open fracture of T1-T6 level with unspecified spinal cord injury

806.31 Open fracture of T1-T6 level with complete lesion of cord

806.32 Open fracture of T1-T6 level with anterior cord syndrome

806.33 Open fracture of T1-T6 level with central cord syndrome

806.34 Open fracture of T1-T6 level with other specified spinal cord injury

806.35 Open fracture of T7-T12 level with unspecified spinal cord injury

806.36 Open fracture of T7-T12 level with complete lesion of cord

806.37 Open fracture of T7-T12 level with anterior cord syndrome

806.38 Open fracture of T7-T12 level with central cord syndrome

806.39 Open fracture of T7-T12 level with other specified spinal cord injury

806.4 Closed fracture of lumbar spine with spinal cord injury

806.5 Open fracture of lumbar spine with spinal cord injury

806.60 Closed fracture of sacrum and coccyx with unspecified spinal cord injury

806.61 Closed fracture of sacrum and coccyx with complete cauda equina lesion

806.62 Closed fracture of sacrum and coccyx with other cauda equina injury

806.69 Closed fracture of sacrum and coccyx with other spinal cord injury

806.70 Open fracture of sacrum and coccyx with unspecified spinal cord injury

806.71 Open fracture of sacrum and coccyx with complete cauda equina lesion

806.72 Open fracture of sacrum and coccyx with other cauda equina injury

806.79 Open fracture of sacrum and coccyx with other spinal cord injury

806.8 Closed fracture of unspecified vertebra with spinal cord injury

806.9 Open fracture of unspecified vertebra with spinal cord injury

807 Fracture of rib(s), sternum, larynx, and trachea

AHA: Sept-Oct, 1985, 3; Q2, 1989, 15; Q2, 1990, 7; Q3, 1990, 5; Q3, 1990, 13; Q4, 1990, 26

Twelve pairs of ribs form the thoracic cage, which protects the critical organs in the thorax and abdomen. The true ribs are the first eight ribs and the false ribs are the last four ribs. The floating ribs are the last two of the false ribs.

All of the ribs, except the floating ribs, are connected to the sternum (the breastbone) with costal cartilage.

Flail chest is one of the most dangerous thoracic injuries, resulting from an injury causing at least four fractured ribs in two locations, and pulmonary contusion, leading to hypoventilation. In flail chest, the movement of the chest is paradoxical (opposite of the natural ventilatory movement). On inhalation, the chest contracts and on expiration the chest expands. Generally, thoracic injuries carry a high mortality risk, with death attributed to hypoxemia, hypovolemia, or myocardial failure.

Fractures of the scapula, the sternum, or the first rib are indicative of applied forces.

When coding rib fractures, review the documentation to capture multiple fractures. In inpatient reimbursement, some payment algorithms are constructed according to the number of ribs fractured, making complete capture of all injuries important in all cases.

The following fifth-digit subclassification is for use with codes 807.0-807.1:

0 rib(s), unspecified
1 one rib
2 two ribs
3 three ribs
4 four ribs
5 five ribs
6 six ribs
7 seven ribs
8 eight or more ribs
9 multiple ribs, unspecified

807.0 5th Closed fracture of rib(s)

807.1 5th Open fracture of rib(s)

807.2 Closed fracture of sternum

 © 2004 Ingenix, Inc.

807.3 Open fracture of sternum

807.4 Flail chest

807.5 Closed fracture of larynx and trachea

807.6 Open fracture of larynx and trachea

808 Fracture of pelvis

AHA: Sept-Oct, 1985, 3; Q2, 1989, 15; Q2, 1990, 7; Q3, 1990, 5; Q3, 1990, 13; Q4, 1990, 26

The pelvis includes the ilium, the ischium, the pubis, and the sacrum, which form a bony circle to protect the pelvic contents, provide stability for the vertebral column, (sacrum) and provide an appropriate surface for femoral articulation for ambulation.

The innominate bone, or hipbone, refers to the three bones making up the hipbone: the pubis, ilium, and ischium. The acetabulum is the socket for the femoral head and is found anterior to the rings of the ischium on the lateral inferior surface of the ilium. When the acetabulum is fractured, the head of the femur functions as a hammer, striking against its socket with undue force.

Note that the term hip fracture, which is often used to describe a fracture of the acetabulum, excludes the femur. A fracture of the shaft of the femur, or of the head of the femur, is anatomically distinct from a disruption of the socket of the femoral head.

Pelvic fractures in an individual age 55 and older are associated with a 9.5 percent mortality rate within one year. In fractures of the pelvic ring (circle), the mortality risk to the patient is quite immediate, due to the hemorrhagic capability of cancellous bone. While the issue of application of external fixation may be debated, all agree that the disruption must be stabilized as soon as possible to ensure a positive outcome.

808.0 Closed fracture of acetabulum

808.1 Open fracture of acetabulum

808.2 Closed fracture of pubis

808.3 Open fracture of pubis

808.41 Closed fracture of ilium

808.42 Closed fracture of ischium

808.43 Multiple closed pelvic fractures with disruption of pelvic circle

808.49 Closed fracture of other specified part of pelvis

808.51 Open fracture of ilium

808.52 Open fracture of ischium

808.53 Multiple open pelvic fractures with disruption of pelvic circle

808.59 Open fracture of other specified part of pelvis

808.8 Unspecified closed fracture of pelvis

808.9 Unspecified open fracture of pelvis

809 Ill-defined fractures of bones of trunk

AHA: Sept-Oct, 1985, 3; Q2, 1989, 15; Q2, 1990, 7; Q3, 1990, 5; Q3, 1990, 13; Q4, 1990, 26

Although this category includes a number of excludes notes, an example is a combination of rib and pelvic fractures, poorly defined in documentation.

809.0 Fracture of bones of trunk, closed

809.1 Fracture of bones of trunk, open

810–819 Fracture of Upper Limb

810 Fracture of clavicle

AHA: Sept-Oct, 1985, 3; Q2, 1989, 15; Q2, 1990, 7; Q3, 1990, 5; Q3, 1990, 13; Q4, 1990, 26

The clavicle, or collarbone, has a shaft and articulating ends — the sternal and acromial ends. The acromial end articulates with the scapula, the shoulder bone.

The following fifth-digit subclassification is for use with category 810:

0 unspecified part

1 sternal end of clavicle

2 shaft of clavicle

3 acromial end of clavicle

810.0 5th Closed fracture of clavicle

810.1 5th Open fracture of clavicle

811 Fracture of scapula

AHA: Sept-Oct, 1985, 3; Q2, 1989, 15; Q2, 1990, 7; Q3, 1990, 5; Q3, 1990, 13; Q4, 1990, 26

The scapula articulates with the clavicle and the humerus, the long bone in the upper arm. Its socket, the glenoid fossa, receives the humoral head. The coracoid process superior to the glenoid fossa provides a surface for attachments of muscles and tendons.

The following fifth-digit subclassification is for use with category 811:

0 unspecified part

1 acromial process

2 coracoid process

3 glenoid cavity and neck of scapula

9 other

811.0 5th Closed fracture of scapula

811.1 5th Open fracture of scapula

800–999

812 *Fracture of humerus*

AHA: Sept-Oct, 1985, 3; Q2, 1989, 15; Q2, 1990, 7; Q3, 1990, 5; Q3, 1990, 13; Q4, 1990, 26

In addition to possession of an anatomical neck, the humerus includes a surgical neck, described as that portion of the anatomical neck most likely to fracture.

812.00	Closed fracture of unspecified part of upper end of humerus
812.01	Closed fracture of surgical neck of humerus
812.02	Closed fracture of anatomical neck of humerus
812.03	Closed fracture of greater tuberosity of humerus
812.09	Other closed fractures of upper end of humerus
812.10	Open fracture of unspecified part of upper end of humerus
812.11	Open fracture of surgical neck of humerus
812.12	Open fracture of anatomical neck of humerus
812.13	Open fracture of greater tuberosity of humerus
812.19	Other open fracture of upper end of humerus
812.20	Closed fracture of unspecified part of humerus
812.21	Closed fracture of shaft of humerus
812.30	Open fracture of unspecified part of humerus
812.31	Open fracture of shaft of humerus
812.40	Closed fracture of unspecified part of lower end of humerus
812.41	Closed fracture of supracondylar humerus
812.42	Closed fracture of lateral condyle of humerus
812.43	Closed fracture of medial condyle of humerus
812.44	Closed fracture of unspecified condyle(s) of humerus
812.49	Other closed fracture of lower end of humerus
812.50	Open fracture of unspecified part of lower end of humerus
812.51	Open fracture of supracondylar humerus
812.52	Open fracture of lateral condyle of humerus
812.53	Open fracture of medial condyle of humerus
812.54	Open fracture of unspecified condyle(s) of humerus
812.59	Other open fracture of lower end of humerus

813 *Fracture of radius and ulna*

AHA: Sept-Oct, 1985, 3; Q2, 1989, 15; Q2, 1990, 7; Q3, 1990, 5; Q3, 1990, 13; Q4, 1990, 26

The radius and ulna operate in tandem, with a hinge-like motion for bending and capabilities for pronation and supination for the hand and wrist. In the anatomical position, the hands are supinated. In the pronated position, the palms are down.

Monteggia's fracture is a common fracture at the proximal end of the ulna, combined with dislocation of the radial head. In a child, closed reduction may suffice, though adults require open reduction and internal fixation (ORIF). Reduction is the repositioning of a bone into proper alignment. Dislocations, which are the disruption of the joint, are also reduced.

Another common fracture is Colles' fracture, which is a transverse fracture of the distal radius, displacing the hand. This injury typically occurs when an individual puts out a hand to break a fall.

813.00	Unspecified fracture of radius and ulna, upper end of forearm, closed
813.01	Closed fracture of olecranon process of ulna
813.02	Closed fracture of coronoid process of ulna
813.03	Closed Monteggia's fracture
813.04	Other and unspecified closed fractures of proximal end of ulna (alone)
813.05	Closed fracture of head of radius
813.06	Closed fracture of neck of radius
813.07	Other and unspecified closed fractures of proximal end of radius (alone)
813.08	Closed fracture of radius with ulna, upper end (any part)
813.10	Unspecified open fracture of upper end of forearm
813.11	Open fracture of olecranon process of ulna
813.12	Open fracture of coronoid process of ulna
813.13	Open Monteggia's fracture
813.14	Other and unspecified open fractures of proximal end of ulna (alone)
813.15	Open fracture of head of radius
813.16	Open fracture of neck of radius
813.17	Other and unspecified open fractures of proximal end of radius (alone)
813.18	Open fracture of radius with ulna, upper end (any part)
813.20	Unspecified closed fracture of shaft of radius or ulna
813.21	Closed fracture of shaft of radius (alone)
813.22	Closed fracture of shaft of ulna (alone)
813.23	Closed fracture of shaft of radius with ulna
813.30	Unspecified open fracture of shaft of radius or ulna
813.31	Open fracture of shaft of radius (alone)
813.32	Open fracture of shaft of ulna (alone)
813.33	Open fracture of shaft of radius with ulna

 © 2004 Ingenix, Inc.

813.40 Unspecified closed fracture of lower end of forearm

813.41 Closed Colles' fracture

813.42 Other closed fractures of distal end of radius (alone)

813.43 Closed fracture of distal end of ulna (alone)

813.44 Closed fracture of lower end of radius with ulna

813.45 Torus fracture of lower end of radius

813.50 Unspecified open fracture of lower end of forearm

813.51 Open Colles' fracture

813.52 Other open fractures of distal end of radius (alone)

813.53 Open fracture of distal end of ulna (alone)

813.54 Open fracture of lower end of radius with ulna

813.80 Closed fracture of unspecified part of forearm

813.81 Closed fracture of unspecified part of radius (alone)

813.82 Closed fracture of unspecified part of ulna (alone)

813.83 Closed fracture of unspecified part of radius with ulna

813.90 Open fracture of unspecified part of forearm

813.91 Open fracture of unspecified part of radius (alone)

813.92 Open fracture of unspecified part of ulna (alone)

813.93 Open fracture of unspecified part of radius with ulna

Coding Scenario

A patient is seen in the emergency department (ED) after falling from a tree. He complains of pain in the right wrist. After x-ray examination, it is determined that the patient has a greenstick break of the upper end of the right radius.

> Code assignment: 813.00 *Unspecified fracture of radius and ulna, upper end of forearm, closed*

A 64-year-old female involved in an automobile accident is seen in the ED. The physician documents that there is a compound fracture of the shaft of the right femur and a fracture of the left shaft of the ulna and radius.

> Code assignment: 821.11 *Fracture of other and unspecified parts of femur, shaft or unspecified part, open, shaft* and 813.23 *Fracture of radius and ulna, shaft, closed, radius with ulna*

814 Fracture of carpal bone(s)

AHA: Sept-Oct, 1985, 3; Q2, 1989, 15; Q2, 1990, 7; Q3, 1990, 5; Q3, 1990, 13; Q4, 1990, 26

The eight carpal bones are functionally linked to the placement of each bone and its articulation with various partners.

Two rows of bones, with the scaphoid bone common to each row, act as a bridge to provide stability. The first row (proximal) is comprised of the scaphoid, lunate, pisiform, and triquetrum. The second row (distal) is comprised of the scaphoid, trapezium, trapezoid, capitate, and hamate.

Fractures of the distal radius and ulna are typically referred to as wrist fractures. They articulate with the proximal carpals, though, technically, they are the bones of the forearm. The carpals, which form the wrist, are considered part of the hand.

Carpal fractures usually occur as a result of extreme dorsiflexion or extension of the wrist and require significant force to happen at all.

814.00 Unspecified closed fracture of carpal bone

814.01 Closed fracture of navicular (scaphoid) bone of wrist

814.02 Closed fracture of lunate (semilunar) bone of wrist

814.03 Closed fracture of triquetral (cuneiform) bone of wrist

814.04 Closed fracture of pisiform bone of wrist

814.05 Closed fracture of trapezium bone (larger multangular) of wrist

814.06 Closed fracture of trapezoid bone (smaller multangular) of wrist

814.07 Closed fracture of capitate bone (os magnum) of wrist

814.08 Closed fracture of hamate (unciform) bone of wrist

814.09 Closed fracture of other bone of wrist

814.10 Unspecified open fracture of carpal bone

814.11 Open fracture of navicular (scaphoid) bone of wrist

814.12 Open fracture of lunate (semilunar) bone of wrist

814.13 Open fracture of triquetral (cuneiform) bone of wrist

814.14 Open fracture of pisiform bone of wrist

814.15 Open fracture of trapezium bone (larger multangular) of wrist

814.16 Open fracture of trapezoid bone (smaller multangular) of wrist

814.17 Open fracture of capitate bone (os magnum) of wrist

814.18 Open fracture of hamate (unciform) bone of wrist

814.19 Open fracture of other bone of wrist

815 Fracture of metacarpal bone(s)

AHA: Sept-Oct, 1985, 3; Q2, 1989, 15; Q2, 1990, 7; Q3, 1990, 5; Q3, 1990, 13; Q4, 1990, 26

The metacarpals are the bones of the hand distal to the carpals and proximal to the phalanges (fingers). The fingers have three joints: the section next to the metacarpals is the proximal phalanx, the midsection is the middle phalanx, and the farthest section is the distal phalanx. The numbering convention selects the thumb as the first metacarpal and the medial finger (pinkie) as the fifth finger.

The anatomy of each phalanx is described in terms of base, body, and head. The base is the end portion closest to the head of the body, the body is the midsection of the bone, and the head is the distal end of the bone. The distal phalanx has an additional descriptor, a tuberosity. Two sesamoid bones are located close to the distal joint of the first metacarpal (thumb).

Because they project and perform many functions, the metacarpals and phalanges account for 10 percent of all fractures, of which 50 percent are work-related.

The following fifth-digit subclassification is for use with category 815:

0 metacarpal bone(s), site unspecified
1 base of thumb [first] metacarpal
2 base of other metacarpal bone(s)
3 shaft of metacarpal bone(s)
4 neck of metacarpal bone(s)
9 multiple sites of metacarpus

815.0 ✓5th Closed fracture of metacarpal bones
815.1 ✓5th Open fracture of metacarpal bones

816 Fracture of one or more phalanges of hand

AHA: Sept-Oct, 1985, 3; Q2, 1989, 15; Q2, 1990, 7; Q3, 1990, 5; Q3, 1990, 13; Q4, 1990, 26

816.00 Closed fracture of unspecified phalanx or phalanges of hand
816.01 Closed fracture of middle or proximal phalanx or phalanges of hand
816.02 Closed fracture of distal phalanx or phalanges of hand
816.03 Closed fracture of multiple sites of phalanx or phalanges of hand
816.10 Open fracture of phalanx or phalanges of hand, unspecified
816.11 Open fracture of middle or proximal phalanx or phalanges of hand
816.12 Open fracture of distal phalanx or phalanges of hand
816.13 Open fractures of multiple sites of phalanx or phalanges of hand

817 Multiple fractures of hand bones

AHA: Sept-Oct, 1985, 3; Q2, 1989, 15; Q2, 1990, 7; Q3, 1990, 5; Q3, 1990, 13; Q4, 1990, 26

Use these categories only if the documentation is extremely sketchy.

817.0 Multiple closed fractures of hand bones
817.1 Multiple open fractures of hand bones

818 Ill-defined fractures of upper limb

AHA: Sept-Oct, 1985, 3; Q2, 1989, 15; Q2, 1990, 7; Q3, 1990, 5; Q3, 1990, 13; Q4, 1990, 26

818.0 Ill-defined closed fractures of upper limb
818.1 Ill-defined open fractures of upper limb

819 Multiple fractures involving both upper limbs, and upper limb with rib(s) and sternum

AHA: Sept-Oct, 1985, 3; Q2, 1989, 15; Q2, 1990, 7; Q3, 1990, 5; Q3, 1990, 13; Q4, 1990, 26

819.0 Multiple closed fractures involving both upper limbs, and upper limb with rib(s) and sternum
819.1 Multiple open fractures involving both upper limbs, and upper limb with rib(s) and sternum

820–829 Fracture of Lower Limb

820 Fracture of neck of femur

AHA: Sept-Oct, 1985, 3; Q2, 1989, 15; Q2, 1990, 7; Q3, 1990, 5; Q3, 1990, 13; Q4, 1990, 26

The proximal femur bears the brunt of accidents leading to fractures, compared to the other bones used for locomotion. Lower extremity fractures in children may suggest child abuse.

Fractures of the femoral shaft are relatively uncommon, while fractures of the neck are among the most frequent. Femoral neck fractures are classified in ICD-9-CM as transcervical, or pertrochanteric, with subdivisions. Radiologists often use the terminology intracapsular and extracapsular. A subcapital or intracapsular fracture of the femoral neck has the highest risk of avascular necrosis, which occurs when a severe injury disrupts the blood supply to the bone. This fracture also is inherently more unstable after surgery than an intertrochanteric fracture since the weakest part of the bone is now supporting the point of greatest stress.

If a clinician reports a proximal femur fracture as opposed to an intertrochanteric, the radiology report will state that the fracture is intertrochanteric. This

© 2004 Ingenix, Inc.

coded information is crucial to achieve an accurate evaluation of patient outcomes and utilization data.

Preferred treatments for the various fractures include the following:

- Shaft fracture — intramedullary nailing; promotes fast weight-bearing capability
- Transcervical fracture — hemiarthroplasty or total hip replacement
- Intertrochanteric fracture — fixation with sliding implant

820.00 Closed fracture of unspecified intracapsular section of neck of femur

820.01 Closed fracture of epiphysis (separation) (upper) of neck of femur

820.02 Closed fracture of midcervical section of femur

820.03 Closed fracture of base of neck of femur

820.09 Other closed transcervical fracture of femur

820.10 Open fracture of unspecified intracapsular section of neck of femur

820.11 Open fracture of epiphysis (separation) (upper) of neck of femur

820.12 Open fracture of midcervical section of femur

820.13 Open fracture of base of neck of femur

820.19 Other open transcervical fracture of femur

820.20 Closed fracture of unspecified trochanteric section of femur

820.21 Closed fracture of intertrochanteric section of femur

820.22 Closed fracture of subtrochanteric section of femur

820.30 Open fracture of unspecified trochanteric section of femur

820.31 Open fracture of intertrochanteric section of femur

820.32 Open fracture of subtrochanteric section of femur

820.8 Closed fracture of unspecified part of neck of femur

820.9 Open fracture of unspecified part of neck of femur

821 Fracture of other and unspecified parts of femur

AHA: Sept-Oct, 1985, 3; Q2, 1989, 15; Q2, 1990, 7; Q3, 1990, 5; Q3, 1990, 13; Q4, 1990, 26

In children and adolescents, whose skeletons are still immature, distal epiphyseal fracture, presenting as valgus instability, results in a significant number of injuries. These fractures occur in normal play and sports activity, and are easy to overlook if the evaluation seems to point to a ligamentous sprain, rather than a physeal fracture.

821.00 Closed fracture of unspecified part of femur

821.01 Closed fracture of shaft of femur

821.10 Open fracture of unspecified part of femur

821.11 Open fracture of shaft of femur

821.20 Closed fracture of unspecified part of lower end of femur

821.21 Closed fracture of femoral condyle

821.22 Closed fracture of lower epiphysis of femur

821.23 Closed supracondylar fracture of femur

821.29 Other closed fracture of lower end of femur

821.30 Open fracture of unspecified part of lower end of femur

821.31 Open fracture of femoral condyle

821.32 Open fracture of lower epiphysis of femur

821.33 Open supracondylar fracture of femur

821.39 Other open fracture of lower end of femur

822 Fracture of patella

AHA: Sept-Oct, 1985, 3; Q2, 1989, 15; Q2, 1990, 7; Q3, 1990, 5; Q3, 1990, 13; Q4, 1990, 26

The anatomy of the knee joint and associated muscles, tendons, and ligaments predispose the occurrence of patellar fractures in conjunction with sprains or ruptures of the ligaments. Typically, injuries are due to direct application of force or twisting. A severely injured knee remains prone to re-injury, instability, or arthritis.

822.0 Closed fracture of patella

822.1 Open fracture of patella

823 Fracture of tibia and fibula

AHA: Sept-Oct, 1985, 3; Q2, 1989, 15; Q2, 1990, 7; Q3, 1990, 5; Q3, 1990, 13; Q4, 1990, 26

The malleolus is the distal end of both the tibia and the fibula and is classified to the ankle in ICD-9-CM. The lateral malleolus is part of the fibula and the medial malleolus is part of the tibia. This category is for fractures of the upper end and shaft of the tibia and fibula, or unspecified parts.

The following fifth-digit subclassification is for use with category 823:

0 tibia alone

1 fibula alone

2 fibula with tibia

823.0 5th Closed fracture of upper end of tibia and fibula

823.1 5th Open fracture of upper end of tibia and fibula

800–999

823.2 ✓5th Closed fracture of shaft of tibia and fibula

823.3 ✓5th Open fracture of shaft of tibia and fibula

823.4 ✓5th Torus fracture of tibia and fibula

823.8 ✓5th Closed fracture of unspecified part of tibia and fibula

823.9 ✓5th Open fracture of unspecified part of tibia and fibula

824 Fracture of ankle

AHA: Sept-Oct, 1985, 3; Q2, 1989, 15; Q2, 1990, 7; Q3, 1990, 5; Q3, 1990, 13; Q4, 1990, 26

A bimalleolar fracture is a fracture of both the lateral and medial aspects of the malleolus. Pott's fracture is any fracture of the malleolus. Dupuytren's fracture is a fracture dislocation of the ankle with the talus downwardly displaced. The talus is one of the major ankle (tarsal) bones. A trimalleolar fracture involves a fracture of the medial malleolus and the fibula with a fracture of the posterior lip of the tibia's articulating surface.

Open reduction and internal fixation is the method of treatment for bimalleolar and trimalleolar fractures.

824.0 Closed fracture of medial malleolus

824.1 Open fracture of medial malleolus

824.2 Closed fracture of lateral malleolus

824.3 Open fracture of lateral malleolus

824.4 Closed bimalleolar fracture

824.5 Open bimalleolar fracture

824.6 Closed trimalleolar fracture

824.7 Open trimalleolar fracture

824.8 Unspecified closed fracture of ankle

824.9 Unspecified open fracture of ankle

825 Fracture of one or more tarsal and metatarsal bones

AHA: Sept-Oct, 1985, 3; Q2, 1989, 15; Q2, 1990, 7; Q3, 1990, 5; Q3, 1990, 13; Q4, 1990, 26

The tarsal bones are the heel bone (calcaneus, os calcis), talus (astragalus), navicular (scaphoid), cuboid, and the lateral, medial, and intermediate cuneiform bones. The metatarsals are the five long bones of the foot extending from the tarsal bones to the phalanges, or toes.

825.0 Closed fracture of calcaneus

825.1 Open fracture of calcaneus

825.20 Closed fracture of unspecified bone(s) of foot (except toes)

825.21 Closed fracture of astragalus

825.22 Closed fracture of navicular (scaphoid) bone of foot

825.23 Closed fracture of cuboid bone

825.24 Closed fracture of cuneiform bone of foot

825.25 Closed fracture of metatarsal bone(s)

825.29 Other closed fracture of tarsal and metatarsal bones

825.30 Open fracture of unspecified bone(s) of foot (except toes)

825.31 Open fracture of astragalus

825.32 Open fracture of navicular (scaphoid) bone of foot

825.33 Open fracture of cuboid bone

825.34 Open fracture of cuneiform bone of foot,

825.35 Open fracture of metatarsal bone(s)

825.39 Other open fractures of tarsal and metatarsal bones

826 Fracture of one or more phalanges of foot

AHA: Sept-Oct, 1985, 3; Q2, 1989, 15; Q2, 1990, 7; Q3, 1990, 5; Q3, 1990, 13; Q4, 1990, 26

826.0 Closed fracture of one or more phalanges of foot

826.1 Open fracture of one or more phalanges of foot

827 Other, multiple, and ill-defined fractures of lower limb

AHA: Sept-Oct, 1985, 3; Q2, 1989, 15; Q2, 1990, 7; Q3, 1990, 5; Q3, 1990, 13; Q4, 1990, 26

Use these categories only if the documentation is extremely sketchy.

827.0 Other, multiple and ill-defined closed fractures of lower limb

827.1 Other, multiple and ill-defined open fractures of lower limb

828 Multiple fractures involving both lower limbs, lower with upper limb, and lower limb(s) with rib(s) and sternum

AHA: Sept-Oct, 1985, 3; Q2, 1989, 15; Q2, 1990, 7; Q3, 1990, 5; Q3, 1990, 13; Q4, 1990, 26

828.0 Multiple closed fractures involving both lower limbs, lower with upper limb, and lower limb(s) with rib(s) and sternum

828.1 Multiple fractures involving both lower limbs, lower with upper limb, and lower limb(s) with rib(s) and sternum, open

829 Fracture of unspecified bones

AHA: Sept-Oct, 1985, 3; Q2, 1989, 15; Q2, 1990, 7; Q3, 1990, 5; Q3, 1990, 13; Q4, 1990, 26

829.0 Closed fracture of unspecified bone

 © 2004 Ingenix, Inc.

829.1 Open fracture of unspecified bone

830–839 Dislocation

Luxation is the term used to describe a complete dislocation, one that has separated the articulating surfaces of the joint. An incomplete dislocation, or subluxation, is one in which the joint surfaces maintain some articulation. A simple dislocation has not penetrated to make a communicating wound. An uncomplicated dislocation is not associated with other important injuries. Open dislocations are subject to infection. They are always compound. Reduction of a dislocation is by manipulation, open or closed. They should be performed immediately, although this does not ensure a good result. Avascular necrosis, traumatic arthritis, and ectopic ossification are considered threats to complete recovery.

Some dislocations are described as anterior and posterior or lateral and medial, which describe the location of the displaced bone in relation to its proper placement. For example, if the bone lies in front of its joint, the dislocation is considered to be anterior.

Dislocation of the acromioclavicular joint ranges in severity according to the degree of damage to the acromioclavicular and coracoclavicular ligaments.

Pubic symphysis and sacroiliac dislocations result from high-energy impact and are associated with other severe pelvic injuries. Regardless of the severity of injuries, a hip dislocation must be reduced first to contain blood loss and to minimize permanent damage to the pelvic structures.

The sternoclavicular joint may sustain anterior or posterior dislocations. While an anterior dislocation is simply remedied, a posterior dislocation poses a grave risk to the patient because of potential risk to critical internal thoracic organs.

Dislocation of the patella is typically lateral. The choice of open or closed reduction depends on the degree of disruption of the nearby ligaments and tendons. Intraarticular dislocations of the patella usually require open reduction. Other dislocations of the knee are serious, requiring immediate surgery to offset the risk of vascular complications.

The ankle is seldom dislocated without an accompanying fracture and is easily reduced.

830 Dislocation of jaw

AHA: Q3, 1990, 12

830.0 Closed dislocation of jaw

830.1 Open dislocation of jaw

831 Dislocation of shoulder

AHA: Q3, 1990, 12

The following fifth-digit subclassification is for use with category 831:

0 shoulder, unspecified
1 anterior dislocation of humerus
2 posterior dislocation of humerus
3 inferior dislocation of humerus
4 acromioclavicular (joint)
9 other

831.0 ✓5th Closed dislocation of shoulder, unspecified

831.1 ✓5th Open dislocation of shoulder

832 Dislocation of elbow

AHA: Q3, 1990, 12

The following fifth-digit subclassification is for use with category 832:

0 elbow, unspecified
1 anterior dislocation of elbow
2 posterior dislocation of elbow
3 medial dislocation of elbow
4 lateral dislocation of elbow
9 other

832.0 ✓5th Closed dislocation of elbow

832.1 ✓5th Open dislocation of elbow

833 Dislocation of wrist

AHA: Q3, 1990, 12

The following fifth-digit subclassification is for use with category 833:

0 wrist, unspecified part
1 radioulnar (joint), distal
2 radiocarpal (joint)
3 midcarpal (joint)
4 carpometacarpal (joint)
5 metacarpal (bone), proximal end
9 other

833.0 ✓5th Closed dislocation of wrist

833.1 ✓5th Open dislocation of wrist

834 Dislocation of finger

AHA: Q3, 1990, 12

The following fifth-digit subclassification is for use with category 834:

0 finger, unspecified part
1 metacarpophalangeal (joint)
2 interphalangeal (joint), hand

800–999

834.0 ✓5th Closed dislocation of finger

834.1 ✓5th Open dislocation of finger

835 Dislocation of hip

AHA: Q3, 1990, 12

The following fifth-digit subclassification is for use with category 835:

0 dislocation of hip, unspecified

1 posterior dislocation

2 obturator dislocation

3 other anterior dislocation

835.0 ✓5th Closed dislocation of hip

835.1 ✓5th Open dislocation of hip

836 Dislocation of knee

AHA: Q3, 1990, 12

836.0 Tear of medial cartilage or meniscus of knee, current

836.1 Tear of lateral cartilage or meniscus of knee, current

836.2 Other tear of cartilage or meniscus of knee, current

836.3 Closed dislocation of patella

836.4 Open dislocation of patella

836.50 Closed dislocation of knee, unspecified part

836.51 Closed anterior dislocation of tibia, proximal end

836.52 Closed posterior dislocation of tibia, proximal end

836.53 Closed medial dislocation of tibia, proximal end

836.54 Closed lateral dislocation of tibia, proximal end

836.59 Other closed dislocation of knee

836.60 Open dislocation of knee unspecified part

836.61 Open anterior dislocation of tibia, proximal end

836.62 Open posterior dislocation of tibia, proximal end

836.63 Open medial dislocation of tibia, proximal end

836.64 Open lateral dislocation of tibia, proximal end

836.69 Other open dislocation of knee

837 Dislocation of ankle

AHA: Q3, 1990, 12

837.0 Closed dislocation of ankle

837.1 Open dislocation of ankle

838 Dislocation of foot

AHA: Q3, 1990, 12

The following fifth-digit subclassification is for use with category 838:

0 foot, unspecified

1 tarsal (bone), joint unspecified

2 midtarsal (joint)

3 tarsometatarsal (joint)

4 metatarsal (bone), joint unspecified

5 metatarsophalangeal (joint)

6 interphalangeal (joint), foot

9 other

838.0 ✓5th Closed dislocation of foot

838.1 ✓5th Open dislocation of foot

839 Other, multiple, and ill-defined dislocations

AHA: Q3, 1990, 12

839.00 Closed dislocation, unspecified cervical vertebra

839.01 Closed dislocation, first cervical vertebra

839.02 Closed dislocation, second cervical vertebra

839.03 Closed dislocation, third cervical vertebra

839.04 Closed dislocation, fourth cervical vertebra

839.05 Closed dislocation, fifth cervical vertebra

839.06 Closed dislocation, sixth cervical vertebra

839.07 Closed dislocation, seventh cervical vertebra

839.08 Closed dislocation, multiple cervical vertebrae

839.10 Open dislocation, unspecified cervical vertebra

839.11 Open dislocation, first cervical vertebra

839.12 Open dislocation, second cervical vertebra

839.13 Open dislocation, third cervical vertebra

839.14 Open dislocation, fourth cervical vertebra

839.15 Open dislocation, fifth cervical vertebra

839.16 Open dislocation, sixth cervical vertebra

839.17 Open dislocation, seventh cervical vertebra

839.18 Open dislocation, multiple cervical vertebrae

839.20 Closed dislocation, lumbar vertebra

839.21 Closed dislocation, thoracic vertebra

839.30 Open dislocation, lumbar vertebra

839.31 Open dislocation, thoracic vertebra

839.40 Closed dislocation, vertebra, unspecified site

839.41 Closed dislocation, coccyx

839.42 Closed dislocation, sacrum

839.49 Closed dislocation, other vertebra

© 2004 Ingenix, Inc.

839.50	Open dislocation, vertebra, unspecified site
839.51	Open dislocation, coccyx
839.52	Open dislocation, sacrum
839.59	Open dislocation, other vertebra
839.61	Closed dislocation, sternum
839.69	Closed dislocation, other location
839.71	Open dislocation, sternum
839.79	Open dislocation, other location
839.8	Closed dislocation, multiple and ill-defined sites
839.9	Open dislocation, multiple and ill-defined sites

840–848 Sprains and Strains of Joints and Adjacent Muscles

A sprain is not identical to a strain and should not be used as a synonym. A sprain is an injury to the ligaments, tough fibrous tissues that bind bones together at joints. A strain is an injury to the muscles or tendons that bind muscles together and does not occur at the joint.

Sprains and strains are graded. A Type I sprain denotes minor ligamentous injury; Type II is an incomplete ligamentous injury; and Type III describes a complete disruption of the ligament. The more ligaments involved in the sprain, the more serious the injury. A Type III strain involves the complete tearing of muscle and separation from its tendon. Both sprains and strains manifest with swelling, pain, and difficulty in using and are best treated according to the RICE therapy — Rest of the affected part, Ice, Compression, and Elevation.

Areas commonly sprained include the ankle, groin, knee, and neck. Ankle sprains seldom require surgery. If the patient suffers repeated injury to the weakened ankle, surgery may be performed. If two or more ligaments are involved in a knee sprain, it is serious and likely to require corrective surgery. A mild sprain may heal in two to six weeks, while a severe sprain may require eight weeks to 10 months to heal.

Whiplash is the sudden and forceful extension and flexion of the neck and can cause death if the movement of the neck injures the brain stem. Arms and shoulders can be affected to the point of paralysis. Whiplash accounts for 10 percent of all long-term disabilities.

Sports Injuries. Acute athletic injuries are those that develop suddenly and last six months or less. Some acute injuries require time to heal, sometimes longer than six months. These include injuries to the musculoskeletal system, especially to the knees and ankles, such as bone fractures, sprains, and muscle strains, and typically result from twisting, tearing, or from lateral force, such as the blows to the side of the knee. Severe acute injuries, such as those to the head or spinal cord, usually result from accidents or extreme overexertion. Chronic athletic injuries include aches and pain of unknown origin, tendonitis, and stress fractures, which are common in athletes who consistently overuse muscles for extended periods. Diagnosis includes visual exam and manipulation of injured joints in concert with more complex procedures, such as arthroscopy for an internal exam of the joints. Common diagnostic imaging techniques include x-rays, computed tomography, ultrasound, and magnetic resonance imaging. Treatments range from cryotherapy and immobilization for simple sprains and strains to surgical procedures for fractures and tears in ligaments or tendons. Rest, physical therapy, and massage are integral to the healing of most injuries. Drugs and corticosteroids can be used to lessen pain and inflammation.

840 Sprains and strains of shoulder and upper arm

840.0	Acromioclavicular (joint) (ligament) sprain and strain
840.1	Coracoclavicular (ligament) sprain and strain
840.2	Coracohumeral (ligament) sprain and strain
840.3	Infraspinatus (muscle) (tendon) sprain and strain
840.4	Rotator cuff (capsule) sprain and strain
840.5	Subscapularis (muscle) sprain and strain
840.6	Supraspinatus (muscle) (tendon) sprain and strain
840.7	Superior glenoid labrum lesions (SLAP)
840.8	Sprain and strain of other specified sites of shoulder and upper arm
840.9	Sprain and strain of unspecified site of shoulder and upper arm

841 Sprains and strains of elbow and forearm

841.0	Radial collateral ligament sprain and strain
841.1	Ulnar collateral ligament sprain and strain
841.2	Radiohumeral (joint) sprain and strain
841.3	Ulnohumeral (joint) sprain and strain
841.8	Sprain and strain of other specified sites of elbow and forearm
841.9	Sprain and strain of unspecified site of elbow and forearm

842 Sprains and strains of wrist and hand

842.00	Sprain and strain of unspecified site of wrist
842.01	Sprain and strain of carpal (joint) of wrist
842.02	Sprain and strain of radiocarpal (joint) (ligament) of wrist
842.09	Other wrist sprain and strain

800–999

842.10 Sprain and strain of unspecified site of hand

842.11 Sprain and strain of carpometacarpal (joint) of hand

842.12 Sprain and strain of metacarpophalangeal (joint) of hand

842.13 Sprain and strain of interphalangeal (joint) of hand

842.19 Other hand sprain and strain

843 Sprains and strains of hip and thigh

843.0 Iliofemoral (ligament) sprain and strain

843.1 Ischiocapsular (ligament) sprain and strain

843.8 Sprain and strain of other specified sites of hip and thigh

843.9 Sprain and strain of unspecified site of hip and thigh

844 Sprains and strains of knee and leg

844.0 Sprain and strain of lateral collateral ligament of knee

844.1 Sprain and strain of medial collateral ligament of knee

844.2 Sprain and strain of cruciate ligament of knee

844.3 Sprain and strain of tibiofibular (joint) (ligament) superior, of knee

844.8 Sprain and strain of other specified sites of knee and leg

844.9 Sprain and strain of unspecified site of knee and leg

845 Sprains and strains of ankle and foot

845.00 Unspecified site of ankle sprain and strain

845.01 Sprain and strain of deltoid (ligament) of ankle

845.02 Sprain and strain of calcaneofibular (ligament)

845.03 Sprain and strain of tibiofibular (ligament)

845.09 Other ankle sprain and strain

845.10 Sprain and strain of unspecified site of foot

845.11 Sprain and strain of tarsometatarsal (joint) (ligament)

845.12 Sprain and strain of metatarsaophalangeal (joint)

845.13 Sprain and strain of interphalangeal (joint), of toe

845.19 Other foot sprain and strain

846 Sprains and strains of sacroiliac region

846.0 Sprain and strain of lumbosacral (joint) (ligament)

846.1 Sprain and strain of sacroiliac (ligament)

846.2 Sprain and strain of sacrospinatus (ligament)

846.3 Sprain and strain of sacrotuberous (ligament)

846.8 Other specified sites of sacroiliac region sprain and strain

846.9 Unspecified site of sacroiliac region sprain and strain

847 Sprains and strains of other and unspecified parts of back

847.0 Neck sprain and strain

847.1 Thoracic sprain and strain

847.2 Lumbar sprain and strain

847.3 Sprain and strain of sacrum

847.4 Sprain and strain of coccyx

847.9 Sprain and strain of unspecified site of back

848 Other and ill-defined sprains and strains

848.0 Sprain and strain of septal cartilage of nose

848.1 Sprain and strain of jaw

848.2 Sprain and strain of thyroid region

848.3 Sprain and strain of ribs

848.40 Sprain and strain of sternum, unspecified part

848.41 Sprain and strain of sternoclavicular (joint) (ligament)

848.42 Sprain and strain of chondrosternal (joint)

848.49 Other sprain and strains of sternum

848.5 Pelvic sprain and strains

848.8 Other specified sites of sprains and strains

848.9 Unspecified site of sprain and strain

850–854 Intracranial Injury, Excluding Those with Skull Fracture

850 Concussion

AHA: Q4, 1990, 24; Q1, 1993, 22; Q2, 1996, 6

850.0 Concussion with no loss of consciousness

850.11 Concussion, with loss of consciousness of 30 minutes or less

850.12 Concussion, with loss of consciousness 31 to 59 minutes

850.2 Concussion with moderate (1-24 hours) loss of consciousness

 © 2004 Ingenix, Inc.

850.3 Concussion with prolonged (more than 24 hours) loss of consciousness and return to pre-existing conscious level

850.4 Concussion with prolonged (more than 24 hours) loss of consciousness, without return to pre-existing conscious level

850.5 Concussion with loss of consciousness of unspecified duration

850.9 Unspecified concussion

Documentation Issues

When coding concussions, the physician must document if the patient has a loss of consciousness; if the loss of consciousness was brief, moderate, or prolonged; and if the patient returned to the previous level of consciousness.

If the concussion is accompanied by cerebral laceration and contusion, the physician should also indicate the site of the laceration and if an open wound is present in addition to the above findings.

When the patient is treated for the symptoms of a concussion within 24 to 48 hours and the diagnosis is identified as "postconcussion syndrome," verify with the physician if the concussion is still in the current stage and should be reported with a code from category 850, rather than as postconcussion syndrome, code 310.2.

Coding Clarification

Also refer to category 800.

Concussion with Cerebral Laceration: Only one code is necessary to indicate a concussion with cerebral laceration. When the documentation states that this condition is present, assign a code from category 851 with a fourth digit indicating the site of the laceration and a fifth digit to identify loss of consciousness and the duration.

Postconcussion syndrome is a term used to describe the symptoms following a concussion, including headache, dizziness, anxiety, fatigue, problems concentrating, and depression. This condition is indicated with code 310.2.

Suspected Concussion: A physician may suspect that a patient has a concussion but may not have confirmed the suspicion. When coding inpatients, the appropriate code from category 850 should be reported.

When coding outpatients, rule-out and suspected conditions cannot be coded. Therefore, the appropriate code indicating the symptoms the patient is having (i.e., headache, dizziness, etc.) should be reported.

851 Cerebral laceration and contusion

AHA: Q4, 1990, 24; Q1, 1993, 22; Q4, 1996, 36

The following fifth-digit subclassification is for use with categories 851-854:

0 unspecified state of consciousness

1 twith no loss of consciousness

2 with brief [less than one hour] loss of consciousness

3 with moderate [1-24 hours] loss of consciousness

4 with prolonged [more than 24 hours] loss of consciousness and return to pre-existing conscious level

5 with prolonged [more than 24 hours] loss of consciousness, without return to pre-existing conscious level

Use fifth-digit five to designate when a patient is unconscious and dies before regaining consciousness, regardless of the duration of the loss of consciousness

6 with loss of consciousness of unspecified duration

9 with concussion, unspecified

851.0 5th Cortex (cerebral) contusion without mention of open intracranial wound

851.1 5th Cortex (cerebral) contusion with open intracranial wound

851.2 5th Cortex (cerebral) laceration without mention of open intracranial wound

851.3 5th Cortex (cerebral) laceration with open intracranial wound

851.4 5th Cerebellar or brain stem contusion without mention of open intracranial wound

851.5 5th Cerebellar or brain stem contusion with open intracranial wound

851.6 5th Cerebellar or brain stem laceration without mention of open intracranial wound

851.7 5th Cerebellar or brain stem laceration with open intracranial wound

851.8 5th Other and unspecified cerebral laceration and contusion, without mention of open intracranial wound

851.9 5th Other and unspecified cerebral laceration and contusion, with open intracranial wound

852 *Subarachnoid, subdural, and extradural hemorrhage, following injury*

AHA: Q1, 1993, 22

The following fifth-digit subclassification is for use with categories 851-854:

0 unspecified state of consciousness

1 twith no loss of consciousness

2 with brief [less than one hour] loss of consciousness

3 with moderate [1-24 hours] loss of consciousness

4 with prolonged [more than 24 hours] loss of consciousness and return to pre-existing conscious level

5 with prolonged [more than 24 hours] loss of consciousness, without return to pre-existing conscious level

Use fifth-digit five to designate when a patient is unconscious and dies before regaining consciousness, regardless of the duration of the loss of consciousness

6 with loss of consciousness of unspecified duration

9 with concussion, unspecified

852.0 ✓5th Subarachnoid hemorrhage following injury without mention of open intracranial wound

852.1 ✓5th Subarachnoid hemorrhage following injury, with open intracranial wound

852.2 ✓5th Subdural hemorrhage following injury without mention of open intracranial wound

852.3 ✓5th Subdural hemorrhage following injury, with open intracranial wound

852.4 ✓5th Extradural hemorrhage following injury without mention of open intracranial wound

852.5 ✓5th Extradural hemorrhage following injury with open intracranial wound

853 *Other and unspecified intracranial hemorrhage following injury*

AHA: Q1, 1993, 22

The following fifth-digit subclassification is for use with categories 851-854:

0 unspecified state of consciousness

1 twith no loss of consciousness

2 with brief [less than one hour] loss of consciousness

3 with moderate [1-24 hours] loss of consciousness

4 with prolonged [more than 24 hours] loss of consciousness and return to pre-existing conscious level

5 with prolonged [more than 24 hours] loss of consciousness, without return to pre-existing conscious level

Use fifth-digit five to designate when a patient is unconscious and dies before regaining consciousness, regardless of the duration of the loss of consciousness

6 with loss of consciousness of unspecified duration

9 with concussion, unspecified

853.0 ✓5th Other and unspecified intracranial hemorrhage following injury, without mention of open intracranial wound

853.1 ✓5th Other and unspecified intracranial hemorrhage following injury with open intracranial wound

854 *Intracranial injury of other and unspecified nature*

AHA: Q2, 1992, 6; Q1, 1993, 22; Q1, 1999, 10

The following fifth-digit subclassification is for use with categories 851-854:

0 unspecified state of consciousness

1 twith no loss of consciousness

2 with brief [less than one hour] loss of consciousness

3 with moderate [1-24 hours] loss of consciousness

4 with prolonged [more than 24 hours] loss of consciousness and return to pre-existing conscious level

5 with prolonged [more than 24 hours] loss of consciousness, without return to pre-existing conscious level

Use fifth-digit five to designate when a patient is unconscious and dies before regaining consciousness, regardless of the duration of the loss of consciousness

6 with loss of consciousness of unspecified duration

9 with concussion, unspecified

854.0 ✓5th Intracranial injury of other and unspecified nature without mention of open intracranial wound

854.1 ✓5th Intracranial injury of other and unspecified nature with open intracranial wound

© 2004 Ingenix, Inc.

860–869 Internal Injury of Thorax, Abdomen, and Pelvis

Internal injuries can result from a blast, blunt trauma, crushing, puncture, rupture, concussion of internal organs, laceration, and hematoma.

Blast injuries result from explosive force capable of generating shock waves that damage the body. The force can emanate from a bomb, a gas leak, or any other explosion. Blast injuries are graded as primary, secondary, tertiary, and miscellaneous. A primary blast injury affects air-filled organs such as the lungs, ears, and bowel. If the tympanic membrane is ruptured, the physician automatically assumes serious organ damage. Secondary injury results from injuries associated with flying objects. Tertiary injuries may result from striking objects while airborne. Morbidity and mortality are greatest if the explosion occurs within a confined space or under water.

The most common fatality associated with blast injury results from injury to the pulmonary system, which can result in pulmonary contusion, air embolism, free radical injury and thrombosis, lipo-oxygenation, and disseminated intravascular coagulation (DIS).

Blunt trauma has two traumatic components: compression and deceleration forces. Compression causes trauma such as rupture of the bowel, which is often a marker for more serious solid organ damage. Deceleration causes stretching and shearing injuries. A common deceleration injury is a hepatic tear along the ligamentum teres. Blunt trauma refers to abdominal injuries. In adults, automobile accidents are to blame for 66 percent of all blunt trauma injuries.

Crush injuries involve smashing, fractures, bleeding, and bruising.

A hematoma is blood that has escaped from the vascular vessels and is free in the tissues (extravascular).

860 Traumatic pneumothorax and hemothorax

AHA: Q2, 1993, 4

Pneumothorax is free gas in the pleural space with lung collapse on the affected side. The medical record may state that a hemothorax is traumatic when arising from a medical procedure, but category 860 for traumatic hemothorax is not to be assigned for the condition arising from the delivery of medical care (998.11).

When hemothorax presents, the clinician suspects further damage to the lungs and heart. An evaluation must assess the integrity of the great vessels (aorta, vena cava, pulmonary artery, and pulmonary vein), as lacerations to these vessels increase mortality risks.

860.0 Traumatic pneumothorax without mention of open wound into thorax

860.1 Traumatic pneumothorax with open wound into thorax

860.2 Traumatic hemothorax without mention of open wound into thorax

860.3 Traumatic hemothorax with open wound into thorax

860.4 Traumatic pneumohemothorax without mention of open wound into thorax

860.5 Traumatic pneumohemothorax with open wound into thorax

861 Injury to heart and lung

861.00 Unspecified injury to heart without mention of open wound into thorax

861.01 Heart contusion without mention of open wound into thorax

861.02 Heart laceration without penetration of heart chambers or mention of open wound into thorax

861.03 Heart laceration with penetration of heart chambers, without mention of open wound into thorax

861.10 Unspecified injury to heart with open wound into thorax

861.11 Heart contusion with open wound into thorax

861.12 Heart laceration without penetration of heart chambers, with open wound into thorax

861.13 Heart laceration with penetration of heart chambers and open wound into thorax

861.20 Unspecified lung injury without mention of open wound into thorax

861.21 Lung contusion without mention of open wound into thorax

861.22 Lung laceration without mention of open wound into thorax

861.30 Unspecified lung injury with open wound into thorax

861.30 Unspecified lung injury with open wound into thorax

861.31 Lung contusion with open wound into thorax

861.32 Lung laceration with open wound into thorax

862 Injury to other and unspecified intrathoracic organs

862.0 Diaphragm injury without mention of open wound into cavity

862.1 Diaphragm injury with open wound into cavity

862.21 Bronchus injury without mention of open wound into cavity

862.22 Esophagus injury without mention of open wound into cavity

800–999

862.29 Injury to other specified intrathoracic organs without mention of open wound into cavity

862.31 Bronchus injury with open wound into cavity

862.32 Esophagus injury with open wound into cavity

862.39 Injury to other specified intrathoracic organs with open wound into cavity

862.8 Injury to multiple and unspecified intrathoracic organs without mention of open wound into cavity

862.9 Injury to multiple and unspecified intrathoracic organs with open wound into cavity

863 Gastrointestinal tract injury

863.0 Stomach injury without mention of open wound into cavity

863.1 Stomach injury with open wound into cavity

863.20 Small intestine injury, unspecified site, without mention of open wound into cavity

863.21 Duodenum injury without mention of open wound into cavity

863.29 Other injury to small intestine without mention of open wound into cavity

863.30 Small intestine injury, unspecified site, with open wound into cavity

863.31 Duodenum injury with open wound into cavity

863.39 Other injury to small intestine with open wound into cavity

863.40 Colon injury unspecified site, without mention of open wound into cavity

863.41 Ascending (right) colon injury without mention of open wound into cavity

863.42 Transverse colon injury without mention of open wound into cavity

863.43 Descending (left) colon injury without mention of open wound into cavity

863.44 Sigmoid colon injury without mention of open wound into cavity

863.45 Rectum injury without mention of open wound into cavity

863.46 Injury to multiple sites in colon and rectum without mention of open wound into cavity

863.49 Other colon and rectum injury, without mention of open wound into cavity

863.50 Colon injury, unspecified site, with open wound into cavity

863.51 Ascending (right) colon injury with open wound into cavity

863.52 Transverse colon injury with open wound into cavity

863.53 Descending (left) colon injury with open wound into cavity

863.54 Sigmoid colon injury with open wound into cavity

863.55 Rectum injury with open wound into cavity

863.56 Injury to multiple sites in colon and rectum with open wound into cavity

863.59 Other injury to colon and rectum with open wound into cavity

863.80 Gastrointestinal tract injury, unspecified site, without mention of open wound into cavity

863.81 Pancreas head injury without mention of open wound into cavity

863.82 Pancreas body injury without mention of open wound into cavity

863.83 Pancreas tail injury without mention of open wound into cavity

863.84 Pancreas injury, multiple and unspecified sites, without mention of open wound into cavity

863.85 Appendix injury without mention of open wound into cavity

863.89 Injury to other and unspecified gastrointestinal sites without mention of open wound into cavity

863.90 Gastrointestinal tract injury, unspecified site, with open wound into cavity

863.91 Pancreas head injury with open wound into cavity

863.92 Pancreas body injury with open wound into cavity

863.93 Pancreas tail injury with open wound into cavity

863.94 Pancreas injury, multiple and unspecified sites, with open wound into cavity

863.95 Appendix injury with open wound into cavity

863.99 Injury to other and unspecified gastrointestinal sites with open wound into cavity

864 Injury to liver

The liver is protected by the fibrous membrane Glisson's capsule. Not all liver injuries need surgical repair. If the patient is stable hemodynamically and has no other intra-abdominal injury that requires surgery, nursing may allow for non-operative management of the injury.

The following fifth-digit subclassification is for use with category 864:

0 unspecified injury

1 hematoma and contusion

2 laceration, minor

3 laceration, moderate

4 laceration, major

5 laceration, unspecified

9 other

 © 2004 Ingenix, Inc.

864.0 ✓5th Liver injury without mention of open wound into cavity

864.1 ✓5th Liver injury with open wound into cavity

865 Injury to spleen

Similar to the liver, the spleen is covered by a thick fibrous membrane, the capsule, which plays a part in grading the severity of splenic injuries.

The following fifth-digit subclassification is for use with category 865:

0 unspecified injury
1 hematoma with rupture of capsule
2 capsular tears, without major disruption of parenchyma
3 laceration extending into parenchyma
4 massive parenchymal disruption
9 other

865.0 ✓5th Spleen injury without mention of open wound into cavity

865.1 ✓5th Spleen injury with open wound into cavity

866 Injury to kidney

The kidney's capsule protects the kidney parenchyma and is part of the injury grading system for the kidney.

The following fifth-digit subclassification is for use with category 866:

0 unspecified injury
1 hematoma without rupture of capsule
2 laceration
3 complete disruption of kidney parenchyma

866.0 ✓5th Kidney injury without mention of open wound into cavity

866.1 ✓5th Kidney injury with open wound into cavity

867 Injury to pelvic organs

Pelvic organs include the bladder, urethra, ureters, uterus, and other specified organs, including the fallopian tubes, ovaries, prostate, seminal vesicles, and vas deferens.

867.0 Bladder and urethra injury without mention of open wound into cavity

867.1 Bladder and urethra injury with open wound into cavity

867.2 Ureter injury without mention of open wound into cavity

867.3 Ureter injury with open wound into cavity

867.4 Uterus injury without mention of open wound into cavity

867.5 Uterus injury with open wound into cavity

867.6 Injury to other specified pelvic organs without mention of open wound into cavity

867.7 Injury to other specified pelvic organs with open wound into cavity

867.8 Injury to unspecified pelvic organ without mention of open wound into cavity

867.9 Injury to unspecified pelvic organ with open wound into cavity

868 Injury to other intra-abdominal organs

The peritoneum is a serous membrane lining the abdominal cavity and reflected over the viscera, the internal organs. The portion covering the viscera is called the omentum (apron). The retroperitoneum lies behind the viscera and outside the cavity. The kidneys are in the retroperitoneum.

The following fifth-digit subclassification is for use with category 868:

0 unspecified intra-abdominal organ
1 adrenal gland
2 bile duct and gallbladder
3 peritoneum
4 retroperitoneum
9 other and multiple intra-abdominal organs

868.0 ✓5th Injury to other intra-abdominal organs without mention of open wound into cavity

868.1 ✓5th Injury to other intra-abdominal organs with open wound into cavity

869 Internal injury to unspecified or ill-defined organs

Use these categories only if the documentation is extremely sketchy.

869.0 Internal injury to unspecified or ill-defined organs without mention of open wound into cavity

869.1 Internal injury to unspecified or ill-defined organs with open wound into cavity

870–879 Open Wound of Head, Neck, and Trunk

A traumatic amputation and an avulsion are essentially the same. Amputation is typically reserved to describe limb injuries and avulsion describes injuries such as the tearing or ripping of fingernails or a portion of an organ, though it can be used in reference to loss of limbs.

When using the term "complicated," described in the fourth-digit of codes 870-897, it includes wounds that have delayed healing, foreign body, infection, or wounds with delayed treatment.

870 Open wound of ocular adnexa

AHA: Q4, 2001, 52

The ocular adnexa are the eyelids, the lacrimal apparatus, the orbit, and the periocular area.

870.0 Laceration of skin of eyelid and periocular area — (Use additional code to identify infection)

870.1 Laceration of eyelid, full-thickness, not involving lacrimal passages — (Use additional code to identify infection)

870.2 Laceration of eyelid involving lacrimal passages — (Use additional code to identify infection)

870.3 Penetrating wound of orbit, without mention of foreign body

870.4 Penetrating wound of orbit with foreign body

870.8 Other specified open wound of ocular adnexa — (Use additional code to identify infection)

870.9 Unspecified open wound of ocular adnexa — (Use additional code to identify infection)

871 Open wound of eyeball

AHA: Q4, 2001, 52

871.0 Ocular laceration without prolapse of intraocular tissue — (Use additional code to identify infection)

871.1 Ocular laceration with prolapse or exposure of intraocular tissue — (Use additional code to identify infection)

871.2 Rupture of eye with partial loss of intraocular tissue — (Use additional code to identify infection)

871.3 Avulsion of eye — (Use additional code to identify infection)

871.4 Unspecified laceration of eye — (Use additional code to identify infection)

871.5 Penetration of eyeball with magnetic foreign body

871.6 Penetration of eyeball with (nonmagnetic) foreign body

871.7 Unspecified ocular penetration — (Use additional code to identify infection)

871.9 Unspecified open wound of eyeball — (Use additional code to identify infection)

872 Open wound of ear

AHA: Q4, 2001, 52

The auricle, or pinna, is another term for the external ear. The ossicles (tiny bones) refer to the three bones facilitating hearing — the malleus, incus, and stapes.

872.00 Open wound of external ear, unspecified site, without mention of complication

872.01 Open wound of auricle, without mention of complication

872.02 Open wound of auditory canal, without mention of complication

872.10 Open wound of external ear, unspecified site, complicated — (Use additional code to identify infection)

872.11 Open wound of auricle, complicated — (Use additional code to identify infection)

872.12 Open wound of auditory canal, complicated — (Use additional code to identify infection)

872.61 Open wound of ear drum, without mention of complication

872.62 Open wound of ossicles, without mention of complication

872.63 Open wound of Eustachian tube, without mention of complication

872.64 Open wound of cochlea, without mention of complication

872.69 Open wound of other and multiple sites, without mention of complication

872.71 Open wound of ear drum, complicated — (Use additional code to identify infection)

872.72 Open wound of ossicles, complicated — (Use additional code to identify infection)

872.73 Open wound of Eustachian tube, complicated — (Use additional code to identify infection)

872.74 Open wound of cochlea, complicated — (Use additional code to identify infection)

872.79 Open wound of other and multiple sites, complicated — (Use additional code to identify infection)

872.8 Open wound of ear, part unspecified, without mention of complication

872.9 Open wound of ear, part unspecified, complicated — (Use additional code to identify infection)

873 Other open wound of head

AHA: Q4, 2001, 52

873.0 Open wound of scalp, without mention of complication

873.1 Open wound of scalp, complicated — (Use additional code to identify infection)

873.20 Open wound of nose, unspecified site, without mention of complication

873.21 Open wound of nasal septum, without mention of complication

873.22 Open wound of nasal cavity, without mention of complication

873.23 Open wound of nasal sinus, without mention of complication

© 2004 Ingenix, Inc.

873.29 Open wound of nose, multiple sites, without mention of complication

873.30 Open wound of nose, unspecified site, complicated — (Use additional code to identify infection)

873.31 Open wound of nasal septum, complicated — (Use additional code to identify infection)

873.32 Open wound of nasal cavity, complicated — (Use additional code to identify infection)

873.33 Open wound of nasal sinus, complicated — (Use additional code to identify infection)

873.39 Open wound of nose, multiple sites, complicated — (Use additional code to identify infection)

873.40 Open wound of face, unspecified site, without mention of complication

873.41 Open wound of cheek, without mention of complication

873.42 Open wound of forehead, without mention of complication

873.43 Open wound of lip, without mention of complication

873.44 Open wound of jaw, without mention of complication

873.49 Open wound of face, other and multiple sites, without mention of complication

873.50 Open wound of face, unspecified site, complicated — (Use additional code to identify infection)

873.51 Open wound of cheek, complicated — (Use additional code to identify infection)

873.52 Open wound of forehead, complicated — (Use additional code to identify infection)

873.53 Open wound of lip, complicated — (Use additional code to identify infection)

873.54 Open wound of jaw, complicated — (Use additional code to identify infection)

873.59 Open wound of face, other and multiple sites, complicated — (Use additional code to identify infection)

873.60 Open wound of mouth, unspecified site, without mention of complication

873.61 Open wound of buccal mucosa, without mention of complication

873.62 Open wound of gum (alveolar process), without mention of complication

873.63 Open wound of tooth (broken), without mention of complication

873.64 Open wound of tongue and floor of mouth, without mention of complication

873.65 Open wound of palate, without mention of complication

873.69 Open wound of mouth, other and multiple sites, without mention of complication

873.70 Open wound of mouth, unspecified site, complicated — (Use additional code to identify infection)

873.71 Open wound of buccal mucosa, complicated — (Use additional code to identify infection)

873.72 Open wound of gum (alveolar process), complicated — (Use additional code to identify infection)

873.73 Open wound of tooth (broken), complicated — (Use additional code to identify infection)

873.74 Open wound of tongue and floor of mouth, complicated — (Use additional code to identify infection)

873.75 Open wound of palate, complicated — (Use additional code to identify infection)

873.79 Open wound of mouth, other and multiple sites, complicated — (Use additional code to identify infection)

873.8 Other and unspecified open wound of head without mention of complication

873.9 Other and unspecified open wound of head, complicated — (Use additional code to identify infection)

874 Open wound of neck

AHA: Q4, 2001, 52

874.00 Open wound of larynx with trachea, without mention of complication

874.01 Open wound of larynx, without mention of complication

874.02 Open wound of trachea, without mention of complication

874.10 Open wound of larynx with trachea, complicated — (Use additional code to identify infection)

874.11 Open wound of larynx, complicated — (Use additional code to identify infection)

874.12 Open wound of trachea, complicated — (Use additional code to identify infection)

874.2 Open wound of thyroid gland, without mention of complication

874.3 Open wound of thyroid gland, complicated — (Use additional code to identify infection)

874.4 Open wound of pharynx, without mention of complication

874.5 Open wound of pharynx, complicated — (Use additional code to identify infection)

874.8 Open wound of other and unspecified parts of neck, without mention of complication

874.9 Open wound of other and unspecified parts of neck, complicated — (Use additional code to identify infection)

875 Open wound of chest (wall)

AHA: Q3, 1993, 17; Q4, 2001, 52

875.0 Open wound of chest (wall), without mention of complication

875.1 Open wound of chest (wall), complicated — (Use additional code to identify infection)

876 Open wound of back

AHA: Q4, 2001, 52

876.0 Open wound of back, without mention of complication

876.1 Open wound of back, complicated — (Use additional code to identify infection)

877 Open wound of buttock

AHA: Q4, 2001, 52

877.0 Open wound of buttock, without mention of complication

877.1 Open wound of buttock, complicated — (Use additional code to identify infection)

878 Open wound of genital organs (external), including traumatic amputation

AHA: Q4, 2001, 52

878.0 Open wound of penis, without mention of complication

878.1 Open wound of penis, complicated — (Use additional code to identify infection)

878.2 Open wound of scrotum and testes, without mention of complication

878.3 Open wound of scrotum and testes, complicated — (Use additional code to identify infection)

878.4 Open wound of vulva, without mention of complication

878.5 Open wound of vulva, complicated — (Use additional code to identify infection)

878.6 Open wound of vagina, without mention of complication

878.7 Open wound of vagina, complicated — (Use additional code to identify infection)

878.8 Open wound of other and unspecified parts of genital organs, without mention of complication

878.9 Open wound of other and unspecified parts of genital organs, complicated — (Use additional code to identify infection)

879 Open wound of other and unspecified sites, except limbs

AHA: Q4, 2001, 52

Flank (879.4) can have two meanings: (1) the part of the body found between the ribs and the uppermost crest of the ilium; or (2) the lateral side of the hip, thigh, and buttock.

When using the term "complicated," described in the fourth-digit of codes 870-897, it includes wounds that have delayed healing, foreign body, infection, or wounds with delayed treatment.

879.0 Open wound of breast, without mention of complication

879.1 Open wound of breast, complicated — (Use additional code to identify infection)

879.2 Open wound of abdominal wall, anterior, without mention of complication

879.3 Open wound of abdominal wall, anterior, complicated — (Use additional code to identify infection)

879.4 Open wound of abdominal wall, lateral, without mention of complication

879.5 Open wound of abdominal wall, lateral, complicated — (Use additional code to identify infection)

879.6 Open wound of other and unspecified parts of trunk, without mention of complication

879.7 Open wound of other and unspecified parts of trunk, complicated — (Use additional code to identify infection)

879.8 Open wound(s) (multiple) of unspecified site(s), without mention of complication

879.9 Open wound(s) (multiple) of unspecified site(s), complicated — (Use additional code to identify infection)

880 Open wound of shoulder and upper arm

AHA: Nov-Dec, 1985, 5; Q4, 2001, 52

The following fifth-digit subclassification is for use with category 880:

0 shoulder region

1 scapular region

2 axillary region

3 upper arm

9 multiple sites

880.0 5th Open wound of shoulder and upper arm, without mention of complication — (Use additional code to identify infection)

880.1 5th Open wound of shoulder and upper arm, complicated — (Use additional code to identify infection)

880.2 5th Open wound of shoulder and upper arm, with tendon involvement

 © 2004 Ingenix, Inc.

881 Open wound of elbow, forearm, and wrist

AHA: Nov-Dec, 1985, 5; Q4, 2001, 52

The following fifth-digit subclassification is for use with category 881:

0 forearm

1 elbow

2 wrist

881.0 [5th] Open wound of elbow, forearm, and wrist, without mention of complication

881.1 [5th] Open wound of elbow, forearm, and wrist, complicated — (Use additional code to identify infection)

881.2 [5th] Open wound of elbow, forearm, and wrist, with tendon involvement — (Use additional code to identify infection)

882 Open wound of hand except finger(s) alone

AHA: Nov-Dec, 1985, 5; Q4, 2001, 52

882.0 Open wound of hand except finger(s) alone, without mention of complication

882.1 Open wound of hand except finger(s) alone, complicated — (Use additional code to identify infection)

882.2 Open wound of hand except finger(s) alone, with tendon involvement

883 Open wound of finger(s)

AHA: Nov-Dec, 1985, 5; Q4, 2001, 52

883.0 Open wound of finger(s), without mention of complication

883.1 Open wound of finger(s), complicated — (Use additional code to identify infection)

883.2 Open wound of finger(s), with tendon involvement

884 Multiple and unspecified open wound of upper limb

AHA: Nov-Dec, 1985, 5; Q4, 2001, 52

884.0 Multiple and unspecified open wound of upper limb, without mention of complication

884.1 Multiple and unspecified open wound of upper limb, complicated — (Use additional code to identify infection)

884.2 Multiple and unspecified open wound of upper limb, with tendon involvement

885 Traumatic amputation of thumb (complete) (partial)

AHA: Nov-Dec, 1985, 5; Q4, 2001, 52

885.0 Traumatic amputation of thumb (complete) (partial), without mention of complication

885.1 Traumatic amputation of thumb (complete) (partial), complicated — (Use additional code to identify infection)

886 Traumatic amputation of other finger(s) (complete) (partial)

AHA: Nov-Dec, 19[illegible]14, 2001, 52

886.0 Traumatic amputation of other finger(s) (complete) (partial), without mention of complication

886.1 Traumatic amputation of other finger(s) (complete) (partial), complicated — (Use additional code to identify infection)

887 Traumatic amputation of arm and hand (complete) (partial)

AHA: Nov-Dec, 1985, 5; Q4, 2001, 52

887.0 Traumatic amputation of arm and hand (complete) (partial), unilateral, below elbow, without mention of complication

887.1 Traumatic amputation of arm and hand (complete) (partial), unilateral, below elbow, complicated — (Use additional code to identify infection)

887.2 Traumatic amputation of arm and hand (complete) (partial), unilateral, at or above elbow, without mention of complication

887.3 Traumatic amputation of arm and hand (complete) (partial), unilateral, at or above elbow, complicated — (Use additional code to identify infection)

887.4 Traumatic amputation of arm and hand (complete) (partial), unilateral, level not specified, without mention of complication

887.5 Traumatic amputation of arm and hand (complete) (partial), unilateral, level not specified, complicated — (Use additional code to identify infection)

887.6 Traumatic amputation of arm and hand (complete) (partial), bilateral (any level), without mention of complication

887.7 Traumatic amputation of arm and hand (complete) (partial), bilateral (any level), complicated — (Use additional code to identify infection)

890–897 Open Wound of Lower Limb

If the patient's injury is both complicated and has tendon involvement, code both conditions to fully describe the condition and the resources used to treat the injury.

Traumatic Amputations: Traumatic amputation injuries are capable of amelioration due to the ability to reattach the severed part. The severed part must be kept on ice to slow the process of decay and the patient must be brought to the operating room within a six- to eight-hour window. The nerves must regrow to the injured part and grow at a rate of about an inch a month.

When using the term "complicated," described in the fourth-digit of codes 870-897, it includes wounds that have delayed healing, a foreign body, infection, or wounds with delayed treatment.

890 Open wound of hip and thigh

AHA: Nov-Dec, 1985, 5; Q4, 2001, 52

890.0 Open wound of hip and thigh, without mention of complication

890.1 Open wound of hip and thigh, complicated — (Use additional code to identify infection)

890.2 Open wound of hip and thigh, with tendon involvement

891 Open wound of knee, leg (except thigh), and ankle

AHA: Nov-Dec, 1985, 5; Q4, 2001, 52

891.0 Open wound of knee, leg (except thigh), and ankle, without mention of complication

891.1 Open wound of knee, leg (except thigh), and ankle, complicated — (Use additional code to identify infection)

891.2 Open wound of knee, leg (except thigh), and ankle, with tendon involvement

892 Open wound of foot except toe(s) alone

AHA: Nov-Dec, 1985, 5; Q4, 2001, 52

892.0 Open wound of foot except toe(s) alone, without mention of complication

892.1 Open wound of foot except toe(s) alone, complicated — (Use additional code to identify infection)

892.2 Open wound of foot except toe(s) alone, with tendon involvement

893 Open wound of toe(s)

AHA: Nov-Dec, 1985, 5; Q4, 2001, 52

893.0 Open wound of toe(s), without mention of complication

893.1 Open wound of toe(s), complicated — (Use additional code to identify infection)

893.2 Open wound of toe(s), with tendon involvement

894 Multiple and unspecified open wound of lower limb

AHA: Nov-Dec, 1985, 5; Q4, 2001, 52

894.0 Multiple and unspecified open wound of lower limb, without mention of complication

894.1 Multiple and unspecified open wound of lower limb, complicated — (Use additional code to identify infection)

894.2 Multiple and unspecified open wound of lower limb, with tendon involvement — (Use additional code to identify infection)

895 Traumatic amputation of toe(s) (complete) (partial)

AHA: Nov-Dec, 1985, 5; Q4, 2001, 52

895.0 Traumatic amputation of toe(s) (complete) (partial), without mention of complication

895.1 Traumatic amputation of toe(s) (complete) (partial), complicated — (Use additional code to identify infection)

896 Traumatic amputation of foot (complete) (partial)

AHA: Nov-Dec, 1985, 5; Q4, 2001, 52

896.0 Traumatic amputation of foot (complete) (partial), unilateral, without mention of complication

896.1 Traumatic amputation of foot (complete) (partial), unilateral, complicated — (Use additional code to identify infection)

896.2 Traumatic amputation of foot (complete) (partial), bilateral, without mention of complication

896.3 Traumatic amputation of foot (complete) (partial), bilateral, complicated — (Use additional code to identify infection)

897 Traumatic amputation of leg(s) (complete) (partial)

AHA: Nov-Dec, 1985, 5; Q4, 2001, 52

897.0 Traumatic amputation of leg(s) (complete) (partial), unilateral, below knee, without mention of complication

897.1 Traumatic amputation of leg(s) (complete) (partial), unilateral, below knee, complicated — (Use additional code to identify infection)

897.2 Traumatic amputation of leg(s) (complete) (partial), unilateral, at or above knee, without mention of complication

897.3 Traumatic amputation of leg(s) (complete) (partial), unilateral, at or above knee, complicated — (Use additional code to identify infection)

© 2004 Ingenix, Inc.

897.4 Traumatic amputation of leg(s) (complete) (partial), unilateral, level not specified, without mention of complication

897.5 Traumatic amputation of leg(s) (complete) (partial), unilateral, level not specified, complicated — (Use additional code to identify infection)

897.6 Traumatic amputation of leg(s) (complete) (partial), bilateral (any level), without mention of complication

897.7 Traumatic amputation of leg(s) (complete) (partial), bilateral (any level), complicated — (Use additional code to identify infection)

900–904 Injury to Blood Vessels

Vascular trauma results from penetrating and blunt injury. A traumatic aneurysm is a weakening in the arterial wall that bulges with the pumping of the blood, posing the threat of rupture. A traumatic fistula is an abnormal communication between an artery and a vein. (These conditions also can arise from a disease process, and are classified elsewhere in ICD 9-CM.)

Not only must the physician accurately assess the extent of trauma, but must control any hemorrhage as soon as possible, as mortality risk is a function of the amount of blood loss. Arterial blood loss manifests as profuse and bright red, while venous loss is steady and dark. Injury to the great vessels that enter and leave the heart is an enormous threat, as are injuries to most arteries.

900 Injury to blood vessels of head and neck

AHA: Q3, 1990, 5

900.00 Injury to carotid artery, unspecified

900.01 Common carotid artery injury

900.02 External carotid artery injury

900.03 Internal carotid artery injury

900.1 Internal jugular vein injury

900.81 External jugular vein injury

900.82 Injury to multiple blood vessels of head and neck

900.89 Injury to other specified blood vessels of head and neck

900.9 Injury to unspecified blood vessel of head and neck

901 Injury to blood vessels of thorax

AHA: Q3, 1990, 5

901.0 Thoracic aorta injury

901.1 Innominate and subclavian artery injury

901.2 Superior vena cava injury

901.3 Innominate and subclavian vein injury

901.40 Injury to unspecified pulmonary vessel(s)

901.41 Pulmonary artery injury

901.42 Pulmonary vein injury

901.81 Intercostal artery or vein injury

901.82 Internal mammary artery or vein injury

901.83 Injury to multiple blood vessels of thorax

901.89 Injury to specified blood vessels of thorax, other

901.9 Injury to unspecified blood vessel of thorax

902 Injury to blood vessels of abdomen and pelvis

AHA: Q3, 1990, 5

902.0 Abdominal aorta injury

902.10 Unspecified inferior vena cava injury

902.11 Hepatic vein injury

902.19 Injury to specified branches of inferior vena cava, other

902.20 Unspecified celiac and mesenteric artery injury

902.21 Gastric artery injury

902.22 Hepatic artery injury

902.23 Splenic artery injury

902.24 Injury to specified branches of celiac axis, other

902.25 Superior mesenteric artery (trunk) injury

902.26 Injury to primary branches of superior mesenteric artery

902.27 Inferior mesenteric artery injury

902.29 Injury to celiac and mesenteric arteries, other

902.31 Injury to superior mesenteric vein and primary subdivisions

902.32 Inferior mesenteric vein injury

902.33 Portal vein injury

902.34 Splenic vein injury

902.39 Injury to portal and splenic veins, other

902.40 Renal vessel(s) injury, unspecified

902.41 Renal artery injury

902.42 Renal vein injury

902.49 Renal blood vessel injury, other

902.50 Unspecified iliac vessel(s) injury

902.51 Hypogastric artery injury

902.52 Hypogastric vein injury

902.53 Iliac artery injury

902.54 Iliac vein injury

902.55 Uterine artery injury

902.56 Uterine vein injury

902.59 Injury to iliac blood vessels, other

© 2004 Ingenix, Inc.

902.81 Ovarian artery injury

902.82 Ovarian vein injury

902.87 Injury to multiple blood vessels of abdomen and pelvis

902.89 Injury to specified blood vessels of abdomen and pelvis, other

902.9 Injury to blood vessel of abdomen and pelvis, unspecified

903 Injury to blood vessels of upper extremity

AHA: Q3, 1990, 5

903.00 Axillary vessel(s) injury, unspecified

903.01 Axillary artery injury

903.02 Axillary vein injury

903.1 Brachial blood vessels injury

903.2 Radial blood vessels injury

903.3 Ulnar blood vessels injury

903.4 Palmar artery injury

903.5 Digital blood vessels injury

903.8 Injury to specified blood vessels of upper extremity, other

903.9 Injury to unspecified blood vessel of upper extremity

904 Injury to blood vessels of lower extremity and unspecified sites

AHA: Q3, 1990, 5

904.0 Common femoral artery injury

904.1 Superficial femoral artery injury

904.2 Femoral vein injury

904.3 Saphenous vein injury

904.40 Unspecified popliteal vessel(s) injury

904.41 Popliteal artery injury

904.42 Popliteal vein injury

904.50 Unspecified tibial vessel(s) injury

904.51 Anterior tibial artery injury

904.52 Anterior tibial vein injury

904.53 Posterior tibial artery injury

904.54 Posterior tibial vein injury

904.6 Deep plantar blood vessels injury

904.7 Injury to specified blood vessels of lower extremity, other

904.8 Injury to unspecified blood vessel of lower extremity

904.9 Injury to blood vessels, unspecified site

905–909 Late Effects of Injuries, Poisonings, Toxic Effects, and Other External Causes

After exiting the acute phase of a closed head injury, the victim faces problems that may be lifelong, including functional cognitive deficits involving working memory, behavioral, affective disorders requiring antipsychotics and antidepressants, and impaired visuospatial ability. Skull fracture injuries pose a higher degree of neuropsychological dysfunction than head trauma without skull fracture. Studies have shown that the ability to find employment is affected by the patient's physical, cognitive, and behavioral functioning from time of admission to discharge, and injury severity as reflected by the initial Glasgow Coma Scale, the highest Glasgow Coma Scale, and the duration of the coma.

Late effects of musculoskeletal injuries include bursitis, traumatic arthritis, joint instability, synovitis, and tenosynovitis.

Late effects of injury to peripheral nerves are quite common, and recovery is very unpredictable. Expert and technically perfect microsurgical repair of a damaged nerve does not predict a full recovery since sensation may not be regained.

Late effects of spinal cord injury include paralysis, loss of bowel and bladder control, muscular atrophy, and limb contracture.

Late effects of burns include scarring, joint immobility, nerve, and psychological damage.

Radiation can result in burns, paralysis, and tissue death.

905 Late effects of musculoskeletal and connective tissue injuries

AHA: Q2, 1994, 3; Q1, 1995, 10

905.0 Late effect of fracture of skull and face bones

905.1 Late effect of fracture of spine and trunk without mention of spinal cord lesion

905.2 Late effect of fracture of upper extremities

905.3 Late effect of fracture of neck of femur

905.4 Late effect of fracture of lower extremities

905.5 Late effect of fracture of multiple and unspecified bones

905.6 Late effect of dislocation

905.7 Late effect of sprain and strain without mention of tendon injury

905.8 Late effect of tendon injury

905.9 Late effect of traumatic amputation

© 2004 Ingenix, Inc.

906 Late effects of injuries to skin and subcutaneous tissues

906.0 Late effect of open wound of head, neck, and trunk

906.1 Late effect of open wound of extremities without mention of tendon injury

906.2 Late effect of superficial injury

906.3 Late effect of contusion

906.4 Late effect of crushing

906.5 Late effect of burn of eye, face, head, and neck

906.6 Late effect of burn of wrist and hand

906.7 Late effect of burn of other extremities

906.8 Late effect of burns of other specified sites

906.9 Late effect of burn of unspecified site

907 Late effects of injuries to the nervous system

907.0 Late effect of intracranial injury without mention of skull fracture

907.1 Late effect of injury to cranial nerve

907.2 Late effect of spinal cord injury

907.3 Late effect of injury to nerve root(s), spinal plexus(es), and other nerves of trunk

907.4 Late effect of injury to peripheral nerve of shoulder girdle and upper limb

907.5 Late effect of injury to peripheral nerve of pelvic girdle and lower limb

907.9 Late effect of injury to other and unspecified nerve

908 Late effect of other and unspecified injury

908.0 Late effect of internal injury to chest

908.1 Late effect of internal injury to intra-abdominal organs

908.2 Late effect of internal injury to other internal organs

908.3 Late effect of injury to blood vessel of head, neck, and extremities

908.4 Late effect of injury to blood vessel of thorax, abdomen, and pelvis

908.5 Late effect of foreign body in orifice

908.6 Late effect of certain complications of trauma

908.9 Late effect of unspecified injury

909 Late effects of other and unspecified external causes

909.0 Late effect of poisoning due to drug, medicinal or biological substance

909.1 Late effect of toxic effects of nonmedical substances

909.2 Late effect of radiation

909.3 Late effect of complications of surgical and medical care

909.4 Late effect of certain other external causes

909.5 Late effect of adverse effect of drug, medical or biological substance

909.9 Late effect of other and unspecified external causes

910 Superficial injury of face, neck, and scalp, except eye

AHA: Q2, 1989, 15

910.0 Face, neck, and scalp, except eye, abrasion or friction burn, without mention of infection

910.1 Face, neck, and scalp except eye, abrasion or friction burn, infected

910.2 Face, neck, and scalp except eye, blister, without mention of infection

910.2 Face, neck, and scalp except eye, blister, without mention of infection

910.3 Face, neck, and scalp except eye, blister, infected

910.4 Face, neck, and scalp except eye, insect bite, nonvenomous, without mention of infection

910.5 Face, neck, and scalp except eye, insect bite, nonvenomous,infected

910.6 Face, neck, and scalp, except eye, superficial foreign body (splinter), without major open wound or mention of infection

910.7 Face, neck, and scalp except eye, superficial foreign body (splinter), without major open wound, infected

910.8 Other and unspecified superficial injury of face, neck, and scalp, without mention of infection

910.9 Other and unspecified superficial injury of face, neck, and scalp, infected

911 Superficial injury of trunk

AHA: Q2, 1989, 15

911.0 Trunk abrasion or friction burn, without mention of infection

911.1 Trunk abrasion or friction burn, infected

911.2 Trunk blister, without mention of infection

911.3 Trunk blister, infected

911.4 Trunk, insect bite, nonvenomous, without mention of infection

911.5 Trunk, insect bite, nonvenomous, infected

911.6 Trunk, superficial foreign body (splinter), without major open wound and without mention of infection

911.7 Trunk, superficial foreign body (splinter), without major open wound, infected

911.8 Other and unspecified superficial injury of trunk, without mention of infection

911.9 Other and unspecified superficial injury of trunk, infected

912 Superficial injury of shoulder and upper arm

AHA: Q2, 1989, 15

912.0 Shoulder and upper arm, abrasion or friction burn, without mention of infection

912.1 Shoulder and upper arm, abrasion or friction burn, infected

912.2 Shoulder and upper arm, blister, without mention of infection

912.3 Shoulder and upper arm, blister, infected

912.4 Shoulder and upper arm, insect bite, nonvenomous, without mention of infection

912.5 Shoulder and upper arm, insect bite, nonvenomous, infected

912.6 Shoulder and upper arm, superficial foreign body (splinter), without major open wound and without mention of infection

912.7 Shoulder and upper arm, superficial foreign body (splinter), without major open wound, infected

912.8 Other and unspecified superficial injury of shoulder and upper arm, without mention of infection

912.9 Other and unspecified superficial injury of shoulder and upper arm, infected

913 Superficial injury of elbow, forearm, and wrist

AHA: Q2, 1989, 15

913.0 Elbow, forearm, and wrist, abrasion or friction burn, without mention of infection

913.1 Elbow, forearm, and wrist, abrasion or friction burn, infected

913.2 Elbow, forearm, and wrist, blister, without mention of infection

913.3 Elbow, forearm, and wrist, blister infected

913.4 Elbow, forearm, and wrist, insect bite, nonvenomous, without mention of infection

913.5 Elbow, forearm, and wrist, insect bite, nonvenomous, infected

913.6 Elbow, forearm, and wrist, superficial foreign body (splinter), without major open wound and without mention of infection

913.7 Elbow, forearm, and wrist, superficial foreign body (splinter), without major open wound, infected

913.8 Other and unspecified superficial injury of elbow, forearm, and wrist, without mention of infection

913.9 Other and unspecified superficial injury of elbow, forearm, and wrist, infected

914 Superficial injury of hand(s) except finger(s) alone

AHA: Q2, 1989, 15

914.0 Hand(s) except finger(s) alone, abrasion or friction burn, without mention of infection

914.1 Hand(s) except finger(s) alone, abrasion or friction burn, infected

914.2 Hand(s) except finger(s) alone, blister, without mention of infection

914.3 Hand(s) except finger(s) alone, blister, infected

914.4 Hand(s) except finger(s) alone, insect bite, nonvenomous, without mention of infection

914.5 Hand(s) except finger(s) alone, insect bite, nonvenomous, infected

914.6 Hand(s) except finger(s) alone, superficial foreign body (splinter), without major open wound and without mention of infection

914.7 Hand(s) except finger(s) alone, superficial foreign body (splinter) without major open wound, infected

914.8 Other and unspecified superficial injury of hand(s) except finger(s) alone, without mention of infection

914.9 Other and unspecified superficial injury of hand(s) except finger(s) alone, infected

915 Superficial injury of finger(s)

AHA: Q2, 1989, 15

915.0 Abrasion or friction burn of finger, without mention of infection

915.1 Finger, abrasion or friction burn, infected

915.2 Finger, blister, without mention of infection

915.3 Finger, blister, infected

915.4 Finger, insect bite, nonvenomous, without mention of infection

915.5 Finger, insect bite, nonvenomous, infected

915.6 Finger, superficial foreign body (splinter), without major open wound and without mention of infection

915.7 Finger, superficial foreign body (splinter), without major open wound, infected

915.8 Other and unspecified superficial injury of finger without mention of infection

915.9 Other and unspecified superficial injury of finger, infected

© 2004 Ingenix, Inc.

916 Superficial injury of hip, thigh, leg, and ankle

AHA: Q2, 1989, 15

916.0 Hip, thigh, leg, and ankle, abrasion or friction burn, without mention of infection

916.1 Hip, thigh, leg, and ankle, abrasion or friction burn, infected

916.2 Hip, thigh, leg, and ankle, blister, without mention of infection

916.3 Hip, thigh, leg, and ankle, blister, infected

916.4 Hip, thigh, leg, and ankle, insect bite, nonvenomous, without mention of infection

916.5 Hip, thigh, leg, and ankle, insect bite, nonvenomous, infected

916.6 Hip, thigh, leg, and ankle, superficial foreign body (splinter), without major open wound and without mention of infection

916.7 Hip, thigh, leg, and ankle, superficial foreign body (splinter), without major open wound, infected

916.8 Other and unspecified superficial injury of hip, thigh, leg, and ankle, without mention of infection

916.9 Other and unspecified superficial injury of hip, thigh, leg, and ankle, infected

917 Superficial injury of foot and toe(s)

AHA: Q2, 1989, 15

917.0 Abrasion or friction burn of foot and toe(s), without mention of infection

917.1 Foot and toe(s), abrasion or friction burn, infected

917.2 Foot and toe(s), blister, without mention of infection

917.3 Foot and toe(s), blister, infected

917.4 Foot and toe(s), insect bite, nonvenomous, without mention of infection

917.5 Foot and toe(s), insect bite, nonvenomous, infected

917.6 Foot and toe(s), superficial foreign body (splinter), without major open wound and without mention of infection

917.7 Foot and toe(s), superficial foreign body (splinter), without major open wound, infected

917.8 Other and unspecified superficial injury of foot and toes, without mention of infection

917.9 Other and unspecified superficial injury of foot and toes, infected

918 Superficial injury of eye and adnexa

AHA: Q2, 1989, 15

918.0 Superficial injury of eyelids and periocular area

918.1 Superficial injury of cornea

918.2 Superficial injury of conjunctiva

918.9 Other and unspecified superficial injuries of eye

919 Superficial injury of other, multiple, and unspecified sites

AHA: Q2, 1989, 15

919.0 Abrasion or friction burn of other, multiple, and unspecified sites, without mention of infection

919.1 Other, multiple, and unspecified sites, abrasion or friction burn, infected

919.2 Other, multiple, and unspecified sites, blister, without mention of infection

919.3 Other, multiple, and unspecified sites, blister, infected

919.4 Other, multiple, and unspecified sites, insect bite, nonvenomous, without mention of infection

919.5 Other, multiple, and unspecified sites, insect bite, nonvenomous, infected

919.6 Other, multiple, and unspecified sites, superficial foreign body (splinter), without major open wound and without mention of infection

919.7 Other, multiple, and unspecified sites, superficial foreign body (splinter), without major open wound, infected

919.8 Other and unspecified superficial injury of other, multiple, and unspecified sites, without mention of infection

919.9 Other and unspecified superficial injury of other, multiple, and unspecified sites, infected

920–924 Contusion with Intact Skin Surface

The skin of the face is vulnerable to severe contusions due to its proximity to unyielding bone. Any blunt trauma to the face may be noticed immediately due to swelling and discoloration.

A black eye can result in permanent vision loss, cataracts, and infection, though these complications are rare.

Gastrocnemius and the quadriceps femoris are the muscle groups most prone to contusions. If a muscle is repeatedly contused, it may become predisposed to developing myositis ossificans in the area of injury.

Hematomas, a large extravascular clot of blood, may require surgical evacuation, though most resorb naturally.

A contusion is a crushing of tissue that causes visible bruising due to trauma and blood leaking from microscopic vessels. A crushing injury occurs when the force deforms tissues beyond their failure limits; the injury may be internal, even though skin surface may be intact. A crushing injury can result in anatomical damage (i.e., fractures), physiologic damage (i.e., central nervous system injury), and death.

Bullets from gunshots injure first by crushing those structures that lie in the bullet path. The extent of injury depends on which structures are penetrated. A Type V fracture is a crushing injury to the end of a tubular bone, which can lead to injury to the vascular supply in the germinal cells of the plate and may not be initially apparent despite x-ray. Premature osseous fusion of the injured portion of the plate may occur. The agricultural industry has a high percentage of deaths due to crushing, as compared to other occupations. For example, an agricultural worker can easily become crushed between a tractor and the machinery being attached when the worker is standing between the tractor and the machine as the operator is backing up the tractor.

920 Contusion of face, scalp, and neck except eye(s) OK

921 Contusion of eye and adnexa

921.0 Black eye, not otherwise specified

921.1 Contusion of eyelids and periocular area

921.2 Contusion of orbital tissues

921.3 Contusion of eyeball

921.9 Unspecified contusion of eye

922 Contusion of trunk

922.0 Contusion of breast

922.1 Contusion of chest wall

922.2 Contusion of abdominal wall

922.31 Contusion of back

922.32 Contusion of buttock

922.33 Contusion of interscapular region

922.4 Contusion of genital organs

922.8 Contusion of multiple sites of trunk

922.9 Contusion of unspecified part of trunk

923 Contusion of upper limb

923.00 Contusion of shoulder region

923.01 Contusion of scapular region

923.02 Contusion of axillary region

923.03 Contusion of upper arm

923.09 Contusion of multiple sites of shoulder and upper arm

923.10 Contusion of forearm

923.11 Contusion of elbow

923.20 Contusion of hand(s)

923.21 Contusion of wrist

923.3 Contusion of finger

923.8 Contusion of multiple sites of upper limb

923.9 Contusion of unspecified part of upper limb

924 Contusion of lower limb and of other and unspecified sites

924.00 Contusion of thigh

924.01 Contusion of hip

924.10 Contusion of lower leg

924.11 Contusion of knee

924.20 Contusion of foot

924.21 Contusion of ankle

924.3 Contusion of toe

924.4 Contusion of multiple sites of lower limb

924.5 Contusion of unspecified part of lower limb

924.8 Contusion of multiple sites, not elsewhere classified

924.9 Contusion of unspecified site

925–929 Crushing Injury

This injury occurs when a body part is subjected to a high degree of force or pressure, typically after being pressed between two heavy or motionless objects. Damage related to crush injury can include lacerations, fractures, bleeding, bruising, and compartment syndrome.

Severe crush injuries cause extensive damage to skin, muscle, nerves, and bone. There may be bleeding, internally and/or externally, or blood supply to extremities may be cut off. Plasma may leak from the blood vessels into the damaged tissues, causing swelling and shock. When the crushed part is released, toxic chemicals produced by damaged muscles get into general circulation, leading to kidney failure in severe cases.

Use an additional code to identify any associated injuries, such as: fractures, 800-829; internal injuries, 860.0-869.1; or intracranial injury, 850.0-854.1.

925 Crushing injury of face, scalp, and neck

AHA: Q2, 1993, 7; Q4, 2003, 77

925.1 Crushing injury of face and scalp — (Use additional code to identify any associated injuries: 800-829, 850.0-854.1, 860.0-869.1)

 © 2004 Ingenix, Inc.

925.2 Crushing injury of neck — (Use additional code to identify any associated injuries: 800-829, 850.0-854.1, 860.0-869.1)

926 Crushing injury of trunk

AHA: Q2, 1993, 7; Q4, 2003, 77

926.0 Crushing injury of external genitalia — (Use additional code to identify any associated injuries: 800-829, 850.0-854.1, 860.0-869.1)

926.11 Crushing injury of back — (Use additional code to identify any associated injuries: 800-829, 850.0-854.1, 860.0-869.1)

926.12 Crushing injury of buttock — (Use additional code to identify any associated injuries: 800-829, 850.0-854.1, 860.0-869.1)

926.19 Crushing injury of other specified sites of trunk — (Use additional code to identify any associated injuries: 800-829, 850.0-854.1, 860.0-869.1)

926.8 Crushing injury of multiple sites of trunk — (Use additional code to identify any associated injuries: 800-829, 850.0-854.1, 860.0-869.1)

926.9 Crushing injury of unspecified site of trunk — (Use additional code to identify any associated injuries: 800-829, 850.0-854.1, 860.0-869.1)

927 Crushing injury of upper limb

AHA: Q2, 1993, 7; Q4, 2003, 77

927.00 Crushing injury of shoulder region — (Use additional code to identify any associated injuries: 800-829, 850.0-854.1, 860.0-869.1)

927.01 Crushing injury of scapular region — (Use additional code to identify any associated injuries: 800-829, 850.0-854.1, 860.0-869.1)

927.02 Crushing injury of axillary region — (Use additional code to identify any associated injuries: 800-829, 850.0-854.1, 860.0-869.1)

927.03 Crushing injury of upper arm — (Use additional code to identify any associated injuries: 800-829, 850.0-854.1, 860.0-869.1)

927.09 Crushing injury of multiple sites of upper arm — (Use additional code to identify any associated injuries: 800-829, 850.0-854.1, 860.0-869.1)

927.10 Crushing injury of forearm — (Use additional code to identify any associated injuries: 800-829, 850.0-854.1, 860.0-869.1)

927.11 Crushing injury of elbow — (Use additional code to identify any associated injuries: 800-829, 850.0-854.1, 860.0-869.1)

927.20 Crushing injury of hand(s) — (Use additional code to identify any associated injuries: 800-829, 850.0-854.1, 860.0-869.1)

927.21 Crushing injury of wrist — (Use additional code to identify any associated injuries: 800-829, 850.0-854.1, 860.0-869.1)

927.3 Crushing injury of finger(s) — (Use additional code to identify any associated injuries: 800-829, 850.0-854.1, 860.0-869.1)

927.8 Crushing injury of multiple sites of upper limb — (Use additional code to identify any associated injuries: 800-829, 850.0-854.1, 860.0-869.1)

927.9 Crushing injury of unspecified site of upper limb — (Use additional code to identify any associated injuries: 800-829, 850.0-854.1, 860.0-869.1)

928 Crushing injury of lower limb

AHA: Q2, 1993, 7; Q4, 2003, 77

928.00 Crushing injury of thigh — (Use additional code to identify any associated injuries: 800-829, 850.0-854.1, 860.0-869.1)

928.01 Crushing injury of hip — (Use additional code to identify any associated injuries: 800-829, 850.0-854.1, 860.0-869.1)

928.10 Crushing injury of lower leg — (Use additional code to identify any associated injuries: 800-829, 850.0-854.1, 860.0-869.1)

928.11 Crushing injury of knee — (Use additional code to identify any associated injuries: 800-829, 850.0-854.1, 860.0-869.1)

928.20 Crushing injury of foot — (Use additional code to identify any associated injuries: 800-829, 850.0-854.1, 860.0-869.1)

928.21 Crushing injury of ankle — (Use additional code to identify any associated injuries: 800-829, 850.0-854.1, 860.0-869.1)

928.3 Crushing injury of toe(s) — (Use additional code to identify any associated injuries: 800-829, 850.0-854.1, 860.0-869.1)

928.8 Crushing injury of multiple sites of lower limb — (Use additional code to identify any associated injuries: 800-829, 850.0-854.1, 860.0-869.1)

928.9 Crushing injury of unspecified site of lower limb — (Use additional code to identify any associated injuries: 800-829, 850.0-854.1, 860.0-869.1)

929 Crushing injury of multiple and unspecified sites

AHA: Q2, 1993, 7; Q4, 2003, 77

929.0 Crushing injury of multiple sites, not elsewhere classified — (Use additional code to identify any associated injuries: 800-829, 850.0-854.1, 860.0-869.1)

929.9 Crushing injury of unspecified site — (Use additional code to identify any associated injuries: 800-829, 850.0-854.1, 860.0-869.1)

930–939 Effects of Foreign Body Entering Through Orifice

Instances of foreign bodies in orifices are one of the most common reasons for emergency department visits. Foreign bodies in the eye are particularly common and only a physician should remove a foreign body in the eye because of the danger of damaging the eye. If the foreign body is not removed, or is improperly removed, infection and permanent vision loss can result.

Children frequently aspirate foreign bodies into the right main bronchus. Often, the act is not observed, and the child may present with pneumonia or a lung abscess if the foreign body has been present for a long time. Hypoxia may result from objects obstructing breathing. Typically, the foreign body is located by use of the flexible bronchoscope and removed in the operating room with a rigid bronchoscope.

Ingested foreign bodies generally do not cause problems unless impacted. An impacted foreign body may erode through the walls of the organ and cause mediastinitis in the chest cavity or peritonitis in the abdominal cavity.

930 Foreign body on external eye

930.0 Foreign body in cornea

930.1 Foreign body in conjunctival sac

930.2 Foreign body in lacrimal punctum

930.8 Foreign body in other and combined sites on external eye

930.9 Foreign body in unspecified site on external eye

931 Foreign body in ear OK

932 Foreign body in nose OK

933 Foreign body in pharynx and larynx

933.0 Foreign body in pharynx

933.1 Foreign body in larynx

934 Foreign body in trachea, bronchus, and lung

934.0 Foreign body in trachea

934.1 Foreign body in main bronchus

934.8 Foreign body in other specified parts of trachea, bronchus, and lung

934.9 Foreign body in respiratory tree, unspecified

935 Foreign body in mouth, esophagus, and stomach

935.0 Foreign body in mouth

935.1 Foreign body in esophagus

935.2 Foreign body in stomach

936 Foreign body in intestine and colon OK

937 Foreign body in anus and rectum OK

938 Foreign body in digestive system, unspecified OK

939 Foreign body in genitourinary tract

939.0 Foreign body in bladder and urethra

939.1 Foreign body in uterus, any part

939.2 Foreign body in vulva and vagina

939.3 Foreign body in penis

939.9 Foreign body in unspecified site in genitourinary tract

940–949 Burns

Burns are classified by the degree of the burn (first degree through fourth degree) and the type of burn such as thermal, chemical, radiation, light, and electrical. The muscles, nerves, bones, blood vessels, respiratory system function, temperature regulation, joint function, fluid/electrolyte balance, physical appearance, and psychological functioning are all affected by a major burn injury.

The impact of burn injuries is magnified according to the amount of body surface burned. Children have much smaller thresholds for what is considered severe. Radiation burns are the most dangerous burns, though they may have a more benign appearance than a third degree thermal burn.

Category 948 classifies the extent of body surface affected by the burn and is useful as an adjunctive set of codes in assessing morbidity and mortality in burn centers. It may also be used when no further information is available, as in a patient who is briefly brought to an emergency department, stabilized, and transported to a specialty unit.

940 Burn confined to eye and adnexa

AHA: March-April, 1986, 9; Q4, 1988, 3; Q2, 1990, 7; Q4, 1994, 22

940.0 Chemical burn of eyelids and periocular area

940.1 Other burns of eyelids and periocular area

940.2 Alkaline chemical burn of cornea and conjunctival sac

940.3 Acid chemical burn of cornea and conjunctival sac

© 2004 Ingenix, Inc.

940.4 Other burn of cornea and conjunctival sac

940.5 Burn with resulting rupture and destruction of eyeball

940.9 Unspecified burn of eye and adnexa

Documentation Issues

For the correct ICD-9-CM code to be assigned, the medical record documentation must contain clear and concise information regarding the site of the burn, the degree of burn, if the burn is healed or nonhealed, any complications existing, and any late effect that may be present.

Coding Clarification

Abrasion Burn: Also indicated as "road rash," abrasion burns, if noted as deep, are not classified as burns, but as open wounds or abrasions. When the medical record documentation indicates that the patient is being treated for deep abrasion burns, indicate the appropriate open wound or abrasion code, not a burn code. If only superficial, code the abrasion burn as a superficial injury.

Infected Burn: When a patient is treated for infected burns, after the initial treatment of burns, two codes are necessary. Indicate the appropriate code for the burn (940-949) and the additional code 958.3 *Posttraumatic wound infection not elsewhere classified* to identify the complication of infection.

Late Effect of Burn: The treatment of current, unhealed burns is classified to categories 940-949. The late effects of burns are coded to subcategories 906.5-906.9. The codes indicate healed burns resulting in sequelae, such as scarring. When coding the late effect of a burn, the appropriate code for describing the late effect itself is coded first, followed by the code identifying it as a late effect of another injury.

Because of the nature of burns, it is possible for a patient to have both healed and nonhealed burns during a single encounter. For this reason, it is appropriate to use a code for currently unhealed burns (940-949) and a code for late effects (906.5-906.9).

Multiple Burns: Patients are often treated with multiple burns. When coding multiple burns, assign separate codes for each burn site. Category 948 is used to classify burns according to the body surface involved. This code is used as an additional code for reporting purposes when there are third-degree burns involving 20 percent or more of the body surface or when further information is needed for evaluating burn mortality.

When there are burns of the same local site (identified by the three-digit category) but of varying degrees, use the fourth digit indicating the highest degree documented in the medical record.

Sequence first the code with the highest degree of burn in cases of multiple burns.

941 Burn of face, head, and neck

AHA: March-April, 1986, 9; Q4, 1988, 3; Q2, 1990, 7; Q4, 1994, 22

The following fifth-digit subclassification is for use with category 941:

0 face and head, unspecified site
1 ear [any part]
2 eye (with any other parts of face, head, and neck)
3 lip(s)
4 chin
5 nose (septum)
6 scalp [any part]
7 forehead and cheek
8 neck
9 multiple sites [except with eye] of face, head, and neck

941.0 5th Burn of face, head, and neck, unspecified degree

941.1 5th Erythema due to burn (first degree) of face, head, and neck

941.2 5th Blisters with epidermal loss due to burn (second degree) of face, head, and neck

941.3 5th Full-thickness skin loss due to burn (third degree nos) of face, head, and neck

941.4 5th Deep necrosis of underlying tissues due to burn (deep third degree) of face, head, and neck without mention of loss of a body part

941.5 5th Deep necrosis of underlying tissues due to burn (deep third degree) of face, head, and neck with loss of a body part

942 Burn of trunk

AHA: March-April, 1986, 9; Q4, 1988, 3; Q2, 1990, 7; Q4, 1994, 22

The following fifth-digit subclassification is for use with category 942:

0 trunk, unspecified site
1 breast
2 chest wall, excluding breast and nipple
3 abdominal wall
4 back [any part]
5 genitalia
9 other and multiple sites of trunk

942.0 5th Burn of trunk, unspecified degree

942.1 5th Erythema due to burn (first degree) of trunk

942.2 5th Blisters with epidermal loss due to burn (second degree) of trunk

800–999

942.3 ✓5th Full-thickness skin loss due to burn (third degree nos) of trunk

942.4 ✓5th Deep necrosis of underlying tissues due to burn (deep third degree) of trunk without mention of loss of a body part

942.5 ✓5th Deep necrosis of underlying tissues due to burn (deep third degree) of trunk with loss of a body part

943 Burn of upper limb, except wrist and hand

AHA: March-April, 1986, 9; Q4, 1988, 3; Q2, 1990, 7; Q4, 1994, 22

The following fifth-digit subclassification is for use with category 943:

0 upper limb, unspecified site
1 forearm
2 elbow
3 upper arm
4 axilla
5 shoulder
6 scapular region
9 multiple sites of upper limb, except wrist and hand

943.0 ✓5th Burn of upper limb, except wrist and hand, unspecified degree

943.1 ✓5th Erythema due to burn (first degree) of upper limb, except wrist and hand

943.2 ✓5th Blisters with epidermal loss due to burn (second degree) of upper limb, except wrist and hand

943.3 ✓5th Full-thickness skin loss due to burn (third degree nos) of upper limb, except wrist and hand

943.4 ✓5th Deep necrosis of underlying tissues due to burn (deep third degree) of upper limb, except wrist and hand, without mention of loss of a body part

943.5 ✓5th Deep necrosis of underlying tissues due to burn (deep third degree) of upper limb, except wrist and hand, with loss of a body part

944 Burn of wrist(s) and hand(s)

AHA: March-April, 1986, 9; Q4, 1988, 3; Q2, 1990, 7; Q4, 1994, 22

The following fifth-digit subclassification is for use with category 944:

0 and, unspecified site
1 single digit [finger (nail)] other than the thumb
2 thumb (nail)
3 two or more digits, not including thumb
4 two or more digits including thumb
5 palm
6 back of hand
7 wrist
8 multiple sites of wrist(s) and hands

944.0 ✓5th Burn of wrist(s) and hand(s), unspecified degree

944.1 ✓5th Erythema due to burn (first degree) of wrist(s) and hand(s)

944.2 ✓5th Blisters with epidermal loss due to burn (second degree) of wrist(s) and hand(s)

944.3 ✓5th Full-thickness skin loss due to burn (third degree nos) of wrist(s) and hand(s)

944.4 ✓5th Deep necrosis of underlying tissues due to burn (deep third degree) of wrist(s) and hand(s), without mention of loss of a body part

944.5 ✓5th Deep necrosis of underlying tissues due to burn (deep third degree) of wrist(s) and hand(s), with loss of a body part

945 Burn of lower limb(s)

AHA: March-April, 1986, 9; Q4, 1988, 3; Q2, 1990, 7; Q4, 1994, 22

The following fifth-digit subclassification is for use with category 945:

0 lower limb (leg), unspecified site
1 toe(s) (nail)
2 foot
3 ankle
4 lower leg
5 knee
6 thigh (any part)
9 multiple sites of lower limb(s)

945.0 ✓5th Burn of lower limb(s), unspecified degree

945.1 ✓5th Erythema due to burn (first degree) of lower limb(s)

945.2 ✓5th Blisters with epidermal loss due to burn (second degree) of lower limb(s)

945.3 ✓5th Full-thickness skin loss due to burn (third degree nos) of lower limb(s)

945.4 ✓5th Deep necrosis of underlying tissues due to burn (deep third degree) of lower limb(s) without mention of loss of a body part

945.5 ✓5th Deep necrosis of underlying tissues due to burn (deep third degree) of lower limb(s) with loss of a body part

946 Burns of multiple specified sites

AHA: March-April, 1986, 9; Q4, 1988, 3; Q2, 1990, 7; Q4, 1994, 22

© 2004 Ingenix, Inc.

946.0 Burns of multiple specified sites, unspecified degree

946.1 Erythema due to burn (first degree) of multiple specified sites

946.2 Blisters with epidermal loss due to burn (second degree) of multiple specified sites

946.3 Full-thickness skin loss due to burn (third degree nos) of multiple specified sites

946.4 Deep necrosis of underlying tissues due to burn (deep third degree) of multiple specified sites, without mention of loss of a body part

946.5 Deep necrosis of underlying tissues due to burn (deep third degree) of multiple specified sites, with loss of a body part

947 Burn of internal organs

AHA: March-April, 1986, 9; Q4, 1988, 3; Q2, 1990, 7; Q4, 1994, 22

947.0 Burn of mouth and pharynx

947.1 Burn of larynx, trachea, and lung

947.2 Burn of esophagus

947.3 Burn of gastrointestinal tract

947.4 Burn of vagina and uterus

947.8 Burn of other specified sites of internal organs

947.9 Burn of internal organs, unspecified site

948 Burns classified according to extent of body surface involved

AHA: Nov-Dec, 1984, 13; March-April, 1986, 9; Q4, 1988, 3; Q2, 1990, 7; Q4, 1994, 22

The rule of nines is a method for rapidly estimating the percent of total body surface area affected by a burn, which, in burn victims, is a strong predictor of the patient's prognosis. This metric helps emergency clinicians to decide whether a patient needs to be transferred to a regional burn center for specialized care and helps in estimating the amount of fluid replacement the patient will need to replace losses through the burned area. The rule of nines derives its name from the fact that an adult body may be divided into anatomic regions that have surface area percentages that are all multiples of 9 percent. According to this system, the head and each limb each account for 9 percent of the body surface area for a total of 45 percent when added together (two legs, two arms, and the head). The genital area accounts for 1 percent, and the back and front of the torso each account for 18 percent of the body surface area.

The following fifth-digit subclassification is for use with category 948 to indicate the percent of body surface with third degree burn; valid digits are in [brackets] under each code:

0 less than 10 percent or unspecified
1 10-19%
2 20-29%
3 30-39%
4 40-49%
5 50-59%
6 60-69%
7 70-79%
8 80-89%
9 90% or more of body surface

948.0 5th Burn (any degree) involving less than 10% of body surface

948.1 5th Burn (any degree) involving 10-19% of body surface

948.2 5th Burn (any degree) involving 20-29% of body surface

948.3 5th Burn (any degree) involving 30-39% of body surface

948.4 5th Burn (any degree) involving 40-49% of body surface

948.5 5th Burn (any degree) involving 50-59% of body surface

948.6 5th Burn (any degree) involving 60-69% of body surface

948.7 5th Burn (any degree) involving 70-79% of body surface

948.8 5th Burn (any degree) involving 80-89% of body surface

948.9 5th Burn (any degree) involving 90% or more of body surface

949 Burn, unspecified site

AHA: March-April, 1986, 9; Q4, 1994, 22

949.0 Burn of unspecified site, unspecified degree

949.1 Erythema due to burn (first degree), unspecified site

949.2 Blisters with epidermal loss due to burn (second degree), unspecified site

949.3 Full-thickness skin loss due to burn (third degree nos), unspecified site

949.4 Deep necrosis of underlying tissue due to burn (deep third degree), unspecified site without mention of loss of body part

949.5 Deep necrosis of underlying tissues due to burn (deep third degree, unspecified site with loss of body part

950–957 Injury to Nerves and Spinal Cord

The body's nerves report to the central nervous system (CNS), which is composed of the brain and the spinal cord. Twelve pairs of cranial nerves originate in the brain, and 31 pairs of spinal nerves emanate from the spinal cord, developing major branches and associated complexes known as peripheral nerves. Every nerve has two roots: sensory and motor. The anatomical arrangement of the spinal

Cranial Nerves	Impairment by Injury to Motor Root
1st - Olfactory	Loss of smell
2nd - Optic	Traumatic blindness
3rd - Oculomotor	Ptosis of eyelid, double vision
4th - Trochlear	Unnatural rotation of eyeball, double vision
5th - Trigeminal	Eccentric jaw alignment, chewing
6th - Abducens	Unnatural rotation of eyeball (outwards); double vision
7th - Facial	Inability to move facial muscles of expression and animation
8th - Vestibulocochlear	Traumatic deafness; loss of balance
9th - Glossopharyngeal	Loss of taste; swallowing difficulty
10th - Vagus	Disturbance of innervation of heart, lungs, digestive organs
11th - Spinal accessory	Inability to rotate head
12th - Hypoglossopharyngeal	Loss of tongue mobility, thick speech or garbled speech

nerve roots places the motor root anteriorly and the sensory root posteriorly.

The table above lists impairments due to injury to specific cranial nerves.

If a nerve is transected, expert and expeditious microsurgery is no guarantee that full functioning will return. Regeneration can lead to appropriate motor and sensory impulses or an aberrant response may later be manifest, such as crying crocodile tears involuntarily when sensing the smell of food.

950 Injury to optic nerve and pathways

950.0 Optic nerve injury

950.1 Injury to optic chiasm

950.2 Injury to optic pathways

950.3 Injury to visual cortex

950.9 Injury to unspecified optic nerve and pathways

951 Injury to other cranial nerve(s)

951.0 Injury to oculomotor nerve

951.1 Injury to trochlear nerve

951.2 Injury to trigeminal nerve

951.3 Injury to abducens nerve

951.4 Injury to facial nerve

951.5 Injury to acoustic nerve

951.6 Injury to accessory nerve

951.7 Injury to hypoglossal nerve

951.8 Injury to other specified cranial nerves

951.9 Injury to unspecified cranial nerve

952 Spinal cord injury without evidence of spinal bone injury

Refer to category 806 for comprehensive descriptions.

952.00 C1-C4 level spinal cord injury, unspecified

952.01 C1-C4 level with complete lesion of spinal cord

952.02 C1-C4 level with anterior cord syndrome

952.03 C1-C4 level with central cord syndrome

952.04 C1-C4 level with other specified spinal cord injury

952.05 C5-C7 level spinal cord injury, unspecified

952.06 C5-C7 level with complete lesion of spinal cord

952.07 C5-C7 level with anterior cord syndrome

952.08 C5-C7 level with central cord syndrome

952.09 C5-C7 level with other specified spinal cord injury

952.10 T1-T6 level spinal cord injury, unspecified

952.11 T1-T6 level with complete lesion of spinal cord

952.12 T1-T6 level with anterior cord syndrome

952.13 T1-T6 level with central cord syndrome

952.14 T1-T6 level with other specified spinal cord injury

952.15 T7-T12 level spinal cord injury, unspecified

952.16 T7-T12 level with complete lesion of spinal cord

952.17 T7-T12 level with anterior cord syndrome

952.18 T7-T12 level with central cord syndrome

952.19 T7-T12 level with other specified spinal cord injury

952.2 Lumbar spinal cord injury without spinal bone injury

952.3 Sacral spinal cord injury without spinal bone injury

952.4 Cauda equina spinal cord injury without spinal bone injury

© 2004 Ingenix, Inc.

952.8 Multiple sites of spinal cord injury without spinal bone injury

952.9 Unspecified site of spinal cord injury without spinal bone injury

953–957 Injury to Nerve Roots, Peripheral, and Superficial Nerves

A plexus or ganglion is a bundle of nerves that serves a particular region of the body. A plexus lies relatively deep in the body as opposed to superficial nerves, which are close to the surface of the skin.

Sympathetic nerves are under the conscious control of the body, whereas parasympathetic nerves are considered to be involuntary, allowing the body to carry on without distraction by routine functions such as breathing, heart beating, digesting, and staying oriented in space. These parasympathetic activities are considered the duties of the autonomic nervous system.

953 Injury to nerve roots and spinal plexus

953.0 Injury to cervical nerve root

953.1 Injury to dorsal nerve root

953.2 Injury to lumbar nerve root

953.3 Injury to sacral nerve root

953.4 Injury to brachial plexus

953.5 Injury to lumbosacral plexus

953.8 Injury to multiple sites of nerve roots and spinal plexus

953.9 Injury to unspecified site of nerve roots and spinal plexus

954 Injury to other nerve(s) of trunk, excluding shoulder and pelvic girdles

954.0 Injury to cervical sympathetic nerve, excluding shoulder and pelvic girdles

954.1 Injury to other sympathetic nerve, excluding shoulder and pelvic girdles

954.8 Injury to other specified nerve(s) of trunk, excluding shoulder and pelvic girdles

954.9 Injury to unspecified nerve of trunk, excluding shoulder and pelvic girdles

955 Injury to peripheral nerve(s) of shoulder girdle and upper limb

955.0 Injury to axillary nerve

955.1 Injury to median nerve

955.2 Injury to ulnar nerve

955.3 Injury to radial nerve

955.4 Injury to musculocutaneous nerve

955.5 Injury to cutaneous sensory nerve, upper limb

955.6 Injury to digital nerve, upper limb

955.7 Injury to other specified nerve(s) of shoulder girdle and upper limb

955.8 Injury to multiple nerves of shoulder girdle and upper limb

955.9 Injury to unspecified nerve of shoulder girdle and upper limb

956 Injury to peripheral nerve(s) of pelvic girdle and lower limb

956.0 Injury to sciatic nerve

956.1 Injury to femoral nerve

956.2 Injury to posterior tibial nerve

956.3 Injury to peroneal nerve

956.4 Injury to cutaneous sensory nerve, lower limb

956.5 Injury to other specified nerve(s) of pelvic girdle and lower limb

956.8 Injury to multiple nerves of pelvic girdle and lower limb

956.9 Injury to unspecified nerve of pelvic girdle and lower limb

957 Injury to other and unspecified nerves

957.0 Injury to superficial nerves of head and neck

957.1 Injury to other specified nerve(s)

957.8 Injury to multiple nerves in several parts

957.9 Injury to nerves, unspecified site

958–959 Certain Traumatic Complications and Unspecified Injuries

A potentially fatal air embolism, whether arterial or venous, may result from a penetrating and blunt chest trauma or from blast injuries. Signs are sudden cardiovascular collapse, air bubbles in arterial blood samples, air bubbles in retinal and coronary arteries, and frothy blood coming from a chest wound. Treatment must commence immediately.

A fat embolism is typically associated with fracture of one of the long bones, especially the femur. Children are vulnerable to throwing multiple fat emboli if subjected to blunt trauma such as in child abuse situations.

Secondary hemorrhage is usually arterial and most often associated with sepsis arising from traumatized tissues that have been repaired. Slipping of a ligature on repaired vessels is the second most frequent cause for secondary hemorrhage.

Posttraumatic wound infection, NEC, includes injuries such as an infected, non-healing burn.

Traumatic shock sets in when the heart fails to deliver oxygenated blood and other nutrients to the body, usually because of a high rate of blood loss. The shock triggers other organ failure, with the kidney among the first affected. Blood volume must be restored as soon as possible to prevent the appearance of shock and its sequelae. Traumatic anuria runs a mortality rate of 60 percent.

Volkmann's ischemic contracture can appear in either the hand or the foot. In the hand, constriction of the radial artery produces the characteristic pronation and flexion. In the foot, a tibial fracture leading to an embolus or thrombus is more likely to be the causative agent.

Traumatic subcutaneous emphysema is tissue rupture that allows gas bubbles to form beneath the skin, a result of a high-pressure injury.

Compartment syndrome is an early complication of trauma, resulting from compression of nerves and tendons. Pain is extreme and is not easily relieved. Any compressive agent such as a cast or splint is immediately removed, though if removal is ineffective, the patient is surgically decompressed.

958 Certain early complications of trauma

958.0 Air embolism as an early complication of trauma

958.1 Fat embolism as an early complication of trauma

958.2 Secondary and recurrent hemorrhage as an early complication of trauma

958.3 Posttraumatic wound infection not elsewhere classified

Coding Clarification
Code 958.3 excludes infected open wounds that should be coded to complicated open wound of the site.

958 Certain early complications of trauma

958.4 Traumatic shock

958.5 Traumatic anuria

958.6 Volkmann's ischemic contracture

958.7 Traumatic subcutaneous emphysema

958.8 Other early complications of trauma

959 Injury, other and unspecified

959.01 Head injury, unspecified

959.09 Injury of face and neck, other and unspecified

959.11 Other injury of chest wall

959.12 Other injury of abdomen

959.13 Other injury, Fracture of corpus cavernosum penis — *a break in the spongy body of the penis; columns of erectile tissue forming the dorsum and the sides of the penis*

959.14 Other injury of external genitals

959.19 Other injury of other sites of trunk

959.2 Injury, other and unspecified, shoulder and upper arm

959.3 Injury, other and unspecified, elbow, forearm, and wrist

959.4 Injury, other and unspecified, hand, except finger

959.5 Injury, other and unspecified, finger

959.6 Injury, other and unspecified, hip and thigh

959.7 Injury, other and unspecified, knee, leg, ankle, and foot

959.8 Injury, other and unspecified, other specified sites, including multiple

959.9 Injury, other and unspecified, unspecified site

960–979 Poisoning by Drugs, Medicinal and Biological Substances

Poisons are chemicals that cause illness, injury, or death when taken in very small quantities. The legal definition of a poison is a chemical that takes less than 50 mg per kilogram of body weight to kill 50 percent of the victims exposed (e.g., about 3/4 of a teaspoon for the average adult and about 1/8 of a teaspoon for a 2-year-old). Symptoms displayed and the systemic effect differ with the type of poison ingested.

Poisoning by drugs, medicinal, and biological substances is the major cause of childhood accidents in the home and can occur by many routes, including oral ingestion, inhalation, dermal absorption, and ocular instillation. Sources of poisoning for children and adults include:

- Acetaminophen overdose, which is rarely fatal. Symptoms are usually mild though prolonged abnormal liver function test results can occur.

- Ingestion of strong acids and alkalis (e.g.., drain and toilet bowl cleaners), which cause burns and damage tissues. Liquid preparations are often more dangerous since they are more often swallowed than the solid preparations and, thus, affect the entire esophagus and stomach. Pain is immediate in severe cases. Initially, the patient may drool, and there may be swelling at the burned areas. The airway may become obstructed. Respiration is shallow and shock is common. Patients who survive the initial poisoning may die of secondary

 © 2004 Ingenix, Inc.

infections, or the esophagus or stomach may perforate after a week or more.

- Exposure to methyl salicylate, which is found in liniments and in solutions used in hot vaporizers and is potentially lethal. The early symptoms are nausea and vomiting, tinnitus, hyperactivity, hyperthermia, and seizures. The central nervous system becomes depressed, followed by lethargy, respiratory failure, and collapse.

Hyperbaric oxygen (HBO) therapy is an accepted form of treatment for a number of serious illnesses including carbon monoxide poisoning. When carbon monoxide is inhaled, the CO combines with the hemoglobin to form carboxyhemoglobin or COHb. The CO displaces the oxygen on hemoglobin and the strong COHb bond makes it difficult for the body to eliminate CO buildups from the bloodstream. Carbon monoxide can poison slowly over a period of several hours, even in low concentrations. Sensitive organs such as the brain, heart, and lungs suffer the most from a lack of oxygen. In HBO therapy, a patient receives pure oxygen by mask, respiratory hood, tent, or endotracheal tube while in a hyperbaric chamber pressurized from two to three atmospheres absolute. HBO accelerates the process to halt carbon monoxide binding to hemoglobin; extra oxygen dissolved in plasma at high oxygen pressure may preserve tissue oxygenation even with lethal levels of carboxyhemoglobin and helps to minimize brain damage that at times accompanies or follows severe poisoning.

960 Poisoning by antibiotics

AHA: Q2, 1990, 11

960.0 Poisoning by penicillins — (Use additional code to specify the effects of the poisoning)

960.1 Poisoning by antifungal antibiotics — (Use additional code to specify the effects of the poisoning)

960.2 Poisoning by chloramphenicol group — (Use additional code to specify the effects of the poisoning)

960.3 Poisoning by erythromycin and other macrolides — (Use additional code to specify the effects of the poisoning)

960.4 Poisoning by tetracycline group — (Use additional code to specify the effects of the poisoning)

960.5 Poisoning of cephalosporin group — (Use additional code to specify the effects of the poisoning)

960.6 Poisoning of antimycobacterial antibiotics — (Use additional code to specify the effects of the poisoning)

960.7 Poisoning by antineoplastic antibiotics — (Use additional code to specify the effects of the poisoning)

960.8 Poisoning by other specified antibiotics — (Use additional code to specify the effects of the poisoning)

960.9 Poisoning by unspecified antibiotic — (Use additional code to specify the effects of the poisoning)

961 Poisoning by other anti-infectives

AHA: Q2, 1990, 11

961.0 Poisoning by sulfonamides — (Use additional code to specify the effects of the poisoning)

961.1 Poisoning by arsenical anti-infectives — (Use additional code to specify the effects of the poisoning)

961.2 Poisoning by heavy metal anti-infectives — (Use additional code to specify the effects of the poisoning)

961.3 Poisoning by quinoline and hydroxyquinoline derivatives — (Use additional code to specify the effects of the poisoning)

961.4 Poisoning by antimalarials and drugs acting on other blood protozoa — (Use additional code to specify the effects of the poisoning)

961.5 Poisoning by other antiprotozoal drugs — (Use additional code to specify the effects of the poisoning)

961.6 Poisoning by anthelmintics — (Use additional code to specify the effects of the poisoning)

961.7 Poisoning by antiviral drugs — (Use additional code to specify the effects of the poisoning)

961.8 Poisoning by other antimycobacterial drugs — (Use additional code to specify the effects of the poisoning)

961.9 Poisoning by other and unspecified anti-infectives — (Use additional code to specify the effects of the poisoning)

962 Poisoning by hormones and synthetic substitutes

AHA: Q2, 1990, 11

962.0 Poisoning by adrenal cortical steroids — (Use additional code to specify the effects of the poisoning)

962.1 Poisoning by androgens and anabolic congeners — (Use additional code to specify the effects of the poisoning)

962.2 Poisoning by ovarian hormones and synthetic substitutes — (Use additional code to specify the effects of the poisoning)

962.3 Poisoning by insulins and antidiabetic agents — (Use additional code to specify the effects of the poisoning)

962.4 Poisoning by anterior pituitary hormones — (Use additional code to specify the effects of the poisoning)

962.5 Poisoning by posterior pituitary hormones — (Use additional code to specify the effects of the poisoning)

962.6 Poisoning by parathyroid and parathyroid derivatives — (Use additional code to specify the effects of the poisoning)

962.7 Poisoning by thyroid and thyroid derivatives — (Use additional code to specify the effects of the poisoning)

962.8 Poisoning by antithyroid agents — (Use additional code to specify the effects of the poisoning)

962.9 Poisoning by other and unspecified hormones and synthetic substitutes — (Use additional code to specify the effects of the poisoning)

963 Poisoning by primarily systemic agents

AHA: Q2, 1990, 11

963.0 Poisoning by antiallergic and antiemetic drugs — (Use additional code to specify the effects of the poisoning)

963.1 Poisoning by antineoplastic and immunosuppressive drugs — (Use additional code to specify the effects of the poisoning)

963.2 Poisoning by acidifying agents — (Use additional code to specify the effects of the poisoning)

963.3 Poisoning by alkalizing agents — (Use additional code to specify the effects of the poisoning)

963.4 Poisoning by enzymes, not elsewhere classified — (Use additional code to specify the effects of the poisoning)

963.5 Poisoning by vitamins, not elsewhere classified — (Use additional code to specify the effects of the poisoning)

963.8 Poisoning by other specified systemic agents — (Use additional code to specify the effects of the poisoning)

963.9 Poisoning by unspecified systemic agent — (Use additional code to specify the effects of the poisoning)

964 Poisoning by agents primarily affecting blood constituents

AHA: Q2, 1990, 11

964.0 Poisoning by iron and its compounds — (Use additional code to specify the effects of the poisoning)

964.1 Poisoning by liver preparations and other antianemic agents — (Use additional code to specify the effects of the poisoning)

964.2 Poisoning by anticoagulants — (Use additional code to specify the effects of the poisoning)

964.3 Poisoning by vitamin K (phytonadione) — (Use additional code to specify the effects of the poisoning)

964.4 Poisoning by fibrinolysis-affecting drugs — (Use additional code to specify the effects of the poisoning)

964.5 Poisoning by anticoagulant antagonists and other coagulants — (Use additional code to specify the effects of the poisoning)

964.6 Poisoning by gamma globulin — (Use additional code to specify the effects of the poisoning)

964.7 Poisoning by natural blood and blood products — (Use additional code to specify the effects of the poisoning)

964.8 Poisoning by other specified agents affecting blood constituents — (Use additional code to specify the effects of the poisoning)

964.9 Poisoning by unspecified agent affecting blood constituents — (Use additional code to specify the effects of the poisoning)

965 Poisoning by analgesics, antipyretics, and antirheumatics

AHA: Q2, 1990, 11

965.00 Poisoning by opium (alkaloids), unspecified — (Use additional code to specify the effects of the poisoning)

965.01 Poisoning by heroin — (Use additional code to specify the effects of the poisoning)

965.02 Poisoning by methadone — (Use additional code to specify the effects of the poisoning)

965.09 Poisoning by opiates and related narcotics, other — (Use additional code to specify the effects of the poisoning)

965.1 Poisoning by salicylates — (Use additional code to specify the effects of the poisoning)

965.4 Poisoning by aromatic analgesics, not elsewhere classified — (Use additional code to specify the effects of the poisoning)

© 2004 Ingenix, Inc.

965.5 Poisoning by pyrazole derivatives — (Use additional code to specify the effects of the poisoning)

965.61 Poisoning by propionic acid derivatives — (Use additional code to specify the effects of the poisoning)

965.69 Poisoning by other antirheumatics — (Use additional code to specify the effects of the poisoning)

965.7 Poisoning by other non-narcotic analgesics — (Use additional code to specify the effects of the poisoning)

965.8 Poisoning by other specified analgesics and antipyretics — (Use additional code to specify the effects of the poisoning)

965.9 Poisoning by unspecified analgesic and antipyretic — (Use additional code to specify the effects of the poisoning)

966 Poisoning by anticonvulsants and anti-Parkinsonism drugs

AHA: Q2, 1990, 11

966.0 Poisoning by oxazolidine derivatives — (Use additional code to specify the effects of the poisoning)

966.1 Poisoning by hydantoin derivatives — (Use additional code to specify the effects of the poisoning)

966.2 Poisoning by succinimides — (Use additional code to specify the effects of the poisoning)

966.3 Poisoning by other and unspecified anticonvulsants — (Use additional code to specify the effects of the poisoning)

966.4 Poisoning by anti-Parkinsonism drugs — (Use additional code to specify the effects of the poisoning)

967 Poisoning by sedatives and hypnotics

AHA: Q2, 1990, 11

967.0 Poisoning by barbiturates — (Use additional code to specify the effects of the poisoning)

967.1 Poisoning by chloral hydrate group — (Use additional code to specify the effects of the poisoning)

967.2 Poisoning by paraldehyde — (Use additional code to specify the effects of the poisoning)

967.3 Poisoning by bromine compounds — (Use additional code to specify the effects of the poisoning)

967.4 Poisoning by methaqualone compounds — (Use additional code to specify the effects of the poisoning)

967.5 Poisoning by glutethimide group — (Use additional code to specify the effects of the poisoning)

967.6 Poisoning by mixed sedatives, not elsewhere classified — (Use additional code to specify the effects of the poisoning)

967.8 Poisoning by other sedatives and hypnotics — (Use additional code to specify the effects of the poisoning)

967.9 Poisoning by unspecified sedative or hypnotic — (Use additional code to specify the effects of the poisoning)

968 Poisoning by other central nervous system depressants and anesthetics

AHA: Q2, 1990, 11

968.0 Poisoning by central nervous system muscle-tone depressants — (Use additional code to specify the effects of the poisoning)

968.1 Poisoning by halothane — (Use additional code to specify the effects of the poisoning)

968.2 Poisoning by other gaseous anesthetics — (Use additional code to specify the effects of the poisoning)

968.3 Poisoning by intravenous anesthetics — (Use additional code to specify the effects of the poisoning)

968.4 Poisoning by other and unspecified general anesthetics — (Use additional code to specify the effects of the poisoning)

968.5 Poisoning by surface (topical) and infiltration anesthetics — (Use additional code to specify the effects of the poisoning)

968.6 Poisoning by peripheral nerve- and plexus-blocking anesthetics — (Use additional code to specify the effects of the poisoning)

968.7 Poisoning by spinal anesthetics — (Use additional code to specify the effects of the poisoning)

968.9 Poisoning by other and unspecified local anesthetics — (Use additional code to specify the effects of the poisoning)

969 Poisoning by psychotropic agents

AHA: Q2, 1990, 11

969.0 Poisoning by antidepressants — (Use additional code to specify the effects of the poisoning)

969.1 Poisoning by phenothiazine-based tranquilizers — (Use additional code to specify the effects of the poisoning)

969.2 Poisoning by butyrophenone-based tranquilizers — (Use additional code to specify the effects of the poisoning)

969.3 Poisoning by other antipsychotics, neuroleptics, and major tranquilizers — (Use additional code to specify the effects of the poisoning)

969.4 Poisoning by benzodiazepine-based tranquilizers — (Use additional code to specify the effects of the poisoning)

969.5 Poisoning by other tranquilizers — (Use additional code to specify the effects of the poisoning)

969.6 Poisoning by psychodysleptics (hallucinogens) — (Use additional code to specify the effects of the poisoning)

969.7 Poisoning by psychostimulants — (Use additional code to specify the effects of the poisoning)

969.8 Poisoning by other specified psychotropic agents — (Use additional code to specify the effects of the poisoning)

969.9 Poisoning by unspecified psychotropic agent — (Use additional code to specify the effects of the poisoning)

Coding Scenario

A patient is seen in the emergency department after ingesting an unknown amount of antidepressants in a suicide attempt. She is in a comatose state.

> Code assignment: 969.0 *Poisoning by psychotropic agents, antidepressants,* 780.01 *Alteration of consciousness, coma,* and E950.3 *Suicide and self-inflicted poisoning by solid or liquid substances, tranquilizers and other psychotropic agents*

A 3-year-old girl is seen in the emergency department after ingesting a single tablet of Amitriptyline found on the floor. She appears sleepy but in no distress and no physiological abnormal findings are noted. She will be observed for the next 24-hours to determine that there are no ill effects.

> Code assignment: 969.0 *Poisoning by psychotropic agents, antidepressants,* 780.7 *Malaise and fatigue,* and E854.0 *Accidental poisoning by other psychotropic agents, antidepressants*

970 Poisoning by central nervous system stimulants

AHA: Q2, 1990, 11

970.0 Poisoning by analeptics — (Use additional code to specify the effects of the poisoning)

970.1 Poisoning by opiate antagonists — (Use additional code to specify the effects of the poisoning)

970.8 Poisoning by other specified central nervous system stimulants — (Use additional code to specify the effects of the poisoning)

970.9 Poisoning by unspecified central nervous system stimulant — (Use additional code to specify the effects of the poisoning)

971 Poisoning by drugs primarily affecting the autonomic nervous system

AHA: Q2, 1990, 11

971.0 Poisoning by parasympathomimetics (cholinergics) — (Use additional code to specify the effects of the poisoning)

971.1 Poisoning by parasympatholytics (anticholinergics and antimuscarinics) and spasmolytics — (Use additional code to specify the effects of the poisoning)

971.2 Poisoning by sympathomimetics (adrenergics) — (Use additional code to specify the effects of the poisoning)

971.3 Poisoning by sympatholytics (antiadrenergics) — (Use additional code to specify the effects of the poisoning)

971.9 Poisoning by unspecified drug primarily affecting autonomic nervous system — (Use additional code to specify the effects of the poisoning)

972 Poisoning by agents primarily affecting the cardiovascular system

AHA: Q2, 1990, 11

972.0 Poisoning by cardiac rhythm regulators — (Use additional code to specify the effects of the poisoning)

972.1 Poisoning by cardiotonic glycosides and drugs of similar action — (Use additional code to specify the effects of the poisoning)

972.2 Poisoning by antilipemic and antiarteriosclerotic drugs — (Use additional code to specify the effects of the poisoning)

972.3 Poisoning by ganglion-blocking agents — (Use additional code to specify the effects of the poisoning)

972.4 Poisoning by coronary vasodilators — (Use additional code to specify the effects of the poisoning)

972.5 Poisoning by other vasodilators — (Use additional code to specify the effects of the poisoning)

972.6 Poisoning by other antihypertensive agents — (Use additional code to specify the effects of the poisoning)

972.7 Poisoning by antivaricose drugs, including sclerosing agents — (Use additional code to specify the effects of the poisoning)

© 2004 Ingenix, Inc.

972.8 Poisoning by capillary-active drugs — (Use additional code to specify the effects of the poisoning)

972.9 Poisoning by other and unspecified agents primarily affecting the cardiovascular system — (Use additional code to specify the effects of the poisoning)

973 Poisoning by agents primarily affecting the gastrointestinal system

AHA: Q2, 1990, 11

973.0 Poisoning by antacids and antigastric secretion drugs — (Use additional code to specify the effects of the poisoning)

973.1 Poisoning by irritant cathartics — (Use additional code to specify the effects of the poisoning)

973.2 Poisoning by emollient cathartics — (Use additional code to specify the effects of the poisoning)

973.3 Poisoning by other cathartics, including intestinal atonia drugs — (Use additional code to specify the effects of the poisoning)

973.4 Poisoning by digestants — (Use additional code to specify the effects of the poisoning)

973.5 Poisoning by antidiarrheal drugs — (Use additional code to specify the effects of the poisoning)

973.6 Poisoning by emetics — (Use additional code to specify the effects of the poisoning)

973.8 Poisoning by other specified agents primarily affecting the gastrointestinal system — (Use additional code to specify the effects of the poisoning)

973.9 Poisoning by unspecified agent primarily affecting the gastrointestinal system — (Use additional code to specify the effects of the poisoning)

974 Poisoning by water, mineral, and uric acid metabolism drugs

AHA: Q2, 1990, 11

974.0 Poisoning by mercurial diuretics — (Use additional code to specify the effects of the poisoning)

974.1 Poisoning by purine derivative diuretics — (Use additional code to specify the effects of the poisoning)

974.2 Poisoning by carbonic acid anhydrase inhibitors — (Use additional code to specify the effects of the poisoning)

974.3 Poisoning by saluretics — (Use additional code to specify the effects of the poisoning)

974.4 Poisoning by other diuretics — (Use additional code to specify the effects of the poisoning)

974.5 Poisoning by electrolytic, caloric, and water-balance agents — (Use additional code to specify the effects of the poisoning)

974.6 Poisoning by other mineral salts, not elsewhere classified — (Use additional code to specify the effects of the poisoning)

974.7 Poisoning by uric acid metabolism drugs — (Use additional code to specify the effects of the poisoning)

975 Poisoning by agents primarily acting on the smooth and skeletal muscles and respiratory system

AHA: Q2, 1990, 11

975.0 Poisoning by oxytocic agents — (Use additional code to specify the effects of the poisoning)

975.1 Poisoning by smooth muscle relaxants — (Use additional code to specify the effects of the poisoning)

975.2 Poisoning by skeletal muscle relaxants — (Use additional code to specify the effects of the poisoning)

975.3 Poisoning by other and unspecified drugs acting on muscles — (Use additional code to specify the effects of the poisoning)

975.4 Poisoning by antitussives — (Use additional code to specify the effects of the poisoning)

975.5 Poisoning by expectorants — (Use additional code to specify the effects of the poisoning)

975.6 Poisoning by anti-common cold drugs — (Use additional code to specify the effects of the poisoning)

975.7 Poisoning by antiasthmatics — (Use additional code to specify the effects of the poisoning)

975.8 Poisoning by other and unspecified respiratory drugs — (Use additional code to specify the effects of the poisoning)

976 Poisoning by agents primarily affecting skin and mucous membrane, ophthalmological, otorhinolaryngological, and dental drugs

AHA: Q2, 1990, 11

976.0 Poisoning by local anti-infectives and anti-inflammatory drugs — (Use additional code to specify the effects of the poisoning)

976.1 Poisoning by antipruritics — (Use additional code to specify the effects of the poisoning)

976.2 Poisoning by local astringents and local detergents — (Use additional code to specify the effects of the poisoning)

976.3 Poisoning by emollients, demulcents, and protectants — (Use additional code to specify the effects of the poisoning)

976.4 Poisoning by keratolytics, keratoplastics, other hair treatment drugs and preparations — (Use additional code to specify the effects of the poisoning)

976.5 Poisoning by eye anti-infectives and other eye drugs — (Use additional code to specify the effects of the poisoning)

976.6 Poisoning by anti-infectives and other drugs and preparations for ear, nose, and throat — (Use additional code to specify the effects of the poisoning)

976.7 Poisoning by dental drugs topically applied — (Use additional code to specify the effects of the poisoning)

976.8 Poisoning by other agents primarily affecting skin and mucous membrane — (Use additional code to specify the effects of the poisoning)

976.9 Poisoning by unspecified agent primarily affecting skin and mucous membrane — (Use additional code to specify the effects of the poisoning)

977 Poisoning by other and unspecified drugs and medicinal substances

AHA: Q2, 1990, 11

977.0 Poisoning by dietetics — (Use additional code to specify the effects of the poisoning)

977.1 Poisoning by lipotropic drugs — (Use additional code to specify the effects of the poisoning)

977.2 Poisoning by antidotes and chelating agents, not elsewhere classified — (Use additional code to specify the effects of the poisoning)

977.3 Poisoning by alcohol deterrents — (Use additional code to specify the effects of the poisoning)

977.4 Poisoning by pharmaceutical excipients — (Use additional code to specify the effects of the poisoning)

977.8 Poisoning by other specified drugs and medicinal substances — (Use additional code to specify the effects of the poisoning)

977.9 Poisoning by unspecified drug or medicinal substance — (Use additional code to specify the effects of the poisoning)

978 Poisoning by bacterial vaccines

AHA: Q2, 1990, 11

978.0 Poisoning by bcg vaccine — (Use additional code to specify the effects of the poisoning)

978.1 Poisoning by typhoid and paratyphoid vaccine — (Use additional code to specify the effects of the poisoning)

978.2 Poisoning by cholera vaccine — (Use additional code to specify the effects of the poisoning)

978.3 Poisoning by plague vaccine — (Use additional code to specify the effects of the poisoning)

978.4 Poisoning by tetanus vaccine — (Use additional code to specify the effects of the poisoning)

978.5 Poisoning by diphtheria vaccine — (Use additional code to specify the effects of the poisoning)

978.6 Poisoning by pertussis vaccine, including combinations with pertussis component — (Use additional code to specify the effects of the poisoning)

978.8 Poisoning by other and unspecified bacterial vaccines — (Use additional code to specify the effects of the poisoning)

978.9 Poisoning by mixed bacterial vaccines, except combinations with pertussis component — (Use additional code to specify the effects of the poisoning)

979 Poisoning by other vaccines and biological substances

AHA: Q2, 1990, 11

979.0 Poisoning by smallpox vaccine — (Use additional code to specify the effects of the poisoning)

979.1 Poisoning by rabies vaccine — (Use additional code to specify the effects of the poisoning)

979.2 Poisoning by typhus vaccine — (Use additional code to specify the effects of the poisoning)

979.3 Poisoning by yellow fever vaccine — (Use additional code to specify the effects of the poisoning)

979.4 Poisoning by measles vaccine — (Use additional code to specify the effects of the poisoning)

979.5 Poisoning by poliomyelitis vaccine — (Use additional code to specify the effects of the poisoning)

979.6 Poisoning by other and unspecified viral and rickettsial vaccines — (Use additional code to specify the effects of the poisoning)

 © 2004 Ingenix, Inc.

979.7 Poisoning by mixed viral-rickettsial and bacterial vaccines, except combinations with pertussis component — (Use additional code to specify the effects of the poisoning)

979.9 Poisoning by other and unspecified vaccines and biological substances — (Use additional code to specify the effects of the poisoning)

980–989 Toxic Effects of Substances Chiefly Nonmedicinal as to Source

The toxicity of a substance is due to its ability to damage or disrupt metabolism. An acutely toxic substance can cause damage as the result of a single or short-duration exposure. A chronically toxic substance causes damage after repeated or long-duration exposure or becomes evident only after a long latency period. Toxicity varies with the route of exposure and the effectiveness at which the material is absorbed. A chemical that enters the body in large quantities but is not easily absorbed is a much lower risk than one that is easily absorbed into the bloodstream.

Skin contact is the most common route of exposure but often the best barrier since the skin guards against the entry of most chemicals. Once a chemical passes through the skin (i.e., through a wound), it enters the bloodstream and is carried to all parts of the body.

Inhalation is the most dangerous route of entry because the lungs are ineffective barriers. Chemicals that pass the lung membrane are absorbed into the bloodstream and carried to all parts of the body. Absorption can be extremely rapid. The rate of absorption depends on the concentration of the toxic substance, its solubility in water, the depth of respiration, and the rate of blood circulation.

Ingested materials are absorbed into the bloodstream anywhere along the gastrointestinal tract. If the material cannot be absorbed, it will be eliminated from the body.

Toxins are not due to absorption of putrified or fermented foodstuffs, nor are they absorbed from the colon in conditions of constipation. A toxic reaction can be similar to an allergic reaction but more severe. If the liver is functioning normally, it may allow a small amount of the toxic material to enter the body, but eliminate the rest. If the liver is not functioning normally, the substance may enter the body and cause a toxic chemical overload that may result in blood poisoning and death. Toxemia is a poisoned condition of the blood caused by the presence of toxic materials, usually bacterial but occasionally chemical or hormonal in nature.

As a general rule, the more known about the poisoning agent, the better the treatment plan and outcome. Poison Control Centers have been invaluable in supplying the health care professional with the exact composition of the thousands of poisonous substances. If the information is unknown, treatment must revolve around general supportive measures.

Treatment includes the use of corticosteroids and mannitol drips to minimize cerebral edema, dialysis to combat renal failure, hasten the excretion of the poison, alkalinization or acidification of the urine, and remove lipid soluble substances from the blood, hemoperfusion, and chelating agents.

980 Toxic effect of alcohol

980.0 Toxic effect of ethyl alcohol — (Use additional code to identify any associated condition: 291.4, 303.0, 305.0)

980.1 Toxic effect of methyl alcohol — (Use additional code to specify the nature of the toxic effect)

980.2 Toxic effect of isopropyl alcohol — (Use additional code to specify the nature of the toxic effect)

980.3 Toxic effect of fusel oil — (Use additional code to specify the nature of the toxic effect)

980.8 Toxic effect of other specified alcohols — (Use additional code to specify the nature of the toxic effect)

980.9 Toxic effect of unspecified alcohol — (Use additional code to specify the nature of the toxic effect)

981 Toxic effect of petroleum products OK

982 Toxic effect of solvents other than petroleum-based

982.0 Toxic effect of benzene and homologues — (Use additional code to specify the nature of the toxic effect)

982.1 Toxic effect of carbon tetrachloride — (Use additional code to specify the nature of the toxic effect)

982.2 Toxic effect of carbon disulfide — (Use additional code to specify the nature of the toxic effect)

982.3 Toxic effect of other chlorinated hydrocarbon solvents — (Use additional code to specify the nature of the toxic effect)

982.4 Toxic effect of nitroglycol — (Use additional code to specify the nature of the toxic effect)

982.8 Toxic effect of other nonpetroleum-based solvents — (Use additional code to specify the nature of the toxic effect)

983 Toxic effect of corrosive aromatics, acids, and caustic alkalis

983.0 Toxic effect of corrosive aromatics — (Use additional code to specify the nature of the toxic effect)

983.1 Toxic effect of acids — (Use additional code to specify the nature of the toxic effect)

983.2 Toxic effect of caustic alkalis — (Use additional code to specify the nature of the toxic effect)

983.9 Toxic effect of caustic, unspecified — (Use additional code to specify the nature of the toxic effect)

984 Toxic effect of lead and its compounds (including fumes)

984.0 Toxic effect of inorganic lead compounds — (Use additional code to specify the nature of the toxic effect)

984.1 Toxic effect of organic lead compounds — (Use additional code to specify the nature of the toxic effect)

984.8 Toxic effect of other lead compounds — (Use additional code to specify the nature of the toxic effect)

984.9 Toxic effect of unspecified lead compound — (Use additional code to specify the nature of the toxic effect)

985 Toxic effect of other metals

985.0 Toxic effect of mercury and its compounds — (Use additional code to specify the nature of the toxic effect)

985.1 Toxic effect of arsenic and its compounds — (Use additional code to specify the nature of the toxic effect)

985.2 Toxic effect of manganese and its compounds — (Use additional code to specify the nature of the toxic effect)

985.3 Toxic effect of beryllium and its compounds — (Use additional code to specify the nature of the toxic effect)

985.4 Toxic effect of antimony and its compounds — (Use additional code to specify the nature of the toxic effect)

985.5 Toxic effect of cadmium and its compounds — (Use additional code to specify the nature of the toxic effect)

985.6 Toxic effect of chromium — (Use additional code to specify the nature of the toxic effect)

985.8 Toxic effect of other specified metals — (Use additional code to specify the nature of the toxic effect)

985.9 Toxic effect of unspecified metal — (Use additional code to specify the nature of the toxic effect)

986 Toxic effect of carbon monoxide OK

987 Toxic effect of other gases, fumes, or vapors

987.0 Toxic effect of liquefied petroleum gases — (Use additional code to specify the nature of the toxic effect)

987.1 Toxic effect of other hydrocarbon gas — (Use additional code to specify the nature of the toxic effect)

987.2 Toxic effect of nitrogen oxides — (Use additional code to specify the nature of the toxic effect)

987.3 Toxic effect of sulfur dioxide — (Use additional code to specify the nature of the toxic effect)

987.4 Toxic effect of freon — (Use additional code to specify the nature of the toxic effect)

987.5 Toxic effect of lacrimogenic gas — (Use additional code to specify the nature of the toxic effect)

987.6 Toxic effect of chlorine gas — (Use additional code to specify the nature of the toxic effect)

987.7 Toxic effect of hydrocyanic acid gas — (Use additional code to specify the nature of the toxic effect)

987.8 Toxic effect of other specified gases, fumes, or vapors — (Use additional code to specify the nature of the toxic effect)

987.9 Toxic effect of unspecified gas, fume, or vapor — (Use additional code to specify the nature of the toxic effect)

988 Toxic effect of noxious substances eaten as food

988.0 Toxic effect of fish and shellfish — (Use additional code to specify the nature of the toxic effect)

988.1 Toxic effect of mushrooms — (Use additional code to specify the nature of the toxic effect)

988.2 Toxic effect of berries and other plants — (Use additional code to specify the nature of the toxic effect)

988.8 Toxic effect of other specified noxious substances — (Use additional code to specify the nature of the toxic effect)

988.9 Toxic effect of unspecified noxious substance — (Use additional code to specify the nature of the toxic effect)

 © 2004 Ingenix, Inc.

Coding Clarification

Category 988 excludes spoiled food that causes illness (food poisoning). The mistletoe berry is an example of poisonous flora belonging in this category.

989 Toxic effect of other substances, chiefly nonmedicinal as to source

989.0 Toxic effect of hydrocyanic acid and cyanides — (Use additional code to specify the nature of the toxic effect)

989.1 Toxic effect of strychnine and salts — (Use additional code to specify the nature of the toxic effect)

989.2 Toxic effect of chlorinated hydrocarbons — (Use additional code to specify the nature of the toxic effect)

989.3 Toxic effect of organophosphate and carbamate — (Use additional code to specify the nature of the toxic effect)

989.4 Toxic effect of other pesticides, not elsewhere classified — (Use additional code to specify the nature of the toxic effect)

989.5 Toxic effect of venom — (Use additional code to specify the nature of the toxic effect)

Each of the 48 contiguous states in the United States harbour at least one species of venomous snake. The pit vipers (copperhead, cottonmouth, and rattlesnakes) and coral snakes are two venomous families widely spread in the United States. Approximately 8,000 of the estimated 45,000 annual snakebites in this country are by poisonous snakes. Snake venoms are rated on a lethality index, with the Mojave rattlesnake having the highest index of any North American snake. Pit viper bites are associated with pain, swelling, and edema. Ecchymosis is common, ranging from moderate to severe. The patient may hemorrhage from the gums and develop hematemesis, melena, and hematuria. The coral snake bite generally produces nerve conduction damage and CNS damage. Annual fatalities are fewer than 15, most of which can be attributed to rattlesnake venom.

Survival often depends on the time it takes until medical help. If the patient is more than 40 minutes from a hospital, an incision over the bite may be made and suction applied. Envenomation must be assessed whenever a patient presents at the medical center with a snake bite since about 20 to 30 percent of all pit viper bites do not involve venom injection, and about 50 percent from the same class as coral snakes does not involve venom injection. Protocol calls for treating snakebites without envenomation as puncture wounds. If envenomation does occur, the patient presents a complex poisoning picture. Depending on the type of snake, the patient may weaken several hours after the bite, experience difficulty salivating or speaking, or experience respiratory distress and cardiovascular failure in fatal cases.

Antivenom is needed in only 60 percent of pit viper bites. The young or elderly require antivenom for copperhead bites. Coral snake envenomation is not typically associated with pain or swelling and three vials of antivenom are routinely administered once envenomation by coral snake bite is determined.

Two lizards, the Gila monster and the beaded lizard, are poisonous. Treatment protocols are similar to those for pit viper bites, though there is no antivenom for these bites.

There are numerous venomous spider species in the United States. Most bites require only local care, although in cases of severe envenomation the victim must be hospitalized for supportive measures. Fatalities are few, with the greatest risk for children and the elderly.

989.6 Toxic effect of soaps and detergents — (Use additional code to specify the nature of the toxic effect)

989.7 Toxic effect of aflatoxin and other mycotoxin (food contaminants) — (Use additional code to specify the nature of the toxic effect)

989.81 Toxic effect of asbestos — (Use additional code to specify the nature of the toxic effect)

989.82 Toxic effect of latex — (Use additional code to specify the nature of the toxic effect)

989.83 Toxic effect of silicone — (Use additional code to specify the nature of the toxic effect)

989.84 Toxic effect of tobacco — (Use additional code to specify the nature of the toxic effect)

989.89 Toxic effect of other substances — (Use additional code to specify the nature of the toxic effect)

989.9 Toxic effect of unspecified substance, chiefly nonmedicinal as to source — (Use additional code to specify the nature of the toxic effect)

990–995 Other and Unspecified Effects of External Causes

990 Effects of radiation, unspecified OK

A substance emitting ionizing radiation is capable of creating radiation sickness. Acute radiation sickness is classified as cerebral, gastrointestinal, or hematopoietic. The cerebral syndrome is fatal within a few hours of exposure to a dose in an amount greater than 30 Gy. The gastrointestinal syndrome involves a dose of at least 4 Gy, with death occurring within two or three weeks. The hematopoietic syndrome is also fatal, with neutropenia the contributing cause of death due to lowered immune resistance. The dose is 2 to 10 Gy.

Recovery from a radiation accident depends on the size of the dose, the rate at which the dose is received, and the distribution of the dose over the body. While a large dose all at once over the entire body is fatal, the same dose administered therapeutically to a small area for a brief period of time may be repeated over time without fear of fatality. Therapeutic doses may cause radiation sickness, involving nausea, vomiting, and diarrhea with malaise and tachycardia. These symptoms decline spontaneously, over time.

991 Effects of reduced temperature

Accidental hypothermia results from conduction, convection, and radiation. Examples of conduction hypothermia are wet clothing and skin freezing upon metal contact. Convection injuries are from wind chill. The body core temperature can drop as low as 79° Fahrenheit. The rule is to resuscitate until the patient is warm. The extremities are at great risk of hypothermia, as well as the nose. They should be warm and dry at all times. While dry, cold injury such as frostbite can result in gangrene, the gangrene is usually superficial, with a large reservoir of intact skin underneath the affected part. Wet, cold injury is more pernicious, leading to wet gangrene. As the patient recovers from frostbite, the skin may slough from the affected part. This skin is treated with burn protocols.

991.0 Frostbite of face

991.1 Frostbite of hand

991.2 Frostbite of foot

991.3 Frostbite of other and unspecified sites

991.4 Effects of immersion of foot

991.5 Effects of chilblains

991.6 Effects of hypothermia

Coding Clarification

This code excludes hypothermia not associated with environmental temperature (780.99).

991.8 Other specified effects of reduced temperature

991.9 Unspecified effect of reduced temperature

992 Effects of heat and light

Heat related illnesses are arranged in order from the most deadly to the mildest. Heat stroke has many names and is a major medical emergency, causing death in 10 percent of its victims.

Heat stroke is partitioned into two categories, equally dangerous — exertional and classic. Classic heat stroke victims typically are older, debilitated from chronic health problems, sedentary, and do not present with major systemic disorders. Exertional heat stroke, which may cause multiple systemic derangement, more often strikes younger, healthier individuals engaged in strenuous activity.

Both types of heat stroke must be treated immediately by immersing the patient in cold water. Water temperature must be monitored to prevent hypothermia. Stroke victims should be transported to the hospital, though prior to summoning help, the patient must be relieved from excessive temperature in the body core greater than 104.9° Fahrenheit.

Heat exhaustion is excessive body core temperature in the range of 100.4° to 104.9° Fahrenheit. The patient must be cooled and orally rehydrated, although there may be gastrointestinal distress necessitating intravenous administration of fluids. The patient generally recovers in two to three hours with appropriate support, though some cases are unresponsive and require hospitalization.

Heat syncope occurs from dehydration, lack of acclimatization to heat when undertaking exercise, and failure to undergo a cool-down period after exercise. Once the patient is prostrate, recovery is immediate.

Heat edema is the swelling of the extremities, typically the legs, in hot weather. Exercise and elevation of the affected parts lessens the swelling.

992.0 Heat stroke and sunstroke

992.1 Heat syncope

992.2 Heat cramps

992.3 Heat exhaustion, anhydrotic

992.4 Heat exhaustion due to salt depletion

992.5 Heat exhaustion, unspecified

992.6 Heat fatigue, transient

992.7 Heat edema

992.8 Other specified heat effects

992.9 Unspecified effects of heat and light

993 Effects of air pressure

993.0 Barotrauma, otitic

Otitic barotrauma can affect aviators, divers, or tunnel workers. Symptoms include pain, hearing loss, rupture of the tympanic membrane, vertigo, and disorientation, which is perhaps the most dangerous manifestation since it can interfere with the ability to move to safety.

993.1 Barotrauma, sinus

Congestion in the sinuses is likely to cause pain and possibly nosebleeds if diving or swift ascent occurs.

993.2 Other and unspecified effects of high altitude

The higher the altitude, the thinner the atmosphere and the greater reduction in oxygen content. The effect is magnified by the proximity of the peak to the earth's poles. At 18,000 feet above sea level, the oxygen content of the atmosphere is reduced by 50 percent and the body must produce a greater number of red blood cells to carry oxygen. Given time to spend at various levels of ascent, most individuals can successfully adapt to the thinner atmosphere.

 © 2004 Ingenix, Inc.

There are three levels of acute mountain sickness: mild, moderate, and severe. If the moderate degree should manifest, the victim must descend 1,000 feet, rest, and adapt. Climbers must take precautions against the severe form of this life-threatening condition, which requires immediate descent of 2,000- to 4000-feet. The moderate to severe forms can alter mental status, change the degree of consciousness, and cause ataxia and shortness of breath with cyanosis, all of which can be fatal if the patient is not removed from the environment.

993.3 Caisson disease

Other common names for this disorder are the bends and decompression sickness. The term "the bends" refers to the pain associated with decompression sickness, though it has become synonymous for the sickness.

Nitrogen gas dissolved in the tissues forms potentially lethal bubbles in the blood. Women who have a higher proportion of fat are at higher risk of decompression sickness than men.

993.4 Effects of air pressure caused by explosion

993.8 Other specified effects of air pressure

993.9 Unspecified effect of air pressure

994 Effects of other external causes

994.0 Effects of lightning

There are an estimated 750 lightning strikes of humans per year, with an associated mortality rate of 3 to 10 percent. Lightning strikes the highest points, so standing in a meadow, standing under a big tree, or carrying an umbrella, increase the chances of a strike. Electrical energy travels along the earth's surface and can enter the human by the leg closest to the strike and exit through the other leg.

The nerves, muscles, and blood vessels are excellent electrical conductors. Once an individual is struck, the results are typically cardiac arrest, respiratory arrest, vascular spasm, neurological damage, and autonomic instability, rather than burns and renal failure.

994.1 Drowning and nonfatal submersion

The great mortality risk in near drowning is posed by respiratory insufficiency leading to hypoxia and respiratory acidosis. These conditions are always addressed first, and aspiration is managed secondarily. Aspiration of seawater is rarely life threatening, although such aspiration can cause mild elevations of sodium and chloride. Aspiration of large quantities of fresh water can cause massive increase of blood volume, life threatening electrolyte imbalance, and hemolysis leading to asphyxia and ventricular fibrillation.

The water temperature and duration of immersion are other factors when predicting survival from immersion. If an individual is exposed to cool water, over time hypothermia will set in, with its attendant problems. However, if the victim is suddenly tipped into cold water, the mammalian diving reflex reduces the body's oxygen need, thus increasing the chance of survival. The rule is to continue resuscitation efforts even if submerged for more than one hour.

994.2 Effects of hunger

994.3 Effects of thirst

994.4 Exhaustion due to exposure

994.5 Exhaustion due to excessive exertion

994.6 Motion sickness

994.7 Asphyxiation and strangulation

994.8 Electrocution and nonfatal effects of electric current

The extent of an injury by electric shock is a function of the amount of voltage delivered, current type, resistance to the current, and the length of contact to the current. If the skin is thick and dry, it will present greater resistance to the current, resulting in extensive burns, though only slight damage to internal organs. Of the two types of current, direct current is the least deadly since it throws the victim, cutting short the exposure to the current. Alternating current is three times more dangerous than direct current since the chances of tetanic contractions multiply threefold. Tetany is likely to occur when the "let-go reflex" is depressed, increasing the victim's length of contact with the current.

994.9 Other effects of external causes

995 Certain adverse effects not elsewhere classified

995.0 Other anaphylactic shock not else where classifed — (Use additional E code to identify external cause: E930-E949)

The key to understanding an allergy is to recognize that the previously sensitized individual has been re-exposed to the dose that begins the allergic reaction. Vasodilation and consequent loss of plasma into the tissues (productive of hives and angioedema) lead to hypovolemia. After receiving the "insult," the agitated system may present with reddened skin, pruritus, laryngeal edema, or bronchospasm. Shock can set in within a short time and, unless the process is arrested, the patient can die of vascular collapse.

995.1 Angioneurotic edema not elsewhere classified

995.2 Unspecified adverse effect of drug medicinal and biological substance, not elsewhere classified

995.3 Allergy, unspecified not elsewhere classified

995.4 Shock due to anesthesia not elsewhere classified

Anesthetic drugs can cause vasodilation, which can lead to hypovolemic shock and vascular collapse. Patients are carefully monitored during anesthesia for any signs of inappropriate vasodilation.

995.50 Child abuse, unspecified

995.51 Child emotional/psychological abuse

995.52 Child neglect (nutritional)

995.53 Child sexual abuse

995.54 Child physical abuse

995.55 Shaken infant syndrome — (Use additional code(s) to identify any associated injuries)

995.59 Other child abuse and neglect

995.60 Anaphylactic shock due to unspecified food

995.61 Anaphylactic shock due to peanuts

995.62 Anaphylactic shock due to crustaceans

995.63 Anaphylactic shock due to fruits and vegetables

995.64 Anaphylactic shock due to tree nuts and seeds

995.65 Anaphylactic shock due to fish

995.66 Anaphylactic shock due to food additives

995.67 Anaphylactic shock due to milk products

995.68 Anaphylactic shock due to eggs

995.69 Anaphylactic shock due to other specified food

995.7 Other adverse food reactions, not elsewhere classified — (Use additional code to identify the type of reaction: 708.0, 786.07)

995.80 Adult maltreatment, usnpecified — (Use additional code to identify any associated injury and perpetrator)

995.81 Adult physical abuse — (Use additional code to identify any associated injury, nature of abuse, and perpetrator)

995.82 Adult emotional/psychological abuse — (Use additional E code to identify perpetrator)

995.83 Adult sexual abuse — (Use additional code to identify any associated injury and perpetrator)

995.84 Adult neglect (nutritional) — (Use additional E code to identify intent of neglect and perpetrator)

995.85 Other adult abuse and neglect — (Use additional code to identify any associated injury, intent of neglect, nature of abuse, and perpetrator)

995.86 Malignant hyperthermia

995.89 Certain adverse effects, not elsewhere classified, other

Hyperthermia and hypothermia due to adverse reaction to anesthesia result from a combination of muscle relaxant and inhalation general anesthetic. When an adverse reaction occurs, the operation must be stopped and a reversal agent such as dantrolene must be administered. Family members should be tested for the same sensitivity.

995.9 [5th] Systemic inflammatory response syndrome (SIRS) — (Code first underlying condition) — *code first underlying condition: 995.91, 995.92. Use additional code to specify organ dysfunction; acute respiratory failure, 518.81; critical illness myopathy, 359.81; critical illness polyneuropathy, 357.82; encephalopathy, 348.31; hepatic failure, 570*
AHA: Q4, 2002, 71

995.90 Systemic inflammatory response syndrome, unspecified — (Code first underlying condition)

995.91 Systemic inflammatory response syndrome due to infectious process without organ dysfunction — (Code first underlying condition)

995.92 Systemic inflammatory response syndrome due to infectious process with organ dysfunction — (Code first underlying condition. Use additional code to specify organ dysfunction: 348.31, 357.82, 359.81, 518.81, 570, 584.5-584.9, 585, 586, 785.52) — *Use an additional code to specify the organ dysfunction, such as: encephalopathy (348.3), heart failure (428.0-428.9) and kidney failure (584.5-584.9, 585, 586)*
AHA: Q4, 2002, 71; Q4, 2003, 73, 79

995.93 Systemic inflammatory response syndrome due to non-infectious process without organ dysfunction — (Code first underlying condition)

995.94 Systemic inflammatory response syndrome due to non-infectious process with organ dysfunction — (Code first underlying condition. Use additional code to specify organ dysfunction: 348.31, 357.82, 359.81, 518.81, 570, 584.5-584.9, 585, 586, 785.52) — *Use an additional code to specify the organ dysfunction, such as: encephalopathy (348.3), heart failure (428.0-428.9) and kidney failure (584.5-584.9, 585, 586)*
AHA: Q4, 2002, 71; Q4, 2003, 79

996–999 Complications of Surgical and Medical Care, NEC

996 Complications peculiar to certain specified procedures

AHA: Q1, 1994, 3

Patients may experience idiosyncratic reactions to the materials used in prostheses, from lens implants to artificial skin. Prostheses can also cause problems when displaced from the site of original insertion.

© 2004 Ingenix, Inc.

Problems classified as mechanical, complications, infectious or inflammatory reactions, or "other" complications include associated pain, embolism, hemorrhage, organ transplant rejections, and complications of reattached extremities or body parts. When the reason for an admission is linked to complications of medical or surgical care, the complication code is listed as the principal diagnosis, with any explanatory codes following. For example, a patient may be readmitted with sepsis following a previous medical contact. In this case, determine if the sepsis is linked to the previous contact since it may be attributable to either an infected line or a postoperative infection.

996.00 Mechanical complication of unspecified cardiac device, implant, and graft

996.01 Mechanical complication due to cardiac pacemaker (electrode)

996.02 Mechanical complication due to heart valve prosthesis

996.03 Mechanical complication due to coronary bypass graft

996.04 Mechanical complication due to automatic implantable cardiac defibrillator

996.09 Mechanical complication of cardiac device, implant, and graft, other

996.1 Mechanical complication of other vascular device, implant, and graft

996.1 Mechanical complication of other vascular device, implant, and graft

996.2 Mechanical complication of nervous system device, implant, and graft

996.30 Mechanical complication of unspecified genitourinary device, implant, and graft

996.31 Mechanical complication due to urethral (indwelling) catheter

996.32 Mechanical complication due to intrauterine contraceptive device

996.39 Mechanical complication of genitourinary device, implant, and graft, other

996.4 Mechanical complication of internal orthopedic device, implant, and graft

996.51 Mechanical complication due to corneal graft

996.52 Mechanical complication due to other tissue graft, not elsewhere classified

996.53 Mechanical complication due to ocular lens prosthesis

996.54 Mechanical complication due to breast prosthesis

996.55 Mechanical complications due to artificial skin graft and decellularized allodermis

996.56 Mechanical complications due to peritoneal dialysis catheter

996.57 Mechanical complication, Due to insulin pump

996.59 Mechanical complication due to other implant and internal device, not elsewhere classified

996.60 Infection and inflammatory reaction due to unspecified device, implant, and graft — (Use additional code to identify specified infections)

996.61 Infection and inflammatory reaction due to cardiac device, implant, and graft — (Use additional code to identify specified infections)

996.62 Infection and inflammatory reaction due to other vascular device, implant, and graft — (Use additional code to identify specified infections)

996.63 Infection and inflammatory reaction due to nervous system device, implant, and graft — (Use additional code to identify specified infections)

996.64 Infection and inflammatory reaction due to indwelling urinary catheter — (Use additional code to identify specified infections: 038.0-038.9, 595.0-595.9)

996.65 Infection and inflammatory reaction due to other genitourinary device, implant, and graft — (Use additional code to identify specified infections)

996.66 Infection and inflammatory reaction due to internal joint prosthesis — (Use additional code to identify specified infections)

996.67 Infection and inflammatory reaction due to other internal orthopedic device, implant, and graft — (Use additional code to identify specified infections)

996.68 Infection and inflammatory reaction due to peritoneal dialysis catheter — (Use additional code to identify specified infections)

996.69 Infection and inflammatory reaction due to other internal prosthetic device, implant, and graft — (Use additional code to identify specified infections)

996.70 Other complications due to unspecified device, implant, and graft

996.71 Other complications due to heart valve prosthesis

996.72 Other complications due to other cardiac device, implant, and graft

996.73 Other complications due to renal dialysis device, implant, and graft

996.74 Other complications due to other vascular device, implant, and graft

996.75 Other complications due to nervous system device, implant, and graft

800–999

996.76 Other complications due to genitourinary device, implant, and graft

996.77 Other complications due to internal joint prosthesis

996.78 Other complications due to other internal orthopedic device, implant, and graft

996.79 Other complications due to other internal prosthetic device, implant, and graft

996.80 Complications of transplanted organ, unspecified site — (Use additional code to identify nature of complication, 078.5)

996.81 Complications of transplanted kidney — (Use additional code to identify nature of complication, 078.5)

996.82 Complications of transplanted liver — (Use additional code to identify nature of complication, 078.5)

996.83 Complications of transplanted heart — (Use additional code to identify nature of complication, 078.5)

996.84 Complications of transplanted lung — (Use additional code to identify nature of complication, 078.5)

996.85 Complications of bone marrow transplant — (Use additional code to identify nature of complication, 078.5)

996.86 Complications of transplanted pancreas — (Use additional code to identify nature of complication, 078.5)

996.87 Complications of transplanted organ, intestine — (Use additional code to identify nature of complication, 078.5)

996.89 Complications of other transplanted organ — (Use additional code to identify nature of complication, 078.5)

996.90 Complications of unspecified reattached extremity

996.91 Complications of reattached forearm

996.92 Complications of reattached hand

996.93 Complications of reattached finger(s)

996.94 Complications of reattached upper extremity, other and unspecified

996.95 Complications of reattached foot and toe(s)

996.96 Complications of reattached lower extremity, other and unspecified

996.99 Complications of other specified reattached body part

Coding Clarification

Acute Coronary Graft Closure: A common complication following coronary bypass surgery is occlusion of the graft. This condition is classified to ICD-9-CM code 996.03 *Mechanical complication of cardiac device, implant and graft, due to coronary bypass graft.*

As noted by the excludes note in the tabular list, this code is not used to indicate atherosclerosis of the graft. When the documentation indicates that this is the cause of the blockage, the appropriate code from 414.02-414.03 should be assigned.

Another common complication following coronary bypass graft is delayed closure of the graft. This is also reported with code 996.03.

Breast Implant Complications: Patients with augmentation mammoplasty may develop complications due to the implant. Such complications may include periprosthetic mammary capsular contracture, rupture, or infection.

When assigning a code to identify periprosthetic mammary capsular contracture, use code 996.79 *Other complications due to other internal prosthetic device, implant and graft.* Code 996.54 classifies the rupture of the implant. Infection or inflammatory reactions to the implant are identified by 996.69 *Infection and inflammatory reaction due to internal prosthetic device, implant, and graft, due to other internal prosthetic device, implant, and graft.*

Complications of Artificial Skin: Advances in the treatment of burns and other severe conditions affecting the skin have provided new technologies that are able to permanently regenerate or replace skin layers. These include artificial skin, decellularized allodermis, and cultured epithelial cells. As with any procedure, complications can occur, mainly infection and mechanical failure.

Complications such as dislodgment, displacement, non-adherence, poor incorporation, shearing or failure are assigned code 996.55. Infection and/or inflammatory reaction to the graft should be assigned code 996.69.

Mechanical Complication of Peritoneal Dialysis Catheter: It is not uncommon for patients with peritoneal dialysis catheters to experience complications associated with the catheter. Such complications include infection or leakage of the catheter. When a complication of a peritoneal dialysis catheter occurs, code 996.56.

Code 996.56 does not indicate a complication of an arteriovenous dialysis catheter. If the complication is of an A-V catheter, code 996.1 should be reported.

Coronary Artery Stent Stenosis: A complication of stent insertion procedures is the formation of scar tissue at the site of the stent. This is not considered to be a mechanical complication of the stent, as the stent is in working order. The scar tissue formation is the body's natural reaction to the introduction of the stent. The scar tissue formed at the stent should not be considered an infection and/or inflammatory reaction to the stent.

© 2004 Ingenix, Inc.

When assigning a code for stenosis of a stent, use a code from subcategory 996.7 *Other complications of internal (biological) (synthetic) prosthetic device, implant, and graft*. In the case of a coronary artery stent stenosis, the fifth-digit code assigned would be 996.72 *Due to other cardiac device, implant, and graft.*

Coding Scenario

A patient is seen by the surgeon due to leakage of the peritoneal dialysis graft.

> Code assignment: 996.56 *Mechanical complication of other specified prosthetic device, implant or graft, due to peritoneal dialysis catheter*

A patient is seen four days post coronary artery bypass graft for blockage of the graft.

> Code assignment: 996.03 *Mechanical complication of cardiac device, implant, and graft, due to coronary bypass graft*

A patient is seen seven years post breast augmentation. She is complaining of pain. The physician documents periprosthetic mammary capsular contracture.

> Code assignment: 996.79 *Other complications of internal (biological) (synthetic) prosthetic device, implant, and graft due to other internal prosthetic device, implant, and graft*

997 Complications affecting specified body systems, not elsewhere classified

AHA: Q1, 1993, 26; Q1, 1994, 4

Complications in the 997 category are organized according to body system. For example, urinary catheterization is an intervention or procedure and a urinary infection attributed to catheterization is coded with the 997.5 subcategory first and the appropriate urinary infection code secondarily. The more typical scenario with postoperative urinary tract infections is that following back, abdominal, or pelvic surgery, the patient is unable to void and, thus, catheterized. The extended period of catheterization leads to a postoperative urinary tract infection, and is coded as such. In all cases, the medical record must clearly link the complication to the procedure. If unclear, the coder should ask the physician to document the existing link in an addendum to the report.

997.00 Unspecified nervous system complication — (Use additional code to identify complications)

997.01 Central nervous system complication — (Use additional code to identify complications)

997.02 Iatrogenic cerebrovascular infarction or hemorrhage — (Use additional code to identify complications)

997.09 Other nervous system complications — (Use additional code to identify complications)

997.1 Cardiac complications — (Use additional code to identify complications)

997.2 Peripheral vascular complications — (Use additional code to identify complications)

997.3 Respiratory complications — (Use additional code to identify complications)

997.4 Digestive system complication — (Use additional code to identify complications)

997.5 Urinary complications — (Use additional code to identify complications)

997.60 Late complications of amputation stump, unspecified — (Use additional code to identify complications)

997.61 Neuroma of amputation stump — (Use additional code to identify complications)

997.62 Infection (chronic) of amputation stump — (Use additional code to identify organism. Use additional code to identify complications)

997.69 Other late amputation stump complication — (Use additional code to identify complications)

997.71 Vascular complications of mesenteric artery — (Use additional code to identify complications)

997.72 Vascular complications of renal artery — (Use additional code to identify complications)

997.79 Vascular complications of other vessels — (Use additional code to identify complications)

997.91 Hypertension — (Use additional code to identify complications)

997.99 Other complications affecting other specified body systems, NEC — (Use additional code to identify complications)

Coding Clarification

Infection of Amputation Stump: Unless it is the original admission for treatment of a current traumatic amputation, a code from subcategory 997.6x should be identified for any type of amputation stump complication. Specifically, code 997.62 *Amputation stump complication, infection* should be identified in this scenario.

Postoperative Urinary Tract Infection: To indicate that a urinary tract infection is a postoperative complication, two codes are necessary. Assign code 997.5 *Urinary complications* first and code 599.0 *Urinary tract infection, site not specified* as a secondary diagnosis.

Postoperative urinary retention following surgery may lead to urinary tract infection. In this instance, one code, 997.5, is indicated on the claim. Likewise,

800–999

© 2004 Ingenix, Inc.

secretion of a decreased amount of urine as opposed to fluid intake can cause a urinary tract infection and also is indicated by code 997.5.

Postoperative Pneumonia: When the physician documents that the patient is being treated for postoperative pneumonia, two codes are necessary. First assign code 997.3 *Complications affecting specified body systems, not elsewhere classified, respiratory complications* followed by the appropriate code from categories 480-487 or 507 for the pneumonia to specify the nature of the complication.

Cholangitis Following Percutaneous Transhepatic Cholangiogram: Cholangitis is an inflammation of the bile duct and can occur following a cholangiogram. Two codes are required to indicate that the condition occurred as a complication to a surgical procedure. First assign code 997.4 *Digestive system complications* to identify that the condition is due to the procedure followed by code 576.1 *Cholangitis* to further elucidate the condition.

Complications Following Bone Marrow Transplant: When complications arise following bone marrow transplant, report with code 996.85 *Complications of transplanted organ, bone marrow* followed by an additional code identifying the nature of the complication such as an infection.

Complications Following Coronary Artery Procedures: Complications resulting from coronary artery procedures generally occur intraoperatively or within the first 24 hours to one week after surgery. The types of complications include thrombus formation, myocardial infarction, graft closures, infection, pulmonary embolism, stroke, and renal failure.

- Thrombus formation: to identify this condition use code 997.2 *Peripheral vascular complication*. If the thrombus is due to an implant or catheter device, code 996.62 should be used.
- Myocardial infarction: When the documentation indicates that the myocardial infarction is a complication from a procedure, report code 997.1 *Cardiac complications*, followed by the appropriate code from category 410 *Acute myocardial infarction* to further identify the specific complication.
- Pulmonary embolism: To report this type of complication, assign codes 997.3 *Respiratory complication* and code 415.11 *Iatrogenic pulmonary embolism and infarction*.
- Stroke: Code 997.9 *Complication affecting other specified body system, not elsewhere classified* and a code from categories 430-435 (describing the cerebral accident) should be assigned when the specific type of stroke is documented. If not, code 997.9 and code 436 *Acute but ill-defined cerebrovascular disease* should be assigned.
- Renal failure: When classifying renal failure following surgery, assign code 997.5 *Urinary complications* and the appropriate code from categories 584-586.

Postoperative Adhesions: Postoperative adhesions are adhesions of the gastrointestinal tract and are attributed to previous abdominal surgery. This condition causes abdominal pain and/or impaired bowel mobility. When the documentation indicates that the adhesions are postoperative, code 997.4 *Digestive System complications* is assigned.

Postoperative Hypertension and Hypotension: Code 997.91 is reported for postoperative hypertension. The physician must state that the hypertension was related to or was a complication of the procedure for this code to be accurately assigned. An additional code from the 401-405 series may be assigned to clarify the nature of the hypertension.

Postoperative Pain: Postoperative pain is assigned to the ICD-9-CM code that describes the pain of the specified site and not to a complication of procedures category.

Postoperative Urinary Retention: When a patient is documented as having postoperative urinary retention, code 997.5 *Urinary complications* and code 778.2x should be reported.

Subhepatic Fluid Accumulation Following Cholecystectomy: When the physician indicates that a subhepatic fluid accumulation resulted following a cholecystectomy, code 997.4 *Digestive System complications* should be assigned.

Report 530.86 for infection of esophagostomy and 530.87 for mechanical complication of esophagostomy.

Coding Scenario

Four days following a hysterectomy, a patient is complaining of urinary frequency and burning. The physician documents that she has a postoperative complication of a UTI and starts her on Bactrim DS, bid.

> Code assignment: 997.5 *Urinary complications* and 599.0 *Urinary tract infection, site unspecified*

Ten days following a below-the-knee amputation, the patient sees her physician. The physician notes that the amputation stump is not healing well and appears to be infected.

> Code assignment: 997.62 *Amputation stump complication, infection*

A 72-year-old female complaining of abdominal pain is seen by her family physician. She has a history of multiple abdominal surgeries including a hysterectomy, appendectomy, bowel resection, and

© 2004 Ingenix, Inc.

cholecystecomy. The physician documents postoperative bowel adhesions.

Code assignment: 997.4 *Digestive system complications*

998 Other complications of procedures, not elsewhere classified

AHA: Q1, 1994, 4

998.0	Postoperative shock, not elsewhere classified
998.11	Hemorrhage complicating a procedure
998.12	Hematoma complicating a procedure
998.13	Seroma complicating a procedure
998.2	Accidental puncture or laceration during procedure
998.31	Disruption of internal operation wound
998.32	Disruption of external operation wound
998.4	Foreign body accidentally left during procedure, not elsewhere classified
998.51	Infected postoperative seroma — (Use additional code to identify organism)
998.59	Other postoperative infection — (Use additional code to identify infection)
998.6	Persistent postoperative fistula, not elsewhere classified
998.7	Acute reaction to foreign substance accidentally left during procedure, not elsewhere classified
998.81	Emphysema (subcutaneous) (surgical) resulting from a procedure
998.82	Cataract fragments in eye following surgery
998.83	Non-healing surgical wound
998.89	Other specified complications
998.9	Unspecified complication of procedure, not elsewhere classified

Coding Clarification

Other Postoperative Infections: When the infection is specified as a seroma, use code 998.51 *Infected postoperative seroma* followed by a code identifying the infectious organism if known.

For other postoperative infections such as stitch abscess, intraabdominal abscess, wound abscess, or septicemia use code 998.59 *Other postoperative infection.* In addition, identify the infectious organism if known.

Postoperative Peritonitis: This condition requires the assignment of two codes. First identify the postoperative infection using code 998.59 *Postoperative infection, other postoperative infection* followed by code 567.2 *Other suppurative peritonitis.*

Coding Scenario

Two days after a bowel resection a patient has a fever and abdominal pain. The physician indicates that the patient is suffering from postoperative peritonitis.

Code assignment: 998.59 *Other postoperative infection* and 567.2 *Other suppurative peritonitis*

999 Complications of medical care, not elsewhere classified

Transfusion reactions, a major complication of medical care, is found in this category. Reaction to dialysis is another common cause of admission to acute care that falls under 999.9.

999.0	Generalized vaccinia as complication of medical care, not elsewhere classified
999.1	Air embolism as complication of medical care, not elsewhere classified
999.2	Other vascular complications of medical care, not elsewhere classified
999.3	Other infection due to medical care, not elsewhere classified
999.4	Anaphylactic shock due to serum, not elsewhere classified
999.5	Other serum reaction, not elsewhere classified
999.6	Abo incompatibility reaction, not elsewhere classified
999.7	Rh incompatibility reaction, not elsewhere classified
999.8	Other transfusion reaction, not elsewhere classified
999.9	Other and unspecified complications of medical care, not elsewhere classified

V01–V84

Supplementary Classification of Factors Influencing Health Status and Contact with Health Services

The Supplementary Classification of Factors Influencing Health Status and Contact with Health Services (V Codes) describes occasions when circumstances other than a disease or an injury justify an encounter with the health care delivery system or influence the patient's current condition.

The V codes are sequenced depending on the circumstance or problem being coded. Some V codes are sequenced first to describe the reason for the encounter, while others are sequenced second because they identify a circumstance that affects the patient's health status but is not in itself a current illness.

The V codes immediately follow the injury and poisoning codes. Only in specific circumstances are these alphanumerical codes listed as the principal diagnosis for inpatient coding or primary diagnosis for outpatient coding based on coding guidelines.

The V codes are divided into three main classifications:

1. **Problem-oriented V Code:** this type of code identifies a circumstance that could affect the patient in the future but is neither a current illness or injury. Use a V code to describe an existing circumstance or problem that may influence future medical care or a patient's health status. Problem-oriented V codes are not usually listed first on the medical claim form because they represent supplemental information. An example of this use would be in the case of a patient with a personal history of cancer. Another example would be in the case of a patient with a family history of ischemic heart disease.
2. **Service-oriented V Code:** this type of code identifies or defines examinations, aftercare, ancillary services, or therapy. Use this type of V code to describe when a person with a known disease or injury, whether it is current or resolving, encounters the health care system for a specific treatment of that disease or injury. Review the outpatient coding guidelines to determine if this type of V code can be used as the primary diagnosis. Examples of when to use a service-oriented V code would be in the case of patient sterilization and in patient orthopaedic aftercare.
3. **Fact-oriented V Code:** this type of code does not describe a problem or a service; it simply states a fact. This type of code generally does not serve as an outpatient or inpatient principal diagnosis. Categories V30-V39 are applied to all live births (fourth and fifth digits) and are always the principal diagnosis if the birth occurred during admission. Categories V40-V49 classify conditions that may influence a patient's health status, such as the presence of a cardiac pacemaker or colostomy.

V01–V06 Persons with Potential Health Hazards Related to Communicable Diseases

This category identifies patients with potential health risks from communicable diseases or diseases that are transferable from one person to another. This includes contact with someone who has the disease, a person who is a carrier of an infectious disease (caused or transferred by infection), or someone in need of preventive immunizations.

Preventive immunizations are the introduction of an immunity and may be active or passive. Active immunizations stimulate the immune system to give protection against disease. Usually this is performed by the administration of a vaccine or toxoid. A passive immunization takes lymphoid cells or serum from immune individuals and administers them to nonimmune individuals to provide specific immune reactivity.

V01 Contact with or exposure to communicable diseases

A communicable disease is an infectious disease that can be transferred from one person to another. In most cases, the patient's immune system can successfully defeat the infective agent. In this instance, the patient may test positive for exposure to

V Codes

the disease but show no symptoms of the active disease. Factors that can influence a person's ability to resist an infection are age, underlying diseases, or some types of current medical treatments. The following codes are used for patients who have been exposed to an infectious disease but have not contracted the condition.

V01.0 Contact with or exposure to cholera — *spread though food, water contaminated with feces of infected person*
AHA: Jan-Feb, 1987, 8

V01.1 Contact with or exposure to tuberculosis — *macrophages, immune cells that detect and destroy foreign matter, ingest the TB bacteria and transport them to the lymph nodes*
AHA: Jan-Feb, 1987, 8

V01.2 Contact with or exposure to poliomyelitis — *polio enters the body through the digestive tract and spreads along nerve cells*
AHA: Jan-Feb, 1987, 8

V01.3 Contact with or exposure to smallpox — *smallpox can be transmitted by infected blankets, linens and clothing*
AHA: Jan-Feb, 1987, 8

V01.4 Contact with or exposure to rubella — *also called German measles*
AHA: Jan-Feb, 1987, 8

V01.5 Contact with or exposure to rabies — *caused by neurotropic virus found in the saliva of rabid animals*
AHA: Jan-Feb, 1987, 8

V01.6 Contact with or exposure to venereal diseases — *caused by sexual contact with infected person or can be transferred from mother to baby*
AHA: Jan-Feb, 1987, 8

V01.71 Contact or exposure to varicella

V01.79 Contact or exposure to other viral diseases

V01.81 Contact with or exposure to anthrax — *can enter the body through a cut in the skin, inhalation, and/or gastrointestinally*
AHA: Jan-Feb, 1987, 8; July-Aug, 1987, 24; Q4, 2002, 70,78

V01.82 Exposure to SARS-associated coronavirus — *Severe Acute Respiratory Syndrome*
AHA: Q4, 2003, 46-47

V01.83 Contact or exposure to Escherichia coli (E. coli)

V01.84 Contact or exposure to meningococcus

V01.89 Contact or exposure to other communicable diseases

V01.9 Contact with or exposure to unspecified communicable disease

Documentation Issues

Documentation should state that the person was exposed to the disease and does not have any acute symptoms at this time.

Coding Clarification

Category V01 codes may be used as the first diagnosis listed or as an additional diagnosis.

These codes exclude V18.8 *Family history of infectious and parasitic diseases* and V12.0 *Personal history of infectious and parasitic diseases.*

Coding Scenario

A patient presents to the physician after traveling to Asia and was exposed to SARS. The patient does not have current symptoms of the disease.

> Code assignment: V01.82 *Exposure to SARS-associated coronavirus*

V02 Carrier or suspected carrier of infectious diseases

A carrier of infectious diseases has a specific disease even though he or she does not exhibit signs or symptoms of the disease. A suspected carrier is one who has been in contact with an individual who has an infectious disease, but does not have signs or symptoms. This person is capable of spreading the disease to others. Some of these diseases can be spread from an asymptomatic mother to an unborn child.

V02.0 Carrier or suspected carrier of cholera — *infection of the bowel caused by Vibrio cholerae*
AHA: Jan-Feb, 1987, 8; Q3, 1994, 4; Q3, 1995, 18

V02.1 Carrier or suspected carrier of typhoid — *systemic bacterial disease caused by the human strain of Salmonella typhi*
AHA: Jan-Feb, 1987, 8; Q3, 1994, 4; Q3, 1995, 18

V02.2 Carrier or suspected carrier of amebiasis — *amebiasis protozoa can live in the large intestine without causing symptoms.*
AHA: Jan-Feb, 1987, 8; Q3, 1994, 4; Q3, 1995, 18

V02.3 Carrier or suspected carrier of other gastrointestinal pathogens

V02.4 Carrier or suspected carrier of diphtheria — *caused by Corynebacterium diphtheriae.*
AHA: Jan-Feb, 1987, 8; Q3, 1994, 4; Q3, 1995, 18

V02.51 Carrier or suspected carrier of Group B streptococcus — *common pharyngeal infection*
AHA: Jan-Feb, 1987, 8; Q3, 1994, 4; Q3, 1995, 18; Q4, 1998, 56; Q1, 2002, 14

© 2004 Ingenix, Inc.

V02.52 Carrier or suspected carrier of other streptococcus

V02.59 Carrier or suspected carrier of other specified bacterial diseases

V02.6 5th Carrier or suspected carrier of viral hepatitis — *can be transmitted through contaminated blood, fecal contamination, and raw shellfish*
AHA: Jan-Feb, 1987, 8; Q3, 1994, 4; Q3, 1995, 18

V02.60 Unspecified viral hepatitis carrier

V02.61 Hepatitis B carrier — *limited to direct contact with blood or blood products or sexual contact*
AHA: Jan-Feb, 1987, 8; Q3, 1994, 4; Q3, 1995, 18; Q4, 1997, 47

V02.62 Hepatitis C carrier — *eighty percent of cases result from blood transfusions*
AHA: Jan-Feb, 1987, 8; Q3, 1994, 4; Q3, 1995, 18; Q4, 1997, 47

V02.69 Other viral hepatitis carrier

V02.7 Carrier or suspected carrier of gonorrhea — *an acute infection caused by Neisseria Gonorrhoeae, usually transmitted sexually*
AHA: Jan-Feb, 1987, 8; Q3, 1994, 4; Q3, 1995, 18

V02.8 Carrier or suspected carrier of other venereal diseases

V02.9 Carrier or suspected carrier of other specified infectious organism

Documentation Issues

Documentation should include that the patient is a confirmed carrier or suspected carrier of the disease.

Coding Clarification

Category V02 codes may be used as the first diagnosis listed or as an additional diagnosis.

Coding Scenario

A heath care worker is suspected of carrying group B streptococcus.

Code assignment: V02.51 *Carrier or suspected carrier of group B streptococcus*

V03 Need for prophylactic vaccination and inoculation against bacterial diseases

Vaccinations help the body fight off specific diseases. The vaccine contains weakened or dead bacteria, viruses, or toxins. Vaccines can be given orally, intramuscularly, or by subcutaneous injection. Once the immunization is given, the body creates antibodies against the vaccine, which provides immunity to the patient. Most immunizations are given during the early childhood years. However, some vaccinations such as for influenza and pneumonia are recommended for adults. Often more than one vaccine is included in one injection.

V03.0 Need for prophylactic vaccination and inoculation against cholera alone — *Vibrio cholerae*
AHA: Jan-Feb, 1987, 8

V03.1 Need for prophylactic vaccination with typhoid-paratyphiod alone (TAB) — *systemic bacterial disease caused by the human strain of Salmonella typhi*
AHA: Jan-Feb, 1987, 8

V03.2 Need for prophylactic vaccination with tuberculosis (BCG) vaccine — *Tuberculin bacillus*
AHA: Jan-Feb, 1987, 8

V03.3 Need for prophylactic vaccination and inoculation against plague — *Yersinia pestis carried by rodents*
AHA: Jan-Feb, 1987, 8

V03.4 Need for prophylactic vaccination and inoculation against tularemia — *Francisella tularensis*
AHA: Jan-Feb, 1987, 8

V03.5 Need for prophylactic vaccination and inoculation against diphtheria alone — *Corynebacterium diphtheria*
AHA: Jan-Feb, 1987, 8

V03.6 Need for prophylactic vaccination and inoculation against pertussis alone — *whooping cough*
AHA: Jan-Feb, 1987, 8

V03.7 Need for prophylactic vaccination with tetanus toxoid alone — *caused by spore-forming bacillus Clostridium tetani, lock jaw*
AHA: Jan-Feb, 1987, 8

V03.81 Need for prophylatic vaccination against Hemophilus influenza type B (Hib) — *can cause meningitis*
AHA: Jan-Feb, 1987, 8

V03.82 Need for prophylatic vaccination against Streptococcus pneumoniae (pneumococcus) — *kills more people a year than any other disease that may be prevented by vaccination*
AHA: Jan-Feb, 1987, 8

V03.89 Need for prophylatic vaccination against other specified vaccination

V03.9 Need for prophylactic vaccination and inoculation against unspecified single bacterial disease

Coding Clarification

If a contraindication is evident in the patient, whether it is because of another condition or the patient's wishes, it should be coded with V64.0 *Vaccination not carried out because of contraindication.* Vaccinations

V Codes

against combinations of diseases should be coded with V06.0-V06.9.

If the disease is currently an active disease, codes 001.0-041.2 should be reported.

Coding Scenario

An elderly woman presents to the physician for her pneumococcal vaccination.

> Code assignment: V03.82 *Need for prophylactic vaccination against Streptococcus pneumoniae (pneumococcus)*

V04 Need for prophylactic vaccination and inoculation against certain viral diseases

V04.0 Need for prophylactic vaccination and inoculation against poliomyelitis — *polio lives in the throat and intestinal tract*
AHA: Jan-Feb, 1987, 8

V04.1 Need for prophylactic vaccination and inoculation against smallpox — *variolae major; variolae minor*
AHA: Jan-Feb, 1987, 8

V04.2 Need for prophylactic vaccination and inoculation against measles alone — *spreads very easily*
AHA: Jan-Feb, 1987, 8

V04.3 Need for prophylactic vaccination and inoculation against rubella alone — *can cause birth defects in unborn children*
AHA: Jan-Feb, 1987, 8

V04.4 Need for prophylactic vaccination and inoculation against yellow fever — *transmitted by mosquitos*
AHA: Jan-Feb, 1987, 8

V04.5 Need for prophylactic vaccination and inoculation against rabies — *causes acute encephalitis*
AHA: Jan-Feb, 1987, 8

V04.6 Need for prophylactic vaccination and inoculation against mumps alone — *spread through the air by coughing, sneezing, or talking*
AHA: Jan-Feb, 1987, 8

V04.7 Need for prophylactic vaccination and inoculation against common cold — *several hundreds of strains of the virus*
AHA: Jan-Feb, 1987, 8

V04.81 Need for prophylactic vaccination and inoculation, Influenza — *can be dangerous for elderly*

V04.82 Need for prophylactic vaccination and inoculation, Respiratory syncytial virus [RSV] — *most children are affected by a mild form of the virus*

V04.89 Need for prophylactic vaccination and inoculation, Other viral diseases

Coding Clarification

If a contraindication is evident in the patient, whether it is because of another condition or the patient's wishes, it should be coded with V64.0 *Vaccination not carried out because of contraindication.* Vaccinations against combinations of diseases should be coded with V06.0-V06.9.

Coding Scenario

A man traveling to South America presents for a yellow fever vaccination.

> Code assignment: V04.4 *Need for prophylactic vaccination and inoculation against yellow fever*

V05 Need for other prophylactic vaccination and inoculation against single diseases

V05.0 Need for prophylactic vaccination and inoculation against arthropod-borne viral encephalitis — *affects animals, wild birds, and transmitted by blood-sucking insects*
AHA: Jan-Feb, 1987, 8

V05.1 Need for prophylactic vaccination and inoculation against other arthropod-borne viral diseases

V05.2 Need for prophylactic vaccination and inoculation against Leishmaniasis — *causes lesions that look like leprosy*
AHA: Jan-Feb, 1987, 8

V05.3 Need for prophylactic vaccination and inoculation against viral hepatitis — *can be caused by IV drug use and unprotected sex*
AHA: Jan-Feb, 1987, 8

V05.4 Need for prophylactic vaccination and inoculation against varicella — *also called chicken pox*
AHA: Jan-Feb, 1987, 8

V05.8 Need for prophylactic vaccination and inoculation against other specified disease

V05.9 Need for prophylactic vaccination and inoculation against unspecified single disease

Coding Clarification

If a contraindication is evident in the patient, whether it is because of another condition or the patient's wishes, it should be coded with V64.0 *Vaccination not carried out because of contraindication.* Vaccinations against combinations of diseases should be coded with V06.0-V06.9.

V Codes

© 2004 Ingenix, Inc.

V06 Need for prophylactic vaccination and inoculation against combinations of diseases

AHA: Jan-Feb, 1987, 8

V06.0 Need for prophylactic vaccination against cholera with typhoid-paratyphoid (cholera + TAB) vaccine — (Use additional single vaccination codes from categories V03-V05 to identify any vaccinations not included in a combination code)

V06.1 Vaccination and inoculation need, prophylactic, combined diphtheria-tetanus-pertussis [DTP] [DTaP] — (Use additional single vaccination codes from categories V03-V05 to identify any vaccinations not included in a combination code)

V06.2 Need for prophylactic vaccination with diptheria-tetanus-pertussis with typhoid-paratyphoid (DTP + TAB) vaccine

V06.3 Need for prophylactic vaccination with diptheria-tetanus-pertussis with poliomyelitis (DTP + polio) vaccine — (Use additional single vaccination codes from categories V03-V05 to identify any vaccinations not included in a combination code)

V06.4 Need for prophylactic vaccination with measles-mumps-rubella (MMR) vaccine — (Use additional single vaccination codes from categories V03-V05 to identify any vaccinations not included in a combination code)

V06.5 Vaccination and inoculation need, prophylactic, tetanus-diphtheria [Td] [DT] — (Use additional single vaccination codes from categories V03-V05 to identify any vaccinations not included in a combination code)

V06.6 Need for prophylactic vaccination with Streptococcus pneumoniae (pneumococcus) and influenza — (Use additional single vaccination codes from categories V03-V05 to identify any vaccinations not included in a combination code)

V06.8 Need for prophylactic vaccination and inoculation against other combinations of diseases — (Use additional single vaccination codes from categories V03-V05 to identify any vaccinations not included in a combination code)

V06.9 Need for prophylactic vaccination with unspecified combined vaccine — (Use additional single vaccination codes from categories V03-V05 to identify any vaccinations not included in a combination code)

Documentation Issues

Combination vaccines should be clearly documented. Some vaccines are administered alone and some are combined into one injection.

Coding Clarification

If any additional vaccinations are given to the patient that are not included in the combination codes, they should be reported separately with V03-V05.

This category excludes V18.8 *Family history of infectious and parasitic diseases* and V12.0 *Personal history of infectious and parasitic diseases.*

Code V06.8 *Need for prophylactic vaccination and inoculation against other combinations of diseases* excludes multiple single-vaccination codes V03.0-V05.9.

Coding Scenario

A patient presents for routine Td administration.

> Code assignment: V06.5 *Vaccination and inoculation need, prophylactic, tetanus-diphtheria [Td] [DT]*

V07–V09 Persons with Need for Isolation, Other Potential Health Hazards and Prophylactic Measures

Isolation is provided to patients in cases where the patient has been exposed to a disease that could be transferred from one person to another or to protect a person from his or her surroundings.

Patients who have allergies to specific items (trees, plants, etc.) are typically given a series of shots over a period of time to improve their immunity or to desensitize their allergies.

Prophylactic measures include the administration of a substance for prevention of certain diseases or conditions, such as antivenin, RhoGAM, or tetanus administration in prophylactic immunotherapy.

V07 Need for isolation and other prophylactic measures

Isolation may be necessary to protect a patient from contamination or to protect other people from a patient who has been exposed to a highly transmissible disease. Isolation is designed to prevent the spread of a disease from one person to another. A person may contract an infectious disease by any of the following ways:

- Inhalation of air-borne evaporated or nonevaporated droplets or dust particles carrying microorganisms or spores, such as a sneeze from an infected patient
- Transmission from one host to another by a carrier of the disease, such as a mosquito

V Codes

- Ingestion of a microorganism transmitted through water, such as when bathing

Some patients are more at risk of infection due to age, current state of health, and indwelling devices, such as catheters. Patients may be put in isolation while conditions are ruled out. Patients who are immunocompromised may be very susceptible to infections. Prophylactic isolation or other measures may be necessary to protect the patient.

V07.0 Need for isolation — *separating a patient from others*
AHA: Jan-Feb, 1987, 8

V07.1 Need for desensitization to allergens — *gradual administration of allergens to prevent severe allergic reactions*
AHA: Jan-Feb, 1987, 8

V07.2 Need for prophylactic immunotherapy — *therapeutic administration of serum containing antibodies to strengthen immune system*
AHA: Jan-Feb, 1987, 8

V07.31 Need for prophylactic fluoride administration — *for the prevention of cavities*
AHA: Jan-Feb, 1987, 8

V07.39 Need for other prophylactic chemotherapy — *may be given for hydatidiform mole*
AHA: Jan-Feb, 1987, 8

V07.4 Hormone replacement therapy (postmenopausal)

V07.8 Need for other specified prophylactic measure

V07.9 Need for unspecified prophylactic measure

Coding Clarification
If the patient is isolated as a result of terrorist acts, report V07.0 *Need for isolation.*

Use V07.2 *Need for prophylactic immunotherapy* for the administration of antivenin, immune sera (gamma globulin) RhoGAM, or tetanus antitoxin.

Coding Scenario
A woman presents to the OB/GYN clinic 48 hours after the birth of her baby for a postpartum injection of RhoGAM.

> Code assignment: V07.2 *Need for prophylactic immunotherapy*

V08 Asymptomatic human immunodeficiency virus (HIV) infection status OK

Human immunodeficiency virus (HIV) is a serious health concern. Two types of HIV are known to exist: HIV-1 and HIV-2. HIV-1 is widespread throughout the world and causes acquired immune deficiency syndrome (AIDS). HIV-2 is found primarily in West Africa and is seldom seen in the United States. Category V08 should be used during the first phase when the patient is asymptomatic. This usually occurs four weeks to six months after infected with HIV-1.

Documentation Issues
Documentation should clearly state that the patient is HIV positive but does not have and has never had any HIV -related illness.

Coding Clarification
Use this code when the patient presents with no HIV symptoms or conditions although the patient tests positive for HIV. If the patient has HIV symptoms or conditions, report 042. For exposure to HIV, use V01.7. For nonspecific serologic evidence of HIV, use 795.71.

Coding Scenario
An asymptomatic 23-year-old male presents for a follow-up of his HIV medication. The patient tested positive for HIV but reports that he has had no symptoms.

> Code assignment: V08 *Asymptomatic human immunodeficiency virus (HIV) infection status*

V09 Infection with drug-resistent microorganisms

AHA: Jan-Feb, 1987, 8; Q4, 1993, 22; Q3, 1994, 4

Since the availability of penicillin and streptomycin, drug-resistance bacteria, parasites, viruses, and fungi have increasingly become a problem. Because of this, many common bacterial infections that were treated with antibiotics may become untreatable. Many of the new drugs used to treat drug-resistant diseases are expensive, which may limit the treatment of some patients. Drug resistance occurs as a result of overuse or underuse of antibiotic drugs, or from patients not completing treatment as prescribed. Health care professionals are more aware of drug resistance and are responding to this problem. New drugs are being developed to help fight these drug-resistant infections.

V09.0 Infection with microorganisms resistant to penicillins — (Use codes from this category as an additional code for infectious conditions classified elsewhere to indicate drug-resistance of the infectious organism)
AHA: Jan-Feb, 1987, 8; Q4, 1993, 22; Q3, 1994, 4; Q4, 2003, 104, 106

V09.1 Infection with microorganisms resistant to cephalosporins and other B-lactam antibiotics — (Use this code as an additional code for infectious conditions classified elsewhere to indicate drug-resistance of the infectious organism)
AHA: Jan-Feb, 1987, 8; Q4, 1993, 22; Q3, 1994, 4

V Codes

 © 2004 Ingenix, Inc.

V09.2 Infection with microorganisms resistant to macrolides — (Use this code as an additional code for infectious conditions classified elsewhere to indicate drug-resistance of the infectious organism)
AHA: Jan-Feb, 1987, 8; Q4, 1993, 22; Q3, 1994, 4

V09.3 Infection with microorganisms resistant to tetracyclines — (Use this code as an additional code for infectious conditions classified elsewhere to indicate drug-resistance of the infectious organism)
AHA: Jan-Feb, 1987, 8; Q4, 1993, 22; Q3, 1994, 4

V09.4 Infection with microorganisms resistant to aminoglycosides — (Use this code as an additional code for infectious conditions classified elsewhere to indicate drug-resistance of the infectious organism)
AHA: Jan-Feb, 1987, 8; Q4, 1993, 22; Q3, 1994, 4

V09.50 Infection with microorganisms resistant to quinolones and fluoroquinolones without mention of resistance to multiple quinolones and fluoroquinolones

V09.51 Infection with microorganisms resistant to quinolones and fluoroquinolones with resistance to multiple quinolones and fluoroquinolones

V09.6 Infection with microorganisms resistant to sulfonamides — (Use this code as an additional code for infectious conditions classified elsewhere to indicate drug-resistance of the infectious organism)
AHA: Jan-Feb, 1987, 8; Q4, 1993, 22; Q3, 1994, 4

V09.70 Infection with microorganisms resistant to other specified antimycobacterial agents without mention of resistance to multiple antimycobacterial agents

V09.71 Infection with microorganisms resistant to other specified antimycobacterial agents with resistance to multiple antimycobacterial agents

V09.80 Infection with microorganisms resistant to other specified drugs without mention of resistance to multiple drugs

V09.81 Infection with microorganisms resistant to other specified drugs with resistance to multiple drugs — (Use this code as an additional code for infectious conditions classified elsewhere to indicate drug-resistance of the infectious organism)

V09.90 Infection with unspecified drug-resistant microorganisms, without mention of multiple drug resistance — (Use this code as an additional code for infectious conditions classified elsewhere to indicate drug-resistance of the infectious organism)

V09.91 Infection with unspecified drug-resistant microorganisms, with multiple drug resistance — (Use this code as an additional code for infectious conditions classified elsewhere to indicate drug-resistance of the infectious organism)

Coding Clarification

The infectious condition should be coded first; category V09 may be used only as a secondary diagnosis.

Code V09.4 *Infection with microorganisms resistant to aminoglycosides* includes amikacin, kanamycin, and streptomycin.

Coding Scenario

A patient is in for a follow-up of lobar pneumonia. A recent sputum culture identified *Streptococcus pneumoniae* as the infecting organism with resistance to penicillin.

> Code assignment: 481 *Pneumococcal pneumonia (Streptococcus pneumoniae pneumonia)* and V09.0 *Infection with microorganisms resistant to penicillins*

V10–V19 Persons with Potential Health Hazards Related to Personal and Family History

Cateogies V10-V19 contain personal and family history codes. Personal history codes include a history of neoplasms, mental disorders, diseases, and allergies. Family history codes include a history of neoplasms and diseases. Personal history codes are often reported to indicate the need for adjunctive surgery and treatment; family history codes are often used to indicate the need for prophylactic surgery and treatment. Family history codes are frequently used with screening codes to justify a test or procedure. This range of codes should be used as secondary codes if the historical condition or family history has an impact on current care or influences treatment.

V10 Personal history of malignant neoplasm

In a malignancy, the neoplasm invades surrounding tissue or sheds cells that seed malignancy in other body sites. Codes in the V10 category describe a personal history of a malignant neoplasm. A personal history of malignant neoplasms identifies a malignancy that has been previously treated or removed but for which there is no current treatment for the condition and no evidence of the disease.

V Codes

V10.0 [5th] Personal history of malignant neoplasm of gastrointestinal tract — *history of conditions reported by 140-159*
AHA: May-June, 1985, 10; Jan-Feb, 1987, 1, 8; Q2, 1990, 9; Q3, 1992, 5; Q1, 1995, 4; Q4, 1998, 69; Q4, 2002, 80

V10.00 Personal history of malignant neoplasm of unspecified site in gastrointestinal tract

V10.01 Personal history of malignant neoplasm of tongue

V10.02 Personal history of malignant neoplasm of other and unspecified parts of oral cavity and pharynx

V10.03 Personal history of malignant neoplasm of esophagus

V10.04 Personal history of malignant neoplasm of stomach

V10.05 Personal history of malignant neoplasm of large intestine

V10.06 Personal history of malignant neoplasm of rectum, rectosigmoid junction, and anus

V10.07 Personal history of malignant neoplasm of liver

V10.09 Personal history of malignant neoplasm of other site in gastrointestinal tract

V10.1 [5th] Personal history of malignant neoplasm of trachea, bronchus, and lung — *history of conditions reported by 162*
AHA: May-June, 1985, 10; Jan-Feb, 1987, 1, 8; Q2, 1990, 9; Q3, 1992, 5; Q1, 1995, 4; Q4, 1998, 69; Q4, 2002, 80

V10.11 Personal history of malignant neoplasm of bronchus and lung

V10.12 Personal history of malignant neoplasm of trachea

V10.2 [5th] Personal history of malignant neoplasm of other respiratory and intrathoracic organs — *history of conditions reported as 160, 161, 163-165*
AHA: May-June, 1985, 10; Jan-Feb, 1987, 1, 8; Q2, 1990, 9; Q3, 1992, 5; Q1, 1995, 4; Q4, 1998, 69; Q4, 2002, 80

V10.20 Personal history of malignant neoplasm of unspecified respiratory organ

V10.21 Personal history of malignant neoplasm of larynx

V10.22 Personal history of malignant neoplasm of nasal cavities, middle ear, and accessory sinuses

V10.29 Personal history of malignant neoplasm of other respiratory and intrathoracic organs

V10.3 Personal history of malignant neoplasm of breast — *history of conditions reported by 174 and 175*
AHA: May-June, 1985, 10; Jan-Feb, 1987, 1, 8; Q1, 1990, 21; Q2, 1990, 9; Q1, 1991, 16; Q3, 1992, 5; Q1, 1995, 4; Q4, 1997, 50; Q4, 1998, 65; Q4, 1998, 69; Q4, 2001, 66; Q4, 2002, 80; Q2, 2003, 5

V10.4 [5th] Personal history of malignant neoplasm of genital organs — *history of conditions reported by 179-187*
AHA: May-June, 1985, 10; Jan-Feb, 1987, 1, 8; Q2, 1990, 9; Q3, 1992, 5; Q1, 1995, 4; Q4, 1998, 69; Q4, 2002, 80

V10.40 Personal history of malignant neoplasm of unspecified female genital organ

V10.41 Personal history of malignant neoplasm of cervix uteri

V10.42 Personal history of malignant neoplasm of other parts of uterus

V10.43 Personal history of malignant neoplasm of ovary

V10.44 Personal history of malignant neoplasm of other female genital organs

V10.45 Personal history of malignant neoplasm of unspecified male genital organ

V10.46 Personal history of malignant neoplasm of prostate

V10.47 Personal history of malignant neoplasm of testis

V10.48 Personal history of malignant neoplasm of epididymis

V10.49 Personal history of malignant neoplasm of other male genital organs

V10.5 [5th] Personal history of malignant neoplasm of urinary organs — *history of conditions reported by 188 and 189*
AHA: May-June, 1985, 10; Jan-Feb, 1987, 1, 8; Q2, 1990, 9; Q3, 1992, 5; Q1, 1995, 4; Q4, 1998, 69; Q4, 2002, 80

V10.50 Personal history of malignant neoplasm of unspecified urinary organ

V10.51 Personal history of malignant neoplasm of bladder

V10.52 Personal history of malignant neoplasm of kidney

V10.53 Personal history of malignant neoplasm, renal pelvis

V10.59 Personal history of malignant neoplasm of other urinary organ

V10.6 [5th] Personal history of leukemia — *history of conditions reported as 204-208*
AHA: May-June, 1985, 10; Jan-Feb, 1987, 1, 8; Q2, 1990, 9; Q4, 1990, 3; Q4, 1991, 26; Q2, 1992, 13; Q3, 1992, 5; Q1, 1995, 4; Q4, 1998, 69; Q4, 2002, 80

V Codes

© 2004 Ingenix, Inc.

V10.60 Personal history of unspecified leukemia

V10.61 Personal history of lymphoid leukemia

V10.62 Personal history of myeloid leukemia

V10.63 Personal history of monocytic leukemia

V10.69 Personal history of other leukemia

V10.7 5th Personal history of other lymphatic and hematopoietic neoplasms — *history of conditions reported as 200-203*
AHA: May-June, 1985, 10; May-June, 1985, 18; Jan-Feb, 1987, 1, 8; Q2, 1990, 9; Q3, 1992, 5; Q1, 1995, 4; Q4, 1998, 69; Q4, 2002, 80

V10.71 Personal history of lymphosarcoma and reticulosarcoma

V10.72 Personal history of Hodgkin's disease

V10.79 Personal history of other lymphatic and hematopoietic neoplasm

V10.8 5th Personal history of malignant neoplasm of other sites — *history of conditions reported by 170-173, 190-195*
AHA: May-June, 1985, 10; Jan-Feb, 1987, 1, 8; Q2, 1990, 9; Q3, 1992, 5; Q1, 1995, 4; Q4, 1998, 69; Q4, 2002, 80

V10.81 Personal history of malignant neoplasm of bone

V10.82 Personal history of malignant melanoma of skin

V10.83 Personal history of other malignant neoplasm of skin

V10.84 Personal history of malignant neoplasm of eye

V10.85 Personal history of malignant neoplasm of brain

V10.86 Personal history of malignant neoplasm of other parts of nervous system

V10.87 Personal history of malignant neoplasm of thyroid

V10.88 Personal history of malignant neoplasm of other endocrine glands and related structures

V10.89 Personal history of malignant neoplasm of other site

V10.9 Unspecified personal history of malignant neoplasm

Documentation Issues

Documentation should include that the malignancy has resolved and there is no further treatment directed at the site.

Coding Clarification

These codes should never be used if active disease is present. When a previously excised malignant neoplasm recurs at the same site, it is still considered a primary malignancy of that site and the history code should not be used. If the malignant neoplasm recurs at a different site, it is reported as a secondary malignant neoplasm and an additional code to identify a history of the malignancy site is reported using category V10.

Report V10.89 for a personal history of a malignant neoplasm of the peripheral, sympathetic, and parasympathetic nerves.

For leukemia in remission, report 204.xx-208.xx. For lymphatic and hematopoietic neoplasms in remission, report 200.xx-203.xx.

Observation of obstetric patients where the malignancy might affect the fetus should be reported with 655.0-655.9.

Coding Scenario

A 70-year-old female patient is admitted for a biopsy of a mass in the right breast. Ten years ago, the patient was treated with lumpectomy and chemotherapy for a malignancy in the left breast. The pathology report stated the right breast mass was benign.

> Code assignment: 217 *Benign neoplasms of the breast* and V10.3 *Personal history of malignant neoplasm of breast*

V11 Personal history of mental disorder

Mental illness covers a broad range of conditions. The causes of mental illness are not well understood. Some believe it is a functioning of the neurotransmitters in the brain; others believe that stress, drugs, and heredity may play a role in mental illness. Because heredity is believed to be a factor in mental illness, code the family history of mental illness when appropriate. Although prescription drugs may help, there is no known cure for these conditions.

V11.0 Personal history of schizophrenia — *withdraw into world of delusions*
AHA: Jan-Feb, 1987, 1, 8

V11.1 Personal history of affective disorder — *pertaining to mood*
AHA: Jan-Feb, 1987, 1, 8

V11.2 Personal history of neurosis — *anxiety, nervous disease*
AHA: Jan-Feb, 1987, 1, 8

V11.3 Personal history of alcoholism — *alcohol addiction*
AHA: Jan-Feb, 1987, 1, 8

V11.8 Personal history of other mental disorder

V11.9 Personal history of unspecified mental disorder

V Codes

Documentation Issues
Documentation should include dates of illness, treatment, and that the illness is no longer present.

Coding Clarification
For patients who have a personal history of schizophrenia, but are in remission, report 295.0x-295.9x with a fifth digit of 5. For patients who have a personal history of manic-depressive psychosis, but are in remission, report 296.0x-296.6x with a fifth digit of 5 or 6.

Category V11 codes may not be listed as the principal or primary diagnosis.

Coding Scenario
A 75-year-old male presents from the nursing home with intermittent altered mental status. Past history includes alcoholism, although the patient went through a treatment program 10 years ago and has been clean and sober since. Blood alcohol is negative.

> Code assignment: 780.02 *Transient alteration of awareness* and V11.3 *Personal history of alcoholism*

V12 Personal history of certain other diseases

This category of codes is used to report that the patient had a particular disease but that the disease is no longer present and the patient is no longer receiving treatment for the illness.

V12.0 5th Personal history of infectious and parasitic diseases — *disease capable of being transmitted from one person to another or disease caused by a parasite*
AHA: Jan-Feb, 1987, 1, 8; Q3, 1992, 11

V12.00 Personal history of unspecified infectious and parasitic disease

V12.01 Personal history of tuberculosis — *infection by Mycobacterium tuberculosis*
AHA: Jan-Feb, 1987, 1, 8; Q3, 1992, 11

V12.02 Personal history of poliomyelitis — *polio enters the body through the digestive tract and spreads along nerve cells*
AHA: Jan-Feb, 1987, 1, 8; Q3, 1992, 11

V12.03 Personal history of malaria — *caused by a parasite*
AHA: Jan-Feb, 1987, 1, 8; Q3, 1992, 11

V12.09 Personal history of other infectious and parasitic disease

V12.1 Personal history of nutritional deficiency — *deprived of nutrition for an extended period of time*
AHA: Jan-Feb, 1987, 1, 8; Q3, 1992, 11

V12.2 Personal history of endocrine, metabolic, and immunity disorders

V12.3 Personal history of diseases of blood and blood-forming organs

V12.40 Unspecified disorer of nervous system and sense organs

V12.41 Benign neoplasm of the brain — *growth in the brain that is not malignant*
AHA: Jan-Feb, 1987, 1, 8; Q3, 1992, 11; Q4, 1997, 48

V12.49 Other disorders of nervous system and sense organs

V12.5 5th Personal history of diseases of circulatory system — *related to blood flow throughout the body*
AHA: Jan-Feb, 1987, 1, 8; Q3, 1992, 11; Q4, 1995, 61

V12.50 Unspecified circulatory disease

V12.51 Venous thrombosis and embolism — *use for pulmonary embolism*
AHA: Jan-Feb, 1987, 1, 8; Q3, 1992, 11; Q4, 1995, 61; Q1, 2002, 15; Q4, 2003, 108

V12.52 Thrombophlebitis — *inflammation of the veins with clot*
AHA: Jan-Feb, 1987, 1, 8; Q3, 1992, 11; Q4, 1995, 61

V12.59 Other diseases of circulatory system

V12.6 Personal history of diseases of respiratory system

V12.70 Personal history of unspecified digestive disease

V12.71 Personal history of peptic ulcer disease — *ulceration of the stomach*
AHA: Jan-Feb, 1987, 1, 8; Q2, 1989, 16; Q3, 1992, 11; Q1, 1995, 3

V12.72 Personal history of colonic polyps — *benign growth in the colon*
AHA: Jan-Feb, 1987, 1, 8; Q2, 1989, 16; Q3, 1992, 11; Q1, 1995, 3; Q3, 2002, 15

V12.79 Personal history of other diseases of digestive disease

Documentation Issues
Category V12 codes should be used when the presence of previous disease may affect the treatment or outcome of a current illness. The history of an illness should always be reported when documented.

Coding Clarification
Report V12.59 *Diseases of circulatory system* only when there are no lasting effects of the condition. If a patient has an old myocardial infarction, report 412; report 411.0 for postmyocardial infarction syndrome.

Coding Scenario
A patient presents to the emergency department with severe left lower abdominal pain. Past history is significant for colon polyps, which were removed a year ago.

 © 2004 Ingenix, Inc.

Code assignment: 789.04 *Pain left lower quadrant* and V12.72 *Personal history of colonic polyps*

V13 Personal history of other diseases

Personal history of other diseases codes are used to report that the patient had a particular disease but that the disease is no longer present. These codes also indicate that the patient is no longer receiving treatment for the illness.

V13.00 Personal history of unspecified urinary disorder

V13.01 Personal history of urinary calculi — *kidney stone*
AHA: Jan-Feb, 1987, 1, 8

V13.09 Personal history of other disorder of urinary system

V13.1 Personal history of trophoblastic disease — *cell layer that erodes the uterine mucosa*
AHA: Jan-Feb, 1987, 1, 8

V13.21 Personal history of pre-term labor — *22 to before 37 completed weeks of gestation*
AHA: Jan-Feb, 1987, 1, 8; Q4, 2002, 78

V13.29 Personal history of other genital system and obstetric disorders

V13.3 Personal history of diseases of skin and subcutaneous tissue

V13.4 Personal history of arthritis — *inflammation of a joint*
AHA: Jan-Feb, 1987, 1, 8

V13.5 Personal history of other musculoskeletal disorders

V13.61 Personal history of hypospadias — *urethra under the penis*
AHA: Jan-Feb, 1987, 1, 8; Q4, 1998, 63

V13.69 Personal history of other congenital malformations

V13.7 Personal history of perinatal problems

V13.8 Personal history of other specified diseases

V13.9 Personal history of unspecified disease

Documentation Issues

Category V13 codes may be documented if the presence of a previous disease may affect the treatment or outcome of a current illness.

Coding Clarification

Category V13 codes may be listed as the primary or secondary diagnosis except for V13.4 *Personal history of arthritis,* V13.61 *Personal history of hypospadias,* and V13.69 *Personal history of congenital malformations,* which can only be listed as secondary diagnoses.

Congenital malformations are typically lifelong problems and do not fall into the definition of "history." Congenital malformations such as hypospadias may be surgically repaired and would then qualify as a history as long as there are no residual or continued problems related to the malformation. Report V13.6x only if it directly affects the care of the patient.

Coding Scenario

A patient presents with right upper quadrant pain. Past medical history is significant for kidney stones, which were treated with lithotripsy.

Code assignment: 789.01 *Abdominal pain right upper quadrant* and V13.01 *Personal history of urinary calculi*

V14 Personal history of allergy to medicinal agents

Drug allergies should not be confused with normal side effects of the drug. Drug allergies can be life threatening. Symptoms of an allergy can be hives, skin rash, itching, wheezing, swelling of lips, tongue, or face, difficulty breathing, and rapid pulse. Allergic reactions are caused by an increased sensitivity of the immune system to the drug. An allergic reaction may not happen the first time the drug is taken, but as the body's immune system creates antibodies against the drug, the allergic reaction may appear in subsequent use of the drug. Treatment may include oral or topical antihistamines, nebulizer treatments, and epinephrine injections.

V14.0 Personal history of allergy to penicillin — *specific type of antibiotic*
AHA: Jan-Feb, 1987, 1, 8

V14.1 Personal history of allergy to other antibiotic agent

V14.2 Personal history of allergy to sulfonamides — *specific type of antibiotic*
AHA: Jan-Feb, 1987, 1, 8

V14.3 Personal history of allergy to other anti-infective agent

V14.4 Personal history of allergy to anesthetic agent — *usually local anesthetic*
AHA: Jan-Feb, 1987, 1, 8

V14.5 Personal history of allergy to narcotic agent

V14.6 Personal history of allergy to analgesic agent — *a chemical that reduces pain*
AHA: Jan-Feb, 1987, 1, 8

V14.7 Personal history of allergy to serum or vaccine

V14.8 Personal history of allergy to other specified medicinal agents

V14.9 Personal history of allergy to unspecified medicinal agent

Documentation Issues

Documentation should include the type and amount of the drug or agent taken and all symptoms the patient is experiencing as a result of the allergic reaction.

Coding Clarification

Codes from this category may only be reported as additional codes.

Coding Scenario

A 21-year-old female presents to the emergency department with a sore throat. A rapid strep test is given and comes up positive. Past medical history is significant for allergy to penicillin.

> Code assignment: 034.0 *Streptococcal sore throat* and V14.0 *Personal history of allergy to penicillin*

V15 Other personal history presenting hazards to health

Food allergies are caused by the body's immune system building up antibodies to the food. Children whose parents both have allergies are more likely to have allergic reactions. The most common foods to cause an allergic reaction are peanuts, milk, eggs, and shellfish. Other reactions include allergies to insect bites, latex, and iodine found in some radiographic dye. Category V15 codes also include a personal history of surgery, abuse, psychological trauma, injury, tobacco use, and exposure to harmful substances that present hazards to the patient's health.

A personal history of extracorporeal membrane oxygenation (ECMO) is also included in category V15. ECMO gives respiratory support by circulating blood through an artificial lung, consisting of two compartments separated by a gas-permeable membrane, with blood on one side and the ventilating gas on the other. This is typically given to babies, but may be used in adults with acute respiratory distress.

V15.01 Personal history of allergy to peanuts

V15.02 Personal history of allergy to milk products

V15.03 Personal history of allergy to eggs

V15.04 Personal history of allergy to seafood — *octopus, squid ink, shellfish*
AHA: Jan-Feb, 1987, 1, 8; Q4, 2000, 42, 49

V15.05 Personal history of allergy to other foods — *food additives, nuts (other than peanuts)*
AHA: Jan-Feb, 1987, 1, 8; Q4, 2000, 42, 49

V15.06 Personal history of allergy to insects — *insect bites and stings*
AHA: Jan-Feb, 1987, 1, 8; Q4, 2000, 42, 49

V15.07 Personal history of allergy to latex — *natural rubber latex allergy, type IV hypersensitivity reaction*
AHA: Jan-Feb, 1987, 1, 8; Q4, 2000, 42, 49

V15.08 Personal history of allergy to radiographic dye — *contrast media used for diagnostic x-rays*
AHA: Jan-Feb, 1987, 1, 8; Q4, 2000, 42, 49

V15.09 Personal history of other allergy, other than to medicinal agents

V15.1 Personal history of surgery to heart and great vessels, presenting hazards to health

V15.2 Personal history of surgery to other major organs, presenting hazards to health

V15.3 Personal history of irradiation, presenting hazards to health — *previous exposure to therapeutic or other ionizing radiation*
AHA: Jan-Feb, 1987, 1, 8

V15.41 Personal history of physical abuse, presenting hazards to health — *rape, domestic violence*
AHA: Jan-Feb, 1987, 1, 8; Q3, 1999, 15

V15.42 Personal history of emotional abuse, presenting hazards to health — *neglect*
AHA: Jan-Feb, 1987, 1, 8; Q3, 1999, 15

V15.49 Other personal history of psychological trauma, presenting hazards to health

V15.5 Personal history of injury, presenting hazards to health

V15.6 Personal history of poisoning, presenting hazards to health

V15.7 Personal history of contraception, presenting hazards to health

V15.81 Personal history of noncompliance with medical treatment, presenting hazards to health

V15.82 Personal history of tobacco use, presenting hazards to health

V15.84 Personal history of exposure to asbestos, presenting hazards to health

V15.85 Personal history of exposure to potentially hazardous body fluids, presenting hazards to health

V15.86 Personal history of exposure to lead, presenting hazards to health

V15.87 History of extracorporeal membrane oxygenation [ECMO]

V15.89 Other specified personal history presenting hazards to health

V15.9 Unspecified personal history presenting hazards to health

Coding Clarification

A patient that has had a past allergic reaction to a substance should always be considered allergic to that agent.

This classification of codes may only be reported as a secondary diagnosis.

Report the medical condition in addition to V15.81 *Personal history of noncompliance with medical treatment, presenting hazards to health* if the condition is caused by noncompliance to medical instructions.

© 2004 Ingenix, Inc.

V Codes

Coding Scenario

A patient presents with a productive cough, which has been present for the past three days. The past medical history is significant for a previous pack-a-day habit. The patient quit smoking one year ago.

> Code assignment: 786.2 *Cough* and V15.82 *Personal history of tobacco use, presenting hazards to health*

V16 Family history of malignant neoplasm

Many people with a family history of cancer have an increased risk of developing cancer. This is particularly true of the most common cancers of the breast, colon, ovary, and prostate. Family history codes are frequently used to indicate the need for prophylactic surgery and treatment.

V16.0 Family history of malignant neoplasm of gastrointestinal tract — *history of conditions reported by 140-159*
AHA: Jan-Feb, 1987, 1, 8; Q1, 1999, 4

V16.1 Family history of malignant neoplasm of trachea, bronchus, and lung — *history of conditions reported by 162*
AHA: Jan-Feb, 1987, 1, 8

V16.2 Family history of malignant neoplasm of other respiratory and intrathoracic organs — *history of conditions reported as 163-165*
AHA: Jan-Feb, 1987, 1, 8

V16.3 Family history of malignant neoplasm of breast — *history of conditions reported by 174*
AHA: Jan-Feb, 1987, 1, 8; Q1, 1992, 11; Q2, 2000, 8; Q2, 2003, 4

V16.4 [5th] Family history of malignant neoplasm of genital organs — *history of conditions reported by 179-187*
AHA: Jan-Feb, 1987, 1, 8; Q4, 1997, 48

V16.40 Family history of malignant neoplasm, unspecified genital organ

V16.41 Family history of malignant neoplasm, ovary

V16.42 Family history of malignant neoplasm, prostate

V16.43 Family history of malignant neoplasm, testis

V16.49 Family history of other malignant neoplasm

V16.5 [5th] Family history of malignant neoplasm of urinary organs — *history of conditions reported by 189*
AHA: Jan-Feb, 1987, 1, 8

V16.51 Family history of malignant neoplasm of kidney

V16.59 Familiy history of malignant neoplasm of other urinary organs

V16.6 Family history of leukemia — *history of conditions reported by 204-208*
AHA: Jan-Feb, 1987, 1, 8

V16.7 Family history of other lymphatic and hematopoietic neoplasms — *history of conditions reported by 200-203*
AHA: Jan-Feb, 1987, 1, 8

V16.8 Family history of other specified malignant neoplasm — *history of conditions reported by 140-199*
AHA: Jan-Feb, 1987, 1, 8

V16.9 Family history of unspecified malignant neoplasm

Documentation Issues

Documentation should include which family member had the cancer, at what age, and the outcome.

Coding Clarification

These codes are often used with screening codes, such as colonoscopy, to justify the test or procedure.

Coding Scenario

A 60-year-old female comes into the office for postmenopausal bleeding. She has a mother who died at the age of 61 of ovarian cancer.

> Code assignment: 627.1 *Postmenopausal bleeding* and V16.42 *Family history of malignant neoplasm, ovary*

V17 Family history of certain chronic disabling diseases

A family history of chronic disabling diseases includes psychiatric conditions, stroke, neurological diseases, ischemic heart disease, other cardiovascular diseases, asthma, other respiratory diseases, arthritis, and other musculoskeletal diseases. Many of these diseases are hereditary. Knowing the family history can help physicians order the appropriate screening or diagnostic tests, and diagnose and treat the patient's condition or symptoms.

V17.0 Family history of psychiatric condition — *history of conditions reported by 18.4*
AHA: Jan-Feb, 1987, 1, 8

V17.1 Family history of stroke (cerebrovascular)

V17.2 Family history of other neurological diseases — *includes epilepsy and Huntington's chorea*
AHA: Jan-Feb, 1987, 1, 8

V17.3 Family history of ischemic heart disease

V17.4 Family history of other cardiovascular diseases

V17.5 Family history of asthma

V17.6 Family history of other chronic respiratory conditions

V Codes

V17.7 Family history of arthritis

V17.8 Family history of other musculoskeletal diseases

V18 Family history of certain other specific conditions

A family history of certain other specific conditions includes diabetes mellitus, other endocrine and metabolic diseases, anemia, other blood disorders, mental retardation, digestive disorders, kidney diseases, other genitourinary diseases, and infectious and parasitic diseases. Knowing the family history can help physicians order the appropriate screening or diagnostic tests, and diagnose and treat the patient's condition or symptoms.

V18.0 Family history of diabetes mellitus

V18.1 Family history of other endocrine and metabolic diseases

V18.2 Family history of anemia

V18.3 Family history of other blood disorders

V18.4 Family history of mental retardation

V18.5 Family history of digestive disorders

V18.61 Family history of polycystic kidney

V18.69 Family history of other kidney diseases

V18.7 Family history of other genitourinary diseases

V18.8 Family history of infectious and parasitic diseases

V19 Family history of other conditions

This category includes a family history of visual loss, other eye disorders, hearing loss, other ear disorders, skin conditions, congenital anomalies, allergic disorders, consanguinity, and other conditions. Knowing the family history can help physicians order the appropriate screening or diagnostic tests, and diagnose and treat the patient's condition or symptoms.

V19.0 Family history of blindness or visual loss

V19.1 Family history of other eye disorders

V19.2 Family history of deafness or hearing loss

V19.3 Family history of other ear disorders

V19.4 Family history of skin conditions

V19.5 Family history of congenital anomalies

V19.6 Family history of allergic disorders

V19.7 Family history of consanguinity — *blood-related kin*
AHA: Jan-Feb, 1987, 1, 8

V19.8 Family history of other condition

V20–V28 Persons Encountering Health Services in Circumstances Related to Reproduction and Development

This section of codes is used to indicate the supervision of an uncomplicated pregnancy and perceived problems which, after evaluation, are determined to be normal states in development (e.g., onset of menses, teething). Codes used to report the outcome of a delivery on the mother's record (used in addition to codes from the obstetric section of ICD-9-CM) are also included.

V20 Health supervision of infant or child

Health supervision of an infant or a child involves medical or nursing care supervision of a healthy infant in cases of: physical or psychiatric maternal illness, adverse condition(s) at home, or too many children at home preventing normal care of the child. These codes include developmental testing of an infant or a child, immunizations appropriate for age, and routine vision and hearing testing.

V20.0 Health supervision of foundling

V20.1 Health supervision of other healthy infant or child receiving care

V20.2 Routine infant or child health check — (Use additional code(s) to identify special screening exams performed: V73.0-V82.9)

Coding Clarification

Category V20 codes may only be reported as the primary diagnosis. Use additional codes to identify any special screening examinations performed.

Code V20.1 *Health supervision of other healthy infant or child receiving care* should not be reported on the baby's record after a routine C-section.

V21 Constitutional states in development

Constitutional states describe developmental conditions of a child during the growth period. This includes rapid growth, puberty, other development of adolescence, and low birth weight. Low birth weight status, which is 2,500 grams (5.59 pounds) or less, may affect the patient's health throughout life.

V21.0 Period of rapid growth in childhood

V21.1 Puberty — *sexual maturity*
AHA: Jan-Feb, 1987, 8

V21.2 Other development of adolescence — *period beginning at puberty and ending at maturity*
AHA: Jan-Feb, 1987, 8

V21.30 Low birth weight status, unspecified

© 2004 Ingenix, Inc.

V21.31 Low birth weight status, less than 500 grams — *1.1 pounds or less*
AHA: Jan-Feb, 1987, 8; Q4, 2000, 51

V21.32 Low birth weight status, 500-999 grams — *1.68-2.23 pounds*
AHA: Jan-Feb, 1987, 8; Q4, 2000, 51

V21.33 Low birth weight status, 1000-1499 grams — *2.24-3.34 pounds*
AHA: Jan-Feb, 1987, 8; Q4, 2000, 51

V21.34 Low birth weight status, 1500-1999 grams — *3.35-4.5 pounds*
AHA: Jan-Feb, 1987, 8; Q4, 2000, 51

V21.35 Low birth weight status, 2000-2500 grams — *4.51-5.58 pounds*
AHA: Jan-Feb, 1987, 8; Q4, 2000, 51

V21.8 Other specified constitutional states in development

V21.9 Unspecified constitutional state in development

Coding Clarification

Do not report status V codes for patients who have a condition that is classifiable to perinatal codes 760-779.

Report low birth weight status codes for patients who no longer have the condition but exhibit the consequences throughout life. Code V21.3 *Low birth weight status* excludes a history of perinatal problems.

V22 Normal pregnancy

Normal pregnancies occur when there is no condition or problem that complicates the pregnancy. Complications may include ectopic and molar pregnancy, hydatidiform mole, spontaneous abortion, ectopic pregnancy, high blood pressure, and excessive vomiting.

Incidental pregnancy is when the patient comes in to see the provider for a reason other than the pregnancy, but the care of the patient may be affected by the pregnancy.

V22.0 Supervision of normal first pregnancy

V22.1 Supervision of other normal pregnancy

V22.2 Pregnant state, incidental

Coding Clarification

If a pregnant patient comes into the hospital for a non-stress test on the baby, V72.8 should be reported as the primary diagnosis with a secondary diagnosis code from category V22 or V23.

Codes V22.0 *Supervision of normal first pregnancy* and V22.1 *Supervision of other normal pregnancy* are generally used in outpatient settings. When a complication of the pregnancy is present, the code for that condition is assigned rather than a code from category V22. These codes are not used with any other pregnancy code.

Coding Scenario

A patient presents to the office for a routine prenatal examination. The patient is 32 weeks along in her first pregnancy. Examination is normal and the patient has not experienced any complications with this pregnancy.

> Code assignment: V22.0 *Supervision of normal first pregnancy*

V23 Supervision of high-risk pregnancy

Trophoblastic disease or hydatidiform mole is an abnormal product of conception in which the epithelial covering of the chorionic villi (the cellular, outmost membrane) disseminates and the avascular stroma of the villi proliferates and has cystic cavitation. The result is a mass of cells that resembles a bunch of grapes. This condition is also called cystic or vesicular mole.

V23.0 Pregnancy with history of infertility

V23.1 Pregnancy with history of trophoblastic disease — *includes hydatidiform mole and vesicular mole*
AHA: Jan-Feb, 1987, 8; Q1, 1990, 10

V23.2 Pregnancy with history of abortion — *history of conditions reported with 634-638*
AHA: Jan-Feb, 1987, 8; Q1, 1990, 10

V23.3 Pregnancy with grand multiparity

V23.4 5th Pregnancy with other poor obstetric history — *history of conditions reported by 630-676*
AHA: Jan-Feb, 1987, 8; Q1, 1990, 10

V23.41 Supervision of pregnancy with history of pre-term labor

V23.49 Supervision of pregnancy with other poor obstetric history

V23.5 Pregnancy with other poor reproductive history — *history of stillbirth or neonatal death*
AHA: Jan-Feb, 1987, 8; Q1, 1990, 10

V23.7 Insufficient prenatal care — *history of little or no prenatal care*
AHA: Jan-Feb, 1987, 8; Q1, 1990, 10

V23.81 Supervision of high-risk pregnancy of elderly primigravida — *age 35 and older*
AHA: Jan-Feb, 1987, 8; Q1, 1990, 10; Q4, 1998, 56,63

V23.82 Supervision of high-risk pregnancy of elderly multigravida — *age 35 and older, 2nd or more pregnancies*
AHA: Jan-Feb, 1987, 8; Q1, 1990, 10; Q4, 1998, 56,63

V Codes

V23.83 Supervision of high-risk pregnancy of young primigravida — *less than 16 years of age*
AHA: Jan-Feb, 1987, 8; Q1, 1990, 10; Q4, 1998, 56,63

V23.84 Supervision of high-risk pregnancy of young multigravida — *less than 16 years of age, 2nd or more pregnancies.*
AHA: Jan-Feb, 1987, 8; Q1, 1990, 10; Q4, 1998, 56,63

V23.89 Supervision of other high-risk pregnancy

V23.9 Unspecified high-risk pregnancy

Documentation Issues

Documentation should include the risk factor of the patient and that there are no current complications of the pregnancy.

Health care providers must define "insufficient" prenatal care (V23.7) and consistently document this for the information to be useful.

Coding Clarification

Category V23 codes provide information on conditions that may add risk to a present pregnancy. A code from Chapter 11 in ICD-9-CM can be assigned with a code from category V23. The codes should be used when there is a history of a complication, but the pregnancy is progressing normally or when the patient's age could affect the pregnancy.

Coding Scenario

A 23-year-old female presents for her 36-week prenatal visit. A past medical history includes a spontaneous abortion at six weeks. This occurred one year ago. The current pregnancy is progressing normally.

> Code assignment: V23.2 *Pregnancy with history of abortion*

V24 Postpartum care and examination

The postpartum period (also called postnatal) of pregnancy begins at the birth of the child and continues for six weeks.

V24.0 Postpartum care and examination immediately after delivery — *care and observation in uncomplicated cases*
AHA: Jan-Feb, 1987, 8

V24.1 Postpartum care and examination of lactating mother — *supervision of lactation*
AHA: Jan-Feb, 1987, 8

V24.2 Routine postpartum follow-up

Coding Clarification

If the mother delivers outside of the hospital and is subsequently admitted for postpartum care, report V24.0 *Postpartum care and examination immediately after delivery.* Category V24 codes are normally used in the outpatient setting. If a postpartum complication is found, the appropriate pregnancy diagnosis codes should be assigned rather than a code from category V24.

Category V24 codes may be used only as the first listed diagnosis.

Coding Scenario

The patient presents for a routine postpartum visit. There are no complications present.

> Code assignment: V24.2 *Routine postpartum follow-up*

V25 Contraceptive management

Contraceptive management is used for patients who are trying to prevent pregnancy. There are many types of contraception, such as oral medication, that stops ovulation with the use of hormones, usually estrogen and/or progesterone; a barrier, such as a diaphragm, that is inserted into the uterus prior to coitus (intercourse), preventing the spermatozoa from entering the endometrial cavity and fallopian tubes; and an intrauterine device (IUD), which is typically a plastic or metal device fitted into the uterus.

Emergency contraceptive counseling is done postcoital (after intercourse), where a medication is prescribed within the first 72 hours after coitus to avoid pregnancy.

Another form of contraception is implantable medication that is inserted under the dermis. This medication is time released and usually lasts for a period of three months.

V25.01 General counseling for prescription of oral contraceptives

V25.02 General counseling for initiation of other contraceptive measures — *diaphragm fitting, prescription of foams, creams, or other agents*
AHA: Jan-Feb, 1987, 8; Q4, 1992, 24; Q3, 1997, 7

V25.03 Encounter for emergency contraceptive counseling and prescription — *morning after pill*
AHA: Q4, 2003, 84

V25.09 Other general counseling and advice for contraceptive management

V25.1 Insertion of intrauterine contraceptive device — *IUD*
AHA: Jan-Feb, 1987, 8; Q4, 1992, 24

V25.2 Sterilization — *admission for tubal ligation or vasectomy*
AHA: Jan-Feb, 1987, 8; Q4, 1992, 24

V25.3 Menstrual extraction — *menstrual regulation*
AHA: Jan-Feb, 1987, 8; Q4, 1992, 24

© 2004 Ingenix, Inc.

V25.40 Unspecified contraceptive surveillance

V25.41 Surveillance of previously prescribed contraceptive pill

V25.42 Surveillance of previously prescribed intrauterine contraceptive device — *checking, reinsertion, or removal of IUD*
AHA: Jan-Feb, 1987, 8; Q4, 1992, 24

V25.43 Surveillance of previously prescribed implantable subdermal contraceptive

V25.49 Surveillance of other previously prescribed contraceptive method

V25.5 Insertion of implantable subdermal contraceptive

V25.8 Other specified contraceptive management — *family planning advice*
AHA: Jan-Feb, 1987, 8; Q4, 1992, 24; Q3, 1996, 9

V25.9 Unspecified contraceptive management

Coding Clarification

Report V45.5 if an intrauterine contraceptive device is already present.

Category V25 codes may be reported as principal or secondary diagnoses.

Coding Scenario

An 18-year-old female presents for prescription of birth control pills.

Code assignment: V25.01 *General counseling for prescription of oral contraceptives*

V26 Procreative management

Procreative management category codes describe health care services related to producing offspring. Services related to genetic testing and infertility services can be described with these codes. Health care encounters for reversal of a previous tubal ligation or vasectomy, artificial insemination, investigation and testing, and genetic counseling are included here.

V26.0 Tuboplasty or vasoplasty after previous sterilization

V26.1 Artificial insemination

V26.21 Fertility testing — *fallopian insufflation, sperm count for fertility testing*
AHA: Jan-Feb, 1987, 8; Q4, 2000, 56

V26.22 Aftercare following sterilization reversal — *fallopian insufflation following sterilization reversal, sperm count following sterilization reversal*
AHA: Jan-Feb, 1987, 8; Q4, 2000, 56

V26.29 Other investigation and testing

V26.3 Genetic counseling and testing

V26.4 General counseling and advice for procreative management

V26.51 Tubal ligation sterilization status

V26.52 Vasectomy sterilization status

V26.8 Other specified procreative management

V26.9 Unspecified procreative management

Coding Clarification

Codes used to describe a person's sterilization status are included here for both men and women. Code V25.2 *Sterilization* is often assigned as an additional diagnosis when a sterilization procedure is performed during the same admission as a delivery. It may also be assigned as a principal diagnosis when the admission is solely for sterilization.

If a failed tubal ligation results in pregnancy, code the pregnancy. If the visit is to evaluate tube patency, report V26.2 *Investigation and testing for procreation management.* Report 628.0-628.9 for infertility not due to previous tubal ligation.

Coding Scenario

A 23-year-old female is admitted as an outpatient for fertility testing by fallopian insufflation.

Code assignment: V26.21 *Fertility testing*

V27 Outcome of delivery

AHA: Jan-Feb, 1987, 8; Q2, 1991, 16

V27.0 Outcome of delivery, single liveborn — (This code is intended for the coding of the outcome of delivery on the mother's record)

V27.1 Outcome of delivery, single stillborn — (This code is intended for the coding of the outcome of delivery on the mother's record)

V27.2 Outcome of delivery, twins, both liveborn — (This code is intended for the coding of the outcome of delivery on the mother's record)

V27.3 Outcome of delivery, twins, one liveborn and one stillborn — (This code is intended for the coding of the outcome of delivery on the mother's record)

V27.4 Outcome of delivery, twins, both stillborn — (This code is intended for the coding of the outcome of delivery on the mother's record)

V27.5 Outcome of delivery, other multiple birth, all liveborn — (This code is intended for the coding of the outcome of delivery on the mother's record)

V27.6 Outcome of delivery, other multiple birth, some liveborn — (This code is intended for the coding of the outcome of delivery on the mother's record)

V27.7 Outcome of delivery, other multiple birth, all stillborn — (This code is intended for the coding of the outcome of delivery on the mother's record)

V27.9 Outcome of delivery, unspecified — (This code is intended for the coding of the outcome of delivery on the mother's record)
AHA: Jan-Feb, 1987, 8; Q2, 1991, 16

Documentation Issues

This category includes an unspecified code (V27.9); however, the health record should be reviewed again for more specific information.

Coding Clarification

Category V27 codes contain an optional code that may be assigned as an additional diagnosis on the mother's health record to indicate whether the outcome of delivery was single or multiple and liveborn or stillborn. These codes are intended for coding the outcome of delivery on the mother's record; the codes should not appear on the baby's record. These codes should also be used on all maternal delivery records. These codes should be reported for an attempted abortion that results in a live birth.

Coding Scenario

A 25-year-old female is admitted for delivery of a full-term live infant.

> Code assignment: 650 *Normal delivery* and V27.0 *Outcome of delivery, single liveborn*

V28 Antenatal screening

Antenatal screening is the testing of a baby before birth for a disease or disease precursors in seemingly well individuals so that early detection and treatment can be provided for those who test positive for the disease.

During amniocentesis, a needle is inserted into the womb and amniotic fluid is withdrawn. A number of tests can be performed on the fluid to confirm or rule out certain conditions.

Isoimmunization is the incompatibility of Rh and ABO between a mother and a fetus. The incompatibility is when an Rh-negative mother carries an Rh-positive fetus. Antibodies that are carried across the placenta into the fetus lead to hemolysis of the fetal blood. Symptoms that typically occur include edema, cardiomegaly, hepatomegaly, splenomegaly, pale skin, and severe generalized edema (hydrops fetalis).

V28.0 Antenatal screening for chromosomal anomalies by amniocentesis — *variation in the DNA strand that carries genetic information*
AHA: Jan-Feb, 1987, 8

V28.1 Antenatal screening for raised alpha-fetoprotein levels in amniotic fluid — *abnormal levels may indicate, neural tube defects, anencephaly, omphalocele*
AHA: Jan-Feb, 1987, 8

V28.2 Other antenatal screening based on amniocentesis

V28.3 Antenatal screening for malformation using ultrasonics — *abnormally formed fetus*
AHA: Jan-Feb, 1987, 8

V28.4 Antenatal screening for fetal growth retardation using ultrasonics — *slow growth of the fetus*
AHA: Jan-Feb, 1987, 8

V28.5 Antenatal screening for isoimmunization — *test for Rh factor*
AHA: Jan-Feb, 1987, 8

V28.6 Screening of Streptococcus B

V28.8 Other specified antenatal screening

V28.9 Unspecified antenatal screening

Coding Clarification

Category V28 codes should only be used if no specific condition is found to exist during the screening process. Code the condition, not the screening, if one is discovered.

Coding Scenario

A 37-year-old female is admitted for an amniocentesis to rule out Down's syndrome.

> Code assignment: V28.0 *Antenatal screening for chromosomal anomalies by amniocentesis*

V29 Observation and evaluation of newborns and infants for suspected condition not found

Observation and evaluation of a newborn and infant are performed when a neonate (the first 28 days of life) is suspected of having a particular condition, resulting from exposure from the mother or birth process, which is ruled out after examination and observation.

V29.0 Observation and evaluation of newborns and infants for suspected infectious condition not found

V29.1 Observation and evaluation of newborns and infants for suspected neurological condition not found

V29.2 Observation and evaluation of newborns and infants for suspected respiratory condition not found

V29.3 Observation for suspected genetic or metabolic condition

© 2004 Ingenix, Inc.

V29.8 Observation and evaluation of newborns and infants for other specified suspected condition not found

V29.9 Observation and evaluation of newborns and infants for unspecified suspected condition not found

Coding Clarification

Category V29 codes may be reported only as primary diagnoses, unless they are documented with codes V30-V39. In this case, category V30-V39 codes will be listed as primary diagnoses and V29 codes will be listed as secondary diagnoses.

Coding Scenario

A five-day-old newborn is admitted to the hospital with suspected sepsis. Following blood cultures, the sepsis is ruled out.

> Code assignment: V29.0 *Observation and evaluation of newborns and infants for suspected infectious condition not found*

V30–V39 Liveborn Infants According to Type of Birth

Category V30-V39 codes are used for the primary diagnosis and describe the type of birth: single or multiple. These codes are used in the inpatient setting for most patients (fourth digit 0) but may be used for those born before admission (fourth digit 1) or not admitted to the hospital (fourth digit 2). The fifth digit identifies whether the delivery was vaginal or cesarean. A cesarean delivery is performed through an incision in the mother's abdomen. Most incisions are performed through a low horizontal incision but a vertical incision may be used in severe fetal distress.

V30 Single liveborn

The following fourth-digit subdivisions are for use with categories V30-V39:

0 Born in hospital

1 Born before admission to hospital

2 Born outside hospital and not hospitalized

The following two fifth-digits are for use with the fourth-digit .0, Born in hospital:

0 delivered without mention of cesarean delivery

1 delivered by cesarean delivery

Cesarean delivery is performed through an incision into the mother's abdomen. Most incisions are performed through a low horizontal incision but a vertical incision may be used in severe fetal distress.

Coding Clarification

Category V30 codes may be used only as the first listed diagnosis and should only be used on the baby's record. If the baby is transferred to another hospital, the receiving hospital should not use this category of codes. The hospital that the baby is transferred to should report the condition of the baby that caused the need for transfer. These codes are intended for the coding of liveborn infants who are consuming health care (e.g., crib or bassinet occupancy).

Coding Scenario

A liveborn male infant is delivered in a hospital via a vaginal delivery.

> Code assignment: V30.00 *Single liveborn, born in hospital, delivered without mention of cesarean delivery*

V31 Twin birth, mate liveborn

Coding Clarification

Category V31 codes may be used only as the first listed diagnosis and should only be used on the baby's record. If the baby is transferred to another hospital, the receiving hospital should not use this category of codes. The hospital that the baby is transferred to should report the condition of the baby that caused the need for transfer. These codes are intended for the coding of liveborn infants who are consuming health care (e.g., crib or bassinet occupancy).

Coding Scenario

Twin live males are born in the hospital by cesarean delivery.

> Code assignment: V31.01 *Twin birth, mate liveborn, born in hospital, delivered by cesarean delivery*

V32 Twin birth, mate stillborn

A stillborn is the delivery of a baby who is dead.

Coding Clarification

Category V32 codes may be used only as the first listed diagnosis and should only be used on the baby's record. If the baby is transferred to another hospital, the receiving hospital should not use this category of codes. The hospital that the baby is transferred to should report the condition of the baby that caused the need for transfer.

V33 Twin birth, unspecified whether mate liveborn or stillborn

Coding Clarification

Category V33 codes may be used only as the first listed diagnosis and should only be used on the baby's record. If the baby is transferred to another hospital, the receiving hospital should not use this category of codes. The hospital that the baby is transferred to should report the condition of the baby that caused the need for transfer. Category V33 codes are intended for the coding of liveborn infants who are

V Codes

consuming health care (e.g., crib or bassinet occupancy).

V34 Other multiple birth (three or more), mates all liveborn

Multiple births with more than three neonates may be a result of heredity or the use of a fertility drug. Typically, the neonates are delivered prematurely and have a low birth weight.

Coding Clarification

Category V34 codes may be used only as the first listed diagnosis and should only be used on the baby's record. If the baby is transferred to another hospital, the receiving hospital should not use these codes. The hospital that the baby is transferred to should report the condition of the baby that caused the need for transfer.

Coding Scenario

Triplets were born via low transverse cesarean section. All babies were liveborn and healthy.

> Code assignment: V34.01 *Other multiple birth, mates all liveborn, born in the hospital, delivered by cesarean delivery*

V35 Other multiple birth (three or more), mates all stillborn

Coding Clarification

Category V35 codes may be used only as the first listed diagnosis and should only be used on the baby's record. If the baby is transferred to another hospital, the receiving hospital should not use these codes. The hospital that the baby is transferred to should report the condition of the baby that caused the need for transfer. Category V35 codes are intended for the coding of liveborn infants who are consuming health care (e.g., crib or bassinet occupancy).

V36 Other multiple birth (three or more), mates liveborn and stillborn

Coding Clarification

Category V36 codes may be used only as the first listed diagnosis and should only be used on the baby's record. If the baby is transferred to another hospital, the receiving hospital should not use these codes. The hospital that the baby is transferred to should report the condition of the baby that caused the need for transfer. Category V36 codes are intended for the coding of liveborn infants who are consuming health care (e.g., crib or bassinet occupancy).

V37 Other multiple birth (three or more), unspecified whether mates liveborn or stillborn

Coding Clarification

Category V37 codes may be used only as the first listed diagnosis and should only be used on the baby's record. If the baby is transferred to another hospital, the receiving hospital should not use these codes. The hospital that the baby is transferred to should report the condition of the baby that caused the need for transfer. Category V37 codes are intended for the coding of liveborn infants who are consuming health care (e.g., crib or bassinet occupancy).

V39 Liveborn, unspecified whether single, twin, or multiple

Coding Clarification

Category V39 codes may be used only as the first listed diagnosis and should only be used on the baby's record. If the baby is transferred to another hospital, the receiving hospital should not use these codes. The hospital that the baby is transferred to should report the condition of the baby that caused the need for transfer. Category V39 codes are intended for the coding of liveborn infants who are consuming health care (e.g., crib or bassinet occupancy).

V40–V49 Persons with a Condition Influencing Their Health Status

Category V40-V49 codes are used to describe circumstances other than a disease or an injury that influences a patient's health status. These codes describe the residual of a past disease or a condition that in some way affects the way the patient's treatment is carried out. The status codes are different from the history codes in that a history code indicates that the patient no longer has the disease. These codes should be used when the condition is documented as a diagnosis or problem.

V40 Mental and behavioral problems

AHA: Jan-Feb, 1987, 8

Mental problems include any conditions that affect the mood or behavior of a person. The conditions may include depression, dysphoria, personality disorder, and phobias. Mental problems may be caused by the malfunction of the brain's neurotransmitters, heredity, stress, or substance abuse.

Behavior problems affect the way people act. Problems include self-injury, aggressive behavior, hostility, and the inability to control actions.

V Codes

 © 2004 Ingenix, Inc.

V40.0 Problems with learning — (This code is intended for use when these conditions are recorded as diagnoses or problems)
AHA: Jan-Feb, 1987, 8

V40.1 Problems with communication (including speech) — (This code is intended for use when these conditions are recorded as diagnoses or problems)

V40.2 Other mental problems — (This code is intended for use when these conditions are recorded as diagnoses or problems)

V40.3 Other behavioral problems — (This code is intended for use when these conditions are recorded as diagnoses or problems)

V40.9 Unspecified mental or behavioral problem — (This code is intended for use when these conditions are recorded as diagnoses or problems)

Coding Clarification

Category V40 codes may be used only as an additional diagnosis.

V41 Problems with special senses and other special functions

AHA: Jan-Feb, 1987, 8

V41.0 Problems with sight — (This code is intended for use when these conditions are recorded as diagnoses or problems)

V41.1 Other eye problems — (This code is intended for use when these conditions are recorded as diagnoses or problems)

V41.2 Problems with hearing — (This code is intended for use when these conditions are recorded as diagnoses or problems)

V41.3 Other ear problems — (This code is intended for use when these conditions are recorded as diagnoses or problems)

V41.4 Problems with voice production — (This code is intended for use when these conditions are recorded as diagnoses or problems)

V41.5 Problems with smell and taste — (This code is intended for use when these conditions are recorded as diagnoses or problems)

V41.6 Problems with swallowing and mastication — (This code is intended for use when these conditions are recorded as diagnoses or problems)
AHA: Jan-Feb, 1987, 8

V41.7 Problems with sexual function — (This code is intended for use when these conditions are recorded as diagnoses or problems)

V41.8 Other problems with special functions — (This code is intended for use when these conditions are recorded as diagnoses or problems)

V41.9 Unspecified problem with special functions — (This code is intended for use when these conditions are recorded as diagnoses or problems)

Coding Clarification

This category of codes is generic. Check in the disease/condition section of ICD-9-CM to verify that no other code better describes the symptoms and/or disease/condition of the patient.

Category V41 codes may be used only as secondary diagnoses.

V42 Organ or tissue replaced by transplant

AHA: Jan-Feb, 1987, 8; Q3, 1998, 3, 4

Patients who require organ transplantation may have a variety or diseases and/or conditions. They may have end-stage renal disease (kidney) or mitral or aortic valve stenosis (heart valve).

V42.0 Kidney replaced by transplant — (This code is intended for use when these conditions are recorded as diagnoses or problems)

V42.1 Heart replaced by transplant — (This code is intended for use when these conditions are recorded as diagnoses or problems)

V42.2 Heart valve replaced by transplant — (This code is intended for use when these conditions are recorded as diagnoses or problems)

V42.3 Skin replaced by transplant — (This code is intended for use when these conditions are recorded as diagnoses or problems)

V42.4 Bone replaced by transplant — (This code is intended for use when these conditions are recorded as diagnoses or problems)

V42.5 Cornea replaced by transplant — (This code is intended for use when these conditions are recorded as diagnoses or problems)

V42.6 Lung replaced by transplant — (This code is intended for use when these conditions are recorded as diagnoses or problems)

V42.7 Liver replaced by transplant — (This code is intended for use when these conditions are recorded as diagnoses or problems)

V42.81 Bone marrow replaced by transplant — (This code is intended for use when these conditions are recorded as diagnoses or problems)

V Codes

V42.82 Peripheral stem cells replaced by transplant — (This code is intended for use when these conditions are recorded as diagnoses or problems)

V42.83 Pancreas replaced by transplant — (This code is intended for use when these conditions are recorded as diagnoses or problems)

V42.84 Organ or tissue replaced by transplant, intestines — (This code is intended for use when these conditions are recorded as diagnoses or problems)

V42.89 Other organ or tissue replaced by transplant — (This code is intended for use when these conditions are recorded as diagnoses or problems)

V42.9 Unspecified organ or tissue replaced by transplant — (This code is intended for use when these conditions are recorded as diagnoses or problems)

Coding Clarification

Category V42 codes should be used for homologous or heterologous (animal) (human) transplant organ status. Transplant status codes indicate that a person has had an organ replaced but there are no current complications with the transplant. Do not report V42 category codes with 996.8 *Complications of a transplanted organ.*

Coding Scenario

A patient presents to the clinic for an annual check of his transplanted kidney. Lab work and examination are normal.

Code assignment: V42.0 *Kidney replaced by transplant*

V43 Organ or tissue replaced by other means

AHA: Jan-Feb, 1987, 8

"Other means" describes anatomical parts that have been replaced with an artificial or mechanical device or prosthesis rather than from another body part or another person.

V43.0 Eye globe replaced by other means — (This code is intended for use when these conditions are recorded as diagnoses or problems)
AHA: Jan-Feb, 1987, 8

V43.1 Lens replaced by other means — (This code is intended for use when these conditions are recorded as diagnoses or problems)
AHA: Jan-Feb, 1987, 8; Q4, 1998, 65

V43.21 Status, Organ or tissue replaced by other means, Heart assist device — (This code is intended for use when these conditions are recorded as diagnoses or problems)

V43.22 Status, Organ or tissue replaced by other means, Fully implantable artificial heart — (This code is intended for use when these conditions are recorded as diagnoses or problems)

V43.3 Heart valve replaced by other means — (This code is intended for use when these conditions are recorded as diagnoses or problems)

V43.4 Blood vessel replaced by other means — (This code is intended for use when these conditions are recorded as diagnoses or problems)

V43.5 Bladder replaced by other means — (This code is intended for use when these conditions are recorded as diagnoses or problems)

V43.60 Unspecified joint replacement by other means — (This code is intended for use when these conditions are recorded as diagnoses or problems)

V43.61 Shoulder joint replacement by other means — (This code is intended for use when these conditions are recorded as diagnoses or problems)

V43.62 Elbow joint replacement by other means — (This code is intended for use when these conditions are recorded as diagnoses or problems)

V43.63 Wrist joint replacement by other means — (This code is intended for use when these conditions are recorded as diagnoses or problems)

V43.64 Hip joint replacement by other means — (This code is intended for use when these conditions are recorded as diagnoses or problems)
AHA: Jan-Feb, 1987, 8

V43.65 Knee joint replacement by other means — (This code is intended for use when these conditions are recorded as diagnoses or problems)

V43.66 Ankle joint replacement by other means — (This code is intended for use when these conditions are recorded as diagnoses or problems)

V43.69 Other joint replacement by other means — (This code is intended for use when these conditions are recorded as diagnoses or problems)

V43.7 Limb replaced by other means — (This code is intended for use when these conditions are recorded as diagnoses or problems)

V43.81 Larynx replaced by other means — (This code is intended for use when these conditions are recorded as diagnoses or problems)
AHA: Jan-Feb, 1987, 8; Q4, 1995, 55

V Codes

© 2004 Ingenix, Inc.

V43.82 Breast replaced by other means — (This code is intended for use when these conditions are recorded as diagnoses or problems)

V43.83 Organ or tissue replaced by artificial skin — (This code is intended for use when these conditions are recorded as diagnoses or problems)

V43.89 Other organ or tissue replaced by other means — (This code is intended for use when these conditions are recorded as diagnoses or problems)

Coding Clarification

Category V43 codes may be reported only as secondary diagnoses except for V43.22, which may be used as either the primary or secondary diagnosis.

Coding Scenario

A patient presents to the emergency department with a closed fracture of the right medial malleolus. A past medical history indicates that the patient had total hip placement on the right side five years ago.

> Code assignment: 824.0 *Fracture of medial malleolus closed* and V43.64 *Hip joint replacement by other means*

V44 Artificial opening status

AHA: Jan-Feb, 1987, 8

A stoma is an artifical opening between the body cavities or organs and the body's surface.

V44.0 Tracheostomy status — (This code is intended for use when these conditions are recorded as diagnoses or problems)
AHA: Jan-Feb, 1987, 8; Q1, 2001, 6; Q4, 2003, 103, 107, 111

V44.1 Gastrostomy status — (This code is intended for use when these conditions are recorded as diagnoses or problems)
AHA: Jan-Feb, 1987, 8; Q1, 1993, 26; Q3, 1997, 12; Q1, 2001, 12; Q4, 2003, 103, 107-108, 110

V44.2 Ileostomy status — (This code is intended for use when these conditions are recorded as diagnoses or problems)
AHA: Jan-Feb, 1987, 8

V44.3 Colostomy status — (This code is intended for use when these conditions are recorded as diagnoses or problems)
AHA: Jan-Feb, 1987, 8; Q4, 2003, 110

V44.4 Status of other artificial opening of gastrointestinal tract — (This code is intended for use when these conditions are recorded as diagnoses or problems)

V44.5 ✓5th Cystostomy status — (This subcategory is intended for use when these conditions are recorded as diagnoses or problems)
AHA: Jan-Feb, 1987, 8

V44.50 Unspecified cystostomy status — (This code is intended for use when these conditions are recorded as diagnoses or problems)

V44.51 Cutaneous-vesicostomy status — (This code is intended for use when these conditions are recorded as diagnoses or problems)
AHA: Jan-Feb, 1987, 8

V44.52 Appendico-vesicostomy status — (This code is intended for use when these conditions are recorded as diagnoses or problems)
AHA: Jan-Feb, 1987, 8

V44.59 Other cystostomy status — (This code is intended for use when these conditions are recorded as diagnoses or problems)

V44.6 Status of other artificial opening of urinary tract — (This code is intended for use when these conditions are recorded as diagnoses or problems)
AHA: Jan-Feb, 1987, 8

V44.7 Artificial vagina status — (This code is intended for use when these conditions are recorded as diagnoses or problems)

V44.8 Other artificial opening status — (This code is intended for use when these conditions are recorded as diagnoses or problems)

V44.9 Unspecified artificial opening status — (This code is intended for use when these conditions are recorded as diagnoses or problems)

Coding Clarification

Category V44 codes should be used when the reason for the visit is for attention or management of an artificial opening such as a tracheostomy, colostomy, or cystostomy and should only be reported as secondary diagnoses.

V45 Other postsurgical states

AHA: Jan-Feb, 1987, 8; Q4, 2003, 85

Acquired absence of an organ indicates that an organ was removed surgically and not as a result of a congenital abnormality.

V45.00 Unspecified cardiac device in situ — (This code is intended for use when these conditions are recorded as diagnoses or problems)

V45.01 Cardiac pacemaker in situ — (This code is intended for use when these conditions are recorded as diagnoses or problems)

V Codes

V45.02 Automatic implantable cardiac defibrillator in situ — (This code is intended for use when these conditions are recorded as diagnoses or problems)

V45.09 Other specified cardiac device in situ — (This code is intended for use when these conditions are recorded as diagnoses or problems)
AHA: Jan-Feb, 1987, 8

V45.1 Renal dialysis status — (This code is intended for use when these conditions are recorded as diagnoses or problems)
AHA: Jan-Feb, 1987, 8; Q2, 2001, 12, 13; Q2, 2003, 7

V45.2 Presence of cerebrospinal fluid drainage device — (This code is intended for use when these conditions are recorded as diagnoses or problems)
AHA: Jan-Feb, 1987, 8; Q4, 2003, 106

V45.3 Intestinal bypass or anastomosis status — (This code is intended for use when these conditions are recorded as diagnoses or problems)

V45.4 Arthrodesis status — (This code is intended for use when these conditions are recorded as diagnoses or problems)
AHA: Nov-Dec, 1984, 18; Jan-Feb, 1987, 8

V45.51 Presence of intrauterine contraceptive device — (This code is intended for use when these conditions are recorded as diagnoses or problems)
AHA: Jan-Feb, 1987, 8

V45.52 Presence of subdermal contraceptive device — (This code is intended for use when these conditions are recorded as diagnoses or problems)
AHA: Jan-Feb, 1987, 8

V45.59 Presence of other contraceptive device — (This code is intended for use when these conditions are recorded as diagnoses or problems)

V45.61 Cataract extraction status — (Use additional code for associated artificial lens staus, V43.1)

V45.69 Other states following surgery of eye and adnexa — (This code is intended for use when these conditions are recorded as diagnoses or problems)

V45.71 Acquired absence of breast — (This code is intended for use when these conditions are recorded as diagnoses or problems)

V45.72 Acquired absence of intestine (large) (small) — (This code is intended for use when these conditions are recorded as diagnoses or problems)

V45.73 Acquired absence of kidney — (This code is intended for use when these conditions are recorded as diagnoses or problems)

V45.74 Acquired absence of organ, other parts of urinary tract — (This code is intended for use when these conditions are recorded as diagnoses or problems)
AHA: Jan-Feb, 1987, 8; Q4, 1997, 50; Q4, 1998, 65; Q4, 2000, 51

V45.75 Acquired absence of organ, stomach — (This code is intended for use when these conditions are recorded as diagnoses or problems)

V45.76 Acquired absence of organ, lung — (This code is intended for use when these conditions are recorded as diagnoses or problems)

V45.77 Acquired absence of organ, genital organs — (This code is intended for use when these conditions are recorded as diagnoses or problems)
AHA: Jan-Feb, 1987, 8; Q4, 1997, 50; Q4, 1998, 65; Q4, 2000, 51; Q1, 2003, 13-14

V45.78 Acquired absence of organ, eye — (This code is intended for use when these conditions are recorded as diagnoses or problems)

V45.79 Other acquired absence of organ — (This code is intended for use when these conditions are recorded as diagnoses or problems)

V45.81 Postsurgical aortocoronary bypass status — (This code is intended for use when these conditions are recorded as diagnoses or problems)
AHA: Jan-Feb, 1987, 8; Q3, 1997, 16; Q3, 2001, 15; Q4, 2003, 105

V45.82 Postsurgical percutaneous transluminal coronary angioplasty status — (This code is intended for use when these conditions are recorded as diagnoses or problems)
AHA: Jan-Feb, 1987, 8

V45.83 Breast implant removal status — (This code is intended for use when these conditions are recorded as diagnoses or problems)

V45.84 Dental restoration status — (This code is intended for use when these conditions are recorded as diagnoses or problems)
AHA: Jan-Feb, 1987, 8; Q4, 2001, 54

V45.85 Insulin pump status — (This code is intended for use when these conditions are recorded as diagnoses or problems)

V45.89 Other postsurgical status — (This code is intended for use when these conditions are recorded as diagnoses or problems)
AHA: Jan-Feb, 1987, 8; Q1, 1995, 11

© 2004 Ingenix, Inc.

Coding Clarification
Category V45 codes may be reported only as secondary diagnoses except for V45.7, which may be reported either as the primary or secondary diagnosis.

For the malfunction of a nervous system device, implant, or graft, report 996.2. For the complication of a contraceptive device, report 996.32.

V46 Other dependence on machines

AHA: Jan-Feb, 1987, 8

Patients who are dependent on machines typically have had a chronic illness in which the disease or condition has decreased their lung capacity or have suffered some form of significant trauma. Hyperbaric chambers reduce hypoxia and edema from injuries, which may include crush injuries and acute traumatic peripheral ischemias.

V46.0 Dependence on aspirator — (This code is intended for use when these conditions are recorded as diagnoses or problems)

V46.1 5th Dependence on respirator — (This code is intended for use when these conditions are recorded as diagnoses or problems)
AHA: Jan-Feb, 1987, 8; Jan-Feb, 1987, 7, 3; Q1, 2001, 12; Q4, 2003, 103

V46.11 Dependence on respirator, status

V46.12 Encounter for respirator dependence during power failure

V46.2 Dependence on machine for supplemental oxygen — (This code is intended for use when these conditions are recorded as diagnoses or problems)
AHA: Jan-Feb, 1987, 8; Q4, 2002, 79; Q4, 2003, 108

V46.8 Dependence on other enabling machine — (This code is intended for use when these conditions are recorded as diagnoses or problems)
AHA: Jan-Feb, 1987, 8

V46.9 Unspecified machine dependence — (This code is intended for use when these conditions are recorded as diagnoses or problems)

Coding Clarification
Category V46 codes may be used only as an additional diagnosis.

V47 Other problems with internal organs

AHA: Jan-Feb, 1987, 8

V47.0 Deficiencies of internal organs — (This code is intended for use when these conditions are recorded as diagnoses or problems)

V47.1 Mechanical and motor problems with internal organs — (This code is intended for use when these conditions are recorded as diagnoses or problems)

V47.2 Other cardiorespiratory problems — (This code is intended for use when these conditions are recorded as diagnoses or problems)

V47.3 Other digestive problems — (This code is intended for use when these conditions are recorded as diagnoses or problems)

V47.4 Other urinary problems — (This code is intended for use when these conditions are recorded as diagnoses or problems)

V47.5 Other genital problems — (This code is intended for use when these conditions are recorded as diagnoses or problems)

V47.9 Unspecified problems with internal organs — (This code is intended for use when these conditions are recorded as diagnoses or problems)

Coding Clarification
This category of codes is generic. Check in the disease/condition section of ICD-9-CM to verify that no other code better describes the symptoms and/or disease/condition of the patient.

Category V47 codes may be used only as an additional diagnosis.

Code V47.2 *Other cardiorespiratory problems* includes cardiovascular exercise intolerance with pain at rest, with less than ordinary activity, and with ordinary activity.

V48 Problems with head, neck, and trunk

AHA: Jan-Feb, 1987, 8

V48.0 Deficiencies of head — (This code is intended for use when these conditions are recorded as diagnoses or problems)

V48.1 Deficiencies of neck and trunk — (This code is intended for use when these conditions are recorded as diagnoses or problems)

V48.2 Mechanical and motor problems with head — (This code is intended for use when these conditions are recorded as diagnoses or problems)

V48.3 Mechanical and motor problems with neck and trunk — (This code is intended for use when these conditions are recorded as diagnoses or problems)

V48.4 Sensory problem with head — (This code is intended for use when these conditions are recorded as diagnoses or problems)

V Codes

V48.5 Sensory problem with neck and trunk — (This code is intended for use when these conditions are recorded as diagnoses or problems)

V48.6 Disfigurements of head — (This code is intended for use when these conditions are recorded as diagnoses or problems)

V48.7 Disfigurements of neck and trunk — (This code is intended for use when these conditions are recorded as diagnoses or problems)

V48.8 Other problems with head, neck, and trunk — (This code is intended for use when these conditions are recorded as diagnoses or problems)

V48.9 Unspecified problem with head, neck, or trunk — (This code is intended for use when these conditions are recorded as diagnoses or problems)

Coding Clarification

This category of codes is generic. Check in the disease/condition section of ICD-9-CM to verify that no other code better describes the symptoms and/or disease/condition of the patient. Category V48 codes may be used only as an additional diagnosis.

Report V48.8 for deficiencies of the ears, eyelids, and nose.

V Codes

V49 Problems with limbs and other problems

AHA: Jan-Feb, 1987, 8

V49.0 Deficiencies of limbs — (This code is intended for use when these conditions are recorded as diagnoses or problems)

V49.1 Mechanical problems with limbs — (This code is intended for use when these conditions are recorded as diagnoses or problems)

V49.2 Motor problems with limbs — (This code is intended for use when these conditions are recorded as diagnoses or problems)

V49.3 Sensory problems with limbs — (This code is intended for use when these conditions are recorded as diagnoses or problems)

V49.4 Disfigurements of limbs — (This code is intended for use when these conditions are recorded as diagnoses or problems)

V49.5 Other problems of limbs — (This code is intended for use when these conditions are recorded as diagnoses or problems)

V49.60 Upper limb amputation, unspecified level — (This code is intended for use when these conditions are recorded as diagnoses or problems)

V49.61 Upper limb amputation, thumb — (This code is intended for use when these conditions are recorded as diagnoses or problems)

V49.62 Upper limb amputation, other finger(s) — (This code is intended for use when these conditions are recorded as diagnoses or problems)

V49.63 Upper limb amputation, hand — (This code is intended for use when these conditions are recorded as diagnoses or problems)

V49.64 Upper limb amputation, wrist — (This code is intended for use when these conditions are recorded as diagnoses or problems)
AHA: Jan-Feb, 1987, 8; Q4, 1994, 39; Q4, 1998, 42

V49.65 Upper limb amputation, below elbow — (This code is intended for use when these conditions are recorded as diagnoses or problems)

V49.66 Upper limb amputation, above elbow — (This code is intended for use when these conditions are recorded as diagnoses or problems)
AHA: Jan-Feb, 1987, 8; Q4, 1994, 39; Q4, 1998, 42

V49.67 Upper limb amputation, shoulder — (This code is intended for use when these conditions are recorded as diagnoses or problems)
AHA: Jan-Feb, 1987, 8; Q4, 1994, 39; Q4, 1998, 42

V49.70 Upper limb amputation, unspecified level — (This code is intended for use when these conditions are recorded as diagnoses or problems)

V49.71 Upper limb amputation, great toe — (This code is intended for use when these conditions are recorded as diagnoses or problems)

V49.72 Upper limb amputation, other toe(s) — (This code is intended for use when these conditions are recorded as diagnoses or problems)

V49.73 Upper limb amputation, foot — (This code is intended for use when these conditions are recorded as diagnoses or problems)

V49.74 Upper limb amputation, ankle — (This code is intended for use when these conditions are recorded as diagnoses or problems)
AHA: Jan-Feb, 1987, 8; Q4, 1994, 39; Q4, 1998, 42

V49.75 Lower limb amputation, below knee — (This code is intended for use when these conditions are recorded as diagnoses or problems)

© 2004 Ingenix, Inc.

V49.76 Lower limb amputation, above knee — (This code is intended for use when these conditions are recorded as diagnoses or problems)
AHA: Jan-Feb, 1987, 8; Q4, 1994, 39; Q4, 1998, 42

V49.77 Upper limb amputation, hip — (This code is intended for use when these conditions are recorded as diagnoses or problems)
AHA: Jan-Feb, 1987, 8; Q4, 1994, 39; Q4, 1998, 42

V49.81 Asymptomatic postmenopausal status (age-related) (natural) — (This code is intended for use when these conditions are recorded as diagnoses or problems)

V49.82 Dental sealant status — (This code is intended for use when these conditions are recorded as diagnoses or problems)

V49.83 Awaiting organ transplant status

V49.89 Other specified conditions influencing health status — (This code is intended for use when these conditions are recorded as diagnoses or problems)

V49.9 Unspecified problems with limbs and other problems — (This code is intended for use when these conditions are recorded as diagnoses or problems)

Coding Clarification

This category of codes is generic. Check in the disease/condition section of ICD-9-CM to verify that no other code better describes the symptoms and/or disease/condition of the patient.

Category V49 codes may be reported only as secondary diagnoses, except for V49.6 and V49.7, which can be reported as either the primary or secondary diagnosis.

V50–V59 Persons Encountering Health Services for Specific Procedures and Aftercare

The codes in this section are used for patients who have already been treated for some disease or injury, but may need aftercare or adjunctive treatment to consolidate the treatment, deal with residual states, or prevent recurrence.

Encounters for plastic surgery are classified in two ways: procedures used for cosmetic surgery or for conditions of a healed injury or operation.

V50 Elective surgery for purposes other than remedying health states

Prophylactic gland, breast, or ovary removal may be performed on a patient with a family or personal history of cancer or another disease.

V50.0 Elective hair transplant for purposes other than remedying health states

V50.1 Other plastic surgery for unacceptable cosmetic appearance — *breast augmentation or reduction, face lift*
AHA: Jan-Feb, 1987, 8

V50.2 Routine or ritual circumcision — *circumcision in the absence of significant medical indication*
AHA: Jan-Feb, 1987, 8

V50.3 Ear piercing

V50.41 Prophylactic breast removal

V50.42 Prophylactic ovary removal

V50.49 Other prophylactic gland removal

V50.8 Other elective surgery for purposes other than remedying health states

V50.9 Unspecified elective surgery for purposes other than remedying health states

Coding Scenario

A patient presents to the plastic surgery clinic for an elective breast augmentation. Her present cup size is a small A. Following the surgery, the patient is a small C cup.

> Code assignment: V50.1 *Other plastic surgery for unacceptable cosmetic appearance*

V51 Aftercare involving the use of plastic surgery

Plastic surgery may be performed on patients who have previously had surgery or had an injury heal in which another procedure is required to put the anatomical site back to its natural state.

Coding Clarification

Plastic surgery as treatment for current injury should be coded to the current condition. Plastic surgery on scar tissue should be coded to the scar, such as a keloid scar.

Code V51 may only be reported as a secondary diagnosis.

V52 Fitting and adjustment of prosthetic device and implant

Fitting and adjustment of prosthetic devices are for devices that have been previously placed in or on the patient.

V52.0 Fitting and adjustment of artificial arm (complete) (partial)

V52.1 Fitting and adjustment of artificial leg (complete) (partial)

V52.2 Fitting and adjustment of artificial eye

V52.3 Fitting and adjustment of dental prosthetic device

V52.4 Fitting and adjustment of breast prosthesis and implant

V52.8 Fitting and adjustment of other specified prosthetic device

V52.9 Fitting and adjustment of unspecified prosthetic device

V53 Fitting and adjustment of other device

Communicating hydrocephalus occurs when there is a slight ventricular enlargement of the cerebrospinal fluid spaces outside of the brain. Shunts are the only treatment for this condition. The shunt has three major components. The first major component is a hollow tube with holes that is inserted through the skull and into the ventricular system where it is connected to the second component, which is a pressure valve that regulates the amount of cerebrospinous fluid that is released. The third component is a distal catheter, which is a long thin tube that attaches to the valve. This is placed under the skin and ends in a distal body cavity, usually in the peritoneum.

A neuropacemaker is an implanted device that is used to relieve nerve injury pain or to help movement disorders. Electrodes are implanted into the brain and attached to a pacemaker that is implanted in the basal ganglia. Electrical pulses are emitted and stimulate the brain.

V53.01 Fitting and adjustment of cerebral ventricular (communicating) shunt

V53.02 Neuropacemaker (brain) (peripheral nerve) (spinal cord)

V53.09 Fitting and adjustment of other devices related to nervous system and special senses — *auditory substitution device, visual substitution device*
AHA: Jan-Feb, 1987, 8; Q4, 1997, 51; Q4, 1998, 66; Q2, 1999, 4

V53.1 Fitting and adjustment of spectacles and contact lenses

V53.2 Fitting and adjustment of hearing aid

V53.3 ✓5th Fitting and adjustment of cardiac device — *reprogramming*
AHA: Nov-Dec, 1984, 18; May-June, 1987, 8; Jan-Feb, 1987, 8; Q1, 1990, 7; Q3, 1992, 3

V53.31 Fitting and adjustment of cardiac pacemaker

V53.32 Fitting and adjustment of automatic implantable cardiac defibrillator

V53.39 Fitting and adjustment of other cardiac device

V53.4 Fitting and adjustment of orthodontic devices

V53.5 Fitting and adjustment of other intestinal appliance

V53.6 Fitting and adjustment of urinary device — *urinary catheter*
AHA: Jan-Feb, 1987, 8

V53.7 Fitting and adjustment of orthopedic device — *orthopedic brace, cast, corset shoes*
AHA: Jan-Feb, 1987, 8

V53.8 Fitting and adjustment of wheelchair

V53.90 Fitting and adjustment, Unspecified device

V53.91 Fitting and adjustment of insulin pump — *insulin pump titration*

V53.99 Fitting and adjustment, Other device

Coding Clarification

For mechanical complications of a cardiac pacemaker, report 996.01.

V54 Other orthopedic aftercare

A fracture is a break or a rupture in a bone. A traumatic fracture is the result of an injury resulting from direct or indirect force against a bone. A pathologic fracture can occur from a weakening of the bone structure due to disease, such as osteoporosis.

V54.01 Encounter for removal of internal fixation device

V54.02 Encounter for lengthening/adjustment of growth rod

V54.09 Other aftercare involving internal fixation device

V54.10 Aftercare for healing traumatic fracture of arm, unspecified

V54.11 Aftercare for healing traumatic fracture of upper arm

V54.12 Aftercare for healing traumatic fracture of lower arm

V54.13 Aftercare for healing traumatic fracture of hip

V54.14 Aftercare for healing traumatic fracture of leg, unspecified

V54.15 Aftercare for healing traumatic fracture of upper leg

V54.16 Aftercare for healing traumatic fracture of lower leg

V54.17 Aftercare for healing traumatic fracture of vertebrae

V54.19 Aftercare for healing traumatic fracture of other bone

V54.20 Aftercare for healing pathologic fracture of arm, unspecified

V54.21 Aftercare for healing pathologic fracture of upper arm

V54.22 Aftercare for healing pathologic fracture of lower arm

V54.23 Aftercare for healing pathologic fracture of hip

 © 2004 Ingenix, Inc.

V54.24 Aftercare for healing pathologic fracture of leg, unspecified

V54.25 Aftercare for healing pathologic fracture of upper leg

V54.26 Aftercare for healing pathologic fracture of lower leg

V54.27 Aftercare for healing pathologic fracture of vertebrae

V54.29 Aftercare for healing pathologic fracture of other bone

V54.81 Aftercare following joint replacement — (Use additional code to identify joint replacement site: V43.60-V43.69)

V54.89 Other orthopedic aftercare

V54.9 Unspecified orthopedic aftercare — *aftercare for healing fracture NOS*
AHA: Jan-Feb, 1987, 8; Q3, 1995, 3

Coding Clarification

Use V54.81 and an additional code from V43.60-V43.69 to identify joint replacement. If there is a malfunction of an internal orthopedic device, report 996.4.

Coding Scenario

A patient presents to the orthopedic clinic for follow-up care of a fracture of the radius and ulna. X-rays are taken and show the fracture to be in alignment.

> Code assignment: V54.12 *Aftercare for healing traumatic fracture of lower arm* and 813.44 *Fracture of radius and ulna, lower end*

V55 Attention to artificial openings

An ostomy refers to an opening that is created in an operation. An ostomy in the following refers to a surgically formed opening connecting the bowel, bladder, or trachea to outside the body.

These codes include the adjustment or repositioning of a catheter, closure, passage of sounds or bougies, reforming, or removal or replacement of a catheter.

V55.0 Attention to tracheostomy

V55.1 Attention to gastrostomy

V55.2 Attention to ileostomy

V55.3 Attention to colostomy

V55.4 Attention to other artificial opening of digestive tract

V55.5 Attention to cystostomy

V55.6 Attention to other artificial opening of urinary tract — *nephrostomy, urethrostomy, ureterostomy*
AHA: Jan-Feb, 1987, 8

V55.7 Attention to artificial vagina

V55.8 Attention to other specified artificial opening

V55.9 Attention to unspecified artificial opening

Coding Clarification

For complications of an external stoma, report from codes 519.00-519.09, 569.60-569.69, 997.4 or 997.5.

V56 Encounter for dialysis and dialysis catheter care

AHA: Jan-Feb, 1987, 8; Q1, 1993, 29; Q4, 1998, 66

Hemodialysis is the removal of toxins in the blood through a semipermeable membrane. In peritoneal dialysis, the peritoneal lining in the peritoneum acts as the membrane. Fluid is infused into the peritoneum through a catheter and drained from the body after absorbing the toxins.

V56.0 Encounter for extracorporeal dialysis — (Use additional code to identify the associated condition)
AHA: Jan-Feb, 1987, 8; Q1, 1993, 29; Q2, 1998, 20; Q3, 1998, 6; Q4, 1998, 66; Q4, 2000, 40

V56.1 Fitting and adjustment of extracorporeal dialysis catheter — (Use additional code for any concurrent extracorporeal dialysis, V56.0. Use additional code to identify the associated condition)
AHA: Jan-Feb, 1987, 8; Q1, 1993, 29; Q2, 1998, 20; Q4, 1998, 66

V56.2 Fitting and adjustment of peritoneal dialysis catheter — (Use additional code for any concurrent peritoneal dialysis, V56.8. Use additional code to identify the associated condition)

V56.31 Encounter for adequacy testing for hemodialysis — (Use additional code to identify the associated condition)

V56.32 Encounter for adequacy testing for peritoneal dialysis — (Use additional code to identify the associated condition)
AHA: Jan-Feb, 1987, 8; Q1, 1993, 29; Q4, 1998, 66; Q4, 2000, 55

V56.8 Encounter other dialysis — (Use additional code to identify the associated condition)
AHA: Jan-Feb, 1987, 8; Q1, 1993, 29; Q4, 1998, 55; Q4, 1998, 66

Coding Clarification

Any concurrent extracorporeal or peritoneal dialysis should be reported in addition to category V56 codes.

V57 Care involving use of rehabilitation procedures

AHA: Sept-Oct, 1986, 3; Jan-Feb, 1987, 8; Q1, 1990, 6; Q3, 1997, 12; Q1, 2002, 19

Rehabilitation is typically needed for patients who after suffering an illness or injury need additional

V Codes

help to return to normal form and/or function or to an optimal functioning level.

In orthoptic training, exercises are performed to adjust the visual axes of one or both eyes. Orthoptic training is conducted in cases where the eyes are not properly coordinated to allow for good vision out of both eyes.

V57.0 Care involving breathing exercises — (Use additional code to identify underlying condition)

V57.1 Other physical therapy — (Use additional code to identify underlying condition)
AHA: Sept-Oct, 1986, 3; Jan-Feb, 1987, 8; Q1, 1990, 6; Q3, 1997, 12; Q4, 1999, 5; Q1, 2002, 19; Q4, 2002, 56

V57.21 Encounter for occupational therapy — (Use additional code to identify underlying condition)

V57.22 Encounter for vocational therapy — (Use additional code to identify underlying condition)
AHA: Sept-Oct, 1986, 3; Jan-Feb, 1987, 8; Q1, 1990, 6; Q3, 1997, 12; Q1, 2002, 19

V57.3 Speech therapy — (Use additional code to identify underlying condition)

V57.4 Orthoptic training — (Use additional code to identify underlying condition)

V57.8 5th Other specified rehabilitation procedure — (Use additional code to identify underlying condition)
AHA: Sept-Oct, 1986, 3; Jan-Feb, 1987, 8; Q1, 1990, 6; Q3, 1997, 12; Q1, 2002, 19

V57.81 Orthotic training — (Use additional code to identify underlying condition)
AHA: Sept-Oct, 1986, 3; Jan-Feb, 1987, 8; Q1, 1990, 6; Q3, 1997, 12; Q1, 2002, 19

V57.89 Other specified rehabilitation procedure — (Use additional code to identify underlying condition)
AHA: Sept-Oct, 1986, 3; Sept-Oct, 1986, 4; Jan-Feb, 1987, 8; Q1, 1990, 6; Q3, 1997, 12; Q3, 1997, 11, 12; Q3, 2001, 21; Q1, 2002, 16; Q1, 2002, 19; Q2, 2003, 16; Q4, 2003, 105-106, 108

V57.9 Unspecified rehabilitation procedure — (Use additional code to identify underlying condition)

Coding Clarification

An additional diagnosis code should be reported indicating the condition requiring the rehabilitative services or therapy (V57.1, V57.2, V57.3, or V57.89).

Coding Scenario

A patient presents for physical therapy after fracturing a hip in a fall.

Code assignment: V57.1 *Care involving use of rehabilitation procedures, other physical therapy* and V54.13 *Aftercare for healing traumatic fracture of the hip*

V58 Encounter for other and unspecified procedure and aftercare

Drug monitory is the measurement of the level of a specific drug in the body or of a specific function. Patients who take a specific drug on a long-term basis oftentimes need to be monitored to evaluate the continued effectiveness of the drug.

V58.0 Radiotherapy — *encounter or admission for radiotherapy*
AHA: Jan-Feb, 1987, 8; Jan-Feb, 1987, 13; Q2, 1990, 7; Q3, 1992, 5

V58.1 Chemotherapy — *encounter or admission for chemotherapy*
AHA: Sept-Oct, 1984, 5; Jan-Feb, 1987, 8; Q2, 1990, 7; Q2, 1991, 17; Q2, 1992, 6; Q3, 1993, 4; Q2, 2003, 16

V58.2 Blood transfusion, without reported diagnosis

V58.3 Attention to surgical dressings and sutures — *change of dressing, removal of sutures*
AHA: Jan-Feb, 1987, 8

V58.41 Planned postoperative wound closure — (This code should be used in conjunction with other aftercare codes to fully identify the reason for the aftercare encounter)

V58.42 Aftercare following surgery for neoplasm — (This code should be used in conjunction with other aftercare codes to fully identify the reason for the aftercare encounter)
AHA: Jan-Feb, 1987, 8; Nov-Dec, 1987, 9; Q4, 1999, 9; Q4, 2002, 80

V58.43 Aftercare following surgery for injury and trauma — (This code should be used in conjunction with other aftercare codes to fully identify the reason for the aftercare encounter)
AHA: Jan-Feb, 1987, 8; Nov-Dec, 1987, 9; Q4, 1999, 9; Q4, 2002, 80

V58.44 Aftercare following organ transplant

V58.49 Other specified aftercare following surgery — (This code should be used in conjunction with other aftercare codes to fully identify the reason for the aftercare encounter)

V58.5 Orthodontics aftercare

V58.61 Encounter for long-term (current) use of anticoagulants

V58.62 Encounter for aftercare for long-term (current) use of antibiotics

V58.63 Long-term (current) use of antiplatelet/antithrombotic

V Codes

© 2004 Ingenix, Inc.

V58.64 Long-term (current) use of nonsteroidal anti-inflammatories

V58.65 Long-term (current) use of steroids

V58.66 Long-term (current) use of aspirin

V58.67 Long-term (current) use of insulin

V58.69 Encounter for long-term (current) use of other medications — *high risk medications*
AHA: Jan-Feb, 1987, 8; Q4, 1995, 61; Q2, 1996, 7; Q1, 1997, 12; Q2, 1999, 17; Q3, 1999, 13; Q2, 2000, 8; Q3, 2002, 15; Q4, 2002, 84; Q1, 2003, 11

V58.71 Aftercare following surgery of the sense organs, NEC — (This code should be used in conjunction with other aftercare codes to fully identify the reason for the aftercare encounter)
AHA: Jan-Feb, 1987, 8; Q4, 2002, 80

V58.72 Aftercare following surgery of the nervous system, NEC — (This code should be used in conjunction with other aftercare codes to fully identify the reason for the aftercare encounter)
AHA: Jan-Feb, 1987, 8; Q4, 2002, 80

V58.73 Aftercare following surgery of the circulatory system, NEC — (This code should be used in conjunction with other aftercare codes to fully identify the reason for the aftercare encounter)
AHA: Jan-Feb, 1987, 8; Q4, 2002, 80; Q4, 2003, 105

V58.74 Aftercare following surgery of the respiratory system, NEC — (This code should be used in conjunction with other aftercare codes to fully identify the reason for the aftercare encounter)
AHA: Jan-Feb, 1987, 8; Q4, 2002, 80

V58.75 Aftercare following surgery of the teeth, oral cavity, and digestive system, NEC — (This code should be used in conjunction with other aftercare codes to fully identify the reason for the aftercare encounter)
AHA: Jan-Feb, 1987, 8; Q4, 2002, 80

V58.76 Aftercare following surgery of the genitourinary system, NEC — (This code should be used in conjunction with other aftercare codes to fully identify the reason for the aftercare encounter)
AHA: Jan-Feb, 1987, 8; Q4, 2002, 80

V58.77 Aftercare following surgery of the skin and subcutaneous tissue, NEC — (This code should be used in conjunction with other aftercare codes to fully identify the reason for the aftercare encounter)
AHA: Jan-Feb, 1987, 8; Q4, 2002, 80

V58.78 Aftercare following surgery of the musculoskeletal system, NEC — (This code should be used in conjunction with other aftercare codes to fully identify the reason for the aftercare encounter)
AHA: Jan-Feb, 1987, 8; Q4, 2002, 80

V58.81 Fitting and adjustment of vascular catheter — *removal or replacement of catheter, toilet or cleaning*
AHA: Jan-Feb, 1987, 8; Q2, 1994, 8; Q4, 1994, 45

V58.82 Encounter for fitting and adjustment of non-vascular catheter NEC — *removal or replacement of catheter, toilet or cleansing*
AHA: Jan-Feb, 1987, 8; Q2, 1994, 8; Q4, 1994, 45

V58.83 Encounter for therapeutic drug monitoring — (Use additional code for any associated long-term current drug use: V58.61-V58.69)

V58.9 Unspecified aftercare

Coding Clarification

When a patient is admitted for radiotherapy or chemotherapy, report V58.0 or V58.1 as the primary diagnosis and the cancer, disease, or condition as a secondary diagnosis. When procedures V58.0 and V58.1 are performed simultaneously, both may be reported on the same record, with either one sequenced first.

Codes V58.2, V58.5, and V58.9 may be reported only as secondary diagnoses.

V59 Donors

This category of codes is used when the sole purpose of the admission of a patient to a hospital is to donate an organ.

V59.01 Whole blood donor

V59.02 Stem cell donor

V59.09 Blood donor, other

V59.1 Skin donor

V59.2 Bone donor

V59.3 Bone marrow donor

V59.4 Kidney donor

V59.5 Cornea donor

V59.6 Liver donor

V59.8 Donor of other specified organ or tissue

V59.9 Donor of unspecified organ or tissue

Documentation Issues

Donor information must be documented in the patient's chart to verify cross-matching of donor parts.

V Codes

Coding Clarification

Category V59 codes may only be reported as primary diagnoses and must report the donor of the tissue only.

For self-donation of an organ or tissue, report the condition.

V60–V68 Persons Encountering Health Services in Other Circumstances

Category V60-V68 codes contain additional information that must be included in the medical record regarding family, household, administrative, follow up, and psychosocial circumstances. Included in this section is category V64 *Persons encountering health services for specific procedures, not carried out.* Code sequencing is dependent upon the reason the procedure was not performed.

V60 Housing, household, and economic circumstances

Housing may pose a problem for a patient. The patient may have no place of residence, or inadequate resources to maintain a household, or be unable to care for self, or may need to be housed in an institution.

Holiday relief care is reported when a patient who normally receives care at home is provided health care in another facility to enable a relative or caretaker to take a vacation.

V60.0 Lack of housing — *hobos, social migrants, tramps, transients, vagabonds*
AHA: Jan-Feb, 1987, 8

V60.1 Inadequate housing — *lack of heating, restricted space, technical defects in home, preventing adequate care*
AHA: Jan-Feb, 1987, 8

V60.2 Inadequate material resources — *economic problem, poverty NOS*
AHA: Jan-Feb, 1987, 8

V60.3 Person living alone

V60.4 No other household member able to render care — *person requiring care (has) (is): family member too handicapped, ill, or otherwise unsuited to render care*
AHA: Jan-Feb, 1987, 8

V60.5 Holiday relief care

V60.6 Person living in residential institution — *boarding school resident*
AHA: Jan-Feb, 1987, 8

V60.8 Other specified housing or economic circumstances

V60.9 Unspecified housing or economic circumstance

Coding Clarification

Category V60 codes may be reported only as secondary diagnoses.

V61 Other family circumstances

Category V61 codes are used to report circumstances for seeking or receiving medical advice or care.

V61.0 Family disruption — *divorce, estrangement*
AHA: Jan-Feb, 1987, 8; Q1, 1990, 9

V61.10 Counseling for marital and partner problems, unspecified — *marital conflict, partner conflict*
AHA: Jan-Feb, 1987, 8; Q1, 1990, 9

V61.11 Counseling for victim of spousal and partner abuse

V61.12 Counseling for perpetrator of spousal and partner abuse

V61.20 Counseling for parent-child problem, unspecified — *concern about behavior of a child, parent-child conflict*
AHA: Jan-Feb, 1987, 8; Q1, 1990, 9

V61.21 Counseling for victim of child abuse — *child battering, child neglect*
AHA: Jan-Feb, 1987, 8; Q1, 1990, 9

V61.22 Counseling for perpetrator of parental child abuse

V61.29 Counseling for perpetrator of parental child abuse — *problem concerning adopted or foster child*
AHA: Jan-Feb, 1987, 8; Q1, 1990, 9; Q3, 1999, 16

V61.3 Problems with aged parents or in-laws

V61.41 Alcoholism in family

V61.49 Other health problem within the family — *care of or presence of sick or handicapped person in family or household*
AHA: Jan-Feb, 1987, 8; Q1, 1990, 9

V61.5 Multiparity — *many children*
AHA: Jan-Feb, 1987, 8; Q1, 1990, 9

V61.6 Illegitimacy or illegitimate pregnancy — *pregnancy without two married parents*
AHA: Jan-Feb, 1987, 8; Q1, 1990, 9

V61.7 Other unwanted pregnancy

V61.8 Other specified family circumstance — *problem with family members NEC*
AHA: Jan-Feb, 1987, 8; Q1, 1990, 9

V61.9 Unspecified family circumstance

Coding Clarification

If the abuse causes injuries, report all current injuries with codes from 995.50-995.59.

© 2004 Ingenix, Inc.

Coding Scenario

A married couple presents for a weekly counseling session.

> Code assignment: V61.10 *Counseling for marital and partner problems, unspecified.*

V62 Other psychosocial circumstances

These codes are used to report circumstances for seeking or receiving medical advice or care.

V62.0 Unemployment

V62.1 Adverse effects of work environment

V62.2 Other occupational circumstance or maladjustment — *career choice problem, dissatisfaction with employment*
AHA: Jan-Feb, 1987, 8

V62.3 Educational circumstance — *dissatisfaction with school, educational handicap*
AHA: Jan-Feb, 1987, 8

V62.4 Social maladjustment — *culture deprivation, political, religious, or sex discrimination, social isolation, persecution*
AHA: Jan-Feb, 1987, 8

V62.5 Legal circumstance — *imprisonment, legal investigation, litigation, prosecution*
AHA: Jan-Feb, 1987, 8

V62.6 Refusal of treatment for reasons of religion or conscience

V62.81 Interpersonal problem, not elsewhere classified

V62.82 Bereavement, uncomplicated

V62.83 Counseling for perpetrator of physical/sexual abuse

V62.89 Other psychological or physical stress, not elsewhere classified — *life circumstance problems, phase of life problems*
AHA: Jan-Feb, 1987, 8

Coding Clarification

Category V62 codes may be reported only as secondary diagnoses.

For circumstances where the main problem is economic inadequacy or poverty, report V60.2.

For bereavement as an adjustment reaction, report 309.0.

V63 Unavailability of other medical facilities for care

Medical facilities may not be accessible to patients for a variety of reasons, such as a patient's resident is too far removed from a health care facility or medical services are not available to a patient at a patient's home. Another reason is a patient is suffering from a disease or condition that requires a specific type of treatment that was unavailable at the time of admission and is awaiting admission to an adequate facility elsewhere.

V63.0 Residence remote from hospital or other health care facility

V63.1 Medical services in home not available

V63.2 Person awaiting admission to adequate facility elsewhere

V63.8 Other specified reason for unavailability of medical facilities — *person on waiting list undergoing social agency investigation*
AHA: Jan-Feb, 1987, 8; Q1, 1991, 21

V63.9 Unspecified reason for unavailability of medical facilities

V64 Persons encountering health services for specific procedures, not carried out

Services and/or procedures may not be carried out due to a condition that renders the patient untreatable (e.g., reaction to anesthesia, extremely high blood pressure) or because the patient refuses treatment.

In certain instances, procedures performed by scopes are converted into open procedures due to the inability to perform the procedure with the scope (e.g., extensive adhesions) or because the procedure is more extensive than originally anticipated.

V64.0 Vaccination not carried out because of contraindication

V64.1 Surgical or other procedure not carried out because of contraindication

V64.2 Surgical or other procedure not carried out because of patient's decision

V64.3 Procedure not carried out for other reasons

V64.41 Laparoscopic surgical procedure converted to open procedure

V64.42 Thorascopic surgical procedure converted to open procedure

V64.43 Arthroscopic surgical procedure converted to open procedure

Documentation Issues

The medical necessity of the conversion from a scope procedure to an open procedure should be well documented in the patient's health record.

Coding Clarification

Category V64 codes may be reported only as secondary diagnoses.

Coding Scenario

A patient is admitted to the ambulatory surgery center for a laparoscopic right inguinal hernia repair. Due to the patient's anatomy, the physician was not able to perform the repair through the scope. The patient was

V Codes

redraped and the hernia repair was performed through an open incision.

> Code assignment: 550.90 *Unilateral inguinal hernia repair unspecified* and V64.41 *Laparoscopic surgical procedure converted to open procedure*

V65 Other persons seeking consultation without complaint or sickness

Insulin pump training is provided to patients who require insulin for diabetes. It is an alternative to daily shots, in which insulin is supplied by a pump worn externally through a tube into the subcutaneous tissue. A large amount of insulin is supplied to the patient prior to mealtime and a continuous amount of insulin is maintained throughout the day.

V65.0 Healthy person accompanying sick person — *boarder*
AHA: Jan-Feb, 1987, 8

V65.11 Pediatric pre-birth visit for expectant mother

V65.19 Other person consulting on behalf of another person

V65.2 Person feigning illness — *malingerer, peregrinating patient*
AHA: Jan-Feb, 1987, 8; Q3, 1999, 20

V65.3 Dietary surveillance and counseling — *colitis, diabetes, allergies, gastritis, high cholesterol, hypoglycemia, obesity*
AHA: Jan-Feb, 1987, 8

V65.4 ✓5th Other counseling, not elsewhere classified — *health advice, education, instruction*
AHA: Jan-Feb, 1987, 8

V65.40 Counseling NOS

V65.41 Excercise counseling — *cardiovascular disease, obesity*
AHA: Jan-Feb, 1987, 8

V65.42 Counseling on substance use and abuse

V65.43 Counseling on injury prevention

V65.44 Human immunodeficiency virus (HIV) counseling

V65.45 Counseling on other sexually transmitted diseases — *herpes simplex, syphilis, gonorrhea, viral hepatitis B*
AHA: Jan-Feb, 1987, 8

V65.46 Encounter for insulin pump training — *diabetes*

V65.49 Other specified counseling

V65.5 Person with feared complaint in whom no diagnosis was made — *feared condition not demonstrated, problem was normal stated, "worried well"*
AHA: Jan-Feb, 1987, 8

V65.8 Other reasons for seeking consultation

V65.9 Unspecified reason for consultation

Coding Clarification

For consultations conducted on behalf of another person, report with codes V65.11-V65.19.

V66 Convalescence and palliative care

Palliative care is given at the end of a person's life, including hospice and terminal care. Palliative care is given to patients whose illness is terminal and the treatment is aimed toward making the patient comfortable rather than treating the illness. It may be used when a patient is admitted for treatment, but during the process of the treatment it is determined that the illness is terminal.

V66.0 Convalescence following surgery

V66.1 Convalescence following radiotherapy

V66.2 Convalescence following chemotherapy

V66.3 Convalescence following psychotherapy and other treatment for mental disorder

V66.4 Convalescence following treatment of fracture

V66.5 Convalescence following other treatment

V66.6 Convalescence following combined treatment

V66.7 Encounter for palliative care — (Code first underlying disease)
AHA: Jan-Feb, 1987, 8; Q4, 1996, 47, 48; Q1, 1998, 11; Q4, 2003, 107

V66.9 Unspecified convalescence

Documentation Issues

The physician must document that admission is for palliative care. Terms meaning the same as palliative care may be hospice, end-of-life, or comfort care. Terms synonymous with palliative care must be well documented in the medical record.

Coding Clarification

Category V66 codes may only be as primary diagnoses except for V66.7, which should be reported as a secondary diagnosis. Report the underlying condition before V66.7.

V67 Follow-up examination

Follow-up treatment may be necessary to check on a patient following surgery, after different types of therapy, or after a fracture has healed to verify the success of treatment.

V67.00 Follow-up examination, following unspecified surgery

V67.01 Following surgery follow-up vaginal pap smear — (Use additional code to identify condition: V10.40-V10.44, V45.77)
AHA: Jan-Feb, 1987, 8; Q3, 1992, 11; Q4, 1994, 48; Q1, 1995, 4; Q2, 1995, 8; Q4, 1997, 50; Q4, 1998, 69; Q4, 2000, 56

 © 2004 Ingenix, Inc.

V67.09 Follow-up examination, following other surgery

V67.1 Radiotherapy follow-up examination

V67.2 Chemotherapy follow-up examination — *cancer chemotherapy follow-up*
AHA: Jan-Feb, 1987, 8; Q4, 1994, 48

V67.3 Psychotherapy and other treatment for mental disorder follow-up examination

V67.4 Treatment of healed fracture follow-up examination

V67.51 Follow-up examination following completed treatment with high-risk medications, not elsewhere classified

V67.59 Other follow-up examination

V67.6 Combined treatment follow-up examination

V67.9 Unspecified follow-up examination

Coding Clarification

Report the acquired absence of uterus (V45.77) and personal history of malignant neoplasm (V10.40-10.44) in addition to V67.01.

Coding Scenario

A 57-year-old female presents to the OB/GYN clinic for a follow-up Pap smear following a total abdominal hysterectomy one year ago with a diagnosis of a malignancy of the cervix. Treatment ended about six months ago and there has been no further sign of the disease.

> Code assignment: V67.01 *Following surgery follow-up vaginal Pap smear;* V10.41 *Personal history of malignant neoplasm, cervix uteri;* and V45.77 *Acquired absence of uterus*

V68 Encounters for administrative purposes

Medical certificates include death certificates, disability papers, and fitness verification. Repeat prescriptions include appliances, orthotics, glasses, and medication.

A request for expert evidence includes medical testimony and depositions.

V68.0 Issue of medical certificates — *cause of death, fitness, incapacity*
AHA: Jan-Feb, 1987, 8

V68.1 Issue of repeat prescriptions

V68.2 Request for expert evidence

V68.81 Referral of patient without examination or treatment

V68.89 Encounters for other specified administrative purpose

V68.9 Encounters for unspecified administrative purpose

Coding Clarification

Category V68 codes may only be reported as primary diagnoses.

V69 Problems related to lifestyle

Some experts agree that lack of exercise can be as damaging as smoking a pack of cigarettes every day. Lack of exercise may contribute to heart disease and increase the risk for diabetes and high blood pressure. Inappropriate diet may also contribute to health related problems.

High-risk sexual behaviors include homosexuality and promiscuity. This behavior puts the patient at risk for sexually transmitted diseases.

V69.0 Problems related to lack of physical excercise — *sedentary*
AHA: Jan-Feb, 1987, 8; Q4, 1994, 48

V69.1 Problems related to inappropriate diet and eating habits — *malnutrition*
AHA: Jan-Feb, 1987, 8; Q4, 1994, 48

V69.2 Problems related to high-risk sexual behavior — *sexually-transmitted diseases*
AHA: Jan-Feb, 1987, 8; Q4, 1994, 48

V69.3 Problems related to gambling and betting — *financial issues*
AHA: Jan-Feb, 1987, 8; Q4, 1994, 48

V69.4 Lack of adequate sleep

V69.8 Other problems related to lifestyle — *self-damaging behavior*
AHA: Jan-Feb, 1987, 8; Q4, 1994, 48

V69.9 Unspecified problems related to lifestyle

Documentation Issues

The health care provider must document that the patient has a risk factor related to lifestyle.

Coding Clarification

Report from codes 260-269.9 for malnutrition and other nutritional deficiencies; 307.1 for anorexia nervosa; and 783.6 for bulimia.

V70–V84 Persons Without Reported Diagnosis Encountered During Examination and Investigation of Individuals and Populations

Category V70-V84 codes represent encounters with health services for general physical and mental examinations, routine tests on specific body systems, and screenings. The special screening codes are used only when screening procedures are done on defined population groups, such as armed forces personnel or pre-employment physicals.

© 2004 Ingenix, Inc.

Observation for suspected condition codes should be reported when a patient presents with a suspected condition but after further examination it is ruled out. This category may be used for administrative or legal observations.

Special investigations and screening codes should be reported for examination of a specific body system or screening for a specific disease that, after examination, is not found to exist. This includes routine eye examination and diabetes screening. If a diagnosis is found or confirmed, assign the code for the disease or illness rather than a V code.

V70 General medical examination

AHA: Jan-Feb, 1987, 8

This section of codes may include a yearly physical, examination for admission to school or camp, receipt of a driver's license, insurance certification, blood alcohol levels, and examination to participate in clinical research or trials. These services may be requested by the patient or could come from another administrative source, such as the military, employer, or legal authority. This also includes special screening studies for potential organ or tissue donors.

V70.0 Routine general medical examination at health care facility — (Use additional code(s) to identify any special screening examination(s) performed: V73.0-V82.9)
AHA: Jan-Feb, 1987, 8

V70.1 General psychiatric examination requested by the authority — (Use additional code(s) to identify any special screening examination(s) performed: V73.0-V82.9)

V70.2 Other and unspecified general psychiatric examination — (Use additional code(s) to identify any special screening examination(s) performed: V73.0-V82.9)

V70.3 Other general medical examination for administrative purposes — (Use additional code(s) to identify any special screening examination(s) performed: V73.0-V82.9)
AHA: Jan-Feb, 1987, 8; Q1, 1990, 6

V70.4 Examination for medicolegal reason — (Use additional code(s) to identify any special screening examination(s) performed: V73.0-V82.9)
AHA: Jan-Feb, 1987, 8

V70.5 Health examination of defined subpopulation — (Use additional code(s) to identify any special screening examination(s) performed: V73.0-V82.9)

V70.6 Health examination in population survey — (Use additional code(s) to identify any special screening examination(s) performed: V73.0-V82.9)
AHA: Jan-Feb, 1987, 8

V70.7 Examination of participant in clinical trial — (Use additional code(s) to identify any special screening examination(s) performed: V73.0-V82.9)
AHA: Jan-Feb, 1987, 8; Q4, 2001, 55

V70.8 Other specified general medical examination — (Use additional code(s) to identify any special screening examination(s) performed: V73.0-V82.9)
AHA: Jan-Feb, 1987, 8

V70.9 Unspecified general medical examination — (Use additional code(s) to identify any special screening examination(s) performed: V73.0-V82.9)

Coding Clarification

Category V70 codes may only be reported as primary diagnoses except for V70.7, which may be reported as either the primary or secondary diagnosis.

Use codes from V73.0-V82.9 in addition to category V70 codes to identify any special screening examinations.

V71 Observation and evaluation for suspected conditions not found

These codes are used when a patient presents with a suspected condition, but after further examination it is ruled out; no further treatment or follow-up is required for the suspected condition. This category may be used for legal and administrative observation.

Antisocial behavior is behavior that is negative and outside what is perceived as normal. This may include irresponsibility, lack of concern for the feelings of others, inability to maintain relationships, easy frustration and aggression, and the inability to learn from experience.

Tuberculosis (TB) is a bacterial infection that usually attacks the lungs, but which may also affect other organs. The disease is caused by *Mycobacterium* tuberculosis. TB is transmitted by inhaling air droplets exhaled by an infected person or, sometimes, the infection is absorbed by the skin.

Observation for suspected abuse and neglect should be reported for adults or children who are examined for abuse but it is ruled out.

With increased threat of terrorism, a code for suspected exposure to anthrax was developed. Anthrax is a potentially deadly bacterial infection that can be transmitted through contact with the skin, inhalation, and eating undercooked meat from infected animals.

V71.0 ✓5th Observation for suspected mental condition — *without manifest psychiatric disorder*
AHA: March-April, 1987, 1; Jan-Feb, 1987, 8; Q2, 1990, 5; Q4, 1994, 47

© 2004 Ingenix, Inc.

V71.01 Observation of adult antisocial behavior — *gang activity in child or adolescent*
AHA: March-April, 1987, 1; Jan-Feb, 1987, 8; Q2, 1990, 5; Q4, 1994, 47

V71.02 Observation of childhood or adolescent antisocial behavior

V71.09 Observation of other suspected mental condition

V71.1 Observation for suspected malignant neoplasm

V71.2 Observation for suspected tuberculosis — *can be spread by close contact to someone who has the disease*
AHA: March-April, 1987, 1; Jan-Feb, 1987, 8; Q2, 1990, 5; Q4, 1994, 47

V71.3 Observation following accident at work

V71.4 Observation following other accident — *includes motor vehicle accident*
AHA: March-April, 1987, 1; Jan-Feb, 1987, 8; Q2, 1990, 5; Q4, 1994, 47

V71.5 Observation following alleged rape or seduction

V71.6 Observation following other inflicted injury

V71.7 Observation for suspected cardiovascular disease

V71.81 Observation for suspected abuse and neglect

V71.82 Observation and evaluation for suspected exposure to anthrax

V71.83 Observation and evaluation for suspected exposure to other biological agent

V71.89 Observation for other specified suspected conditions

V71.9 Observation for unspecified suspected condition

Coding Clarification

Category V71 codes may only be reported as primary diagnoses. Conditions that coexist at the time of observation for a suspected condition may be reported and sequenced after the V71 category codes.

Observation codes for alleged rape or seduction or following an injury may be used for the victim or the suspect.

Report from codes 995.80-995.85 for adult abuse and neglect and 995.50-995.59 for child abuse and neglect.

Code V71.81 should not be reported on an inpatient following outpatient surgery if a symptom or condition exists that can be coded, such as nausea and vomiting.

Report V29.9 for a baby less than 29 days old observed for a suspected condition that is ruled out.

Coding Scenario

A patient is admitted to the emergency department following a motor vehicle accident for observation of suspected head and internal injuries. After a thorough check, all injuries are ruled out.

Code assignment: V71.4 *Observation following other accident*

V72 Special investigations and examinations

AHA: Jan-Feb, 1987, 8

Preoperative clearance exams are performed prior to surgery to ensure the patient is healthy enough to undergo anesthesia and surgical procedures. This category includes routine examininations or exams performed in the absence of symptoms.

V72.0 Examination of eyes and vision — (Use additional code(s) to identify any special screening examination(s) performed: V73.0-V82.9)

V72.1 Examination of ears and hearing — (Use additional code(s) to identify any special screening examination(s) performed: V73.0-V82.9)

V72.2 Dental examination — (Use additional code(s) to identify any special screening examination(s) performed: V73.0-V82.9)

V72.3 5th Gynecological examination — (Use additional code to identify routine vaginal pap smear, V76.47.)
AHA: Jan-Feb, 1987, 8

V72.31 Routine gynecological examination

V72.32 Encounter for Papanicolaou cervical smear to confirm findings of recent normal smear following initial abnormal smear

V72.4 5th Pregnancy examination or test, pregnancy unconfirmed — (Use additional code(s) to identify any special screening examination(s) performed: V73.0-V82.9)
AHA: Jan-Feb, 1987, 8

V72.40 Pregnancy examination or test, pregnancy unconfirmed

V72.41 Pregnancy examination or test, negative result

V72.5 Radiological examination, not elsewhere classified — (Use additional code(s) to identify any special screening examination(s) performed: V73.0-V82.9)
AHA: Jan-Feb, 1987, 8; Q1, 1990, 19

V72.6 Laboratory examination — (Use additional code(s) to identify any special screening examination(s) performed: V73.0-V82.9)

V Codes

V72.7 Diagnostic skin and sensitization tests — (Use additional code(s) to identify any special screening examination(s) performed: V73.0-V82.9)
AHA: Jan-Feb, 1987, 8

V72.81 Pre-operative cardiovascular examination — (Use additional code(s) to identify any special screening examination(s) performed: V73.0-V82.9)

V72.82 Pre-operative respiratory examination — (Use additional code(s) to identify any special screening examination(s) performed: V73.0-V82.9)

V72.83 Other specified pre-operative examination — (Use additional code(s) to identify any special screening examination(s) performed: V73.0-V82.9)

V72.84 Unspecified pre-operative examination — (Use additional code(s) to identify any special screening examination(s) performed: V73.0-V82.9)

V72.85 Other specified examination — (Use additional code(s) to identify any special screening examination(s) performed: V73.0-V82.9)

V72.9 Unspecified examination — (Use additional code(s) to identify any special screening examination(s) performed: V73.0-V82.9)

Coding Clarification

Category V72 codes may only be reported as primary diagnoses and should only be used when there is not a symptom or confirmed condition that can be coded.

V73 Special screening examination for viral and chlamydial diseases

Viruses are pathogens that can attach to the cell membrane and take over cell functions. They can only grow and reproduce after infecting a host. There are more than 400 types of viruses that cause a variety of diseases ranging from the common cold to hemorrhagic fever. Viruses may immediately cause a disease or remain dormant for several years.

Chlamydial infections are classified as bacterial. They only grow inside a cell and are responsible for causing a variety of diseases including pneumonia and genital infections in men and women.

Poliomyelitis is an infectious viral disease of the central nervous system that sometimes results in paralysis. The World Health Organization (WHO) declared the Western Hemisphere polio-free in 1994. Today polio is most prevalent in areas of Africa, the Middle East and South Asia.

Smallpox is a highly contagious human disease caused by the virus variolae, of which there are two strains: variolae major, which has severe symptoms and a mortality rate of 20 to 40 percent; and variolae minor, which has less severe symptoms and a 1 percent mortality rate. The disease can be spread from person to person and through infected blankets, linens, and clothing.

Measles is an acute infection caused by paramyxovirus and presents with a hacking cough, rash, and fever.

Rubella or German measles is a highly contagious virus, but the symptoms are mild and short-lived in most people. Symptoms include malaise, arthralgia, rash, headache, and fever. Rubella during pregnancy can result in abortion, stillbirth, or congenital defects.

Yellow fever is transmitted from mosquito to man. In cities, the bite of an Aedes aegypti mosquito causes the infection; in the jungle, Haemagogus and other forest canopy mosquitoes acquire the virus from jungle primates and transmit the virus to man. In the United States, cases of yellow fever are usually limited to people who have been abroad.

Trachoma is caused by infection with the organism *Chlamydia trachomatis*. It begins slowly as a mild conjunctivitis that develops into a severe onset infection.

V73.0 Screening examination for poliomyelitis — *viral disease of the central nervous system*
AHA: Jan-Feb, 1987, 8

V73.1 Screening examination for smallpox — *caused by virus variolae*
AHA: Jan-Feb, 1987, 8

V73.2 Screening examination for measles — *caused by paramyxovirus*
AHA: Jan-Feb, 1987, 8

V73.3 Screening examination for rubella — *German measles*
AHA: Jan-Feb, 1987, 8

V73.4 Screening examination for yellow fever — *transmitted from mosquito to man*
AHA: Jan-Feb, 1987, 8

V73.5 Screening examination for other arthropod-borne viral diseases — *dengue fever, viral encephalitis, hemorrhagic fever*
AHA: Jan-Feb, 1987, 8

V73.6 Screening examination for trachoma — *caused by chlamydia trachomatis*
AHA: Jan-Feb, 1987, 8

V73.88 Special screening examination for other specified chlamydial diseases

V73.89 Special screening examination for other specified viral diseases

V73.98 Special screening examination for unspecified chlamydial disease

V73.99 Special screening examination for unspecified viral disease

© 2004 Ingenix, Inc.

Coding Clarification

Category V73 codes may be reported as primary or secondary diagnoses. Screening codes should not be used for patients who have signs, symptoms, or a history of a disease. If a condition is found during the screening, code the condition and do not use the screening codes.

V74 Special screening examination for bacterial and spirochetal diseases

Bacterial and spirochetal diseases include diagnostic skin tests for the diseases. Bacteria are one-cell organisms that cause a wide variety of diseases. A bacterium is capable of undergoing mutations, which makes fighting diseases caused by bacteria an ongoing battle.

A spiral shaped bacterium causes a spirochetal infection. It is responsible for diseases such as syphilis and Lyme disease.

V74.0 Screening examination for cholera — *infectious disease of the bowel*
AHA: Jan-Feb, 1987, 8

V74.1 Screening examination for pulmonary tuberculosis — *caused by Mycobacterium tuberculosis*
AHA: Jan-Feb, 1987, 8

V74.2 Screening examination for leprosy (Hansen's disease) — *highest incidence in India and Brazil*
AHA: Jan-Feb, 1987, 8

V74.3 Screening examination for diphtheria — *caused by Corynebacterium diphtheriae*
AHA: Jan-Feb, 1987, 8

V74.4 Screening examination for bacterial conjunctivitis — *pink eye*
AHA: Jan-Feb, 1987, 8

V74.5 Screening examination for venereal disease — *sexually transmitted diseases*
AHA: Jan-Feb, 1987, 8

V74.6 Screening examination for yaws — *infectious nonvenereal disease*
AHA: Jan-Feb, 1987, 8

V74.8 Screening examination for other specified bacterial and spirochetal diseases

V74.9 Screening examination for unspecified bacterial and spirochetal diseases

Coding Clarification

Category V74 codes may be reported as primary or secondary diagnoses. Screening codes should not be used for patients who have signs, symptoms, or a history of a disease. If a condition is found during the screening, code the condition and do not use the screening codes.

Coding Scenario

A patient presents to the clinic for a routine TB test. The test is read as negative.

> Code assignment: V74.1 *Screening examination for pulmonary tuberculosis*

V75 Special screening examination for other infectious diseases

An infectious disease is caused by a microorganism that can be transmitted with or without contact. A parasite is an organism that attacks a host but does not contribute to the survival of a host.

Rickettsial diseases include Rocky Mountain spotted fever, catscratch disease, Q fever, louse-born typhus, and rickettsial pox and are caused by the microorganism rickettsiae. The organism is somewhere between a virus and a bacterium. The diseases can be serious and various organs and tissues can be affected.

Malaria is a parasite that is transmitted by an infected mosquito. It is a potentially deadly disease that affects 300-500 million people. There are about 1,200 cases each year, mostly contracted by immigrants and people who have traveled to malaria-risk areas.

Leishmaniasis is a disease caused by a parasite. It is transmitted by the bite of infected sand flies. It occurs most often in developing countries and found more in rural than urban areas.

A fungus causes mycotic infections. It can affect a variety of body systems including the skin.

Schistosomiasis, also know as bilharzia or blood fluke, is a water-borne parasitic disease carried by water snails. The disease is caused by infested water. The eggs of the schistomosomes in the excreta of an infected host open on contact with water and release a parasite, the miracidium, which seeks a fresh water snail. Once it has found its snail host, the miracidium produces thousands of new parasites. The snail excretes the parasites into the surrounding water.

Filarial infections are roundworms that are transmitted through the bites of arthropods. The larvae travel through the body to sites such as lymphatic vessels, lymph nodes, subcutaneous tissue, and body cavities and surrounding tissue.

Helminthiases are parasitic worms that can be found in the gastrointestinal tract or under the skin.

V75.0 Screening examination for rickettsial diseases — *most common is Rocky Mountain spotted fever*
AHA: Jan-Feb, 1987, 8

V75.1 Screening examination for malaria — *less than 1000 are diagnosed in the United States each year*
AHA: Jan-Feb, 1987, 8

V Codes

V75.2 Screening examination for leishmaniasis — *seen most in developing nations*
AHA: Jan-Feb, 1987, 8

V75.3 Screening examination for trypanosomiasis — *disease can affect the central nervous system and major organs and can be fatal*
AHA: Jan-Feb, 1987, 8

V75.4 Screening examination for mycotic infections — *condition that is caused by a fungus*
AHA: Jan-Feb, 1987, 8

V75.5 Screening examination for schistosomiasis — *caused by a parasite*
AHA: Jan-Feb, 1987, 8

V75.6 Screening examination for filariasis — *caused by filarial parasites*
AHA: Jan-Feb, 1987, 8

V75.7 Screening examination for intestinal helminthiasis

V75.8 Screening examination for other specified parasitic infections

V75.9 Screening examination for unspecified infectious disease

Coding Clarification

Category V75 codes may be reported as primary or secondary diagnoses. Screening codes should not be used for patients who have signs, symptoms, or a history of a disease. If a condition is found during the screening, code the condition, not the screening codes.

V76 Special screening for malignant neoplasms

This category is broken down by body site, such as breast, bladder, skin, and cervix. It is used for routine screenings or for patients who present without any signs, symptoms, or history of the disease.

V76.0 Special screening for malignant neoplasm of the respiratory organs

V76.10 Unspecified breast screening — *manual breast exam*
AHA: Jan-Feb, 1987, 8; Q4, 1998, 67

V76.11 Screening mammogram for high-risk patient

V76.12 Other screening mammogram

V76.19 Other screening breast examination

V76.2 Screening for malignant neoplasm of the cervix — *routine cervical Pap smear*
AHA: Jan-Feb, 1987, 8

V76.3 Screening for malignant neoplasm of the bladder

V76.41 Screening for malignant neoplasm of the rectum

V76.42 Screening for malignant neoplasm of the oral cavity

V76.43 Screening for malignant neoplasm of the skin

V76.44 Special screening for malignant neoplasm of prostate

V76.45 Special screening for malignant neoplasm of testis

V76.46 Special screening for malignant neoplasms, ovary

V76.47 Special screening for malignant neoplasms, vagina — (Use additional code to identify acquired absence of uterus, V45.77)

V76.49 Special screening for malignant neoplasms, other sites

V76.50 Special screening for malignant neoplasms, intestine, unspecified

V76.51 Special screening for malignant neoplasms, colon

V76.52 Special screening for malignant neoplasms, small intestine

V76.81 Special screening for malignant neoplasms, nervous system

V76.89 Special screening for other malignant neoplasm

V76.9 Screening for unspecified malignant neoplasm

Coding Clarification

Screening codes should not be used for patients who have signs, symptoms, or a history of a disease. If a condition is found during the screening, code the condition, not the screening codes.

Category V76 codes are used to report special screening for malignant neoplasms. Report a code for the risk factor as well as the screening mammogram if no pathology is found after the exam.

Coding Scenario

A screening cervical Pap smear specimen is sent to the pathologist for reading. The specimen is normal.

> Code assignment: V76.2 *Screening for malignant neoplasm of the cervix*

V77 Special screening for endocrine, nutritional, metabolic, and immunity disorders

Endocrine glands are ductless glands, such as the thyroid and pancreas, that secrete directly into the blood system. Nutritional deficiencies include deficiencies in vitamins, minerals, and protein-calorie malnutrition. Metabolic disorders are when the body is not able to break down or utilize certain nutrients. This includes problems with amino-acid transport, carbohydrate transport, lipoid metabolism, and gout.

The thyroid is an organ located in the front of the neck that excretes hormones into the blood stream.

 © 2004 Ingenix, Inc.

The main hormones released are thyroxine (T4) and triiodothyronine (T3). Symptoms of thyroid disorders can include nervousness, irritability, feeling hot or cold, weight loss or gain, and loss of energy.

Diabetes mellitus is a condition in which the body does not produce enough insulin or does not correctly use the insulin it does produce. The body needs insulin to convert sugars and starches into energy.

Malnutrition results from inadequate intake or malabsorption of nutrients. Infants and children are at the highest risk for malnutrition, since there is a high demand for nutrients during the growth years. Pregnancy and old age also pose other significant risks for malnutrition.

Phenylketonuria (PKU) is an inherited error of metabolism affecting phenylalanine. This condition is a failure to break down amino acids found in many foods. This can cause mental retardation and hyperphenylalaninemia.

Galactosemia is a congential condition marked by the body's inability to break down galactose. This is due to an absence of enzymes needed to convert galactose to glucose.

Gout is caused by deposits of monosodium urate or monohydrate crystals. The most common site for these deposits is around the joints, especially around the big toe.

Cystic fibrosis is caused by a defect in the manufacture of cystic fibrosis transmembrane conductance regulator (CFTR). Normally, CFTR forms a channel through which chloride ions transverse the cells lining in the lungs, pancreas, sweat glands, and small intestine. Cystic fibrosis causes a thick, sticky mucus that blocks the airway and can interfere with enzyme production in the pancreas.

Obesity is defined as a condition in which the body weight of the patient is at least 30 percent above the ideal weight as seen on standardized weight charts.

Lipoid disorders are disorders of lipoproteins. There are three types of lipoproteins that carry cholesterol through the bloodstream including high-density lipoproteins (HDL), also known as good cholesterol; low-density lipoproteins (LDL), also know as bad cholesterol; and very low-density lipoproteins (VLDL), also known as very bad cholesterol.

V77.0 Screening for thyroid disorder — *hypothyroid, hyperthyroid*
AHA: Jan-Feb, 1987, 8

V77.1 Screening for diabetes mellitus — *body does not produce enough insulin*
AHA: Jan-Feb, 1987, 8

V77.2 Screening for malnutrition

V77.3 Screening for phenylketonuria (PKU) — *failure to break down an amino acid found in many food products*
AHA: Jan-Feb, 1987, 8

V77.4 Screening for galactosemia — *failure to break down galactose*
AHA: Jan-Feb, 1987, 8

V77.5 Screening for gout — *monosodium crystals in the joint*
AHA: Jan-Feb, 1987, 8

V77.6 Screening for cystic fibrosis — *mucoviscidosis*
AHA: Jan-Feb, 1987, 8

V77.7 Screening for other inborn errors of metabolism — *defective proteins, metabolism, cholesterol, lipoprotein, amino acids, fatty acids, and nucleotide*
AHA: Jan-Feb, 1987, 8

V77.8 Screening for obesity

V77.91 Screening for lipoid disorders — *cholesterol level, hypercholesterolemia, hyperlipidemia*
AHA: Jan-Feb, 1987, 8; Q4, 2000, 53

V77.99 Other and unspecified endocrine, nutritional, metabolic, and immunity disorders

Coding Clarification

Screening codes should not be used for patients who have signs, symptoms, or a history of a disease. If a condition is found during the screening, code the condition, not the screening codes.

V78 Special screening for disorders of blood and blood-forming organs

The term anemia refers to a lower than normal erythrocyte count or level of hemoglobin in the circulating blood. Iron deficiency anemia is almost always caused by blood loss in adults.

Sickle-cell anemia is a severe, chronic, and incurable form of anemia occurring in patients who inherit hemoglobin S genes from both parents. Less severe variations of the disease occur when the patient inherits one hemoglobin S gene from one parent and one hemoglobin C, D, or E gene from the other.

V78.0 Screening for iron deficiency anemia

V78.1 Screening for other and unspecified deficiency anemia

V78.2 Screening for sickle-cell disease or trait — *highest among African-Americans, native African, and Mediterranean cultures*
AHA: Jan-Feb, 1987, 8

V78.3 Screening for other hemoglobinopathies

V78.8 Screening for other disorders of blood and blood-forming organs

V78.9 Screening for unspecified disorder of blood and blood-forming organs

Coding Clarification

Category V78 codes may be reported as primary or secondary diagnoses. Screening codes should not be used for patients who have signs, symptoms, or a history of a disease. If a condition is found during the screening, code the condition, not the screening codes.

V79 Special screening for mental disorders and developmental handicaps

Depression is marked by a loss of interest in activities and feeling sad for long periods of time. There are several kinds of depression that affects more than 20 million people in the United States.

Alcoholism is both a mental and physical condition, resulting from excessive alcohol consumption. It is characterized by behavioral and other responses that always include a compulsion to take alcohol on a continuous or periodic basis in order to experience its psychic effects and sometimes to avoid the discomfort of its absence; tolerance may or may not be present.

Mental retardation is defined as general intellectual functioning at least two standard deviations below the norm as measured in a standardized intelligence test. It must be accompanied by significant limitation in communication, self care, home living, interpersonal skills, self-direction, work, leisure, health, or safety. This onset must occur before adulthood.

A developmental delay is the failure to obtain developmental milestones that are related to a specific age. This may include sitting, crawling, and walking.

V79.0	Screening for depression
V79.1	Screening for alcoholism
V79.2	Screening for mental retardation
V79.3	Screening for developmental handicaps in early childhood
V79.8	Screening for other specified mental disorders and developmental handicaps
V79.9	Screening for unspecified mental disorder and developmental handicap

Coding Clarification

Category V79 codes may be reported as primary or secondary diagnoses. These codes should not be used for patients who have signs, symptoms, or a history of a disease. If a condition is found during the screening, code the condition, not the screening codes.

Coding Scenario

A mother of a one-year-old male presents to the pediatric clinic with concerns that the child is not walking. After examination and testing it is determined that there is no problem with the child.

Code assignment: V79.3 *Screening for developmental handicaps in early childhood*

V80 Special screening for neurological, eye, and ear diseases

Neurological conditions are those that affect the central nervous system. This can include epilepsy, dementia, migraines, and neuromuscular diseases.

Glaucoma is an increase in intraocular pressure due to an abnormal aqueous humor outflow from the anterior chamber or, rarely, from an above normal rate of aqueous humor production by the ciliary body. If untreated, glaucoma ultimately leads to optic nerve damage and loss of vision.

V80.0	Screening for neurological conditions
V80.1	Screening for glaucoma
V80.2	Screening for other eye conditions — *cataract, senile macular lesions* **AHA:** Jan-Feb, 1987, 8
V80.3	Screening for ear diseases

Coding Clarification

Category V80 codes may be reported as primary or secondary diagnoses. Screening codes should not be used for patients who have signs, symptoms, or a history of a disease. If a condition is found during the screening, code the condition, not the screening codes.

V81 Special screening for cardiovascular, respiratory, and genitourinary diseases

Ischemic heart disease is an inadequate flow of blood through the coronary arteries to the tissue of the heart. The predominant etiology of the ischemia is arteriosclerosis. Partially obstructed coronary artery blood flow can manifest in angina pectoris; complete obstruction results in an infarction of the myocardium.

Hypertension is a condition in which the diastolic pressure exceeds 100 mm Hg in persons 60 years of age and older or 90 mm Hg in persons younger than 60 years of age. WHO defines hypertension as pressures exceeding 160/90 mm Hg, but studies have shown that increased morbidity and mortality are associated with diastolic pressures of just 85 mm Hg. It is generally asymptomatic until complications develop. Complications may include retinal changes, loud aortic sounds, and early systolic ejection click heard on auscultation, headache, tinnitus, and palpations.

Bronchitis is defined as a persistent cough with sputum production occurring on most days for at least three months of the year for at least two years.

© 2004 Ingenix, Inc.

Emphysema refers to any condition in which air is present in a small area of an organ or tissue. This causes over inflation of the lungs. The most common cause of emphysema is smoking; however, environmental factors may have an influence.

Nephropathy refers to diseases of the kidney. Included in this are nephritis and sclerotic lesions of the kidney.

V81.0 Screening for ischemic heart disease

V81.1 Screening for hypertension

V81.2 Screening for other and unspecified cardiovascular conditions

V81.3 Screening for chronic bronchitis and emphysema

V81.4 Screening for other and unspecified respiratory condition

V81.5 Screening for nephropathy — *asymptomatic bacteruria*
AHA: Jan-Feb, 1987, 8

V81.6 Screening for other and unspecified genitourinary condition

Coding Clarification

Category V81 codes may be reported as primary or secondary diagnoses. Screening codes should not be used for patients who have signs, symptoms, or a history of a disease. If a condition is found during the screening, code the condition, not the screening codes.

Coding Scenario

A 65-year-old male presents to the family practice clinic for a routine blood pressure check. The patient has no history of hypertension.

> Code assignment: V81.1 *Screening for hypertension*

V82 Special screening for other condition

Rheumatoid arthritis is a chronic, systemic inflammatory disease of unknown etiology, characterized by a variable but prolonged course with swelling. In early stages, the disease attacks the joints of the hands and feet. As the disease progresses, more joints become involved. Also known as primary progressive arthritis and proliferative arthritis, the disease often leads to progressive deformities, which may develop rapidly and cause permanent disability.

Congenital dislocation of the hip is caused by failure of the hip joint to form correctly. This is characterized by a hip click that can be heard when the leg is moved.

Chromosomal anomalies are either lack of genetic material or extra genetic material. Mothers can pass genetic anomalies to their children without having the specific disease. Genetic anomalies can also occur at conception when genetic material from the mother and father are joined.

Multiphasic screening refers to multiple tests that are used to identify illness or disease.

Osteoporosis is generalized bone disease characterized by decreased osteoblastic formation of matrix combined with increased osteoclastic resorption of bone, resulting in a marked decrease in bone mass.

V82.0 Screening for skin condition

V82.1 Screening for rheumatoid arthritis

V82.2 Screening for other rheumatic disorder

V82.3 Screening for congenital dislocation of hip

V82.4 Maternal postnatal screening of chromosomal anomalies

V82.5 Screening for chemical poisoning and other contamination

V82.6 Multiphasic screening

V82.81 Special screening for osteoporosis — (Use additional code to identify postmenopausal status: V07.4, V49.81)

V82.89 Special screening for other specified conditions

V82.9 Screening for unspecified condition

Coding Clarification

Category V82 codes may reported as primary or secondary diagnoses. Screening codes should not be used for patients who have signs, symptoms, or a history of a disease. If a condition is found during the screening, code the condition, not the screening codes.

Report V07.4 for postmenopausal hormone replacement therapy status or V49.81 for postmenopausal (age-related) (natural) status in addition to V82.81.

V83 Genetic carrier status

Category V83 codes are used to report genetic carrier status. The codes are mainly used for women who are pregnant or are considering pregnancy and are known carriers of a disease. The codes listed are for asymptomatic carriers except for V83.02, which is for carriers of hemophilia A, who have trouble with blood coagulation.

Hemophilia A is abnormal coagulation characterized by subcutaneous and intramuscular hemorrhage and caused by a mutant gene on the X chromosome.

Cystic fibrosis is caused by a defect in the manufacture of cystic fibrosis transmembrane conductance regulator (CFTR). Normally, CFTR forms a channel through which chloride ions transverse the cells lining in the lungs, pancreas, sweat glands, and small intestine. Cystic fibrosis causes a thick, sticky mucus that blocks the airway and can interfere with enzyme production in the pancreas.

V83.01 Asymptomatic hemophilia A carrier

V83.02 Symptomatic hemophilia A carrier

V83.81 Cystic fibrosis gene carrier

V83.89 Other genetic carrier status

Coding Clarification

Screening codes should not be used for patients who have signs, symptoms, or a history of a disease.

If a condition is found during the screening, code the condition, not the screening codes.

V84 Genetic susceptibility to diseases

Having a genetic susceptibility to a disease, in particular a malignancy, is not the same as being a carrier of a disease, that may be passed on to offspring. Those people who are genetically susceptibility is a red flag a person is at higher risk and has a greater chance of getting a disease or malignant growth because of their inborn predisposition. These patients sometimes request to have the particular organ at risk removed prophylactically in the hope that taking such a step will prevent the disease from occurring. Most of these requests are for prophylactic breast or ovary removal.

V84.01 Genetic susceptibility to malignant neoplasm of breast

V84.02 Genetic susceptibility to malignant neoplasm of ovary

V84.03 Genetic susceptibility to malignant neoplasm of prostate

V84.04 Genetic susceptibility to malignant neoplasm of endometrium

V84.09 Genetic susceptibility to other malignant neoplasm

V84.8 Genetic susceptibility to other disease

V Codes

© 2004 Ingenix, Inc.

E800–E999

Supplementary Classification of External Causes of Injury and Poisoning

E codes are used to indicate how an accident occurred, what caused an injury, whether a drug overdose was accidental, an adverse drug reaction, or the location of an injury. This information can be used by payers to determine if another insurance company (e.g., automobile insurance) should be billed, but the primary intent is to gather information for injury research and prevention. These codes are used as an additional diagnosis and should never be listed first; the most serious condition or injury should be coded as the primary diagnosis.

When accidents involve more than one motor vehicle, the following order should be used:

- Aircraft and spacecraft (E840-E845)
- Watercraft (E830-E838)
- Motor vehicle (E810-E825)
- Railway (E800-E807)
- Other road vehicles (E826-E829)
- If injuries are sustained from more than one cause, report as many E codes as necessary. The codes should be listed in the following order:
- E codes for abuse
- E codes for terrorism
- E codes for catastrophe or natural disaster
- E codes for transport accidents
- Assign the code for the most serious injuries in each category first.

Transport accidents (E800-E848) involve a vehicle that is primarily used to transport people or products. Agriculture and construction vehicle accidents are considered transport accidents if the machinery is under its own power on a highway.

E800–E807 Railway Accidents

Railway accidents involve vehicles that travel on rails and transport people or products. Use this category whether or not the train is moving. A train is defined as an electric car or a street car that is operated on its own right-of-way and is not open to other traffic, a railway train, a car on a flexible cable either monorail or two rail, a subway or elevated train and any other vehicle designed to run on a railway track. Excluded from this category are interurban electric cars (streetcars) specified to be operating on a street that forms part of the public street or highway.

According to ICD-9-CM guidelines, a railway or railroad is a right-of-way designed for traffic on rails, which is used by carriages or wagons transporting passengers or freight, and by other rolling stock, and which is not open to other public vehicular traffic.

A passenger on the train is any authorized person traveling on the train. Use fourth digit .8 *Other specified person,* for passengers waiting to get on the train or unauthorized riders.

The following fourth-digit subdivisions are for use with categories E800-E807 to identify the injured person:

0 Railway employee
1 Passenger on railway
2 Pedestrian
3 Pedal cyclist
8 Other specified person
9 Unspecified person

E800 [5th] Railway accident involving collision with rolling stock

Rolling stock is any kind of car or vehicle that travels on a track. Included in this code category is any kind of collision that involves a railway train or railway vehicle, a collision not otherwise specified (NOS) on railway, or a derailment with preceding collision with rolling stock.

A railway accident is one that involves a train and another vehicle that travels on rails.

An antecedent collision with derailment means the engine collides with an object causing the train to derail.

E Codes

Coding Clarification

Category E800 codes may only be reported as a secondary diagnosis.

E code reporting varies from state to state and hospital to hospital. Check with payers and hospital policies to determine if E codes should be reported.

Use an additional code from category E849 to identify the place of occurrence.

E801 5th Railway accident involving collision with other object

Included in this code category is the collision of a railway train with buffers, which includes fallen trees or rocks on the railway, a gate, a platform, a streetcar, a bicycle, or any other object that is not a motorized vehicle.

Coding Clarification

Category E801 codes may only be reported as a secondary diagnosis.

Use an additional code from category E849 to identify the place of occurrence.

Coding Scenario

A train engineer presented to the emergency department with a left radial and ulnar shaft fracture after the train he was driving hit a tree that had fallen on to the track.

> Code assignment: 813.2 *Closed fracture of shaft of the radius and ulna,* E800.0 *Railway accident involving collision with other object, railroad employee,* E849.8 *Place of occurrence, other specified place.*

E802 5th Railway accident involving derailment without antecedent collision

Railway accidents involving derailment without antecedent collision means a train derailment that is not caused by the engine hitting an object.

Coding Clarification

Category E802 codes may only be reported as a secondary diagnosis.

Use an additional code from category E849 to identify the place of occurrence.

E803 5th Railway accident involving explosion, fire, or burning

A railway accident that is caused by or involves a type of fire or explosion may be a mechanical issue related to the train's engine, a fire in a commuter train caused by an individual or cooking vessel, or other flammable items.

Coding Clarification

Category E803 codes may only be reported as a secondary diagnosis.

Report the code for the injury sustained in the accident before the E code.

Use an additional code from category E849 to identify the place of occurrence.

E804 5th Fall in, on, or from railway train

Category E804 codes are used to report a fall in, on, or from the railway train, which includes a fall while getting on or off the train. Report the ICD-9-CM code for the injury before the E code.

Coding Clarification

Category E804 codes may only be reported as a secondary diagnosis.

Use an additional code from category E849 to identify the place of occurrence.

Coding Scenario

A 54-year-old female presents to the emergency department with pain in the right ankle. She fell while stepping off the train at the station. X-rays show no fracture. The final diagnosis is a sprained right ankle.

> Code assignment: 845.00 *Unspecified site of ankle sprain and strain,* E804.1 *Fall in, on, or from railway train, passenger on railway*, E849.8 *Place of occurrence, other specified place*

E805 5th Hit by rolling stock

Category E805 codes are used to describe railway accidents caused by a hit to rolling stock. Rolling stock is defined as anything that travels on the track. These kinds of accidents include persons being crushed, injured, killed, knocked down, or run over stock by a railway train or part.

Coding Clarification

Category E805 codes may only be reported as a secondary diagnosis.

Use an additional code from category E849 to identify the place of occurrence.

E806 5th Other specified railway accident

Category E806 codes are used to describe any other specified railway accident. This code category includes an object falling on and hitting a pedestrian in the railway train, pedestrian injuries caused by a door or window on a railway train, an object set in motion by a railway train hitting a non-motor-road vehicle or pedestrian, or falling earth NOS, a rock, a tree, or other object hitting a railway train.

Coding Clarification

Category E806 codes may only be reported as a secondary diagnosis.

Use an additional code from category E849 to identify the place of occurrence.

© 2004 Ingenix, Inc.

Coding Scenario

A 48-year-old male was found on a railroad track with a severe laceration to the thigh. He could not provide any details of the accident.

> Code assignment: 890.0 *Open wound of the thigh without mention of complication* and E806.9 *Railway accident of unspecified nature, unspecified person*

E807 ✓5th Railway accident of unspecified nature

Category E807 codes are used to report an unspecified railway accident. Included in these types of accidents are a person found dead or injured on the railway right-of-way and a railway accident NOS.

Coding Clarification

Category E807 codes may only be reported as a secondary diagnosis.

Use an additional code from category E849 to identify the place of occurrence.

E810–E819 Motor Vehicle Traffic Accidents

According to ICD-9-CM guidelines, a motor vehicle accident is a transport accident involving a vehicle that is motorized. A motor vehicle accident is an accident that occurs on the highway and is assumed to have occurred on the highway unless otherwise specified. An accident that involves an off-road vehicle, such as an ATV or a snowmobile, is considered a nontraffic accident unless otherwise specified. All codes require fourth digits.

A motor vehicle is defined as a self-powered device intended to move people or objects. Motor vehicles travel on the highway and not on rails. Included in this category are automobiles, buses, construction machinery, farm and industrial machinery, steam rollers, tractors, army tanks, highway graders or similar vehicles on wheels or treads while in transport under its own power, fire engines, motorcycles, motorized bicycles, mopeds, scooters, trolley buses (not operating on rails), trucks, and vans.

A driver is considered the occupant of a car who is operating the vehicle. All other occupants are considered passengers.

A pedal cycle is any vehicle operated solely by pedal power. A pedal cyclist includes any person riding on a pedal cycle, including a passenger.

A pedestrian is defined as a person not riding in a vehicle, on a motorcycle, or on an animal. A pedestrian can be a person changing a tire, operating a pedestrian conveyance, fixing a vehicle, or traveling on foot.

The following fourth-digit subdivisions are for use with categories E810-E819 to identify the injured person:

0 Driver of motor vehicle other than motorcycle

1 Passenger in motor vehicle other than motorcycle

2 Motorcyclist

3 Passenger on motorcycle

4 Occupant of streetcar

5 Rider of animal; occupant of animal-driven vehicle

6 Pedal cyclist

7 Pedestrian

8 Other specified person

9 Unspecified person

E810 ✓5th Motor vehicle traffic accident involving collision with train

Category E810 codes are used to report an accident involving a motor vehicle and a train.

Coding Clarification

Category E810 codes may only be reported as a secondary diagnosis.

Use an additional code from category E849 to identify the place of occurrence.

E811 ✓5th Motor vehicle traffic accident involving re-entrant collision with another motor vehicle

Category E811 is used to report a motor vehicle traffic accident involving a re-entrant collision with another motor vehicle. A re-entry accident includes the collision between two motor vehicles caused by one motor vehicle accidentally leaving the roadway and then re-entering the same roadway or a motor vehicle that crosses over to the opposite roadway or a divided highway.

Coding Clarification

Category E811 codes may only be reported as a secondary diagnosis.

Use an additional code from category E849 to identify the place of occurrence.

E812 ✓5th Other motor vehicle collision with unmoving motor vehicle

Category E812 codes are used to report a motor vehicle accident involving a collision with another motor vehicle. This code category includes the collision of one motor vehicle with another motor vehicle that is parked, stopped, stalled, disabled, or abandoned on the highway and a motor vehicle collision NOS.

Coding Clarification

Category E812 codes may only be reported as a secondary diagnosis.

Use an additional code from category E849 to identify the place of occurrence.

E813 ✓5th Motor vehicle collision with nonmotor transport vehicle

Category E813 codes are used to report a motor vehicle collision with another vehicle. This includes a collision between a motor vehicle of any kind and other road (non-motor-transport) vehicles, such as an animal carrying a person, an animal-drawn vehicle, a pedal cycle, or a streetcar.

Coding Clarification

Category E813 codes may only be reported as a secondary diagnosis.

Use an additional code from category E849 to identify the place of occurrence.

Coding Scenario

A 21-year-old female was brought into the emergency department following a car vs. bicycle accident. The patient was riding her bike in the street and was hit by a car from behind. The patient complains of pain in her right wrist. X-rays were negative for a fracture. The final diagnosis is sprain of the right wrist.

> Code assignment: 842.00 *Sprain and strain of unspecified part of the wrist*, E813.3 *Motor vehicle traffic accident involving collision with other vehicle, Pedal cyclist*, and E849.5 *Place of occurrence street and highway*

E814 ✓5th Motor vehicle collision with pedestrian

Category E14 codes identify a motor vehicle collision with a pedestrian. This code category includes all kinds of motor vehicles. A pedestrian dragged, hit, or run over by a motor vehicle is included in this category.

Coding Clarification

Category E814 codes may only be reported as a secondary diagnosis.

Use an additional code from category E849 to identify the place of occurrence.

E815 ✓5th Other motor vehicle collision with object on the highway

Category E815 codes are used to report other motor vehicle collisions on the highway. This code category includes a collision due to loss of control on the highway between a motor vehicle and an abutment (a structure that receives force or pressure), a bridge, an overpass, an animal, fallen stone, a traffic sign, a tree, a utility pole, a guard rail, a fence, a highway divider, a landslide (not moving), an object set in motion by a railway train or road vehicles, fixed, moveable, or moving object thrown in front of motor vehicle safety island, a temporary traffic signs or markers, or walls.

Coding Clarification

Category E815 codes may only be reported as a secondary diagnosis.

Report E816.0-E816.9 for collision with any object that normally would have been off the highway and is not stated as having been on it.

Use an additional code from category E849 to identify the place of occurrence.

E816 ✓5th Motor vehicle traffic accident due to loss of control, without collision on the highway

Category E816 codes are used to report traffic accidents due to loss of control of a motor vehicle without collision on the highway. This code category includes a motor vehicle that fails to make a curve, a motor vehicle going out of control due to a tire blowout, the driver falling asleep, the driver not paying attention, excessive speeding, or the failure of mechanical parts. This type of accident also includes an out-of-control vehicle colliding with an object off the highway, overturning the car, and stopping abruptly off the highway.

Coding Clarification

Category E816 codes may only be reported as a secondary diagnosis.

Use an additional code from category E849 to identify the place of occurrence.

Coding Scenario

A 16-year-old male is brought into the emergency department following a one-car rollover accident. He went out of control after overcorrecting on a turn. He complains of left elbow pain. There are no other injures. The final diagnosis is a fracture of the distal humerus.

> Code assignment: 812.4 *Fracture lower end of humerus*, E816.0 *Motor vehicle traffic accident due to loss of control without collision on the highway, driver* , E849.5 *Place of occurrence, street and highway*

E817 ✓5th Noncollision motor vehicle traffic accident while boarding or alighting

Category E817 codes are used to report non-collision, motor-vehicle-traffic accidents while boarding or alighting (getting out of the car). This code category includes a fall while getting on or off a bus, a fall getting in or out of a car, an injury by a moving part of a vehicle, or a passenger trapped by the door of a bus.

Coding Clarification

Category E817 codes may only be reported as a secondary diagnosis.

Use an additional code from category E849 to identify the place of occurrence.

E Codes

© 2004 Ingenix, Inc.

E818 5th Other noncollision motor vehicle traffic accident

Category E818 codes are used to report other noncollision motor vehicle traffic accidents. This code category includes most accidents that are not caused by one vehicle colliding with another vehicle. Examples of this are accidental poisoning from exhaust gas; falling, jumping, or being accidentally pushed from a moving car; a fire starting in a moving car; and an injury from being hit by an object thrown into or on a moving vehicle.

A traffic accident is one that occurs on a public highway. A motor vehicle accident is assumed to have occurred on the highway unless otherwise specified.

Coding Clarification

Category E818 codes may only be reported as a secondary diagnosis.

Use an additional code from category E849 to identify the place of occurrence.

E819 5th Motor vehicle traffic accident of unspecified nature

Category E819 codes are used to report motor vehicle accidents of an unspecified nature. This code category includes motor vehicle traffic accidents NOS and traffic accidents NOS.

A traffic accident is one that occurs on a public highway. A motor vehicle accident is assumed to have occurred on the highway unless otherwise specified.

A motor vehicle is one that is mechanically or electrically powered and primarily used on a highway. Any object being towed by the motor vehicle is considered a part of the vehicle.

Coding Clarification

Category E819 codes may only be reported as a secondary diagnosis.

Use an additional code from category E849 to identify the place of occurrence.

Coding Scenario

An 18-year-old male is brought into the emergency department following a motor vehicle accident with another car at an intersection. He is the restrained driver. The patient has a small laceration on his forehead. No other injuries were found.

> Code assignment: 873.42 *Open wound, forehead, without complication*, E819.0 *Motor vehicle traffic accident of unspecified nature, driver of motor vehicle other than motorcycle*, and E849.5 *Place of occurrence, street and highway*

E820–E825 Motor Vehicle Nontraffic Accidents

Category E820-E825 codes are used to report nontraffic accidents. Nontraffic accidents are defined as those that occur in a place other than a public highway. This code category includes snowmobile accidents, off-road vehicle accidents, and collisions with stationary objects. Also included in this category is an accident while boarding and alighting a vehicle not on a public highway. Accidents that involve off-road vehicles, such as all-terrain vehicles (ATVs) and snowmobiles, are assumed to be nontraffic accidents unless otherwise specified. Fourth digits are required for all of the codes.

A driver is considered the occupant of a car who is operating the vehicle. All other occupants are considered passengers.

A pedal cycle is any vehicle operated solely by pedal power. A pedal cyclist includes any person riding on a pedal cycle, including a passenger.

A pedestrian is defined as a person not riding in a vehicle, on a motorcycle, or on an animal. A pedestrian can be a person changing a tire, operating a pedestrian conveyance, fixing a motor vehicle, or traveling on foot.

A pedestrian conveyance is defined as a device powered by a human to transport a person other than by walking. This includes a baby carriage, coaster wagon, ice skates, perambulator, pushcart, pushchair, roller skates, scooter, skateboard, skis, sled, or wheelchair. For coding purposes, a person in or on a pedestrian conveyance is considered a pedestrian.

A streetcar is a vehicle that normally runs on rails but is subject to traffic signals and forms part of the traffic way. A trailer being towed by a streetcar is considered part of the streetcar.

Accidents involving off-road vehicles are assumed to be nontraffic accidents unless otherwise specified.

The following fourth-digit subdivisions are for use with categories E820-E825 to identify the injured person:

0 Driver of motor vehicle other than motorcycle
1 Passenger in motor vehicle other than motorcycle
2 Motorcyclist
3 Passenger on motorcycle
4 Occupant of streetcar
5 Rider of animal; occupant of animal-drawn vehicle
6 Pedal cyclist
7 Pedestrian
8 Other specified person
9 Unspecified person

E Codes

E820 5th Nontraffic accident involving motor-driven snow vehicle

Category E820 codes are used to report nontraffic accidents involving motor-driven snow vehicles. This code category is used to report an injury from falling off of or being dragged by a snowmobile. Also included in this code category is any injury caused by a rough landing of the snow vehicle.

Alcohol and excessive speed contribute to the majority of snowmobile injuries and death.

Nontraffic accidents are those that occur any place other than a public highway. Off-road vehicle accidents are considered nontraffic accidents unless otherwise specified.

Coding Clarification

Category E820 codes may only be reported as a secondary diagnosis.

Use an additional code from category E849 to identify the place of occurrence.

E821 5th Nontraffic accident involving other off-road motor vehicle

Category E821 codes are used to report nontraffic accidents involving other off-road motor vehicles. An off-road motor vehicle is one specially designed to negotiate rough or soft terrain (e.g., vehicles that are high in construction, have special wheels and tires, or are driven by treads). A non-motor-vehicle accident is one that occurs any place other than a public highway. Off-road vehicle accidents are considered nontraffic accidents unless otherwise specified.

Coding Clarification

Category E821 codes may only be reported as a secondary diagnosis.

Use an additional code from category E849 to identify the place of occurrence.

Coding Scenario

A 45-year-old male is brought into the emergency department with an abrasion to the right hip after falling off the ATV he was driving. X-rays are negative for a fracture. The final diagnosis is an abrasion the right hip.

> Code assignment: 916.0 *Hip, thigh, and ankle abrasion or friction burn without mention of infection*, E821.0 *Nontraffic accident involving other off-road motor vehicle, driver*

E822 5th Other motor vehicle nontraffic accident involving collision with moving object

Category E822 codes are used to report other motor vehicle accidents involving collision with a moving object. This code category includes collision between a motor vehicle and an animal, a non-motor-vehicle, another motor vehicle, a pedestrian, a train, or another moving object. A non-motor-vehicle accident is one that occurs any place other than a public highway. Do not use this code for off-road motor vehicles.

Coding Clarification

Category E822 codes may only be reported as a secondary diagnosis.

Use an additional code from category E849 to identify the place of occurrence.

E823 5th Other motor vehicle nontraffic accident involving collision with stationary object

Category E823 codes are used to report a nontraffic collision between a motor vehicle and any other object that is not moving. This type of accident includes collisions with objects that are fixed or moveable. Nontraffic accidents are those that occur any place other than a public highway. Do not use this code for off-road motor vehicles. A motor vehicle is one that is mechanically or electrically powered and primarily used on a highway. Any object being towed by the motor vehicle is considered a part of the vehicle.

Coding Clarification

Category E823 codes may only be reported as a secondary diagnosis.

Use an additional code from category E849 to identify the place of occurrence.

Coding Scenario

A 17-year-old female is admitted to the emergency department with a suspected head injury after the ATV she was driving hit a rock and flipped her out. All x-rays and tests are negative for a head injury and she is sent home.

> Code assignment: V71.4 *Observation following other accident* and E823.0 *Other motor vehicle nontraffic accident involving collision with stationary object, driver of motor vehicle other than motorcycle*

E824 5th Other motor vehicle nontraffic accident while boarding and alighting

Category E824 codes are used to report injuries while getting in or out of a motor vehicle or on or off a motorcycle. This code category also includes injury from any moving part of the vehicle or being trapped by the door of the vehicle. Codes in this category are used to report an injury that occurs when the vehicle is not moving. Do not use this code for off-road motor vehicles. An off-road motor vehicle is one specifically designed to negotiate rough or soft terrain (e.g., vehicles that are high in construction, have special wheels and tires, or driven by treads). A motor vehicle is one that is mechanically or electrically powered and primarily used on a highway. Any object being towed by the motor vehicle is considered a part of the vehicle.

© 2004 Ingenix, Inc.

Coding Clarification
Category E824 codes may only be reported as a secondary diagnosis.

Use an additional code from category E849 to identify the place of occurrence.

E825 ✓5th Other motor vehicle nontraffic accident of other and unspecified nature

Category E825 codes are used to report other and unspecified injuries sustained as a result of a nontraffic accident. A nontraffic accident is one that occurs any place other than on a public highway. Unspecified injuries include injury from accidental carbon monoxide poisoning and injury from a part of a moving vehicle. Also included is injury that occurs when from falling, jumping, or being accidentally pushed from a moving vehicle. This category also includes an injury sustained from an object thrown into a moving vehicle.

Coding Clarification
Category E825 codes may only be reported as a secondary diagnosis.

Use an additional code from category E849 to identify the place of occurrence.

E826–E829 Other Road Vehicle Accidents

Other road vehicle accidents are those that involve any device other than motor vehicles. This type of accident includes those that occur while a person is riding on an animal, and any accident that involves an animal-drawn carriage, a bicycle, a tricycle, or a streetcar.

A pedestrian is defined as a person not riding in a vehicle, on a motorcycle, or on an animal. A pedestrian can be a person changing a tire, operating a pedestrian conveyance, fixing a motor vehicle, or traveling on foot.

A streetcar is a vehicle that normally runs on rails but is subject to traffic signals and forms part of the traffic way. A trailer being towed by a streetcar is considered part of the streetcar.

The following fourth-digit subdivisions are for use with categories E826-E829 to identify the injured person:

0 Pedestrian

1 Pedal cyclist

2 Rider of animal

3 Occupant of animal-drawn vehicle

4 Occupant of streetcar

8 Other specified person

9 Unspecified person

E826 ✓5th Pedal cycle accident

Category E826 codes are used to report an accident involving a pedal cycle. A pedal cycle is defined as any vehicle that is run solely by pedal power. A pedal cyclist is any person riding a pedal cycle or riding in a sidecar. This code category includes most injuries caused by parts of the cycle or by a person becoming entangled in a part. Also included in this code category is injury sustained from a fall off of the cycle or from an object thrown at the cycle.

Coding Clarification
Category E826 codes may only be reported as a secondary diagnosis.

Use an additional code from category E849 to identify the place of occurrence.

Coding Scenario
A 34-year-old male, riding in the street, fell off his bicycle and sustained a laceration to his right hand.

> Code assignment: 882.0 *Open wound to hand alone*, E826.1 *Pedal cycle accident, pedal cyclist*, and E849.5 *Place of occurrence, street and highway*

E827 ✓5th Animal-drawn vehicle accident — *carriage, sled*

Animal-drawn-vehicle accidents include those caused by a breakage of any part of the vehicle. Included in this category are injuries sustained from a collision with an animal-drawn vehicle and an animal, a nonmotor vehicle, a pedestrian, or a pedestrian conveyance. Also included in this category is an injury sustained by falling off of or being thrown from an animal-drawn vehicle. This does not include an accident between an animal-drawn-vehicle and a pedal cycle. A non-motor-vehicle accident is one that occurs any place other than on a public highway.

A pedestrian is defined as a person not riding in a vehicle, on a motorcycle, or on an animal. A pedestrian can be a person changing a tire, operating a pedestrian conveyance, fixing a vehicle, or traveling on foot. A pedestrian conveyance is defined as a device powered by a human to transport a person other than by walking, which includes a baby carriage, a coaster wagon, ice skates, a perambulator, a pushcart, a pushchair, roller skates, a scooter, a skateboard, skis, a sled, or a wheelchair. For coding purposes, a person in or on a pedestrian conveyance is considered a pedestrian.

Coding Clarification
Category E827 codes may only be reported as a secondary diagnosis.

Use an additional code from category E849 to identify the place of occurrence.

© 2004 Ingenix, Inc.

Only fourth digits 0, 2-4, 8, and 9 may be used with category E827.

Coding Scenario

A 10-year-old female is admitted to the emergency department with a left arm injury. The girl was ice skating on a frozen lake and was hit and knocked down by a horse-drawn sleigh. The final diagnosis is a sprain of the left wrist.

> Code assignment: 842.00 *Sprain and strain of unspecified site of wrist*, E 827.0 *Animal-drawn vehicle accident, pedestrian*, and E849.4 *Place of occurrence, place for recreation and sport*

E828 ✓5th Accident involving animal being ridden

Category E828 codes are used to report accidents that involve an animal being ridden. This type of accident includes a collision with another animal, a nonmotor vehicle except pedal cycle, an animal-drawn vehicle, a pedestrian, or a pedestrian conveyance. Also included in this category are injuries caused by a fall from, being knocked down by, being thrown from, or being trampled by an animal.

A non-motor-vehicle accident is one that occurs any place other than a public highway. A pedestrian is defined as a person not riding in a vehicle, on a motorcycle, or on an animal. A pedestrian can be a person changing a tire, operating a pedestrian conveyance, fixing a motor vehicle, or traveling on foot. A pedestrian conveyance is defined as a device powered by a human to transport a person other than by walking, which includes a baby carriage, a coaster wagon, ice skates, a perambulator, a pushcart, a pushchair, roller skates, a scooter, a skateboard, skis, a sled, or a wheelchair. For coding purposes, a person in or on a pedestrian conveyance is considered a pedestrian.

Coding Clarification

Category E828 codes may only be reported as a secondary diagnosis.

Use an additional code from category E849 to identify the place of occurrence.

Only fourth digits 1, 2, 4, 8, and 9 may be used with category E828.

E829 ✓5th Other road vehicle accidents

Category E828 codes are used to report accidents that involve an animal being ridden. This type of accident includes a collision with another animal, a nonmotor vehicle except pedal cycle, an animal-drawn vehicle, a pedestrian, or a pedestrian conveyance. Also included in this category are injuries caused by a fall from, being knocked down by, being thrown from, or being trampled by an animal.

A non-motor-vehicle accident is one that occurs any place other than a public highway. A pedestrian is defined as a person not riding in a vehicle, on a motorcycle, or on an animal. A pedestrian can be a person changing a tire, operating a pedestrian conveyance, fixing a motor vehicle, or traveling on foot. A pedestrian conveyance is defined as a device powered by a human to transport a person other than by walking, which includes a baby carriage, a coaster wagon, ice skates, a perambulator, a pushcart, a pushchair, roller skates, a scooter, a skateboard, skis, a sled, or a wheelchair. For coding purposes, a person in or on a pedestrian conveyance is considered a pedestrian.

Coding Clarification

Category E829 codes may only be reported as a secondary diagnosis.

Use an additional code from category E849 to identify the place of occurrence.

Only fourth digits 0, 4, 8, and 9 may be used with category E829.

Coding Scenario

A 65-year-old woman presents to the emergency room after getting her hand caught in the door of a streetcar. The diagnosis is a fracture at the base of the third metacarpal.

> Code assignment: 815.02 *Closed fracture base of other metacarpal*, E829.4 *Other road vehicle accidents, occupant of streetcar*, and E849.5 *Place of occurrence, street and highway*

E830–E838 Water Transport Accidents

Water transport accidents involve vehicles that travel in the water and are used for transporting people or products. This definition includes recreational boating.

A small boat is defined as a boat propelled by paddles, oars, or a small engine that carries fewer than 10 people. Small boats can be canoes, cobles, dinghies, punts, rafts, rowboats, rowing shells, sculls, skiffs, and small motorboats. Excluded from this definition are barges, lifeboats, rafts (anchored), and yachts.

The crew of a watercraft is defined as people who are working on a boat or ship, which includes ship operators, people providing passenger services, entertainment personnel, and shop operators.

Dockers and stevedores are longshoreman employed on the dock and work loading and unloading a ship.

E Codes

© 2004 Ingenix, Inc.

The following fourth-digit subdivisions are for use with categories E830-E838 to identify the injured person:

0 Occupant of small boat, unpowered

1 Occupant of small boat, powered

2 Occupant of other watercraft - crew

3 Occupant of other watercraft - other than crew

4 Water skier

5 Swimmer

6 Dockers, stevedores

8 Other specified person

9 Unspecified person

E830 5th Accident to watercraft causing submersion

Category E830 codes are used to report injuries sustained from an overturned or sinking watercraft, which include submerging and drowning, falling or jumping from a boat that is on fire, or falling or jumping from a crushed watercraft.

Drowning is death from suffocation after submersion that occurs within 24 hours of injury. At first a person holds his or her breath and carbon dioxide levels increase and hypoxia progresses. There are then two types of drowning: wet drowning, when water is taken into the lungs and dry drowning, when the patient experiences a laryngospasm. Near drowning is now more commonly referred to as a submersion accident.

A watercraft is a device traveling on the water that transports goods or people.

Coding Clarification

Category E830 codes may only be reported as a secondary diagnosis.

Use an additional code from category E849 to identify the place of occurrence.

E831 5th Accident to watercraft causing other injury

Category E831 codes are used to report any injury, except sinking and drowning, that involves a watercraft. Use these codes to report burns sustained from a ship fire, and injuries from being crushed between ships during a collision, or by a lifeboat after abandoning ship. Also included are injuries sustained from a colliding watercrafts, falling objects during a watercraft accident, and falling or jumping from a damaged boat and being struck by another boat or part of a boat.

A watercraft is a device traveling on the water that transports goods or people.

Coding Clarification

Category E831 codes may only be reported as a secondary diagnosis.

Use an additional code from category E849 to identify the place of occurrence.

E832 5th Other accidental submersion or drowning in water transport accident

Category E832 codes are used to report accidental submerging or drowning in a watercraft accident other than from the boat sinking, which includes injuries sustained from falling from the boat, falling overboard, or falling from the gangplank. Also included are injuries from being thrown overboard by the motion of the boat or being washed overboard.

Drowning is death from suffocation after submersion that occurs within 24 hours of injury. At first a person holds his or her breath and carbon dioxide levels increase and hypoxia progresses. There are then two types of drowning: wet drowning, when water is taken into the lungs and dry drowning, when the patient experiences a laryngospasm. Near drowning is now more commonly referred to as a submersion accident.

Coding Clarification

Category E832 codes may only be reported as a secondary diagnosis.

Use an additional code from category E849 to identify the place of occurrence.

E833 5th Fall on stairs or ladders in water transport

Category E833 codes are used to report a fall on stairs or a ladder of a boat or ship. This includes slipping, tripping, and falling. Excluded from this section are falls due to an accident of the watercraft.

Coding Clarification

Category E833 codes may only be reported as a secondary diagnosis.

Use an additional code from category E849 to identify the place of occurrence.

Coding Scenario

A 38-year-old male is admitted to the emergency department with a 4.0 cm laceration to his right knee. The patient was climbing up the ladder in his motorboat and slipped and hit his leg on the ladder.

> Code assignment: 891.1 *Open wound knee, without mention of complication*, E833.1 *Fall on stairs or ladders in water transport, occupant of small boat, powered*, and E849.8 *Place of occurrence, other specified place*

E834 5th Other fall from one level to another in water transport

Category E834 codes are used to report injury from a fall from one level to another in a watercraft, such as falling from the deck to the lower cabin. Excluded from this code category is a fall that is the result of a watercraft accident.

A watercraft is a device traveling on the water that transports goods or people.

E Codes

Coding Clarification

Category E834 codes may only be reported as a secondary diagnosis.

Use an additional code from category E849 to identify the place of occurrence.

E835 ✓5th Other and unspecified fall in water transport

Category E835 codes are used to report other and unspecified falls in water transport. Excluded from this code is a fall caused by an accident in a watercraft.

A watercraft is a device traveling on the water that transports goods or people.

Coding Clarification

Category E835 codes may only be reported as a secondary diagnosis.

Use an additional code from category E849 to identify the place of occurrence.

Coding Scenario

An 8-year-old boy is admitted to the emergency department with an injured wrist. He was at the lake on a scout activity and slipped and fell in the canoe. The diagnosis is a sprained right wrist.

> Code assignment: 842.00 *Sprain or strain unspecified part of wrist*, E835.0 *Other and unspecified fall in water transport, occupant of a small boat, unpowered*, and E849.8 *Place of occurrence, other specified place*

E836 ✓5th Machinery accident in water transport

Category E836 codes are used to report machinery accidents in water transport. This includes injuries caused by machinery on the deck, machinery in the engine room, galley, or laundry room, and loading machinery onto the ship.

Coding Clarification

Category E836 codes may only be reported as a secondary diagnosis.

Use an additional code from category E849 to identify the place of occurrence.

E837 ✓5th Explosion, fire, or burning in watercraft

Category E837 codes are used to report the explosion, fire, or burning of a watercraft, which includes localized fire on a watercraft and explosion of a boiler. Excluded from this category are fires caused by collision or explosion that results in sinking, submerging, or other injury. Near drowning is now more commonly referred to as a submersion accident.

A watercraft is a device traveling on the water that transports goods or people.

Coding Clarification

Category E837 codes may only be reported as a secondary diagnosis.

Use an additional code from category E849 to identify the place of occurrence.

Coding Scenario

A 39-year-old female chef on a cruise ship suffered second degree burns to her right hand when a small fire started on the stove.

> Code assignment: 944.20 *Second degree burn, unspecified part of hand*, E837.2 *Explosion, fire, or burning in watercraft, occupant of watercraft, crew*, and E849.8 *Place of occurrence, other specified place*

E838 ✓5th Other and unspecified water transport accident

Category E838 codes are used to report other and unspecified water transport accidents. This category includes a person crushed between the dock and the watercraft, a person crushed by a falling object while loading or unloading the ship, or a person hit by a boat while water-skiing. Also included in this category are injuries caused by being struck by boat or part of a boat, accidental poisoning by gas or fumes, or atomic power plant malfunction on the ship. Note that fourth category .4 identifies a water skier. Transport accidents are those involving a vehicle being used primarily for transporting people or goods from one place or another.

Coding Clarification

Category E838 codes may only be reported as a secondary diagnosis.

Use an additional code from category E849 to identify the place of occurrence.

E840–E845 Air and Space Transport Accidents

The chances of being in an airline-related accident while traveling on one of the top 25 airlines are one in 3.72 million. Rubrics E840-E845 describe air- and space-transport accidents. An aircraft is a vehicle that transports products or people by air. This includes commercial or noncommercial flights. Categories E840-E845 include accidents during take off and landing, accidents to unpowered aircraft, falls in, on, or from an aircraft, and accidents involving spacecraft.

E Codes

© 2004 Ingenix, Inc.

The following fourth-digit subdivisions are for use with categories E840-E845 to identify the injured person. Valid fourth digits are in [brackets] under codes E842-E845.

0 Occupant of spacecraft

1 Occupant of military aircraft, any

2 Crew of commercial aircraft (powered) in surface to surface transport

3 Other occupant of commercial aircraft (powered) in surface to surface transport

4 Occupant of commercial aircraft (powered) in surface to air transport

5 Occupant of other powered aircraft

6 Occupant of unpowered aircraft, except parachutist

7 Parachutist (military) (other)

8 Ground crew, airline employee

9 Other person

E840 ✓5th Accident to powered aircraft at takeoff or landing

Category E840 codes are used to report aircraft accidents during takeoff or landing, which includes the collision of a plane with any object, a crash, an explosion, a fire, or a forced landing.

An aircraft is a device traveling in the air that transports goods or people.

Coding Clarification

Category E840 codes may only be reported as a secondary diagnosis.

Use an additional code from category E849 to identify the place of occurrence.

Coding Scenario

A patient is admitted to the emergency room following a plane crash while the plane was taking off. The patient has an open femur fracture.

Code assignment: 821.1 *Open fracture, unspecified part of femur*, E840.3 *Accident to powered aircraft at takeoff or landing, other occupant of commercial aircraft (powered) in surface to surface transport*, and E849.8 *Place of occurrence, other specified places*

E841 ✓5th Accident to powered aircraft, other and unspecified

Category E841 codes are used to report accidents to powered aircraft. Included in this category are aircraft accidents NOS, an aircraft crash or wreck NOS, collisions with other aircraft or another object, aircraft explosions while traveling, or a fire on the aircraft. Use this category for an accident when it is not specified that the accident took place during take off, landing, or in transit.

An aircraft is a device traveling in the air that transports goods or people.

Coding Clarification

Category E841 codes may only be reported as a secondary diagnosis.

Use an additional code from category E849 to identify the place of occurrence.

E842 ✓5th Accident to unpowered aircraft

Category E842 codes are used to report accidents to unpowered aircraft except for collision with a powered aircraft. Unpowered aircraft include hot air balloons, gliders, hang gliders, or a kite carrying a person.

Coding Clarification

Category E842 codes may only be reported as a secondary diagnosis.

Use an additional code from category E849 to identify the place of occurrence.

Only fourth digits 6-9 may be used with category E842.

E843 ✓5th Fall in, on, or from aircraft

Category E843 codes describe falls in, on, or from an aircraft. This code category includes falls that occur when people are getting on or off an aircraft, and falling in, on, or from an aircraft while traveling, taking off, or landing, except as a result of an aircraft accident.

An aircraft is a device traveling in the air that transports goods or people.

Coding Clarification

Category E843 codes may only be reported as a secondary diagnosis.

Use an additional code from category E849 to identify the place of occurrence.

E844 ✓5th Other specified air transport accidents

Category E844 codes describe other specified air transport accidents. This code category includes injuries sustained from a wide variety of causes such as an injury from an object that falls from the aircraft, an injury from machinery on the aircraft, an injury from a rotating propeller, or an injury involving a voluntary parachute descent. Also included in this category is poisoning by carbon monoxide while traveling on an aircraft. All of the previously mentioned causes are without accident to the aircraft. Excluded from this category is airsickness, effects of high altitude or pressure change, and injury to a parachutist due to an accident to the aircraft.

An aircraft is a device traveling in the air that transports goods or people. Transport accidents are those involving a vehicle being used primarily for transporting people or goods from one place or another.

Coding Clarification

Category E844 codes may only be reported as a secondary diagnosis.

Use an additional code from category E849 to identify the place of occurrence.

E845 5th Accident involving spacecraft

Category E845 codes include accidents involving spacecraft. Excluded from this category is the effect of weightlessness in a spacecraft.

Coding Clarification

Category E845 codes may only be reported as a secondary diagnosis.

Use an additional code from category E849 to identify the place of occurrence.

Only fourth digits 0, 8, and 9 may be used with category E845.

E846–E848 Vehicle Accidents Not Elsewhere Classifiable

Codes in this rubric are assigned for vehicle accidents that are not well described by other categories. This code category includes accidents that involve vehicles used exclusively in commercial buildings or premises, accidents that involve cable cars not on rails, and accidents that involve other types of vehicles such as yachts.

E846 Accidents involving powered vehicles used solely within the buildings and premises of industrial or commercial establishment

Code E846 is used to report accidents that involve vehicles used solely within the building or premises of an industrial or a commercial establishment. Included in E846 are accidents involving battery powered airport passenger vehicles, battery powered trucks, coal cars, or trams, trucks or tubs used in a mine or quarry. This may involve a collision with a pedestrian or another vehicle. This code category also includes explosion of, fall from, overturning of, or being struck by an industrial or commercial powered vehicle. Excluded from E846 is accidental poisoning by exhaust gas and injury by a crane, forklift, or an elevator.

A pedestrian is defined as a person who is not riding in a vehicle, on a motorcycle, or on an animal. A pedestrian can be a person changing a tire, operating a pedestrian conveyance, fixing a motor vehicle, or traveling on foot.

Coding Clarification

Code E846 may only be reported as a secondary diagnosis.

Use an additional code from category E849 to identify the place of occurrence.

E847 Accidents involving cable cars not running on rails

Code E847 is used to report accidents involving cable cars not running on rails, ski chair lifts, ski lifts with gondolas, or teleferique (means transfer on the ground). This code also is used to report accidents caused by a broken cable.

Coding Clarification

Code E847 may only be reported as a secondary diagnosis.

Use an additional code from category E849 to identify the place of occurrence.

Coding Scenario

A 25-year-old male presents to the emergency department with left knee pain. The patient says that he jumped off a ski lift after missing the exit. He fell a distance of about six feet. He is diagnosed with a tear of the medial meniscus on the left knee.

> Code assignment: 836.0 *Tear of medial cartilage of the knee, current injury*, E847 *Accident involving cable cars not running on rails*, and E849.4 *Place of occurrence, places for recreation and sport*

E848 Accidents involving other vehicles, not elsewhere classifiable

Code E848 is used to report accidents involving other vehicles, not elsewhere classified. This code category includes accidents involving yachts that have the capacity to carry more than 10 people and vehicles not otherwise specified.

A watercraft is a device traveling on the water that transports goods or people.

Coding Clarification

Use an additional code from category E849 to identify the place of occurrence.

E849 Place of occurrence

Category E849 codes are used to identify where the injury or poisoning occurred. The place of occurrence should describe where the accident happened and not what the patient was doing at the time of the accident.

A home is defined as an apartment, a boarding house, a farmhouse, a noninstitutional place of residence, a private driveway, a private garage, a garden home, or a yard. Report a home under construction but not yet occupied with E849.3. Report an institutional place of residence with E849.7.

A farm includes farm buildings and land under cultivation.

A quarry and mine include gravel pits, sand pits, and any tunnel under construction.

 © 2004 Ingenix, Inc.

An industrial place includes a building under construction, a dockyard, a dry dock, a factory, an industrial yard, a shop, a warehouse, and a loading platform.

A place for recreation and sports includes an amusement park, a baseball field, a basketball court, a football field, a golf course, a gymnasium, a hockey field, a skating rink, a resort, a playground, a public park, a stadium, and a tennis court.

A public building includes an airport, a bank, a cafe, a casino, a church, a hotel, a store, a theater, a nightclub, a office building, a post office, and a school.

A residential institution includes a children's home, a dormitory, a hospital, a jail, a retirement home, an orphanage, a prison, and a reform school.

Other specified places include a beach, desert, dock, forest, harbor, hill, lake, mountain, parking lot, pond, river, sea, stream, swamp, and trailer court.

E849.0 Place of occurrence, home

E849.1 Place of occurrence, farm

E849.2 Place of occurrence, mine and quarry

E849.3 Place of occurrence, industrial places and premises

E849.4 Place of occurrence, place for recreation and sport

E849.5 Place of occurrence, street and highway

E849.6 Place of occurrence, public building

E849.7 Place of occurrence, residential institution

E849.8 Other specified place of occurrence

E849.9 Unspecified place of occurrence

Coding Clarification

According to ICD-9-CM guidelines, code E849.9 should not be used if the place of occurrence is not stated.

Guidelines pertaining to place of occurrence codes may vary by payer and hospital policy. Check with payers to determine if E849 codes are required.

Coding Scenario

A patient presents with a sprained right ankle after falling at home.

> Code assignment: 845.00 *Sprain, unspecified part of ankle*, E888.9 *Unspecified fall*, and E849.0 *Place of occurrence, home*

E850–E858 Accidental Poisoning by Drugs, Medicinal Substances, and Biologicals

Poisoning by drugs, medicinal, and biological substances is the major cause of childhood accidents in the home and can occur by many routes, including oral ingestion, inhalation, dermal absorption, and ocular instillation.

Accidental poisoning codes identify accidental overdose of a drug, a wrong substance given or taken, a drug taken inadvertently, and accidents in the use of drugs and biologicals in medical and surgical procedures. The alphabetical index of ICD-9-CM can give a more complete list of specific drugs classified under a fourth-digit category; however, codes should not be assigned directly from the table of drugs and chemicals. Always consult the tabular section of ICD-9-CM before assigning the accidental poisoning codes. Many of the common medications can be found in the pharmacological listings found in the back of ICD-9-CM.

As a general rule, the more known about the poisoning agent, the better the treatment plan and outcome. Poison control centers have been invaluable in supplying the health care professional with the exact composition of the thousands of poisonous substances. If the information is unknown, treatment must revolve around general supportive measures.

E850 Accidental poisoning by analgesics, antipyretics, and antirheumatics

Category E850 codes are used to report accidental poisoning by analgesics, antipyretics and antirheumatics. An analgesic medication is one that provides pain relief or reduces pain. An antipyretic is a medication that is used to eliminate or reduce a fever. An antirheumatic is an anti-inflammatory medication.

Heroin is a highly addictive drug. It can be injected, snorted or smoked. Accidental overdoses can occur as a result of varying strength of the street drug. Drug users are not always sure of the purity of the drug. Heroin is usually mixed with other substances. Drug users may experience an accidental overdose using the same amount of heroin because of the purity.

Methadone is a synthetic form of heroin. It blocks the effects of heroin which results in a reduced craving. Methadone overdose is a serious medical condition that usually affects people who are using the drug illegally. Symptoms of methadone overdose include muscle spasm, difficulty breathing, pin point pupils and death.

© 2004 Ingenix, Inc.

Opiates are drugs derived from a Papaver somniferum plant. Common names are opium, codeine, morphine, Dilaudid, Percodan, Vicodin, Demerol, and fentanyl. Symptoms of overdose include decreased respiration, clammy skin, coma and possible death.

Salicylates are found in many commonly used drugs. Aspirin is the most common salicylate. Because aspirin is found in many common drugs, accidental overdose can occur from taking more than one medication that includes salicylates.

Aromatic analgesics include acetaminophen, acetanilid and acetophenetidin. Tylenol is a common form of aromatic analgesic.

Pyrazole is a non-narcotic pain reliever and fever reducer that includes aminophenazone and phenylbutazone.

Antirheumatics include gold salts and indomethacin. Excluded in this section are salicylates and steroids. Symptoms of overdose may include ringing in ears, blurred vision, nausea and vomiting.

E850.0 Accidental poisoning by heroin

E850.1 Accidental poisoning by methadone

E850.2 Accidental poisoning by other opiates and related narcotics

E850.3 Accidental poisoning by salicylates

E850.4 Accidental poisoning by aromatic analgesics, not elsewhere classified

E850.5 Accidental poisoning by pyrazole derivatives

E850.6 Accidental poisoning by antirheumatics (antiphlogistics)

E850.7 Accidental poisoning by other non-narcotic analgesics

E850.8 Accidental poisoning by other specified analgesics and antipyretics

E850.9 Accidental poisoning by unspecified analgesic or antipyretic

Coding Clarification

If a reaction is the result of medicine and alcohol, assign a code for each drug and/or the alcohol.

Apply each E code only once even if the agent is responsible for more than one adverse reaction.

When coding accidental poisoning use as many codes as necessary to completely describe the drug, medicinal, or biological poisoning. Sequence poisoning first, manifestation second, and the E code third. Assign an additional code for drug dependency, if applicable.

When assigning codes for the late effect of a poisoning, code the nature of the late effect first, the cause of the late effect second, and then the applicable E code describing the cause of the poisoning.

Use a secondary E code from category E849 to identify the place of occurrence.

E851 Accidental poisoning by barbiturates OK

Barbiturates are depressant type drugs used for sleep and relaxation. Most barbiturate overdoses are combinations such as barbiturates and alcohol. For combination overdoses, use as many E codes as necessary to describe the overdose. There are no antidotes to barbiturate overdoses. Maintenance of airway and drugs to make the urine less acidic can be used to treat barbiturate overdose.

Coding Clarification

Code E851 codes may only be reported as a secondary diagnosis.

Use a secondary E code from category E849 to identify the place of occurrence.

E852 Accidental poisoning by other sedatives and hypnotics

Sedatives are agents used to calm and quiet the body. Several types and compounds of sedatives are available for use today. Accidental overdose can occur when a patient forgets that he or she has taken a dose or accidentally takes too much medication.

Chloral hydrate is the oldest sleep medication. It may still be used for children prior to dental or medical procedures. Mixed with alcohol, it produces the infamous knockout drops, or Mickey. Symptoms of an overdose include gastrointestinal (GI) irritation, vomiting, GI bleed, and a pear like odor of the breath.

Paraldehyde is used to treat certain convulsive disorders. It may also be used in the treatment of alcoholism and used to calm or relax patients. The medication should be taken with a metal spoon because paraldehyde tends to react with plastic. The medication will cause the patient to have bad breath. Signs of overdose are confusion, muscle tremors, nausea, vomiting, stomach cramps, weakness, depressed breathing, and slow heartbeat. This medication has generally been replaced by safer and more effective drugs.

Bromine compounds are central nervous center depressants and are mixed with other drugs to form compound drugs. They have a tranquilizing effect on the body.

E852.0 Accidental poisoning by chloral hydrate group

E852.1 Accidental poisoning by paraldehyde

E852.2 Accidental poisoning by bromine compounds

E852.3 Accidental poisoning by methaqualone compounds

E Codes

 © 2004 Ingenix, Inc.

E852.4 Accidental poisoning by glutethimide group

E852.5 Accidental poisoning by mixed sedatives, not elsewhere classified

E852.8 Accidental poisoning by other specified sedative and hypnotic

E852.9 Accidental poisoning by unspecified sedative or hypnotic

Coding Clarification

Category E852 codes may only be reported as a secondary diagnosis.

Use a secondary E code from category E849 to identify the place of occurrence.

Coding Scenario

A 75-year-old male is brought into the emergency department following an accidental overdose of Ambien. The patient misunderstood the dosage and took additional medication. The patient is experiencing nausea and vomiting.

> Code assignment: 967.8 *Poisoning by other sedatives and hypnotics*, 787.01 *Nausea and vomiting*, and E852.8 *Accidental poisoning by other specified sedative or hypnotic*

E853 Accidental poisoning by tranquilizers

Tranquilizers are antianxiety medications used to calm a patient. Phenothiazine-based tranquilizers include chlorpromazine, fluphenazine, prochlorperazine and promazine. Butyrophenone-based tranquilizers include haloperidol, spiperone, and trifluperidol . Other specified tranquilizers include hydroxyzine and meprobamate.

E853.0 Accidental poisoning by phenothiazine-based tranquilizers

E853.1 Accidental poisoning by butyrophenone-based tranquilizers

E853.2 Accidental poisoning by benzodiazepine-based tranquilizers

E853.8 Accidental poisoning by other specified tranquilizers

E853.9 Accidental poisoning by unspecified tranquilizer

Coding Clarification

Category E853 codes may only be reported as a secondary diagnosis.

Use a secondary E code from category E849 to identify the place of occurrence.

E854 Accidental poisoning by other psychotropic agents

Category E854 codes describe accidental poisoning by antidepressants, psychodysleptics, psychostimulants, and central nervous system stimulants.

Antidepressants are used to treat mood disorders. Symptoms of mood disorders include sadness, loss of appetite, sleep problems, hopelessness, helplessness, guilt, loss of energy, agitation, and lack of pleasure. Overdoses of antidepressants can cause central nervous symptom problems, cardiovascular symptoms, and parasympathetic nervous system symptoms.

Psychodysleptics are hallucinogenic drugs that include cannabis derivatives, LSD, marihuana derivatives, mescaline, psilocin, and psilocybin.

Psychostimulants include amphetamine and caffeine. Psychostimulants are often used to treat children with attention deficit hyperactivity disorder (ADHD).

Central nervous system stimulants include analeptics and opiate antagonists. Central nervous system stimulants speed up the mental and physical processes. They are used to treat children with ADHD and other people with attention span disorders. Opiate antagonists reduce the affects of opiates.

E854.0 Accidental poisoning by antidepressants

E854.1 Accidental poisoning by psychodysleptics (hallucinogens)

E854.2 Accidental poisoning by psychostimulants

E854.3 Accidental poisoning by central nervous system stimulants

E854.8 Accidental poisoning by other psychotropic agents

Coding Clarification

Category E854 codes may only be reported as a secondary diagnosis.

Use a secondary E code from category E849 to identify the place of occurrence.

E855 Accidental poisoning by other drugs acting on central and autonomic nervous system

Category E855 codes are used to report accidental poisoning by other drugs acting on the central nervous system, which includes anti-Parkinsonism drugs, central nervous system depressants, anesthetics, parasympatholytics, sympathomimetics, and sympatholytics.

Parkinson's disease is a progressive neurologic disease that affects walking, talking, and movement. Symptoms of the disease include tremors, stiffness, and slow movement. The cause of Parkinson's disease is not known. The disease causes a degeneration of nerves in the brain that produce a chemical called dopamine. There is no treatment for the disease; however, medications are used to decrease the symptoms.

Anesthetics can be used to produce a loss of consciousness or a local pain blocking effect. Overdose can cause reduced cardiac output and arrhythmias.

Parasympathomimetics are drugs that produce the effects of parasympathetic nerve stimulation. Therapeutic use of the drugs includes stimulation and motility of the GI tract and bladder following surgery, glaucoma, diagnosis of myasthenia gravis, and treatment of delayed gastric emptying time.

Parasympatholytics relax smooth muscles. Drugs in this category include atropine, homatropine, hyoscine, and quaternary ammonium derivatives.

Sympathomimetic agents are used to increase myocardial contractility, increase blood pressure, maintain blood pressure, treat bronchospasm, reduce systemic local anesthetic absorption, and manage severe allergic reactions. Drugs in this category include epinephrine and levarterenol.

Sympatholytics stimulate smooth muscles. This category of drugs is used to treat hypertension, angina, glaucoma, and to prevent migraines. Medications include phenoxybenzamine and tolazoline hydrochloride.

E855.0 Accidental poisoning by anticonvulsant and anti-Parkinsonism drugs

E855.1 Accidental poisoning by other central nervous system depressants

E855.2 Accidental poisoning by local anesthetics

E855.3 Accidental poisoning by parasympathomimetics (cholinergics)

E855.4 Accidental poisoning by parasympatholytics (anticholinergics and antimuscarinics) and spasmolytics

E855.5 Accidental poisoning by sympathomimetics (adrenergics)

E855.6 Accidental poisoning by sympatholytics (antiadrenergics)

E855.8 Accidental poisoning by other specified drugs acting on central and autonomic nervous systems

E855.9 Accidental poisoning by unspecified drug acting on central and autonomic nervous systems

Coding Clarification

Category E855 codes may only be reported as a secondary diagnosis.

Use a secondary E code from category E849 to identify the place of occurrence.

Coding Scenario

A 10-year-old female presents to the emergency department with an accidental overdose of Dilantin. The young girl suffers from a seizure disorder. The patient's mother forgot when the medication was given and administered two extra doses to the child. The child has nystagmus on examination.

> Code assignment: 966.1 *Poisoning by hydantoin derivatives*, 379.50 *Unspecified nystagmus*, 780.39 *Other convulsions*, and E855.0 *Accidental poisoning by anticonvulsant and anti-Parkinsonism drugs*

E856 Accidental poisoning by antibiotics OK

Antibiotics are used to fight infections including pneumonia, cystitis, strep infections, and ear infections. They can be administered topically, intravenously (IV), intramuscularly (IM), and orally. Overuse of antibiotics has lead to a decrease in their effectiveness. Symptoms of an overdose can include decreased respiration, tightness in the chest, low blood pressure, and unconsciousness.

Coding Clarification

Code E856 codes may only be reported as a secondary diagnosis.

Use a secondary E code from category E849 to identify the place of occurrence.

Coding Scenario

A 2-year-old female presents to the emergency department with diaphoresis after getting into the ampicillin prescribed for her brother. The diagnosis is diaphoresis and ampicillin poisoning.

> Code assignment: 960.0 *Poisoning by penicillins*, 780.8 *Hyperhidrosis*, and E856 *Accidental poisoning by antibiotics*

E857 Accidental poisoning by other anti-infectives OK

Anti-infectives include medications such as sulfonamides, arsenical anti-infectives, heavy metal anti-infectives, hydroxyquinoline derivatives, antimalarials, antiprotozoal drugs, anthelmintics, antiviral drugs, and drugs acting on other blood forming protozoa.

Coding Clarification

Code E857 codes may only be reported as a secondary diagnosis.

Use a secondary E code from category E849 to identify the place of occurrence.

E Codes

© 2004 Ingenix, Inc.

E858 Accidental poisoning by other drugs

Category E858 codes are used to report accidental poisoning by the following kinds of drugs: hormones, synthetic substitutes, and systemic agents. Also included are drugs that affect the following systems: blood constituents, cardiovascular system, gastrointestinal system, uric acid metabolism, smooth and skeletal muscles, and respiratory system. Additionally, agents that affect skin, mucous membranes, eyes, ears, nose, throat and mouth are included in this category.

Poisoning by hormones and synthetic substitutes include adrenal cortical steroids, androgens and anabolic congeners, ovarian hormones, insulin and antidiabetic agents, anterior pituitary hormones, posterior pituitary hormones, parathyroid and parathyroid derivatives, thyroid and thyroid derivatives, and antithyroid agents.

E858.0 Accidental poisoning by hormones and synthetic substitutes

E858.1 Accidental poisoning by primarily systemic agents

E858.2 Accidental poisoning by agents primarily affecting blood constituents

E858.3 Accidental poisoning by agents primarily affecting cardiovascular system

E858.4 Accidental poisoning by agents primarily affecting gastrointestinal system

E858.5 Accidental poisoning by water, mineral, and uric acid metabolism drugs

E858.6 Accidental poisoning by agents primarily acting on the smooth and skeletal muscles and respiratory system

E858.7 Accidental poisoning by agents primarily affecting skin and mucous membrane, ophthalmological, otorhinolaryngological, and dental drugs

E858.8 Accidental poisoning by other specified drugs — *central appetite depressants*

E858.9 Accidental poisoning by unspecified drug

Coding Clarification

Category E858 codes may only be reported as a secondary diagnosis.

Use a secondary E code from category E849 to identify the place of occurrence.

E860–E869 Accidental Poisoning by Other Solid and Liquid Substances, Gases, and Vapors

The toxicity of a substance is due to its ability to damage or disrupt the metabolism. An acutely toxic substance can cause damage as the result of a single- or short-duration exposure. A chronically toxic substance causes damage after repeated or long-duration exposure or becomes evident only after a long latency period. Toxicity varies with the route of exposure and the effectiveness at which the material is absorbed. A chemical that enters the body in large quantities, but is not easily absorbed, is a much lower risk than one that is easily absorbed into the bloodstream.

Ingested materials are absorbed into the bloodstream anywhere along the gastrointestinal tract. If the material cannot be absorbed, it will be eliminated from the body.

A toxic reaction can be similar to an allergic reaction, but more severe. If the liver is functioning normally, it may allow a small amount of the toxic material to be absorbed into the body, but eliminate the rest. If the liver is not functioning normally, the substance may be absorbed and cause a toxic chemical overload that may result in blood poisoning and death. Toxemia is a poisoned condition of the blood caused by the presence of toxic materials, usually bacterial but occasionally chemical or hormonal in nature.

Skin contact can be a common route of exposure but the skin acts as a barrier against the entry of most chemicals. Once a chemical passes through the skin (i.e., through a wound), it enters the bloodstream and is carried to all parts of the body.

Inhalation can be the most dangerous route of entry because the lungs are ineffective barriers. Chemicals that pass the lung membrane are absorbed into the bloodstream and carried to all parts of the body. Absorption can be extremely rapid. The rate of absorption depends on the concentration of the toxic substance, its solubility in water, the depth of respiration, and the rate of blood circulation.

Treatment includes the use of corticosteroids and mannitol drips to minimize cerebral edema dialysis to combat renal failure and hasten the excretion of the poison, and removal of lipoid soluble substances from the blood by hemoperfusion and chelating agents.

Categories E860-E869 are primarily used to indicate the cause of poisoning (980-989), however, they may also be used to indicate the cause of a localized reaction (001-799).

E860 Accidental poisoning by alcohol, not elsewhere classified

Alcohol poisoning occurs from consuming too much alcohol. Factors that affect alcohol poisoning are the strength or concentration of alcohol in a drink, how fast it is consumed, and the amount of food in the system. Combining certain drugs, such as sedatives, tranquilizers, pain medication, and certain anti-seizure medication, can be harmful if consumed in addition to alcohol. The signs and symptoms of alcohol intoxication include giddiness, slurred speech, uninhibited behavior, and coordination problems. Signs and symptoms of alcohol poisoning or ethanol overdose are mental confusion, vomiting, seizures, slow or irregular breathing, paleness, bluish skin, and unconsciousness. If a reaction is the result of medicine and alcohol, assign the codes for both.

Wood alcohol and methanol is a common substance found in paint thinner and antifreeze. Methanol poisoning can cause serious kidney damage and blindness. This can be absorbed by skin contact or inhalation but is far more serious when ingested. Symptoms include headache, nausea, vomiting, ringing in the ears, diarrhea, constipation, lethargy, central nervous system depression, stupor, cerebral edema, coma, and profound metabolic acidosis.

Rubbing alcohol consists mainly of isopropyl alcohol. Poisoning from this substance can occur from skin contact, inhalation, and ingestion. Symptoms include headache, dizziness, mental depression, nausea, vomiting, and coma.

Fuel oil is irritating to the mucous membranes. Symptoms of overdose include headache, dizziness, pungent taste, nausea, vomiting, diarrhea, delirium, and central nervous center depression.

E860.0 Accidental poisoning by alcoholic beverages

E860.1 Accidental poisoning by other and unspecified ethyl alcohol and its products

E860.2 Accidental poisoning by methyl alcohol

E860.3 Accidental poisoning by isopropyl alcohol

E860.4 Accidental poisoning by Fuel oil

E860.8 Accidental poisoning by other specified alcohols

E860.9 Accidental poisoning by unspecified alcohol

Coding Clarification

When coding accidental poisoning use as many codes as necessary to completely describe the drug, medicinal, or biological poisoning.

Coding Scenario

A 21-year-old male college student is brought to the emergency department by his friends for nausea and vomiting and confusion. This patient has been drinking vodka for the last eight hours. The diagnosis is acute alcohol toxicity, intoxication, and confusion.

> Code assignment: 980.0 *Toxic effects of alcohol*, 305.0 *Alcohol intoxication*, 787.01 *Nausea and vomiting*, 298.2 *Reactive confusion*, and E860.0 *Accidental poisoning by alcoholic beverages*

E861 Accidental poisoning by cleansing and polishing agents, disinfectants, paints, and varnishes

Poisoning continues to be one of the leading causes of pediatric admission. Although the numbers have declined, this is still a significant threat. The second most common cause of poisoning is from cleaning supplies. Keeping cleaning supplies out of children's reach is the most effective way of preventing poisoning. Treatment for poisoning includes ipecac syrup, gastric lavage, medication to increase GI motility, and administration of activated charcoal.

Lead is a highly toxic metal that was used for many years in paint and other products found around the home. Lead poisoning has steadily decreased over the years. In 1978 there were three to four million children with lead in their blood. In the 1990s the number has dropped to 434,000. Lead poisoning usually happens slowly and most children show no symptoms. Children between the ages of one to two, when they are crawling, learning to walk, and putting things in their mouth, are most likely to get lead poisoning. Many older homes were painted with lead-based paint. These paint chips and dust can poison a child. Acute lead poisoning is rare but it can cause abdominal pain, vomiting, diarrhea, weakness in the extremities, behavioral problems, seizures, coma, and death. This would only occur if a person ingested a large amount of lead at once. If the lead level in a child is high, a treatment called chelation can be used to bind the lead and help the body pass it through the urine. Report E866.4 for poisoning from lead and its compounds and fumes other than paint.

E861.0 Accidental poisoning by synthetic detergents and shampoos

E861.1 Accidental poisoning by soap products

E861.2 Accidental poisoning by polishes

E861.3 Accidental poisoning by other cleansing and polishing agents

E861.4 Accidental poisoning by disinfectants — *excludes carbolic acid or phenol*

E861.5 Accidental poisoning by lead paints

E861.6 Accidental poisoning by other paints and varnishes

E861.9 Accidental poisonings by unspecified cleansing and polishing agents, disinfectants, paints, and varnishes

Coding Clarification

Category E861 codes may only be reported as a secondary diagnosis.

Use a secondary E code from category E849 to identify the place of occurrence.

E Codes

© 2004 Ingenix, Inc.

E862 Accidental poisoning by petroleum products, other solvents and their vapors, not elsewhere classified

Petroleum products include solvents, fuels, cleaners, oils, and wax. Symptoms of poisoning are anal seepage and irritation, lipid granuloma, lipid pneumonia, eczematous dermatitis, and melanosis. Vomiting is generally not recommended for petroleum product ingestion as vomiting causes an increased risk of pneumonia.

E862.0 Accidental poisoning by petroleum solvents

E862.1 Accidental poisoning by petroleum fuels and cleaners

E862.2 Accidental poisoning by lubricating oils

E862.3 Accidental poisoning by petroleum solids

E862.4 Accidental poisoning by other specified solvents

E862.9 Accidental poisoning by unspecified solvent

Coding Clarification

Category E862 codes may only be reported as a secondary diagnosis.

Use a secondary E code from category E849 to identify the place of occurrence.

E863 Accidental poisoning by agricultural and horticultural chemical and pharmaceutical preparations other than plant foods and fertilizers

Pesticides can readily be absorbed through the skin or cause harm from ingestion or inhalation. Death from insecticide poisoning can occur between five minutes and 24 hours after ingestion. The most common cause of death is respiratory failure. Symptoms include headache, nausea, pupil dilation, excessive sweating, salivation, respiratory distress, and death.

Rodenticides are one of the most toxic substances found in the home. Until 20 years ago, arsenic was the main ingredient. Most rodenticides today contain an anticoagulant. They are toxic to almost every organ system in the body. Most accidental poisoning by rodenticides affects children. Adults who ingest this substance are usually attempting suicide. Symptoms include abdominal pain, shortness of breath, nausea, vomiting, abdominal pain, dizziness, hair loss, muscle pain or twitching, facial grimace, pulmonary edema, and a garlic taste in the mouth. Patients may require dialysis or blood transfusions. Activated charcoal is usually given to inhibit additional absorption of the toxin.

E863.0 Accidental poisoning by insecticides of organochlorine compounds

E863.1 Accidental poisoning by insecticides of organophosphorus compounds

E863.2 Accidental poisoning by carbamates

E863.3 Accidental poisoning by mixtures of insecticides

E863.4 Accidental poisoning by other and unspecified insecticides

E863.5 Accidental poisoning by herbicides

E863.6 Accidental poisoning by fungicides

E863.7 Accidental poisoning by rodenticides

E863.8 Accidental poisoning by fumigants

E863.9 Accidental poisoning by other and unspecified agricultural and horticultural chemical and pharmaceutical preparations other than plant foods and fertilizers

Coding Clarification

Category E863 codes may only be reported as a secondary diagnosis.

Use a secondary E code from category E849 to identify the place of occurrence.

E864 Accidental poisoning by corrosives and caustics, not elsewhere classified

A corrosive is a substance that destroys living tissue. The most common types of corrosives are hydrochloric acid, sulfuric acid, nitric acid, acetic acid, phosphoric acid, oxalic acid, chronic acid, formic acid, and boric acid. These corrosives are commonly found in metal cleaners, toilet and drain cleaners, batteries, and antirust compounds. Symptoms of ingestion include a severe burning pain in the mouth, throat, and abdomen; dysphagia; vomiting; diarrhea; and cold, clammy skin. Symptoms will usually begin immediately after swallowing. Symptoms of inhalation include cough, dyspnea, pleuritic chest pain, pulmonary edema, and frothy sputum. These symptoms could be delayed several hours. Eye exposure can cause burning, irritation and swelling eyes, photophobia, corneal erosion, and perforation of the conjunctiva and cornea.

E864.0 Accidental poisoning by corrosive aromatics not elsewhere classified

E864.1 Accidental poisoning by acids not elsewhere classified

E864.2 Accidental poisoning by caustic alkalis not elsewhere classified

E864.3 Accidental poisoning by other specified corrosives and caustics not elsewhere classified

E864.4 Accidental poisoning by unspecified corrosives and caustics not elsewhere classified

Coding Clarification

Category E864 codes may only be reported as a secondary diagnosis.

Use a secondary E code from category E849 to identify the place of occurrence.

E865 Accidental poisoning from poisonous foodstuffs and poisonous plants

Category E865 codes identify poisoning from food and plants. This type of poisoning does not include bacterial food poisoning or toxic reactions to venomous plants. This category does include poisoning from food or plants that should not be eaten, such as a child ingesting plants or berries that are poisonous to humans.

The four main types of toxic shellfish poisoning are paralytic, amnesic, neurotoxic, and diarrhetic. Paralytic shellfish poisoning differs in effect based on the species of shellfish and the species of algae producing the toxin. Symptoms of amnesic poisoning are neurological in nature and usually begin within 24 to 48 hours. Neurotoxic shellfish toxins affect the nervous system. Symptoms, which will appear within 24 hours, include difficulty swallowing, double vision, tremor, nausea, diarrhea, vomiting, numbness, and tingling in the mouth, lips, and extremities. Diarrhetic shellfish poisoning cause GI problems such as nausea, vomiting, diarrhea, and abdominal pain.

Relatively few plants are fit for human consumption. Many have toxins that are designed to deter predators from eating them. Many of these forms of toxic plants are houseplants or plants that are commonly found in people's flower gardens. Some plants, such as herbs, spices, and condiments are safe to eat in small quantities. Polluted water may add to the toxicity of plants. Examples of toxic plants are hyacinth, daffodil, oleander, larkspur, iris, bleeding heart, rhubarb leaf blades, daphne berries, jasmine berries, mistletoe berries, and jimson weed. Toadstools that are commonly found outside are also toxic. Some types of poisoning cause mild GI symptoms and some can be fatal.

E Codes

E865.0 Accidental poisoning by meat

E865.1 Accidental poisoning by shellfish

E865.2 Accidental poisoning from other fish

E865.3 Accidental poisoning from berries and seeds

E865.4 Accidental poisoning from other specified plants

E865.5 Accidental poisoning from mushrooms and other fungi

E865.8 Accidental poisoning from other specified foods

E865.9 Accidental poisoning from unspecified foodstuff or poisonous plant

Coding Clarification

Category E865 codes may only be reported as a secondary diagnosis.

Use a secondary E code from category E849 to identify the place of occurrence.

E866 Accidental poisoning by other and unspecified solid and liquid substances

Category E866 codes are used to report poisoning by other and unspecified solid or liquid substances. Excluded from this section are substances as components of medicines, paints, pesticides, petroleum fuels, lead paint, and fertilizers mixed with herbicides.

E866.0 Accidental poisoning by lead and its compounds and fumes

E866.1 Accidental poisoning by mercury and its compounds and fumes

E866.2 Accidental poisoning by antimony and its compounds and fumes

E866.3 Accidental poisoning by arsenic and its compounds and fumes

E866.4 Accidental poisoning by other metals and their compounds and fumes

E866.5 Accidental poisoning by plant foods and fertilizers

E866.6 Accidental poisoning by glues and adhesives

E866.7 Accidental poisoning by cosmetics

E866.8 Accidental poisoning by other specified solid or liquid substances

E866.9 Accidental poisoning by unspecified solid or liquid substance

Coding Clarification

Category E866 codes may only be reported as a secondary diagnosis.

Use a secondary E code from category E849 to identify the place of occurrence.

E867 Accidental poisoning by gas distributed by pipeline OK

The most common poisoning by gas distributed by pipeline is from carbon monoxide poisoning. Carbon monoxide is produced whenever pipeline gas is burned. The amount produced is usually not hazardous. Improper ventilation and malfunctioning equipment can result in a deadly amount of carbon monoxide emitted into the air. Although the lead in gas has decreased over the years, gasoline fumes can also cause short- or long-term health problems.

© 2004 Ingenix, Inc.

Coding Clarification

Code E867 codes may only be reported as a secondary diagnosis.

Use a secondary E code from category E849 to identify the place of occurrence.

E868 Accidental poisoning by other utility gas and other carbon monoxide

Carbon monoxide poisoning can be deadly. There is no smell and it can't been seen, but it can kill in just a matter of minutes. If appliances that burn fuel are not properly working, toxic levels of carbon monoxide can be produced. Accidental carbon monoxide poisoning kills hundreds of people each year. Symptoms of carbon monoxide poisoning include severe headache, dizziness, mental confusion, nausea, and fainting. Since the symptoms are similar to many other causes, carbon monoxide poisoning has been hard to diagnose. Use of carbon monoxide alarms has greatly reduced the mortality rate from carbon monoxide poisoning.

E868.0 Accidental poisoning by liquefied petroleum gas distributed in mobile containers

E868.1 Accidental poisoning by other and unspecified utility gas

E868.2 Accidental poisoning by motor vehicle exhaust gas

E868.3 Accidental poisoning by carbon monoxide from incomplete combustion of other domestic fuels

E868.8 Accidental poisoning by carbon monoxide from other sources

E868.9 Accidental poisoning by unspecified carbon monoxide

Coding Clarification

Category E868 codes may only be reported as a secondary diagnosis.

Use a secondary E code from category E849 to identify the place of occurrence.

Coding Scenario

A 57-year-old male presents to the emergency department with a severe headache. It is found that the man was in his barn working on his tractor engine with all doors and windows closed. The tractor had been running for several minutes. The diagnosis is carbon monoxide poisoning.

> Code assignment: 986 *Toxic effect of carbon monoxide*, E868.2 *Accidental poisoning by motor vehicle exhaust gas*, and E849.1 *Place of occurrence, farm*

E869 Accidental poisoning by other gases and vapors

Symptoms from exposure to gas and vapors can range from mild to severe. These include headache, nausea, vomiting, eye irritation, pulmonary edema, confusion, drowsiness, loss of consciousness, shortness of breath, cough, and bronchospasm. Life-threatening symptoms may appear as late as several weeks after exposure to some gases.

E869.0 Accidental poisoning by nitrogen oxides

E869.1 Accidental poisoning by sulfur dioxide

E869.2 Accidental poisoning by freon

E869.3 Accidental poisoning by lacrimogenic gas (tear gas)

E869.4 Accidental poisoning by second-hand tobacco smoke

E869.8 Accidental poisoning by other specified gases and vapors

E869.9 Accidental poisoning by unspecified gases and vapors

Coding Clarification

Category E869 codes may only be reported as a secondary diagnosis.

Use a secondary E code from category E849 to identify the place of occurrence.

E870–E876 Misadventures to Patients During Surgical and Medical Care

Many people are incapacitated as a result of medical errors. As many people as 98,000 Americans die each year as a result of medical errors, approximately the eighth leading cause of death. These errors increase health care costs significantly. The following kinds of errors unfortunately are often made: prescribing the wrong medication, administering an anesthetic improperly, operating a mechanical device incorrectly, causing an infection by improper wound treatment, contaminating blood or other pathological tests, completing a surgical procedure incorrectly.

E870 Accidental cut, puncture, perforation, or hemorrhage during medical care

Category E870 codes are used to report accidental puncture, perforation, or hemorrhage during medical care. Procedures where these accidents might take place are surgery, infusion or transfusion, dialysis, perfusion, injection or vaccination, endoscopic exam, aspiration of fluid or tissue, puncture, catheterization, heart catheterization, and administration of an enema. One study indicates that 3.29 out of 1,000 discharges and 31.17 per 100,000 people experience a complication from an accidental puncture, perforation, or hemorrhage.

Hemodialysis is the use of an artificial kidney to clear waste products from the blood when the patient's own kidneys are not functioning. Risk of accidental perforation could happen when connecting the dialysis machine to the catheter implanted in the patient.

Accidental laceration, when performing an endoscopy, was the second highest complication reported by ambulatory surgery centers in 1999. During the endoscopy, the physician's field is closed and the physician's view is limited to what is in the camera's line of site. Most physicians are proficient in performing endoscopic procedures; however, the closed surgical field increases the chance of puncturing a structure.

Accidental dural puncture during an epidural is one of the most common complications of that procedure. Symptoms may include a severe headache. An epidural blood patch may be necessary to treat the dural puncture.

During a cardiac catheterization a puncture is made in a blood vessel in the groin and a catheter is fed through this to the heart. Different vessels of the heart are imaged and often a repair can be made at the same time as the diagnosis. One risk of the procedure is an inadvertent puncture of an artery.

Enemas are performed to evacuate the bowel or in some instances to instill radio opaque dye to image the bowel. There is a slight risk that the bowel may be punctured during the process.

E870.0 Accidental cut, puncture, perforation, or hemorrhage during surgical operation

E870.1 Accidental cut, puncture, perforation, or hemorrhage during infusion or transfusion

E870.2 Accidental cut, puncture, perforation, or hemorrhage during kidney dialysis or other perfusion

E870.3 Accidental cut, puncture, perforation, or hemorrhage during injection or vaccination

E870.4 Accidental cut, puncture, perforation, or hemorrhage during endoscopic examination

E870.5 Accidental cut, puncture, perforation, or hemorrhage during aspiration of fluid or tissue, puncture, and catheterization

E870.6 Accidental cut, puncture, perforation, or hemorrhage during heart catheterization

E870.7 Accidental cut, puncture, perforation, or hemorrhage during administration of enema

E870.8 Accidental cut, puncture, perforation, or hemorrhage during other specified medical care

E870.9 Accidental cut, puncture, perforation, or hemorrhage during unspecified medical care

Documentation Issues

The physician should document clearly that a misadventure occurred and the nature of the complication.

Rubrics E870-E876 must be assigned if documented by the physician. Office or hospital policies cannot state that these codes never be used.

Coding Clarification

Category E870 codes may only be reported as a secondary diagnosis.

Do not assign traumatic injury codes (800-959) in addition to 998.2 *Accidental puncture or laceration during a procedure.*

Report a code from the E878-E879 rubric for an abnormal reaction or later complication of a procedure that the physician does not document as a misadventure. Codes E870-E876 should be assigned if the physician documents the misadventure.

Coding Scenario

A 23-year-old female suffers a puncture into the dura during an epidural injection.

> Code assignment: 998.2 *Accidental puncture or laceration during a procedure* and E870.5 *Accidental cut, puncture, perforation, or hemorrhage during aspiration of fluid or tissue, puncture, and catheterization*

E871 Foreign object left in body during procedure

Category E871 codes are used to report foreign objects left in the body during surgery. This set of codes should not be used if the foreign body was left in intentionally. Foreign bodies include sponges, needles, catheters, instruments, and any other object not intended to remain in the patient.

E871.0 Foreign object left in body during surgical operation

E871.1 Foreign object left in body during infusion or transfusion

E871.2 Foreign object left in body during kidney dialysis or other perfusion

E871.3 Foreign object left in body during injection or vaccination

E871.4 Foreign object left in body during endoscopic examination

E871.5 Foreign object left in body during aspiration of fluid or tissue, puncture, and catheterization

E871.6 Foreign object left in body during heart catheterization

E Codes

© 2004 Ingenix, Inc.

E871.7 Foreign object left in body during removal of catheter or packing

E871.8 Foreign object left in body during other specified procedure

E871.9 Foreign object left in body during unspecified procedure

Documentation Issues

The physician should document clearly that a misadventure occurred and the nature of the complication.

Coding Clarification

Category E871 codes may only be reported as a secondary diagnosis.

Codes E870-E876 should be assigned if the physician documents the misadventure.

Report a code from the E878-E879 rubric for an abnormal reaction or later complication of a procedure that the physician does not document as a misadventure.

E872 Failure of sterile precautions during procedure

Category E872 codes are used to report failure of sterile precautions during a procedure. Sterile technique is the process of keeping the operating area free from all germs. This involves ensuring that anything that will be used during the procedure is sterile. This is primarily done by autoclaving the instruments.

An autoclave is a machine that heats instruments to a high enough temperature to kill bacteria. Color change indicators wrapped with the instruments show operating room personnel that the sterilization process was successful.

All surgeons and scrub personnel are responsible for maintaining a sterile field. This is accomplished by wearing sterile gowns and gloves and by the use of sterile drapes and instruments. These should be carefully inspected to ensure that there are no cuts or holes in the attire or in the packages in which the instruments are wrapped. Even the smallest hole will breach the integrity of the sterile field.

The surgical site should only be touched by items that are sterile. Each member of the surgical team has the responsibility to ensure that there is not a break in the sterile technique. A break in sterile technique may go unnoticed, but it is the responsibility of all operating room personnel to report any problem with sterile technique so it can be quickly corrected.

E872.0 Failure of sterile precautions during surgical operation

E872.1 Failure of sterile precautions during infusion or transfusion

E872.2 Failure of sterile precautions during kidney dialysis and other perfusion

E872.3 Failure of sterile precautions during injection or vaccination

E872.4 Failure of sterile precautions during endoscopic examination

E872.5 Failure of sterile precautions during aspiration of fluid or tissue, puncture, and catheterization

E872.6 Failure of sterile precautions during heart catheterization

E872.8 Failure of sterile precautions during other specified procedure

E872.9 Failure of sterile precautions during unspecified procedure

Coding Clarification

Category E872 codes may only be reported as a secondary diagnosis.

Codes E870-E876 should be assigned if the physician documents the misadventure.

Report a code from the E878-E879 rubric for an abnormal reaction or later complication of a procedure that the physician does not document as a misadventure.

E873 Failure in dosage

Category E873 codes are used to report failure in dosage. This could mean excessive fluid or blood administration, which can cause heart failure or electrolyte imbalance in the patient or an excess amount of iron in the blood in the case of excessive blood transfusion.

Excess radiation can cause short-term effects such as burns on the skin to long-term effects such as cancer and birth defects. Radiation is commonly used to treat certain types of cancer.

Drug administration errors can include giving the patient too much medication, not enough medication, or failing to give an ordered drug.

E873.0 Excessive amount of blood or other fluid during transfusion or infusion

E873.1 Incorrect dilution of fluid during infusion

E873.2 Overdose of radiation in therapy

E873.3 Inadvertent exposure of patient to radiation during medical care

E873.4 Failure in dosage in electroshock or insulin-shock therapy

E873.5 Inappropriate (too hot or too cold) temperature in local application and packing

E873.6 Nonadministration of necessary drug or medicinal substance

E873.8 Other specified failure in dosage

E873.9 Unspecified failure in dosage

Coding Clarification

Category E873 codes may only be reported as a secondary diagnosis.

Codes E870-E876 should be assigned if the physician documents the misadventure.

Report a code from the E878-E879 rubric for an abnormal reaction or later complication of a procedure that the physician does not document as a misadventure.

E874 Mechanical failure of instrument or apparatus during procedure

Category E874 codes are used to report the mechanical failure of an instrument or apparatus during a procedure, which includes the malfunction of instruments or equipment used during a surgical procedure. Procedures during which equipment malfunctions might occur include infusion, transfusion, dialysis, perfusion, endoscopy, aspiration, puncture, catheterization, heart catheterization, and other procedures. The practice of testing equipment and instrumentation will help eliminate problems in this area.

E874.0 Mechanical failure of instrument or apparatus during surgical operation

E874.1 Mechanical failure of instrument or apparatus during infusion and transfusion

E874.2 Mechanical failure of instrument or apparatus during kidney dialysis and other perfusion

E874.3 Mechanical failure of instrument or apparatus during endoscopic examination

E874.4 Mechanical failure of instrument or apparatus during aspiration of fluid or tissue, puncture, and catheterization

E874.5 Mechanical failure of instrument or apparatus during heart catheterization

E874.8 Mechanical failure of instrument or apparatus during other specified procedure

E874.9 Mechanical failure of instrument or apparatus during unspecified procedure

Coding Clarification

Category E874 codes may only be reported as a secondary diagnosis.

Codes E870-E876 should be assigned if the physician documents the misadventure.

Report a code from the E878-E879 rubric for an abnormal reaction or later complication of a procedure that the physician does not document as a misadventure.

E875 Contaminated or infected blood, other fluid, drug, or biological substance

Blood can be transfused as whole blood, red blood cells, plasma, cryoprecipitated AHF, platelets, white blood cells, and plasma derivatives. Blood can be stored from five days to 10 years depending on the component of the blood being stored. Currently blood is tested for Hepatitis B surface antigen, Hepatitis B core antibody, Hepatitis C virus antibody, HIV-1 antibody, HIV 2 antibody, HTLV-I antibody, HTLV-II antibody, syphilis, and nucleic acid amplification. Nucleic acid amplification testing, which detects the genetic material of viruses, is also performed. These tests are all considered screening tests. The tests are sensitive and may result in false positives. Confirmatory tests can be done to confirm a positive result. The Food and Drug Administration (FDA) allows investigational tests for the West Nile virus, which can be transmitted through a blood transfusion.

E875.0 Contaminated substance transfused or infused

E875.1 Contaminated substance injected or used for vaccination

E875.2 Contaminated drug or biological substance administered by other means

E875.8 Other contamination of patient during medical care

E875.9 Unspecified contamination of patient during medical care

Coding Clarification

Category E875 codes may only be reported as a secondary diagnosis.

Codes E870-E876 should be assigned if the physician documents the misadventure.

Report a code from the E878-E879 rubric for an abnormal reaction or later complication of a procedure that the physician does not document as a misadventure.

E876 Other and unspecified misadventures during medical care

A patient given the incorrect blood type can suffer clotting problems, kidney failure, and death. A blood type is the presence or absence of certain proteins on the red blood cells. If the wrong blood type is given, the body's immune system would try to fight off the unfamiliar virus.

An endotracheal tube (ET) is placed into a patient's trachea to provide ventilation. Often the patient is paralyzed before the procedure so the patient is completely dependent on the ET tube to provide

E Codes

© 2004 Ingenix, Inc.

oxygen to the body. If this tube is incorrectly placed into the esophagus, the patient can die from lack of oxygen.

The Joint Commission on Accreditation of Healthcare Organizations (JCAHO) states that since 1996 more than 150 cases of wrong-site surgery has occurred. This means the physician operated on the wrong side or wrong body part. There are also incidences where surgery was performed on the wrong patient.

E876.0 Mismatched blood in transfusion

E876.1 Wrong fluid in infusion

E876.2 Failure in suture and ligature during surgical operation

E876.3 Endotracheal tube wrongly placed during anesthetic procedure

E876.4 Failure to introduce or to remove other tube or instrument

E876.5 Performance of inappropriate operation

E876.8 Other specified misadventure during medical care

E876.9 Unspecified misadventure during medical care

Coding Clarification

Category E876 codes may only be reported as a secondary diagnosis.

Codes E870-E876 should be assigned if the physician documents the misadventure.

Report a code from the E878-E879 rubric for an abnormal reaction or later complication of a procedure that the physician does not document as a misadventure.

E878–E879 Surgical and Medical Procedures as the Cause of Abnormal Reaction of Patient or Later Complication, Without Mention of Misadventure at the Time of Procedure

Rubric E878-E879 codes are used to report abnormal reactions that patients have following surgical and medical procedures. These codes can also be used to report a later complication of a misadventure that occurred at the time of a procedure. Examples of these kinds of procedures are those that cause an abnormal reaction such as displacement or malfunction of a prosthetic device, liver or renal failure, malfunction of an external stoma, postoperative intestinal obstruction, or rejection of a transplanted organ. Excluded from this category are anesthetic management properly carried out as the cause of an adverse effect and infusion and transfusion without mention of misadventure in the technique. These codes should be used when a physician documents that an abnormal reaction or later complication is a result of a medical or surgical procedure, but does not mention any misadventure at the time of the procedure.

E878 Surgical operation and other surgical procedures as the cause of abnormal reaction of patient, or of later complication, without mention of misadventure at the time of operation

Transplanted organs are rejected because the body's immune system sees the transplanted organ as a potentially harmful foreign body. Although tissue typing is performed prior to the transplant, no two people (except identical twins) have the same tissue antigens. Other than with corneal transplants, patients have to be on immunosuppressive drugs all of their lives. Symptoms of organ rejection include the following:

- Organ does not function properly
- General feeling of uneasiness or illness
- Fever and pain or swelling at the organ site

A stoma is an artificial opening from an internal organ to outside the body. A gastrostomy is an opening from the stomach to the skin. This allows feeding directly into the stomach. A jejunostomy is an opening from the first portion of the bowel to outside the body, which also can be used for feeding. An ileostomy is an opening from the small bowel to outside the body, which allows feces to leave the body without passing through the large intestine. A colostomy is an opening from the large bowel to outside the body, which allows feces to be eliminated from the body bypassing the anus. A urostomy is a connection between the urinary system and the abdominal wall. This procedure also may be referred to as a urinary conduit. Some stomas may be temporary and will require another surgery to close them.

Also included in this category are surgical procedures to remove a limb or organ, such as an amputated limb and a cholecystectomy.

E878.0 Surgical operation with transplant of whole organ causing abnormal patient reaction, or later complication, without mention of misadventure at time of operation

E878.1 Surgical operation with implant of artificial internal device causing abnormal patient reaction, or later complication, without mention of misadventure at time of operation

© 2004 Ingenix, Inc.

E878.2 Surgical operation with anastomosis, bypass, or graft, with natural or artificial tissues used as implant causing abnormal patient reaction, or later complication, without mention of misadventure at time of operation

E878.3 Surgical operation with formation of external stoma causing abnormal patient reaction, or later complication, without mention of misadventure at time of operation

E878.4 Other restorative surgery causing abnormal patient reaction, or later complication, without mention of misadventure at time of operation

E878.5 Amputation of limb(s) causing abnormal patient reaction, or later complication, without mention of misadventure at time of operation

E878.6 Removal of other organ (partial) (total) causing abnormal patient reaction, or later complication, without mention of misadventure at time of operation

E878.8 Other specified surgical operation and procedure causing abnormal patient reaction, or later complication, without mention of misadventure at time of operation

E878.9 Unspecified surgical operation and procedure causing abnormal patient reaction, or later complication, without mention of misadventure at time of operation

Coding Clarification

Category E878 codes may only be reported as a secondary diagnosis.

Report a code from the E878-E879 rubric for an abnormal reaction or later complication of a procedure that the physician does not document as a misadventure.

For misadventures during a surgical or medical procedure, report E870-E876.

Coding Scenario

A patient who has undergone appendectomy experiences a dehiscence of the skin wound. The patient is taken back to the operating room and the wound is repaired. There is no sign of infection.

> Code assignment: 998.32 *Dehiscence of external wound*, and E878.6 *Removal of other organ (partial) (total) causing abnormal patient reaction, or later complication, without mention of misadventure at time of operation*

E879 Other procedures, without mention of misadventure at the time of procedure, as the cause of abnormal reaction of patient, or of later complication

During a cardiac catheterization a puncture is made into a blood vessel in the groin and a catheter is fed through this to the heart. Different vessels of the heart are imaged and often a repair can be made at the same time as the diagnosis.

Hemodialysis is the use of an artificial kidney to clear waste products from the blood when the patient's own kidneys are not functioning.

Between 100,000 to 150,000 patients are given electroconvulsive therapy (shock therapy) every year to treat schizophrenia and depression. Anesthetic and muscle relaxants are given to the patient prior to the administration of the therapy.

E879.0 Cardiac catheterization as the cause of abnormal reaction of patient, or of later complication, without mention of misadventure at time of procedure

E879.1 Kidney dialysis as the cause of abnormal reaction of patient, or of later complication, without mention of misadventure at time of procedure

E879.2 Radiological procedure and radiotherapy as the cause of abnormal reaction of patient, or of later complication, without mention of misadventure at time of procedure

E879.3 Shock therapy as the cause of abnormal reaction of patient, or of later complication, without mention of misadventure at time of procedure

E879.4 Aspiration of fluid as the cause of abnormal reaction of patient, or of later complication, without mention of misadventure at time of procedure

E879.5 Insertion of gastric or duodenal sound as the cause of abnormal reaction of patient, or of later complication, without mention of misadventure of time of procedure

E879.6 Urinary catheterization as the cause of abnormal reaction of patient, or of later complication, without mention of misadventure at time of procedure

E879.7 Blood sampling as the cause of abnormal reaction of patient, or of later complication, without mention of misadventure at time of procedure

E879.8 Other specified procedure as the cause of abnormal reaction of patient, or of later complication, without mention of misadventure at time of procedure

© 2004 Ingenix, Inc.

E879.9 Unspecified procedure as the cause of abnormal reaction of patient, or of later complication, without mention of misadventure at time of procedure

Coding Clarification
Category E879 codes may only be reported as a secondary diagnosis.

Report a code from the E878-E879 rubric for an abnormal reaction or later complication of a procedure that the physician does not document as a misadventure.

E880–E888 Accidental Falls

Accidental fall codes are one of the most frequently assigned series of E codes. A fall is the most common cause of fatal injury in the elderly and a common cause of injury in children.

Accidental falls are broken down into specific types depending on whether the fall was from a bed, a chair, a ladder, the toilet, or the sidewalk curb. Also included in this category is a fall that results in the person striking against an object.

Excluded from this rubric is a fall in or from a burning building; into a fire; into water with submerging and drowning; in or from operating machinery; on an edged, painted, or sharp object; and in or from a transport or other vehicle.

E880 Accidental fall on or from stairs or steps

Category E880 codes describe falls from an escalator, a sidewalk curb, stairs, or steps. An escalator is defined as mechanically moving stairs or steps. This category does not include moving sidewalks.

E880.0 Accidental fall on or from escalator

E880.1 Accidental fall on or from sidewalk curb

E880.9 Accidental fall on or from other stairs or steps

Coding Clarification
Category E880 codes may only be reported as a secondary diagnosis.

Use a secondary E code from category E849 to identify the place of occurrence.

E881 Accidental fall on or from ladders or scaffolding

Category E881 codes are used to report falls from a ladder or scaffolding. A scaffolding is a temporary platform used to stand on when performing tasks above the ground.

E881.0 Accidental fall from ladder

E881.1 Accidental fall from scaffolding

Coding Clarification
Category E881 codes may only be reported as a secondary diagnosis.

Use a secondary E code from category E849 to identify the place of occurrence.

E882 Accidental fall from or out of building or other structure OK

Code E882 is used to report falls from out of a building or other structure. Included in this category is a fall from a turret, viaduct, wall, window, balcony, bridge, building, flagpole, tower, and a fall through the roof. Excluded from this category is a fall or jump from a burning building or a fall due to a collapse of a building.

Coding Clarification
Code E882 codes may only be reported as a secondary diagnosis.

Use a secondary E code from category E849 to identify the place of occurrence.

E883 Accidental fall into hole or other opening in surface

Category E883 codes are used to report a fall into a hole or opening in the surface. This includes a hole, pit quarry, shaft, and tank. There are specific codes for accidents caused by diving or jumping into water, falling into a well, and falling into a storm drain or manhole.

E883.0 Accident from diving or jumping into water (swimming pool)

E883.1 Accidental fall into well

E883.2 Accidental fall into storm drain or manhole

E883.9 Accidental fall into other hole or other opening in surface

Coding Clarification
Category E883 codes may only be reported as a secondary diagnosis.

Use a secondary E code from category E849 to identify the place of occurrence.

Coding Scenario
A 29-year-old male presents to the emergency department with a neck injury. The patient was diving into a pool in his back yard and hit his head on the bottom. The diagnosis is a strained neck.

> Code assignment: 847.0 *Neck strain or sprain*, E883.0 *Accident from diving or jumping into water*, and E849.0 *Place of occurrence, home*

E Codes

E884 Other accidental fall from one level to another

Category E884 codes are used to report any fall from one level to another. Specific codes are available to report a fall from playground equipment, a cliff, chair, wheelchair, bed, other furniture, and a commode.

Many playground accidents involve falls from playground equipment onto hard surfaces. This is one of the major types of falls for children ages 5 to 14.

E884.0 Accidental fall from playground equipment
E884.1 Accidental fall from cliff
E884.2 Accidental fall from chair
E884.3 Accidental fall from wheelchair
E884.4 Accidental fall from bed
E884.5 Accidental fall from other furniture
E884.6 Accidental fall from commode
E884.9 Other accidental fall from one level to another

Coding Clarification
Category E884 codes may only be reported as a secondary diagnosis.

Use a secondary E code from category E849 to identify the place of occurrence.

E885 Accidental fall on same level from slipping, tripping, or stumbling

Category E885 codes are used to describe falls on the same level. This code category includes falls from scooters, roller skates, skateboards, skis, snowboards, or from slipping, tripping, and stumbling.

E885.0 Fall on same level from (nonmotorized) scooter
E885.1 Fall from roller skates
E885.2 Fall from skateboard
E885.3 Fall from skis
E885.4 Fall from snowboard
E885.9 Fall from other slipping, tripping, or stumbling

Coding Clarification
Category E885 codes may only be reported as a secondary diagnosis.

Use a secondary E code from category E849 to identify the place of occurrence.

E886 Accidental fall on same level from collision, pushing, or shoving, by or with other person

Category E886 codes are used to describe falls from the same level due to a collision, push, or shove, by or with another person. Code E886.0 is used to report colliding, pushing, or shoving injuries that occur in sports. Code 886.9 includes a fall from or a collision with a pedestrian conveyance. A pedestrian conveyance is a device that is human powered and used to move a pedestrian, which includes a baby carriage, coaster wagon, ice skates, pushcart, and pushchair.

E886.0 Accidental fall on same level from collision, pushing, or shoving, by or with other person in sports
E886.9 Other and unspecified accidental falls on same level from collision, pushing, or shoving, by or with other person

Coding Clarification
Category E886 codes may only be reported as a secondary diagnosis.

Use a secondary E code from category E849 to identify the place of occurrence.

Coding Scenario
A 17-year-old male presents to the emergency department with a dislocated right shoulder. The patient was playing in a high school football game and was tackled landing on his right shoulder. The diagnosis is a closed dislocation of the right shoulder.

> Code assignment: 831.0 *Closed dislocation of shoulder*, E886.0 *Accidental fall on same level from collision, pushing, or shoving, by or with other person in sports*, and E849.4 *Place of occurrence, place for recreation and sport*

E887 Fracture in accidental fall, cause unspecified OK

Code E887 is used to report a fracture caused by a fall when the cause of the fall is not specified. This code should only be used if the information cannot be obtained from the patient or the physician.

Coding Clarification
Code E887 codes may only be reported as a secondary diagnosis.

Use a secondary E code from category E849 to identify the place of occurrence.

E888 Other and unspecified accidental fall

Category E888 codes are used to report other and unspecified falls. Specific codes in this category are for falls that result in striking against a sharp object and falls that result in striking against other objects.

E888.0 Fall resulting in striking against sharp object
E888.1 Fall resulting in striking against other object
E888.8 Other fall

E Codes

 © 2004 Ingenix, Inc.

E888.9 Unspecified fall

Coding Clarification
Category E888 codes may only be reported as a secondary diagnosis.

Use an additional E code from category E920 to identify the sharp object.

Use a secondary E code from category E849 to identify the place of occurrence.

E890–E899 Accidents Caused by Fire and Flames

Rubrics E890-E899 are used to describe accidents caused by fire and flames. This code category includes asphyxia or poisoning due to fire. Asphyxia is suffocation or lack of oxygen intake, which can occur in a very short amount of time. In the United States, fires are the third leading cause of accidental death, with the number one cause being smoke inhalation. Smoke contents are heated particles and gases. The exact composition of smoke and the toxicity are dependent on the material that is on fire.

E890 Conflagration in private dwelling

Category E890 codes are used to report conflagration in a private dwelling. A private dwelling is defined as an apartment, a boarding house, camping place, farmhouse, house, mobile home, or private garage. Conflagration is a widespread, general burning. One of the harmful gases that can be generated in a fire is polyvinylchloride (PVC). PVC is a flame and water-resistant plastic material that can be found in communication and building cables.

E890.0 Explosion caused by conflagration in private dwelling

E890.1 Fumes from combustion of polyvinylchloride (PVC) and similar material in conflagration in private dwelling

E890.2 Other smoke and fumes from conflagration in private dwelling

E890.3 Burning caused by conflagration in private dwelling

E890.8 Other accident resulting from conflagration in private dwelling

E890.9 Unspecified accident resulting from conflagration in private dwelling

Coding Clarification
Category E890 codes may only be reported as a secondary diagnosis.

Use a secondary E code from category E849 to identify the place of occurrence.

E891 Conflagration in other and unspecified building or structure

Category E891 codes are used to report conflagration in a structure other than a private dwelling. A nonprivate dwelling is defined as a barn, church, retirement home, factory, hospital, hotel, school, store, or theater. Conflagration is a widespread, general burning. One of the harmful gases that can be generated in a fire is PVC. PVC is a flame- and water-resistant plastic material that can be found in communication and building cables.

E891.0 Explosion caused by conflagration in other and unspecified building or structure

E891.1 Fumes from combustion of polyvinylchloride (PVC) and similar material in conflagration in other and unspecified building or structure

E891.2 Other smoke and fumes from conflagration in other and unspecified building or structure

E891.3 Burning caused by conflagration in other and unspecified building or structure

E891.8 Other accident resulting from conflagration in other and unspecified building or structure

E891.9 Unspecified accident resulting from conflagration of other and unspecified building or structure

Coding Clarification
Category E891 codes may only be reported as a secondary diagnosis.

Use a secondary E code from category E849 to identify the place of occurrence.

E892 Conflagration not in building or structure OK

Code E892 is used to report conflagration not in a building or structure, which includes forest, grass, and lumber fires. This code category also includes fire in a transport vehicle when the vehicle is not moving. Conflagration is a widespread, general burning.

Coding Clarification
Code E892 codes may only be reported as a secondary diagnosis.

Use a secondary E code from category E849 to identify the place of occurrence.

E893 Accident caused by ignition of clothing

Category E893 codes are used to describe accidents caused by ignition of clothing. The United States government issued regulations to restrict the use of flammable materials in children's clothing. Legislation classifies clothing into the following three different categories:

E Codes

- Class one is normal flammability. These are textiles without raised fiber in which flames spread in four seconds or more.
- Class two is intermediate flammability. These are textiles having raised fiber in which flames spread between four and seven seconds.
- Class three is rapid and intense burning. These are textiles without raised fiber in which flames spread in less than four seconds.

E893.0 Accident caused by ignition of clothing from controlled fire in private dwelling

E893.1 Accident caused by ignition of clothing from controlled fire in other building or structure

E893.2 Accident caused by ignition of clothing from controlled fire not in building or structure

E893.8 Accident caused by ignition of clothing from other specified sources

E893.9 Accident caused by ignition of clothing by unspecified source

Coding Clarification

Category E893 codes may only be reported as a secondary diagnosis.

Use a secondary E code from category E849 to identify the place of occurrence.

Coding Scenario

A 40-year-old male is admitted to the emergency department with second-degree burns of his upper arm. The patient was using a torch at work and his shirt was ignited.

> Code assignment: 942.23 *Second degree burn of upper arm*, E893.8 *Accident caused by ignition of clothing from other specified source*, and E849.3 *Place of occurrence, industrial place and premises*

E894 Ignition of highly inflammable material OK

Code E894 is used to report ignition of clothing by highly inflammable material. These are materials such as gasoline, fat, kerosene, paraffin, and benzine. Excluded from this category is ignition of highly inflammable materials with conflagration or explosion. Conflagration is a widespread burning.

Coding Clarification

Code E894 codes may only be reported as a secondary diagnosis.

Use a secondary E code from category E849 to identify the place of occurrence.

E895 Accident caused by controlled fire in private dwelling OK

Code E895 is used to describe accidents caused by a controlled fire in a private dwelling. The definition of a private dwelling is an apartment, a boarding house, camping place, caravan, farmhouse, house, lodging house, mobile home, private garage, rooming house, and tenement. Examples of controlled burns are those in a brazier, fireplace, furnace, and stove. A brazier is a device that holds coal or charcoal and is used to heat food.

Coding Clarification

Code E895 codes may only be reported as a secondary diagnosis.

Use a secondary E code from category E849 to identify the place of occurrence.

E896 Accident caused by controlled fire in other and unspecified building or structure OK

Code E896 is used to report accidents caused by a controlled fire in other and unspecified buildings or structures. The following are kinds of buildings or structures: a barn, church, convalescent home, residential home, dormitory, factory, any type of farm outbuilding, hospital, hotel, school, store, and theater. Examples of controlled burns are those in a brazier, fireplace, furnace, and stove. A brazier is a device that holds coal or charcoal and is used to heat food.

Coding Clarification

Code E896 codes may only be reported as a secondary diagnosis.

Use a secondary E code from category E849 to identify the place of occurrence.

E897 Accident caused by controlled fire not in building or structure OK

Code E897 is used to report accidents caused by a controlled fire not in a building or structure. Examples of this type of controlled fire include a bonfire, brazier fire, trash fire, and campfire. A brazier is a device that holds coal or charcoal and is used to heat food.

Coding Clarification

Code E897 codes may only be reported as a secondary diagnosis.

Use a secondary E code from category E849 to identify the place of occurrence.

E Codes

© 2004 Ingenix, Inc.

E898 Accident caused by other specified fire and flames

Burning bedclothes can be the cause of flashover. Flashover is a temperature that is so intense it causes everything in the room to burst into flames. This happens at a heat-release rate of about 1,000 kilowatts. King-size bedclothes can contribute to more than 400 kilowatts and a mattress and box spring can contribute to more than 500 kilowatts.

E898.0 Accident caused by burning bedclothes

E898.1 Accident caused by other burning materials

Coding Clarification

Category E898 codes may only be reported as a secondary diagnosis.

Use a secondary E code from category E849 to identify the place of occurrence.

E899 Accident caused by unspecified fire OK

Code E899 is used to describe fires of an unspecified nature. This should only be used if more specific information cannot be obtained from the physician or patient.

Coding Clarification

Code E899 codes may only be reported as a secondary diagnosis.

Use a secondary E code from category E849 to identify the place of occurrence.

E900–E909 Accidents due to Natural and Environmental Factors

E900 Accident caused by excessive heat

Sunstroke is a rise in temperature caused by exposure to the sun, hot climates, overcrowding, and poor ventilation. It may also be called siriasis. Symptoms of heatstroke include heat syncope, sudden seizure, flushed face, quick pulse, gasping or sighing respiration, headache, vomiting, nausea, and thermic fever, which is a body temperature of 110 degrees or more.

E900.0 Accident due to excessive heat weather conditions

E900.1 Accident due to excessive heat, man-made origin

E900.9 Accident due to excessive heat, unspecified origin

Coding Clarification

Category E900 codes may only be reported as a secondary diagnosis.

Use a secondary E code from category E849 to identify the place of occurrence.

E901 Accident due to excessive cold

Chilblains are painful, small, itchy, red areas of the skin that appear on the skin after exposure to cold temperature. They are more common in cold, humid climates. Chilblains are most common on the toes but can appear on the fingers, nose, and ears also. The skin breaks down and ulcers and infection can occur. Chilblains are more common in females and can be recurrent for the rest of the patient's life or last only a few years.

Immersion foot occurs when the feet have been submerged or subjected to wet conditions for long periods of time. It is less serious than frost bite but can cause gangrene and necrosis.

E901.0 Accident due to excessive cold, weather conditions

E901.1 Accident due to excessive cold, man-made origin

E901.8 Accident due to excessive cold, other specified origin

E901.9 Accident due to excessive cold, unspecified origin

Coding Clarification

Category E901 codes may only be reported as a secondary diagnosis.

Use a secondary E code from category E849 to identify the place of occurrence.

E902 Accident due to high and low air pressure and changes in air pressure

Altitude sickness can occur when people are above 6,000 to 8,000 feet. Susceptibility to altitude sickness does not seem to be affected by training or the physical condition of the patient. The three types of altitude sickness are:

- Acute mountain sickness (AMS). This is the most common type. It can occur in altitudes as low as 4,000 to 6,000 feet but most often occurs in rapid ascents to greater than 9,000 feet. Symptoms include headache, fatigue, loss of appetite, nausea, and vomiting. Symptoms can occur between six and 24 hours after ascent.
- High-altitude cerebral edema (HACE). This is a severe progression of AMS. The patient may have the symptoms of AMS plus profound confusion and ataxia during a tandem gait test. A tandem gait test is walking heel to toe in a straight line. A person who fails the tandem gait test has HACE and should descend immediately.

E Codes

- High-altitude pulmonary edema (HAPE). This can occur by itself or in conjunction with high-altitude cerebral edema. Symptoms include increased breathlessness with exertion and eventually increased loss of breath at rest. If the increased loss of breath continues after several minutes at rest, the patient should descend immediately.

The bends or diver's sickness is caused by nitrogen bubble formation in the blood and tissues. This is usually caused by a diver ascending to the surface too fast. The symptoms include headache, vertigo, disturbed sensation, paralysis, and death.

E902.0	Accident due to residence or prolonged visit at high altitude
E902.1	Accident due to changes in airpressure in aircraft
E902.2	Accident due to changes in air pressure due to diving
E902.8	Accident due to changes in air pressure due to other specified cause
E902.9	Accident due to changes in air pressure from unspecified cause

Coding Clarification

Category E902 codes may only be reported as a secondary diagnosis.

Use a secondary E code from category E849 to identify the place of occurrence.

E903 Accident due to travel and motion OK

Motion sickness is caused by a disturbance in the balance center in the middle ear. Many people will experience motion sickness when there is increased turbulence. Symptoms include dizziness, nausea, and vomiting.

Coding Clarification

Code E903 codes may only be reported as a secondary diagnosis.

Use a secondary E code from category E849 to identify the place of occurrence.

Coding Scenario

A 42-year-old female traveling by air from Salt Lake City to Cincinnati experiences nausea and vomiting. She presents to the emergency department for treatment. The diagnosis is nausea and vomiting due to motion sickness.

> Code assignment: 787.01 *Nausea and vomiting*, E903 *Accidents due to travel and motion*, and E849.8 *Place of occurrence, other specified place*

E904 Accident due to hunger, thirst, exposure, and neglect

Malnutrition results from inadequate intake of nutrients. Infants and children are at the highest risk for malnutrition, since there is a high demand for nutrients during the growth years. Pregnancy and old age also pose other significant risks for malnutrition. Malnutrition as the result of abandonment and neglect should be reported with E904.0. When neglect is determined to be due to abandonment or neglect, E904.0 should be the first listed E code.

Dehydration is the depletion of total body water and sodium. This can be caused by profuse sweating and not replacing the fluid adequately.

E904.0	Accident due to abandonment or neglect of infant and helpless person
E904.1	Accident due to lack of food
E904.2	Accident due to lack of water
E904.3	Accident due to exposure (to weather conditions), not elsewhere classifiable
E904.9	Accident due to unqualified privation

Coding Clarification

Category E904 codes may only be reported as a secondary diagnosis.

Use a secondary E code from category E849 to identify the place of occurrence.

E905 Venomous animals and plants as the cause of poisoning and toxic reactions

Each of the 48 contiguous states in the United States harbors at least one species of venomous snake. The pit vipers (copperhead, cottonmouth, and rattlesnakes) and coral snakes are two venomous families widely spread throughout the United States. Approximately 8,000 of the estimated 45,000 annual snakebites in this country are by poisonous snakes. Snake venoms are rated on a lethality index, with the Mojave rattlesnake having the highest index of any North American snake. Pit viper bites are associated with pain, swelling, and edema. Ecchymosis is common, ranging from moderate to severe. The patient may hemorrhage from the gums and develop hematemesis, melena, and hematuria. The coral snake bite generally produces nerve conduction damage and central nervous system (CNS) damage. Annual fatalities are fewer than 15, most of which can be attributed to rattlesnake venom.

Two lizards, the Gila monster and the bearded lizard, are poisonous. There is currently no antivenom for these bites.

There are numerous venomous spider species in the United States. Most bites require only local care, although in cases of severe envenomation, the victim

 © 2004 Ingenix, Inc.

must be hospitalized for supportive measures. Fatalities are few, with the greatest risks for children and elderly.

As many as 85 percent of all people will develop a reaction if exposed to poison ivy, poison oak, or poison sumac. It may take several exposures to develop a sensitivity or the effects may appear with the initial contact. Although the toxin is only found in the sap of the plant, they are fragile and are often damaged causing the sap to come to the surface.

E905.0 Venomous snakes and lizards as the cause of poisoning and toxic reactions

E905.1 Venomous spiders as the cause of poisoning and toxic reactions

E905.2 Scorpion sting as the cause of poisoning and toxic reactions

E905.3 Sting of hornets, wasps, and bees as the cause of poisoning and toxic reactions

E905.4 Centipede and venomous millipede (tropical) bite as the cause of poisoning and toxic reactions

E905.5 Other venomous arthropods as the cause of poisoning and toxic reactions

E905.6 Venomous marine animals and plants as the cause of poisoning and toxic reactions

E905.7 Poisoning and toxic reactions caused by other plants

E905.8 Poisoning and toxic reactions caused by other specified animals and plants

E905.9 Poisoning and toxic reactions caused by unspecified animals and plants

Coding Clarification

Category E905 codes may only be reported as a secondary diagnosis.

Use a secondary E code from category E849 to identify the place of occurrence.

E906 Other injury caused by animals

There are an estimated 4.7 million people bitten by dogs each year. Injuries can range from minor and superficial to vicious, harmful attacks. There are steps people can take to avoid being bitten, such as staying away from unfamiliar dogs, not running from dogs, slowly backing away from a dog once it loses interest, and, if knocked down by a dog, rolling into a ball and staying motionless.

Although instances of rat bites are on the decline, children in poverty stricken areas are still at risk. There is a high probability of transmission of disease with wild rat bites. Diseases include streptobacillary rat-bite fever and spirillary rat-bite fever.

There are approximately 94 out of 120 snakes found in the United States that are not venomous. Bites from nonvenomous snakes are more common than venomous types. Nonvenomous snakebites are treated much like any other puncture wound.

E906.0 Dog bite

E906.1 Rat bite

E906.2 Bite of nonvenomous snakes and lizards

E906.3 Bite of other animal except arthropod

E906.4 Bite of nonvenomous arthropod

E906.5 Bite by unspecified animal

E906.8 Other specified injury caused by animal

E906.9 Unspecified injury caused by animal

Coding Clarification

Category E906 codes may only be reported as a secondary diagnosis.

Use a secondary E code from category E849 to identify the place of occurrence.

E907 Accident due to lightning OK

Lightning strikes can cause a wide variety of injuries. Many people struck by lightning suffer temporary paralysis that is distinctive to a lightning strike. Cardiac injuries such as cardiac arrest, arrhythmias, and infarction, as well as superficial burns and neurologic injuries, can occur as a result of lightning strikes. The eardrum is commonly ruptured causing hearing loss and pain.

Coding Clarification

Code E907 codes may only be reported as a secondary diagnosis.

Use a secondary E code from category E849 to identify the place of occurrence.

E908 Accident due to cataclysmic storms, and floods resulting from storms

A cataclysmic event is one that is caused by the force of nature. Hurricanes, tornadoes, floods, blizzards, and dust storms are considered cataclysmic events.

Hurricanes are storms containing two parts, an eye or calm portion in the middle and a wall of clouds that surround the eye. Hurricanes can be several hundred feet in diameter. A hurricane can maintain winds of 74 miles per hour or higher.

There are approximately 1,200 tornadoes each year causing more than 1,500 injuries and 80 deaths. A tornado is a violent storm that consists of a column of air that rotates violently. Tornadoes can range in speed from 30 to 70 miles per hour.

E908.0 Accident due to hurricane

E908.1 Accident due to tornado

E Codes

E908.2 Accident due to floods

E908.3 Accident due to blizzard (snow) (ice)

E908.4 Accident due to dust storm

E908.8 Accident due to other cataclysmic storms

E908.9 Accident due to unspecified cataclysmic storms and floods resulting from storms

Coding Clarification

Category E908 codes may only be reported as a secondary diagnosis.

Use a secondary E code from category E849 to identify the place of occurrence.

E codes for cataclysmic events take priority over all other E codes except child and adult abuse and terrorism.

E909 Accident due to cataclysmic earth surface movements and eruptions

A cataclysmic event is one that is caused by the force of nature. Category E909 codes include earthquakes, volcanic eruptions, avalanches, landslides or mudslides, collapse of dams or man-made structures, and tidal waves caused by earthquakes.

Earthquakes are caused by shifting of the earth because of faults or a pre-existing weakness in the earth. Earthquakes are measured on a Richter scale. If the earthquake registers at less than a 3.5 on the scale, the earthquake is generally not felt, 3.5 to 5.4 and the earthquake can be felt but generally does not cause damage, 5.5 to 6.0 may cause damage to poorly constructed buildings, 6.1 to 6.9 can cause damage, 7.0 to 7.9 is a major earthquake and can cause major damage over large areas, and 8.0 is a great earthquake that can cause damage to areas more than 100 kilometers.

Volcanic eruptions do both harm and good. An eruption can destroy hundreds of acres of land but is key in forming land masses, such as the islands of Hawaii. Geologists are still unsure of exactly how volcanoes work but continue to study them. By learning how they work, scientists may better learn how to predict their eruption.

E909.0 Earthquakes

E909.1 Volcanic eruptions

E909.2 Avalanche, landslide, or mudslide

E909.3 Collapse of dam or man-made structure

E909.4 Tidalwave caused by earthquake

E909.8 Other cataclysmic earth surface movements and eruptions

E909.9 Unspecified cataclysmic earth surface movements and eruptions

Coding Clarification

Category E909 codes may only be reported as a secondary diagnosis.

Use a secondary E code from category E849 to identify the place of occurrence.

E codes for cataclysmic events take priority over all other E codes except child and adult abuse and terrorism.

E910–E915 Accidents Caused by Submersion, Suffocation, and Foreign Bodies

Rubric E910-E915 is used to report accidents caused by submersion, suffocation, and foreign bodies. The great mortality risk in near drowning is posed by respiratory insufficiency leading to hypoxia and respiratory acidosis. Aspiration of large quantities of fresh water can cause massive increase of blood volume, life-threatening electrolyte imbalance, and hemolysis leading to asphyxia and ventricular fibrillation. Near drowning is now more commonly referred to as a submersion accident.

The water temperature and duration of immersion are factors when predicting survival from immersion. If an individual is exposed to cool water, over time hypothermia will set in, with its attendant problems.

E910 Accidental drowning and submersion

Drowning can cause serious long-term effects such as brain damage or death. Alcohol and drugs contribute to drowning and near drowning, now more commonly referred to as a submersion accident. Nearly three-fourths of boating-related deaths are a result of drowning. More than one-third of adults are unable to swim.

Drowning is the third leading cause of death in children younger than five years of age. Children can drown in only a few inches of water and in a short period of time. Children should never be left unattended in the bathtub for any reason.

E910.0 Accidental drowning and submersion while water-skiing

E910.1 Accidental drowning and submersion while engaged in other sport or recreational activity with diving equipment

E910.2 Accidental drowning and submersion while engaged in other sport or recreational activity without diving equipment

E910.3 Accidental drowning and submersion while swimming or diving for purposes other than recreation or sport

© 2004 Ingenix, Inc.

E910.4 Accidental drowning and submersion in bathtub

E910.8 Other accidental drowning or submersion

E910.9 Unspecified accidental drowning or submersion

Coding Clarification

Category E910 codes may only be reported as a secondary diagnosis.

Use a secondary E code from category E849 to identify the place of occurrence.

E911 Inhalation and ingestion of food causing obstruction of respiratory tract or suffocation OK

Inhalation of food or a foreign object can cause obstruction of the airway. This can be caused by talking and eating at the same time, drinking alcohol and talking, and in older people due to dentures. Dentures do not have the chewing power of natural teeth, which can cause the patient to try to swallow larger pieces of food that get lodged in the airway.

People who are choking usually have a look of panic on their face. Their face may turn red or purple. The universal signal for someone choking is putting their hands to their throat. Using the Heimlich maneuver will help to dislodge an item blocking the airway by using the air already in the lungs to push the foreign body out.

Coding Clarification

Code E911 codes may only be reported as a secondary diagnosis.

Use a secondary E code from category E849 to identify the place of occurrence.

E912 Inhalation and ingestion of other object causing obstruction of respiratory tract or suffocation OK

In 2001, there were more than 17,000 visits to the emergency department due to choking in children 0 to 14 years of age. The highest incidence is for children younger than age one because they tend to put everything in their mouths. This includes small toys and coins. Of the children treated in 2001 for choking incidences, 10.5 percent were admitted or transferred to another facility.

Coding Clarification

Coded E912 codes may only be reported as a secondary diagnosis.

Use a secondary E code from category E849 to identify the place of occurrence.

E913 Accidental mechanical suffocation

Accidental mechanical suffocation codes are used for suffocation on items other than food. Specific codes exist for suffocation in a bed or cradle, by a plastic bag, due to lack of air in a closed in place, such as a refrigerator, and by falling earth or other substance.

Shopping bags, dry cleaning bags, and even mattress bags can cause instances of suffocation in children. All items that could cause airway obstruction in children should be kept out of their reach.

E913.0 Accidental mechanical suffocation in bed or cradle

E913.1 Accidental mechanical suffocation by plastic bag

E913.2 Accidental mechanical suffocation due to lack of air (in closed place)

E913.3 Accidental mechanical suffocation by falling earth or other substance

E913.8 Accidental mechanical suffocation by other specified means

E913.9 Accidental mechanical suffocation by unspecified means

Coding Clarification

Category E913 codes may only be reported as a secondary diagnosis.

Use a secondary E code from category E849 to identify the place of occurrence.

E914 Foreign body accidentally entering eye and adnexa OK

A foreign body in the eye can cause anything from a minor irritation to a serious penetrating eye trauma. The eye's natural tears remove many foreign bodies. Those that aren't removed require medical treatment. Most foreign bodies can be removed using a slit lamp for vision and sometimes a special instrument. Symptoms of a foreign body in the eye include, irritation, pain, redness, tearing, decreased vision, itching, and sensitivity to light.

Coding Clarification

Code E914 codes may only be reported as a secondary diagnosis.

Use a secondary E code from category E849 to identify the place of occurrence.

E915 Foreign body accidentally entering other orifice OK

Foreign bodies accidentally entering another orifice include a foreign body in the ear, genitourinary tract, or the gastrointestinal tract. Children may put things like toys, food, or other small objects in their ear.

Adults can have things such as a hearing aid battery, insect, or even a lost button in their ear. Symptoms include pain, decreased hearing, and strange sounds. Many people do not know they have a foreign body in their ear until they have a foul-smelling discharge from the ear.

Coding Clarification

Code E915 codes may only be reported as a secondary diagnosis.

Use a secondary E code from category E849 to identify the place of occurrence.

E916–E928 Other Accidents

Rubric E916-E928 identifies other accidents. Accidents in this code category include being struck accidentally by a falling object, striking against an object or a person, and being caught accidentally in or between objects. Also included are accidents caused by machinery, cutting instruments, explosion of a pressure vessel (i.e., a boiler), guns, explosives, corrosive materials, electricity, and radiation. Environmental accidents, vibration, human bite, and constriction caused by hair are also types of accidents in this code category.

E916 Struck accidentally by falling object OK

Code E916 is used to report injuries caused by a falling object. Injuries from cataclysmic events take priority over other E codes except for terrorism and adult and child abuse. For example, if a piece of a building falls and injures a person during a hurricane, the code for the hurricane would be used rather than E916.

Coding Clarification

Code E916 codes may only be reported as a secondary diagnosis.

Use a secondary E code from category E849 to identify the place of occurrence.

E Codes

E917 Striking against or struck accidentally by objects or persons

Category E917 codes are used to describe accidents caused by striking against an object or person without a subsequent fall. The appropriate code from the fall category (E888) should be used if the collision with an object or person causes a subsequent fall or if the fall is from an object.

E917.0 Striking against or struck accidentally by objects or persons in sports

E917.1 Striking against or struck accidentally by crowd, by collective fear or panic

E917.2 Striking against or struck accidentally in running water

E917.3 Strike against or struck accidentally by furniture without subsequent fall

E917.4 Strike against or struck accidentally by other stationary object without subsequent fall

E917.5 Strike against or struck accidentally by other object in sports with subsequent fall

E917.6 Strike against or struck accidentally by crowd, by collective fear or panic with subsequent fall

E917.7 Strike against or struck accidentally by furniture with subsequent fall

E917.8 Strike against or struck accidentally by other stationary object with subsequent fall

E917.9 Other accident caused by striking against or being struck accidentally by objects or persons

Coding Clarification

Category E917 codes may only be reported as a secondary diagnosis.

Use a secondary E code from category E849 to identify the place of occurrence.

Coding Scenario

A 16-year-old female injured her right ankle playing soccer for the school team. Another girl stepped on her and her right ankle twisted. She felt pain immediately. The diagnosis is a sprained deltoid ligament of the right ankle.

> Code assignment: 845.01 *Sprain or strain of the deltoid ligament ankle*, E917.0 *Striking against or struck accidentally by objects or person in sports, without subsequent fall*, and E849.4 *Place of occurrence, place for recreation and sport*

E918 Caught accidentally in or between objects OK

Code E918 is used to report a mishap caused by a person accidentally caught in an object or between objects, which includes moving objects such as an escalator, folding doors, and sliding doors. Pinching injuries often happen to the hands and fingers but can occur anywhere on the body.

Coding Clarification

Code E918 codes may only be reported as a secondary diagnosis.

Use a secondary E code from category E849 to identify the place of occurrence.

E919 Accident caused by machinery

Category E919 codes are used to report accidents caused by machinery. Accidents caused by machinery under their own power on a highway are classified as transport accidents. Transport accidents are those involving a vehicle being used primarily for transporting people or goods from one place or another.

Pinching injuries are when body parts or clothing are caught between two pieces of machinery, at least one of them moving. Wrapping injuries are caused by machinery parts that are rotating. Body parts or clothing can be caught and wrapped around the rotating part. Cutting injuries are caused by sharp parts of machinery, such as blades. These pieces can cut or even sever limbs. Crushing injuries are caused by machinery rolling or falling on a person or body part. Also included in this category are injuries by an object being thrown from machinery, such as a rock.

E919.0 Accident caused by agricultural machines

E919.1 Accident caused by mining and earth-drilling machinery

E919.2 Accident caused by lifting machines and appliances

E919.3 Accident caused by metalworking machines

E919.4 Accident caused by woodworking and forming machines

E919.5 Accident caused by prime movers, except electrical motors

E919.6 Accident caused by transmission machinery

E919.7 Accident caused by earth moving, scraping, and other excavating machines

E919.8 Accident caused by other specified machinery

E919.9 Accident caused by unspecified machinery

Coding Clarification

Category E919 codes may only be reported as a secondary diagnosis.

Use a secondary E code from category E849 to identify the place of occurrence.

E920 Accident caused by cutting and piercing instruments or objects

Lawn mowers are considered one of the most dangerous pieces of equipment around the home. They can cause minor cuts, broken bones, and severed fingers and toes. Many of these injuries can be prevented by simple precautions: wear heavy duty shoes when mowing and make sure the engine is off, the spark plug is removed, and the blades have stopped completely before removing debris.

Needle stick injuries are one of the most common injuries in the health care field. Injuries by hypodermic needle punctures can increase the risk of disease as well as HIV. In 1991, OSHA issued standards regulating the exposure to blood-borne pathogens, which has greatly reduced the risk of workers contracting a blood-borne disease while working.

E920.0 Accident caused by powered lawn mower

E920.1 Accident caused by other powered hand tools

E920.2 Accident caused by powered household appliances and implements

E920.3 Accident caused by knives, swords, and daggers

E920.4 Accident caused by other hand tools and implements

E920.5 Accident caused by hypodermic needle

E920.8 Accident caused by other specified cutting and piercing instruments or objects

E920.9 Accident caused by unspecified cutting and piercing instrument or object

Coding Clarification

Category E920 codes may only be reported as a secondary diagnosis.

Use a secondary E code from category E849 to identify the place of occurrence.

E921 Accident caused by explosion of pressure vessel

Category E921 codes are used to report injuries as a result of accidents caused by the explosion of a pressure vessel, which includes boilers and gas cylinders, such as air tanks, aerosol cans, and pressure cookers.

E921.0 Accident caused by explosion of boilers

E921.1 Accident caused by explosion of gas cylinders

E921.8 Accident caused by explosion of other specified pressure vessels

E921.9 Accident caused by explosion of unspecified pressure vessel

Coding Clarification

Category E921 codes may only be reported as a secondary diagnosis.

Use a secondary E code from category E849 to identify the place of occurrence.

E922 Accident caused by firearm, and air gun missiles

Paintball gun injuries have increased over the past several years. Paintballs can travel up to 300 feet per second. Eye injuries are the most serious cause of injury from a paintball and can cause permanent damage. These most often occur when people do not wear protective eye gear when using the paintball guns.

Although most injuries are unintentional, as many as 30,00 people are injured each year by BB guns and pellet guns.

E Codes

E922.0 Accident caused by handgun

E922.1 Accident caused by shotgun (automatic)

E922.2 Accident caused by hunting rifle

E922.3 Accident caused by military firearms

E922.4 Accident caused by air gun

E922.5 Accident caused by paintball gun

E922.8 Accident caused by other specified firearm missile

E922.9 Accident caused by unspecified firearm missile

Coding Clarification

Category E922 codes may only be reported as a secondary diagnosis.

Use a secondary E code from category E849 to identify the place of occurrence.

E923 Accident caused by explosive material

Many fireworks can be used with relative safety. However, all fireworks are potentially hazardous and can cause injury. Some states allow all types of fireworks, some limit fireworks, and some do not allow any type of consumer fireworks. The following safety precautions should be observed when lighting any kind of fireworks: have a bucket of water handy; all children should be supervised by an adult; make sure the area is free from debris, such as dry leaves or grass; if a firework does not light, do not try to relight it; and make sure everyone is clear before lighting.

E923.0 Accident caused by fireworks

E923.1 Accident caused by blasting materials

E923.2 Accident caused by explosive gases

E923.8 Accident caused by other explosive materials

E923.9 Accident caused by unspecified explosive material

Coding Clarification

Category E923 codes may only be reported as a secondary diagnosis.

Use a secondary E code from category E849 to identify the place of occurrence.

E924 Accident caused by hot substance or object, caustic or corrosive material, and steam

Skin exposed to 140-degree water for three seconds or less may be seriously burned. Children and the elderly have skin that is more sensitive to burns. Steps can be taken to reduce the risk of scalding burns. Turn the temperature down on the water heater, install faucets with scald prevention technology, always check the water temperature before entering the bath or shower or putting a child in the tub, keep hot liquids away from a counter edge and table, keep pan handles out of a child's reach, and remove lids from hot foods carefully to avoid steam burns.

E924.0 Accident caused by hot liquids and vapors, including steam

E924.1 Accident caused by caustic and corrosive substances

E924.2 Accident caused by hot (boiling) tap water

E924.8 Accident caused by other hot substance or object

E924.9 Accident caused by unspecified hot substance or object

Coding Clarification

Category E924 codes may only be reported as a secondary diagnosis.

Use a secondary E code from category E849 to identify the place of occurrence.

Coding Scenario

An 11-year-old female is admitted to the emergency department with third-degree burns on her left knee. The young girl was home carrying a pan of bacon from the stove to the table and the pan slipped spilling hot grease onto her leg. The diagnosis is a third-degree burn to the left knee.

> Code assignment: 945.35 *Third degree burn, left knee*, E924.0 *Accident caused by liquids and vapors, including steam*, and E849.0 *Place of occurrence, home*

E925 Accident caused by electric current

Faulty wiring, malfunctioning appliances, or loose connectors can cause electric injuries. Approximately one person a day dies from electrocution at work. This is the fourth leading cause of death from work accidents. Because the body is made mostly of water, it is susceptible to injuries from electrical currents. Electrical injuries may result in burns and respiratory or heart failure.

E925.0 Electrical accident caused by domestic wiring and appliances

E925.1 Electrical accident caused by electric current in electric power generating plants, distribution stations, transmission lines

E925.2 Electrical accident caused by industrial wiring, appliances, and electrical machinery

E925.8 Accident caused by other electric current

E925.9 Accident caused by unspecified electric current

Coding Clarification

Category E925 codes may only be reported as a secondary diagnosis.

E Codes

© 2004 Ingenix, Inc.

Use a secondary E code from category E849 to identify the place of occurrence.

E926 Exposure to radiation

The sun is the primary source of ultra violet radiation. About 10 percent of ultra violet radiation from the sun reaches the earth. However, artificial sources such as tanning beds, sun lamps, welders, and lasers also produce ultra violet radiation. A sunburn is a reaction to overexposure of this radiation. The effects of a sunburn may not be felt until eight to 10 hours after exposure. The intensity of ultra violet radiation from the sun can vary based on time of day, time of year, cloud cover, and proximity to the equator. Symptoms of sunburn are redness, blisters, swelling, pain, fever, chills, and weakness. Sunburned skin may peel several days after the burn.

E926.0	Exposure to radiofrequency radiation
E926.1	Exposure to infrared radiation from heaters and lamps
E926.2	Exposure to visible and ultraviolet light sources
E926.3	Exposure to x-rays and other electromagnetic ionizing radiation
E926.4	Exposure to lasers
E926.5	Exposure to radioactive isotopes
E926.8	Exposure to other specified radiation
E926.9	Exposure to unspecified radiation

Coding Clarification
Category E926 codes may only be reported as a secondary diagnosis.

Use a secondary E code from category E849 to identify the place of occurrence.

Assign E926.2 for welder's flash burns.

E927 Overexertion and strenuous movements OK

Overexertion and strenuous movements may cause small tears in the muscle, which are referred to as muscle strain. This occurs when the muscle is suddenly stretched beyond its limit. Muscle strains are graded according to their severity. Muscle strains can heal rapidly in the cases of mild strain or take months to heal for more severe strains. Standard treatment for muscle strains is rest, ice, compression, and elevation. Properly warming up, using correct body mechanics, strengthening muscles, and regular exercise can prevent muscle strains.

Coding Clarification
Code E927 codes may only be reported as a secondary diagnosis.

Use a secondary E code from category E849 to identify the place of occurrence.

Coding Scenario
A 45-year-old male presents to the emergency department with back pain. The patient was helping his son move over the weekend and slowly developed back pain. The diagnosis is back strain due to heavy lifting.

> Code assignment: 847.9 *Strains and sprains of unspecified part of back*, E927 *Overexertion and strenuous movements*, and E849.0 *Place of occurrence, home*

E928 Other and unspecified environmental and accidental causes

Loss of hearing due to noise can be the result of one loud exposure. However, the most common cause is an accumulation of noise over a period of time. Loss of hearing is caused by damage to the nerve cells in the ear and progresses with exposure. Hearing loss onset is often subtle. It is recommended that workers exposed to noise levels higher than 85 decibels wear ear protection.

E928.0	Prolonged stay in weightless environment
E928.1	Exposure to noise
E928.2	Accident caused by vibration
E928.3	Accidental human bite
E928.4	External constriction caused by hair
E928.5	External constriction caused by other object
E928.8	Other accident
E928.9	Unspecified accident

Coding Clarification
Category E928 codes may only be reported as a secondary diagnosis.

Use a secondary E code from category E849 to identify the place of occurrence.

E929 Late Effects of Accidental Injury

A late effect is the residual effect that remains after the acute phase of an illness or injury has terminated. Terminology that may be found in diagnostic statements that indicate a late effect include residuals of, old, sequela of, late, and due to or following previous illness or injury. There are late-effect E codes for injuries and poisonings. There are no late-effect E codes for the adverse effects of drugs, misadventures, and surgical complications.

Late effects of accidents are used for the presence of a residual condition caused by the accident. Examples of this category are scars, nonunion of fractures, functional and cognitive deficits, behavioral disorders, bursitis, traumatic arthritis, joint instability, paralysis, muscular atrophy, contracture, nerve damage, and psychological damage. Category E929 codes should be used to report the cause of the accident that resulted in late effects.

E929.0 Late effects of motor vehicle accident

E929.1 Late effects of other transport accident

E929.2 Late effects of accidental poisoning

E929.3 Late effects of accidental fall

E929.4 Late effects of accident caused by fire

E929.5 Late effects of accident due to natural and environmental factors

E929.8 Late effects of other accidents

E929.9 Late effects of unspecified accident

Coding Clarification
Do not use a late effect E code with a related current injury code.

Coding Scenario
A patient has a scar on the hand secondary to a laceration sustained in an automobile accident.

> Code assignment: 709.2 *Scar conditions and fibrosis of skin*, 906.1 *Late effect of open wound of extremities, without mention of tendon injuries*, E929.0 *Late effects of motor vehicle accident*, and E849.5 *Place of occurrence, street and highway*

E930–E949 Drugs, Medicinal and Biological Substances Causing Adverse Effects in Therapeutic Use

Rubric E930-E949 is used to report adverse reactions causing adverse reaction in therapeutic dose. This category is not used to report overdoses but rather allergic reaction or hypersensitivity. Symptoms can range from hives or skin rash to anaphylactic shock. Anaphylaxis is a severe allergic reaction and, in some cases, can produce bronchospasm and laryngeal edema, which can be deadly.

E930 Antibiotics causing adverse effects in therapeutic use

An adverse effect in antibiotics is any unintentional, unwanted reaction that is caused when the drug is taken at the appropriate dose. Because antibiotic allergic reactions can be the same as those of the disease being treated, such as rash, some patients may be labeled as having an allergic reaction where none exists.

E930.0 Penicillins causing adverse effect in therapeutic use

E930.1 Antifungal antibiotics causing adverse effect in therapeutic use

E930.2 Chloramphenicol group causing adverse effect in therapeutic use

E930.3 Erythromycin and other macrolides causing adverse effect in therapeutic use

E930.4 Tetracycline group causing adverse effect in therapeutic use

E930.5 Cephalosporin group causing adverse effect in therapeutic use

E930.6 Antimycobacterial antibiotics causing adverse effect in therapeutic use

E930.7 Antineoplastic antibiotics causing adverse effect in therapeutic use

E930.8 Other specified antibiotics causing adverse effect in therapeutic use

E930.9 Unspecified antibiotic causing adverse effect in therapeutic use

Coding Clarification
Category E930 codes may only be reported as a secondary diagnosis.

E931 Other anti-infectives causing adverse effect in therapeutic use

Anti-infectives cover medications such as sulfonamides, arsenical anti-infectives, heavy metal anti-infectives, quinoline and hydroxyquinoline derivatives, antimalarials and drugs acting on other blood forming protozoa, antiprotozoal drugs, anthelmintics, and antiviral drugs. Therapeutic use is taking the drug as prescribed to treat a disease.

E931.0 Sulfonamides causing adverse effect in therapeutic use

E931.1 Arsenical anti-infectives causing adverse effect in therapeutic use

E931.2 Heavy metal anti-infectives causing adverse effect in therapeutic use

E931.3 Quinoline and hydroxyquinoline derivatives causing adverse effect in therapeutic use

E931.4 Antimalarials and drugs acting on other blood protozoa causing adverse effect in therapeutic use

E931.5 Other antiprotozoal drugs causing adverse effect in therapeutic use

E931.6 Anthelmintics causing adverse effect in therapeutic use

E931.7 Antiviral drugs causing adverse effect in therapeutic use

E931.8 Other antimycobacterial drugs causing adverse effect in therapeutic use

E931.9 Other and unspecified anti-infectives causing adverse effect in therapeutic use

Coding Clarification
Category E931 codes may only be reported as a secondary diagnosis.

E Codes

© 2004 Ingenix, Inc.

E932 Hormones and synthetic substitutes causing adverse effect in therapeutic use

A hormone is a substance in a gland or organ that, when released, stimulates a part of the body to decrease or increase function. Examples of this include growth hormones, hormones that stimulate the beginning of puberty, digestive hormones, and pancreatic hormones.

E932.0 Adrenal cortical steroids causing adverse effect in therapeutic use

E932.1 Androgens and anabolic congeners causing adverse effect in therapeutic use

E932.2 Ovarian hormones and synthetic substitutes causing adverse effect in therapeutic use

E932.3 Insulins and antidiabetic agents causing adverse effect in therapeutic use

E932.4 Anterior pituitary hormones causing adverse effect in therapeutic use

E932.5 Posterior pituitary hormones causing adverse effect in therapeutic use

E932.6 Parathyroid and parathyroid derivatives causing adverse effect in therapeutic use

E932.7 Thyroid and thyroid derivatives causing adverse effect in therapeutic use

E932.8 Antithyroid agents causing adverse effect in therapeutic use

E932.9 Other and unspecified hormones and synthetic substitutes causing adverse effect in therapeutic use

Coding Clarification

Category E932 codes may only be reported as a secondary diagnosis.

E933 Primarily systemic agents causing adverse effect in therapeutic use

Antineoplastic drugs are those that fight cancer. They can have many side effects such as nausea, vomiting, and hair loss. Antineoplastic drugs can also weaken the immune system as they are destroying the cancer cells. Cancer cells and hair cells are both fast growing. Many antineoplastic drugs attack fast growing cells, which is why many people lose their hair when on chemotherapy. Gastrointestinal (GI) squamous cells and bone marrow cells are also fast growing and may be affected by chemotherapy.

E933.0 Antiallergic and antiemetic drugs causing adverse effect in therapeutic use

E933.1 Antineoplastic and immunosuppressive drugs causing adverse effect in therapeutic use

E933.2 Acidifying agents causing adverse effect in therapeutic use

E933.3 Alkalizing agents causing adverse effect in therapeutic use

E933.4 Enzymes, not elsewhere classified, causing adverse effect in therapeutic use

E933.5 Vitamins, not elsewhere classified, causing adverse effect in therapeutic use

E933.8 Other systemic agents, not elsewhere classified, causing adverse effect in therapeutic use

E933.9 Unspecified systemic agent causing adverse effect in therapeutic use

Coding Clarification

Category E933 codes may only be reported as a secondary diagnosis.

E934 Agents primarily affecting blood constituents causing adverse effect in therapeutic use

Anticoagulants are used to prevent blood clots from forming or reduce blood clots that are already present. One of the biggest problems with anticoagulants is regulating the dosages. Patients have to be monitored regularly to ensure that the levels are high enough to be effective but not high enough to cause bleeding.

E934.0 Iron and its compounds causing adverse effect in therapeutic use

E934.1 Liver preparations and other antianemic agents causing adverse effect in therapeutic use

E934.2 Anticoagulants causing adverse effect in therapeutic use

E934.3 Vitamin K (phytonadione) causing adverse effect in therapeutic use

E934.4 Fibrinolysis-affecting drugs causing adverse effect in therapeutic use

E934.5 Anticoagulant antagonists and other coagulants causing adverse effect in therapeutic use

E934.6 Gamma globulin causing adverse effect in therapeutic use

E934.7 Natural blood and blood products causing adverse effect in therapeutic use

E934.8 Other agents affecting blood constituents causing adverse effect in therapeutic use

E934.9 Unspecified agent affecting blood constituents causing adverse effect in therapeutic use

Coding Clarification

Category E934 codes may only be reported as a secondary diagnosis.

E935 Analgesics, antipyretics, and antirheumatics causing adverse effect in therapeutic use

An analgesic medication is one that provides pain relief or reduces pain. An antipyretic is a medication that is used to eliminate or reduce a fever. An antirheumatic is an anti-inflammatory medication.

Methadone is a synthetic form of heroin. It blocks the effects of heroin, which results in a reduced craving.

Opiates are drugs derived from a Papaver somniferum plant. Common names are opium, codeine, morphine, Dilaudid, Percodan, Vicodin, Demerol, and fentanyl.

Salicylates are found in many commonly used drugs. Aspirin is the most common salicylate.

Aromatic analgesics include acetaminophen, acetanilid, and acetophenetidin. Tylenol is a common form of aromatic analgesic.

Pyrazole is a non-narcotic pain reliever and fever reducer, which includes aminophenazone and phenylbutazone.

E935.0 Heroin causing adverse effect in therapeutic use

E935.1 Methadone causing adverse effect in therapeutic use

E935.2 Other opiates and related narcotics causing adverse effect in therapeutic use

E935.3 Salicylates causing adverse effect in therapeutic use

E935.4 Aromatic analgesics, not elsewhere classified, causing adverse effect in therapeutic use

E935.5 Pyrazole derivatives causing adverse effect in therapeutic use

E935.6 Antirheumatics (antiphlogistics) causing adverse effect in therapeutic use

E935.7 Other non-narcotic analgesics causing adverse effect in therapeutic use

E935.8 Other specified analgesics and antipyretics causing adverse effect in therapeutic use

E935.9 Unspecified analgesic and antipyretic causing adverse effect in therapeutic use

Coding Clarification

Category E935 codes may only be reported as a secondary diagnosis.

E936 Anticonvulsants and anti-Parkinsonism drugs causing adverse effect in therapeutic use

Parkinson's disease is a progressive neurologic disease that affects walking, talking, and moving. Symptoms of the disease include tremors, stiffness, and slow movement. The cause of Parkinson's disease is not known. The disease causes a degeneration of nerves in the brain that produces a chemical called dopamine. There is no treatment for the disease; however, medications are used to decrease the symptoms.

E936.0 Oxazolidine derivatives causing adverse effect in therapeutic use

E936.1 Hydantoin derivatives causing adverse effect in therapeutic use

E936.2 Succinimides causing adverse effect in therapeutic use

E936.3 Other and unspecified anticonvulsants causing adverse effect in therapeutic use

E936.4 Anti-Parkinsonism drugs causing adverse effect in therapeutic use

Coding Clarification

Category E936 codes may only be reported as a secondary diagnosis.

E937 Sedatives and hypnotics causing adverse effect in therapeutic use

Sedatives are agents used to calm and quiet the body. Several types and compounds of sedatives are available for use today.

Chloral hydrate is the oldest sleep medication. It may still be used for children prior to dental or medical procedures. Mixed with alcohol, it produces the infamous knockout drops, also called a Mickey.

Paraldehyde is used to treat certain convulsive disorders. It may also be used in the treatment of alcoholism and used to calm or relax patients. The medication should be taken with a metal spoon because paraldehyde tends to react with the plastic. The medication will cause the patient to have bad breath.

Bromine compounds are central nervous center depressants and are mixed with other drugs to form compound drugs. They have a tranquilizing effect on the body.

E937.0 Barbiturates causing adverse effect in therapeutic use

E937.1 Chloral hydrate group causing adverse effect in therapeutic use

E937.2 Paraldehyde causing adverse effect in therapeutic use

E937.3 Bromine compounds causing adverse effect in therapeutic use

E937.4 Methaqualone compounds causing adverse effect in therapeutic use

E937.5 Glutethimide group causing adverse effect in therapeutic use

 © 2004 Ingenix, Inc.

E937.6 Mixed sedatives, not elsewhere classified, causing adverse effect in therapeutic use

E937.8 Other sedatives and hypnotics causing adverse effect in therapeutic use

E937.9 Unspecified sedatives and hypnotics causing adverse effect in therapeutic use

Coding Clarification

Category E937 codes may only be reported as a secondary diagnosis.

E938 Other central nervous system depressants and anesthetics causing adverse effect in therapeutic use

Anesthetics can be used to produce a loss of consciousness or a local pain blocking effect. Side effects of anesthesia drugs include nausea, vomiting, urinary retention, myalgia, pruritus, alteration of mental status, and vasodilation. Vasodilatation can lead to hypovolemic shock and vascular collapse. Patients are carefully monitored during anesthesia for any signs of inappropriate vasodilation.

E938.0 Central nervous system muscle-tone depressants causing adverse effect in therapeutic use

E938.1 Halothane causing adverse effect in therapeutic use

E938.2 Other gaseous anesthetics causing adverse effect in therapeutic use

E938.3 Intravenous anesthetics causing adverse effect in therapeutic use

E938.4 Other and unspecified general anesthetics causing adverse effect in therapeutic use

E938.5 Surface and infiltration anesthetics causing adverse effect in therapeutic use

E938.6 Peripheral nerve- and plexus-blocking anesthetics causing adverse effect in therapeutic use

E938.7 Spinal anesthetics causing adverse effect in therapeutic use

E938.9 Other and unspecified local anesthetics causing adverse effect in therapeutic use

Coding Clarification

Category E938 codes may only be reported as a secondary diagnosis.

E939 Psychotropic agents causing adverse effect in therapeutic use

Tranquilizers are antianxiety medications used to calm a patient. Phenothiazine-based tranquilizers include chlorpromazine, fluphenazine, prochlorperazine, and promazine. Butyrophenone-based tranquilizers include haloperidol, spiperone, and trifluperidol. Benzodiazepine-based tranquilizers include haloperidol, spiperone, and trifluperidol. Other specified tranquilizers include hydroxyzine and meprobamate.

E939.0 Antidepressants causing adverse effect in therapeutic use

E939.1 Phenothiazine-based tranquilizers causing adverse effect in therapeutic use

E939.2 Butyrophenone-based tranquilizers causing adverse effect in therapeutic use

E939.3 Other antipsychotics, neuroleptics, and major tranquilizers causing adverse effect in therapeutic use

E939.4 Benzodiazepine-based tranquilizers causing adverse effect in therapeutic use

E939.5 Other tranquilizers causing adverse effect in therapeutic use

E939.6 Psychodysleptics (hallucinogens) causing adverse effect in therapeutic use

E939.7 Psychostimulants causing adverse effect in therapeutic use

E939.8 Other psychotropic agents causing adverse effect in therapeutic use

E939.9 Unspecified psychotropic agent causing adverse effect in therapeutic use

Coding Clarification

Category E939 codes may only be reported as a secondary diagnosis.

E940 Central nervous system stimulants causing adverse effect in therapeutic use

An analeptic is a drug that stimulates the central nervous system. One of the uses is for ventilatory failure in patients who have chronic obstructive airway disease. Some side effects may include epilepsy and liver impairment. This type of drug is given only with strict supervision.

E940.0 Analeptics causing adverse effect in therapeutic use

E940.1 Opiate antagonists causing adverse effect in therapeutic use

E940.8 Other specified central nervous system stimulants causing adverse effect in therapeutic use

E940.9 Unspecified central nervous system stimulant causing adverse effect in therapeutic use

Coding Clarification

Category E940 codes may only be reported as a secondary diagnosis.

E941 Drugs primarily affecting the autonomic nervous system causing adverse effect in therapeutic use

Parasympathomimetics are drugs that produce the affects of parasympathetic nerve stimulation. Therapeutic use of the drugs includes stimulation and motility of the GI tract and bladder following surgery, glaucoma, diagnosis of myasthenia gravis, and treatment of delayed gastric emptying syndrome.

Parasympatholytics relax smooth muscles. Drugs in this category include atropine, homatropine, hyoscine, and quaternary ammonium derivatives.

Sympathomimetic agents are used to increase myocardial contractility, increase blood pressure, maintain blood pressure, treat bronchospasm, reduce systemic local anesthetic absorption, and manage severe allergic reactions. Drugs in this category include epinephrine and levarterenol.

Sympatholytics stimulate smooth muscles. This category of drugs is used to treat hypertension, angina, glaucoma, and to prevent migraines. Medications include phenoxybenzamine, and tolazoline hydrochloride.

E941.0 Parasympathomimetics (cholinergics) causing adverse effect in therapeutic use

E941.1 Parasympatholytics (anticholinergics and antimuscarinics) and spasmolytics causing adverse effect in therapeutic use

E941.2 Sympathomimetics (adrenergics) causing adverse effect in therapeutic use

E941.3 Sympatholytics (antiadrenergics) causing adverse effect in therapeutic use

E941.9 Unspecified drug primarily affecting the autonomic nervous system causing adverse effect in therapeutic use

Coding Clarification

Category E941 codes may only be reported as a secondary diagnosis.

E942 Agents primarily affecting the cardiovascular system causing adverse effect in therapeutic use

Vasodilators are medications that widen the blood vessels. They allow blood to flow through the blood vessels more easily and are used to treat high blood pressure. Untreated blood pressure increases the risk of heart disease, stroke, and heart failure. Side effects of these medications include headaches and dizziness.

E942.0 Cardiac rhythm regulators causing adverse effect in therapeutic use

E942.1 Cardiotonic glycosides and drugs of similar action causing adverse effect in therapeutic use

E942.2 Antilipemic and antiarteriosclerotic drugs causing adverse effect in therapeutic use

E942.3 Ganglion-blocking agents causing adverse effect in therapeutic use

E942.4 Coronary vasodilators causing adverse effect in therapeutic use

E942.5 Other vasodilators causing adverse effect in therapeutic use

E942.6 Other antihypertensive agents causing adverse effect in therapeutic use

E942.7 Antivaricose drugs, including sclerosing agents, causing adverse effect in therapeutic use

E942.8 Capillary-active drugs causing adverse effect in therapeutic use

E942.9 Other and unspecified agents primarily affecting the cardiovascular system causing adverse effect in therapeutic use

Coding Clarification

Category E942 codes may only be reported as a secondary diagnosis.

E943 Agents primarily affecting gastrointestinal system causing adverse effect in therapeutic use

An ulcer is a sore in the lining of the stomach that is usually caused by the bacteria *Helicobacter pylori* and can be treated in a couple of weeks with antibiotics. Some ulcers can be due to the use of anti-inflammatory medications. In all of these cases, bacteria, medication, or cancer weaken the mucous lining of the stomach and the stomach acid irritates the lining and causes an ulcer. One symptom of an ulcer is dull, gnawing ache. It may come and go for several weeks. It usually occurs a couple of hours after a meal and it is worse at night or when the stomach is empty. Other symptoms may include weight loss, poor appetite, bloating, burping, nausea, and vomiting.

E943.0 Antacids and antigastric secretion drugs causing adverse effect in therapeutic use

E943.1 Irritant cathartics causing adverse effect in therapeutic use

E943.2 Emollient cathartics causing adverse effect in therapeutic use

E943.3 Other cathartics, including intestinal atonia drugs, causing adverse effect in therapeutic use

E943.4 Digestants causing adverse effect in therapeutic use

E943.5 Antidiarrheal drugs causing adverse effect in therapeutic use

E Codes

© 2004 Ingenix, Inc.

E943.6 Emetics causing adverse effect in therapeutic use

E943.8 Other specified agents primarily affecting the gastrointestinal system causing adverse effect in therapeutic use

E943.9 Unspecified agent primarily affecting the gastrointestinal system causing adverse effect in therapeutic use

Coding Clarification

Category E943 codes may only be reported as a secondary diagnosis.

E944 Water, mineral, and uric acid metabolism drugs causing adverse effect in therapeutic use

Diuretics stimulate the kidney to produce more urine. Diuretics also reduce the amount of minerals, such as sodium, in the body. Diuretics are used to treat high blood pressure, congestive heart failure, and edema. Side effects of the drug may include numbness, tingling, or burning in the hands, feet, fingers, and toes, potassium deficiency, and increased blood sugar in diabetics.

E944.0 Mercurial diuretics causing adverse effect in therapeutic use

E944.1 Purine derivative diuretics causing adverse effect in therapeutic use

E944.2 Carbonic acid anhydrase inhibitors causing adverse effect in therapeutic use

E944.3 Saluretics causing adverse effect in therapeutic use

E944.4 Other diuretics causing adverse effect in therapeutic use

E944.5 Electolytic, caloric, and water-balance agents causing adverse effect in therapeutic use

E944.6 Other mineral salts, not elsewhere classified, causing adverse effect in therapeutic use

E944.7 Uric acid metabolism drugs causing adverse effect in therapeutic use

Coding Clarification

Category E944 codes may only be reported as a secondary diagnosis.

E945 Agents primarily acting on the smooth and skeletal muscles and respiratory system causing adverse effect in therapeutic use

Muscle relaxants are medications that relax certain muscles in the body. They are used to treat muscle strain and muscle spasms. They do not cure the muscle injury but help reduce the pain by reducing the muscle spasms. Side effects may include drowsiness, confusion, and light-headedness.

E945.0 Oxytocic agents causing adverse effect in therapeutic use

E945.1 Smooth muscle relaxants causing adverse effect in therapeutic use

E945.2 Skeletal muscle relaxants causing adverse effect in therapeutic use

E945.3 Other and unspecified drugs acting on muscles causing adverse effect in therapeutic use

E945.4 Antitussives causing adverse effect in therapeutic use

E945.5 Expectorants causing adverse effect in therapeutic use

E945.6 Anti-common cold drugs causing adverse effect in therapeutic use

E945.7 Antiasthmatics causing adverse effect in therapeutic use

E945.8 Other and unspecified respiratory drugs causing adverse effect in therapeutic use

Coding Clarification

Category E945 codes may only be reported as a secondary diagnosis.

E946 Agents primarily affecting skin and mucous membrane, ophthalmological, otorhinolaryngological, and dental drugs causing adverse effect in therapeutic use

Keratolytics are medications that loosen and soften the tough outer layer of the skin. These are topical solutions applied directly to the skin. They are normally used for about six weeks. Adverse reactions may include discoloration of the treated area, peeling, blistering, swelling, and skin irritation.

E946.0 Local anti-infectives and anti-inflammatory drugs causing adverse effect in therapeutic use

E946.1 Antipruritics causing adverse effect in therapeutic use

E946.2 Local astringents and local detergents causing adverse effect in therapeutic use

E946.3 Emollients, demulcents, and protectants causing adverse effect in therapeutic use

E946.4 Keratolytics, keratoplastics, other hair treatment drugs and preparations causing adverse effect in therapeutic use

E946.5 Eye anti-infectives and other eye drugs causing adverse effect in therapeutic use

E946.6 Anti-infectives and other drugs and preparations for ear, nose, and throat causing adverse effect in therapeutic use

E946.7 Dental drugs topically applied causing adverse effect in therapeutic use

E946.8 Other agents primarily affecting skin and mucous membrane causing adverse effect in therapeutic use

E946.9 Unspecified agent primarily affecting skin and mucous membrane causing adverse effect in therapeutic use

Coding Clarification

Category E946 codes may only be reported as a secondary diagnosis.

E947 Other and unspecified drugs and medicinal substances causing adverse effect in therapeutic use

Lipotropics prevent abnormal accumulation of fat in the liver. They help keep cholesterol more soluble and reduce the build up in the blood stream.

E947.0 Dietetics causing adverse effect in therapeutic use

E947.1 Lipotropic drugs causing adverse effect in therapeutic use

E947.2 Antidotes and chelating agents, not elsewhere classified, causing adverse effect in therapeutic use

E947.3 Alcohol deterrents causing adverse effect in therapeutic use

E947.4 Pharmaceutical excipients causing adverse effect in therapeutic use

E947.8 Other drugs and medicinal substances causing adverse effect in therapeutic use

E947.9 Unspecified drug or medicinal substance causing adverse effect in therapeutic use

Coding Clarification

Category E947 codes may only be reported as a secondary diagnosis.

E948 Bacterial vaccines causing adverse effect in therapeutic use

Tuberculosis (TB) is a bacterial infection that usually attacks the lungs, but which may also affect other organs. The disease is caused by *Mycobacterium tuberculosis*. TB is transmitted by inhaling air droplets exhaled by an infected person or, sometimes, the infection is absorbed through the skin.

Vaccinations prevent a patient from getting a disease. Although there are small risks with every vaccine, the benefits far outweigh the risks.

E948.0 Bcg vaccine causing adverse effect in therapeutic use

E948.1 Typhoid and paratyphoid vaccines causing adverse effect in therapeutic use

E948.2 Cholera vaccine causing adverse effect in therapeutic use

E948.3 Plague vaccine causing adverse effect in therapeutic use

E948.4 Tetanus vaccine causing adverse effect in therapeutic use

E948.5 Diphtheria vaccine causing adverse effect in therapeutic use .

E948.6 Pertussis vaccine, including combinations with pertussis component, causing adverse effect in therapeutic use

E948.8 Other and unspecified bacterial vaccines causing adverse effect in therapeutic use

E948.9 Mixed bacterial vaccines, except combinations with pertussis component, causing adverse effect in therapeutic use

Coding Clarification

Category E948 codes may only be reported as a secondary diagnosis.

E949 Other vaccines and biological substances causing adverse effect in therapeutic use

Measles is an acute infection caused by paramyxovirus and presents with a hacking cough, rash, and fevers. Measles are usually transmitted from person to person via airborne respiratory droplets. Pharyngitis is common. Koplik's spots are white, grainy spots that can occur in the buccal mucosa and are an early symptom of measles. In the United States, measles outbreaks have been greatly reduced by government immunization programs. Measles has a low mortality rate in healthy individuals.

Vaccinations prevent a patient from getting a disease. Although there are small risks with every vaccine, the benefits far outweigh the risks.

E949.0 Smallpox vaccine causing adverse effect in therapeutic use

E949.1 Rabies vaccine causing adverse effect in therapeutic use

E949.2 Typhus vaccine causing adverse effect in therapeutic use

E949.3 Yellow fever vaccine causing adverse effect in therapeutic use

E949.4 Measles vaccine causing adverse effect in therapeutic use

E949.5 Poliomyelitis vaccine causing adverse effect in therapeutic use

E949.6 Other and unspecified viral and rickettsial vaccines causing adverse effect in therapeutic use

E949.7 Mixed viral-rickettsial and bacterial vaccines, except combinations with pertussis component, causing adverse effect in therapeutic use

© 2004 Ingenix, Inc.

E949.9 Other and unspecified vaccines and biological substances causing adverse effect in therapeutic use

Coding Clarification

Category E949 codes may only be reported as a secondary diagnosis.

E950–E959 Suicide and Self–Inflicted Injury

Rubric E950-E959 is used to report suicide and self-inflicted injury, which includes injury and suicide by self-inflicted poisoning, hanging, strangulating, suffocating, shooting, submerging and drowning, and cutting or piercing. Near drowning is now more commonly referred to as a submersion accident.

If the intent is not specified, is unknown, or documented as questionable, probable, or suspected, assign the E code for cause undetermined.

Suicide is the third leading cause of death among people ages 15 to 24 and is the 11th leading cause of death for all Americans.

The following signs may be observed in a person thinking about suicide:

- Talks about or has tried suicide before
- Experiences disturbances in sleeping and eating
- Exhibits a drastic behavior change
- Withdraws from life
- Loses interest in hobbies, work, school
- Writes a will or makes final arrangements
- Seems preoccupied with death and dying
- Increases use of alcohol and drugs
- Loses interest in personal appearance

E950 Suicide and self-inflicted poisoning by solid or liquid substances

Attempted suicides are classified as one third of all drug abuse incidences. Females are more likely to attempt suicide by overdose than males. Alcohol consumption is commonly used in suicides and suicide attempts.

E950.0 Suicide and self-inflicted poisoning by analgesics, antipyretics, and antirheumatics

E950.1 Suicide and self-inflicted poisoning by barbiturates

E950.2 Suicide and self-inflicted poisoning by other sedatives and hypnotics

E950.3 Suicide and self-inflicted poisoning by tranquilizers and other psychotropic agents

E950.4 Suicide and self-inflicted poisoning by other specified drugs and medicinal substances

E950.5 Suicide and self-inflicted poisoning by unspecified drug or medicinal substance

E950.6 Suicide and self-inflicted poisoning by agricultural and horticultural chemical and pharmaceutical preparations other than plant foods and fertilizers

E950.7 Suicide and self-inflicted poisoning by corrosive and caustic substances

E950.8 Suicide and self-inflicted poisoning by arsenic and its compounds

E950.9 Suicide and self-inflicted poisoning by other and unspecified solid and liquid substances

Coding Clarification

Category E950 codes may only be reported as a secondary diagnosis.

E951 Suicide and self-inflicted poisoning by gases in domestic use

Symptoms of inhaling natural gas are dizziness and vomiting. Natural gas does have an odor and this type of suicide may be interrupted before it is completed.

E951.0 Suicide and self-inflicted poisoning by gas distributed by pipeline

E951.1 Suicide and self-inflicted poisoning by liquefied petroleum gas distributed in mobile containers

E951.8 Suicide and self-inflicted poisoning by other utility gas

Coding Clarification

Category E951 codes may only be reported as a secondary diagnosis.

E952 Suicide and self-inflicted poisoning by other gases and vapors

Carbon monoxide poisoning can be deadly. There is no smell and it cannot be seen but it can kill in just a matter of minutes. Symptoms of carbon monoxide poisoning include severe headache, dizziness, mental confusion, nausea, and fainting. Since the symptoms are similar to many other causes, carbon monoxide poisoning has been hard to diagnose.

E952.0 Suicide and self-inflicted poisoning by motor vehicle exhaust gas

E952.1 Suicide and self-inflicted poisoning by other carbon monoxide

E952.8 Suicide and self-inflicted poisoning by other specified gases and vapors

E952.9 Suicide and self-inflicted poisoning by unspecified gases and vapors

Coding Clarification

Category E952 codes may only be reported as a secondary diagnosis.

E953 Suicide and self-inflicted injury by hanging, strangulation, and suffocation

Suicide by hanging is on the increase. Men are more likely than women to commit suicide by hanging. Hangings can be categorized as complete where the body is totally suspended and does not touch the floor, or incomplete where some part of the body is touching the floor. The human neck is susceptible to injury due to the location of the spinal cord, airway, and major blood vessels.

Suffocation deprives the body of oxygen and can quickly cause death. Symptoms include venous obstruction, arterial and airway obstruction, low cerebral blood flow, and collapse.

E953.0 Suicide and self-inflicted injury by hanging

E953.1 Suicide and self-inflicted injury by suffocation by plastic bag

E953.8 Suicide and self-inflicted injury by other specified means

E953.9 Suicide and self-inflicted injury by unspecified means

Coding Clarification

Category E953 codes may only be reported as a secondary diagnosis.

E954 Suicide and self-inflicted injury by submersion (drowning) OK

Drowning is death from suffocation after submersion that occurs within 24 hours of injury. At first the person holds his or her breath and carbon dioxide levels increase and hypoxia progresses. There are then two types of drowning: wet drowning when water is taken into the lungs and dry drowning when the patient experiences a laryngospasm. Near drowning is now more commonly referred to as a submersion accident.

E Codes

Coding Clarification

Code E954 codes may only be reported as a secondary diagnosis.

E955 Suicide and self-inflicted injury by firearms, air guns and explosives

It is estimated that in 2001, 55 percent of all suicides were committed with guns. Suicide is the leading cause of death from firearms. Unlike other forms of suicide, most suicide attempts with guns are successful. Suicide from handguns is usually to the head. Suicides by more than one shot are uncommon. However, the victim may test fire the gun before the suicide.

E955.0 Suicide and self-inflicted injury by handgun

E955.1 Suicide and self-inflicted injury by shotgun

E955.2 Suicide and self-inflicted injury by hunting rifle

E955.3 Suicide and self-inflicted injury by military firearms

E955.4 Suicide and self-inflicted injury by other and unspecified firearm

E955.5 Suicide and self-inflicted injury by explosives

E955.6 Suicide and self-inflicted injury by air gun

E955.7 Suicide and self-inflicted injury by paintball gun

E955.9 Suicide and self-inflicted injury by firearms and explosives, unspecified

Coding Clarification

Category E955 codes may only be reported as a secondary diagnosis.

E956 Suicide and self-inflicted injury by cutting and piercing instrument OK

This category includes suicide and self-inflicted injury by cutting and piercing with sharp instruments. This includes self-mutilation. Self-mutilation is cutting the skin enough to damage the tissue, which is done in an attempt to change the mood or state. It is not considered self-harming if it is done to fit in with a crowd, as a part of tattooing or piercing, for sexual gratification, or as a ritual.

Coding Clarification

Code E956 codes may only be reported as a secondary diagnosis.

Coding Scenario

A 17-year-old female is brought to the emergency department for lacerations of the left forearm. The patient has a history of depression and gets a sense of relief from cutting herself with a razor blade. The diagnosis is a laceration of the left forearm and depression.

> Code assignment: 881 *Laceration of wrist, forearm, elbow without mention of complication*, 311 *Depressive disorder NOS*, and E956 *Suicide and self inflicted injury by cutting and piercing instrument*

E957 Suicide and self-inflicted injuries by jumping from high place

Category E957 codes are used to describe suicide or self-inflicted injuries by jumping from high places. This includes residential premises, other man-made

© 2004 Ingenix, Inc.

structures such as bridges or commercial buildings, or natural structures.

E957.0 Suicide and self-inflicted injuries by jumping from residential premises

E957.1 Suicide and self-inflicted injuries by jumping from other man-made structures

E957.2 Suicide and self-inflicted injuries by jumping from natural sites

E957.9 Suicide and self-inflicted injuries by jumping from unspecified site

Coding Clarification

Category E957 codes may only be reported as a secondary diagnosis.

E958 Suicide and self-inflicted injury by other and unspecified means

Category E958 codes describe other suicide and self-inflicted injuries. This includes jumping or lying before a moving object, burning, scalding, freezing, electrocuting, crashing a motor vehicle, crashing an aircraft, or injury caused by caustic substance, except poisoning.

E958.0 Suicide and self-inflicted injury by jumping or lying before moving object

E958.1 Suicide and self-inflicted injury by burns, fire

E958.2 Suicide and self-inflicted injury by scald

E958.3 Suicide and self-inflicted injury by extremes of cold

E958.4 Suicide and self-inflicted injury by electrocution

E958.5 Suicide and self-inflicted injury by crashing of motor vehicle

E958.6 Suicide and self-inflicted injury by crashing of aircraft

E958.7 Suicide and self-inflicted injury by caustic substances, except poisoning

E958.8 Suicide and self-inflicted injury by other specified means

E958.9 Suicide and self-inflicted injury by unspecified means

Coding Clarification

Category E958 codes may only be reported as a secondary diagnosis.

E959 Late effects of self-inflicted injury OK

Code E959 is used to describe a late effect of a self-inflicted injury. A late effect is the residual effect that remains after the acute phase of an illness or injury has terminated. A residual is the temporary or permanent health care problem that follows the acute phase of an illness or injury. Terminology that may be found in diagnostic statements that indicate a late effect include residuals of, old, sequela of, late, due to, or following previous illness or injury. The late-effect E codes should be used with any report of a late effect. Do not use a late-effect E code with a related current injury code.

Coding Clarification

Code E959 codes may only be reported as a secondary diagnosis.

E960–E969 Homicide and Injury Purposely Inflicted by Other Persons

This section includes fights, rape, assault by corrosive substance, assault by poisoning, and assault by firearm. Also included in this section are codes to describe the perpetrator of child and adult abuse.

E codes for child and adult abuse take priority over all other E codes. An E code for the type of abuse should be listed first, followed by the code for perpetrator. Report an accidental neglect code first if the intent is an accidental abandonment of an adult or a child.

If the intent is not specified, unknown, or documented as questionable, probable, or suspected, assign the E code for cause undetermined.

E960 Fight, brawl, rape

Rape is sexual contact without consent. Rape is usually an act of power and is not related to sexual desire. Many sexual assault victims report that the attack occurred in their own home, home of a friend, or home of a neighbor. Some rapes happen because the victim is under the influence of alcohol or drugs. However, it is still a crime and should be reported as such. A sexual assault should be reported with E968.8.

E960.0 Unarmed fight or brawl

E960.1 Rape

Coding Clarification

Category E960 codes may only be reported as a secondary diagnosis.

E961 Assault by corrosive or caustic substance, except poisoning OK

Code E961 is used to report assault by corrosive or caustic substances, except poisoning, which includes acid, corrosive substance, and vitriol. Burns from hot liquids and chemical burns from swallowing a corrosive substance are excluded from this code.

Coding Clarification

Code E961 codes may only be reported as a secondary diagnosis.

E Codes

E962 Assault by poisoning

Poisons are chemicals that cause illness, injury, or death when taken in very small quantities. The legal definition of a poison is a chemical that takes less than 50 mg per kilogram of body weight to kill 50 percent of the victims exposed (e.g., about three-fourths of a teaspoon for the average adult and about one-eighth of a teaspoon for a two-year-old child). Symptoms displayed and the systemic effect differs with the type of poison ingested.

E962.0 Assault by drugs and medicinal substances
E962.1 Assault by other solid and liquid substances
E962.2 Assault by other gases and vapors
E962.9 Assault by unspecified poisoning

Coding Clarification
Category E962 codes may only be reported as a secondary diagnosis.

E963 Assault by hanging and strangulation OK

Hangings can be categorized as complete where the body is totally suspended and does not touch the floor, or incomplete where some part of the body is touching the floor. The human neck is susceptible to injury due to the location of the spinal cord, airway, and major blood vessels.

Coding Clarification
Code E963 codes may only be reported as a secondary diagnosis.

E964 Assault by submersion (drowning) OK

Drowning is death from suffocation after submersion that occurs within 24 hours of injury. At first a person holds his or her breath and carbon dioxide levels increase and hypoxia progresses. There are then two types of drowning: wet drowning when water is taken into the lungs and dry drowning when the patient experiences a laryngospasm. Near drowning is now more commonly referred to as a submersion accident.

Coding Clarification
Code E964 codes may only be reported as a secondary diagnosis.

E965 Assault by firearms and explosives

There are a wide variety of firearms such as, handguns, single shot pistols, Derringers, revolvers, rifles, shotguns, submachine guns, and machine guns. As the primer strikes the primer compound, a fire is ignited, which starts the gunpowder burning, and changes it into a gas. This causes pressure to build up in the cartridge and forces the bullet down the barrel. The bullet explodes out of the gun.

E965.0 Assault by handgun
E965.1 Assault by shotgun
E965.2 Assault by hunting rifle
E965.3 Assault by military firearms
E965.4 Assault by other and unspecified firearm
E965.5 Assault by antipersonnel bomb
E965.6 Assault by gasoline bomb
E965.7 Assault by letter bomb
E965.8 Assault by other specified explosive
E965.9 Assault by unspecified explosive

Coding Clarification
Category E965 codes may only be reported as a secondary diagnosis.

E966 Assault by cutting and piercing instrument OK

The following sharp objects are used as weapons in an assault: glass, sword, razor, switchblade, butterfly knife, automatic knife, kitchen knife, military knife, survival knife, stiletto, tonto knife, and pair of scissors. There are different types of wounds that can be caused by these various devices. An incised wound is a sharp cutting injury, usually made with a knife or broken glass, etc. In a slash wound, the length is greater than the depth. In a stab wound, the depth is greater than the length. The seriousness of the wound can range from a scratch to deep, life threatening wounds.

Coding Clarification
Code E966 codes may only be reported as a secondary diagnosis.

E967 Child and adult battering and other maltreatment

Category E967 codes are used to report the perpetrator of child or adult abuse. This code selection should be based on the relationship of the perpetrator and the victim. If the intent of the assault is not known, code the intent with the undetermined cause E codes. Codes E960-E968 should be the first listed E codes, followed by a code from category E967. Codes for child and adult abuse take priority over all other E codes.

E967.0 Child and adult battering and other maltreatment by father or stepfather
E967.1 Child and adult battering and other maltreatment by other specified person
E967.2 Child and adult battering and other maltreatment by mother or stepmother

© 2004 Ingenix, Inc.

E967.3 Child and adult battering and other maltreatment by spouse or partner

E967.4 Child and adult battering and other maltreatment by child

E967.5 Child and adult battering and other maltreatment by sibling

E967.6 Child and adult battering and other maltreatment by grandparent

E967.7 Child and adult battering and other maltreatment by other relative

E967.8 Child and adult battering and other maltreatment by non-related caregiver

E967.9 Child and adult battering and other maltreatment by unspecified person

Coding Clarification

Category E967 codes may only be reported as a secondary diagnosis.

Coding Scenario

A 1-year-old child is brought into the emergency department with burns on both feet. The mother plunged the baby into a hot bath when the baby wouldn't stop crying. The diagnosis is a second-degree burn on both feet caused by child abuse by mother.

> Code assignment: 945.22 *Blister with epidermal loss due to burns, feet*, 995.54 *Child maltreatment syndrome, child physical abuse*, E978.3 *Assault by hot liquid*, and E967.2 *Child and adult battering and other maltreatment by mother or stepmother*

E968 Assault by other and unspecified means

Category E968 codes are used to identify assault by other and unspecified means. This category includes injuries sustained from the following malicious acts: being burned by an intentionally set fire or with a hot liquid, being pushed from a high place, and being struck by blunt or thrown object. Also included is criminal neglect, which includes abandonment of child, infant, or other helpless person with intent to injure or kill. Also included in this category is assault by an air gun, a human bite, and a transport vehicle.

E968.0 Assault by fire

E968.1 Assault by pushing from high place

E968.2 Assault by striking by blunt or thrown object

E968.3 Assault by hot liquid

E968.4 Criminal neglect

E968.5 Assault by transport vehicle

E968.6 Assault by air gun

E968.7 Assault by human bite

E968.8 Assault by other specified means

E968.9 Assault by unspecified means

Coding Clarification

Category E968 codes may only be reported as a secondary diagnosis.

E969 Late effects of injury purposely inflicted by other person OK

Code E969 is used to describe a late effect of an injury purposely inflicted by another person. A late effect is the residual effect that remains after the acute phase of an illness or injury has terminated. A residual is the temporary or permanent health care problem that follows the acute phase of an illness or injury. Terminology indicating a late effect that may be found in diagnostic statements includes residuals of, old, sequela of, late, due to, or following previous illness or injury. The late-effect E codes should be used with any report of a late effect. Do not use a late-effect E code with a related current injury code.

Coding Clarification

Code E969 codes may only be reported as a secondary diagnosis.

E970–E978 Legal Intervention

Rubric E970-E978 is used to report legal intervention injuries. These are injuries inflicted by police, law enforcement, or military police officers while arresting criminals or suspected criminals, suppressing disturbances, maintaining order, or during other legal action.

E970 Injury due to legal intervention by firearms OK

There are a wide variety of firearms such as, handguns, Derringers, revolvers, rifles, lever action, bolt action, pump action, auto-loading, shotguns, submachine guns, and machine guns. As the primer strikes the primer compound, a fire is ignited, which starts the gunpowder burning and changes it into a gas. This causes pressure to build up in the cartridge and forces the bullet down the barrel. The bullet explodes out of the gun.

Coding Clarification

Code E970 codes may only be reported as a secondary diagnosis.

E971 Injury due to legal intervention by explosives OK

Code E971 is used to report legal intervention by explosives. This includes injury by dynamite, explosive shell, grenade, and mortar bomb. Injuries sustained by civilians during a war should be reported by E990-E999.

E Codes

Coding Clarification
Code E971 codes may only be reported as a secondary diagnosis.

E972 Injury due to legal intervention by gas OK

When used correctly, there are no lasting effects of tear gas. It is used by legal authorities to control civilian crowds and subdue criminals. The two most widely used forms of tear gas are chlorobenzylidenemalononitrile and chloroacetophenone. Although tear gas causes only temporary disability, injuries from a tear bomb explosion have been reported.

Coding Clarification
Code E972 codes may only be reported as a secondary diagnosis.

E973 Injury due to legal intervention by blunt object OK

A nightstick is a short, club like instrument used by police in close combat to subdue a suspect.

Coding Clarification
Code E973 codes may only be reported as a secondary diagnosis.

E974 Injury due to legal intervention by cutting and piercing instrument OK

The following sharp objects are used as weapons during a legal intervention: glass, sword, razor, switchblade, butterfly knife, automatic knife, kitchen knife, military knife, survival knife, stiletto, tonto knife, and pair of scissors. There are different types of wounds that can be caused by these various devices. An incised wound is a sharp cutting injury, usually made with a knife or broken glass, etc. In a slash wound, the length is greater than the depth. In a stab wound, the depth is greater than the length. The seriousness of the wound can range from a scratch to deep, life threatening wounds.

Coding Clarification
Code E974 codes may only be reported as a secondary diagnosis.

E975 Injury due to legal intervention by other specified means OK

Code E975 is used to report an injury due to legal intervention by other specified means. Use this code if the other legal intervention codes do not apply. This includes injuries by a blow or by manhandling.

Coding Clarification
Code E975 codes may only be reported as a secondary diagnosis.

E976 Injury due to legal intervention by unspecified means OK

Use this code as a last resort if the method of injury is not documented or cannot be obtained.

Coding Clarification
Code E976 codes may only be reported as a secondary diagnosis.

E977 Late effects of injuries due to legal intervention OK

A late effect is the residual effect that remains after the acute phase of an illness or injury has terminated. A residual is the temporary or permanent health care problem that follows the acute phase of an illness or injury. Terminology that may be found in diagnostic statements that indicate a late effect include residuals of, old, sequela of, late, due to, or following previous illness or injury. The late effect E codes should be used with any report of a late effect. Do not use a late effect E code with a related current injury code. This code should be used to indicate circumstances classifiable to E970-E976.

Coding Clarification
Code E977 codes may only be reported as a secondary diagnosis.

E978 Legal execution OK

A legal execution is one that is performed at the direction of the judiciary or ruling authority. Methods can include asphyxiating by gas, decapitating, electrocuting, hanging, shooting, administering lethal injection, or other specified means.

Many states use a three-drug cocktail to perform lethal injections. First a drug that renders the prisoner unconscious is administered, followed by a muscle relaxant that paralyzes the diaphragm and lungs. Finally, a drug is administered that causes cardiac arrest.

Coding Clarification
Code E978 codes may only be reported as a secondary diagnosis.

E979 Terrorism

Due to the events of September 11, 2001, new codes were developed to track injuries as a result of terrorism. The cause of the injury attributed to terrorism must by identified by the FBI as terrorism. Terrorism is defined as injuries resulting from the unlawful use of force or violence against persons or property to intimidate or coerce a government, the civilian population, or any segment, in furtherance of political or social objective.

E Codes

© 2004 Ingenix, Inc.

If terrorism is suspected, category E979 codes should not be used. Assign an E code based on the documentation and the facts that are known. Terrorism codes take priority over all other E codes except child and adult abuse.

E979.0 Terrorism involving explosion of marine weapons

E979.1 Terrorism involving destruction of aircraft

E979.2 Terrorism involving other explosions and fragments

E979.3 Terrorism involving fires, conflagration and hot substances

E979.4 Terrorism involving firearms

E979.5 Terrorism involving nuclear weapons

E979.6 Terrorism involving biological weapons

E979.7 Terrorism involving chemical weapons

E979.8 Terrorism involving other means

E979.9 Terrorism, secondary effects

Coding Clarification

Category E979 codes may only be reported as a secondary diagnosis.

E980–E989 Injury Undetermined Whether Accidentally or Purposely Inflicted

If the intent of an injury, a suicide, or an assault is undetermined or unspecified, use rubric E980-E989.

E980 Poisoning by solid or liquid substances, undetermined whether accidentally or purposely inflicted

An analgesic medication is one that provides pain relief or reduces pain. An antipyretic is a medication that is used to eliminate or reduce a fever. An antirheumatic is an anti-inflammatory medication.

Barbiturates are drugs used to treat convulsions, anxiety, and aid in sleep.

Sedatives are agents used to calm and quiet the body. Several types and compounds of sedatives are available for use today.

A tranquilizer helps reduce tension and anxiety. Tranquilizers may cause dependence or addiction.

A corrosive is a substance that destroys living tissue. The most common types of corrosives are hydrochloric acid, sulfuric acid, nitric acid, acetic acid, phosphoric acid, oxalic acid, chronic acid, formic acid, and boric acid. These corrosives are commonly found in metal cleaners, toilet and drain cleaners, batteries, and antirust compounds. Symptoms of ingestion include severe burning pain in the mouth, throat, and abdomen; dysphagia; vomiting; diarrhea; and cold, clammy skin. Symptoms will usually begin immediately after swallowing. Symptoms of inhalation include cough, dyspnea, pleuritic chest pain, pulmonary edema, and frothy sputum. These symptoms could be delayed several hours. Eye exposure can cause burning, irritation, and swelling eyes; photophobia; corneal erosion; and perforation of the conjunctiva and cornea.

E980.0 Poisoning by analgesics, antipyretics, and antirheumatics, undetermined whether accidentally or purposely inflicted

E980.1 Poisoning by barbiturates, undetermined whether accidentally or purposely inflicted

E980.2 Poisoning by other sedatives and hypnotics, undetermined whether accidentally or purposely inflicted

E980.3 Poisoning by tranquilizers and other psychotropic agents, undetermined whether accidentally or purposely inflicted

E980.4 Poisoning by other specified drugs and medicinal substances, undetermined whether accidentally or purposely inflicted

E980.5 Poisoning by unspecified drug or medicinal substance, undetermined whether accidentally or purposely inflicted

E980.6 Poisoning by corrosive and caustic substances, undetermined whether accidentally or purposely inflicted

E980.7 Poisoning by agricultural and horticultural chemical and pharmaceutical preparations other than plant foods and fertilizers, undertermined whether accidentally or purposely inflicted

E980.8 Poisoning by arsenic and its compounds, undetermined whether accidentally or purposely inflicted

E980.9 Poisoning by other and unspecified solid and liquid substances, undetermined whether accidentally or purposely inflicted

Coding Clarification

Category E980 codes may only be reported as a secondary diagnosis.

E981 Poisoning by gases in domestic use, undetermined whether accidentally or purposely inflicted

The most common poisoning by gas distributed by pipeline is from carbon monoxide poisoning. Carbon monoxide is produced whenever pipeline gas is burned. The amount produced is usually not hazardous. Improper ventilation and malfunctioning equipment can result in a deadly amount of carbon monoxide emitted into the air. Although the lead in gas has decreased over the years, gasoline fumes can also cause short- or long-term health problems.

E981.0 Poisoning by gas distributed by pipeline, undetermined whether accidentally or purposely inflicted

E981.1 Poisoning by liquefied petroleum gas distributed in mobile containers, undetermined whether accidentally or purposely inflicted

E981.8 Poisoning by other utility gas, undetermined whether accidentally or purposely inflicted

Coding Clarification

Category E981 codes may only be reported as a secondary diagnosis.

E982 Poisoning by other gases, undetermined whether accidentally or purposely inflicted

Carbon monoxide poisoning can be deadly. It cannot be seen or smelled, but it can kill in just a matter of minutes. If appliances that burn fuel are not properly working, toxic levels of carbon monoxide can be produced. Accidental carbon monoxide poisoning kills hundreds of people each year. Symptoms of carbon monoxide poisoning include severe headache, dizziness, mental confusion, nausea, and fainting. Since the symptoms are similar to many other causes, carbon monoxide poisoning has been hard to diagnose. Use of carbon monoxide alarms has greatly reduced the mortality from carbon monoxide poisoning.

E982.0 Poisoning by motor vehicle exhaust gas, undetermined whether accidentally or purposely inflicted

E982.1 Poisoning by other carbon monoxide, undetermined whether accidentally or purposely inflicted

E982.8 Poisoning by other specified gases and vapors, undetermined whether accidentally or purposely inflicted

E982.9 Poisoning by unspecified gases and vapors, undetermined whether accidentally or purposely inflicted

Coding Clarification

Category E982 codes may only be reported as a secondary diagnosis.

E983 Hanging, strangulation, or suffocation, undetermined whether accidentally or purposely inflicted

Hangings can be categorized as complete where the body is totally suspended and does not touch the floor, or incomplete where some part of the body is touching the floor. The human neck is susceptible to injury due to the location of the spinal cord, airway, and major blood vessels.

E983.0 Hanging, undetermined whether accidentally or purposely inflicted

E983.1 Suffocation by plastic bag, undetermined whether accidentally or purposely inflicted

E983.8 Strangulation or suffocation by other specified means, undetermined whether accidentally or purposely inflicted

E983.9 Strangulation or suffocation by unspecified means, undetermined whether accidentally or purposely inflicted

Coding Clarification

Category E983 codes may only be reported as a secondary diagnosis.

E984 Submersion (drowning), undetermined whether accidentally or purposely inflicted OK

Drowning is death from suffocation after submersion that occurs within 24 hours of injury. At first a person holds his or her breath and carbon dioxide levels increase and hypoxia progresses. There are then two types of drowning: wet drowning when water is taken into the lungs and dry drowning when the patient experiences a laryngospasm. Near drowning is now more commonly referred to as a submersion accident.

Coding Clarification

Code E984 codes may only be reported as a secondary diagnosis.

E985 Injury by firearms, air guns and explosives, undetermined whether accidentally or purposely inflicted

There are a wide variety of firearms such as handguns, Derringers, revolvers, rifles, shotguns, submachine guns, and machine guns. As the primer strikes the primer compound, a fire is ignited that starts the gunpowder burning and changes it into a gas. This causes pressure to build up in the cartridge and forces the bullet down the barrel. The bullet explodes out of the gun.

Paintballs can travel up to 300 feet per second. The increased used of paintball guns over the past few years has increased the incidence of injuries. Eye injuries are the most serious and can cause permanent damage.

E985.0 Injury by handgun, undetermined whether accidentally or purposely inflicted

E985.1 Injury by shotgun, undetermined whether accidentally or purposely inflicted

E985.2 Injury by hunting rifle, undetermined whether accidentally or purposely inflicted

E985.3 Injury by military firearms, undetermined whether accidentally or purposely inflicted

E Codes

© 2004 Ingenix, Inc.

E985.4 Injury by other and unspecified firearm, undetermined whether accidentally or purposely inflicted

E985.5 Injury by explosives, undetermined whether accidentally or purposely inflicted

E985.6 Injury by air gun, undetermined whether accidental,or purposefully inflicted

E985.7 Injury by paintball gun, undetermined whether accidentally or purposefully inflicted

Coding Clarification

Category E985 codes may only be reported as a secondary diagnosis.

E986 Injury by cutting and piercing instruments, undetermined whether accidentally or purposely inflicted OK

The following sharp objects can cause either accidental or purposeful injury: glass, sword, razor, switchblade, butterfly knife, automatic knife, kitchen knife, military knife, survival knife, stiletto, tonto knife, and pair of scissors. There are different types of wounds that can be caused by these various devices. An incised wound is a sharp cutting injury, usually made with a knife or broken glass, etc. In a slash wound, the length is greater than the depth. In a stab wound, the depth is greater than the length. The seriousness of the wound can range from a scratch to deep, life threatening wounds.

Coding Clarification

Code E986 codes may only be reported as a secondary diagnosis.

E987 Falling from high place, undetermined whether accidentally or purposely inflicted

Category E987 codes are used to describe falling from high places, when the cause is undetermined to be accidental or purposely inflicted. This includes falls from residential premises, other man made structures, natural sites, or an unspecified site.

E987.0 Falling from high place on residential premises, undetermined whether accidentally or purposely inflicted

E987.1 Falling from high place on other man-made structures, undetermined whether accidentally or purposely inflicted

E987.2 Falling from high place on natural sites, undetermined whether accidentally or purposely inflicted

E987.9 Falling from unspecified high place, undetermined whether accidentally or purposely inflicted

Coding Clarification

Category E987 codes may only be reported as a secondary diagnosis.

E988 Injury by other and unspecified means, undetermined whether accidentally or purposely inflicted

Chilblains are painful, small, itchy, red areas of the skin that appear on the skin after exposure to cold temperature. They are more common in cold, humid climates. Chilblains are most common on the toes but can also appear on the fingers, nose, and ears. The skin breaks down and ulcers and infection can occur. Chilblains are more common in females and can be recurrent for the rest of the patient's life or last only a few years.

Skin exposed to 140-degree water for three seconds or less may be seriously burned. Children and the elderly have skin that is more sensitive to burns.

Electrocution can cause burns and the heart to stop. High voltage contact can cause death instantly.

E988.0 Injury by jumping or lying before moving object, undetermined whether accidentally or purposely inflicted

E988.1 Injury by burns or fire, undetermined whether accidentally or purposely inflicted

E988.2 Injury by scald, undetermined whether accidentally or purposely inflicted

E988.3 Injury by extremes of cold, undetermined whether accidentally or purposely inflicted

E988.4 Injury by electrocution, undetermined whether accidentally or purposely inflicted

E988.5 Injury by crashing of motor vehicle, undetermined whether accidentally or purposely inflicted

E988.6 Injury by crashing of aircraft, undetermined whether accidentally or purposely inflicted

E988.7 Injury by caustic substances, except poisoning, undetermined whether accidentally or purposely inflicted

E988.8 Injury by other specified means, undetermined whether accidentally or purposely inflicted

E988.9 Injury by unspecified means, undetermined whether accidentally or purposely inflicted

Coding Clarification

Category E988 codes may only be reported as a secondary diagnosis.

E989 Late effects of injury, undetermined whether accidentally or purposely inflicted OK

A late effect is the residual effect that remains after the acute phase of an illness or injury has terminated. A residual is the temporary or permanent health care problem that follows the acute phase of an illness or injury. Terminology that may be found in diagnostic statements indicating a late effect include residuals of, old, sequela of, late, due to, or following previous illness or injury. There are late-effect E codes for injuries and poisonings. There are not late effect E codes for the adverse effects of drugs, misadventures, and surgical complications. The late-effect E codes should be used with any report of a late effect. Do not use a late-effect E code with a related current injury code. This code should be used to indicate circumstances classifiable to E980-E988.

Coding Clarification
Code E989 codes may only be reported as a secondary diagnosis.

E990–E999 Injury Resulting from Operations of War

Rubric E990-E999 is used to report injury resulting from operations of war. Operations of war are injuries to military personnel and civilians caused by war and civil revolt and occurring during the time of war. Excluded from this rubric are accidents during training of military personnel, manufacture of war material, and transport, unless attributable to enemy action.

E990 Injury due to war operations by fires and conflagrations

Category E990 codes are used to report fires and conflagration due to war. Conflagration is a widespread, general burning. This includes asphyxia, burns, or other injury originating from fire caused by a fire-producing device or indirectly by any conventional weapon.

E990.0 Injury due to war operations from gasoline bomb

E990.9 Injury due to war operations from other and unspecified source

Coding Clarification
Category E990 codes may only be reported as a secondary diagnosis.

E991 Injury due to war operations by bullets and fragments

Category E991 codes are used to report injuries due to war operations by bullets and fragments. Bullets and fragments are defined as rubber bullets, pellets, machine gun bullets, pistol bullets, rifle bullets, shotgun bullets, antipersonnel bomb fragments, fragments from artillery shells, bombs, grenades, guided missiles, land mines, rockets, shells, and shrapnel.

E991.0 Injury due to war operations from rubber bullets (rifle)

E991.1 Injury due to war operations from pellets (rifle)

E991.2 Injury due to war operations from other bullets

E991.3 Injury due to war operations from antipersonnel bomb (fragments)

E991.9 Injury due to war operations from other and unspecified fragments

Coding Clarification
Category E991 codes may only be reported as a secondary diagnosis.

E992 Injury due to war operations by explosion of marine weapons OK

Code E992 is used to report an injury due to war operations by explosion of marine weapons. This includes depth charge, mine explosions at sea or in a harbor, sea-based artillery shell, torpedo, and underwater blasts.

Coding Clarification
Code E992 codes may only be reported as a secondary diagnosis.

E993 Injury due to war operations by other explosion OK

Code E993 is used to report an injury due to war operations by other explosions. This includes accidental explosion of munitions being used in war, accidental explosion of weapons, air blast, explosion of artillery shell, breechblock, cannon block, mortar bomb, and weapon burst.

Coding Clarification
Code E993 codes may only be reported as a secondary diagnosis.

E994 Injury due to war operations by destruction of aircraft OK

Code E994 is used to report an injury due to war operations by destruction of aircraft. This includes the burning or exploding of an airplane, an airplane being shot down, and being crushed by a falling airplane.

Coding Clarification
Code E994 codes may only be reported as a secondary diagnosis.

E Codes

© 2004 Ingenix, Inc.

E995 Injury due to war operations by other and unspecified forms of conventional warfare OK

Code E995 is used to report an injury due to war operations by other and unspecified forms of conventional warfare. This includes battle wounds, bayonet injuries, and drowning in war operations.

Coding Clarification
Code E995 codes may only be reported as a secondary diagnosis.

E996 Injury due to war operations by nuclear weapons OK

Code E996 is used to report an injury due to war operations by nuclear weapons. Nuclear weapons have four major destructive effects: blast, thermal radiation, initial nuclear radiation, and fallout. Blasts cause an energy explosion that creates great pressure. The pressure can be equal to several thousand pounds per square inch. It crushes and destroys objects, including the human lungs. Thermal radiation includes light and heat. There is a huge amount of light emitted from a nuclear explosion. It is bright enough to blind people many miles away and burn skin. Initial nuclear radiation contains gamma rays and neutrons. These can enter the body directly and cause radiation exposure. This will kill a person within about six to seven weeks. Fallout consists of particles from objects that become irradiated by the explosion and can lodge in different parts of the body.

Coding Clarification
Code E996 codes may only be reported as a secondary diagnosis.

E997 Injury due to war operations by other forms of unconventional warfare

A laser is an acronym for light amplification by stimulated emission of radiation. It emits intense heat and power but is only effective at close range.

Biologic warfare is intentionally using viruses, bacteria, fungi, or toxins to kill or harm people, animals, or plants.

E997.0 Injury due to war operations by lasers

E997.1 Injury due to war operations by biological warfare

E997.2 Injury due to war operations by gases, fumes, and chemicals

E997.8 Injury due to other specified forms of unconventional warfare

E997.9 Injury due to unspecified form of unconventional warfare

Coding Clarification
Category E997 codes may only be reported as a secondary diagnosis.

E998 Injury due to war operations but occurring after cessation of hostilities OK

Code E998 is used to report injuries due to war operations but occurring after cessation of hostilities. This includes injuries by explosion of bombs or mines placed in the course of operations of war, if the explosion occurred after the hostilities cease.

Coding Clarification
Code E998 codes may only be reported as a secondary diagnosis.

E999 Late effect of injury due to war operations and terrorism

A late effect is the residual effect that remains after the acute phase of an illness or injury has terminated. A residual is the temporary or permanent health care problem that follows the acute phase of an illness or injury. Terminology found in diagnostic statements that indicate a late effect include residuals of, old, sequela of, late, due to, or following previous illness or injury. The late-effect E codes should be used with any report of a late effect. Do not use a late-effect E code with a related current injury code. This code should be used to indicate circumstances classifiable to E979 and E990-E998.

E999.0 Late effect of injury due to war operations

E999.1 Late effect of injury due to terrorism

Coding Clarification
Category E999 codes may only be reported as a secondary diagnosis.

© 2004 Ingenix, Inc.